Pelvic Ring Fractures

Axel Gänsslen • Jan Lindahl
Stephan Grechenig • Bernd Füchtmeier
Editors

Pelvic Ring Fractures

Springer

Editors
Axel Gänsslen
Department of Trauma Surgery, Orthopedics and Hand Surgery
Hospital Wolfsburg
Wolfsburg
Germany

Stephan Grechenig
Klinik für Unfallchirurgie
Krankenhaus Barmherzige Brüder
Regensburg
Bayern
Germany

Jan Lindahl
Orthopaedics and Trauma Surgery
Helsinki University Hospital
Helsinki
Finland

Bernd Füchtmeier
Klinik für Unfallchirurgie
Krankenhaus Barmherzige Brüder
Regensburg
Bayern
Germany

ISBN 978-3-030-54729-5 ISBN 978-3-030-54730-1 (eBook)
https://doi.org/10.1007/978-3-030-54730-1

This Springer imprint is published by the registered company Springer Nature Switzerland AG
The registered company address is: Gewerbestrasse 11, 6330 Cham, Switzerland

Preface

High-energy pelvic fractures continue to present a serious challenge to trauma care. Over the last five decades, our knowledge has increased on the assessment, trauma mechanisms, classification, and management protocols for this particular, potentially lethal injury.

During the 1970s, the patho-anatomical pattern of a lethal vascular injury was revealed in post-mortem studies by Huittinen and Slätis in 1973. At the same time (1972), the first case report by Margolies et al. was published on the use of angiographic embolization in the emergency treatment of pelvic fracture-related arterial bleeding. The last decades have been a time of rapid progress in the control of pelvic fracture-related mortality and morbidity. A better understanding of the anatomic features of these fractures and an awareness of potential major, exsanguinating arterial hemorrhage have led to multidisciplinary approaches for controlling bleeding and temporarily stabilizing the pelvic ring.

After the wide adoption and successful outcomes of external skeletal fixation devices for the treatment of extremity injuries, interest was focused on the use of these devices in pelvic fracture management first by Carabalona et al. (1973) and Slätis and Karaharju (1975). In the 1980s, the concept of internal fixation was introduced, for both anterior and posterior aspects of the pelvis, based on previous biomechanical studies.

The mechanical understanding of the pelvic ring structure, estimated direction of the major force vector, and the degree of pelvic instability lead to the current comprehensive classification system of pelvic ring injuries, which combines the AO classification and the Orthopaedic Trauma Association's (OTA) classification system with the Tile classification.

The highly difficult pelvic area, including the special three-dimensional bone structure and the pelvic organs and the intrapelvic neurovascular structures, needs a comprehensive understanding to the peri- and intrapelvic anatomy.

Therefore, the ***connection of anatomy and surgery*** is the predominant basis of adequately treating patients with pelvic ring injuries.

At the entrance of the Institute of Anatomy in Graz, two relevant statements accompany every participant before entering the dissection area. These statements have influenced the authors in numerous courses and ultimately to a significant increase of knowledge in pelvic ring injury treatment:

> "Ärzte ohne anatomische Kenntnisse gleichen Maulwürfen: Sie arbeiten im Dunkeln und ihrer Hände Tagewerk sind – ERDHÜGEL"
> "Surgeons without anatomy are like moles: They work in the dark and their hands work are EARTH HILLS."
> (Tiedemann)

> "Anatomie ohne Klinik ist tot – Klinik ohne Anatomie ist tödlich"
> "Anatomy without clinic is dead—Clinic without anatomy is deadly."
> (Platzer)

Historically, Albin Lambotte (1907 and 1913) was the first who proposed several options for the surgical treatment of different fractures of the anterior and posterior pelvic ring including screw, plate, and wire stabilization techniques. For symphysis pubis, Lambotte described both screw and plate fixation techniques, and for sacral fractures open posterior iliosacral screw fixation and sacral bar fixation techniques. Today, it is widely accepted that internal fixation of all unstable injuries in the anterior and posterior pelvic ring provides superior stability for the whole pelvis and better anatomical results as determined by the quality of reduction and lower malunion rate.

The treatment of injuries of the posterior pelvic ring need a demanding understanding of the posterior pelvic ring anatomy, even for experienced surgeons, due to different fracture morphology. The close relationship of relevant neurovascular structures and the biomechanical significance of the posterior pelvic ring requires a maximum of anatomical and surgical knowledge in order to achieve an optimal long-term outcome, as mild persistent malhealing can lead to relevant clinical impairments.

The development of special preoperative, intraoperative, and post-operative radiological techniques now allows a much better understanding of this region for the treating surgeon.

Overall, treating a patient with a pelvic ring injury should lead the surgeon to focus on mechanical and hemodynamic stabilization.

Therefore, sophisticated clinical–radiological diagnostics with the appropriate evaluation of parameters for an optimal, individual indication, pelvic ring region-specific approaches, and a detailed understanding of detailed reduction and fixation techniques are necessary.

During the last decade, a trend to more less invasive techniques can be drawn from the literature. Accordingly, an emphasis in this book was placed on stabilization techniques of specific fracture locations, the relevant intraoperative imaging techniques in a practice-oriented manner and their results of treatment.

In addition, specific problems in age extremes (paediatric and geriatric) and in osteoporosis as well as the current knowledge of late deformities are presented in detail. We felt that a textbook that provides a comprehensive overview of these injuries would provide a practical approach to the learner as well as the experienced orthopaedic trauma surgeon.

Wolfsburg, Germany — Axel Gänsslen
Helsinki, Finland — Jan Lindahl
Regensburg, Germany — Stephan Grechenig
Regensburg, Germany — Bernd Füchtmeier

Acknowledgements

The authors would like to thank the whole team of the Institute of Anatomy of the Medical University of Graz for years of help and their outstanding anatomical and surgical expertise.

In particular, our very special thanks are given to Professor Wolfgang Grechenig, Graz University Hospital and Professor Friedrich Anderhuber (†), former Chair of the Institute of Anatomy, Medical University of Graz, Austria, for having the opportunity to perform anatomical studies with their cadavers and to teach pelvic surgery on their courses with practical exercises on human specimens during the last two decades.

Additionally, we would like to thank our friends Peter Tesch, Andreas Weiglein, and Georg Feigl.

The frequent outstanding discussions and the didactic presentations of the anatomical basis at the institute have considerably enlarged our knowledge in this field and became the basis of our daily practice.

Special thanks also to our European friends, especially the support by Bore Bakota, and Mario Steresinic, which led to our increasing knowledge in the field of pelvic ring surgery.

It is a great pleasure for us to know you all and to work with you.

Contents

About the Editors

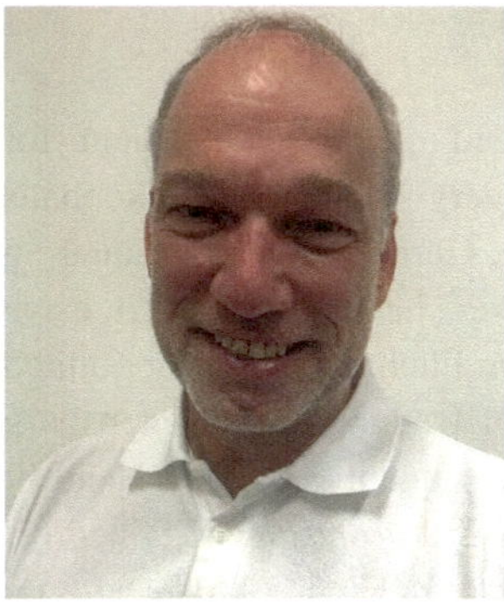

Axel Gänsslen, MD is a Consultant in Trauma Surgery in the Trauma Department, Wolfsburg General Hospital Wolfsburg, Germany. Since 2012, he has also been Chairman of the AO Trauma Course—Pelvis and Acetabulum in the Department of Anatomy, University of Graz, Austria. Dr. Gänsslen graduated from Hannover Medical School (MHH) in 1993 and subsequently undertook a number of residencies in trauma surgery before becoming a Consultant in Trauma Surgery in the Trauma Department of Hannover Medical School in 2006. Since 1994, he has been Regional/International Faculty on more than 100 AO Trauma courses. He is the author of numerous papers in peer-reviewed journals as well as 5 books and more than 50 book chapters.

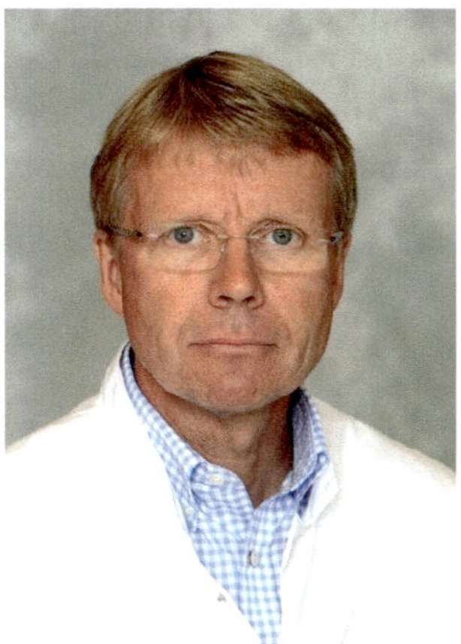

Jan Lindahl, MD, PhD is Head of the Pelvis and Lower Extremity Orthopaedic and Trauma Surgery Ward at Helsinki University Hospital and Adjunct Professor (Docent) in Orthopaedics and Traumatology at the University of Helsinki, Finland. He graduated from the University of Tampere in 1986 and subsequently completed specializations in Orthopaedics and Traumatology and General Surgery at the University of Helsinki before taking up his current post in 2000. Dr. Lindahl has been chairman of AO Trauma, Finland, since 2010 and is a past president of the Finnish Trauma Association, of which he was a founding member. He has received various awards, including the Hughston Award for best paper published in the American Journal of Sports Medicine in 2006. He is the author of almost 50 original articles and more than 30 book chapters, predominantly on management of injuries of the pelvic ring and acetabulum, fractures of the lower extremities, and knee injuries.

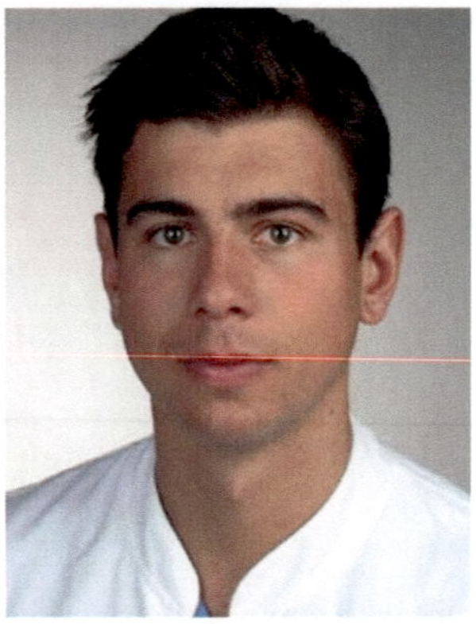

Stephan Grechenig, MD, Priv. Doz. Dr. Med. Univ. is a resident in Orthopaedic and Trauma Surgery at the Clinic for Trauma Surgery, Orthopaedics and Sports Medicine, Krankenhaus Barmherzige Brüder, Regensburg, Germany. He graduated from Medical School at the University of Graz, Austria, in 2013 and subsequently was a post-doc in Musculoskeletal Biomechanics at the AO Research Institute, Davos, Switzerland, and a resident in Trauma Surgery at the University Medical Center, Regensburg, Germany. He is a member of AO Trauma, the AO Faculty Group, and the German Society for Trauma Surgery (DGU) and is the author of almost 50 PubMed-listed articles.

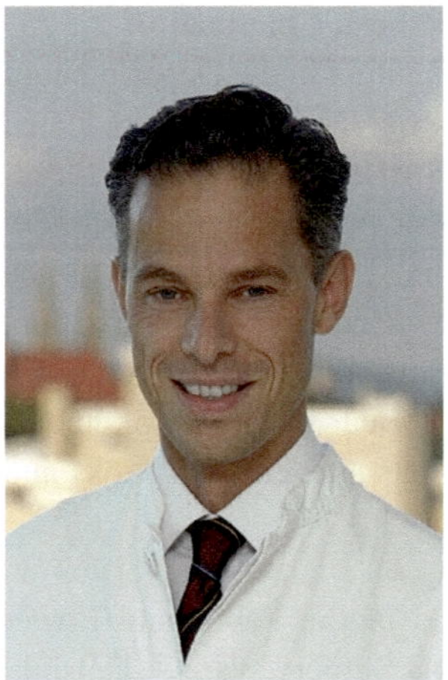

Bernd Füchtmeier, MD is Head of the Department for Trauma and Orthopaedic Surgery at the Krankenhaus Barmherzige Brüder, Regensburg, Germany. After graduating from Medical School in Hannover, he undertook extensive training in orthopaedic surgery. Dr. Füchtmeier was appointed as a consultant in the Department of Traumatology, Regensburg University Clinic in 2001 and subsequently became Head of the Section of Pelvic Surgery and Arthroplasty. He gained his habilitation in trauma surgery in 2007. In 2008, he was appointed senior consultant in the Clinic for Trauma Surgery, Orthopaedics, and Sports Medicine at Krankenhaus Barmherzige Brüder. Prior to taking up his current position, he was a consultant at the Center for Musculoskeletal Surgery, Charité University Clinic, Berlin. In 2011, Dr. Füchtmeier was appointed Associate Professor in the Medical Faculty, University of Regensburg. He is a member of the Advisory Board for AO Trauma, Germany.

Part I

Introduction

The History of Pelvic Fracture Treatment

1

Axel Gänsslen and Jan Lindahl

First experiences with pelvic ring fractures were reported in the nineteenth century by analysis of clinical courses and autopsy findings [1–7].

1.1 Malgaigne´s Fractures

It was not until Malgaigne in 1847, who reported ten pelvic fracture cases (Fig. 1.1) and defined the double vertical fracture of the pelvis [8]. A detailed description of pelvic ring injuries was reported. He distinguished between the following injuries:

- Sacrum fractures
- Iliac crest fractures
- Pubic fracture
- Fractures of the ischium
- Double vertical fractures of the pelvis

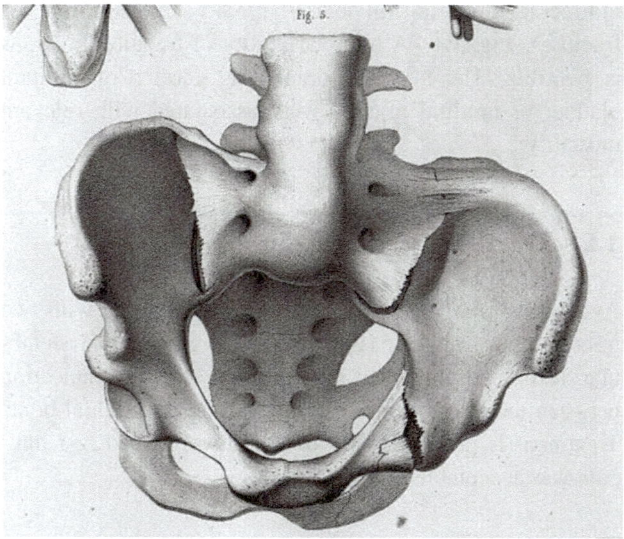

Fig. 1.1 Dysmorphic sacral bone and left anterior ring fracture from Malgaigne´s textbook

1.2 Sacrum Fractures

Only one case was seen in a group of 2358 patients. Two possible fracture types were distinguished:

- Isolated sacral fractures
- Sacral fractures as part of a pelvic ring injury

Isolated sacral fractures most commonly were the result of a direct blow from a fall and hit against the distal sacrum, which resulted in an angular deformity of the fracture with an open anterior angle. Malgaigne treated three of these cases [9].

Closed digital reduction was recommended by fracture manipulation using a finger inserted into the rectum. Additionally, a wooden cylinder or comparable measures can be introduced into the rectum for temporary stabilization of the fracture.

More complex injuries of the sacrum as part of a pelvic ring injury were associated with a high mortality rate. Malgaigne cited a case from Guérétin with a horizontal fracture and two vertical fractures, potentially representing the first described lumbo-pelvic dissociation injury. Additionally, he observed one case of a coccyx fracture.

A. Gänsslen (✉)
Department of Trauma Surgery, Orthopedics and Hand Surgery, Hospital Wolfsburg, Wolfsburg, Germany

J. Lindahl
Orthopaedics and Trauma Surgery, Helsinki University Hospital, Helsinki, Finland
e-mail: jan.lindahl@hus.fi

A. Gänsslen et al. (eds.), *Pelvic Ring Fractures*, https://doi.org/10.1007/978-3-030-54730-1_1

1.3 Iliac Crest Fractures

Iliac crest fractures are the result of a direct blow against the ilium. These fractures were often undisplaced or showed intrapelvic displacement. Manual direct or indirect manipulation was recommended for reduction. The prognosis was mainly influenced by accompanying injuries of the pelvic region.

1.4 Pubic Fractures

The most common mechanism is a direct injury with different forces acting on the pubic region, but sometimes also an indirect mechanism (fall on the buttock) can result in pubic fractures (Fig. 1.1). A high variability of fracture locations is possible. The healing potential is good. Concomitant bladder or urethral injuries were associated with relevant mortality.

1.5 Fractures of the Ischium

Avulsion injuries and complete ischium fractures with two fracture lines were discussed: one fracture below the acetabular level and the other fracture line at the connection between the inferior pubic ramus and the true ischial bone. Treatment is predominantly conservative by bed rest until pain was acceptable to allow walking.

1.6 Double Vertical Fracture

Malgaigne was the first to describe this special entity of pelvic ring injuries and recognized that these injuries merit special attention in respect to diagnosis, prognosis, and treatment. Double vertical fractures of the pelvis were defined as multiple pelvic fractures. Typically, two vertical fracture components are present on one pelvic side, separating the hip joint (floating acetabulum), leading to hemipelvic cranialization and internal rotation deformity with resulting leg length inequality.

The anterior ring injury was usually an upper and lower pubic rami fracture, while the posterior injury most often was a complete ilium fracture or rarely a sacrum fracture or a sacroiliac (SI) joint injury.

Compared to the other pelvic injury types, higher forces acted on the pelvis (fall from height, pelvic crush mechanisms, etc.). Variable displacement and clinical deformity were observed. Treatment was stated more difficult in trying to correct the deformity, which sometimes was performed using traction methods.

1.7 Knowledge on Pelvic Fracture Treatment Before X-Ray Availability

Gurlt reported first epidemiological data on pelvic ring injuries in 1862 [10]. In an analysis of 22,616 fractures, treated at the London Hospital between 1842 and 1862, 70 pelvic fractures were reported (0.31%).

Rose described eight cases with pelvic ring injuries in a group of 800 adult patients with fractures [11]. Thus, 1% of all fractures are pelvic ring fractures. Considering also iliac crest fractures, acetabular rim fractures, transverse fractures of the sacrum and coccyx, and one case with a bullet fracture, 2% of all fractures were pelvic fractures.

Leisrink analyzed 470 fractures and reported on five pelvic injuries (1.1%) [12].

In a further analysis from 1880 by Gurlt, 51,938 fractures were analyzed from the years 1842–1877 [13]. One hundred forty-two pelvic fractures (0.273%) and 15 coccyx fractures (0.028%) were treated. The majority of these fractures were admitted to a hospital (91.7%).

> Pelvic ring injuries are rare with an expected incidence of 0.3–1% in historical analyses.

1.8 Mechanism of Injury

Typical injury mechanisms included roll-over injuries, crush mechanisms, and fall from a great height [14]. Crush injuries were frequently observed from train or mining injuries.

1.9 Pathoanatomy

Rose stated, according to Malgaigne, that every pelvic fracture consists of at least two parallel fracture lines in the pelvis axis [11]. Of these, often, one vertical split is running through the symphysis or SI joint. The majority of detected injuries before his analysis consisted of non-survivors, and the type of pelvic injury was described during autopsy.

Theodor Billroth reported on 43 fractures of the pelvis [15]. Of these, 28 patients survived. He reported one case of a traumatic hemicorporectomy after a train roll-over injury in a 6-year-old child, who died within 1 h after the injury. No relevant bleeding was observed from the transected pelvic vessels. The majority of patients died due to septical problems. Billroth described the clinical diagnostics in detail.

Clinically, a lateral pelvic compression, pressure to the symphysis, and rectal exploration allow for detection of bony instability and local pelvic pain. Additionally, after exclusion of relevant accompanying injuries, further signs, indicative of a pelvic injury after major forces acting to the pelvic region, include impossible standing and walking. Bladder voiding disturbances were frequently observed, and Billroth expected a temporary paralysis of the bladder detrusor nerves and muscles.

Suspected injury mechanisms included forces, acting by anterior-posterior or lateral compression to the pelvic area, crush mechanisms from heavy loads, and a fall from a great height.

Pathoanatomical observations presented typical pelvic injury types:

- Symphyseal disruption
- Ilium fractures
- Uni- or bilateral double vertical (anterior and posterior) fractures
- Hemipelvic dislocations

Pelvic injuries with additional pelvic organ injuries were associated with a high mortality rate.

Conservative treatment is usually necessary for 4–8 weeks, and despite some mal-healing, most often, no relevant subjective complaints were reported.

> Theodor Billroth already in 1869 described clinical examination techniques, typical injury mechanisms, fracture types, and risk factors of mortality, which are still valid today [15].

Several case descriptions were reported in the literature after this overview, and an increasing rate of survivors was reported. Interesting results included:

- Complex pelvic trauma with urethral disruption and a lateral compression type C injury with bilateral pubic rami fractures, symphyseal disruption, and a complete transforaminal sacrum fracture; death [16].
- Open spino-pelvic dissociation injury (symphyseal disruption, crescent fracture, contralateral sacrum fracture with a transverse component at the S1 level); death [17].
- Complete posterior hemipelvic dislocation injury after crush injury mechanism [18].
- Complete anterior hemipelvic dislocation after a hit by a heavy load from posterior and lateral [19]; four of six cases in the analyzed literature died (concomitant pelvic organ injuries).
- A postpartum symphyseal widening after primary delivery [20].
- Symphyseal disruption during labor/sport after forceful adductor contraction [21].
- Geriatric fracture after simple fall on the left body resulting in left pubic rami fractures with accompanying obturator vein injury (cause of death) [22].

Areilza (1891) reported on 13 cases after lateral compression forces [23]. These injuries were associated with four urethral stretch injuries and three urethral disruptions (all three patients died).

In 1895, Katzenelson analyzed part of the literature and distinguished between five possible injury mechanisms [24]:

- Eleven cases after frontal force transmission: seven deaths (63.6%), five urethral and two bladder lacerations; 60% of urethral lesions survived.
- Four cases after anterior sagittal force transmission: two deaths (50%), one urethral laceration and two bladder lacerations.
- Four cases after lateral force transmission to the hemipelvis: 2× type A2, 2× type C1.2 injuries; three deaths (75%), two urethral and two bladder lacerations.
- Six cases after posterior sagittal force transmission: four deaths (66.6%), two urethral and two bladder lacerations.
- Five cases after muscular contraction: one death (20%) after a fall from 12 m height with bladder laceration (pubic avulsion), all others with uneventful course.

1.10 Clinical Diagnostics

Drechsler summarized the knowledge from the nineteenth century in 1891 [25]. Typical clinical signs, indicative of pelvic fractures/injuries according to Rose, included:

- Localized pain on palpation
- Bladder voiding disturbance
- Iliopsoas pain and functional disturbance

Additionally, Drechsler recommended further potential signs of a pelvic ring injury:

- Local ecchymosis
- Bowel disturbances

Classical fracture signs, e.g., displacement and crepitation, were infrequently observed due to the soft tissue mantle around the pelvis.

1.11 Experimental Analyses

Fere performed experimental side impacts on whole body cadavers from a height of 50–60 cm. In elderly cadavers, anterior ring lesions were frequently observed; sometimes, a symphyseal disruption occurred; with increasing forces, a second injury site was detected at the posterior pelvic ring (ilium, sacrum, or SI joint). In younger cadavers, no injuries were detected [22].

Kusmin performed experimental studies on cadaver pelves based on classical clinical injury mechanisms derived from the literature [14].

Anterior-posterior/posterior-anterior compression forces resulted in (Fig. 1.2a):

- Upper pubic ramus fractures at the level of the pubic tubercle or at the iliopectineal eminence close to or involving the acetabular cavity.

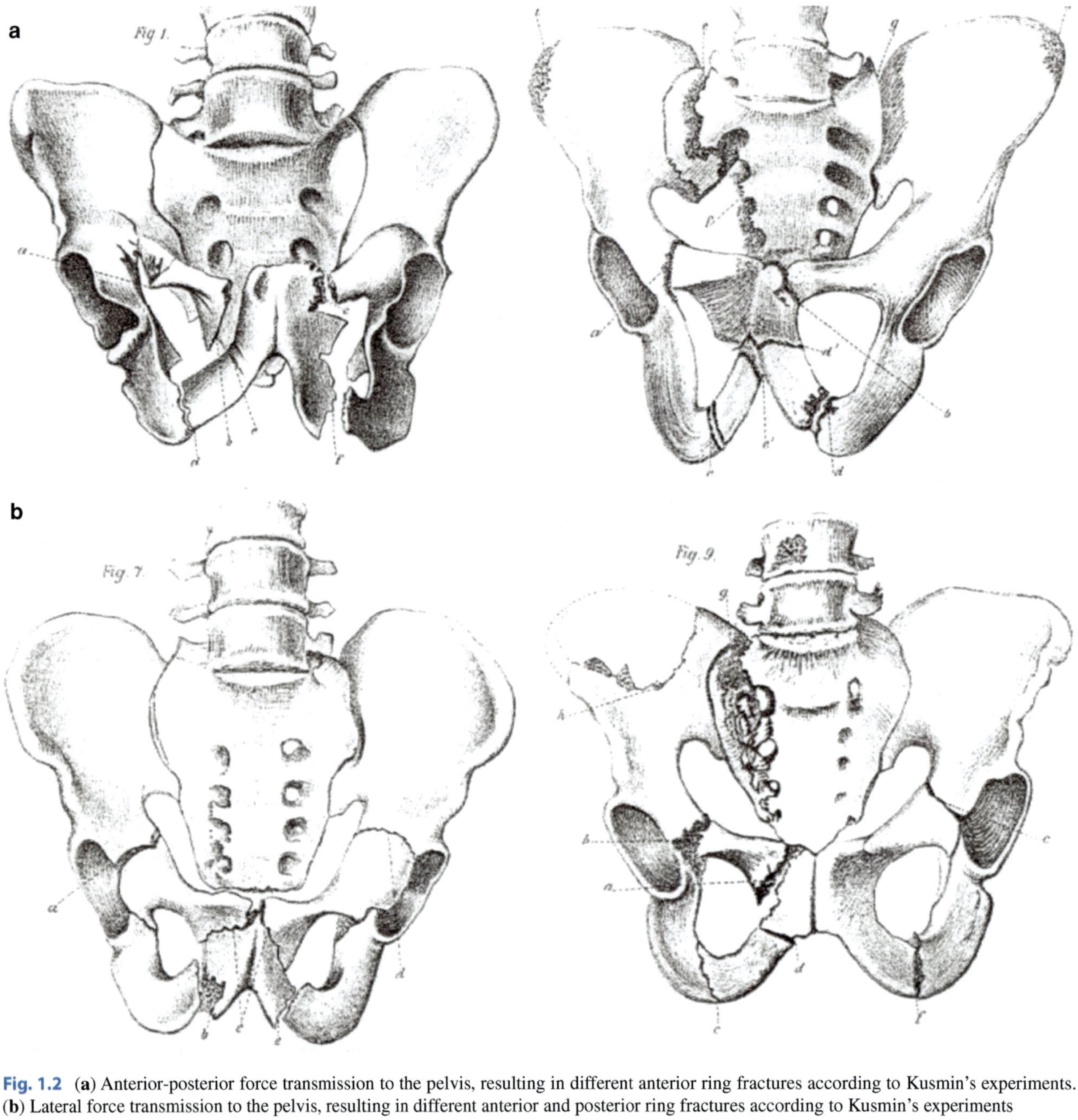

Fig. 1.2 (**a**) Anterior-posterior force transmission to the pelvis, resulting in different anterior ring fractures according to Kusmin's experiments. (**b**) Lateral force transmission to the pelvis, resulting in different anterior and posterior ring fractures according to Kusmin's experiments

- Lower pubic ramus fractures near the ischial tuberosity.

Fractures were predominantly observed at thze thin area of the rami or even at their thicker parts.

Excessive expanding forces often (lateral compression forces) resulted in (Fig. 1.2b):

- Anterior SI joint injuries, sometimes associated with an anterior or cranial sacrum displacement.
- Lateral foraminal fractures of the sacrum.
- Lateral sacral avulsion fractures (pelvic floor ligamentous avulsions).

Forces acting on the ilium resulted in:

- Anterior ring fractures with/without accompanying uni- or bilateral sacrum fractures.
- Anterior ring fractures with/without accompanying uni- or bilateral sacrum fractures and additional posterior ilium fracture.

In fresh cadavers, lateral compression was simulated by Areilza [23, 26]. With 100–300 kg, a combined symphyseal disruption with ipsilateral pubic rami fractures and secondary SI joint disruption was frequently observed. After force reduction, elasticity of the pelvic girdle led to near anatomic reduction. Additionally, isolated symphyseal disruptions, unilateral pubic rami fractures, and ilium fractures were observed.

Areilza further analyzed the effect on pelvic organ injuries. Lateral compression forces can result in urethral lesions, especially at the level of the pars membranacea, by tensioning near the pubic aponeurosis.

1.12 Pelvic Ring Stabilization

Richardson described a 5-year-old girl after a roll-over injury with open pelvic injury, consisting of a vaginal laceration and separation of the pubic bones (symphyseal disruption), which was treated by pubic wiring. Recovery was uneventful [27].

The potential first pelvic surgery in a fracture case was performed already in the eighteenth century by J. Ph. Maret (1705–1780), but no clear data are available [28].

1.13 Prognosis

The prognosis of pelvic fractures was mainly influenced by additional organ injuries. Especially urethral disruption was associated with a high mortality [29].

Historically, the prognosis of pelvic injuries was based on concomitant injuries. The presence of additional intrapelvic organ and neurovascular injuries often influenced mortality [4, 30].

> In the pre-radiographic era, pelvic fractures were rarely observed and were associated with a high mortality rate due to concomitant injuries [8, 11, 31].
> Clinically diagnosed injuries, fractures identified during autopsy examination, and experimental studies identified already the classical injury mechanisms and injury pattern [14, 15, 22, 23].
> Richardson first reported a symphyseal wire stabilization in 1887 [27].
> A hemipelvic dislocation was identified as a high-risk injury.

1.14 Knowledge on Pelvic Fracture Treatment After X-Ray Availability

The discovery of X-rays by Wilhelm Conrad Röntgen in 1895 led to a complete new understanding of injuries.

Visualization of the pelvic injury was now possible, and therefore, treatment changes were introduced and analysis of comparable cases was possible. Additionally, ideas on operative treatment were increasingly published.

> The discovery of X-rays led to the development of surgical pelvic injury stabilization techniques.

Shortly after the introduction of X-rays, the gold standard in treating pelvic injuries was still conservative treatment, which was described in detail by Cheyne in his book *A Manual of Surgical Treatment* in 1900 [32].

For the next decade, no clear ideas on surgical stabilization were presented. Pelvic X-rays led more to a better understanding of injury mechanism and injury pathologies. Fischer in 1909 presented an atypical injury with six persons sustaining different injuries after a sledge trauma during winter time [33]. These six persons were sitting on a sledge while hitting a tree. The first person immediately died at the scene, while the second and third persons died at day 1 and day 9, respectively. The others survived. Fischer analyzed the dead patients 2 and 3 and could identify the typical anterior-posterior compression injury with bilateral posterior hemipelvic dislocations.

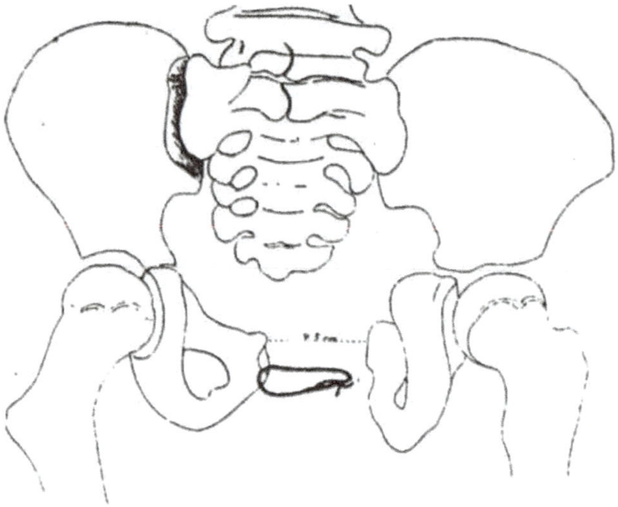

Fig. 1.3 Hirschberg's drawing of a symphyseal wire stabilization

Otto Hirschberg in 1911 described a hemipelvic dislocation, which was treated by a metallic sling around the pubic bones for symphyseal stabilization [34], comparable to the technique described by Richarson in 1887 (Fig. 1.3).

Finsterer in 1911 treated a 12-year-old boy in the same way [35]. He described the technique of osteosynthesis in detail. A Pfannenstiel incision was used. After periosteal dissection, reduction was manually achieved and stabilization was performed using an aluminum bronze wire. The periosteum was sutured, and after fascial reconstruction, the skin was closed. After treatment consisted of a pelvic sling and bed rest for 6 weeks.

Original text:

Querschnitt über die Symphyse von einem Leistenring zum anderen reichend; Freilegen des oberen Randes der Schambeine, Incision und Abheben des Periostes auf der vorderen und hinteren Fläche. Das rechte Schambein stellt etwas nach rückwärts, aber beide gleich hoch. Es zeigt sich, daß die Trennungslinie, die durch lockeres Bindegewebe verschlossen ist, im unteren Teile in der Mitte der Symphyse entsprechend dem Gelenkspalt verläuft, während sie an der oberen Seite durch den Knorpel nach rechts bis zur Knochen-Knorpel-Grenze zieht; der Knochen selbst ist intakt. Es wird nun das rechte Schambein nach vorn gezogen, der Spalt angefrischt, dann durch beide Schambeinäste eine Aluminumbronzedrahtnaht gelegt und fest zusammengeknüpft. Naht des Periostes, der Fascie und der Haut.

Anlegen eines Beckengurtes, der durch seitliche Gewichte das Becken zusammenschnürt. Reaktionsloser Verlauf; Heilung per primam. Bettruhe durch weitere sechs Wochen. Bei der Entlassung zeigt das Becken wieder normale Form, keine Verkürzung. Gang frei, ohne Schmerzen.

Albin Lambotte (1907 and 1913) was the first who proposed several options for the surgical treatment of different fractures including screw, plate, and wire stabilization techniques. For pelvic fractures and symphyseal disruptions, the following stabilization techniques were proposed [36, 37]:

- Screw stabilization of transverse sacral fractures (Fig. 1.4).
- Copper-wire stabilization of the pubic symphysis (after reduction) (Fig. 1.5).
- Screw osteosynthesis of the pubic symphysis (Fig. 1.5).
- Plate stabilization of the pubic symphysis.
- Screw stabilization of pubic rami fractures (Fig. 1.4).
- Open iliosacral screw fixation (entry point definition in Fig. 1.4).
- Sacral bar fixation of the posterior pelvis (Fig. 1.6).
- Wire or screw fixation of iliac crest fractures (Fig. 1.6).

It took some time until these ideas were taken over by others.

Lane in 1914 still did not focus on pelvic stabilizations [38], and in 1916, Hey-Grooves published extensive ideas in treating fractures of the upper and lower extremities, but options for pelvic fractures were not described [39]. And even Geiger in 1918, who developed the first fracture table (Fig. 1.7), which could be used even for traction of pelvic injuries, did not describe pelvic fracture stabilizations [40].

Between 1920 and 1922, Block and Haumann proposed iliac wing traction for hemipelvic dislocations [41, 42] (Fig. 1.8).

Bauer in 1927 described the treatment of pelvic fractures [43]. It was stated that no specific treatment is necessary for simple fractures as muscular forces support dynamic stabilization and 4–6 weeks of supine bed rest is supposed to be sufficient.

Undisplaced pelvic ring fractures can be treated by towel slinging around the pelvis.

In displaced fractures, traction or leg pulling is indicated. A detailed description of conservative treatment of concomitant bladder or urethral injuries using a catheter was proposed. In some urethral injuries, direct urethral reconstruction was favored.

The majority of pelvic injuries will heal uneventful equal to a complete restitution. In particular, patients with posterior pelvic ring fractures and acetabular fractures more often complained of remaining disturbances. Mal-healing was stated to be relevant in pregnant women.

Westerborn performed an extensive literature review and analyzed 306 cases in detail with different pelvic and acetabular fractures [44]. Surgical pelvic ring stabilization was only discussed for symphyseal separations, and it was stated that "the surgical treatment of symphyseal disruption as recommended by Lambotte is simple, but normally not necessary" ("Die operative Behandlung der Symphysenruptur, die

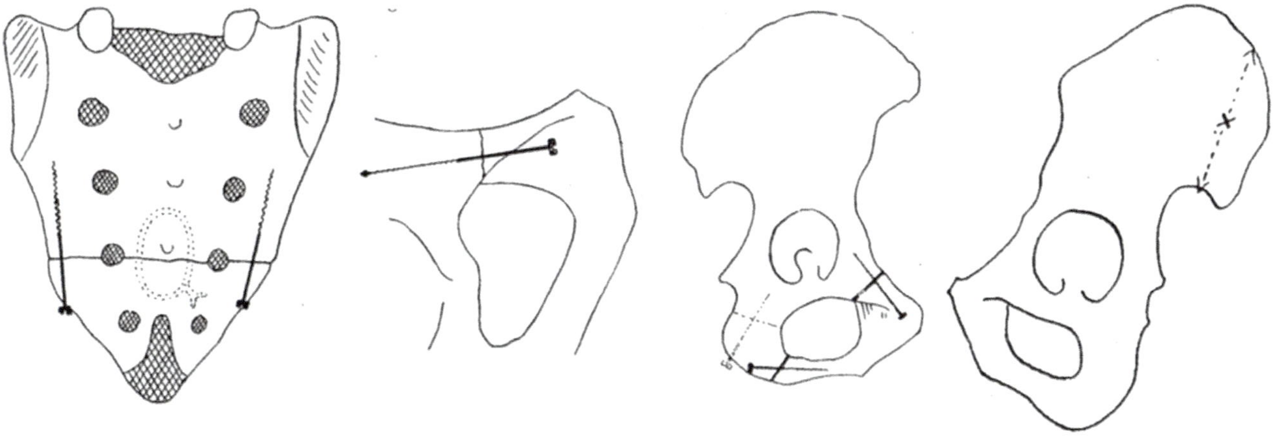

Fig. 1.4 Drawings from Albin Lambotte: screw fixation techniques for transverse sacral fractures, pubic rami fractures, and definition of the entry point for iliosacral screw fixation

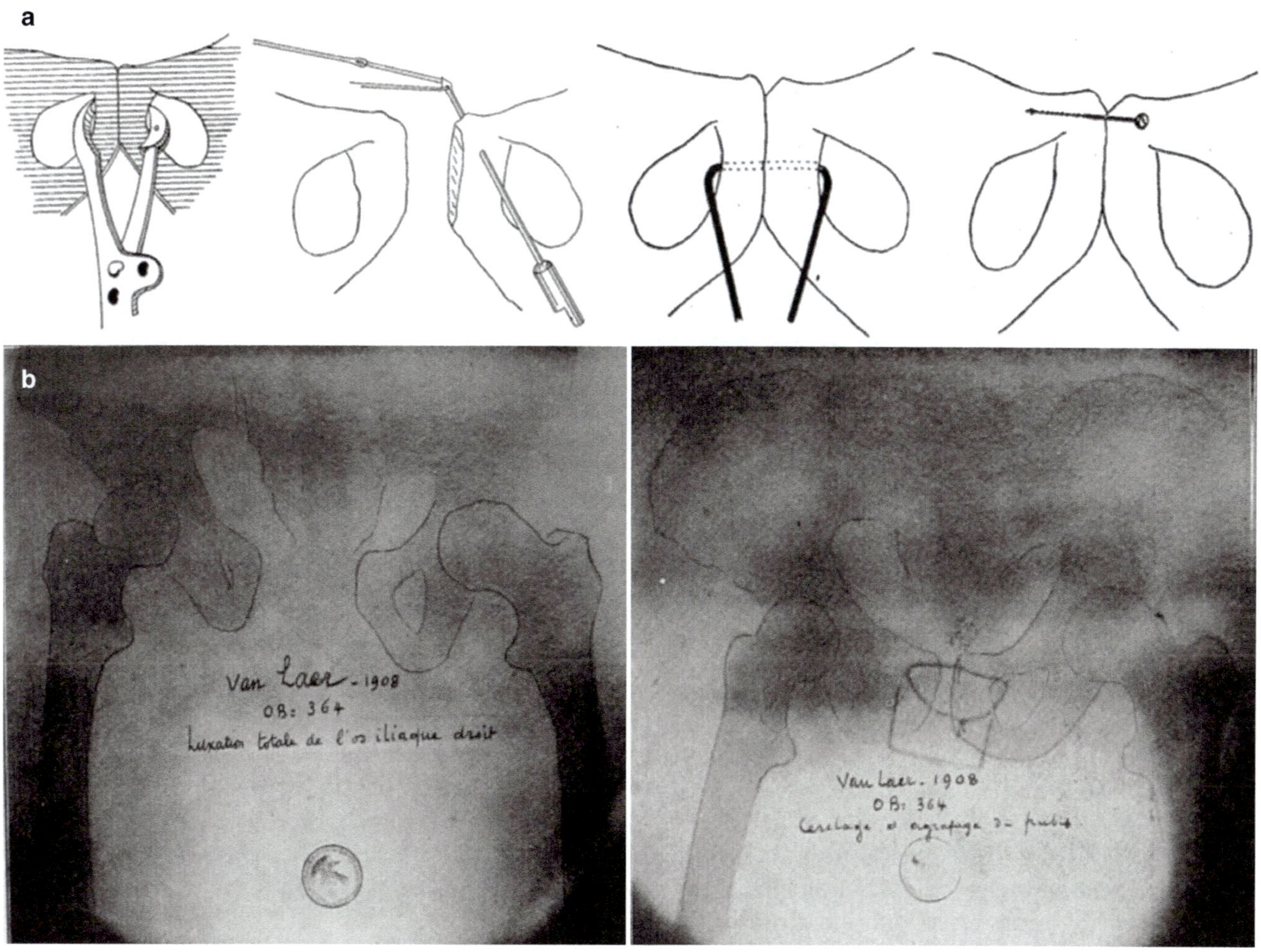

Fig. 1.5 (**a**) Drawings from Albin Lambotte: reduction and fixation techniques for symphyseal separations. (**b**) X-ray from Albin Lambotte: wire fixation of a disrupted pubic symphysis

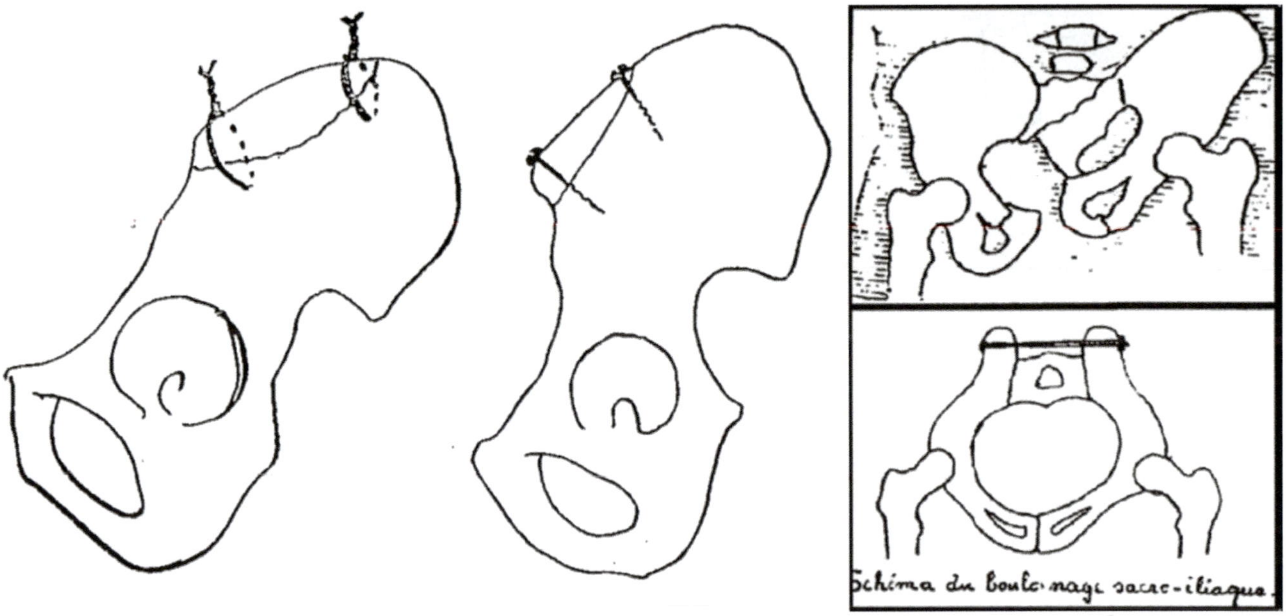

Fig. 1.6 Drawings from Albin Lambotte: fixation techniques for iliac wing fractures and sacral fractures

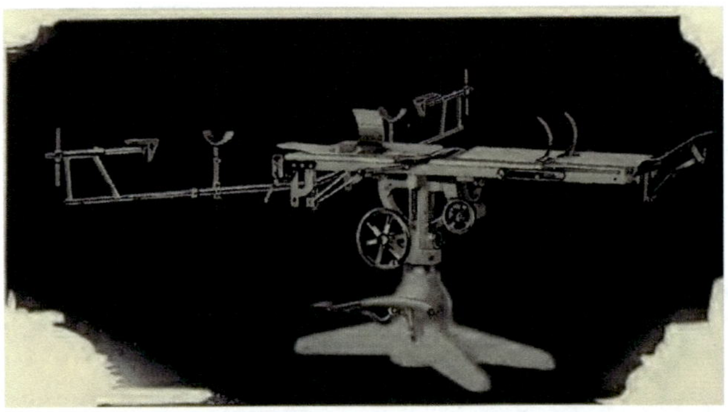

Fig. 1.7 Geiger´s traction table, also for reduction of pelvic fractures

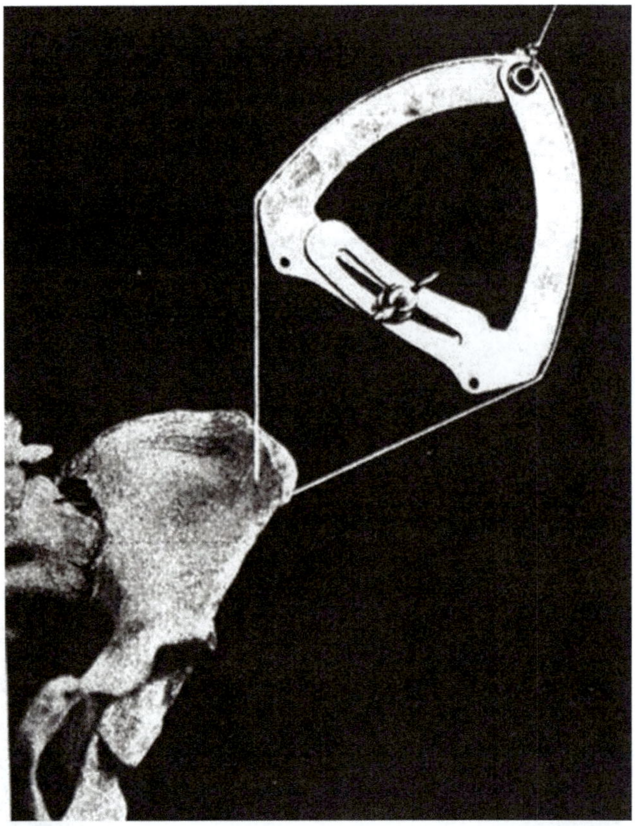

Fig. 1.8 Pelvic traction technique according to Block, directly at the ilium

u.a. von Lambotte empfohlen wird, ist einfach, aber meist unnötig").

The first larger series on pelvic ring injuries was published in 1930 by Wakeley in the *British Journal of Surgery* still performing conservative treatment [45]. Further results were reported by Magnus (1210 cases) [46] and Noland (185 cases) [47]. The treatment was conservative by traction devices (Fig. 1.9) as also recommended in the book by Hermann Matti on "Die Knochenbrüche und Ihre Behandlung" (Fractures and Their Treatment) [48].

Stabilization of the disrupted SI joint was probably first described by Lehmann in 1934, who presented a case with a screw stabilization [49].

After closed reduction maneuvers, open reduction in the prone position was performed using a posterior curved approach along the posterior iliac crest with mobilization of the gluteus maximus muscle. Under direct visualization, a screw was inserted respecting the upper neuroforamina, resulting in a screw orientation, which was rated non-optimal regarding biomechanical principles.

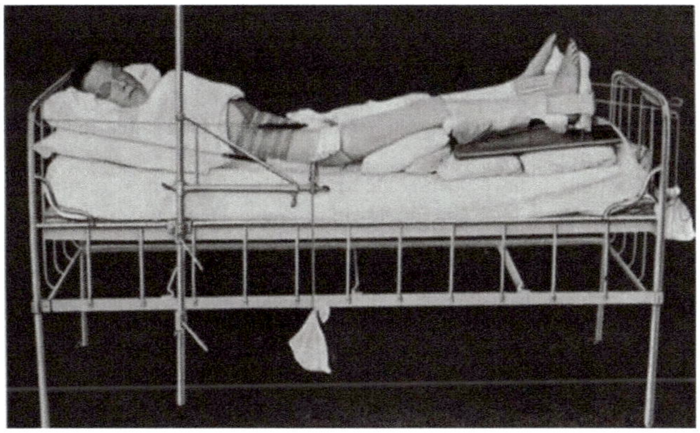

Fig. 1.9 In bed traction proposed by Matti in 1931

Original text:

Technik: Extensionstisch, Bauchlage. Direkter Zug mit Extensionszange an den Femurcondylen der verletzten Seite und—da an der zerrissenen Symphyse ein Gegenlager nicht angebracht werden konnte—direkter Gegenzug mit Kirschnerdraht am entgegengesetzten Beckenkamm. Nach Anziehen der Extensionsspindel Röntgenkontrolle. Dann Freilegen der Synchondrosis mit einem flachen Bogenschnitt unter teilweisem Ablösen des Glut. max. Nun konnte man bei direkter Sicht die gelungene Reposition kontrollieren. Bei der Verschraubung wurde Rücksicht auf die Zwischenwirbellöcher mit ihren Nerven genommen. Die Richtung der Schraube wurde dadurch im mechanischen Sinne nicht einwandfrei. Trotzdem erfüllte die Schraube ihren Zweck, das gute Repositionsergebnis zu erhalten [49].

Meyer-Burgdorf reported two further cases with open ("bloody") reduction, without describing the technique in detail [50].

For the next two decades, still conservative treatment was proposed [51].

Since the ideas of open reduction and internal fixation of pelvic injuries in 1913, during the next four decades, conservative treatment was still the predominant treatment.

It took until 1953 when Gordon Whiston published five cases with open reduction and internal fixation of pelvic fractures in the *American Journal of Bone and Joint Surgery* [52]. The potential techniques were identical to the descriptions by Albin Lambotte.

In 1965, Maurice Müller, Martin Allgöwer, and Hans Willenegger published the work *Technique of Internal Fixation of Fractures* [53].

One part was dealing with "Fractures of the Pelvis" but only described the technique of open reduction and internal fixation using screws of acetabular rim fractures.

The first and second AO Manuals were published in 1970 and 1977 and were still focusing on acetabular fracture stabilization and hip joint arthrodesis [54, 55].

Since Malgaigne's analysis of pelvic fracture types, over the next 100 years, primarily pathological-anatomical analyses and descriptions of the injuries were reported, and clinical results were almost exclusively published after nonoperative therapy.
Until the 1970s, nonsurgical therapy consisted predominantly of bed rest, manual reduction, and retention in a belt-shaped bandage with or without the use of compression or even in the pelvic cast. In addition, so-called Beckenschwebe or traction devices were used.

Johannes Poigenfürst summarized the nonoperative treatment concepts from the first half of the twentieth century [56]:

- Isolated functional treatment [46, 57, 58].
- Use of a specially designed compression apparatus [59, 60].
- Cast fixations [57, 58, 61].
- Reduction and fixation (pull—counter pull) and pelvic sling (Beckenschwebe) [57, 58].
- Pelvic traction [41, 62].
- Pelvic transfixation (cited in [56]).

Dommisse in 1960 performed wire wrapping of the pubic symphysis. For this purpose, a metal wire was attached around two screws inserted parallel to the symphysis plane to allow for dynamic stabilization [63].

Due to rather poor results after nonoperative treatment [64–66], surgical stabilization was now increasingly favored. Plate osteosynthesis of the pubic symphysis was increasingly performed [64, 67–69]. Schweiberer stated in 1978 that posterior deformities after insufficient reduction should be surgically exposed and stabilized with short plates [70].

First attempts were made to stabilize the pubic symphysis using plates.

It was the merit of Raoul Hoffmann in 1941 to develop the concept of osteotaxis and external fixation [71, 72]. George Pennal reported already in 1958 on the use of external fixation in pelvic fractures. Carabalona reported their first results in 1973 [73]. Slätis experimentally analyzed various pelvic external fixator constructs [74]. In 1980, clinical results were presented [75]. In the 1980s and 1990s, external fixation was increasingly used as a standard procedure for pelvic ring injuries [76–78].

External fixation of pelvic ring injuries became popular during the 1970s and 1980s.

Overall, internal osteosynthesis was infrequently used. In the late 1970s and 1980s, some surgeons started to perform plate and screw stabilizations [68, 79–84].

In 1978, Emile Letournel gave some basic recommendations regarding operative treatment of pelvic fractures [85]:

- "The external fixator achieves a good reduction more dependably than conservative methods" … "secondary displacement seems to be uncommon."
- Operative treatment.
  - "Allows an anatomical reduction" … "and a rigid fixation can be obtained to eliminate the need for postoperative immobilization"
  - "Provides relief of pain and discomfort after the first 2 days".

The following concepts were proposed by Letournel:

- An absolute indication is either an injury of the SI joint or the pubic symphysis.
- The symphysis is fixed by a plate.
- In the presence of additional rami fractures, the plate is extended to these fracture areas.
- Sacroiliac injuries should also be accurately repaired.
- The SI joint is approached from posterior using a vertical incision with detachment of the gluteus maximus muscle from the sacral crest.
- For combined symphyseal and sacroiliac injuries, first, the SI joint is stabilized, and after repositioning of the patient, the pubic symphysis is addressed.
- Pure anterior fractures should be treated conservatively.
- Transiliac or transsacral fractures "were neglected too long and are most often incompletely reduced."
- In transiliac or transsacral fractures, the surgeon should choose between external and internal stabilization methods according to his experience.

Letournel concluded that "the need to obtain the best possible reduction of unstable fractures of the pelvis seems to have become more generally accepted."

In 1980, Marvin Tile stated [86]:

> In most cases where an adequate posterior reduction cannot be obtained by closed means or maintained with external fixators, open reduction has been advocated. As mentioned previously, in fractures that occur through the ilium in a patient who is able to withstand surgical intervention, open reduction and rigid fixation of the iliac fracture will restore anatomic configuration, compression and stability to the pelvic ring and are desirable. If the fracture is in the sacrum or the sacroiliac joint, open reduction is more difficult.
>
> Attempts have been made to use cancellous type screws in that situation, but as previously indicated, the techniques are difficult and cannot be recommended at this time.

During the next years, based on biomechanical studies performed in Toronto by the group of Marvin Tile, it became clear that anterior and posterior internal stabilization was associated with optimal results [84].

In 1988, Marvin Tile published his landmark paper "Pelvic ring fractures: should they be fixed?" in the *British Journal of Bone and Joint Surgery* [87].

Several internal stabilization methods were described, and the following statements can be cited:

- In open book injuries, a two to four-hole plate should be placed on the superior surface and fixed with fully threaded cancellous screws.
- For unstable type C injuries, where no posterior fixation is planned, two plates at 90° to each other should be used.
- For sacral fractures, two sacral bars from one posterior iliac spine to the other will provide good stability and compression of the sacral fracture, at no risk to the neural structures.
- For sacroiliac dislocations, with or without an iliac fracture, we favor an anterior approach to the joint, with plates across the sacroiliac joint and any iliac fracture.
- Iliac fractures may be fixed by plates using standard techniques of interfragmental compression; an anterior approach is preferred, especially if a sacroiliac dislocation is present.

In 1988, Marvin Tile recommended a clear concept addressing the anterior and posterior pelvic ring for partially and completely unstable pelvic ring injuries.

In 1989, Joel Matta and Tomas Saucedo added a detailed description of useful approaches to address the anterior and posterior pelvic areas and standardized the concept of iliosacral screw fixation as an additional possible procedure for posterior ring stabilization [88].

Tile and Matta are the pioneers for open reduction and internal fixation of pelvic ring injuries. The concepts, which were developed in the late 1980s, are still today of substantial value.

References

1. Baker. Dislocation of the ossa innominata, vol. 7. London: Medical Gazette; 1830. p. 115–6.
2. Cameron T. An account of the death of the reverend Dr. Greene. Philos Trans R Soc Lond A. 1747;484:609–12.
3. Dieckmann E. Ueber Beckenfractur. Berlin: Friedrich-Wilhelms-Universität; 1877.
4. Drechsler O. Beitrag zur Geschichte und Casuistik der Beckenfrakturen. Berlin: Friedrich-Wilhelms-Universität; 1890.
5. Hall. Fractured pelvis, with laceration of the bladder. Am J Med Sci. 1844;8:248.
6. Layard D. A letter from Mr. D.P. Layard, Surgeon to C. Mortimer, M. D. Secr. R. S. inclosing an account of a fracture of the os ilium, and its cure. Philos Trans R Soc Lond A. 1745;43:537–9.
7. Riedinger. Ueber Beckenfracturen. Arch Klin Chir. 1876;20:446–53.
8. Malgaigne J. Traites des fractures et des luxations. Paris: J.B. Balliere; 1847.
9. Malgaigne J. Mémoire sur les fractures du sacrum et du coccyx. J Chir. 1846;
10. Gurlt E. Eine Normal-Statistik für die relative Frequenz der Knochenbrüche. Arch Klin Chir. 1862;III:393–7.
11. Rose E. Zur Diagnostik der einfachen Beckenfrakturen. Charité Annalen. 1865;13:19–66.
12. Leisrink H. Studien über Fracturen aus dem Hamburger allgemeinen Krankenhause. Arch Klin Chir. 1872:47–76.
13. Gurlt E. Beiträge zur chirurgischen Statistik. Arch Klin Chir. 1880:466–9.
14. Kusmin W. Ueber Beckenfracturen—Experimentelle Untersuchung. Wiener Med Jahrbücher. 1882;1:105–41.
15. Billroth T. Becken- und Lumbalgegend. Arch Klin Chir. 1869;10:561–5.
16. Augier. Triple fracture verticale du bassin par compression.—Dechirure de Turetlire.—Infiltration d'urine. Mort sept jours apres l'accident. Societe Anatomique, seance du 27. nov. 1874. Progr Med. 1875;1875:11; cited in: Zentralbl Chir.
17. Kirmisson. Disjonction des symphyses du bassin; fractures de Tos iliaque et du sacrum. Societe anatomique, searice du 13. nov. 1874. Progres Medical. 1875. 9; cited in:b 1875 Zentralbl Chir.
18. Dupont. Luxation complete de la moitie droite du bassin. Arch Med Belg. 1875;7:1; cited in: 1875 Zentralbl Chir.
19. Varrailhon. Luxation traumatique des sympliyses pubiennes et sousiliaquen droite. Rev Chir. 1886:10; cited in: Zentralbl Chir 1988.
20. Adams L. Case of rupture of the symphysis pubis during labor. Bost Med Surg J. 1876;2:4; cited in: Zentralbl Chir 1876.
21. Gallez. Deux cas de luxations fort rares. de Belgique Tome: Bulletin de Pacademie Royale de Medecine; 1876. p. 2; cited in: Zentralbl Chir 1876.
22. Fere. Fractures du bassin. de Paris: Bulletin de la soc. anatomique; 1876. p. 123; cited in: Zentralbl Chir 1877.
23. Areilza E. Resultados ecxperimentales y clinicos de las présiones transversales de la pelvis. Dt Zeitschr Chir. 1891;613:616.
24. Katzenelson M. Ueber die fracturen des beckenringes. Dtsch Z Chir. 1895;41:473–512.
25. Drechsler O. Beitrag zur Geschichte und casuistik der Beckenfrakturen. Inaugural-Dissertation welche zur Erlangung der Doctorwürde in der Medicin und Chirurgie mit Zustimmung der Medicinischen Fakultät der Friedrich-Wilhelms-Universität zu Berlin am 20. Mai 1890ß nebst den angefeügten Thesen öffentlich vertheidigen wird; 1890.
26. Areilza E. Resultados ecxperimentales y clinicos de las présiones transversales de la pelvis. Zentralbl Chir. 1891;41:806–7.
27. Richardson. Cited in: Ann Surg 1888. Bost Med Surg J. 1887.
28. Povacz F. Geschichte der Unfallchirurgie. 2. Auflage. Berlin, Heidelberg, New York: Springer-Verlag; 2011.
29. Rose E. Zwei Fälle von Blasenruptur. Dt Zeitschr Chir. 1891;XXXI:347–69.
30. Rust J. Handbuch der Chirurgie. Bd VII. 1832.
31. Duverney J. Traite de maladies des os, vol. 1. Paris: Bure l'Aiine; 1751. p. 285.
32. Cheyne W, Burghard F. A manual of surgical treatment. Part III. Chapter V.—Fractures of the Pelvis. 1900. pp. 103–8.
33. Fischer A. Über schwere beckenluxationen und verletzungen der umgebenden weichteile: typische rodelverletzungen. Zentbl Chir. 1909;36:1313–9.
34. Hirschberg O. Isolierte luxation einer beckenhälfte und technik der reposition. Dtsch Med Wochenschr. 1911;33:904.
35. Finsterer H. Über Beckenluxationen. Dtsch Z Chir. 1911;110:191–210.
36. Lambotte A. L'Intervention Opératoire dans les fractures récentes et anciennes. Bruxelles, Henri Lamertin, Libraire-Editeur. 20. Rue du Marché-au-Bois. 1907;20:133–7.
37. Lambotte A. Chirurgie opératoire des fractures. Paris: Masson & Cie, Éditeurs Libraires De L'académie De Médecine 120, Boulevard Saint-Gërmain; 1913. p. 126–44.
38. Lane W. The operative treatment of fractures. 2nd Ed. London: The Medical Publishing Company, Limited. 23, Bartholomew Close, E.G.; 1914.
39. Hey Groves E. On modern methods of treating fractures. New York: William Wood and Company; 1916.
40. Geiger C. Operative bone surgery with special reference to the treatment of fractures. Philadelphia, PA: Davis Company Publishers; 1918.
41. Block W. Arch Klin Chir. Drahtextension am Beckenkamm. 1922;120:410–4.
42. Haumann W. Ueber die halbseitige Beckenverrenkung. Bruns Beitr Klin Chir. 1921;123:278–307.
43. Bauer K. Fraktruren und Luxationen. Berlin: Verlag von Julius Springer; 1927.
44. Westerborn A. Beiträge zur Kenntnis der der Beckenbrüche und Beckenluxationen. Acta Chir Scand Suppl. 1928;63:8.
45. Wakeley C. Fractures of the pelvis: an analysis of 100 cases. Br J Surg. 1930;17:22–9.
46. Magnus G. Über Beckenbrüche, Behandlung und Resultate. Mitteilung von 1210 Fällen. Arch Klin Chir. 1931:667–70.
47. Noland L, Conwell H. Fractures of the pelvis. Surg Gynecol Obstet. 1933;56:522–5.
48. Matti H. Die Knochenbrüche und ihre Behandlung. Berlin: Verlag Julius Springer; 1931.
49. Lehmann J. Luxation einer Beckenhälfte. Zentralbl Chir. 1934;37:2149–52.
50. Meyer-Burgdorff G. Über Beckenbrüche. Zentralbl Chir. 1936;63:1016.
51. Holdsworth F. Dislocation and fracture-dislocation of the pelvis. J Bone Joint Surg. 1948;30-B(3):461–6.
52. Whiston G. Internal fixation for fractures and dislocations of the pelvis. J Bone Joint Surg. 1953;35-A:701–6.
53. Müller M, Allgöwer M, Willenegger H. Technique of internal fixation of fractures. Berlin, Heidelberg, New York: Springer-Verlag; 1965.
54. Müller M, Allgöwer M, Schneider R, Willenegger H. Manual der osteosynthese. AO-Technik. Berlin, Heidelberg, New York: Springer-Verlag; 1977.
55. Müller M, Allgöwer M, Willenegger H. Manual of internal fixation. Technique Recommended by the AO-Group. Berlin, Heidelberg, New York: Springer-Verlag; 1970.
56. Poigenfürst J. Beckenbrüche. In: Nigst H, editor. Spezielle Frakturen- und Luxationslehre. Stuttgart: Thieme; 1972. p. 141–228.
57. Böhler L. Die Technik der Knochenbruchbehandlung. Wien: Verlag Wilhelm Maudrich; 1954. p. 12–3.

58. Böhler L. Die Technik der Knochenbruchbehandlung, Ergänzungsband. Wien: Verlag Wilhelm Maudrich; 1963. p. 12–3.
59. Narat J. New splint for pelvic fractures. Am J Surg. 1938;42:443.
60. Vorschütz. Schraubenzwingenbehandlung bei Symphysenspaltung. Zentbl Chir. 1937;48:2755–66.
61. Curry G. Fractures of the pelvis. J Bone Joint Surg. 1939;21-A: 384–6.
62. Block W. Beitrag zur halbseitigen Beckenluxation nebst Vorschlägen zur Drahtextension am Beckenkamm. Dtsch Z Chir. 1920;160:113–22.
63. Domisse G. Diametric fractures of the pelvis. JBJS. 1960;42(B):432–4443.
64. Fink D, Möseneder H. Offene Symphysensprengung mit primärer Verplattung. Hefte zur Unfallheilkunde. 1974;Heft 124: 292–3.
65. Möseneder H, Fink A, Lippert K. Ergebnisse der konservativen Behandlung der Symphysenzerreißung. Hefte zur Unfallheilkunde. 1974;Heft 124:207–9.
66. Slätis P, Huittinen V. Double vertical fractures of the pelvis: a report on 163 patients. Acta Chir Scand. 1972;138:799–807.
67. Beck E. Beckenfrakturen und Luxationen. Hefte zur Unfallheilkunde. 1974;124:156–66.
68. Dolati B. Die operative Versorgung der Symphysenruptur. Unfallchirurgie. 1985;11:223–7.
69. Jenkins D, Young M. The operative treatment of sacro-iliac subluxation and disruption of the symphysis pubis. Injury. 1978;10:139–41.
70. Schweiberer L, Scheib D. Retroperitoneale Verletzungen: Wirbelsäule und Beckenfraktur. Langenbecks Arch Chir. 1978;347:177–86.
71. Hoffmann R. Perkutane Frakturbehandlung. Chirurg. 1941;13:101–12.
72. Hoffmann R. Ostéotaxis, ostéosynthèse externe par fiches et rotoules. Acta Chir Scand. 1954;107:72–88.
73. Carabalona P, Rabichong P, Bonnel F, Peruchon E, Peguret F. Apports du fixateur externe dans le disjonctions du pubis and de l'articulation sacro-iliaque. Montpell Chir. 1973;19:61–70.
74. Slätis P, Karaharju E. External fixation of the pelvic girdle with a trapezoid compression frame. Injury. 1975;7:53–6.
75. Slätis P, Kraharju E. External fixation of unstable pelvic fractures: experiences in 22 patients treated with a trapezoid compression frame. Clin Orthop. 1980;151:73–9.
76. Mears D, Fu F. External fixation in pelvic fractures. Orthop Clin North Am. 1980;11:465–79.
77. Mears D, Fu F. Modern concepts of external skeletal fixation of the pelvis. Clin Orthop. 1980;151:65–72.
78. Rubash H, Mears D. External fixation of the pelvis. AAOS Instr Course Lect. 1984;32:329–49.
79. Berner W, Oestern H-J, Sorge J. Ligamentäre Beckenringverletzungen. Behandlung und Spätergebnisse Unfallheilkunde. 1982;85:377–87.
80. Ecke H, Burger H, Hofmann D, Nazari P, Maier K. Stabilitätsprüfung verschiedener osteosyntheseverfahren nach symphysenruptur und sprengung der ileosacralfuge. Langenbecks Arch Chir. 1984;84:195–9.
81. Ecke H, Hagen P. Operative Möglichkeitenzur Behandlung von Verletzungen des Beckenrings. Krankenhausarzt. 1984;53: 346–52.
82. Ecke H, Hofmann D. Indikation und Technik der Osteosynthese bei Beckenringverletzungen: Zuggurtung. Hefte Unfallheilkunde. 1986;181:581–2.
83. Goldstein A, Phillips T, Sclafani S, Scalea T, Duncan A, Goldstein J, Panetta T, Shaftan G. Early open reduction and internal fixation of the disrupted pelvic ring. J Trauma. 1986;26(4):325–33.
84. Tile M. Fractures of the pelvis and acetabulum. Baltimore: Williams & Wilkings; 1984.
85. Letournel E. Annotation to pelvic fractures. Injury. 1978;10: 145–8.
86. Tile M, Pennal G. Pelvic disruptions: principles of management. Clon Orthop. 1980;151:56–64.
87. Tile M. Pelvic ring fractures: should they be fixed? J Bone Joint Surg. 1988;70-B:1–12.
88. Matta J, Saucedo T. Internal fixation of pelvic ring fractures. Clin Orthop. 1989;242:83–97.

Surgical Anatomy of the Pelvis

2

Norbert Peter Tesch, Axel Gänsslen, Jan Lindahl,
Wolfgang Grechenig, and Georg Feigl

The anatomy of the pelvic region is complex due to the involved structures, including bones, ligaments, joints, muscles, pelvic organs, and neurovascular structures.

For the treatment of pelvic ring injuries, the relevant surgical anatomy is of major importance, while detailed anatomical descriptions of all possible anatomical structures are clinically irrelevant.

Thus, the focus of this chapter is to deal with the main surgical structures, which have to be considered during open, minimal invasive (percutaneous), and even conservative treatment of pelvic ring injuries.

2.1 Osseous Anatomy

The bony pelvic ring consists of the two innominate bones, resulting from fusion of the pubis, the ilium, and the ischium and the sacrum with the coccyx (Fig. 2.1). A more detailed description of the osseous anatomy during growth is given in the chapter of pediatric pelvic ring injuries.

N. P. Tesch · G. Feigl
Division of Macroscopic and Clinical Anatomy,
Medical University of Graz, Graz, Austria
e-mail: norbert.tesch@medunigraz.at; georg.feigl@medunigraz.at

A. Gänsslen (✉)
Department of Trauma Surgery, Orthopedics and Hand Surgery,
Hospital Wolfsburg, Wolfsburg, Germany

J. Lindahl
Orthopaedics and Trauma Surgery,
Helsinki University Hospital, Helsinki, Finland

W. Grechenig
Department of Orthopaedics and Trauma,
Medical University of Graz, Graz, Austria
e-mail: wolfgang.grechenig@medunigraz.at

The elastic nature of the pelvic ring structure is based on three joints, anterior of the pubic symphysis and posterior of bilateral sacroiliac joints (SI joints).

These structures are relevant for load transmission from the lower extremities via the hip joints to the sacrum and the spine.

The pure osseous anatomy is the basic construct for static stability of the pelvic ring structure, while the joints, together with peripelvic muscles and ligaments, act as dynamic stabilizers.

Due to the presence of the large iliac wings, a false pelvis is distinguished from the true pelvis (Fig. 2.2), the latter surrounding the pelvic organs, the sacral plexus, and the relevant vascular structures.

2.1.1 Hemipelvis ("Innominate Bone")

The hemipelvis consists of three bones (Fig. 2.3), which fuse during puberty and early adulthood. Their connection is the triangular cartilage, which fuses to the bony acetabulum, typically during the 14th–16th year of age. Details regarding acetabular development is extensively described elsewhere [1–3].

The hemipelvic development is supported by additional epiphyseal and apophyseal growth. In the developing skeleton, apophyses serve as secondary ossification centers, which develop during the second decade of life. They serve as origin and insertion sites of muscles and tendons [1–3].

The iliac crest apophysis consists of the anterior superior iliac spine apo-/epiphysis; the true anterior iliac crest epiphysis, which extends to approximately one-half of the whole iliac crest; and the posterior iliac crest apophysis, which develops from the posterior superior iliac spine apophysis [4]. The true iliac crest epiphyses (anterior and posterior) typically join close to the middle of the iliac crest.

A. Gänsslen et al. (eds.), *Pelvic Ring Fractures*, https://doi.org/10.1007/978-3-030-54730-1_2

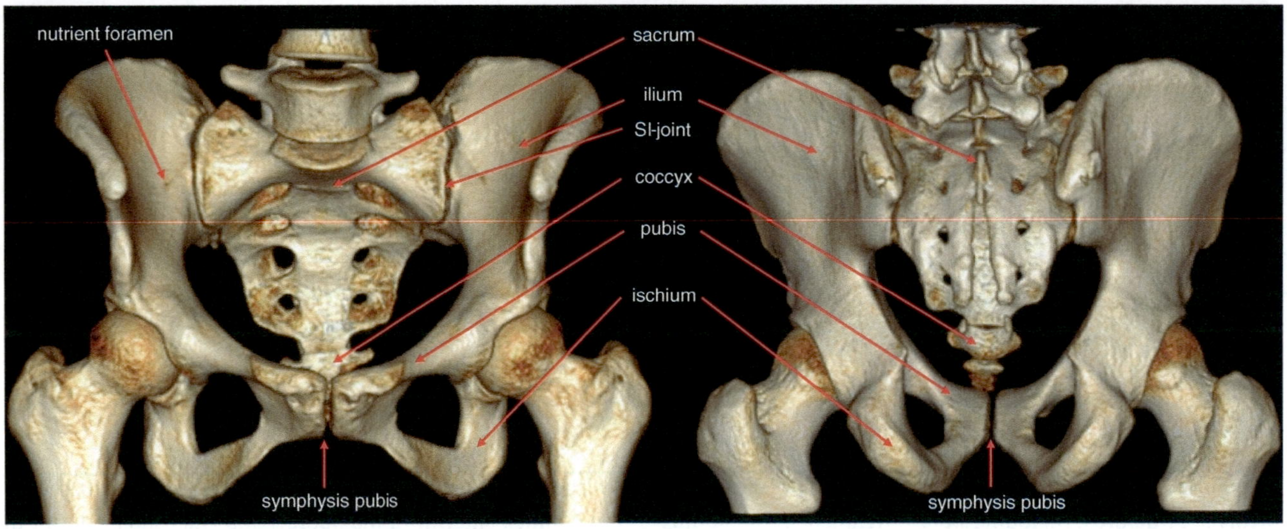

Fig. 2.1 Bony and articular contributions to the pelvic ring anatomy, the pelvis can be divided into two innominate bones and the sacrococcygeal bone connected by bilateral sacroiliac joints (SI joint) posterior and the symphysis pubis anterior

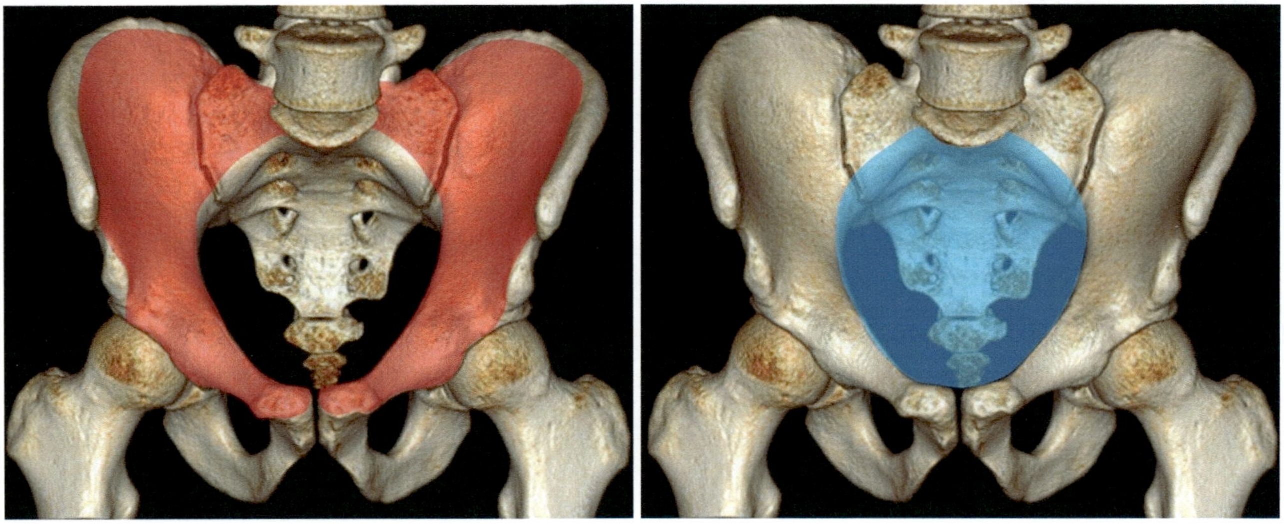

Fig. 2.2 The whole pelvis can be distinguished into the false pelvis (red) and the true pelvis (blue), the latter contains the relevant pelvic the latter surrounding the pelvic organs and neurovascular structures

The iliac crest apophysis develops in male patients between 12 and 15 years (median 14 years), and closure is observed between 16 and 23.9 years (median 21.6 years). In females, the apophysis appears between 11.3 and 15.9 years (median 14.4 years), and closure is found at an age of 15.8–25.8 years (median 23.3 years) [5]. Ossification typically starts from anterior to posterior [6, 7].

The apophysis of the anterior superior iliac spine (ASIS) normally develops at the 16th year of age and fuses around the 25th year of age [8].

The apophysis of the anterior inferior iliac spine (AIIS) normally develops between the 11th and 15th year of age and fuses between the 16th and 18th year of age [9, 10].

The ischial tuberosity apophysis initiates between 13 and 16 years of age, while fusion occurs between 16 and 18 years of age with complete union between 20 and 23 years of age [11].

Data on fusion of the posterior iliac spines are missing.

Clinical Relevance

Thus, in skeletally immature patients, especially in young athletes at the age of 14–17 years, there is a risk of injury to these areas, as the physes are the most vulnerable areas of the musculotendinous connection to the bone due to perpendicular acting forces on the apophyses.

Morphologically, the fully developed innominate bone corresponds to the shape of a figure of eight according to Mollier [12]. Between the perpendicular orientation of the iliac wing plane and the obturator foramen, the acetabulum is integrated. Gänsslen et al. extended this view and proposed a three-ring structure of the hemipelvis [13]. The periphery of these rings allows implant anchorage.

2.1.1.1 Ilium

The ilium is the most superior part of the three hemipelvic bones (Fig. 2.4). An upper part and a lower part can be distinguished, separated by a ridge on the medial (inner) surface. This ridge is termed the arcuate line in its anterior part, which here forms part of the linea terminalis and the pelvic brim [5].

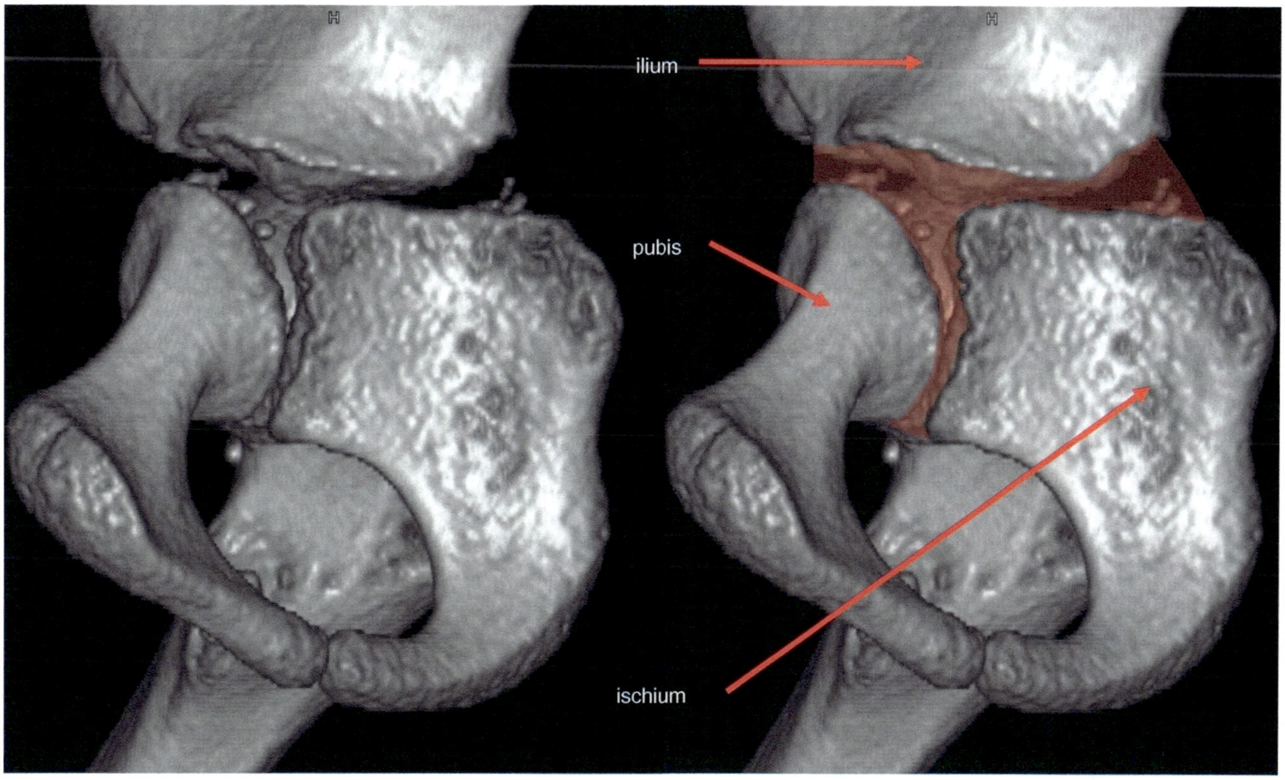

Fig. 2.3 The hemipelvis fuses during puberty and early adulthood. The medial view of a 7-year-old girl shows the triradiate cartilage formation connecting the pubis, the ischium, and the ilium

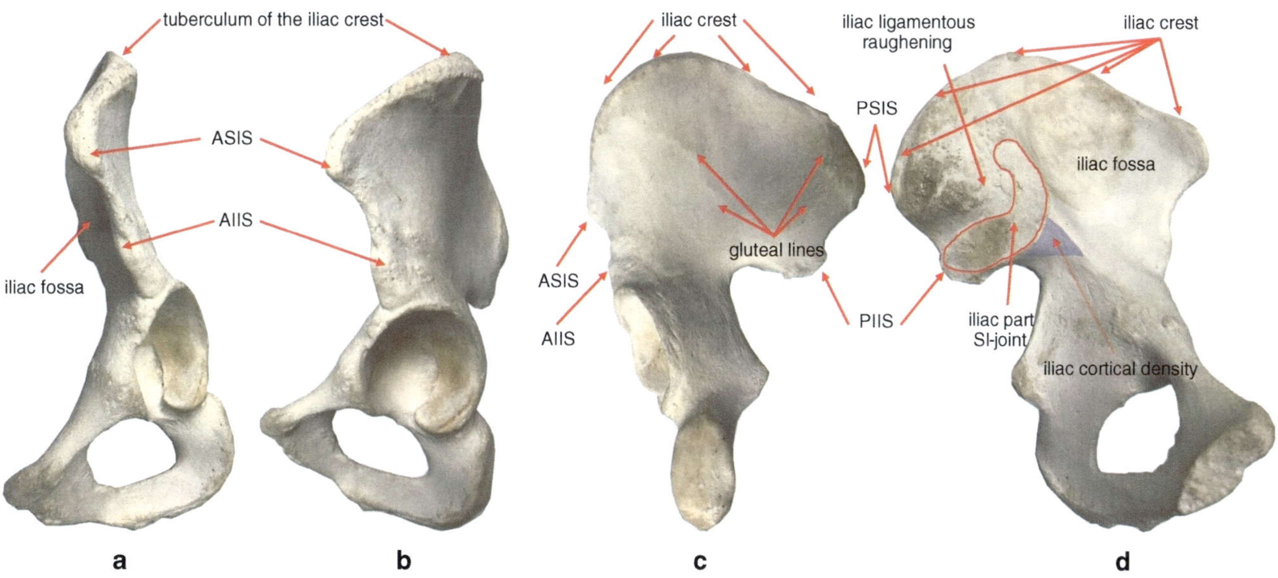

Fig. 2.4 Relevant bony landmarks of the iliac bone

The upper part of the ilium (Fig. 2.3c, d), belonging to the false pelvis, presents as a flat, fan-shaped wing-structure and serves as an origin of essential muscle groups for the movement of the lower leg (abductors, gluteus maximus, iliacus muscle).

The inner (medial) surface of the wing is concave (iliac fossa), which is covered by the iliacus muscle. Near the SI joint, a large nutrient foramen is present (Fig. 2.1). During surgery, relevant bleeding can occur from here.

Ebraheim et al. analyzed the location of this foramen and reported its location approximately 12.5 mm lateral to the anterosuperior sacroiliac joint line and 23.5 mm perpendicular to this line along the pelvic brim parallel to the sacroiliac joint line [14]. In a further analysis, the nutrient artery was found to cross the SI joint. In average, the nutrient foramen was identified 88.1 mm medial to ASIS, 20.1 mm above the pelvic brim, and 20.1 mm lateral to SI joint [15].

At the posterior ilium, a ridge is found directly superior to the articulating area with the sacrum. Within the true pelvis, the iliac L-shaped articular surface of the SI joint becomes visible. More posterior, a roughened area for attachment of interosseous and posterior sacroiliac ligaments is present.

The external (gluteal) surface of the iliac wing presents with some bony margins (gluteal lines) and roughenings, indicating muscular attachments. The abductors originate along the anterior and inferior gluteal line, the gluteus maximus muscle to a large extent along the posterior gluteal line.

The superior margin of the ilium is thickened and forms the iliac crest for muscular and fascial attachments of lumbar, abdominal, and lower leg muscles and fascias. Anterior and posterior, the iliac crest ends at the ASIS and posterior superior iliac spine (PSIS), respectively. The shape of the iliac crest is convex on the outer side (Fig. 2.5). Approximately 4–8 cm posterior to the ASIS, a prominent tubercle, the tuberculum of the iliac crest, becomes visible. This area is relatively thick and includes a slightly angulated bone corridor, running from the iliac crest to the supraacetabular region (Fig. 2.5, blue). This landmark is of surgical relevance during pelvic ring external fixation techniques. Here, the strong bone structure allows sufficient holding forces for pin application in an iliac external fixator [16].

Inferior to the ASIS at the anterior margin of the ilium, the anterior inferior iliac spine (AIIS), the attachment area of the rectus femoris muscle is an important landmark.

Along the plane from the AIIS to the posterior inferior iliac spine (PSIS), a long bone corridor is present (Fig. 2.5, red), which forms the inferior part of the ilium [16], integrating the acetabular roof. More posterior, the upper margin of the greater sciatic notch represents its inferior base.

Clinical Relevance

Several investigators analyzed the bone corridor between the AIIS and PSIS for posterior and anterior stabilization techniques using different orientations [16–21]. Its length is between 10 and 15 cm with a width of 11.4 mm and a height of 23 mm.

Parallel and anterior to the SI joint, the strongest bone structure, the "iliac cortical density" is a relevant structure

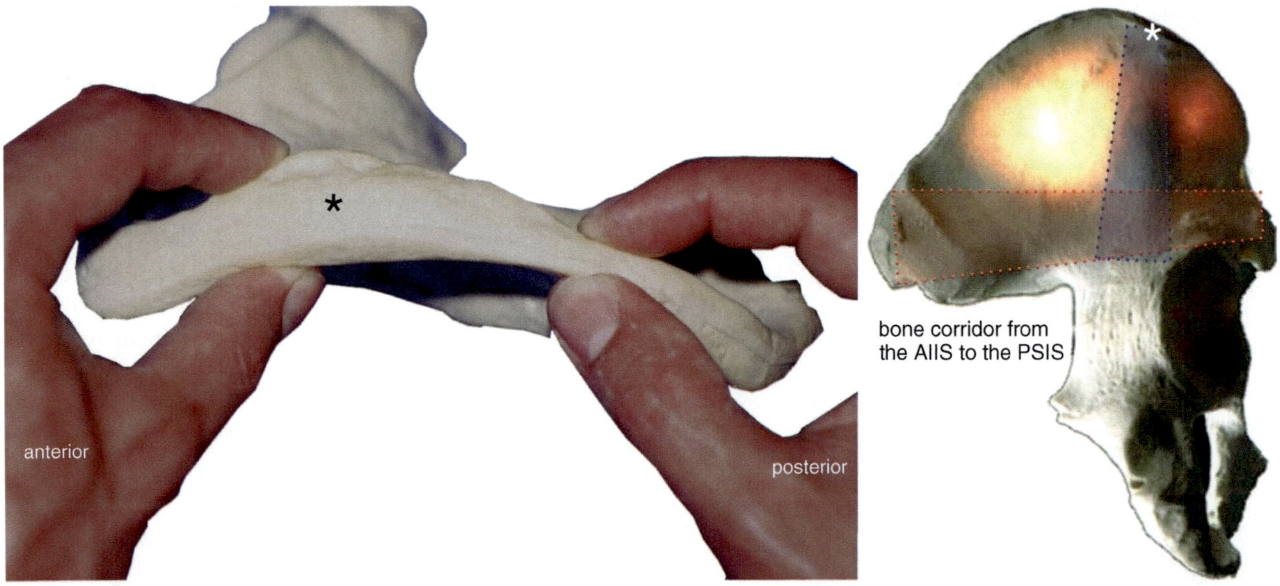

Fig. 2.5 Anatomy of the iliac crest with the tuberculum of the iliac crest (*). The lateral view confirms the localization of two relevant bone corridors: supraacetabular corridor (red) and vertical bone corridor (blue), starting at the tuberculum of the iliac crest

for implant fixation. The iliac cortical density is almost always caudal and posterior to the sacral alar slope [22].

The corpus and iliac wing form an angle of approximately 60° in the frontal plane on the inner side of the pelvis. On the outer side, this angle is reduced to 20°–30° due to the more prominent posterior wall and the posterior column of the acetabulum [23].

2.1.1.2 Ischium

The ischium is the posterior and inferior part of the hemipelvis and consists of a large body that joins with the ilium and the superior ramus of the pubis, and an anterior extension from the ischial tuberosity, which joins with the inferior ramus of the pubis to form the posterior-inferior border of the obturator foramen [5]. The large ischium body comprises about 2/5 of the acetabular surface, including the acetabular fossa. It is a relevant static stabilizer (Fig. 2.6).

At its posterior margin, which is part of the posterior acetabular column, the ischial spine separates the lesser sciatic notch from the greater sciatic notch due to the insertion of the sacrospinous ligament.

The ischial tuberosity is important for load transfer during and to support sitting and is the important origin of the hamstring muscles.

2.1.1.3 Pubis

The pubis is the anterior and inferior part of the hemipelvis with its symphysis body and the superior and inferior rami (Fig. 2.7).

The superior pubic ramus is orientated posterior-laterally from the body and joins the acetabular cavity creating the anterior acetabular wall. On top of the superior ramus, several surgical landmarks are relevant (Fig. 2.7c–e):

- Pubic tubercle: a prominent anterior projected tubercle on the upper border of the medial superior ramus portion, where the inguinal ligament inserts.
- Pecten pubis: a sharp superior margin, which forms part of the pelvic brim, arising from the pubic tubercle and runs posterior-medial to form the iliopectineal line together with the more posterior arcuate line; it creates the medial border to the true pelvis.
- Iliopectineal eminence: medial border of the groove, where the iliacus and psoas major muscles run over the inguinal region to the minor trochanter of the femur; it marks the union point of the superior pubic ramus and the ilium; the psoas minor inserts at its medial border (pectineal line/pectin pubis).
- Pubic crest: it extends from pubic tubercle to the medial upper border of the pubic symphysis; the conjoined tendon of the rectus abdominis, the abdominal external oblique muscle, and the pyramidalis muscle insert at this area.

The strong pectineal ligament ("Cooper's ligament") extends from the pubic tubercle to the iliopectineal eminence (Fig. 2.7c). Part of the inguinal ligament, the iliopectineal arch separates the lacuna musculorum from the lacuna

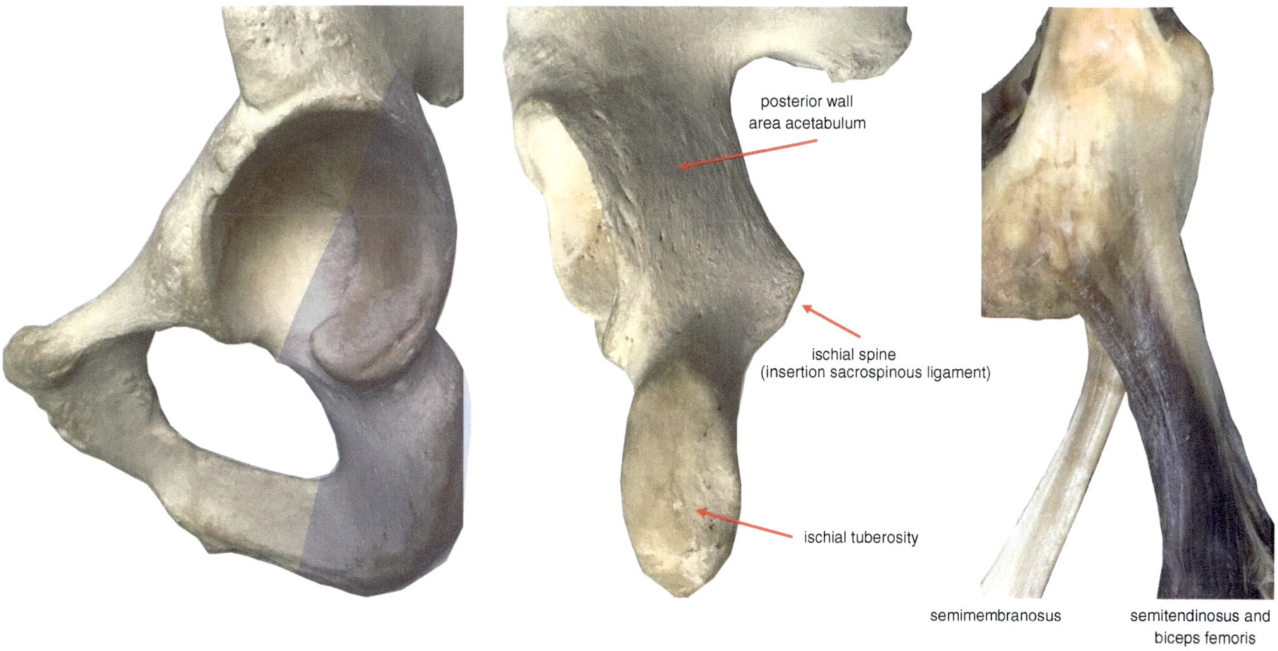

Fig. 2.6 Bone anatomy of the ischium with the hamstring origins

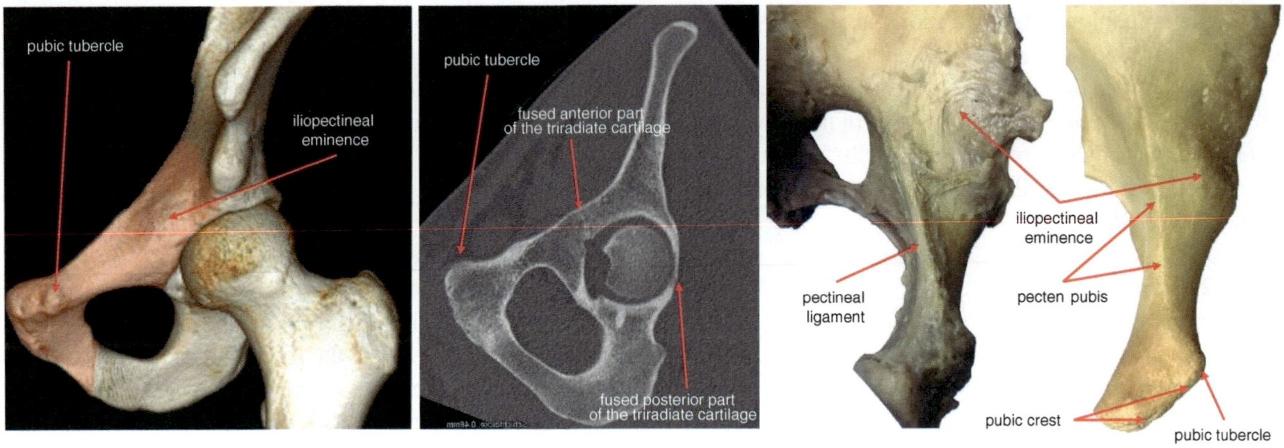

Fig. 2.7 Anatomical landmarks of the pubic bone

vasorum and strengthens the pectineal ligament distally and medially. Lateral to the iliopectineal eminence, the posterior part of the iliopsoas fascia closes off the entrance to the pelvis.

Together with the inferior pubic ramus and the ischial body, the superior ramus creates a major part of the obturator foramen.

At the lateral upper margin of the obturator foramen, a bony groove, the obturator sulcus can be detected, which forms the bony, upper border of the obturator canal. The obturator neurovascular structures pass from inside the pelvis to the thigh.

The thin and flat inferior ramus is directed lateral and inferior from the medial end of the superior ramus to join with the ramus of the ischium. The anterior surface is rough, where the gracilis, the obturator externus, and the adductor brevis and magnus muscles originate. The smooth posterior, internal surface is the origin of the obturator internus muscle.

The superior and inferior pubic rami are therefore surrounded by the muscular sling of the obturator muscles, which allow, together with the thick superior periosteum, fast healing of anterior pelvic ring fractures (Fig. 2.8).

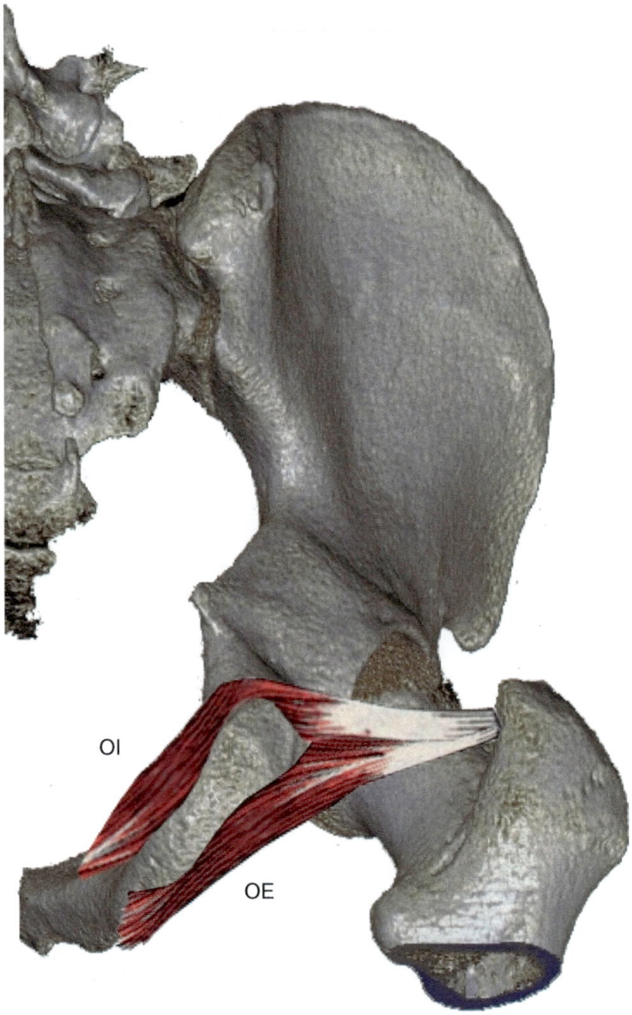

Fig. 2.8 Muscular sling around the obturator foramen consisting of the obturator internus (OI) and externus (OE) muscles

2.1.2 Anatomy of the Sacrum

The sacrum is a complex anatomical structure [24], which is formed by fusion of normally five sacral vertebrae, creating a large triangular bone (Fig. 2.9). Overall, the sacrum develops from 58 to 60 sacral ossification centers [25]. The definitive shape and fusion develop during puberty at the age of 16–18 years and is completed between 25 and

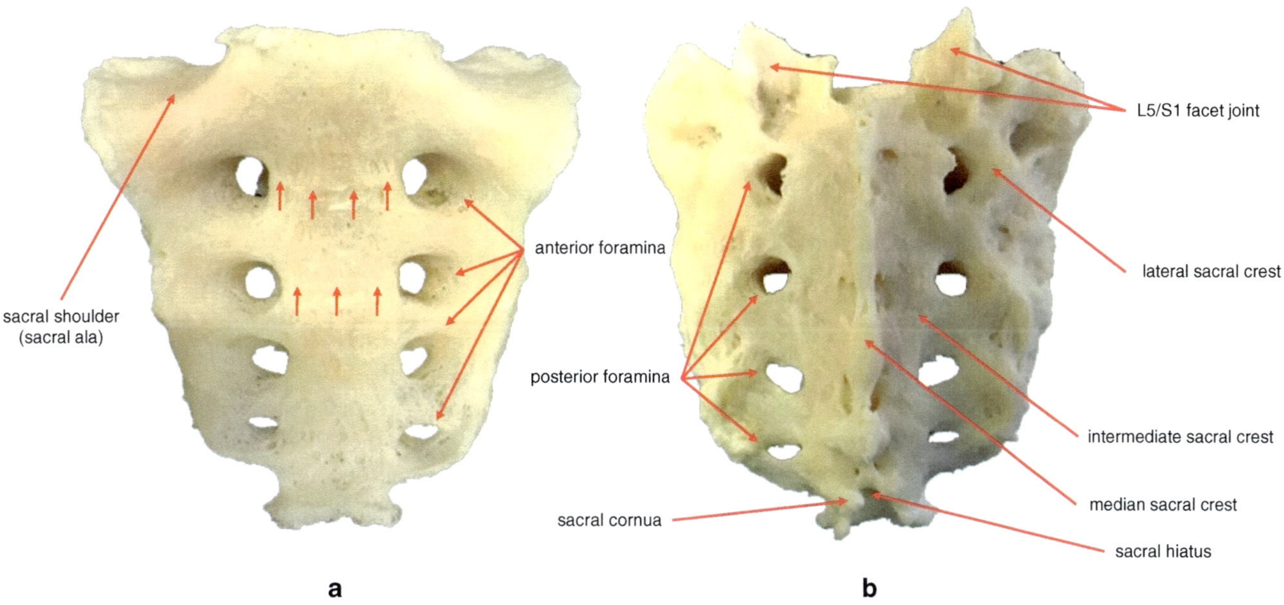

Fig. 2.9 Anterior (**a**) and posterior (**b**) sacral surface. Lateral to the anterior transverse fusion lines of the former vertebral bodies (arrows), the four pairs of anterior sacral foramina are located. Posteriorly, several sacral crests and bony protuberances can be identified

34 years [26–29]. Fusion occurs along the intervertebral disks [26–28], starting inferiorly [30].

Clinical Relevance
A persisting intervertebral disk can be sometimes observed between the S1 and S2 vertebrae (Fig. 2.10).

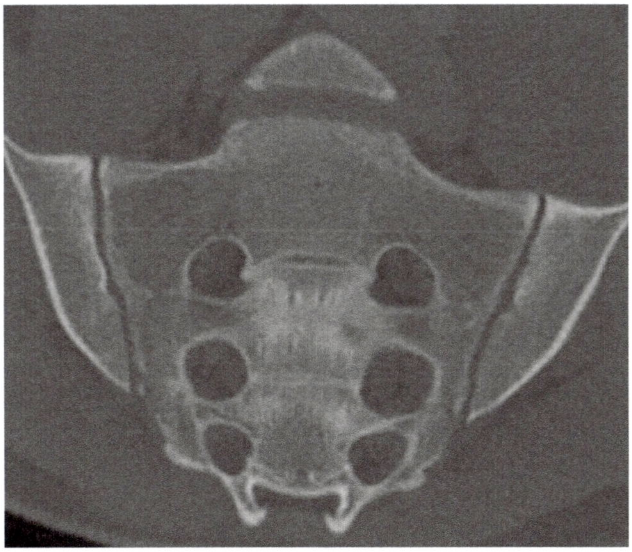

Fig. 2.10 Persisting intervertebral disk between the S1 and S2 body, indicating a dysmorphic sacrum

The sacrum articulates with the fifth lumbar vertebra, both innominate bones via the sacroiliac joint and distal with the coccyx.

The sacrum shows four anterior and posterior sacral foramina. The S1–S4 nerve roots exit through their corresponding foramen, while the S5 nerve root exits between the sacrum and coccyx [31]. The anterior foramina are larger than the posterior foramina, as the anterior nerve root diameter is larger [31].

2.1.2.1 Surface Anatomy

The bony shape of the postmature sacrum shows a concave anterior pelvic surface and a corresponding posterior convex surface. The lateral sacral surface is broader in the superior area and narrows in direction to the coccyx. Its broad base is directed upward and forward, and the tapered apex is directed downward. The bony architecture consists of a high amount of cancellous bone, which is enveloped by a thin layer of cortical bone. The sacrum has a height and width of 10–11 cm [32].

Anterior Sacral Surface

The anterior concave sacral surface is relatively smooth and represents the posterior border of the true pelvis. It shows fusion lines of the former vertebral bodies (ridges), which are recognizable as transverse lines (Fig. 2.9a). Typically, four pairs of anterior sacral foramina are present, which decrease in size from proximal to distal [33], allowing the passage of the anterior nerve roots creating the sacral plexus and the lateral sacral arteries. These foramina are located on each side of the corresponding transverse ridge. The foraminal orientation is slightly anterolateral. The anterior foramina are larger than the posterior foramina, as the anterior nerve root diameter is larger [31].

At the superior lateral anterior sacrum, parts of the iliacus muscle arise from its surface. Lateral to the foramina, the piriformis muscle arises.

Posterior Sacral Surface

The posterior sacral surface is convex and highly irregular [34, 35]. The posterior elements of the former sacral vertebrae create several longitudinal crests (Fig. 2.9b).

The prominent median sacral crest shows proximally a more prominent S1 tubercle (old spinal process), while the S2–S5 tubercles are less prominent. At the inferior part of the median crest, often, the fifth sacral lamina shows no fusion in the midline, creating an opening, termed the sacral hiatus. Different variations of the hiatus location exist [36, 37].

The fused lamina follows lateral to these spinal processes. The irregularity of the further lateral posterior sacral area is based on the fused articular processes, presenting as an intermediate crest. Its most inferior part forms an osseous protuberance, the sacral cornua, which connect to the coccyx.

Further lateral, four pairs of dorsal foramina are present, which decrease in size from proximal to distal [33], for passage of the posterior divisions of the sacral nerves, which exit at the whole lateral foraminal border [38]. At the inferior lateral quadrant of the foramina, a foraminal branch of the lateral sacral artery is typically present medial to the nerve root. An accompanying venous plexus is typically missing [39].

Intraoperatively, these are relevant landmarks for control of fracture reduction. Compared to the anterior foramina, the posterior foramina are much smaller and less regular [29, 31]. The orientation between the anterior and posterior foramina shows a Y shape (Fig. 2.11) where the anterior foramen forms the base with two limbs orientating medially into the sacral vertebral canal and posterior to the posterior foramina [40].

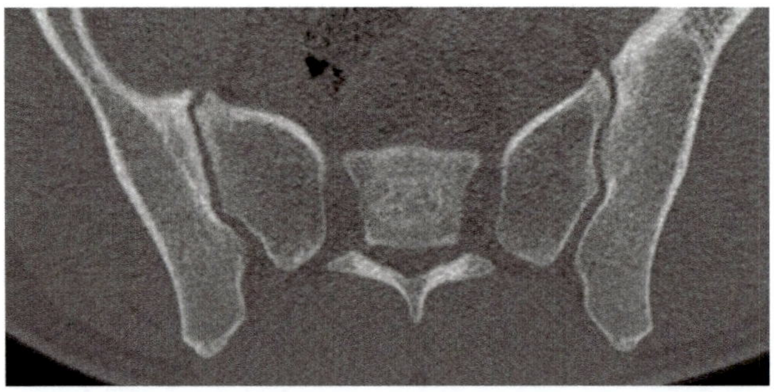

Fig. 2.11 Y-shaped configuration of the sacral nerve root canal with the exiting anterior and posterior nerve roots

Clinical Relevance

Farrell et al. analyzed the course of the upper sacral nerve root tunnel (Fig. 2.12) on standard intraoperative images [41]. It was visible in 100%, 21%, and 91% in the outlet view, inlet view, and true lateral view, respectively.

The morphological association between the second posterior sacral foramen and the PSIS can be of surgical relevance during fracture fixation for control of reduction. The second foramen is normally located approximately 2–3 cm medial to the PSIS in a 45° inferior angulation from the PSIS [42].

The fused transverse processes represent the most lateral part of the posterior surface. Here, the posterior iliosacral ligaments have their origins.

Posterior muscular attachments include parts of the gluteus maximus lateral just below the SI joint and the multifidus, sacrospinalis, and erector spinae muscles, which originate from the sacral grooves medial to the median crest.

Lateral Sacral Surface

The lateral sacral surface with its triangular shape presents with the sacral articular part of the SI joint (Fig. 2.13). The L-shaped articular surface presents with superior and inferior limbs, nearly rectangular to each other [43], and is located at the anterior border of the sacrum, while the posterior border is non-articular due to the insertion of the interosseous iliosacral ligaments. The length of the superior, longitudinal limb is between 3.7 and 4.4 cm, while the inferior, horizontal limb has a 5.6-cm dimension [32, 43]. The auricular surface of the sacrum has a mean surface area of 18.4 cm^2 [44].

Superior Sacral Surface

The superior sacral surface consists of the sacral promontory (anterior portion of the first sacral vertebra) and the sacral ala (Fig. 2.13). Posterior to the S1 body, a triangular opening represents the entrance of the sacral canal. Medial to the sacral canal, the superior facets of the lumbosacral facet joint are prominent with a posterior-medial orientation. The pedicle area of S1 is located directly lateral to the sacral canal with its cephalad margin located under the most anterior aspect of the superior facet [29]. The medial margin represents the lateral edge of the sacral canal [45], while no clear anatomical location is known for the lateral margin [29].

The sacral mass (sacral ala) follows the pedicle laterally and consists of fused costal elements and transverse processes [29].

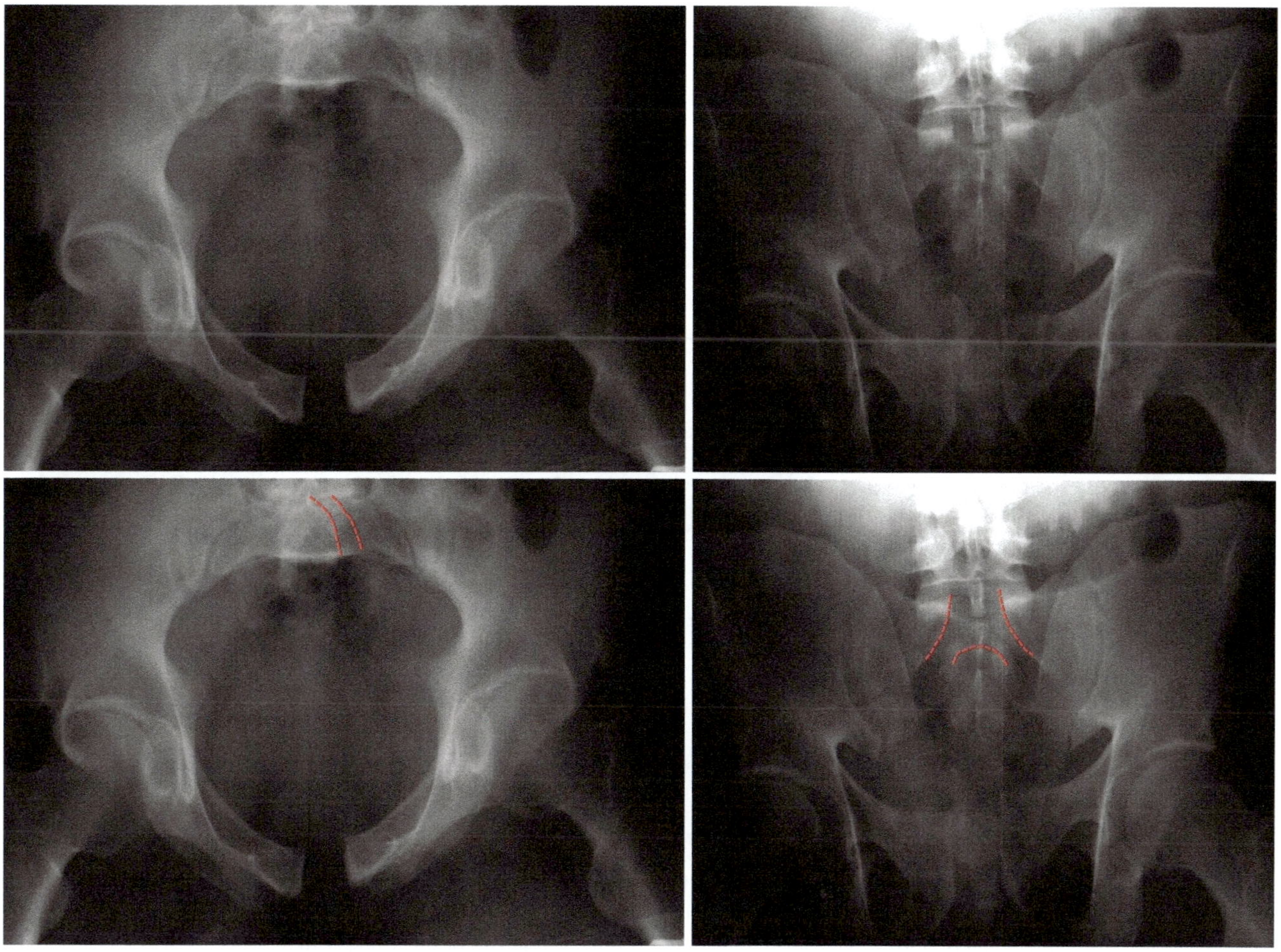

Fig. 2.12 Upper sacral nerve root tunnel on inlet and outlet views

Routt et al. proposed the concept of the sacral alar slope [22], which is defined as the plane difference between the promontory and the sacral ala (Fig. 2.14). A resulting angle is orientated approximately 30° caudal to the frontal plane [46].

Attachments on the sacral ala include the iliolumbar ligament and the lumbosacral ligament.

2.1.2.2 Anatomical Variations

The lumbosacral junction is a highly variable region with common anatomical variations (Fig. 2.15). Here, especially a sixth lumbar vertebra or a six-bone sacrum is of surgical relevance.

Atypical morphology of the upper sacral bone is observed in 30–55% [22, 47–50]. Compared to the normal sacrum, the resultant upper additional fifth sacral foramen is larger, noncircular, misshapen, and irregular [51]. Often, a residual disk space can be observed, especially on the outlet view or computed tomography (CT) scan, transecting the dysmorphic upper part and the original second sacral segment. Additionally, the cross-sectional area of the dysmorphic sacral bone can be 36% smaller than in the normal S1 body, making a horizontal screw orientation impossible [48].

Pathoanatomically, a relatively high position of the sacral wing in relation to the iliac crest is found, as well as the presence of mammillary processes and joint connections between lumbar and sacral transverse processes [22]. In addition, lumbarization or sacralization may occur [52].

Surgical Relevance

A dysmorphic upper sacrum is associated with a different screw pathway for iliosacral screw fixation. The osseous pathways are narrowed and obliquely oriented. In 80%, the S2 sacral segment safe zone is larger than the S1 sacral segment safe zone [51, 53], so the S2 level is safer and therefore recommended to use. This results in a different screw orientation in the dysmorphic sacrum [48].

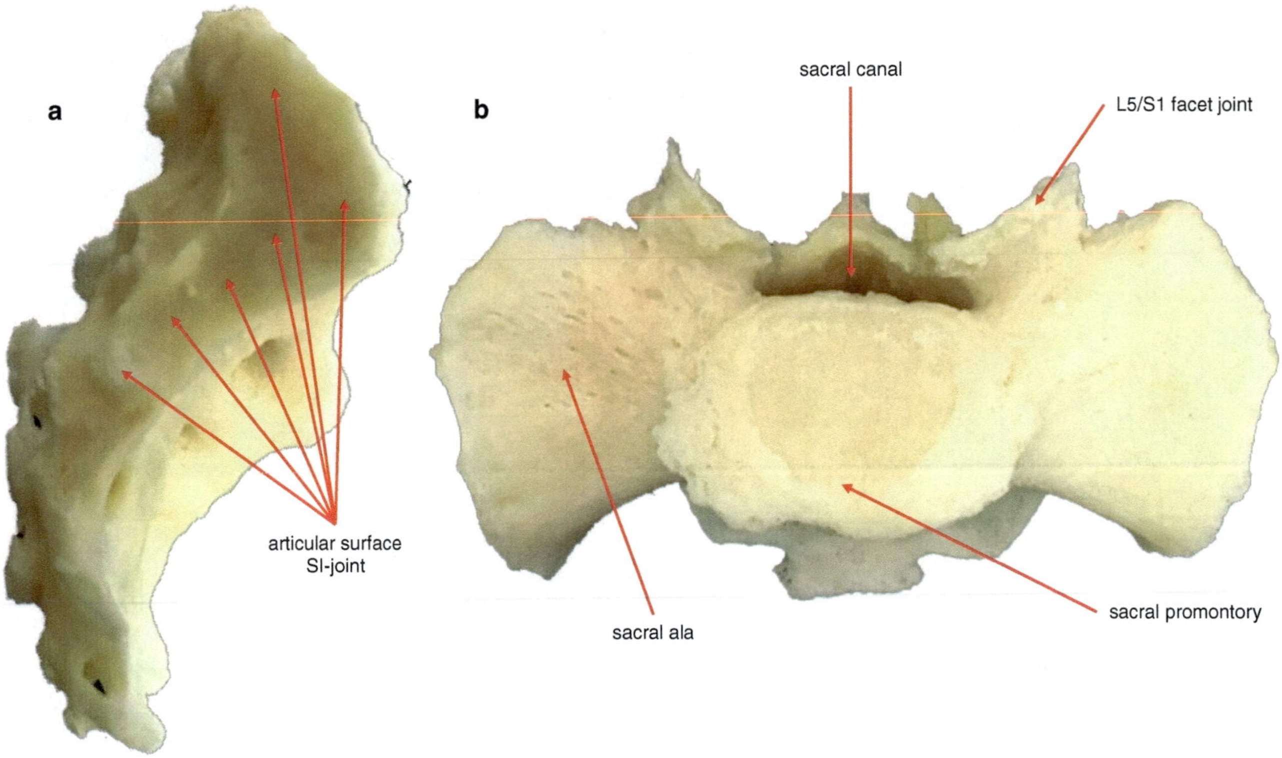

Fig. 2.13 Lateral (**a**) and superior (**b**) sacral surface

Routt et al. described morphological abnormalities including a more cephalic position of the sacral ala relative to the iliac crests, the presence of additional sacral alar mammillary processes, and articulations of both lumbar and sacral transverse processes with the true ala [22].

Kaiser et al. described several types of sacral dysmorphism and correlated these findings with the use of iliosacral screw fixation [50]. The frequency of five clinically relevant morphological abnormalities was analyzed (Fig. 2.16):

- 33% upper sacral segment not recessed in the pelvis
- 52.5% existence of mammillary processes
- 35.5% acute alar slope
- 35.5% residual disk between the first and second sacral segments
- 29.5% noncircular upper sacral neural foramina

Pohlemann et al. analyzed the safe zones for screw insertion from the posterior sacral aspect [54–56]. The junction between the posterior sacral pedicle and the vertebral body is considered a safe zone [54–57].

Ebraheim et al. reported an optimal medial screw path at S1 starting just lateral and inferior to the superior facet and angling 30° anteromedially or anterolaterally [58]. For S2, the optimal screw orientation starts at the posterior midpoint of the medial mass.

2.1.2.3 Internal Sacral Architecture

The bone mineral density of the sacrum is irregular depending on specific bone zones (Fig. 2.17).

Ebraheim et al. reported the weakest bone zones to be in the lateral sacral alar of S1 and at the level of the junction of S2 and S3, while the strongest bone zone was observed between the S1 and S2 foramina [59].

A CT analysis of the normal sacrum revealed a reduced bone density in typical sacral regions, with lowest bone density paraforaminal lateral and between S1 and S2 [60, 61].

The mean bone mineral density (BMD) of the S1 was found to be 31.9% higher than that of the sacral alar, and the highest bone mineral density is typically observed near the lateral posterior and lateral anterior part of the S1 body [62].

A DEXA scan analysis found highest cancellous BMD in the anterior two-thirds of the S1 body, while the highest cortical BMD was observed anteriorly [63].

> **Clinical Relevance**
> The internal bone density can explain specific fracture patterns in traumatic and fragility fractures of the sacrum [64], and therefore, specific screw pathways can be recommended.

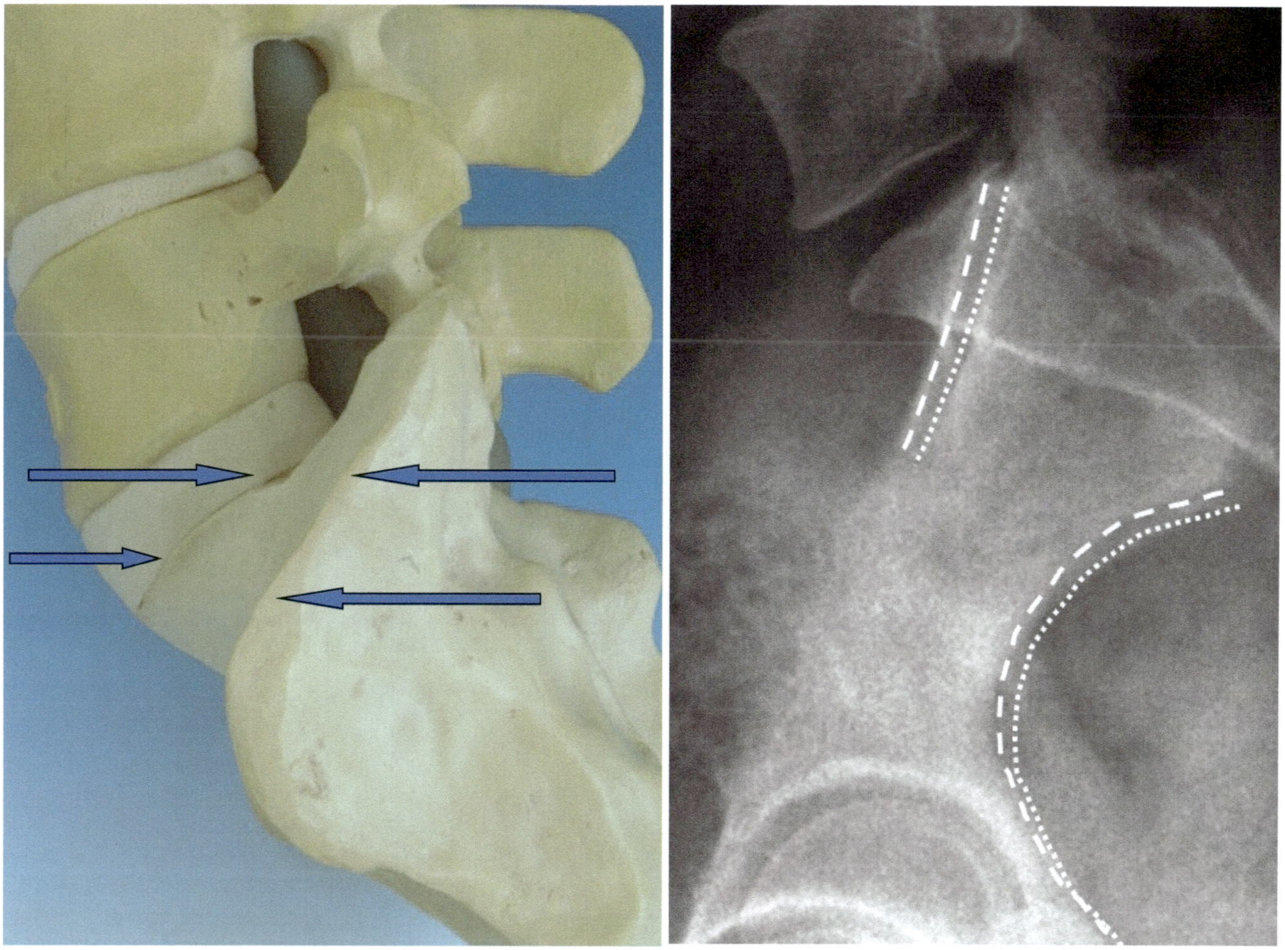

Fig. 2.14 Sacral alar slope on a plastic model and corresponding on a true lateral sacral X-ray view, which is the angulation between the upper sacral ala and the superior surface of the S1 sacral body (promontory)

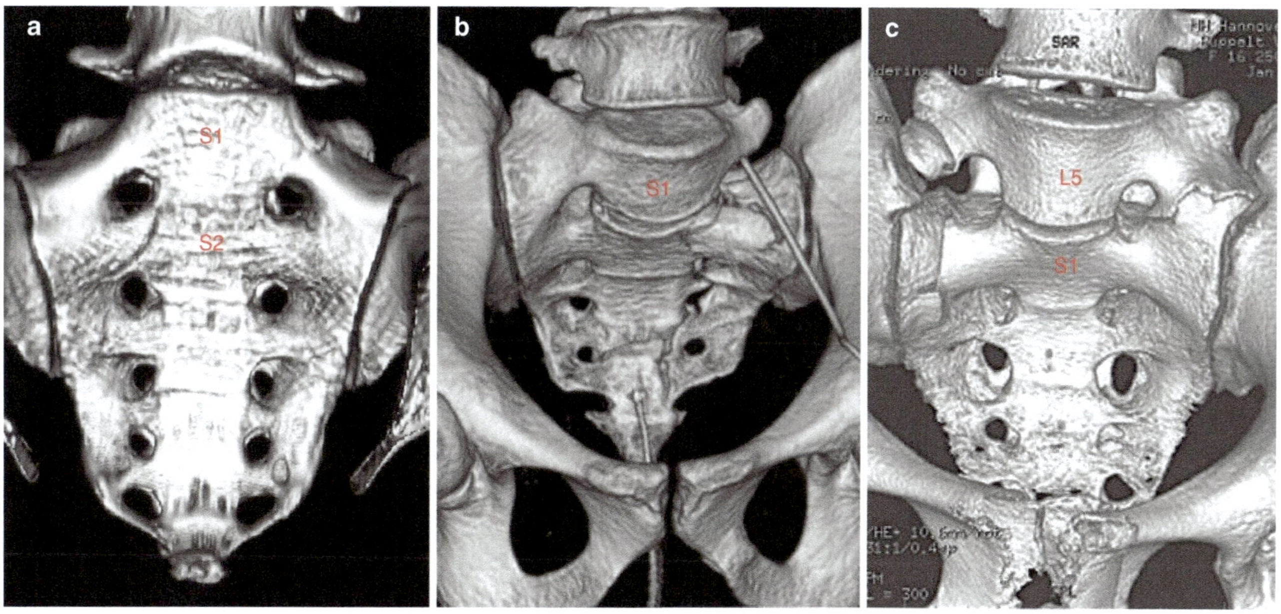

Fig. 2.15 Atypical sacral morphology: sacral dysmorphism (**a**), right hemisacralization (**b**) of the S1-vertebra and left incomplete sacralization with a dysmorphic fifth lumbar spine (**c**)

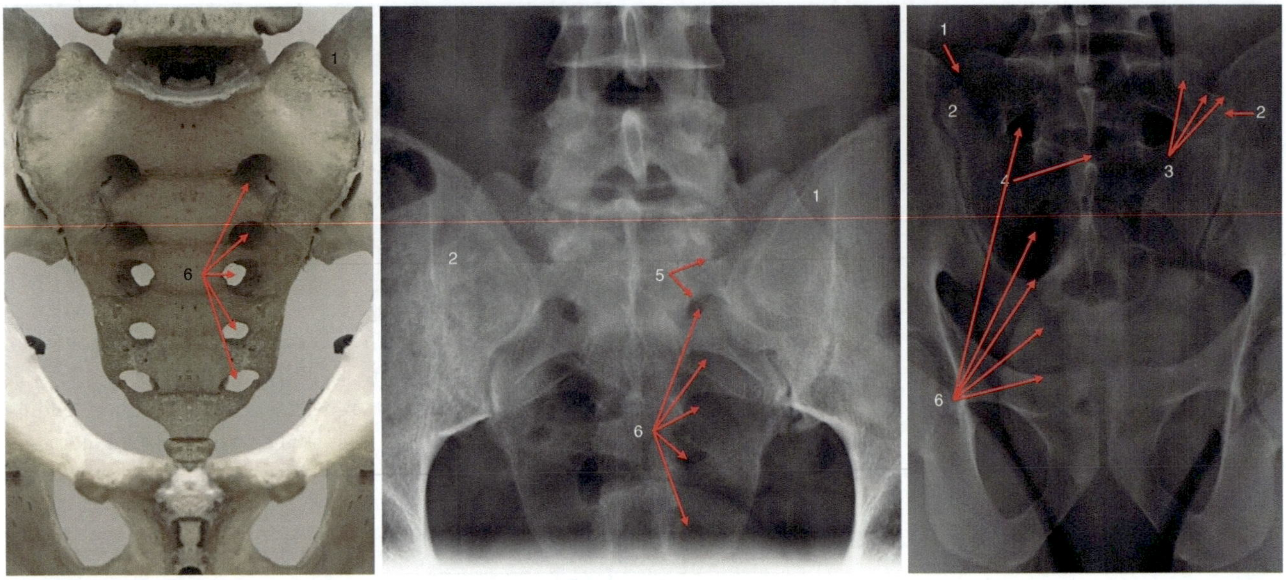

Fig. 2.16 Radiological-anatomical signs of sacral dysmorphism: upper sacral segment not recessed in the pelvis (*1*), existence of mammillary processes (*2*), acute alar slope (*3*), residual disk between the first and second sacral segments (*4*), noncircular upper sacral neural foramina (*5*), and five sacral foramina (*6*)

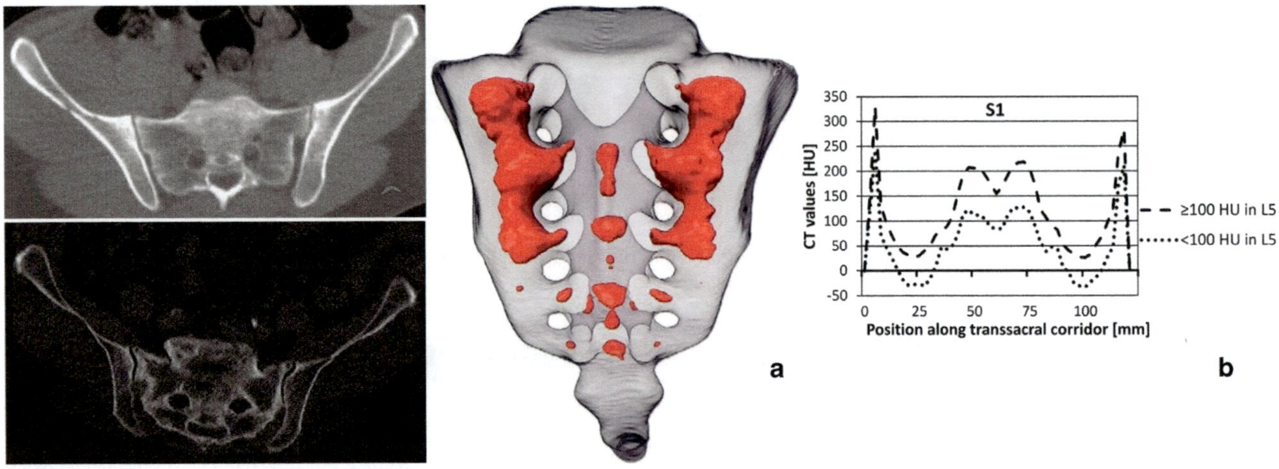

Fig. 2.17 Internal osseous anatomy of the sacrum: a weak area is located in the foraminal zone (CT of a 24-year-old male and an 87-year-old female). The corresponding Houndsfield units were analyzed by Wagner et al. Source: Wagner D, Kamer L, Rommens PM. Chapter 4: Bone Mass Distribution in the Sacrum. p. 35–42; in: Rommens PM, Hofmann A (eds.) Fragility fractures of the Pelvis. doi:10.1007/978-3-319-66572-6, Springer International Publishing AG 2017

A typical internal trabecular pattern of the upper sacrum was found by Pal et al., which shows strong trabeculae running from the superior surface of the S1 body to the articular surface of the SI joint, from the articular process and the S1 pedicle to the SI joint, from the posterolateral angle of the ala (attachment site of the lumbosacral ligament) to the S1 body, and from the lateral portion of the laminae to the auricular surface [44].

The vertebral canal is triangular in shape, and its posterior wall is often incomplete in the inferior part from undeveloped laminae and spinous processes. It contains typically four foramina on each side for transmitting the anterior and posterior sacral nerves.

The dural sac in 84% terminates at the level of S2. The diameter of the nerve roots S1 and S2 is approximately 1/3 to 1/4 of the diameter of the surrounding bony foramen, whereas at the level of S3 and S4, the diameter of the nerve roots was only 1/6 of the foraminal diameter [65].

The cross-section of the S2–S5 roots was found to be 80%, 60%, 20%, and 15% of the cross-section of the S1 nerve root [65]. Fractures involving the S1 and S2 foramina are thus more vulnerable for accompanying nerve injury than more distal fractures.

The so-called vestibule concept considers the special bony anatomy of the S1 pedicle, which rises slightly in the frontal plane and is perpendicular in the horizontal

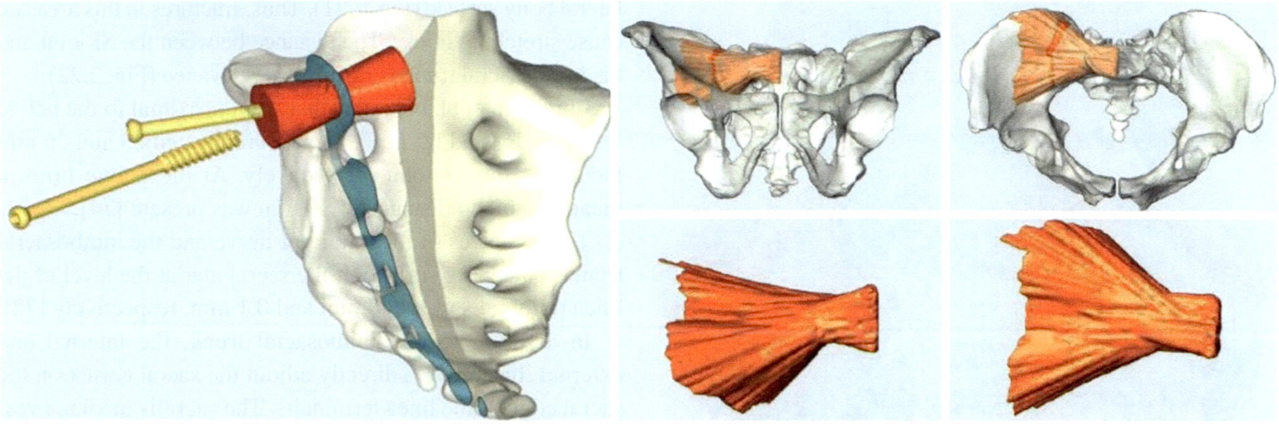

Fig. 2.18 Vestibule concept of the S1 architecture (figures with permission from: Mendel T, Appelt K, Kuhn P, Suhm N: Der sakroiliakale Knochenkorridor. Unfallchirurg 1: 19–26 (2008)

plane (Fig. 2.18). The tube-shaped channel for a screw is smallest in diameter at the level of the neural foramina but then develops into a skittle shape laterally and medially [66, 67].

The size of the vestibule at S1 was analyzed by different groups:

- Carlson et al. reported an average square area of the vestibule of 534 mm^2 in males and 450 mm^2 in females with a larger anteroposterior diameter of the outlet than the superoinferior diameter [66].
- Noojin et al. performed a CT analysis and found an average vestibular width of 28 mm and a height of 27.7 mm [68].
- In an analysis of Chinese adults, the vestibular width was 25 mm, and the height was 20.94 mm, representing a mean vestibular size of 400 mm^2. Males presented with a large vestibule than females [69].

Clinical Relevance
The anatomy of the S1 vestibule should be considered during iliosacral screw orientation.

2.1.2.4 Sagittal Orientation

In the sagittal plane, an anterior angulation averaging 20° at birth increases during adulthood up to 70° [52].

The sacral slope [22], the angle between the promontory and the horizontal plane, is approximately 40° in young adults [70, 71].

2.1.2.5 Neurovascular Topographical Anatomy

The anterior lumbosacral anatomy is highly variable with different important structures located in this region. The most relevant structures include the common and internal iliac vessels, the lumbosacral and obturator trunk, and parts of the rectosigmoid [72].

The sigmoid colon is located directly anterior to the anterior sacral surface, where it is highly mobile. At the S3 level, it becomes complete retroperitoneal with direct contact to the anterior cortex [72].

The common iliac vessels bifurcate at the lumbosacral junction arising to the internal and external iliac vessels. The veins are always located closer to the bony surface than the corresponding arteries (Fig. 2.19). At the upper sacrum, the internal iliac veins are in close relationship to the bone, medial to the SI joints and with contact to the sacral alar, running in a superior-medial direction. In contrast, the corresponding artery is located anterolateral to the vein, without bone contact [72]. The distances of the internal iliac vein and the internal iliac artery to the bony surface of the sacral ala at the level of the linea terminalis were 2.4 mm and 11.4 mm, respectively [72]. Thus, the latter is not in relevant danger during local dissection. The external iliac arteries are separated from the sacrum by the psoas muscles [73].

The sacral plexus leaves the sacrum through the anterior sacral foramen (Fig. 2.20). The main senso-motoric nerve root functions of the sacral plexus are as follows:

- L5 nerve root: dermatome, dorsal foot to great toe; myotome, extensor hallucis longus, gluteus medius; reflex, medial hamstring reflex.
- S1 nerve root: dermatome, lateral and plantar foot; myotome, gastrocnemius, soleus; reflex, Achilles.
- S2–S5 nerve roots: bowel and bladder function; unilateral preservation normally adequate for control.

The lumbosacral trunk, which consists normally of parts of the L4 and L5 nerve roots, runs on the sacral alar medial to the SI joint and lateral to the internal iliac vein [72]. The lumbosacral trunk (nerve root L4/L5) is located close to the superior-

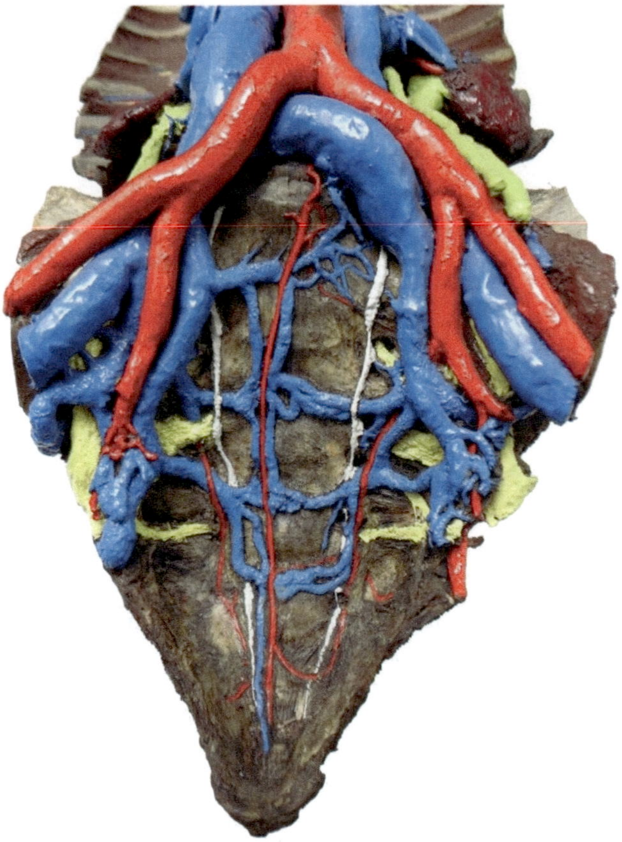

Fig. 2.19 Vascular anatomy anterior to the sacrum, showing the more closed relationship of the venous vessels closed to the bone compared to the arteries. The presacral venous plexus is visible with a ladder-shaped configuration

lateral bony surface (Fig. 2.21). Thus, fractures in this area can cause stretching injury. The distance between the SI joint and the lumbosacral trunk is of surgical relevance (Fig. 2.22).

Ebraheim et al. observed that 4 cm proximal to the pelvic brim, the L4 and L5 nerve roots were located 23 and 26 mm medial to the SI joint, respectively. At the pelvic brim, a mean combined distance of 10 mm was present [74].

The distances of the obturator nerve and the lumbosacral trunk to the bony surface of the sacral alar at the level of the linea terminalis were 9.7 mm and 0.1 mm, respectively [72].

In addition to the lumbosacral trunk, the internal and external iliac arteries directly adjoin the sacral cortex on the sacral edge of the linea terminalis. The sacralis mediana vessels and the sympathetic sacral nerves are located close to the promontory [72].

The internal iliac artery and the lumbosacral trunk are as close as 5 mm to the anterior sacral cortex (Fig. 2.23).

The left common iliac vein is located 2 mm closer to the anterior wall than the right common iliac vein [75], while the common iliac arteries are more anterior to the veins [76]. The first sacral nerve was located just behind the layer of parietal fascia covering the piriformis muscle, thus outside the presacral space [76]. The distance from the midsacral promontory to the internal iliac artery, the common iliac vein, and the common iliac artery was approximately 22 mm, 21 mm, and 23 mm, respectively [76].

The star-like presacral venous plexus is located directly anterior to the sacrum and is formed from branches and anastomoses between the two lateral veins, the median sacral

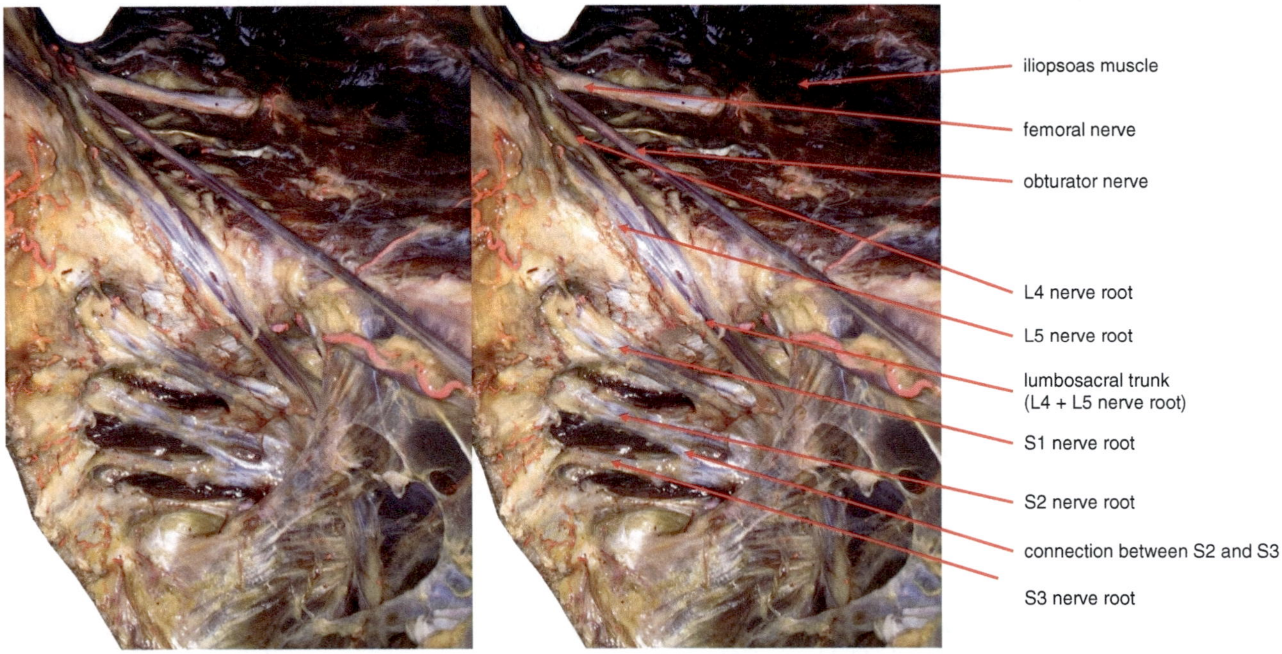

Fig. 2.20 Lumbosacral plexus in relation to the iliopsoas and the anterior sacral area

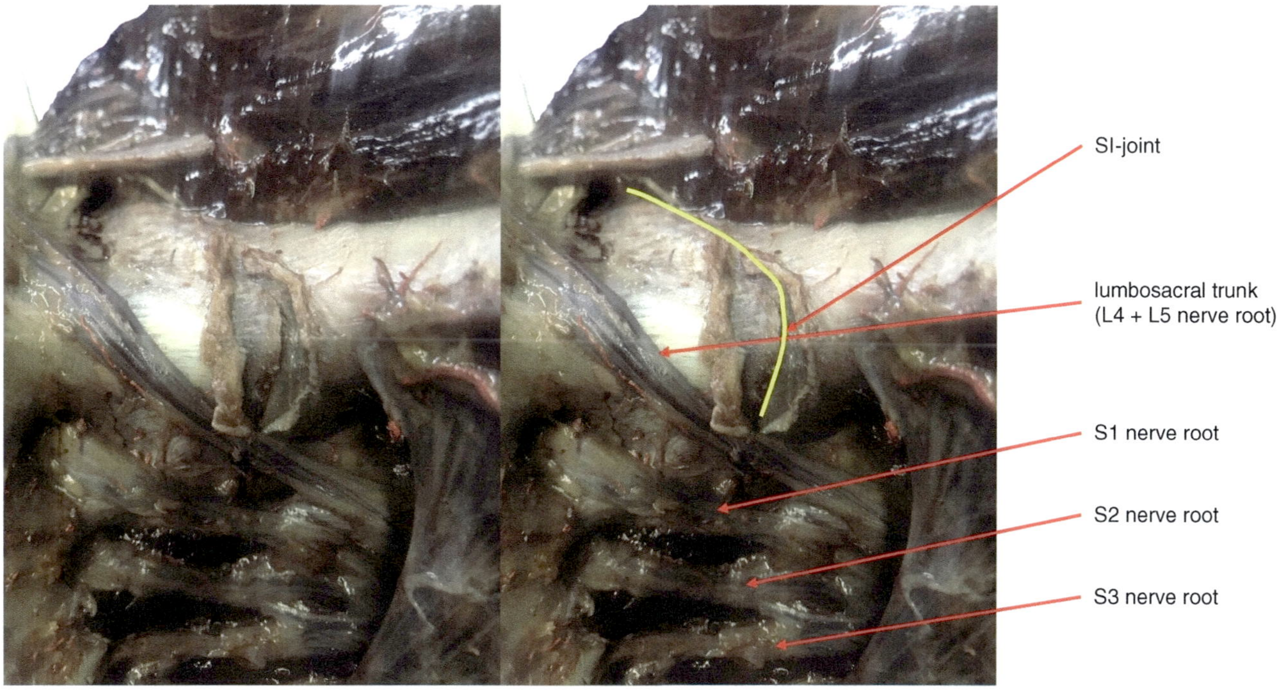

Fig. 2.21 Lumbosacral plexus anterior to the iliosacral region, consisting of the lumbosacral trunk, and the S1–S3 nerve roots, forming the sciatic nerve after running through the greater sciatic notch

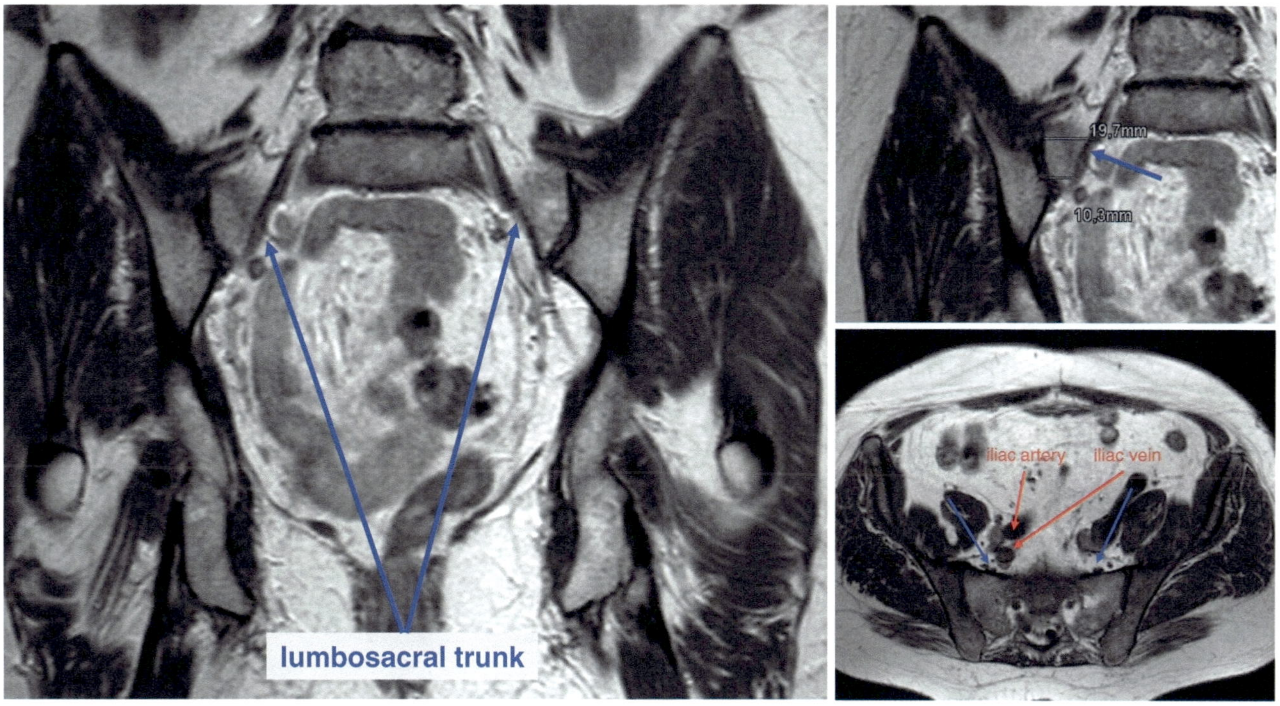

Fig. 2.22 MR-topography of the lumbosacral trunk and its relation to the SI joint and iliac vessels

vein and communicating veins between the former ones (Figs. 2.19 and 2.23). Additional communication exists to the internal sacral bone venous system via the sacral foramina [77].

The presacral venous plexus extends with venous communications to the piriformis and coccygeal muscle fascia and the sacrospinous ligament [78]. The main part of the venous plexus contribution of the lateral veins runs in the anterior foraminal zone of the sacrum [78].

> **Clinical Relevance**
> Injuries to the presacral venous plexus may cause hemodynamic instability.

The dural sac in 84% terminates at the level of S2. The diameter of the nerve roots S1 and S2 is approximately 1/3 to 1/4 of the diameter of the surrounding bony foramen, whereas at the level of S3 and S4, the diameter of the nerve roots was only 1/6 of the foraminal diameter [65].

The cross-section of the S2–S5 roots was found to be 80%, 60%, 20%, and 15% of the cross-section of the S1 nerve root [65].

> **Clinical Relevance**
> Fractures involving the S1 and S2 foramina are more vulnerable for accompanying nerve injury than more distal fractures.

2.1.2.6 Musculo-Ligamentous Topographical Anatomy

Several ligaments are attached to the sacral surface. The anterior longitudinal ligament of the spine has connections to the sacral promontory, while the posterior longitudinal ligament passes posteriorly over the vertebral bodies and at the inner surface of the spinal canal [73].

Further relevant ligaments include the sacroiliac ligaments, the iliolumbar ligament complex, and the pelvic floor ligaments.

The Sacroiliac Ligamentous Complex

It consists of the anterior, interosseous, and posterior ligaments (Fig. 2.24).

- The sacral origin of the anterior sacroiliac ligaments is the anterior-inferior part of the upper sacrum at the SI joint; these ligaments are supposed to be a thickening of the fibrous membrane of the joint capsule [5]; they act as a posterior tension band stabilization system and opposes axial translation of sacrum and therefore separation of the SI joint [79].
- The interosseous sacroiliac ligament is located posterosuperior to the joint and is the largest and strongest sacroiliac ligament; it attaches to adjacent expansive roughened areas on the ilium and sacrum, filling the gap between the two bones [5].
- The posterior sacroiliac ligament runs posterior to the interosseous sacroiliac ligament and tightens during counternutation [79].

The Iliolumbar Ligament Complex

The iliolumbar ligament complex (Fig. 2.25) shows a wide anatomical variety [80] and consists of the true iliolumbar ligament and the lumbosacral ligament [5]. It takes part in

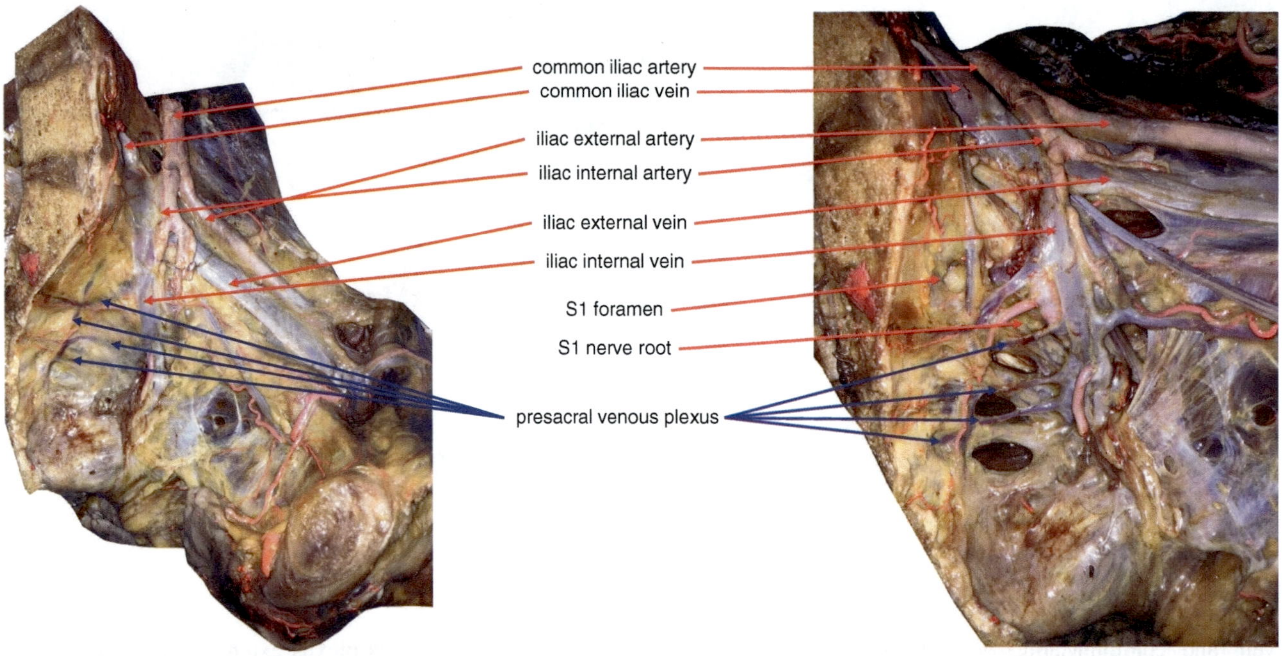

Fig. 2.23 Relationship between the neural and vascular structures at the anterior iliosacral region. Note the more closed relationship of the venous vessels closed to the bone compared to the arteries

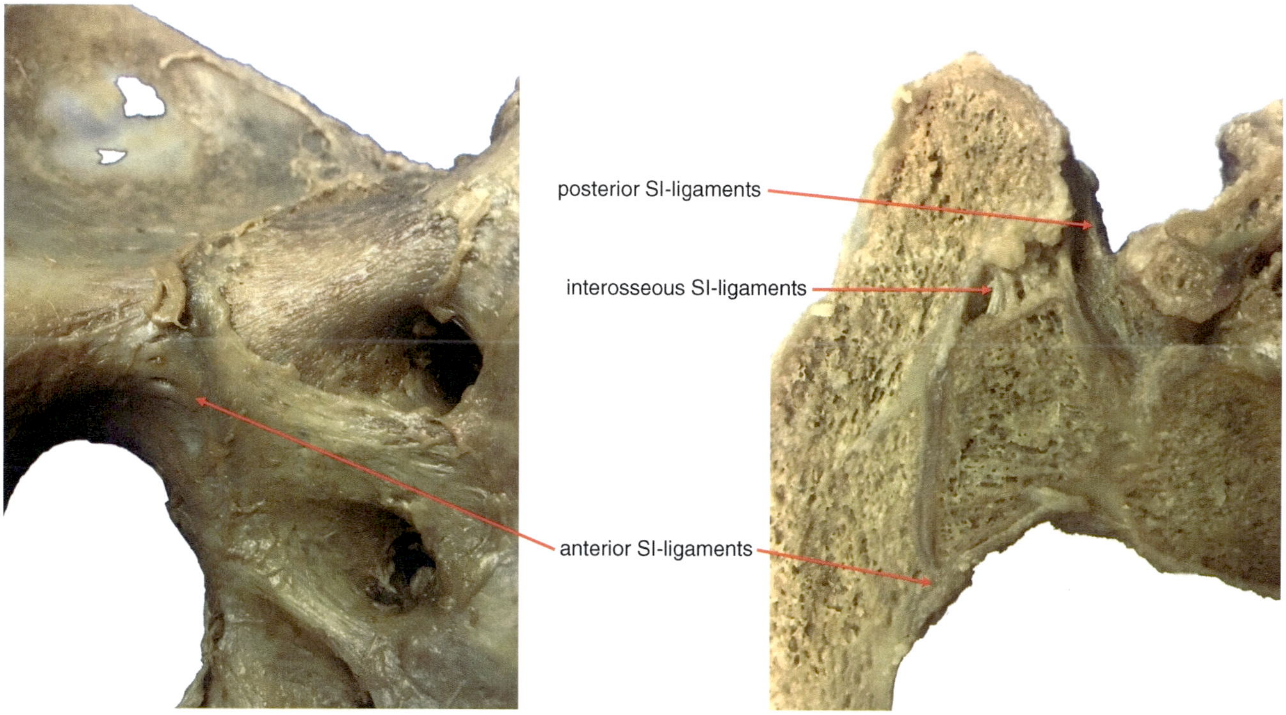

Fig. 2.24 Ligamentous sacroiliac joint complex: the hemipelvis is connected to the sacrum via the thin anterior sacroiliac ligaments, the strong interosseous ligaments, and posterior sacroiliac ligaments

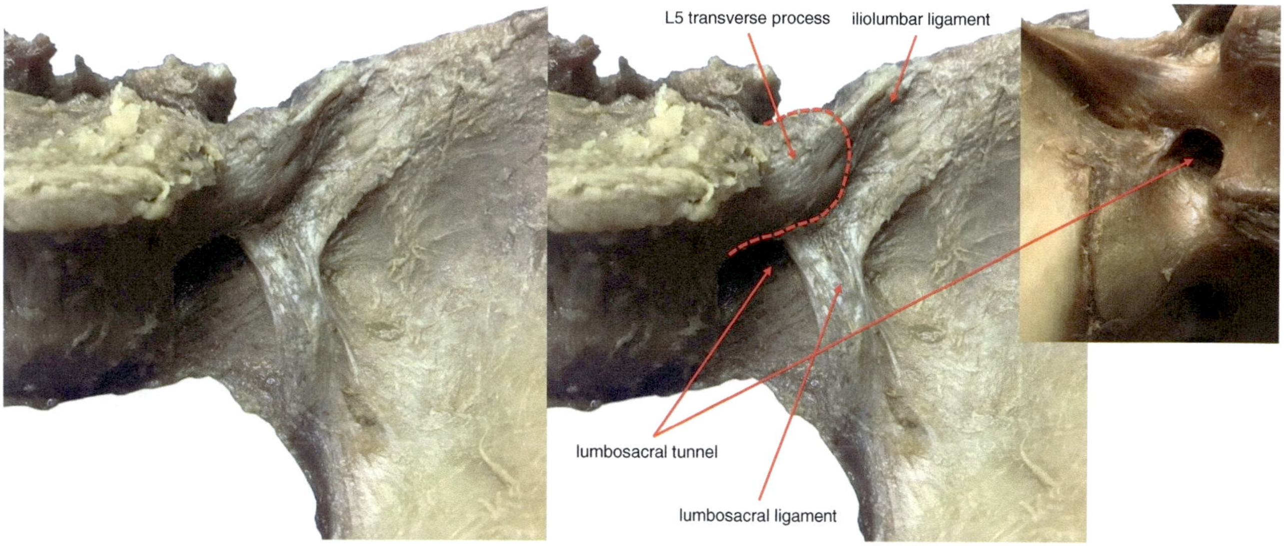

Fig. 2.25 Iliolumbar ligament complex consisting of the true iliolumbar ligament and the lumbosacral ligament creating the lumbosacral tunnel

stabilizing the lumbosacral spinal region [81–83]. The fan-shaped iliolumbar ligament most often arises from the fourth and/or fifth lumbar transverse process to insert at the posterior iliac crest and the SIJ capsule on top of the sacrum [82, 84]. Its lumbosacral ligament portion arises from the fifth lumbar transverse process to insert on the sacral alar [80, 85].

The true iliolumbar ligament presents with a more horizontal course, arising from the tip of the fifth transverse process to insert at various positions at the iliac crest, while the lumbosacral ligament arises from the inferior part of the L5 transverse process to origin at the anterior surface of the SI joint. This ligament complex limits axial rotation and anterior displacement of the fifth lumbar spine [79].

The lumbosacral ligament, together with the sacral ala and the L5 body/L5-S1 disk medial, creates the lumbosacral tunnel [86]. The tunnel boundaries include the floor represented by sacral alar; the roof, which is only present proximal at the inferior surface of the L5 transverse process; the medial border (the L5 body/L5-S1 disk); and the lateral border, formed by the lumbosacral ligament.

The lumbosacral ligament arises from the inferior L5 transverse process, about 1 cm lateral from the base, in a variable angle <45°. The mean ligament length was found to be 32.5 mm [86].

Clinical Relevance

The lumbosacral ligament together with the sacral alar, the L5 transverse process, and the anterior-superior sacroiliac ligaments forms a bony-ligamentous tunnel, which integrates the lumbosacral trunk [86]. Additional tissue connections can further decrease this tunnel [87], which can lead to strain injuries of the lumbosacral trunk.

The Pelvic Floor Ligaments

The pelvic floor ligaments (Fig. 2.26) include the sacrotuberous and sacrospinous ligaments, which have a crossing area of up to 2.4 cm^2 [88] and therefore have different functions.

The sacrotuberous ligament has a triangular shape, arises broad at the posterolateral sacrum from the transverse tubercles of the sacrum and the upper aspect of the coccyx [89], and is superficial to the sacrospinous ligament. It resists shearing and flexion.

The triangular-shaped sacrospinous ligament arises from the anterior sacrum and coccyx [5]. It resists external rotation.

No muscles directly act on the SI joint to produce active physiologic movements. On the posterior part of the sacrum, the multifidus, responsible for some nutational sacral movement, passes above the interosseous sacroiliac ligament to insert onto sacrum, the iliac crest, and the sacrotuberous ligaments.

Activation of the erector spinae muscle leads to spinal and pelvic extension via sacral locking during nutation movement due to ligamentous tightening. Additionally, the transverse abdominal muscle performs a core stabilization of the spine and pelvis.

2.1.2.7 Coccyx

The os coccyx consists of three or four fused coccygeal vertebrae, which develops from eight ossification centers [25]. It is attached to the distal sacrum via the sacral cornu. This articulation can be a symphysis or a synovial joint [90].

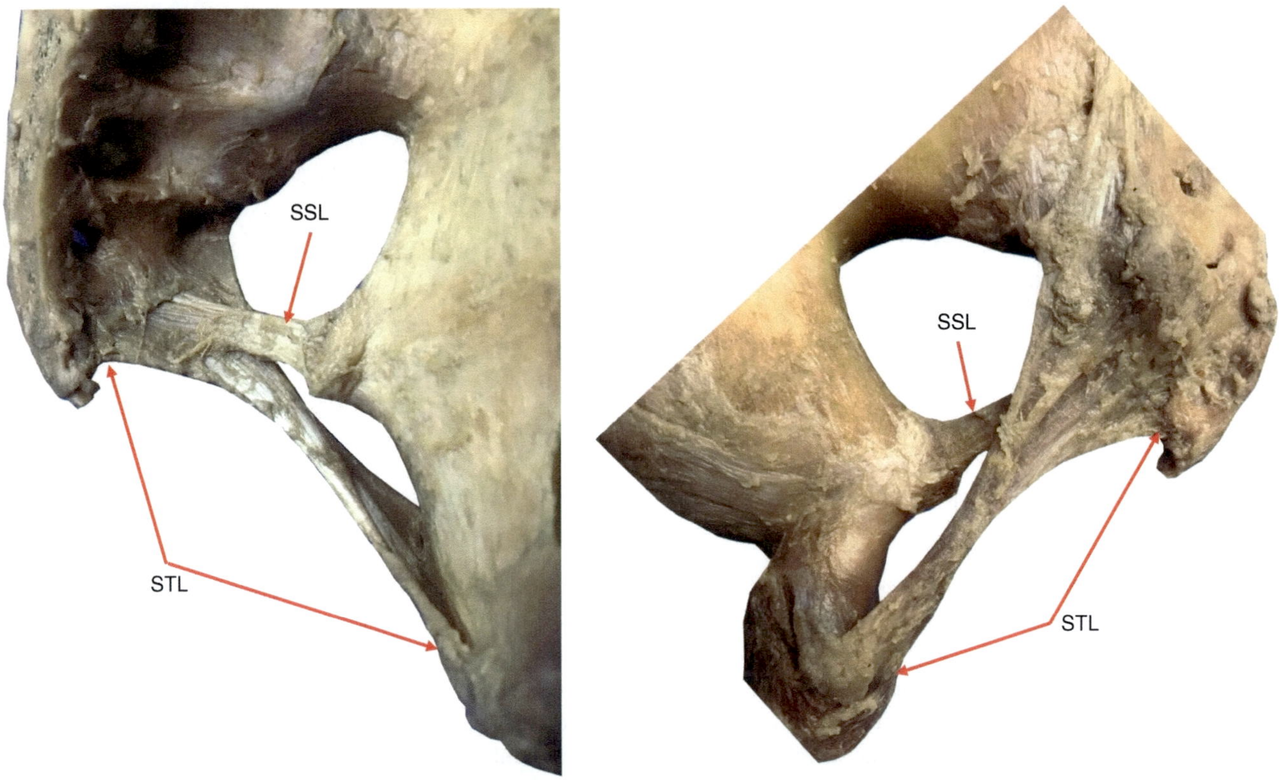

Fig. 2.26 Pelvic floor ligaments: sacrotuberous (STL) and sacrospinal ligaments (SSL)

The coccyx has a triangular shape and is often a complete bone, while sometimes the first coccygeal segment is not fused with the distal parts. Additionally, sacrococcygeal fusion can be present in up to 57% [91, 92].

The most common coccyx types are type 1 coccyx with a slightly curved coccyx pointing downward and type 2 coccyx with a more curved coccyx pointing forward [91, 92].

Attachments of the coccyx include the gluteus maximus muscle, the coccygeal muscle, and the anococcygeal ligament.

2.1.3 Pelvic Articular Joints

There are four joints connecting the pelvic bones. At the anterior pelvic ring, the pubic symphysis joins both pubic bones. At the posterior pelvic ring, both SI joints connect the sacrum with each hemipelvis. The fourth joint is the described connection between the sacrum and the coccyx.

2.1.3.1 The Pubic Symphysis

The present basic anatomical understanding of the pubic symphysis is described in detail in the work by Becker et al. [93]. Knowledge of the following surgical anatomical details is relevant for fracture treatment.

The pubic symphysis is defined as a secondary cartilaginous [94, 95] or fibrocartilaginous joint [96].

The joint partners consist of the medial part of both pubic bones connected by a fibrocartilaginous disk, which shows fiber orientations indicating compressive and tensile acting forces (Fig. 2.27). The disk is more broader superior and inferior than in the mid-symphysis [97, 98]. In clinical practice, a posterior bulge (retropubic eminence; [99, 100]) can often be palpated to identify the midline during anterior approaches to the retropubic space.

The disk can contain a cavity (cleft), most often in its superior and posterior part [99–103]. The presence of the cleft is in coincidence with the described posterior bulge [102, 104].

The articular surfaces have a mean length of 30–35 mm and a width of 10–12 mm and are oval in shape [97, 99, 105]. The symphyseal space is radiographically often parallel, especially in its posterior part, while sometimes an anterior, superior, and inferior widening can be observed. Especially in women, some asymmetry can be present.

The articular hyaline cartilage has a thickness between 0.5 and 3 mm [97, 101, 106–109], which decreases with age [104].

In young adults, the subchondral bone is irregular due to bony ridges. This can be identified on conventional radiography, becomes more smooth in the third decade of life, and shows degenerative changes in the sixth decade of life [97, 99, 102, 109, 110].

A 55° orientation of the pubic symphysis body with respect to the coronal plane was observed in a CT analysis [111].

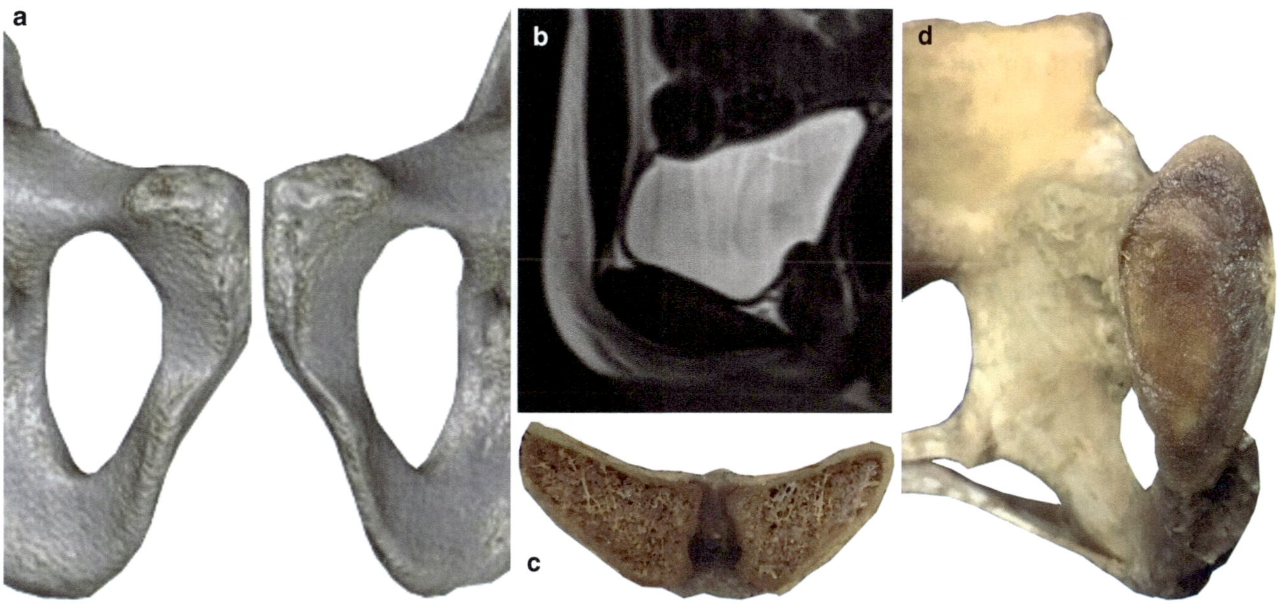

Fig. 2.27 Anatomy of the pubic symphysis: the bony configuration (**a**) shows the pubic tubercle, the pubic crest, and the parallel orientation of the rami; The insertion of the rectus abdominis muscle is at its anterior border (**b**); the close relationship to the bladder is shown (**b**); the transverse anatomical dissection reveals the anterior opening of the symphyseal cleft and the anterior and posterior symphyseal ligaments (**c**); the cadaveric dissection (**d**) shows the oval-shaped configuration

Pubic Ligaments

Overall, there are four periarticular ligaments at the pubic symphysis (Fig. 2.27), listed with decreasing strength of each ligament [112, 113]:

- Anterior pubic ligament: it connects anteriorly pubic bones, inserts at the periosteum [97, 99, 100], and is supposed to be the main stabilizer of the joint [99, 105, 112]; its thickness is approximately 5–12 mm [97, 99, 105, 106]; it consists of several different orientated fiber layers, responsible for the biomechanical forces acting on the symphysis [100, 105]; recently, its connections to the pyramidalis muscle and the adductor muscles [97, 99, 105, 114] were confirmed with the pyramidalis muscle as the only anterior pubic bone muscle arising from and the adductor longus attaching at this ligament [115].
- Superior pubic ligament: it connects the superior pubic ramus bilaterally, starting from even the pubic tubercles and the upper pubic rami periosteum [99, 108] with some fibers inserting at the interpubic disk, the pectineal ligament, and the linea alba [97, 99, 101, 105]; its clinical relevance is not clear.
- Inferior pubic ligament (arcuate pubic ligament): it connects the inferior parts of pubic rami in an arch-shaped manner [96, 99, 107] and is stronger than the superior ligament [100, 105, 112].
- Posterior pubic ligament: only few fibers of this ligament can be identified; it was considered a thickening of the posterior periosteum [93].

Width of the Pubic Symphysis

In trauma practice, it is of relevance to identify injuries. Thus, the normal, age-dependent width of the pubic symphysis is important.

Consensus exists that the symphysis is wider anteriorly than posteriorly [104, 108, 116, 117]. An age and sex dependency of the pubic symphysis width is present.

Kraus already in 1930 reported that the width decreases continuously from approximately 10 mm in the toddler age to 2 mm in the older age of 50 years [118]. Patel and Chapman observed a width of 7.4 mm in the first months of life, which decreases to 5.4 mm at the age of 16 [119].

During the last decade, several investigations analyzed especially CT data in patients of different age for standard measurements of the symphysis width (Fig. 2.28).

- Alicioglu et al. performed a CT analysis on adult patients >16 years of age in 278 women and 264 men [120]. They reported a constant narrowing of the anterior and posterior part of the symphyseal width, while the middle part showed no significant changes, independent from the number of birth and the body mass index. Female patients were associated with larger values anterior and in the middle.
- McAlister et al. measured the symphyseal width using standard radiographs in 316 consecutive pediatric patients (165 boys, 151 girls), who were separated by gender and divided into three age groups: 2–6 years, 7–10 years, and 11–14 years [121]. Normal values between 5.2 and 8.4 mm were observed with an average width of 6.8 mm. Interestingly, a subsequent widening was observed within the three age groups: 6.6 mm, 6.8 mm, and 7.2 mm, respectively. It was concluded that a width >8.4 mm should lead to further evaluation for pathology.
- Bayer et al. analyzed 350 CT scans of children in different age groups: 0–6 years, 7–11 years, 12–15 years, and 16–17 years. The mean width in these age groups was 5.4 mm, 5.3 mm, 4.1 mm, and 3.5 mm in girls and 5.9 mm, 5.4 mm, 5.2 mm, and 4.0 mm in boys, respectively [122].
- A further CT analysis of 1020 CT axial scans in pediatric patients (2–18 years) revealed an average pubic symphyseal width at 2-year-old boys of 6.35 mm and 5.85 mm in girls. A decrease to 3.68 mm in boys and 3.92 mm in girls at an age of 18 years was observed [123].

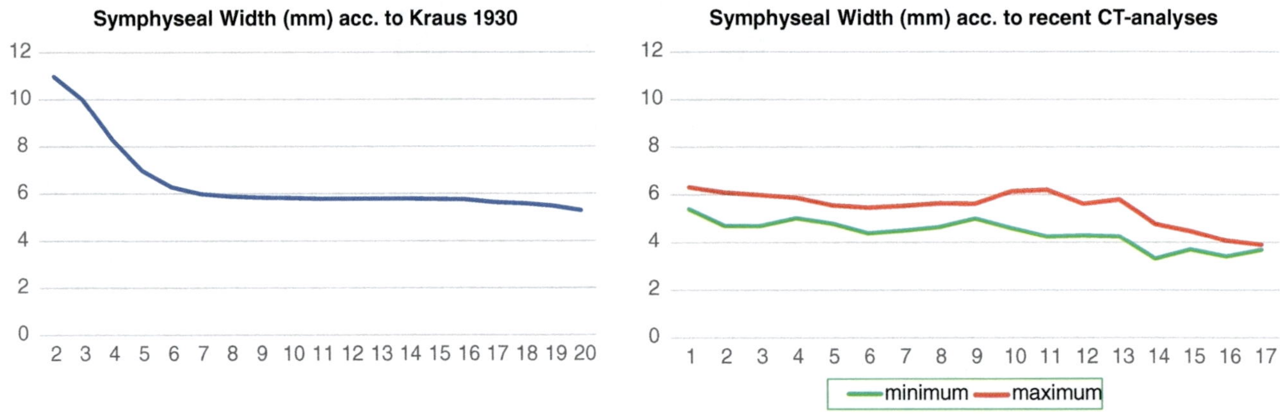

Fig. 2.28 Age-dependent symphyseal width

- Recently, data on 811 CT measurements of the pubic symphysis were analyzed, stating that from age 2–16 years, the average pubic symphysis width decreased from 5.55 to 3.69 mm [124].

Clinical Relevance

The width of the pubic symphysis decreases from 5–6 mm 2 years after birth to 3–4 mm in early adulthood using CT analyses.

In pediatric trauma patients <10 years of age, a symphyseal width >10 mm should lead to suspicion of injury [123].

Additionally, symphyseal widening occurs under labor [125].

Topographical Anatomy

Topographical analyses found a strong relationship of muscle attachment to the anterior pubic symphysis.

Gamble et al. already stated that the pyramidalis, the rectus abdominis, the gracilis, the adductors, the obturator, and the levator ani muscles contribute to the anatomic area around the pubic symphysis [108].

In a cadaver analysis, the adductor longus and rectus abdominis regularly showed connection to the symphysis pubis capsule and even to the disk of the symphysis pubis. More infrequently, the adductor brevis and rarely the gracilis muscle inserted at the capsule [114].

Recently, the pyramidalis muscle was found to be the only abdominal muscle, which runs anterior to the pubic symphysis. This muscle had its origin at the pubic crest and the anterior pubic ligament running superiorly to insert at the medial border of the rectus sheath at the linea alba. Fibers of the external abdominal oblique aponeurosis are also connected with the anterior pubic ligament. The adductor longus also arises from the pubic crest and from the anterior pubic ligament [115].

It is well known that the rectus abdominis inserts at the anterior and cranial border of the pubic crest.

During surgery of symphyseal disruptions, dissection is usually necessary up to the pubic tubercles or, when using the intrapelvic approach, further along the linea terminalis.

The spermatic cord is at risk during dissection due to its extremely near relationship to the pubic tubercles. The spermatic cord is located directly lateral and immediately adjacent to the pubic tubercle after it exits the inguinal canal with an average distance of 0.8 mm [126].

Clinical Relevance

During open reduction and internal fixation of symphyseal disruptions, the plate should be positioned posterior to rectus insertion to avoid pressure necrosis.

2.1.3.2 The SI Joint

The anatomical basis of the SI joint is described in detail by Vleeming et al. [80]. Knowledge of the following surgical anatomical details is relevant for fracture treatment. The SI joint is the largest axial joint [127, 128] and is surrounded by muscles and ligaments. The innervation is received from the lateral branches of the posterior rami L4–S3 and an anterior innervation from the L2–L3 segments [129–132].

The SI joint is considered a true joint containing a joint cavity between two bones with synovial fluid, cartilage, ligaments, and a fibrous capsule [132–135]. Recently, a histological analysis classified the SI joint as a symphysis with only few classical joint characteristics [136].

The SI joint is usually composed of the first three sacral vertebrae in males, while in females, the S3 vertebra often only partially contributes to the joint area [137].

The shape of the SI joint is highly variable [138]. It consists of two articular surfaces. The sacral part is concave, while the iliac part is slightly convex. It is usually an L-shaped joint, comparable to an auricular-, C-, or crescent-like shape, which changes during development until adulthood [139, 140]. A near perpendicular orientation of a shorter longitudinal/cranial and a longer horizontal/transverse arm is present (Fig. 2.4). A synovial membrane surrounds this true joint, and a capsular contribution follows the articular surface. Cole et al. stated that only the lower portion of the longitudinal limb and the caudal limb is synovial in construction, while the upper part is more fibrous [141].

The SI joint has oblique orientation to the sagittal plane [132, 139, 140]. During standing, the S1 part is orientated vertically in a craniolateral to caudomedial direction. The mean joint angle decreases from 40° at S1 to 25° at S2 and 10° at S3 [128, 132, 142].

The surface of the SI joint consists of three parts (three sacral vertebrae) with a decrease of their sizes from S1 cranially to S3 caudally. Especially in males, an intra-articular bony tubercle is frequently present in the middle part of the articular sacral surface. Cartilage covers the joint surfaces. It is thicker and smoother at the sacral than at the iliac surface [135, 143]. The joint has an average surface area of 17.5 cm^2 (1). The average auricular surface area is reported to range between 18 and 23 cm^2 [135, 144].

Degenerative changes of the SI joint are common. Sacroiliac bridging was predominantly observed in males vs. females: 12.27% vs. 1.83%, respectively. It was present bilaterally in 38.6% and associated with increasing age [145]. In the majority of males (97%), bridging was extra-articular, while all females showed intra-articular bridging [146].

SI Joint Ligaments

Besides capsular structures, the main SI joint ligaments (Figs. 2.24 and 2.29) include the anterior, posterior, and interosseous ligaments [147].

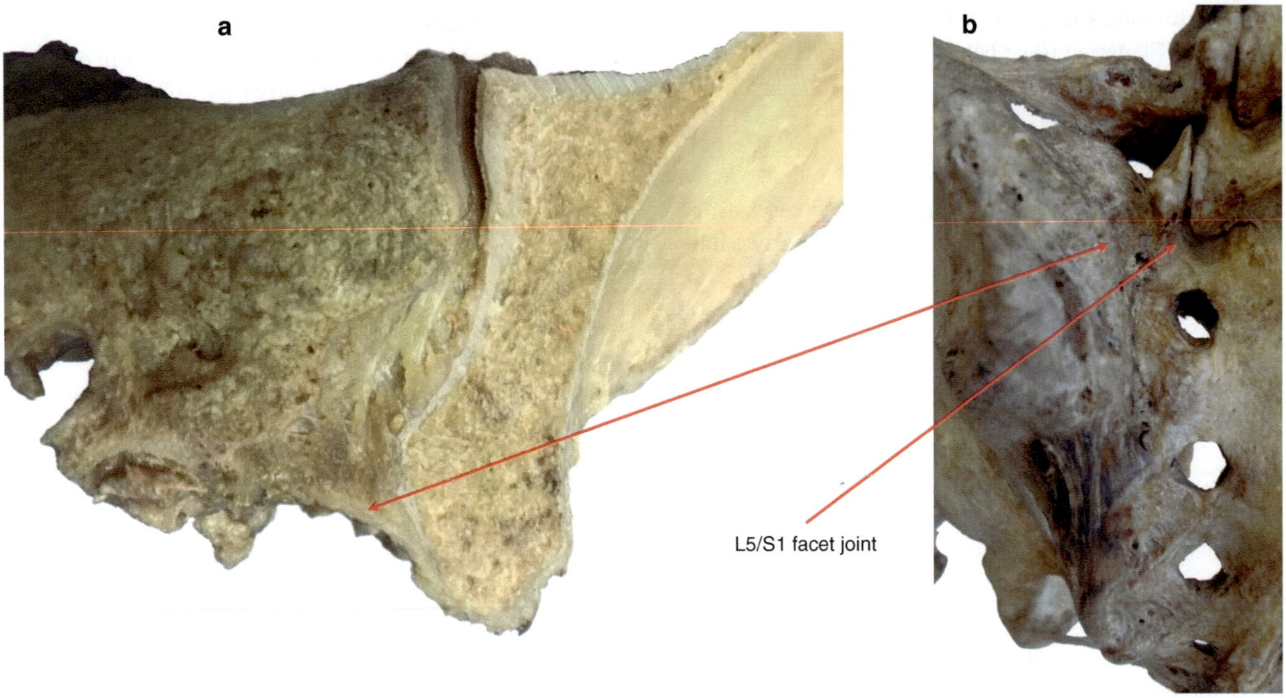

Fig. 2.29 Anatomy of the SI joint: one-third of the SI joint area represents the true joint part with cartilage formation of the corresponding joint partners (**a**); the posterior area is filled with the strong interosseous ligaments and the smaller posterior ligaments (**a**); the posterior view (**b**) shows the ligamentous coverage of the SI joint area

Anterior Sacroiliac Ligament

The anterior sacroiliac ligament corresponds to the anterior thickening of the joint capsule, which is reinforced by a caudal extension of the lumbosacral ligament of the iliolumbar ligament complex inserting on the sacral alar. The inferior part of the anterior capsule contains parts of the sacrospinous ligament. The lumbosacral trunk and the iliac vessels are closely related to these structures. The ligament (capsule) is thin and often presents with some defects [148].

Interosseous Sacroiliac Ligament

The interosseous ligament bridges the irregular space between sacrum and ilium directly posterior-superior to the articular surface at the level of S1 and S2. It is the strongest part of the three ligaments, with the most largest origin area and overall volume [149]. It is larger in females than in males [149]. A deep part can be distinguished from a more superficial part. The latter unites partially with the posterior sacroiliac ligament. Variable moderate to extensive ridging is observed at the sacrum and ilium, and frequently ligamentous ossification can be present [150].

Posterior Sacroiliac Ligament

The strong posterior sacroiliac ligament lies posterior to the interosseous sacroiliac ligament and originates from the posterior superior iliac spine (PSIS) and the inner part of the iliac crest to insert in an oblique direction at the median and lateral crests of the sacrum [151, 152]. It consists of different fascicles, which create superficial and deep ligament layers. Its lateral part unites with fibers of the sacrotuberous ligament; other fibers attach to the erector spinae and multifidus muscle and the posterior lumbar fascia [80]. This ligament is larger in males [149]. During counternutation, this ligament is tensioned [152].

Pelvic Floor Ligaments

The pelvic floor ligaments, the sacrotuberous and sacrospinous ligaments, are also labeled as accessory ligaments [153]. The latter divides the greater sciatic notch into a greater, superior and a lesser, inferior foramen (Fig. 2.26).

Sacrotuberous Ligament

The sacrotuberous ligament has a triangular shape and arises broad from the posterior iliac spines, the lower part of the sacrum (transverse tubercles), and the upper part of the coccyx to insert in an oblique descending direction at the medial ischial tuberosity [89]. It is located superficial to the sacrospinous ligament. Muscle fibers and fascial adhesions of the gluteus maximus, the thoracolumbar fascia, and the multifidus muscle can be present. Infrequently, adhesions from the long head of biceps femoris can be present, indicating the ligament as the degenerated biceps tendon [154]. Additionally, a membranous (falciform) segment extending to the ischioanal fossa is often observed, which can clinically be a cause of pudendal nerve entrapment [155]. The average length was reported to be between 68 and 86 mm [89, 155] with an average width of 63 mm (range, 50–80 mm) [89]. The ligament surface is approximately 18.5 cm^2 [88].

Sacrospinous Ligament

The thinner triangular-shaped sacrospinous ligament arises from the lateral sacral and coccygeal margins anterior to the sacrotuberous ligament, to course in a lateral, caudal, and anterior direction to insert at the spine of the ilium. The ligament surface is approximately 7–8 cm^2 [88].

SI Joint Width

Recently, the radiological age-dependent physiological width of the joint was analyzed using CT data (Fig. 2.30).

In a CT analysis by Oetgen et al., in 821 pediatric patients without bony or ligamentous injury aged 2–16 years, the average SI joint widths decreased from 3.11 to 1.80 mm [124].

A further CT analysis on 1020 CT data observed an average width of 4.4–4.5 mm in 2-year-old children to decrease to 2.0–2.3 mm in 18-year-olds [123]. Girls presented with slightly larger widths with increasing age.

> **Clinical Relevance**
>
> In pediatric trauma patients <10 years of age, a width of the SI joint >8 mm should lead to suspicion of sacroiliac injury [123].

Topographic Anatomy

Several muscles surround the sacroiliac joint complex. No direct muscular insertions are present at the sacroiliac joint. Thus, active SI joint motion is impossible.

The surrounding muscles include the erector spinae, psoas, quadratus lumborum, piriformis, abdominal oblique, gluteal, and hamstring muscles, which act on hip and lumbar spine movement. Activation of the erector spinae and multifidi muscles results in sacral nutation, while the gluteus maximus leads to lateral pulling of the sacrum [140]. The forces created by these muscles are called force closure.

- Gluteus maximus: SI joint compression; strong connection to sacrotuberous and sacrospinous ligaments [156].
- Hamstrings: tension/stretching of the sacrotuberous ligament by attached fibers [156, 157].
- Piriformis muscle: SI joint compression; dorsal fascia continuous with sacrotuberous ligament [156].
- Multifidus: nutation.
- Erector spinae: nutation (locking).
- Transverse abdominal muscle: core stabilization.

The proximity of lumbosacral trunk and the SI joint is surgically relevant during treatment of SI joint (fracture) dislocations.

The lumbosacral trunk crosses the sacral alar medial to the SI joint in a close relationship to a superior-lateral bony surface of 0.1 mm [72].

Ebraheim et al. analyzed the distance between the L4 and L5 nerve roots relative to the SI joint and reported a 23 and 26 mm distance 4 cm proximal to the pelvic brim, while at the pelvic brim (anterior joint), this distance was reduced to 10 mm [74].

In a recent combined CT and cadaver analysis, Bai et al. specified these results [158]. The distance of the L4 and L5 nerve roots to the highest point, the midpoint, and the lowest point of the sacroiliac joint line was measured. The distance to the L4 nerve root was 2.1 cm, 1.7 cm, and 1.2 cm, respectively, the distance to the L5 nerve root was 2.6 cm, 2.2 cm, and 1.5 cm, respectively.

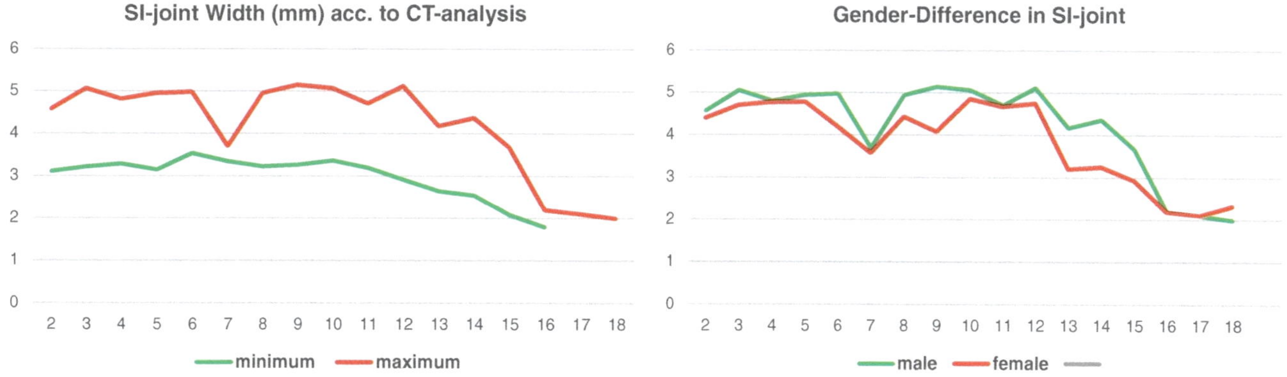

Fig. 2.30 Age-dependent width of the SI joint. Females present with slightly smaller width

Using the anterior-lateral approach in SI joint (fracture) dislocations for plate stabilization, cadaver dissections revealed that the lumbosacral trunk can nearly always be visualized [159].

Clinical Relevance
Direct subperiosteal dissection on the sacral ala using the anterior approach along the iliac crest to the SI joint can avoid injury to the lumbosacral trunk. The proximity between both structures should be considered. Near the anterior border of the joint, the safe zone is only 1.2 cm (Fig. 2.13).

The Iliolumbar Ligament

The iliolumbar ligament (ILL) (Fig. 2.25) has a variable course [84]. It arises from the L5 transverse process [160] and also more infrequently from the L4 transverse process [161] to insert at the iliac crest.

It contributes to SI joint and lumbosacral stability [83, 162] and resists lateral pelvic bending [81, 103].

Typically, two major bands can be identified: an anterior (upper) band and a posterior (lower) band [81, 84] with the following characteristics [163, 164]:

- Anterior iliolumbar band: flat structure; length, 30–40 mm long; width, 5–10 mm; diameter, 2–3 mm; origin, anterior-inferior-lateral portion of L5 transverse process; insertion, anterior part of the iliac tuberosity.
- Posterior iliolumbar band: round structure; length, 10–12 mm long; diameter, 5–7 mm; origin, tip of the L5 transverse process; insertion, superior and apex of the iliac crest/anterior portion of the iliac tuberosity.

Avulsion of the L5 transverse process is supposed to be a marker of posterior pelvic ring instability.

In an analysis of 80 patients with 45 stable and 35 unstable fractures according to the Young-Burgess classification, the prevalence of transverse process fracture in stable fractures was 6.7% vs. 40% in unstable fractures. The calculated odds ratio in unstable fracture to present with a fracture of the L5 transverse process was 9.3, and the relative risk was 2.5 [165].

Maqungo et al. reported a difference of prevalence in stable type A injuries according to Tile vs. type B and C injuries of 19% vs. 12%, respectively, and stated that the presence of an L5 transverse process fracture is strongly associated with a pelvic fracture, without distinguishing stable or unstable fracture pattern [166].

A systematic review and meta-analysis only stated that present data only allow the conclusion that a fractured L5 transverse process is a potential sign of high-energy trauma and not of unstable pelvic injury [167].

Clinical Relevance
A fracture of the transverse process of L5 should lead to suspicion of an unstable pelvic fracture.

2.1.4 Lumbosacral Plexus

Knowledge of the anatomy of the lumbosacral plexus is important to understand concomitant injuries of pelvic ring fractures (Figs. 2.20 and 2.21).

2.1.4.1 Lumbar Plexus

The lumbar plexus is formed by the anterior rami of the L1–L4 nerve roots and constitutes the iliohypogastric, ilioinguinal, genitofemoral, lateral cutaneous femoral, femoral, and obturator nerves. Several variants exist [168].

The size of the lumbar plexus nerve roots increases from L1 to L4 with L1 4.1 mm, L2 4.8 mm, L3 5.2 mm, and L4 5.5 mm [169].

The ilioinguinal nerve is running within the inguinal canal below the spermatic cord or the round ligament [170].

The lateral cutaneous femoral, femoral, and obturator nerves are of major surgical importance when treating pelvic ring fractures and thus are discussed more in detail.

Lateral Femoral Cutaneous Nerve (LFCN)

The LFCN (L2, L3 nerve roots) shows high anatomic variability, when leaving the pelvic cavity, as it passes through or behind the inguinal ligament [171–175] between the superior and inferior anterior iliac spines. Typically, the nerve is dissected under the inguinal ligament outside the pelvis approximately 15–20 mm medial to the anterior superior iliac spine (ASIS). Below the inguinal ligament, the nerve trunk runs lateral to the sartorius border to divide into several branches around 5 cm below the level of the ASIS [174, 176, 177].

The mean diameter of the LFCN is 1.8 mm [169].

The LFCN is at risk of damage when performing the first window of the ilioinguinal approach to the SI joint due to its close proximity to the anterior superior iliac spine (ASIS). Here, the nerve can course up to 5 cm lateral to the ASIS through the abdominal wall [178–180].

Femoral Nerve

The femoral nerve (L2–L4) follows a protected course within the fibrous fascia of the iliopsoas muscle, leaving the pelvis through the muscular lacuna, directly lateral to the iliopectineal fascia [181].

Identification of the femoral nerve is possible on a half line medial to the ASIS on a half line between the ASIS and the pubic symphysis [182].

The mean diameter of the femoral nerve is 2.6 mm [169].

A potential risk of damage to the nerve exists using anterior approaches during iliopsoas mobilization.

Obturator Nerve

The obturator nerve (L2–L4) descends through the psoas major muscle. In the pelvic cavity, the nerve runs near the SI joint, with an acceptable distance to the superior sacral ala, in contact with the bone of the anterior column, before it enters the true pelvis and leaving it through the obturator foramen. Its course is superior and in front of the obturator artery and vein and therefore is the most superior visible structure at the obturator canal [181].

At the level of the SI joint and sacral alar, the nerve passes anterior to the L5 transverse process and the iliolumbar ligament medial to the lumbosacral trunk and behind the common iliac vessels to reach the anterior SI joint [170].

In one-fourth of cases, the nerve trunk has already divided into two main branches before entering the obturator canal [183, 184].

The mean diameter of the obturator nerve is 1.6 mm [169].

There is a potential risk of nerve damage during anterior approaches including the intrapelvic approach.

2.1.4.2 Lumbosacral Trunk

The lumbosacral trunk presents as the link between the lumbar and the sacral plexus. It is partially formed by the anterior part of the L4 nerve root and the complete L5 nerve root, joining the S1 nerve root anterior to the SI joint and the sacrum (Fig. 2.13).

The course of the lumbosacral trunk starts medial to the psoas major, running on top of the sacral alar over the pelvic brim to the first sacral foramen.

The length of the lumbosacral trunk was analyzed by Ebraheim et al., who reported a range between 21 and 38 mm and a width of 4–4.4 mm [185]. The union between the L4 and L5 nerve roots can occur above, below, or directly at the anterior SI joint [186].

The localization of the lumbosacral trunk in relation to the SI joint is of major importance during the anterior approach to the SI joint for plate osteosynthesis.

Atlihan et al. reported an average distance between the trunk and the superior aspect of the SI joint of 11.5 mm, whereas directly anterior, near the pelvic brim, this distance was 5.3 mm [187].

Ebraheim et al. reported a distance of 23 mm for the L4 root and a distance of 26 mm 4 cm proximal and medial to the SI joint at the pelvic brim, decreasing to 10 mm near the pelvic brim [74].

The lumbosacral trunk is fixed to the sacral ala with fibrous tissue [185].

2.1.4.3 Sacral Plexus

The sacral plexus is formed by the anterior rami S1–S4 nerve roots. These anterior nerves converge in front of the sacrum to a large band located in front of the piriformis muscle and behind the internal iliac vessels and the ureter [170]. The main nerves, resulting from the sacral plexus, include the sciatic nerve and the pudendal nerve.

The largest nerve root is the S1 nerve root with a width of 8.6–9.8 mm [185].

The different nerve roots of the sacral plexus were analyzed in relation (mean distance) to the most inferior part of the SI joint [186]:

- S1 nerve root: 2.18 mm in the coronal and 8.16 mm in the sagittal plane.
- S2 nerve root: 16.88 mm in the coronal and 9.33 mm in the sagittal plane.
- S3 nerve root: 24.01 mm in the coronal and 8.89 mm in the sagittal plane.

Sciatic Nerve

The sciatic nerve consists of two main nerve branches: the common peroneal nerve and the tibial nerve. The lateral portion of the sciatic nerve is always the common peroneal nerve. The nerve leaves the pelvis through the infrapiriform foramen below the piriformis muscle (infrapiriform foramen) in approximately 80% of patients. Variations include nerve penetration through the piriformis muscle with one branch passing through the piriformis fibers in up to 20% of patients, a pure suprapiriform course, and others [188–190].

Superior Gluteal Nerve

The superior gluteal nerve is the most cranial branch of the sacral plexus. The nerve runs anterior to the SI joint to leave the true pelvis through the suprapiriform foramen between the upper edge of the piriformis muscle and the bony border of the greater sciatic together with the superior gluteal vessels [181]. Besides a common nerve trunk, a spray pattern is often present [191–195]. The nerve branches are located on the gluteus minimus between the medius and the minimus.

Application of the pelvic C-clamp or percutaneous iliosacral screw fixation can potentially endanger this nerve when a wrong entry point is used.

In a cadaver analysis of iliosacral screw fixation, Collinge et al. observed an 18% injury rate to the superior gluteal nerve and/or vessels. The mean distance between the screw head and the nerve was 9.1 mm [196].

Inferior Gluteal Nerve

The inferior gluteal nerve exits the pelvis through the infrapiriform foramen below the piriformis muscle belly close and medial to the sciatic nerve [197].

Pudendal Nerve

The pudendal nerve (S2–S4) leaves the true pelvis between the piriformis muscle and the sacrospinal ligament through the greater sciatic notch running around the sciatic spine to penetrate the gluteal region.

2.1.5 Vascular Anatomy

The pelvis is surrounded by a dense network of arterial and venous vessels with an adequate collateral supply to the pelvic organs, which makes surgical bleeding control sometimes difficult (Figs. 2.19 and 2.23). Even more pronounced is the collateralization of the dense venous plexus. Therefore, venous bleeding can be often only controlled by tamponades.

2.1.5.1 Arterial Vascular System

The vascular supply of the lower limb is provided from the common iliac artery. Anterior to the SI joint, the common iliac artery divides into the internal iliac artery, which supplies the pelvic organs in the true pelvis, and the external iliac artery to supply the leg. The external iliac artery is located in the connective tissue medial to the iliopsoas fascia. Before passing through the lacuna vasorum, the epigastric inferior and the iliac profunda arteries leave the main arterial trunk. After passage through the lacuna vasorum, the vessel is called the femoral artery. A more detailed anatomical description of the vascular system with its anastomoses is well stated in the anatomical literature [9, 26, 94, 95].

All pelvic organs, except the testes, which historically have a different source of arterial blood supply, are supplied by branches of the internal iliac artery (Fig. 2.31). The internal iliac artery divides at the level of the linea terminalis into posterior and anterior main trunks.

The posterior trunk gives branches for supply of the abdominal and truncal wall [23]:

- Iliolumbar artery (psoas major, iliacus, quadratus lumborum muscle).
- Lateral sacral artery (anterior sacral surface, lateral to the foraminal area).
- Superior gluteal artery: it exits the true pelvis through the greater sciatic notch proximal to the piriformis muscle and divides into two major branches, the superficial branch and deep branch, which supply the abductors [198–201]; anastomoses are observed with the superficial and deep circumflex iliac arteries, with branches of the iliolumbar artery and branches of the ascending branch of the lateral circumflex femoral artery (LCFA) [181].

The anterior main trunk with its intestinal branches submits the bladder, rectum, and genitals. Relevant branches include:

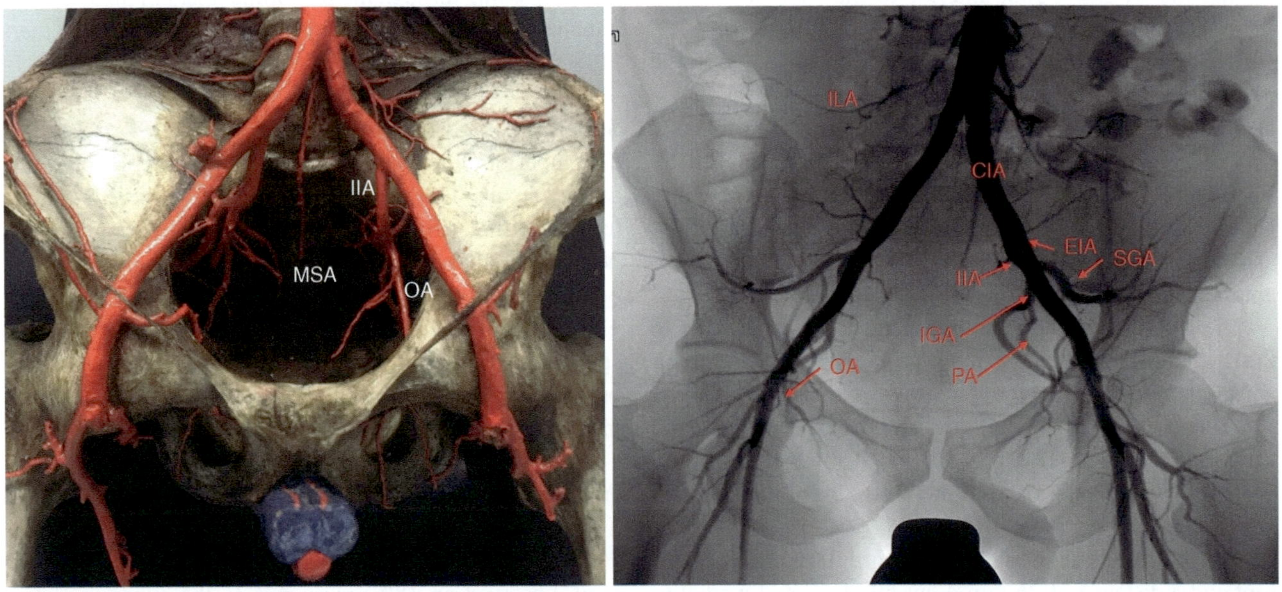

Fig. 2.31 Arterial pelvic network: *CIA* common iliac artery, *IEA* iliac external artery, *IIA* iliac internal artery, *ILA* iliolumbar artery, *SGA* superior gluteal artery, *IGA* inferior gluteal artery, *IPA* internal pudendal artery, *OA* obturator artery, and *MSA* median sacral artery

- Inferior gluteal artery: it exits the pelvis through the infrapiriform foramen, supplying the gluteus maximus and piriformis muscles, and the sciatic nerve [181].
- Internal pudendal artery: it leaves the true pelvis together with the pudendal plexus through the infrapiriform foramen, running medially to the ischial spine to enter the Alcock's canal, running around the sciatic spine through the lesser sciatic notch to reenter the true pelvis.
- Obturator artery: it typically arises from the main anterior branch of the internal iliac artery, but variably it can arise from the external iliac artery or even the inferior epigastric artery [201] to supply the quadrilateral surface, leaving the true pelvis through the obturator canal supplying muscles of the medial compartment of the thigh.

2.1.5.2 Corona Mortis

A relevant vascular anastomosis is the "corona mortis," which refers to any connection between the obturator vessels and the iliac external or inferior epigastric vessels [181].

These anastomoses can be present as purely arterial, purely venous, or combined arterial and venous (overview in: [181]).

Clinical data indicate an overall less relevance of the corona mortis. These vessels were observed in 41% after different surgical approaches were used for treating pelvic ring and acetabular fractures [202]. In contrast, sometimes, massive hemorrhage from these vessels is reported [203–205].

2.1.5.3 Venous Vascular System

The venous system mainly consists of large venous plexus, which enters into the common iliac vein. Additional portocaval anastomoses exist via rectal veins.

Surgically significant plexuses of the true pelvis include:

- Venous plexus between the symphysis, and bladder ("cavum Retzii").
- Rectal venous plexus.
- Presacral venous plexus (Figs. 2.19 and 2.23).

During emergency treatment of unstable pelvic ring fractures, relevant bleeding predominantly occurs from the presacral venous plexus.

Retrosymphyseal Venous Plexus

The (pre)vesical venous plexus (Fig. 2.32) surrounds the lower part of the urinary bladder and in men additionally the base of prostate [206].

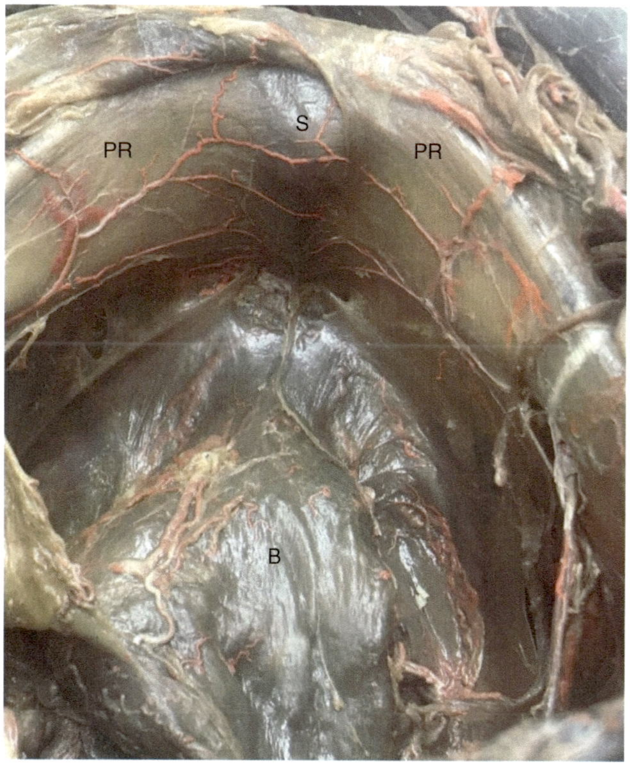

Fig. 2.32 Retrosymphyseal arterial network at the pubic rami *PR*, the symphysis *S* and the anterior wall of the bladder *B*

It typically includes two to five rows of veins that coursed within the paravaginal tissue parallel to the bladder and drained into the internal iliac veins [207].

Presacral Venous Plexus

The bilateral symmetric sacral venous plexus is located caudal to the lumbosacral junction, presenting as a hexagonal venous system draining into the lateral branch of the hypogastric vein [208]. The caudal part consists of bilateral ladder-type longitudinal veins, which anastomoses by transverse veins with the midline longitudinal medial sacral veins (Figs. 2.19 and 2.23).

Thus, the main venous contribution to this plexus results from two lateral sacral veins, the middle sacral vein and the communicating veins [78]. Anastomoses further exist to the internal vertebral venous system through basivertebral veins, which pass through the sacral foramina [77].

The presacral venous plexus covers the anterior sacral body underneath the presacral fascia in direct relation to the piriformis and coccygeal muscle fascia, and the sacrospinous ligament [78].

Thus, any injury to the anterior sacrum can result in relevant bleeding.

References

1. Bucholz R, Ezaki M, Ogden J. Injury of the acetabular triradiate physeal cartilage. J Bone Joint Surg. 1982;64-A(4):600–9.
2. Ponseti I. Growth and development of the acetabulum in the normal child. J Bone Joint Surg. 1978;60-A(5):575–85.
3. Watts H. Fractures of the pelvis in children. Orthop Clin North Am. 1976;7(3):615–24.
4. Stevenson P. Age order of epiphyseal union in man. Am J Phys Anthropol. 1924;7:53–93.
5. Drake R, Vogl W, Mitchell A. Chapter 5: Pelvis and perineum. In: Gray's anatomy for students, Third Edition. Amsterdam: Elsevier Inc.; 2015.
6. Lombardo S, Retting A, Kerlan R. Radiographic abnormalities of the iliac apophysis in adolescent athletes. J Bone Joint Surg Am. 1983;65:444–6.
7. Risser J. The iliac apophysis; an invaluable sign in the management of scoliosis. Clin Orthop. 1958;11:111–9.
8. Parvaresh K, Upasani V, Bomar J, Pennock A. Secondary ossification center appearance and closure in the pelvis and proximal femur. J Pediatr Orthop. 2018;38(8):418–23.
9. Gray. In: Warwick R, Williams PL, editors. Gray's anatomy. 35th ed. Edinburgh: Longmon; 1973.
10. Steinbrück K, Krahl H. Apophysäre Frakturen am Becken beim Jugendlichen. In: Pförringer W, Rosemeyer B, editors. Die Epiphysenfugen. München: Perimed Fachbuch-Verlagsgesellschaft mbH Erlangen; 1987. p. 182–94.
11. Scheuer L, Black S. The juvenile skeleton. Cambridge, MA: Academic Press; 2004.
12. Mollier S. Plastische anatomie. 2. Auflage, unveränderter Neudruck 1967 ed. München: J.F.Bergmann; 1938.
13. Gänsslen A, Hildebrand F, Klebingat M, Nerlich M, Lindahl J. Chapter 22: Special screws and views. In: Gänsslen A, et al., editors. Acetabular fractures: diagnosis, indications, treatment strategies. Stuttgart: Thieme; 2017. ISBN-13: 978-3132415607.
14. Ebraheim N, Lu J, Biyani A, Yang H. Anatomic considerations of the principal nutrient foramen and artery on internal surface of the ilium. Surg Radiol Anat. 1997;19:237–9.
15. Alla S, Roberts C, Ojike N. Vascular risk reduction during anterior surgical approach sacroiliac joint plating. Injury. 2013;44:175–7.
16. Gänsslen A, Pohlemann T, Krettek C. A simple supraacetabular external fixation for pelvic ring fractures. Oper Orthop Traumatol. 2005;17:296–312.
17. Berry J, Stahurski T, Asher M. Morphometry of the supra sciatic notch intrailiac implant anchor passage. Spine. 2001;26:E143–8.
18. Gras F, Hillmann S, Rausch S, Klos K, Hofmann G, Marintschev I. Biomorphometric analysis of Ilio-sacro-iliacal corridors for an intra-osseous implant to fix posterior pelvic ring fractures. J Orthop Res. 2015;33:254–60.
19. Lidder S, Heidari N, Gänsslen A, Grechenig W. Radiological landmarks for the safe extra-capsular placement of supra-acetabular half pins for external fixation. Surg Radiol Anat. 2013;35:131–5.
20. Schildhauer T, McCulloch P, Chapman J, Mann F. Anatomic and radiographic considerations for placement of transiliac screws in lumbopelvic fixations. J Spinal Disord Tech. 2002;15:199–205.
21. Tian X, Li J, Sheng W, Qu D, Ouyang J, Xu D, Chen S, Ding Z. Morphometry of iliac anchorage for transiliac screws: a cadaver and CT study of the eastern population. Surg Radiol Anat. 2010;32:455–62.
22. Routt MJ, Simonian P, Agnew S, Mann F. Radiographic recognition of the sacral alar slope for optimal placement of iliosacral screws: a cadaveric and clinical study. J Orthop Trauma. 1996;10:171–7.
23. Pohlemann T. Chapter 1.2: Chirurgische Anatomie. In: Tscherne H, Pohlemann T, editors. Tscherne Unfallchirurgie: Becken und Acetabulum. Spirnger Verlag: Berlin, Heidelberg, New York; 1998.
24. Wagner D, Kamer L, Sawaguchi T, Richards R, Noser H, Hofmann A, Rommens P. Morphometry of the sacrum and its implication on trans-sacral corridors using a computed tomography data-based three-dimensional statistical model. Spine J. 2017;17:1141–7.
25. Broome D, Hayman L, Herrick R, Braverman R, Glass R, Fahr L. Postnatal maturation of the sacrum and coccyx: MR imaging, helical CT, and conventional radiography. AJR Am J Roentgenol. 1998;170:1061–6.
26. Agur A. Grant's Atlas of anatomy. ed 10. Philadelphia: Lippincott Williams & Wilkins; 1999.
27. Esses S, Botsford D. Surgical anatomy and operative approaches to the sacrum. In: Frymoyer JW, Ducker TB, Hadler NM, et al., editors. The adult spine: principles and practice, ed. 2. Philadelphia: Lippincott-Raven; 1997. p. 2329–41.
28. Gray H. Anatomy of the human body. Philadelphia: Lea & Febiger; 1918.
29. Xu R, Ebraheim N, Gove N. Surgical anatomy of the sacrum. Am J Orthop. 2008;37:E177–81.
30. Rios L, Weissensee K, Rissech C. Sacral fusion as an aid in age estimation. For Sci Int. 2008;180(2–3):111.e1–7.
31. Whelan M, Gold R. Computed tomography of the sacrum: 1. Normal anatomy. AJR Am J Roentgenol. 1982;139:1183–90.
32. Başaloğlu H, Turgut M, Taşer F, Ceylan T, Başaloğlu H, Ceylan A. Morphometry of the sacrum for clinical use. Surg Radiol Anat. 2005;27:467–71.
33. Arman C, Naderi S, Kiray A, Aksu F, Yilmaz H, Tetik S, Korman E. The human sacrum and safe approaches for screw placement. J Clin Neurosci. 2009;16:1046–9.
34. Rajangam S, Khan S, Jayakaran F. Features on the dorsal surface of the sacrum. J Mahatma Ghandi Inst Med Si. 2014;19:112–8.
35. Vasuki A, Sundaram K, Nirmaladevi M, Jamuna M, Hebzibah D, Fenn T. Anatomical variations of sacrum and its clinical significance. Int J Anat Res. 2016;4:1859–63.
36. Bagheri H, Govsa F. Anatomy of the sacral hiatus and its clinical relevance in caudal epidural block. Surg Radiol Anat. 2017;39:943–51.
37. Nagendrappa R, Jayanthi K. Study of dorsal wall of sacrum. Int J Res Med Sci. 2014;2:1325–8.
38. Cox R, Fortin J. The anatomy of the lateral branches of the sacral dorsal rami: implications for radiofrequency ablation. Pain Phys. 2014;17:459–64.
39. Liguoro D, Viejo-Fuertes D, Midy D, Guerin J. The posterior sacral foramina: an anatomical study. J Anat. 1999;195:301–4.
40. Jackson H, Burke J. The sacral foramina. Skelet Radiol. 1984;11:282–8.
41. Farrell E, Gardner M, Krieg J, Routt MJ. The upper sacral nerve root tunnel: an anatomic and clinical study. J Orthop Trauma. 2009;23:333–9.
42. McGrath M, Stringer M. Bony landmarks in the sacral region: the posterior superior iliac spine and the second dorsal sacral foramina: a potential guide for sonography. Surg Radiol Anat. 2011;33:279–86.
43. Waldrop J, Ebraheim N, Yeasting R, Jackson W. The location of the sacroiliac joint on the outer table of the posterior ilium. J Orthop Trauma. 1993;7:510–3.
44. Pal G. Weight transmission through the sacrum in man. J Anat. 1989;162:9–17.
45. Zindrick M. Pedicle screw fixation. In: Weilstein SL, editor. The pediatric spine: principles and practice. New York, NY: Raven Press; 1994. p. 1698.
46. Xu R, Ebraheim N, Robke J, Yeasting R. Radiologic evaluation of iliosacral screw placement. Spine. 1996;21:582–8.
47. Bron J, van Royen B, Wuisman P. The clinical significance of lumbosacral transitional anomalies. Acta Orthop Belg. 2007;73:687–95.

48. Gardner M, Morshed S, Nork S, Ricci W, Routt MJ. Quantification of the upper and second sacral segment safe zones in normal and dysmorphic sacra. J Orthop Trauma. 2010;24:622–9.
49. Hasenboehler E, Stahel P, Williams A, Smith W, Newman J, Symonds D, Morgan S. Prevalence of sacral dysmorphia in a prospective trauma population: Implications for a "safe" surgical corridor for sacro-iliac screw placement. Patient Saf Surg. 2011;5:8. https://doi.org/10.1186/1754-9493-5-8.
50. Kaiser S, Gardner M, Liu J, Routt MJ, Morshed S. Anatomic determinants of sacral Dysmorphism and implications for safe Iliosacral screw placement. J Bone Joint Surg Am. 2014;96:e120.
51. Miller A, Routt MJ. Variations in sacral morphology and implications for iliosacral screw fixation. J Am Acad Orthop Surg. 2012;20:8–16.
52. Cheng J, Song J. Anatomy of the sacrum. Neurosurg Focus. 2003;15:1–4.
53. Conflitti J, Graves M, Routt MJ. Radiographic quantification and analysis of dysmorphic upper sacral osseous anatomy and associated iliosacral screw insertions. J Orthop Trauma. 2010;24:630–6.
54. Pohlemann T, Angst M, Schneider E, Ganz R, Tscherne H. Fixation of transforaminal sacrum fractures: a biomechanical study. J Orthop Trauma. 1993;7(2):107–17.
55. Pohlemann T, Culemann U, Tscherne H. Vergleichende biomechanische Untersuchungen zur internen Stabilisierung der transforaminalen Sakrumfraktur. Orthopade. 1992;21:413–21.
56. Pohlemann T, Gänsslen A, Tscherne H. Sacral fractures. In: Tile M, Helfet DL, Kellam JF, editors. Fractures of the pelvis and acetabulum. 3rd ed. Philadelphia: Lippincot Williams & Wilkins; 2003. p. 294–322.
57. Ebraheim N, Lin D, Xu R, Yeasting R. Evaluation of the upper sacrum by three dimensional computed tomography. Am J Orthop. 1999;28:578–82.
58. Ebraheim N, Xu R, Li J, Yeasting R. Computed tomographic considerations of dorsal sacral screw placement. J Spinal Disord. 1998;11:71–4.
59. Ebraheim N, Sabry F, Nadim Y, Xu R, Yeasting R. Internal architecture of the sacrum in the elderly. An anatomic and radiographic study. Spine. 2000;25:292–7.
60. Wagner D, Kamer L, Rommens P, Sawaguchi T, Richards R, Noser H. 3D statistical modeling techniques to investigate the anatomy of the sacrum, its bone mass distribution, and the trans-sacral corridors. J Orthop Res. 2014;32:1543–8.
61. Wagner D, Kamer L, Sawaguchi T, Richards R, Noser H, Rommens P. Sacral bone mass distribution assessed by averaged three-dimensional CT models: implications for pathogenesis and treatment of fragility fractures of the sacrum. J Bone Joint Surg Am. 2016;98:584–90.
62. Zheng Y, Lu W, Zhu Q, Qin L, Zhong S, Leong J. Variation in bone mineral density of the sacrum in young adults and its significance for sacral fixation. Spine. 2000;25:353–7.
63. Richards A, Coleman N, Knight T, Belkoff S, Mears S. Bone density and cortical thickness in normal, osteopenic, and osteoporotic sacra. J Osteoporos. 2010;2010:1. https://doi.org/10.4061/2010/504078.
64. Waites M, Mears S, Mathis J, Belkoff S. The strength of the osteoporotic sacrum. Spine. 2007;32:E652–5.
65. Denis F, Steven D, Comfort T. Sacral fractures: an important problem, retrospective analysis of 236 cases. Clin Orthop. 1988;227:67–81.
66. Carlson DA, Scheid DK, Maar DC, Baele JR, Kaehr DM. Safe placement of S1 and S2 iliosacral screws: the "vestibule" concept. J Orthop Trauma. 2000;14(4):264–9.
67. Day CS, Prayson MJ, Shuler TE, Towers J, Gruen GS. Transsacral versus modified pelvic landmarks for percutaneous iliosacral screw placement—a computed tomographic analysis and cadaveric study. Am J Orthop. 2000;29(9 Suppl):16–21.
68. Noojin F, Malkani A, Haikal L, Lundquist C, Voor M. Cross-sectional geometry of the sacral ala for safe insertion of iliosacral lag screws: a computed tomography model. J Orthop Trauma. 2000;14:31–5.
69. Dong Q, Tian W, Ma B. Evaluation and clinical application of sacral S1 vestibule measurements in Chinese adults. Int J Morphol. 2014;32:202–7.
70. Marty C, Boisaubert B, Descamps H, Montigny J, Hecquet J, Legaye J, Duval-Beaupère G. The sagittal anatomy of the sacrum among young adults, infants, and spondylolisthesis patients. Eur Spine J. 2002;11:119–25.
71. Peleg S, Dar G, Steinberg N, Peled N, Hershkovitz I, Masharawi Y. Sacral orientation revisited. Spine. 2007;32:E397–404.
72. Mirkovic S, Abitol J, Steinmann J, Edwards C, Schaffler M, Massie J, Garfin S. Anatomic consideration for sacral screw placement. Spine. 1991;16(6):289–94.
73. Bydon M, Fredrickson V, De la Garza-Ramos R, Li Y, Lehman RJ, Trost G, Gokaslan Z. Sacral fractures. Neurosurg Focus. 2014;37:E12.
74. Ebraheim N, Padanilam T, Waldrop J, Yeasting R. Anatomic consideration in the anterior approach to the sacro-iliac joint. Spine. 1994;19(6):721–5.
75. Akhgar J, Terai H, Suhrab Rahmani M, Tamai K, Suzuki A, Toyoda H, Hoshino M, Abdullah Ahmadi S, Hayashi K, Nakamura H. Anatomical location of the common iliac veins at the level of the sacrum: relationship between perforation risk and the trajectory angle of the screw. Biomed Res Int. 2016;2016:1. https://doi.org/10.1155/2016/1457219.
76. Florian-Rodriguez M, Hamner J, Corton M. First sacral nerve and anterior longitudinal ligament anatomy: clinical applications during sacrocolpopexy. Am J Obstet Gynecol. 2017;217:607.e1–607.e4.
77. Gillot C. Le système cave inférieur. In: Chevrel JP, editor. Anatomie clinique. Berlin, Heidelberg, New York: Springer; 1994. p. 441–53.
78. Baqué P, Karimdjee B, Iannelli A, Benizri E, Rahili A, Benchimol D, Bernard J, Sejor E, Bailleux S, de Peretti F, Bourgeon A. Anatomy of the presacral venous plexus: implications for rectal surgery. Surg Radiol Anat. 2004;26:355–8.
79. Tilvawala K, Kothari K, Patel R. Sacroiliac joint: a review. Indian J Pain. 2018;32:4–15.
80. Vleeming A, Schuenke M, Masi A, Carreiro J, Danneels L, Willard F. The sacroiliac joint: an overview of its anatomy, function and potential clinical implications. J Anat. 2012;221:537–67.
81. Butt A, Gill C, Demerdash A, Watanabe K, Loukas M, Rozzelle C, Tubbs R. A comprehensive review of the sub-axial ligaments of the vertebral column: part I anatomy and function. Childs Nerv Syst. 2015;31:1037–59.
82. Luk K, Ho H, Leong J. The iliolumbar ligament. A study of its anatomy, development and clinical significance. J Bone Joint Surg (Br). 1986;68:197–200.
83. Pool-Goudzwaard A, Hoek van Dijke A, Mulder P, Spoor C, Snijders C, Stoeckart R. The iliolumbar ligament: its influence on stability of the sacroiliac joint. Clin Biomech (Bristol, Avon). 2002;18:99–105.
84. Hanson P, Sonesson B. The anatomy of the iliolumbar ligament. Arch Phys Med Rehabil. 1994;75:1245–6.
85. Pool-Goudzwaard A, Hoek van Dijke G, Mulder P, Spoor C, Snijders C, Stoeckart R. The iliolumbar ligament: its influence on stability of the sacroiliac joint. Clin Biomech (Bristol, Avon). 2003;18:99–105.
86. Zoccali C, Skoch J, Patel A, Walter C, Avila M, Martirosyan N, Demitri S, Baaj A. The surgical anatomy of the lumbosacroiliac triangle: a cadaveric study. World Neursurg. 2016;88:36–40.

87. Kleihues H, Albrecht S, Noack W. Topographic relations between the neural and ligamentous structures of the lumbosacral junction: in-vitro investigation. Eur Spine J. 2001;10:124–32.
88. Seizeur R, Forlodou P, Person H, Morin J, Sénécail B. The morphometric study of the sacrospinal and sacrotuberal ligaments correlated with the morphometry of the pelvis. Surg Radiol Anat. 2005;27:517–23.
89. Lai J, du Plessis M, Wooten C, Gielecki J, Tubbs R, Oskouian R, Loukas M. The blood supply to the sacrotuberous ligament. Surg Radiol Anat. 2017;39:953–9.
90. Fogel G, Cunningham PR, Esses S. Coccygodynia: evaluation and management. J Am Acad Orthop Surg. 2004;12:49–54.
91. Woon J, Perumal V, Maigne J, Stringer M. CT morphology and morphometry of the normal adult coccyx. Eur Spine J. 2013;22:863–70.
92. Yoon M, Moon M, Park B, Lee H, Kim D. Analysis of sacrococcygeal morphology in Koreans using computed tomography. Clin Orthop Surg. 2016;8:412–9.
93. Becker I, Woodley S, Stringer M. The adult human pubic symphysis: a systematic review. J Anat. 2010;217:475–87.
94. McMinn R. Last's Anatomy. Regional and applied. 9th edn. Edinburgh: Churchill Livingstone; 1994. p. 414.
95. Standring S. Gray's anatomy: the anatomical basis of clinical practice. 40th ed. New York: Churchill Livingstone, Elsevier; 2008. p. 1365.
96. Rosse C, Gaddum-Rosse P. Hollinshead's textbook of anatomy. 5th ed. New York: Lippincott-Raven; 1997. p. 313.
97. Luschka H. Die Anatomie des menschlichen Beckens. Tübingen: Verlag der Laupp'schen Buchhandlung; 1864.
98. Weber E. Handbuch der Anatomie des Menschen—Beschreibung des Knochensystems, des Muskelsystems under der Haut. 4th ed. Verlag der Schulbuchhandlung: Braunschweig; 1830. p. 187–8.
99. Fick R. Handbuch der Anatomie und Mechanik der Gelenke unter Berücksichtigung der bewegenden Muskeln. Erster Teil: Anatomie der Gelenke. Verlag von Gustav Fischer: Jena; 1904. p. 303–11.
100. Knox R. A system of human anatomy: on the basis of the "Traite d'anatomie descriptive" of M.H. Cloquet. 2nd edn. MacLachlan and Stewart: Edinburgh; 1831. p. 196–8.
101. Frick H, Leonhardt H, Starck H. Human anatomy 1. 3rd edn. Stuttgart: Georg Thieme Verlag; 1991. p. 309–10.
102. Putschar W. The structure of the human symphysis pubis with special consideration of parturition and its sequelae. Am J Phys Anthropol. 1976;45:589–94.
103. Zulauf C. Die Höhlenbildung im Symphysenknorpel. Archiv Anat Physiol. 1901;1:95–116.
104. Loeschcke H. Untersuchungen über die Entstehung und Bedeutung der Spaltbildungen in der Symphyse, sowie über physiologische Erweiterungsvorgaenge am Becken Schwangerer und Gebärender. Archiv Gynaek. 1912;96:525–60.
105. Testut J, Latarjet A. Traite d'Anatomie Humaine. 8th ed. Paris: Gaston Doin & Co.; 1928. p. 663–9.
106. Aeby C. Über die Symphysis Ossium Pubis des Menschen nebst Beiträgen zur Lehre vom hyalinen Knorpel und seiner Verknöcherung. Z Ration Med. 1858;4:1–25.
107. Frazer J. The human anatomy of the skeleton. 2nd edn. London: J & A Churchill; 1920. p. 134–5.
108. Gamble JG, Simmons SC, Freedman M. The symphysis pubis anatomic and pathologic considerations. Clin Orthop. 1986;203:261–72.
109. Sutro C. The pubic bones and their symphysis. Arch Surg. 1936;32:823–41.
110. Todd T. Age changes in the pubic bone. VIII: Roentgenographic differentiation. Am J Phys Anthropol. 1930;14:255–71.
111. Link B, Ha N, Solomon L, Rickman M. Defining the pubic symphysis angle with respect to the coronal plane—clinical and biomechanical considerations. Injury. 2017;48:1714–6.
112. Dolati B. Kapitel 3: Biomechanik. Becken und Acetabulumchirurgie. In: Weller S, Hierholzer G, editors. Traumatologie aktuell Band 10. Stuttgart, New York: Thieme; 1993. p. 19–23.
113. Ibrahim A, El-Sherbini A. The different ligaments of the symphysis pubis in the pregnant and the non-pregnant state. J Obstet Gynaecol Br Emp. 1961;68:592–6.
114. Robinson P, Salehi F, Grainger A, Clemence M, Schilders E, O'Connor P, Agur A. Cadaveric and MRI study of the musculotendinous contributions to the capsule of the symphysis pubis. AJR Am J Roentgenol. 2007;188:W440–5.
115. Schilders E, Bharam S, Golan E, Dimitrakopoulou A, Mitchell A, Spaepen M, Beggs C, Cooke C, Holmich P. The pyramidalis-anterior pubic ligament-adductor longus complex (PLAC) and its role with adductor injuries: a new anatomical concept. Knee Surg Sports Traumatol Arthrosc. 2017;25:3969–77.
116. Björklund K, Bergström S, Lindgren P, Ulmsten U. Ultrasonographic measurement of the symphysis pubis: a potential method of studying symphyseolysis in pregnancy. Gynecol Obstet Investig. 1996;42:151–3.
117. Vix V, Ryu C. The adult symphysis pubis: normal and abnormal. Am J Roentgenol Radium Therapy, Nucl Med. 1971;112:517–25.
118. Krauss F. Über Symphysensprengung. Zentbl Chir. 1930;3:134–5.
119. Patel K, Chapman S. Normal symphysis width in children. Clin Radiol. 1993;47:56–7.
120. Alicioglu B, Kartal O, Gurbuz H, Sut N. Symphysis pubis distance in adults: a retrospective computed tomography study. Surg Radiol Anat. 2008;30:153–7.
121. McAlister D, Webb H, Wheeler P, Shinault K, Teague D, Fish J, Beall D. Pubic symphyseal width in pediatric patients. J Pediatr Orthop. 2005;25:725–7.
122. Bayer J, Neubauer J, Saueressig U, Südkamp N, Reising K. Age- and gender-related characteristics of the pubic symphysis and triradiate cartilage in pediatric computed tomography. Pediatr Radiol. 2016;46:1705–12.
123. Kalenderer Ö, Turgut A, Bacaksız T, Bilgin E, Kumbaracı M, Akkan H. Evaluation of symphysis pubis and sacroiliac joint distances in skeletally immature patients: a computerized tomography study of 1020 individuals. Acta Orthop Traumatol Turc. 2017;51:150–4.
124. Oetgen M, Andelman S, Martin B. Age-based normative measurements of the pediatric pelvis. J Orthop Trauma. 2017;31:e205–9.
125. Rustamova S, Predanic M, Sumersille M, Cohen W. Changes in symphysis pubis width during labor. J Perinat Med. 2009;37:370–3.
126. Collinge C, Beltran M. Anatomic relationship between the spermatic cord and the pubic tubercle: are our clamps injuring the cord during symphyseal repair? J Orthop Trauma. 2015;29:290–4.
127. Bernard T, Kirkaldy-Willis W. Recognizing specific characteristics of nonspecific low back pain. Clin Orthop. 1987;217:266–80.
128. Dijkstra P, Vleeming A, Stoeckart R. Complex motion tomography of the sacroiliac joint. An anatomical and roentgenological study. ROFO. 1989;150:635–42.
129. Bernard T, Cassidy J. The sacroiliac joint syndrome. Pathophysiology, diagnosis and management. In: Frymoyer JW, editor. The adult spine: principles and practice. New York: Raven Press; 1991. p. 2107–30.
130. Grob K, Neuhuber W, Kissling R. Innervation of the sacroiliac joint of the human. Z Rheumatol. 1995;54:117–22.
131. McGrath M, Zhang M. Lateral branches of dorsal sacral nerve plexus and the long posterior sacroiliac ligament. Surg Radiol Anat. 2005;27:327–30.

132. Solonen K. The sacroiliac joint in the light of anatomical, roentgenological and clinical studies. Acta Orthop Scand. 1957;Suppl. 27:1–127.
133. Albee F. A study of the anatomy and the clinical importance of the sacroiliac joint. JAMA. 1909;53:1273–6.
134. Brooke R. The sacro-iliac joint. J Anat Physiol. 1924;58:299–305.
135. Sashin D. A critical analysis of the anatomy and the pathologic changes of the sacroiliac joints. JBJS. 1930;28:891–910.
136. Egund N, Jurik A. Anatomy and histology of the sacroiliac joints. Semin Musculoskelet Radiol. 2014;18:332–40.
137. Vleeming A, Stoeckart R. The role of the pelvic girdle in coupling the spine and the legs: a cinical-anatomical perspective on pelvic stability. In: Vleeming A, Mooney V, Stoeckart R, editors. Movement, stability and lumbopelvic pain: integration and research. Edinburgh: Churchill Livingstone; 2007. p. 113–37.
138. Schuncke G. The anatomy and development of the sacroiliac joint in man. Anat Rec. 1938;72:313–31.
139. Bowen V, Cassidy J. Macroscopic anatomy of the sacro-iliac joint from embryonic life until the eighth decade. Spine. 1981;6:620–8.
140. Vleeming A, Stoeckaert R, Volkers A, Snijders C. Relation between form and function in the sacro-iliac joint. Part I: Clinical anatomical aspects. Spine. 1990;15:130–2.
141. Cole J, Blum D, Ansel L. Outcome after fixation of unstable posterior pelvic ring injuries. Clin Orthop. 1996;329:160–79.
142. Vleeming A, van Wingerden J, Dijkstra P, Stoeckart R, Snijders C, Stijnen T. Mobility in the sacroiliac joints in the elderly: a kinematic and radiological study. Clin Biomech (Bristol, Avon). 1992;7:170–6.
143. Walker J. The sacroiliac joint: a critical review. Phys Ther. 1992;72:903–16.
144. Miller J, Schultz A, Andersson G. Load-displacement behavior of sacroiliac joints. J Orthop Res. 1987;5:92–101.
145. Dar G, Peleg S, Masharawi Y, Steinberg N, Rothschild B, Peled N, Hershkovitz I. Sacroiliac joint bridging: demographical and anatomical aspects. Spine. 2005;30:E429–32.
146. Dar G, Hershkovitz I. Sacroiliac joint bridging: simple and reliable criteria for sexing the skeleton. J Forensic Sci. 2006;51:480–3.
147. Soames R. Skeletal system. In: Bannister LH, editor. Gray's anatomy. Edinburgh: Churchill Livingstone; 1995. p. 425–900.
148. Fortin J, Kissling R, O'Connor B, Vilensky J. Sacroiliac joint innervation and pain. Am J Orthop. 1999;28:687–90.
149. Steinke H, Hammer N, Slowik V, Stadler J, Josten C, Böhme J, Spanel-Borowski K. Novel insights into the sacroiliac joint ligaments. Spine. 2010;35:257–63.
150. Rosatelli A, Agur A, Chhaya S. Anatomy of the interosseous region of the sacroiliac joint. J Orthop Sports Phys Ther. 2006;36: 200–8.
151. Moore A, Jeffery R, Gray A. An anatomical ultrasound study of the long posterior sacro-iliac ligament. Clin Anat. 2010;23:971–7.
152. Vleeming A, Pool-Goudzwaard A, Hammudoghlu D, Stoeckart R, Snijders C, Mens J. The function of the long dorsal sacroiliac ligament: its implication for understanding low back pain. Spine. 1996;21:556–62.
153. Palastanga N, Field D, Soames R. Anatomy and human movement: structure and function. Butterworth Heinemann: Oxford, UK; 1998.
154. Sinnatamby C. Last's anatomy regional and applied. 10th ed. Edinburgh: Churchill Livingstone; 1999. p. 315–6.
155. Loukas M, Louis RJ, Hallner B, Gupta A, White D. Anatomical and surgical considerations of the sacrotuberous ligament and its relevance in pudendal nerve entrapment syndrome. Surg Radiol Anat. 2006;28:163–9.
156. Vleeming A, Stoeckart R, Snijders C. The sacrotuberous ligament: a conceptual approach to its dynamic role in stabilizing the sacroiliac joint. Clin Biomech (Bristol, Avon). 1989;4:201–3.
157. Barker P, Briggs C, Bogeski G. Tensile transmission across the lumbar fasciae in unembalmed cadavers: effects of tension to various muscular attachments. Spine. 2004;29:129–38.
158. Bai Z, Gao S, Liu J, Liang A, Yu W. Anatomical evidence for the anterior plate fixation of sacroiliac joint. J Orthop Sci. 2018;23:132–6.
159. Phelps K, Ming B, Fox W, Bellamy N, Sims S, Karunakar M, Hsu J. A quantitative exposure planning tool for surgical approaches to the sacroiliac joint. J Orthop Trauma. 2016;30:319–24.
160. Aihara T, Takahashi K, Ogasawara A, Itadera E, Ono Y, Moriya H. Intervertebral disc degeneration associated with lumbosacral transitional vertebrae: a clinical and anatomical study. J Bone Joint Surg (Br). 2005;87:687–91.
161. Pool-Goudzwaard A, Kleinrensink G, Snijders C, Entius C, Stoeckart R. The sacroiliac part of the iliolumbar ligament. J Anat. 2001;199:457–63.
162. Viehofer A, Shinohara Y, Sprecher C, Boszczyk B, Buettner A, Benjamin M, Milz S. The molecular composition of the extracellular matrix of the human iliolumbar ligament. Spine. 2015;15:1325–31.
163. Basadonna P, Gasparini D, Rucco V. Iliolumbar ligament insertions. In vivo anatomic study. Spine. 1996;21:2313–6.
164. Sims J, Moorman S. The role of the iliolumbar ligament in low back pain. Med Hypothesis. 1996;46:511–5.
165. Starks I, Frost A, Wall P, Lim J. Is a fracture of the transverse process of L5 a predictor of pelvic fracture instability? J Bone Joint Surg (Br). 2011;93:967–9.
166. Maqungo S, Kimani M, Chhiba D, McCollum G, Roche S. The L5 transverse process fracture revisited. Does its presence predict the pelvis fracture instability? Injury. 2015;46:1629–30.
167. Nasef H, Elhessy A, Abushaban F, Alhammoud A. Pelvic fracture instability-associated L5 transverse process fracture, fact or myth? A systematic review and meta-analysis. Eur J Orthop Surg Traumatol. 2018;28:885–91.
168. Matejcík V. Anatomical variations of lumbosacral plexus. Surg Radiol Anat. 2010;32:409–14.
169. Izci Y, Gürkanlar D, Ozan H, Gönül E. The morphological aspects of lumbar plexus and roots. Turk Neurosurg. 2005;15:87–92.
170. Dietemann J, Sick H, Wolfram-Gabel R, Cruz da Silva R, Koritke J, Wackenheim A. Anatomy and computed tomography of the normal lumbosacral plexus. Neuroradiology. 1987;29:58–68.
171. Kosiyatrakul A, Nuansalee N, Luenam S, Koonchornboon T, Prachaporn S. The anatomical variation of the lateral femoral cutaneous nerve in relation to the anterior superior iliac spine and the iliac crest. Musculoskelet Surg. 2010;94:17–20.
172. Majkrzak A, Johnston J, Kacey D, Zeller J. Variability of the lateral femoral cutaneous nerve: an anatomic basis for planning safe surgical approaches. Clin Anat. 2010;23:304–11.
173. Ropars M, Morandi X, Huten D, Thomazeau H, Berton E, Darnault P. Anatomical study of the lateral femoral cutaneous nerve with special reference to minimally invasive anterior approach for total hip replacement. Surg Radiol Anat. 2009;31:199–204.
174. Sürücü H, Tanyeli E, Sargon M, Karahan S. An anatomic study of the lateral femoral cutaneous nerve. Surg Radiol Anat. 1997;19:307–10.
175. Üzel M, Akkin S, Tanyeli E, Koebke J. Relationships of the lateral femoral cutaneous nerve to bony landmarks. Clin Orthop. 2011;469:2605–11.
176. de Ridder VA, de Lange S, Popta JV. Anatomical variations of the lateral femoral cutaneous nerve and the consequences for surgery. J Orthop Trauma. 1999;13(3):207–11.
177. Hospodar P, Ashman E, Traub J. Anatomic study of the lateral femoral cutaneous nerve with respect to the ilioinguinal surgical dissection. J Orthop Trauma. 1999;13:17–9.

178. Aszmann OC, Dellon ES, Dellon AL. Anatomical course of the lateral femoral cutaneous nerve and its susceptibility to compression and injury. Plast Reconstr Surg. 1997;100(3):600–4.
179. Mears DC, Velyvis JH, Chang CP. Displaced acetabular fractures managed operatively: indicators of outcome. Clin Orthop. 2003;407:173–86.
180. Rommens P, Broos P, Vanderschot P. Vorbereitung und Technik der operativen Behandlung von 225 Acetabulumfrakturen Zweijahresergebnisse in 175 Fällen. Unfallchirurg. 1997;100:338–48.
181. Tesch N, Gänsslen A, Anderhuber F, Grechenig W, Grechenig S. Chapter 1: Surgical anatomy. In: Gänsslen A, et al., editors. Acetabular fractures. Stuttgart: Thieme; 2017. p. 1–18.
182. Gustafson K, Pinault G, Neville J, Syed I, Davis JJ, Jean-Claude J, Triolo R. Fascicular anatomy of human femoral nerve: implications for neural prostheses using nerve cuff electrodes. J Rehabil Res Dev. 2009;46:973–84.
183. Anagnostopoulou S, Kostopanagiotou G, Paraskeuopoulos T, Chantzi C, Lolis E, Saranteas T. Anatomic variations of the obturator nerve in the inguinal region: implications in conventional and ultrasound regional anesthesia techniques. Reg Anesth Pain Med. 2009;34:33–9.
184. Anagnostopoulou S, Mavridis I. Human obturator nerve: gross anatomy. World J Neurol. 2013;3:62–6.
185. Ebraheim N, Lu J, Biyani A, Huntoon M, Yeasting R. The relationship of lumbosacral plexus to the sacrum and the sacroiliac joint. Am J Orthop. 1997;26:105–10.
186. Waikakul S, Chandraphak S, Sangthongsil P. Anatomy of L4 to S3 nerve roots. J Orthop Surg. 2010;18:352–5.
187. Atlihan D, Tekdemir I, Ateŝ Y, Elhan A. Anatomy of the anterior sacroiliac joint with reference to lumbosacral nerves. Clin Orthop. 2000;376:236–41.
188. Anbumani T, Thamarai Selvi A, Anthony Ammal S. Sciatic nerve and its variations: an anatomical study. Int J Anat Res. 2015;3:1121–7.
189. Bergmann R, Uz A, Ozmen M. Compendium of human anatomis variation. Baltimore: Urban & Schwarzenberg; 1988. p. 164.
190. Kanawati A. Variations of the sciatic nerve anatomy and blood supply in the gluteal region: a review of the literature. ANZ J Surg. 2014;84:816–9.
191. Apaydin N, Kendir S, Loukas M, Tubbs R, Bozkurt M. Surgical anatomy of the superior gluteal nerve and landmarks for its localization during minimally invasive approaches to the hip. Clin Anat. 2013;26:614–20.
192. Basarir K, Ozsoy M, Erdemli B, Bayramoglu A, Tuccar E, Dincel V. The safe distance for the superior gluteal nerve in direct lateral approach to the hip and its relation with the femoral length: a cadaver study. Arch Orthop Trauma Surg. 2008;128:645–50.
193. Diop M, Parratte B, Tatu L, Vuillier F, Faure A, Monnier G. Anatomical bases of superior gluteal nerve entrapment syndrome in the suprapiriformis foramen. Surg Radiol Anat. 2002;24:155–9.
194. Ray B, D'Souza A, Saxena A, Nayak D, Sushma R, Shetty P, Pugazhendi B. Morphology of the superior gluteal nerve: a study in adult human cadavers. Bratisl Lek Listy. 2013;114:409–12.
195. Stecco C, Macchi V, Baggio L, Porzionato A, Berizzi A, Aldegheri R, De Caro R. Anatomical and CT angiographic study of superior gluteal neurovascular pedicle: implications for hip surgery. Surg Radiol Anat. 2013;35:107–13.
196. Collinge C, Coons D, Aschenbrenner J. Risks to the superior gluteal neurovascular bundle during percutaneous iliosacral screw insertion: an anatomical cadaver study. J Orthop Trauma. 2005;19:96–101.
197. Ling Z, Kumar V. The course of the inferior gluteal nerve in the posterior approach to the hip. J Bone Joint Surg. 2006;88B:1580–3.
198. Beck M, Leunig M, Ellis T, Sledge JB, Ganz R. The acetabular blood supply: implications for periacetabular osteotomies. Surg Radiol Anat. 2003;25(5–6):361–7.
199. Feugier P, Fessy MH, Bejui J, Bouchet A. Acetabular anatomy and the relationship with pelvic vascular structures. Implications in hip surgery. Surg Radiol Anat. 1997;19(2):85–90.
200. Juliano P, Bosse M, Edwards K. The superior gluteal artery in complex acetabular procedures. J Bone Joint Surg. 1994;76-A(2):244–8.
201. Katthagen BD, Spies H, Bachmann G. Arterial vascularization of the bony acetabulum. Z Orthop Ihre Grenzgeb. 1995;133(1):7–13.
202. Jensen K, Sprengel K, Mica L, Somlyay L, Jentzsch T, Werner C. Surgical relevance of corona mortis and clinical outcome in pelvic trauma. Austin J Anat. 2015;2:1033. ISSN: 2381-8921
203. Henning P, Brenner B, Brunner K, Zimmermann H. Hemodynamic instability following an avulsion of the corona mortis artery secondary to a benign pubic ramus fracture. J Trauma. 2007;62:E14–7.
204. Kong W, Sun C, Tsai I. Delayed presentation of hypovolemic shock after a simple pubic ramus fracture. Am J Emerg Med. 2012;30:1–4.
205. Wong T, Chan W, Wu W. Life threatening stable pubic rami fracture. Injury. 2005;36:300–2.
206. Kachlik T, Pechacek V, Musil V, Baca V. The venous system of the pelvis: new nomenclature. Phlebology. 2010;25:162–73.
207. Pathi S, Castellanos M, Corton M. Variability of the retropubic space anatomy in female cadavers. Am J Obstet Gynecol. 2009;201:e15.
208. Zeit R, Cop C. Anatomy of the sacral venous plexus. AJR Am J Roentgenol. 1983;140:143–4.

Biomechanics of the Pelvis

3

Peter Grechenig, Axel Gänsslen, Stephan Grechenig, and Bernd Füchtmeier

Knowledge of the basic biomechanics of the pelvic ring is essential for diagnosis and treatment of pelvic ring injuries.

The bony pelvis consists of three bones (e.g., both hemipelves and the sacrum) and three joints (e.g., both sacroiliac (SI) joints and the pubic symphysis), forming a ring structure (Fig. 3.1).

As only minor movements are possible in these three joints, the pelvic ring of the adult is a relatively rigid ring structure, making movements only possible within the elastic modulus of the bone. A key role in load transfer is attributed to the posterior part of this ring structure.

Dolati also considered the fifth lumbar spine to be a relevant functional part of the pelvis due to its ligamentous connections to the posterior pelvis [1]. The fifth lumbar vertebra is connected to the posterior pelvis by:

- Anterior: anterior longitudinal ligament.
- Lateral: iliolumbar ligaments.
- Posterior: myofascial parts of the erector trunci muscle.

The anatomy of this ring structure is based on a static and dynamic stability:

- *Static stabilizers* are the bony structures (injuries involving bony structures will lead to static instability).
- *Dynamic stabilizers* include ligaments, muscles, and tendons (injuries to the joints will result in dynamic instability):
  - Ligamentous dynamic stabilizers include the ligaments of the joints and the pelvic floor ligaments (sacrotuberous and sacrospinal ligaments) and the iliolumbar ligaments.
  - Fascial dynamic stabilizers include the obturator segment fascia, pelvic floor fascia, etc.
  - Myofascial stabilizers include the abdominal wall, pelvic compartments, posterior truncal muscles, etc.

From the practical perspective, often, a combination of static and dynamic instability will be present in pelvic ring injuries.

External load on a bone results in internal and external reactions, which lead to some deformation or even a fracture. A load-deformation curve can therefore be calculated [2].

The practical effect of bone loading is an anisotropic effect (change of bone behavior depending on load vector) and a viscoelastic effect (a load-speed and load-duration dependent behavior: a slow load application can result in earlier fracture) [3].

Additionally, bone has an elastic response (accepted deformation up to 3%, with complete recovery of the deformation) and a plastic response (above 3% deformity, a resultant persistent deformity will be observed) [2].

Possible forces acting on the bone can be tensile forces, compressive forces, bending forces, friction forces, and torsion forces. At the pelvis, often, a combination of these forces will lead to a bony or ligamentous injury.

From a morphological point of view, relevant elements only include the bones, ligaments, and musculature, which are responsible purely for passive compression and tensile forces. Additionally, muscle contraction should be considered when analyzing pelvic stability. Overall, very little is known about

P. Grechenig
Division of Macroscopic and Clinical Anatomy, Medical University of Graz, Graz, Austria
e-mail: peter.grechenig@stud.medunigraz.at

A. Gänsslen (✉)
Department of Trauma Surgery, Orthopedics and Hand Surgery, Hospital Wolfsburg, Wolfsburg, Germany

S. Grechenig
Department of Orthopedics and Trauma Surgery, AUVA Trauma Hospital Klagenfurt, Klagenfurt, Austria

Department of Trauma Surgery, University Hospital Regensburg, Regensburg, Germany

B. Füchtmeier
Department of Trauma Surgery, Hospital Barmherzige Brüder, Regensburg, Germany
e-mail: Bernd.Fuechtmeier@barmherzige-regensburg.de

A. Gänsslen et al. (eds.), *Pelvic Ring Fractures*, https://doi.org/10.1007/978-3-030-54730-1_3

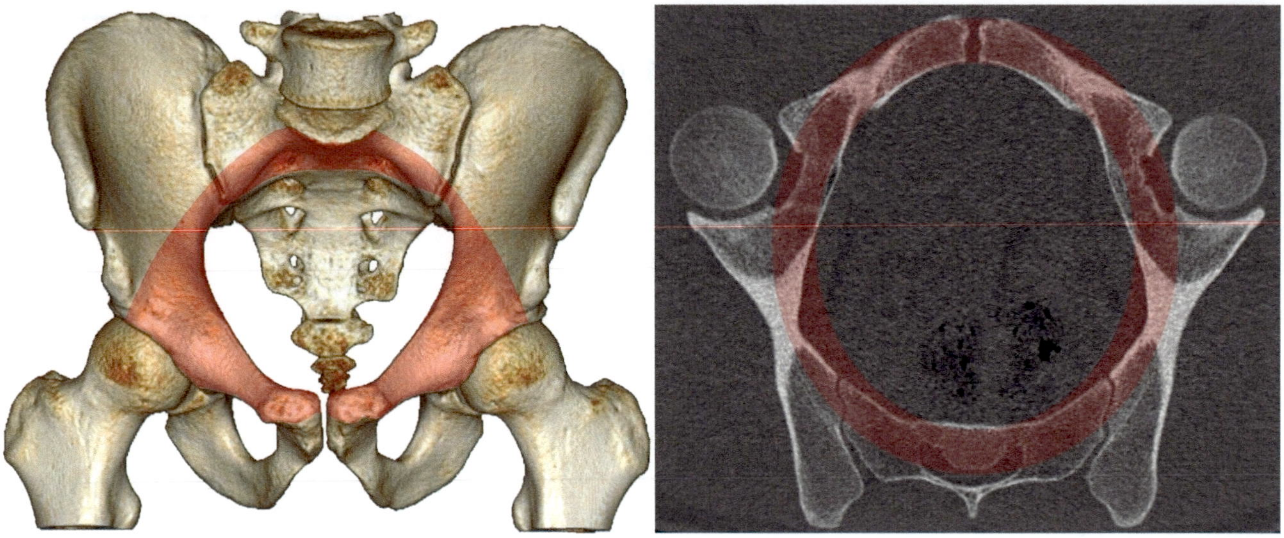

Fig. 3.1 Ring structure of the pelvis

these dynamic responses to pelvic stability. Relevant muscle groups include the erector spinae muscle, the superficial and deep low back muscles, and the iliopsoas muscle.

3.1 Ring Structure of the Pelvis

The pelvis is a true ring structure comparable to an inclined ring, starting with the pubic bones along the pelvic brim (linea terminalis) to the first sacral vertebra (Fig. 3.1). Pelvic parts not integrated into this basic ring structure are the lower part of the sacrum, the coccyx, and the iliac wings.

The present basic understanding on pelvic trauma biomechanics is based on the extended work of Marvin Tile's group.

In his leading paper on pelvic ring fractures, he stated that [4]:

- "The pelvis is a ring structure, and if the ring is broken in one area and the fragments displaced, then there must be a fracture or dislocation in another portion of the ring."
- "The stability of the pelvic ring depends upon the integrity of the posterior weight-bearing sacroiliac complex, with the major sacroiliac, sacrotuberous and sacrospinous ligaments. The extremely strong posterior sacroiliac ligaments maintain the normal position of the sacrum in the pelvic ring and the entire complex has the appearance of a suspension bridge."
- "The sacrospinous ligaments join the lateral edge of the sacrum to the ischial spine and resist external rotation of the hemipelvis, whereas the sacrotuberous ligaments resist both rotational forces and shearing forces in the vertical plane."
- "The major forces acting upon a hemipelvis are external rotation, internal rotation (compression from the lateral side) and vertical shear."

Prior to the computed tomography (CT) era, often, isolated injuries to the anterior pelvic ring (pubic area) were described, but bone scan analyses and autopsy results already described additional posterior ring injuries [5, 6].

This lead to the term "pretzel theory" of pelvic ring injuries [7]:

- Only a fresh pretzel (children) can be cracked at one point.
- "Older" pretzels nearly always crack at two points.

The posterior pelvis is the relevant part of the ring structure for load transfer from the trunk to the extremities [1, 4, 8].

The posterior pelvis was considered the key element to provide structural support with its stabilizing structures, whereas the anterior ring with the pubic symphysis contributes only little to the intrinsic stability of the ring [9]. Tile compared the posterior pelvis, with its ligamentous and bony structures, with a suspension bridge [4, 8, 10, 11]. Under loading, the strong posterior sacroiliac ligaments tension the posterior SI joint complex, suspending the posterior superior iliac spines.

The surrounding muscles and ligaments significantly contribute to the overall stability of the ring structure, as the three bony components of the pelvic ring alone, the sacrum and both innominate bones (hemipelves), have no intrinsic stability.

Thus, the posterior pelvic segment is less anatomical than a functional segment. Complete posterior ring disintegration results in complete posterior, static instability.

3.2 Keystone Theory

The load transfer from the trunk during standing runs along the spinal column to the lower extremities, through the sacrum, the sacroiliac joints, and the posterior acetabular column. Thus, for optimal force transmission, the integrity of the posterior pelvic ring is of major relevance.

The posterior pelvic ring, with both hemipelves, creates a vault with the sacrum integrated as a keystone of a Roman arch [12, 13].

Due to the sacral bony shape and the spatial orientation of the articular surfaces of the SI joints, this concept shows some limitations.

In the pelvic outlet plane, the sacrum has the shape of a true keystone (Fig. 3.2) and is wedged between the two hemipelves. However, in the inlet plane, which is near perpendicular to the pelvic outlet, the sacrum presents with an opposite shape, not able to shrink within the vault (Fig. 3.3). The joint line of both SI joints presents with an open anterior angle of about 15°, representing posterior convergence (Fig. 3.3).

Due to the different sacral planes, the biomechanical consequences depend on the plane of the whole pelvis [8]:

- In the inlet position, the sacrum is orientated as a reverse keystone (instability).
- In the outlet position, the sacrum is orientated as a "true" keystone (stability).

During walking, there is tendency for anterior displacement of the sacrum within both hemipelves due to its posterior narrowing. Accordingly, the sacrum does not work as a self-blocking system. Anterior displacement is protected by the tension effect of posterior iliosacral ligaments (Fig. 3.4).

Tile developed the concept of the posterior ligamentous support comparable to a suspension bridge [8]. The posterior superior iliac spines were considered the pillars of the bridge; the interosseous sacroiliac ligaments, strongest ligaments of the body, act as suspension bars, and the sacrum represents the true bridge (Fig. 3.4). The relevance of the iliolumbar ligaments was stated as a further suspensory mechanism [8].

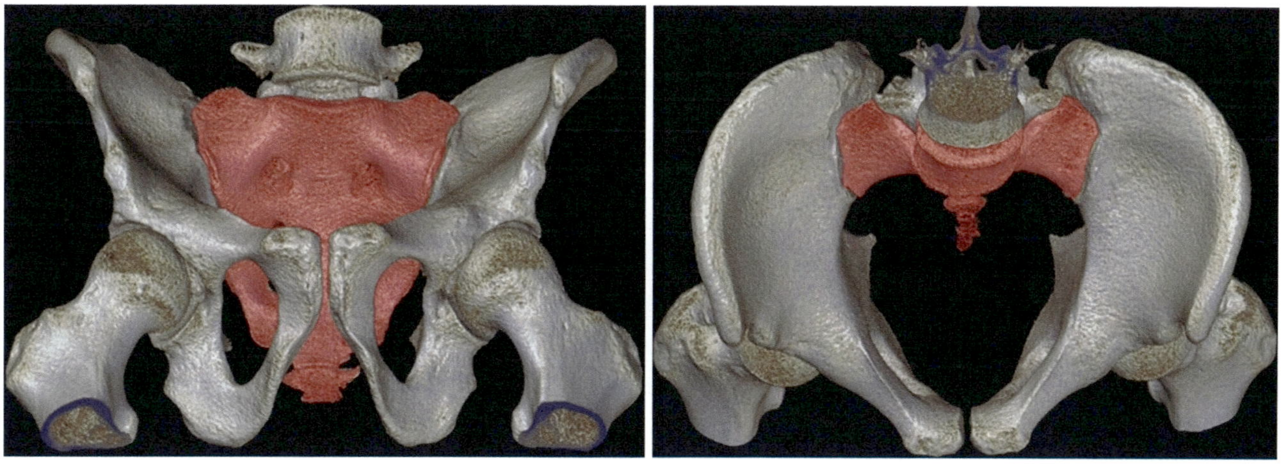

Fig. 3.2 Keystone theory of the sacrum within the posterior pelvis

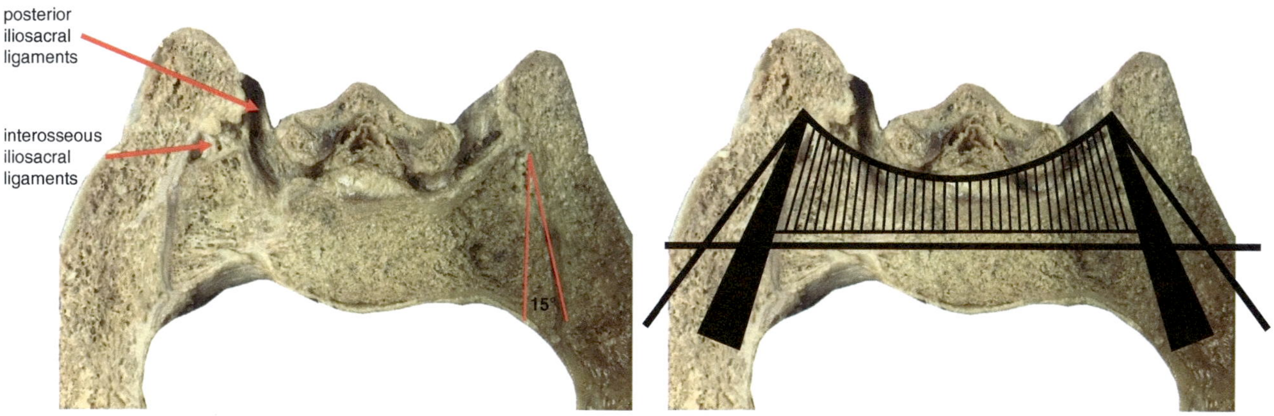

Fig. 3.3 Suspension bridge concept of the posterior pelvic ring with the posterior sacroiliac ligaments acting as dynamic stabilizers presented on an anatomic specimen

They stabilize the connection of the whole spine into the pelvic ring by tensioning during anterior flexion of the spine.

In contrast, the anterior pelvic ring with the pubic symphysis and the pubic arch acts as a pull bar (strut) to prevent lateral spreading (Fig. 3.5) [8].

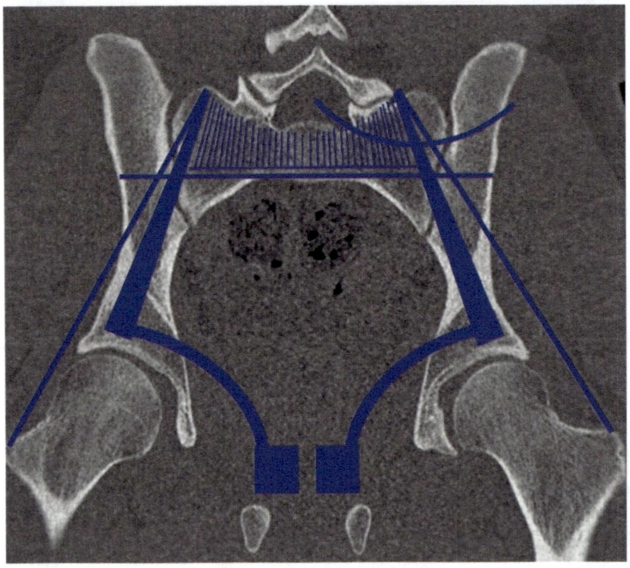

Fig. 3.4 Suspension bridge concept drawn into a CT-plane of the pelvis

Strong ligamentous structures are necessary to stabilize the sacrum within the ring structure of the pelvis. The most relevant ligaments are the posterior sacral ligaments [14].

Overall, the sacral orientation has a deficit in the upright stand, whereas for quadripedals, the sacrum really acts as a keystone.

3.3 Biomechanics of the Bones

Mechanical forces acting on the pelvic bone are primarily transferred on cortical structures. The cancellous bone distributes the resulting shear and pressure forces to reduce the force maxima. According to Wolff's law, the resulting trabecular orientation corresponds to the natural strains within the hemipelvis [15, 16].

Euler performed an analysis using polarized light (PhotoStress method) to detect surface tension behavior of the hemipelvis under load [17]. A tension center was identified on the inner pelvic surface close to the SI joint around the pelvic brim (corresponding to the iliac cortical density). This area corresponds to bone mineral density distribution using CT densitometry [18].

Poigenfürst et al. proposed that a slowly directed static load can lead to a deformation of the entire pelvic ring (hemipelvis) with resulting bending forces at the points of greatest deformation, whereas dynamic loading (acute impact against

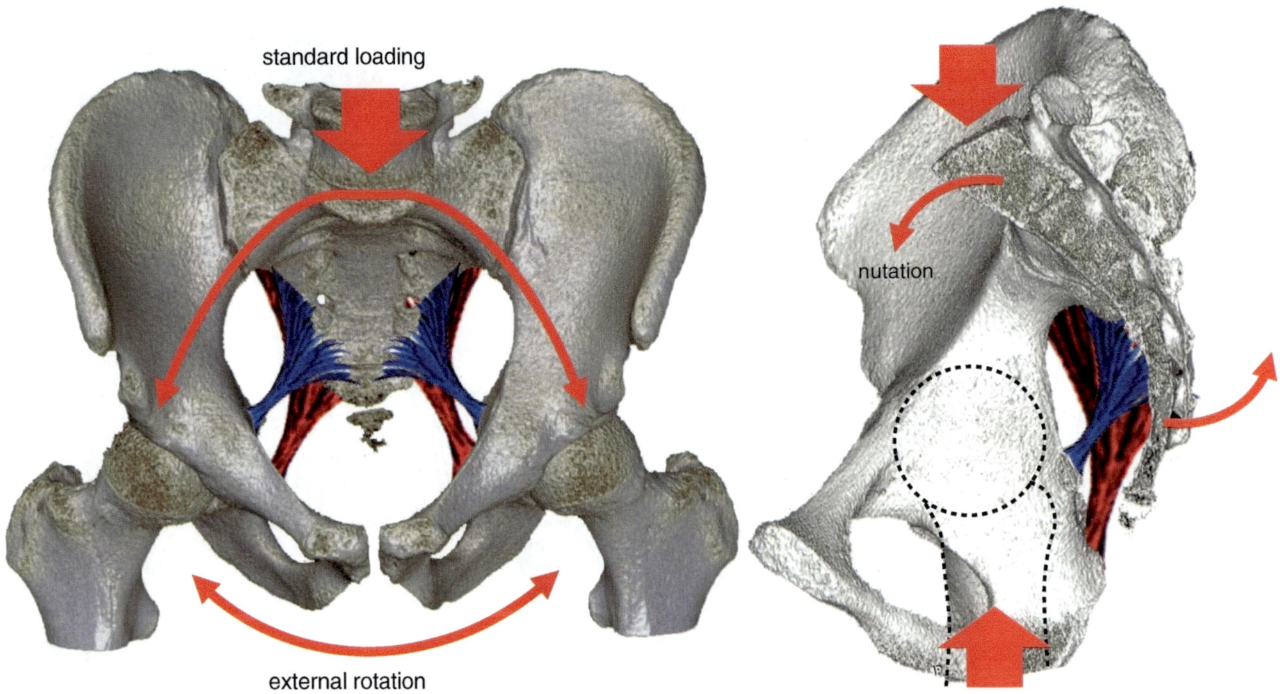

Fig. 3.5 Anterior ring pull bar concept acting against external rotation during axial loading (left). Nutation of the sacrum under axial loading (right)

the pelvis) only leads to a deformation at the direct force application area [19]. The ongoing impulse results in shear stresses at distant pelvic areas. Thus, considerable forces can be absorbed without harming the bone/joints. It was stated that the first fracture usually occurs at the anterior ring, while with ongoing force transmission, due to hemipelvic rotation around an axis near the SI joint, posterior injuries and secondary further anterior injuries can be expected [19].

Due to the bipedal weight bearing in humans with vertical sacral loading, the fusion of the sacral segments can be explained [20].

According to the pelvic ring structure, the lower sacral segments are not contributing to load bearing [21–24].

Linstrom et al. performed a finite element (FE) analysis to detect typical load pattern of the pelvis [25].

During standing, the maximum stress was observed at the lateral S1 body. Walking led to a bilateral vertical stress distribution along the sacral ala and along the iliac cortical density to the posterior acetabular column. A peak load transfer was observed during single-leg stance at the ipsilateral medial sacral shoulder.

Pal et al. stated that the lumbosacral facet joints contribute to the overall load transmission to the pelvis by 21%, while load transfer via the sacrum occurs with 67% [22]. Alterations of lumbosacral biomechanics after fractures can therefore be associated with lumbar instability and low back pain like in degenerative pathologies [26].

The deformation of the uninjured pelvis is elastic under axial force, e.g., reducing the applied load results in near anatomical re-orientation of the whole pelvis. Thus, no physiological load limits are exceeded [27].

In the uninjured pelvis, mobility is only possible at the SI joints and the symphysis pubis. Thus, knowledge of their behavior during physiological loading is the basis of understanding injury mechanics.

3.4 Biomechanics of the Pubic Symphysis

Historical anatomic and biomechanic analyses proved that in addition to the assumed tensile loads, compressive and shear forces are present at the pubic symphysis [28–32].

> Biomechanical forces acting on the pubic symphysis mainly include tension, shearing, and compression forces.

Recent biomechanical analyses resulted in a better understanding of these forces.

Walheim analyzed volunteers in the supine and standing position and reported on average translational movements of 1 mm and rotations in the frontal and sagittal planes <1.5°. Vertical movements showed a maximum of 2 mm [33]. The symphyseal mobility was largest in the cranio-caudal direction within the symphyseal plane. No effective mobility in the horizontal direction was observed.

In a further roentgen stereophotogrammetric analysis of two volunteers, maximum translations at the pubic symphysis of 2 mm and rotations of 3° were observed [34].

3.4.1 Single-Leg Stance

- Ulmer et al. observed that in the majority of pelves, compressive forces act on the pubic symphysis which were caused by an approximation of the pubic rami to a maximum of 1.4 mm; also, an internal rotation of the hemipelvis of maximum 1.7° was observed; in the sagittal plane, an anterior rotation of 0.8° occurred, resulting in shear forces on the symphysis [27].
- Walheim analyzed the effect of the one-leg stance and reported a mobility of up to 2.6 mm in the vertical direction and 1.3 mm in the sagittal direction; comparable mobility was reported during walking with 2.2 mm and 1.3 mm, respectively [33].
- Meissner et al. examined ten fresh cadaver anterior pelvic ring parts and reported on mean forces of 169 N (maximum 398 N) in the vertical plane and 148 N in the sagittal direction [35] to induce mobility; during walking, vertical tension was possible at 120 N (maximum 333 N) and sagittal tensioning at 68 N (maximum 136 N).
- In a cadaver simulating one-leg-standing, narrowing of the symphysis was observed indicating compressive forces combined with caudal rotation on the contralateral side [36].

3.4.2 Double-Leg Stance

- Under loading, the symphysis was subjected to pressure due to approximation of the pubic rami in the horizontal plane with additional slight internal rotation of both hemipelves [27].
- Meissner et al. reported on distraction and shearing forces at the pubic symphysis in the double-leg stance, while compressive forces were not observed [37].
- Double-leg-standing cadaveric simulation showed an equal and uniform widening of the symphyseal space, indicating tensile forces acting at the joint [36].

3.4.3 Sitting

- Ulmer et al. reported a tensile force at the symphysis resulting predominantly in a divergence of the pubic rami up to 0.5 mm and an external rotation of the hemipelves of approximately 0.5° [27].

> Under physiological loading, anterior and internal rotation forces <2° act at the pubic symphysis. Depending on the type of loading (single, double-leg stance, sitting), tensile (double-leg stance), compression (single-leg stance), and shearing forces (double-leg stance, sitting) act on the pubic symphysis.

3.5 Biomechanics of the SI Joint

The exact physiological mechanics of the SI joint is not fully understood. Hippocrates and Vesalius believed that the SI joint is completely immobile and only during pregnancy a mobility is present [38]. Paré confirmed some mobility even in males [38].

Historically, a complex, multidimensional movement under physiological loads was supposed, based on experimental studies and theoretical considerations not sufficiently described with a single horizontal axis [12, 39–48].

An estimated rotational axis was considered posterior to the SI joint at the transition between the first and second sacral vertebrae, which changes its location during movements [48, 49].

As a result of bipedal movements, the sagittal sacral orientation allows optimal nutation and counter-nutation movements [21, 50–52].

Under loading, the sacrum performs a combined anterior rotation and "inferior" translational movement ("nutation") of variable extent [49], depending on several factors including amount of applied load, gender, age, and the individual anatomical shape of the SI joint [53].

Walker in 1992 summarized the existing literature (different clinical and experimental setups) regarding movements of the SI joint and reported on the following physiological movements [54]:

- 1–12° rotation
- 0.5–7.25 mm translation

It is well known that the SI joint mobility is increased in females and during pregnancy, whereas mobility decreases with older age [55].

Several investigations focused on the amount of rotation and translation. Different results were obtained, depending on the chosen biomechanical setup.

Coalchis et al. were one of the first to perform clinical investigations of SI joint movements in volunteers. K-wires were used to detect mobility, and interindividual differences of very slight movements were reported [38].

In an analysis of isolated SI joints, tensile forces resulting in horizontal displacements of up to 2.7 mm were reversible, indicating elastic deformities of the SI joint without ligament disruption [56, 57]. Ligamentous injury was seen at mean translational movements of 5.1 mm and rotations of up to 11°.

Stability testing of the isolated SI joint was performed by Rothkötter et al. using a hemipelvic model with the attached sacrum. Transverse traction resulted in SI joint disruption at an average of 3368 N (5.5 mm displacement); dorso-cranial joint failure occurred at 5150 N (6.6 mm displacement) and anterior-cranial failure at 4933 N [58]. Frictional stability was higher in the posterior-cranial direction than in the anterior-cranial direction.

Several investigations distinguished between single- and double-leg standing and even sitting position to analyze the resulting forces acting on the SI joint.

3.5.1 Single-Leg-Stance

- In a single-leg stance model with abductor muscle simulation, a nutation movement of 1.3° and a maximum translation of 1.6 mm were recorded [59].
- Ulmer et al. reported a posterior widening of the SI joint on the standing leg resulting in anterior SI joint compression and therefore wedging of the sacrum between both hemipelves; a nutation movement of 1–2 ° was observed [27].
- In a simulated static load analysis of SI joint cadavers in eight adult specimens with translational and rotational loading along the central S1 endplate [60], mean sacral displacements were highest in anterior direction with a mean of 2.74 mm; the main rotations occurred as joint torsion with 6.21°, whereas flexion of 2.68° and extension (contranutation) of 3.52° were observed; the SI joint resisted loads between 500 N and 1440 N, and 42 N to 160 Nm without joint failure, respectively.

3.5.2 Double-Leg Stance

- Under loading, a relative cranialization of the hemipelvis due to caudalization of the sacrum was observed, combined with posterior SI joint widening, which was restricted by the posterior SI joint ligaments; a nutation movement of maximum 1.5° with resulting hyperlordosis of the lumbar spine and an anterior translation of 1–2 mm were detected [27].
- In a simulated static load analysis of SI joint cadavers in eight adult specimens with translational and rotational loading along the central S1 endplate [60], mean sacral displacements in bilateral fixed iliac conditions were minor than for the simulated single-leg stance with

translational movements of maximum 0.53 mm and rotations of maximum 2°.

- Wilke et al. performed clinical measurements using a posterior external fixator in healthy patients in the prone position; rotational movements <2° and maximal translational movements of 1 mm were observed [61].
- In four fresh female cadaver specimens, eccentric compressive forces (60% body weight) were applied to the sacrum, and relative SI joint movements were recorded; a maximum rotation of 1.2° (superior external rotation + nutation) and 0.9 mm translation were measured; a 10% increase of rotation was observed after cutting the anterior or posterior ligaments and a 30% increase when all ligaments were dissected [62].

3.5.3 Sitting

- Ulmer et al. found comparable movements in the SI joint as for double-leg stance while simulating sitting conditions with slight nutation and anterior translation [27].

3.6 Biomechanics of the Ligaments

Relevant ligaments include the pelvic floor ligaments as well as the inguinal ligament, which have a preloading effect to gain further stability [19].

Tile stated that the integrity of the pelvic floor ligaments is of major relevance [8]. The sacrospinous ligament has a horizontal orientation, whereas the sacrotuberous ligament is vertically orientated. Both are in a perpendicular orientation to each other. Thus, the sacrotuberous ligament resists vertical displacement, whereas the sacrospinous ligament resists external rotation.

For men, the sacrotuberous and the sacrospinous ligaments have a mean length of 64 and 38 mm, respectively. For women, lengths of 70 and 46 mm were measured for the sacrotuberous and sacrospinous ligaments [63].

Vrahas et al. performed a biomechanical study on ligamentous contributions to pelvic stability. Thirteen fresh frozen cadaver pelves were axially loaded. Stability significantly dropped after cutting the pubic symphysis under constant loading (21% decreased stability), resulting in only 1 mm maximum displacement at the symphysis under an axial load of 600 N. Isolated anterior SI joint ligament cutting led to a 91% stability compared to the intact pelvis, whereas isolated cutting of the posterior SI joint ligaments led to a 15% reduction of intact pelvic stability. If the pubic symphysis was dissected, the pelvic floor ligaments (sacrotuberous and sacrospinous ligaments) contributed little to overall pelvic stability [64].

An experimental biomechanical study stated that the pelvic floor ligaments did not add any stability to the SI joint mechanics [65], which could be confirmed by Vrahas et al. [64]. After dissecting the pubic symphysis, the pelvic floor ligaments (sacrotuberous and sacrospinous ligaments) contributed little to overall pelvic stability.

Varga et al. used the biomechanical setup of Marvin Tile, simulating a bilateral stance model, and analyzed the isolated effect of the pelvic floor ligaments on pelvic stability [66]. Dissection of one ligament (either sacrotuberous or sacrospinous ligament) resulted in a mean axial stiffness reduction of 4.8%, whereas dissection of both ligaments resulted in a 5.2% stiffness reduction. Resulting displacements were minor with a maximum of <4 μm.

In a recently developed FE model of the pelvis, several investigations were performed on pelvic stability [49].

To analyze the effect of posterior pelvic ring ligaments on pelvic stability, a vertical load of 600 N was simulated in standing and sitting positions. Either tensile and compressive forces were observed at the SI joint and the pubic symphysis. The posterior pelvic ring cartilage and the posterior ligaments significantly contributed to pelvic stability [49].

In contrast, pelvic floor ligaments contributed significantly to ligamentous stability of the pelvis [49].

> Under physiological loading, a slight anterior rotation of the sacrum of approximately 2° relative to the hemipelvis has to be expected (nutation movement) in combination with slight translational movements below 2 mm. Thus, an isolated axis of movement is not present.
>
> Depending on the type of loading (single, double-leg stance, sitting), varying forces are acting on the SI joint. Anterior compression and posterior distraction are the typical deformity types.
>
> The stabilizing effect of the sacrotuberous or sacrospinous ligaments is presently not fully understood.

3.7 Ligamentous Contributions to Pelvic Stability

Several ligaments are supposed to act on pelvic stability, e.g., symphyseal ligaments, pelvic floor ligaments, iliosacral ligaments, and iliolumbar ligaments.

Several authors investigated the effect on pelvic instability after sequential dissection of the symphyseal, the pelvic floor, and iliosacral ligaments to produce an anterior external rotation deformity of the pelvis. This led to an understanding of ligamentous contribution of pelvic stability.

Fundamental studies were performed by Marvin Tile's group using a step-by-step instability model [8, 10, 11, 67]:

- Isolated transection of the pubic symphysis led to a maximum diastasis of 2.5 cm; the remaining structures compensated rotational and translational movements.
- Additional transection of the pelvic floor ligaments (sacrospinous and sacrotuberous ligaments) markedly increased "instability"; only the anterior SI joint ligaments provided some remaining resistance against rotational (horizontally directed) forces.
- Transection of the anterior SI joint ligaments resulted in complete rotation of the hemipelvis around a "hinge" through the posterior sacroiliac ligaments; translational movements were prevented by the remaining iliosacral and iliolumbar ligamentous structures.
- Complete transection of the sacroiliac joint ligament complex made translational movements possible.

The amount of external rotational forces acting on the pelvis therefore results in the corresponding pelvic instability.

In the ligamentous dissection analysis by Krueger et al. [68], the main results showed that:

- Isolated dissection of the symphysis led to hemipelvic external rotation and opening of the pubic symphysis up to 2.5 cm without vertical displacement.
- Additional dissection of the sacroiliac ligaments results in a strong cranial shift of the hemipelvis.
- Further transection of pelvic floor ligaments results in extended external rotation without relevant increase of vertical displacement.

A comparable analysis was performed by Dolati et al. with progressive external rotation movements resulting in up to 18 cm symphyseal diastasis. Four degrees of instability were observed [69]:

- Symphyseal widening of 3–4 cm did not result in injury to the SI joint ligaments.
- Symphyseal widening of 5 cm resulted in anterior SI joint ligament injury.
- Symphyseal widening of 8 cm resulted in anterior and interosseous SI joint ligament injury with a possible rotational instability around a transverse axis; all pelves showed elastic deformity, leading to some reduction after reduction of the forces.
- Symphyseal widening of >13 cm resulted in anterior and interosseous SI joint ligament injury.

Simonian et al. performed ligamentous transections on seven fresh-frozen non-embalmed cadavers [70]. In a double-leg stance model, vertical loading was performed on intact pelves, and thereafter, sequential dissection of the pubic symphysis, the anterior and intraosseous sacroiliac ligaments, and the sacrospinous/sacrotuberous ligaments was performed.

The following displacements were observed:

- Dissection of the symphyseal ligaments: 1.2 mm symphyseal gap, no SI joint displacement, no change of SI joint angulation (0.43°).
- Additional anterior and intraosseous sacroiliac ligament dissection: 1.1 mm symphyseal gap, 0.4 mm SI joint displacement, 0.8° SI joint angulation.
- Additional sacrospinous/sacrotuberous ligament dissection: 1.5 mm symphyseal gap, 0.3 mm SI joint displacement, 1.05° SI joint angulation.

Simonian et al. reported results on fresh-frozen non-embalmed cadaver vertical loading in a biomechanical double-leg stance model [70].

The maximum symphyseal diastasis under 400 N loading was 0.03 mm, displacement of the SI joint was 0.04 mm, and the SI joint flexion angle was 0.43°. Lateral bending resulted in comparable motions with 0.05 mm symphyseal displacement, 0.06 mm SI joint displacement, and 0.43° SI joint rotation.

Abdelfattah et al. performed fluoroscopy-based instability testing by manual external rotational force application on six cadaver pelves [71]:

- Dissection of the symphyseal ligaments resulted in a mean horizontal displacement of 11.8 mm and a mean vertical displacement of 6.3 mm.
- Dissection of the pelvic floor ligaments showed no relevant displacement change (12.1 mm horizontal, 7.4 mm vertical displacement).
- Further dissection of the SI joint ligaments resulted in a significantly mean horizontal and vertical increase of displacement to 38.4 mm and 20 mm, respectively.
- Primary dissection off the SI joint ligaments led to 42.1 mm horizontal and 18.4 mm vertical displacement.
- Secondary pelvic floor ligament dissection resulted in no further instability.

Abdelfattah et al. concluded that the sacrospinous and sacrotuberous ligaments had only minor influence on anterior-posterior stability [71].

Böhme et al. simulated an anterior-posterior compression injury type II according to Young-Burgess loaded in a double-leg stance using an FE model [72].

The intact pelvis revealed that >95% of the total load was distributed through the posterior pelvic ring ligaments with relevant strain to the pelvic floor, iliolumbar, and sacroiliac ligaments, whereas the anterior pelvic ligaments (e.g., inguinal ligament, obturator membrane) together with the interosseous and posterior sacroiliac ligaments accounted for <5% of the total load. The pubic symphysis ligaments showed no relevant loading [72].

After symphyseal transection simulation, 831 N force was necessary to create a symphyseal widening of 10 cm. Unphysiological ligament loading was observed with 80% of the total load transferred to the anterior iliosacral ligaments and 17% to the sacrotuberous ligaments. Peak loads were found in the anterior-cranial part of the anterior iliosacral ligament. The ligament load was ten times higher than in the intact situation. Simulation additionally revealed that the pelvic floor ligaments and the interosseous iliosacral ligaments remained intact in this APC II injury. Overall, an APC II injury shows horizontal instability, but no vertical instability, as a type B injury according to Tile.

The posterior pelvic ligaments mainly stabilize the pelvis against horizontal forces [14].

Pelvic floor ligaments compensate vertical displacement forces and the nutation movement of the sacrum. Thus, elastic cushioning of the trunk is reduced [14].

The interosseous iliosacral ligaments are anatomically the most strong parts within the SI joint ligament complex, which is supported by FE analyses as highest ligamentous strains occur during classical nutation movements [73].

3.8 The Iliolumbar Ligament

The iliolumbar ligament (ILL) is one of the three vertebro-pelvic ligaments and therefore takes part in stabilizing the lumbosacral spinal region [74–76].

The iliolumbar ligament is a large fan-shaped ligament, which most often arises from the fourth and/or fifth lumbar transverse process to insert at the posterior iliac crest and the SIJ capsule on top of the sacrum [75, 77]. Part of this ligament was named the lumbosacral ligament [55, 78, 79], which arises from the fifth lumbar transverse process to insert on the sacral ala. A wide variety of its anatomy is reported in the literature [55].

As the lumbosacral ligament is much stronger, it was expected that more load is transferred by this ligamentous part. This could be proven, as the most trabecular structures were observed at the inferior part of the L5 transverse process [80].

Several subligamentous structures are described, especially an anterior part inserting at the anterior part of the posterior iliac crest and a corresponding posterior part inserting posterior at the iliac crest sacrum [75, 77]. In contrast, Basadonna et al. reported a crossing of the anterior and posterior bands [81].

The ligament has a length of approximately 32 mm in Caucasian, whereas in African Americans, the length is nearly doubled with approximately 61 mm [82].

Due to its anatomical course, the ILL stabilizes the fourth and fifth lumbar vertebrae to the pelvis and can resist movement of lateral side bending of the pelvis up to 29% [83–85].

Transectional analyses revealed that the ILL contributes to lumbosacral stability by restriction of lateral bending, some flexion and extension, and rotational movement of the lumbosacral junction [78, 85].

- Yamamoto et al. performed a biomechanical analysis and stated that bilateral dissection of the ligaments resulted in an increase of rotation around a vertical body axis of 18% (0.3°), pelvic extension of 20% (1.1°), flexion of 23% (1.7°), and lateral bending of 29% (1.2°) [85]; isolated dissection had no relevant influence on instability.
- Pool-Goudzward et al. analyzed the effect of dissecting several parts of the ILL in 12 human cadavers. The anterior bands were found to be the main stabilizers of the lumbosacral region, whereas the posterior and sacroiliac parts had no influence on instability [78].

3.9 Biomechanics of Myofascial Structures

The peripelvic muscles are supposed to stiffen the pelvic joints.

In a clinical analysis in 13 healthy volunteers, the transverse abdominis muscle contraction led to a better stability of the SI joints than activation of lateral abdominal wall muscles [86].

In contrast, an experimental setup using 15 embalmed specimens detected no change of the stiffness of the pubic symphysis and the hemipelvis under transverse abdominis muscle activation [87]. This was consistent with recent findings, where, despite some flexibility of the SI joint (bigger during anterior vs. posterior rotation of the hemipelvis), activation of the transverse abdominis muscle had no influence on pelvic stiffness [88].

Tensioning the pelvic floor muscles resulted in an 8.5% stiffening of the SI joints in females, whereas in males, no change could be detected. It was assumed that the more mobile SI joints in females were responsible for these results [89].

3.10 Pathomechanics of the Pelvic Ring

A variety of different injury mechanisms can exceed the elastic structure of the pelvic ring. Uniform injury patterns were identified, depending on the extent and direction of the resulting force vectors and the individual "biological situation" of the patient.

Typical force vectors resulting in pelvic ring injuries are typically indirect force transmissions via the femur and the hip from anterior, direct lateral impacts and in more rare situations extreme hyperflexion of the lumbar spine.

The individual extent of the energy leading to a disruption of the ring structure is still unknown, as investigations reported a high variance of the measured values.

The present understanding of pelvic injury mechanism is based on early clinical, experimental, and cadaver dissection (autopsy) analyses and later on more detailed analyses of theoretical and clinical accident data analyses and finite element (FE) analyses.

3.10.1 Early Clinical Results

Historically, several attempts tried to identify injury mechanism resulting in pelvic ring disruptions on a clinical basis:

- Already in 1847, Malgaigne analyzed ten patients after severe trauma and reported on the two main clinical injury mechanisms [90, 91]: anterior-posterior force transmissions lead to anterior and posterior pelvic fractures, and sagittal forces lead to pubic fractures and pelvic joint dislocations.
- Fisher in 1909 reported on a sledge injury, where six people, sitting in a row, suffered a high velocity injury when struck against a tree; three of these patients immediately died at the scene; this anterior-posterior injury mechanism resulted predominantly in SI joint dislocations [92].
- Haumann analyzed 18 patients sustaining pelvic injuries in the early mining industry; detailed descriptions of the injury mechanism identified anterior-posterior compression mechanisms and shear mechanisms as the main causes of injury, whereas lateral compression injuries were uncommon [93].
- Hirsch in 1924 analyzed mining industry injuries in 102 patients and stated that the direction and magnitude of the suspected forces determined the injury characteristics; direct, local forces led to iliac wing fractures; anterior-posterior compression forces led to fractures at the anterior pelvic ring, occasionally with incomplete SI joint involvement; and forces in the sagittal or frontal direction led to anterior ring disruptions combined with sacral and posterior iliac fractures [94].
- Watson-Jones analyzed 18 unstable pelvic fractures and identified two main injury mechanisms: lateral compression forces resulted in anterior pelvic ring disruptions, whereas anterior-posterior compression forces led to combined anterior and posterior ring disruptions [95].

> Already one century ago, the typical injury mechanisms resulting in pelvic ring injuries were anterior-posterior or lateral compression mechanisms.

3.10.2 Experimental Results

Even during these early decades, experimental analyses were performed:

- Messerer carried out experimental studies on pelvic injury mechanics in 1880 and confirmed the clinical injury mechanisms described by Malgaigne [96].
- Kusmin in 1882 performed static and impact loadings on complete cadaver bodies and pelvic specimens in various positions; specific injury combinations were defined after anterior-posterior and lateral force transmissions [97]; Katzenelson clinically confirmed the latter experimental results [98].

> Experimental results from the late nineteenth century confirmed the clinical proven injury mechanisms.

Newer experimental analyses focused on forces resulting in specific injury locations.

- Berner examined isolated posterior pelvic ring specimens and reported on SI joint disruptions at loads of 4933 ± 1038 N and fractures at loads of 3313 ± 469 N after translational forces; torque forces of 120 Nm resulted in ligamentous disruption, while sacral fractures were produced with maximum torque forces of 149 Nm [56, 57].
- Stuhler performed anterior-posterior loadings on pediatric pelvic specimens [99]:
  - In young pelves (age 1 year), only plastic deformation without fractures was observed, despite forces of up to 10,000 N.
  - In pelves 12 years of age, the first structure involved was the acetabulum (triradiate cartilage) at 2300 N, followed by disruption of the SI joint at 8000 N and the pubic symphysis at 10,000 N; no bone fracture occurred in this age group.
  - In the age of 14 years after acetabular injury and/or SI joint injury at 2000–3000 N, pubic fractures were

observed at 4000 N and disruption of the pubic symphysis at 6000 N.

3.10.3 Autopsy Results

Further information on potential injury mechanisms was obtained from autopsy studies of accident victims.

- Voigt described 27 different fracture patterns resulting from different "axes of rotation" [100].
- Buchholz analyzed 47 trauma victims and reported on three major injury types [5]:
  1. Isolated anterior pelvic ring injury, intact posterior pelvic ring.
  2. Additional injury to the sacroiliac and sacrotuberous ligaments without posterior instability.
  3. Complete disruption of the posterior sacroiliac ligaments.

3.11 Accident Simulations

Investigations with whole human cadaver bodies, simulating typical injury situations, showed large interindividual differences of forces required for fracture development.

In general, frontal and side impact can be distinguished.

3.11.1 Experimental Lateral Impact Studies

Data from the 1980s, where cars had insufficient side protections, revealed that lateral compression car-to-car impacts could result in pelvic fractures/injuries after forces of 4000 N in women and 10,000 N in men in the middle age range, while with older ages, lower forces resulted in pelvic injuries [101]. Fleischer et al. reported on quantitative data resulting in pelvic fractures. Lateral compression forces of 7.8–14.9 kN or force peaks of 6.5–11 kN over a period of 3 ms were necessary to result in pelvic fractures [101].

Several investigations used models with different parameters, e.g., impactors, accelerations, speeds, etc.

Fayon et al. performed lateral-side directed free-fall experiments involving 18 human cadaver subjects from a drop height between 0.5 and 3 m. Pelvic injuries were rare. Only after 3 m simulations in three of six cadavers, pelvic fractures occurred. Injuries to the anterior rami were observed (AIS 2–3). The fracture threshold was above accelerations of 50 g over 3 ms [102]. Comparable results were presented by Tarriere et al., with a higher reported tolerance level for pelvic fractures (80–90 g during 3 ms) [103].

Cesari et al. performed a pendulum impaction aimed to the greater trochanter and most commonly observed multiple fractures of the pubic rami. Male pelves fractured between 4.9 and 11.9 kN, female pelves between 4.4 and 8.2 kN with an average force for an AIS 2 or 3 pelvic injuries of 8.6 kN and 5.6 kN, respectively. The proposed tolerance force was calculated to be 10 kN for a 75-kg person [104].

Nusholtz et al. performed pendulum tests simulating a lateral impact on the greater trochanter of pelvic specimens. Fractures occurred only after loadings of 45 kN, whereas loads below 26 kN resulted in no pelvic bony injury [105]. Peak accelerations ranged from 38 to 135 g with a resulting peak force between 3.2 and 14 kN. Six of twelve cadavers sustained pelvic fractures, four of which were to the pubic rami. No correlation between fracture and acceleration or force levels was detected.

Viano experimentally reported on tolerance values of 27% maximum pelvic compression resulting in a 25% probability of pelvic fractures [106], and Cavanaugh et al. revealed a fracture tolerance value of 32.6% [107].

Zhu et al. proposed a 25% probability of pelvic injuries of >AIS 2 with a force injury criterion of 5.0 kN [108].

Molz et al. suggested that a 4.5 m/s lateral impact speed with a 25.2-kg impactor was just below the fracture tolerance of human pelvis [109]. In the analysis by Guillemot et al., a controlled falling mass of 3.68 kg at a speed of 4 m/s resulted in 83% fracture incidence in 12 cadaver pelves, presenting with a wide variety of fracture types. A relatively low energy threshold of 30 J was calculated [110].

Bouquet et al. found a 50% probability of AIS 2+ injuries to the pelvis after an applied force of 7.6 kN [111], whereas Matsui et al. reported a 50% pelvic fracture risk at 9.6 kN [112].

Beason et al. found commonly (medially displaced) pubic rami fractures, followed by lateral sacral fractures and iliac wing and lower pubic ramus fractures as a result of lateral impact loading [113]. Pubic rami fractures occurred at peak loads of approximately 3500 N. Additionally, a correlation between total hip bone mineral density (DEXA measurement) and fracture loads/maximum pelvic compression was detected.

Comparing mean fracture loads, different results with different experimental setups were presented in the literature. Overall, in unpadded lateral compression loading, the mean fracture loads ranged between 3.86 and 11.7 kN, whereas padded loading showed mean fracture loads ranged between 2.29 and 13 kN (literature in [113]).

In a porcine cadaver model, anterior-posterior loading resulted in type C injuries with classical unilateral or Malgaigne-fracture-type injuries after a minimal loading of 4030 N [114].

Salzar et al. distinguished the location of the lateral impact. A more posterior impact at the ilium led the symphysis to fracture at 420 N and the sacrum at 3110 N, whereas for a direct acetabular impact, the fracture load was 1910 N at the pubic symphysis and 1020 N at the sacrum [115].

A low bone mineral density and a low trabecular bone density were associated with the risk of sustaining pelvic fractures in lateral impacts [116].

In free-fall (drop) tests, the pelvic fracture tolerance ranged from 80 to 90 g [102, 103].

Yoganandan (2001) observed a pelvic tolerance decrease to 6.8 kN with a flexion-adduction position of the hip-femur-knee complex, while in a straight leg position, femoral fractures resulted after 10 kN [117].

3.11.2 Experimental Frontal Impact Studies

Fleischer et al. reported on quantitative data resulting in pelvic fractures. Anterior-posterior quasi-static loads of 4.7–10 kN resulted in pelvic ring fractures [101].

Patrick et al. performed frontal impacts on ten unrestrained, embalmed cadavers of advanced age, reporting a fracture tolerance below 6.2–11.8 kN. Due to the high age of the cadavers, the fracture loads were considered conservative [118].

Melvin analyzed only six unembalmed cadavers after knee loading and measured pelvic accelerations. Combined knee loads of 8.9–25.6 kN were responsible for pelvic fractures [119]. In a following analysis of 37 pelves, no pelvic fractures were detected after forces of up to 37 kN [120].

In a whole-body analysis of Brun-Cassan et al., only one of ten cadavers showed a pelvic fracture after a load of 8.8 kN [121].

Patrick et al. in a seat-belted dummy analysis of 128 frontal collisions observed no pelvic fractures [122].

King et al. stated from these analyses that a 10 kN frontal femoral load seems to adequately protect the pelvis [123].

3.12 Computed Accident Analysis

Analyses of "real" accidents, combined with medical findings, provide additional information about pelvic bone "limits."

- McCoy et al. investigated 40 resulting pelvic fractures [124]; frontal car collisions resulted in shearing injuries of the pelvic ring and acetabular fractures (with posterior dislocation), while side impacts resulted in classical "lateral compression injuries"; a relative speed of >35 miles/h (56 km/h) resulted in a 40% chance of suffering a pelvic fracture or hip dislocation as an unrestrained front passenger.
- Siegel et al. prospectively analyzed 121 patients with multiple injuries after head-on collisions and side impacts [125]; a significantly higher risk of pelvic fractures after side impact was calculated (56%; most commonly pubic fractures, sacrum fractures, and acetabular fractures); a frontal impact most likely resulted in acetabular fractures; no clear correlation between injury mechanism and type of pelvic fractures could be observed; lateral crashes resulted in 53% pelvic fractures compared to 23% after frontal crashes.
- In a combined technical and medical analysis in restrained vehicle occupants, pelvic ring injuries mostly occurred after a delta-v of >30 km/h, whereas in unrestrained occupants, pedestrians, and cyclists, lower delta-v or collision speeds resulted in pelvic fractures; higher vehicle velocities resulted in higher percentages of type B and C injuries [126, 127]; approximately 75.5% of pelvic fractures occurred at a relative speed between 20 and 59 km/h, while for type C injuries, the speed values increased to 40–79 km/h; 75% of all pelvic fractures were observed at a calculated energy level of up to 5000 kJ, with no correlation to the observed fracture type [128].
- The use of safety belts led to a dramatic decrease of unstable and even stable pelvic ring injuries [129]. A 2.83-fold reduction of unstable pelvic fractures and a 1.5-fold reduction of potentially stable pelvic ring injuries could be observed.

The effect of tension of the pelvic floor muscles on stiffness of the pelvic ring was analyzed by Pool-Goudzwaard et al. in 18 embalmed specimens during simulation of sagittal rotation [89]. A gender difference was reported with stiffening of the SI joints in females but without effects in males, while females SI joint showed more mobility. Additionally, a backward rotation of the sacrum was observed in both sexes. It was concluded that pelvic floor muscles in females can increase the stiffness of the pelvic ring.

Hefzy et al. analyzed the biomechanical consequences of an open book injury of the pelvis under biomechanical loading in the prone position under posterior sacral loading [130]. As in clinical experience, the pubic bone on the injured side rotates/displaces inferiorly, while the SI joint showed no vertical shearing.

A clinical analysis confirmed that lateral impacts have the highest probability of sustaining pelvic fractures. Interestingly, seat belts and airbags were not protective against pelvic ring injuries, while the crash severity was a more predictive factor [131]. Lateral impact resulted in a 35.2% incidence of pelvic fractures and a higher injury severity sclae (ISS) in contrast to 7.7% after frontal impacts, despite a lower mean crash severity.

Pel et al. analyzed the effect of muscle innervation of SI joint stability in a 3-D simulation model [132]. A maximal vertical shear SI joint force of 563 N was calculated in the stance position. Reducing these shear forces by 20% led to a 70% increase in compressive SI joint forces by activation of hip flexors and counteracting hip extensors. A 40% reduction of shear forces further increased compression forces by 400%. This increase was found to be the result of clamping the sacrum between both hemipelves by transverse abdominis muscle and pelvic floor muscle activation.

3.13 Finite Element Analyses

Li et al. developed an FE model of the pelvis [133] and simulated side impacts to the pubic symphysis [134]. During lateral loading, highest stresses were observed at the contralateral superior pubic ramus, followed by the ipsilateral superior and contralateral inferior ramus. A deformation with a tendency to symphyseal overlapping was observed with a mean of 3.9 mm in the sagittal, 2.7 mm in the vertical, and 1.4 mm in the transverse symphyseal plane. The posterior symphyseal ligament was under tension, whereas the inferior ligament showed compressive strains.

The pelvis can be injured during lateral impacts due to stiff bonnet edges or bonnet tops as a result of compressive forces to the upper femur and pelvis.

The most common sites of lateral side impact injuries in pedestrians hit by a car were the head, the chest, and the lower extremities. The most frequently injured structures are the pelvis, which was observed between 4.5% and 9.2% (average, 7.3%), the pubic symphysis, and the pubic rami (2005 Int J Vehicle Safety Yang).

The risk of pedestrians hit by a car sustaining pelvic injuries was analyzed by Otte et al. in a combined medical and technical analysis (Otte IRCOBI 2001). Pelvic fractures most often occur during primary impact (direct hit by the car, five times more) than during second impact (fall on the ground). Higher impact speeds (41–70 km/h) of the car resulted in more bony pelvic injuries than low-velocity injuries (20–40 km/h).

References

1. Dolati B. Kapitel 3: Biomechanik. Becken und Acetabulumchirurgie. In: Weller S, Hierholzer G, editors. Traumatologie aktuell Band 10. Stuttgart, New York: Thieme; 1993. p. 19–23.
2. Holtrop M. The ultra structure of bone. Ann Clin Lab Sci. 1975;5:264.
3. Bankoff A. Morfologia e Cinesiologia Aplicada ao Movimento Humano. Rio de Janeiro, Brasil: Editora Guanabara Koogan; 2007.
4. Tile M. Pelvic ring fractures: should they be fixed ? J Bone Joint Surg. 1988;70-B:1–12.
5. Bucholz R. The pathological anatomy of malgaigne fracture-dislocations of the pelvis. J Bone Joint Surg. 1981;63-A(3):400–4.
6. Gertzbein S, Chenoweth D. Occult injuries of the pelvic ring. Clin Orthop. 1977;128:202–7.
7. Tile M. Personal communication. 2005.
8. Tile M. Fractures of the pelvis and acetabulum. Baltimore: Williams & Wilkings; 1984.
9. Khurana B, Sheehan S, Sodickson A, Weaver M. Pelvic ring fractures: what the orthopedic surgeon wants to know. Radiographics. 2014;34:1317–33.
10. Tile M. Fractures of the pelvis and acetabulum. 2nd ed. Baltimore: Williams & Wilkings; 1995.
11. Tile M, Helfet D, Kellam J. Fractures of the pelvis and acetabulum. Philadelphia: Lippincott Williams and Williams; 2003.
12. Fick R. Spezielle Gelenk- und Muskelmechanik (3.Teil). In: Handbuch der Anatomie und Mechanik der Gelenke unter Berücksichtigung der bewegenden Muskeln. Jena: Fischer; 1911. p. 443.
13. Waldeyer W. In: Joessel G, editor. Das Becken, in Lehrbuch der apographisch-chirurgischen Anatomie. Bonn: Friedrich Cohen Verlag; 1899.
14. Böhme J, Steinke H, Huelse R, Hammer N, Klink T, Slowik V, Josten C. Complex ligament instabilities after "open book"-fractures of the pelvic ring—finite element computer simulation and crack simulation. Z Orthop Unfall. 2011;149:83–9.
15. Holm N. The internal stress pattern of the os coxae. Acta Orthop Scand. 1980;51:421–8.
16. Wolff J. Das Gesetz der Transformation der Knochen. Berlin: Hirschwald; 1892.
17. Euler E. Das Becken—Ein Beitrag zur Anatomie, Biomechanik, Habilitationsschrift. 1993.
18. Euler E, Heining S, Kotsianos D, Müller-Gerbl M. Anatomie und Biomechanik des Beckens. Trauma Berufskrankh. 2000;2:2–10.
19. Poigenfürst J. Beckenbrüche. In: Nigst H, editor. Spezielle Frakturen- und Luxationslehre. Stuttgart: Thieme; 1972. p. 141–228.
20. Abitbol M. Evolution of the lumbosacral angle. Am J Phys Anthropol. 1987;72:361–72.
21. Dar G, Peleg S, Masharawi Y, Steinberg N, Rothschild B, Peled N, Hershkovitz I. Sacroiliac joint bridging: demographical and anatomical aspects. Spine. 2005;30:E429–32.
22. Pal G. Weight transmission through the sacrum in man. J Anat. 1989;162:9–17.
23. Snijders C, Vleeming A, Stoeckart R. Transfer of lumbosacral load to iliac bones and legs part 1: biomechanics of selfbracing of the sacroiliac joints and its significance for treatment and exercise. Clin Biomech. 1993;8:285–94.
24. Snijders C, Vleeming A, Stoeckart R. Transfer of lumbosacral load to iliac bones and legs part 2: loading of the sacroiliac joints when lifting in a stooped posture. Clin Biomech. 1993;8:295–301.
25. Linstrom N, Heiserman J, Kortman K, Crawford N, Baek S, Anderson R, Pitt A, Karis J, Ross J, Lekovic G, Dean B. Anatomical and biomechanical analyses of the unique and consistent locations of sacral insufficiency fractures. Spine. 2009;34:309–15.
26. Mahato N. Implications of structural variations in the human sacrum: why is an anatomical classification crucial? Surg Radiol Anat. 2016;38:947–54.
27. Ulmer J, Lange S, Kunze K. Verformung der Beckenhalbgelenke im kontrollierten Belastungstest. In: Szyszkowitz R, Seggl W, editors. Verrenkungsbrüche der Hüftpfanne und Beckenverletzungen. Bern, Göttingen, Toronto, Seattle: Verlag Hand Huber; 1993. p. 100–7.
28. Lühken H. Die Statik des menschlichen Beckens. Anat Entwickl Gesch. 1935;104:729–38.
29. Meyer H. Lehrbuch der anatomie des beckens. Leipzig: W Engelmann; 1873.
30. Pauwels F. Gesammelte Abhandlungen zur funktionellen Anatomie des Bewegungsapparates. Berlin, Heidelberg, New York: Springer-Verlag; 1965.

31. Pauwels F. Atlas zur Biomechanik der gesunden und kranken Hüfte. Berlin, Heidelberg, New York: Springer-Verlag; 1973.
32. Schmidt H. Die funktionelle Struktur der Symphyse im Erwachsenenalter. Anat Anz. 1956;102:135–52.
33. Walheim G, Olerud S, Ribbe T. Mobility of the pubic symphysis. Measurements by an electromechanical method. Acta Orthop Scand. 1984;55:203–8.
34. Walheim G, Selvik G. Mobility of the pubic symphysis. In vivo measurements with an electromechanic method and a roentgen stereophotogrammetric method. Clin Orthop. 1984;191: 129–35.
35. Meißner A, Fell M, Wilk R, Boenick U, Rahmanzadeh R. Zur Biomechanik der Symphyse. Welche Kräfte führen zur Mobilität der Symphyse unter physiologischen Bedingungen ? Unfallchirurg. 1996;99(6):415–21.
36. Icke C, Koebke J. Normal stress pattern of the pubic symphysis. Anat Cell Biol. 2014;47:40–3.
37. Meißner A, Breyer H, Ramanzadeh R. Experimentelle Untersuchungen zur Beweglichkeit in der Symphyse. Hefte Unfallheilk. 1986;181:79–82.
38. Colachis SJ, Worden R, Bechtol C, Strohm B. Movement of the sacro-iliac joint in the adult male; a preliminary report. Arch Physical Med Rehab. 1963;44:490–8.
39. Balandic. Über die Beweglichkeit in den Gelenken des schwangeren Beckens. Tageblatt der 44. Vers. dtsch. Naturforscher und Ärzte. Rostock. 1871.
40. Brooke R. The sacro-iliac joint. J Anat Physiol. 1924;58: 299–305.
41. Duncan J. The behaviour of the pelvic articulations in the mechanism of parturition. Dublin Q J Med Sci. 1854;18:60–9.
42. Feneis H. Experimentelle Beiträge zur Beckenmechanik. Anat Anz. 1939;88:187–97.
43. Klein G. Zur Biomechanik des Iliosakralgelenkes. Zeitschrift fGebh u Gynäk. 1891;21:74–118.
44. Luschka H. Die Kreuzdarmbeinfuge und die Schambeinfuge des Menschen. Arch f Path Anatomie u Physiologie f Klin Medizin. 1854;7:299–316.
45. Merk A. Die Veränderlichkeit der Beckenmasse und deren Ursache. Würzburg: Universität Würzburg; 1880.
46. Meyer G. Der Mechanismus der symphysis sacro-iliaca. Archiv für Anatomie und Physiologie. 1878;2:1–19.
47. Sashin D. A critical analysis of the anatomy and the pathologic changes of the sacroiliac joints. JBJS. 1930;28:891–910.
48. Winkel D. Das Sakroiliakalgelenk. Stuttgart, Jena, New York: Fischer; 1992.
49. Hammer N, Steinke H, Lingslebe U, Bechmann I, Josten C, Slowik V, Böhme J. Ligamentous influence in pelvic load distribution. Spine J. 2013;13:1321–30.
50. Dar G, Hershkovitz I. Sacroiliac joint bridging: simple and reliable criteria for sexing the skeleton. J Forensic Sci. 2006;51:480–3.
51. Dar G, Peleg S, Masharawi Y, Steinberg N, Rothschild B, Hershkovitz I. The association of sacroiliac joint bridging with other enthesopathies in the human body. Spine. 2007;32:E303–8.
52. Peleg S, Dar G, Medlej B, Steinberg N, Masharawi Y, Latimer B, Jellema L, Peled N, Arensburg B, Hershkovitz I. Orientation of the human sacrum: anthropological perspectives and methodological approaches. Am J Phys Anthropol. 2007;133:967–77.
53. Vleeming A, Stoeckart R, Volkers A, Snijders C. Relation between form and function in the sacroiliac joint. Part I: anatomical aspects. Spine. 1990;15(2):130–2.
54. Walker J. The sacroiliac joint: a crital review. Phys Ther. 1992;72:903–16.
55. Vleeming A, Schuenke M, Masi A, Carreiro J, Danneels L, Willard F. The sacroiliac joint: an overview of its anatomy, function and potential clinical implications. J Anat. 2012;221:537–67.
56. Berner W., Biomechanische Untersuchungen am Sakroiliakalgelenk, Topographie, Beanspruchung und operative Stabilisierung. Habilitationsschrift, Hannover. 1986.
57. Berner W, Rothkötter H, Hoyer H, Tscherne H. Biomechanische Untersuchungen am Ileosacralgelenk. In: Stelzner F, editor. Chirugisches Forum 85 g. experm. u. klinische Forschung. Berlin, Heidelberg, New York, Tokio: Springer; 1985. p. S1–4.
58. Rothkötter H, Berner W. Failure load and displacement of the human sacroiliac joint under in vitro loading. Arch Orthop Trauma Surg. 1988;107:283–7.
59. Gänsslen A, Pohlemann T, Culemann U, Krettek C, von Samson F, Tscherne H. Vergleichende dreidimensionale Stabilitätsprüfung verschiedener Osteosynthesen zur SI-Gelenks-Stabilisierung. Swiss Surg. 1996;Suppl. 2:43.
60. Miller J, Schultz A, Andersson G. Load-displacement behavior of sacroiliac joints. J Orthop Res. 1987;5:92–101.
61. Wilke H, Fischer K, Jeanneret B, Claes L, Magerl F. In-vivo-Messung der dreidimensionalen Bewegung des Iliosakralgelenks. Z Orthop. 1997;135:550–6.
62. Wang M, Dumas GA. Mechanical behavior of the female sacroiliac joint and influence of the anterior and posterior sacroiliac ligaments under sagittal loads. Clin Biomech. 1998;13(4–5):293–9.
63. Hammer N, Steinke H, Slowik V, Josten C, Stadler J, Böhme J, Spanel-Borowski K. The sacrotuberous and the sacrospinous ligament—a virtual reconstruction. Ann Anat. 2009;191:417–25.
64. Vrahas M, Hern T, Diangelo D, Kellam J, Tile M. Ligamentous contributions to pelvic stability. Orthopedics. 1995;18:271–4.
65. Philippeau J, Hamel O, Pecot J, Robert R. Are sacrospinal and sacrotuberal ligaments involved in sacro-iliac joint stability? Morphology. 2008;92:16–30.
66. Varga E, Dudas B, Tile M. Putative proprioceptive function of the pelvic ligaments: biomechanical and histological studies. Injury. 2008;39:858–64.
67. Tile M, Pennal G. Pelvic disruptions: principles of management. Clon Orthop. 1980;151:56–64.
68. Krueger P, Euler E, Raderschadt M, Wischhöfer E, Hartge S, Weimann E, Schweiberer L. Vergleichende experimentelle und klinische Untersuchungen verschiedener stabilisierender Osteosynthesetechniken im dorsalen Beckenbereich. Hefte Unfallheilkd. 1986;181:625–6.
69. Dolati B. Becken und Acetabulumchirurgie. In: Weller S, Hierholzer G, editors. Traumatologie aktuell Band 10. Stuttgart, New York: Thieme; 1993. p. 21, 28–29.
70. Simonian PT, Routt ML Jr, Harrington RM, Mayo KA, Tencer AF. Biomechanical simulation of the anteroposterior compression injury of the pelvis. An understanding of instability and fixation. Clin Orthop. 1994;309:245–56.
71. Abdelfattah A, Moed B. Ligamentous contributions to pelvic stability in a rotationally unstable open-book injury: a cadaver study. Injury. 2014;45:1599–603.
72. Böhme J, Lingslebe U, Steinke H, Werner M, Slowik V, Josten C, Hammer N. The extent of ligament injury and its influence on pelvic stability following type II anteroposterior compression pelvic injuries—a computer study to gain insight into open book trauma. J Orthop Res. 2014;32:873–9.
73. Eichenseer P, Sybert D, Cotton J. A finite element analysis of sacroiliac joint ligaments in response to different loading conditions. Spine. 2011;36:E1446–52.
74. Butt A, Gill C, Demerdash A, Watanabe K, Loukas M, Rozzelle C, Tubbs R. A comprehensive review of the sub-axial ligaments of the vertebralcolumn: part I anatomy and function. Childs Nerv Syst. 2015;31:1037–59.
75. Luk KD, Ho HC, Leong JC. The iliolumbar ligament. A study of its anatomy, development and clinical significance. J Bone Joint Surg (Br). 1986;68(2):197–200.

76. Pool-Goudzwaard A, Hoek van Dijke A, Mulder P, Spoor C, Snijders C, Stoeckart R. The iliolumbar ligament: its influence on stability of the sacroiliac joint. Clin Biomech. 2002;18: 99–105.
77. Hanson P, Sonesson B. The anatomy of the iliolumbar ligament. Arch Phys Med Rehabil. 1994;75:1245–6.
78. Pool-Goudzwaard A, Hoek van Dijke G, Mulder P, Spoor C, Snijders C, Stoeckart R. The iliolumbar ligament: its influence on stability of the sacroiliac joint. Clin Biomech. 2003;18: 99–105.
79. Williams P, Warwick R. Gray's Anatomy. 36th ed. Edinburgh: Longman; 1980. p. 414.
80. Pal G, Cosio L, Routal R. Trajectory architecture of the trabecular bone between the body and the neural arch in human vertebrae. Anat Rec. 1988;222:418–25.
81. Basadonna P, Gasparini D, Rucco V. Iliolumbar ligament insertions. In vivo anatomic study. Spine. 1996;21:2313–6.
82. Hanson P, Magnusson S, Sorensen H, Simonsen E. Differences in the iliolumbar ligament and the transverse process of the L5 vertebra in young white and black people. Acta Anat. 1998;163: 218–23.
83. Chow DH, Luk KD, Leong JC, Woo CW. Torsional stability of the lumbosacral junction. Significance of the iliolumbar ligament. Spine. 1989;14(6):611–5.
84. Leong J, Luk K, Chow D, Woo C. The biomechanical functions of the iliolumbar ligament in maintaining stability of the lumbosacral junction. Spine. 1987;12:669–74.
85. Yamamoto I, Panjabi M, Oxland T, Crisco J. The role of the iliolumbar ligament in the lumbosacral junktion. Spine. 1990;15(11):1138–41.
86. Richardson C, Snijders C, Hides J, Damen L, Pas M, Storm J. The relation between the transversus abdominis muscles, sacroiliac joint mechanics, and low back pain. Spine. 2002;27: 399–405.
87. Pool-Goudzwaard A, Gnat R, Spoor K. Deformation of the innominate bone and mobility of the pubic symphysis during asymmetric moment application to the pelvis. Man Ther. 2012;17: 66–70.
88. Gnat R, Spoor K, Pool-Goudzwaard A. The influence of simulated transversus abdominis muscle force on sacroiliac joint flexibility during asymmetric moment application to the pelvis. Clin Biomech. 2015;30:827–31.
89. Pool-Goudzwaard A, van Dijke G, van Gurp M, Mulder P, Snijders C, Stoeckart R. Contribution of pelvic floor muscles to stiffness of the pelvic ring. Clin Biomech. 2004;19:564–71.
90. Malgaigne J. Traites des fractures et des luxations. Paris: J.B. Balliere; 1847.
91. Malgaigne J. In: Bearbeitet von Burger C, editor. Die Knochenbrüche und Verrenkungen für praktische Aerzte, Wundärzte und Studirende. Erster Band: Knochenbrüche. (deutsche Übersetzung der französischen Ausgabe von 1847). Stuttgart: Rieger'sche Verlagsbuchhandlung; 1850.
92. Fischer A. Über schwere Beckenluxationen und Verletzungen der umgebenden Weichteile: Typische Rodelverletzungen. Zentbl Chir. 1909;36:1313–9.
93. Haumann W. Ueber die halbseitige Beckenverrenkung. Bruns Beitr Klin Chir. 1921;123:278–307.
94. Hirsch L. Ueber Beckenfrakturen. Bruns Beitr Klin Chir. 1924;132:441–65.
95. Watson-Jones R. Dislocations and fracture-dislocations of the pelvis. Br J Surg. 1938;25:773–81.
96. Messerer O. Über Elasticität und Festigkeit der menschlichen Knochen. Stuttgart: Verlag der J.G. Cotta'schen Buchhandlung; 1880.
97. Kusmin W. Ueber Beckenfracturen—Experimentelle Untersuchung. Wiener Med Jahrbücher. 1882;1:105–41.
98. Katzenelson M. Ueber die Fracturen des Beckenringes. Dtsch Z Chir. 1895;41:473–512.
99. Stuhler T, Stankovic P, Krause P, Koch A. Kindliche Beckenfrakturen: Klinik, Spätergebnisse. Biomechanik Arch Orthop Unfall-Chir. 1977;90:187–98.
100. Voigt G. Untersuchungen zur Mechanik der Beckenfrakturen und Luxationen. Hefte Unfallheilk. 1965;85:1–92.
101. Fleischer G, Kallieris D, Käppner R, Schmidt G. Zur quantitativen Traumatomechanik der Beckenfraktur. Unfallchirurg. 1995;98(7):398–4405.
102. Fayon A, Tarrièree C, Walfisch G, Got C, Patel A. Contribution to defining the human tolerance to perpendicular side impact. IRCOBI Conference, Munich, 1977.
103. Tarriere C, Walfisch G, Fayon A, Got C, Guillon F. Synthesis of human impact tolerance obtained from lateral impact simulations. Washington, DC: 7th International Tech Conference on Experimental Safety Vehicles; 1979. p. 359–73.
104. Cesari D, Ramet M, Bouquet R. Tolerance of human pelvis to fracture and proposed pelvic protection criterion to be measured on side impact dummies. Proceedings of the International Technical Conference on the Enhanced Safety of Vehicles, 9th, Kyoto, Japan; 1983. pp. 261–269.
105. Nusholtz G, Kaiker P. Pelvic stress. J Biomech. 1986;19(12):1003–14.
106. Viano D, Lau I, Asbury C, King A, Begeman P. Biomechanics of the human chest, abdomen, and pelvis in lateral impact. Accid Anal Prev. 1989;21:553–74.
107. Cavanaugh J, Huang Y, Zhu Y, King A. Regional tolerance of the shoulder, thorax, abdomen and pelvis to padding in side impact. Stapp Car Crash Conference; San Antonio, TX, 1993: p. 973–980.
108. Zhu Y, Cavanaugh J, King A. Pelvic biomechanical response and padding benefits in side impact based on a cadaveric test series. Stapp Car Crash Conference; San Antonio, TX, 1993. pp. 223–233.
109. Molz, F., George, P. and Bidez, M., Simulated automotive side impact on the isolated human pelvis: phase 1: development of a containment device. phase 2: analysis of pubic symphysis motion and overall pelvic compression. Paper Presented at: 41st Stapp Car Crash Conference; November 13–1, Orlando, FL, 1997.
110. Guillemot H, Lasasu J, Le Coz Y, Robin S, Lavaste F. Pelvic behavior in side collisions: static and dynamic tests on isolated pelvic bones. International Technical Conference on Experimental Safety Vehicles. Sixteenth. Proceedings. Volume II. Washington, DC: NHTSA; 1998. p. 1412–24.
111. Bouquet R, Ramet M, Bermond F, Vyes C. Pelvic Human Response to Lateral Impact. 16th International Technical Conference on the Enhanced Safety of Vehicles, Paper No. 98-S7-W-16. Windsor: National Highway Traffic Administration; 1998.
112. Matsui Y, Wittek A, Ishikawa H. Injury pattern and tolerance of human pelvis under lateral loading simulating car–pedestrian impact. Warrendale, PA: SAE; 2003. SAE Paper 2003-01-0165, 2003
113. Beason D, Dakin G, Lopez R, Alonso J, Bandak F, Eberhardt A. Bone mineral density correlates with fracture load in experimental side impacts of the pelvis. J Biomech. 2003;36:219–27.
114. Krappinger D, Schubert H, Wenzel V, Rieger M, Stadlbauer K, Blauth M, Schmoelz W. A pelvic fracture model for the assessment of treatment options in a laboratory environment. Injury. 2007;38:1151–7.
115. Salzar R, Genovese D, Bolton J. Load path distribution within the pelvic structure under lateral loading. Int J Crashworthiness. 2009;14:99–110.

116. Snedeker J, Walz F, Muser M, Schroeder G, Mueller T, Müller R. Microstructural insight into pedestrian pelvic fracture as assessed by high-resolution computed tomography. J Biomech. 2006;39:2709–13.
117. Yoganandan N, Pintar F, Gennarelli T, Maltese M, Eppinger R. Mechanisms and factors involved in hip injuries during frontal crashes. Stapp Car Crash J. 2001;45:437–48.
118. Patrick L, Kroell C, Merrz H. Forces on the human body in simulated crashes. In: Cragun MK, editor. Proceedings of the 9th Stapp Car Crash Conference. MN: Minneapolis; 1965. p. 237–59.
119. Melvin J, Nusholtz G. Tolerance and response of the knee-femur-pelvis complex to axial impacts. Rep. No. UMHSRI-80–27. Ann Arbor: University of Michigan, Highway Safety Research Institute; 1980.
120. Nusholtz, G., Alem, N. and Melvin, J., Impact response and injury to the pelvis. Proceedings of Stapp Conference, 26th, Ann Arbor, MI, Pap. No. 821160. Warrendale, PA: Society *of* Automotive Engineers, 1982.
121. Brun-Cassan, F., Leung, Y., Tarriere, C., Fayon, A. and Patel, A., Determination of knee-femur-pelvis tolerance from the simulation of car frontal impacts. Proc. Int. Conf. Biokinetics Impacts, 7th, Cologne, Germany, pp. 101–115. Bron, France: International Research Council on Biomechanics of Impact; 1982.
122. Patrick, L. and Andersson, A., Threepoint harness accident and laboratory data comparison. Proceedings of Stapp Conference, 18th, Ann Arbor, MI, Pap. No. 741181. Warrendale, PA: Society of Automotive Engineers, 1974.
123. King A. Fundamentals of impact biomechanics: part 2—biomechanics of the abdomen, pelvis, and lower extremities. Annu Rev Biomed Eng. 2001;3:27–55.
124. McCoy GF, Johnstone RA, Kenwright J. Biomechanical aspects of pelvic and hip injuries in road traffic accidents. J Orthop Trauma. 1989;3(2):118–23.
125. Siegel J, Dalal S, Burgess A, Young J. Pattern of organ injuries in pelvic fracture: impact force implications for survival and death in motor vehicle injuries. Accid Anal Prev. 1990;22(5):457–66.
126. Pohlemann T, Richter M, Otte D, Gänsslen A, Bartram H, Tscherne H. Mechanism of pelvic girdle injuries in street traffic. Medical-technical accident analysis. Unfallchirurg. 2000;103:267–74.
127. Richter M, Otte D, Gänsslen A, Bartram H, Pohlemann T. Injuries of the pelvic ring in road traffic accidents: a medical and technical analysis. Injury. 2001;32:123–8.
128. Pohlemann T, Otte D, Bartram H, Tscherne H. The ralevance of accident mechanisms in "real accidents" for fracture pattern and classification of pelvis fractures. USA: International Conference on Pelvic and Lower Extremity Injuries; 1995. p. 329.
129. Teifke AV, Degreif J, Geist M, Schild H, Strunk H, Schunk K. Der Sicherheitsgurt: Auswirkungen auf das Verletzungsmuster von Autoinsassen. ROFÖ. 1993;159(3):278–83.
130. Hefzy M, Ebraheim N, Mekhail A, Caruntu D, Lin H, Yeasting R. Kinematics of the human pelvis following open book injury. Med Eng Phys. 2003;25:259–74.
131. Rowe S, Sochor M, Staples K, Wahl W, Wang S. Pelvic ring fractures: implications of vehicle design, crash type, and occupant characteristics. Surgery. 2004;136:842–7.
132. Pel J, Spoor C, Pool-Goudzwaard A, Hoek van Dijke G, Snijders C. Biomechanical analysis of reducing sacroiliac joint shear load by optimization of pelvic muscle and ligament forces. Ann Biomed Eng. 2008;36:415–24.
133. Li Z, Alonso J, Kim J, Davidson J, Etheridge B, Eberhardt A. Three-dimensional finite element models of the human pubic symphysis with viscohyperelastic soft tissues. Ann Biomed Eng. 2006;34:1452–62.
134. Li Z, Eberhardt A. Finite element modeling of the human pelvis, vol. 34. Saarbrücken, Germany: Verlag Dr. Müller; 2008. p. 1452–62.

Classification of Pelvic Ring Injuries

4

Christoph Grechenig, Stephan Grechenig, Gloria Hohenberger, Axel Gänsslen, and Jan Lindahl

When considering classification of pelvic injuries, besides the pure osteoligamentous injury, additional peripelvic injuries and their consequences, e.g., relevant soft tissue injuries including open fractures, pelvic organ lesion, neurovascular injuries, and potential accompanying hemodynamic instability, which are summarized under the term "complex pelvic trauma" should be considered.

The primary basis of decision-making is the osteoligamentous injury, which most often guides treatment decision in terms of stabilization necessity, while additional injuries of the pelvic region lead to time-dependent decisions.

C. Grechenig
Department of Ophthalmology, Medical University of Vienna, Wien, Austria
e-mail: christoph.grechenig@meduniwien.ac.at

S. Grechenig
Department of Orthopedics and Trauma Surgery, AUVA Trauma Hospital Klagenfurt, Klagenfurt, Austria

Department of Trauma Surgery, University Hospital Regensburg, Regensburg, Germany

G. Hohenberger
Department of Orthopaedics and Trauma, Medical University of Graz, Graz, Austria
e-mail: gloria.hohenberger@medunigraz.at

A. Gänsslen (✉)
Department of Trauma Surgery, Orthopedics and Hand Surgery, Hospital Wolfsburg, Wolfsburg, Germany

J. Lindahl
Orthopaedics and Trauma Surgery, Helsinki University Hospital, Helsinki, Finland

4.1 Osteoligamentous Pelvic Ring Classifications

Several classifications of pelvic ring injuries are in clinical use. The most frequently used classifications of the osteoligamentous injury are the Young-Burgess classification, which is based on the main force vector acting on the whole pelvis; the Tile classification, which is based on the amount of pelvic instability; and the AO/OTA classification, which is based on the Tile classification.

Further classifications analyze subtypes of these classifications including sacral fracture classifications due to their prognostic and therapeutic relevance, sacroiliac (SI) joint injury classification, and age-related classifications, including geriatric pelvic fracture and pediatric classifications.

4.1.1 Tile Classification

Based on the main injury mechanisms acting on the pelvis (anterior-posterior compression, lateral compression, and vertical shear), reported early in the 1980s [1, 2], Tile developed his instability-based classification [3], which is focused on the involvement and integrity of the posterior pelvic ring structures.

This classification consists of three main fracture/injury types, type A, B, and C, with increasing mechanical instability of the pelvic ring:

- Type A: minimally displaced, stable fractures.
- Type B: rotational instability, vertical stability.
- Type C: vertical instability.

A further subclassification of these fracture types was performed, depending on pelvic injury severity.

A. Gänsslen et al. (eds.), *Pelvic Ring Fractures*, https://doi.org/10.1007/978-3-030-54730-1_4

4.1.1.1 Type A: Stable, Minimally Displaced

Type A injuries were subdivided into:

- Type A1: no pelvic ring involvement (isolated iliac wing fractures, avulsion fractures).
- Type A2: undisplaced, stable ring fractures.

4.1.1.2 Type B: Rotationally Unstable, Vertically Stable

Type B injuries were subdivided according to the main injury mechanisms: external rotation (open book injury) and internal rotation (lateral compression injury) [3].

Type B1 open book injuries are a result of external rotation with most often symphyseal disruption. This group consists of three stages, depending on the transferred force to the pelvis:

- Type B1.1: symphyseal separation <2.5 cm on pelvic a.p. X-ray, no posterior pelvic ring lesion.
- Type B1.2: symphyseal separation >2.5 cm on pelvic a.p. X-ray; unilateral disruption of the anterior sacroiliac ligament and a suspected injury of the sacrospinous ligament.
- Type B1.3: symphyseal separation >2.5 cm on pelvic a.p. X-ray; bilateral posterior injury with disruption of the anterior sacroiliac ligaments and suspected injury of both sacrospinous ligaments.

Types B2 and B3 are both the result of lateral compression/internal rotation. The posterior ring complex shows impaction without translational deformity:

- Type B2 injuries present with an ipsilateral anterior pubic rami fracture and a posterior crush injury (anterior sacral fracture); rarely, an overlapping pubic symphysis or a combined symphyseal injury with a pubic rami fracture is observed, the latter sometimes creating a "tilt fracture" (pubic spike).
- Type B3 injuries are caused by a direct blow to the iliac crest resulting in a contralateral injury (bucket handle: anterior-superior hemipelvic rotation); the anterior ring involvement is typically contralateral to the posterior lesion but can be observed even bilaterally.

4.1.1.3 Type C: Rotationally and Vertically Unstable

The definition of type C injuries includes suspected complete disruption of the pelvic floor ligaments (sacrospinous/sacrotuberous ligaments) and complete posterior pelvic ring disruption with a hemipelvic displacement >1 cm, avulsion of the L5 transverse process (iliolumbar ligament), and/or bony avulsion at the lateral sacrum or ischial tuberosity (pelvic floor ligaments) [3]. Three subgroups were distinguished:

- Type C1: unilateral posterior C-type injury.
- Type C2: bilateral posterior C-type injury.
- Type C3: type C injury with an associated acetabular fracture.

With increasing understanding of the injury mechanism and the stability-based concept of the pelvic ring, this primary classification scheme was changed [4–6] resulting in the comprehensive AO and OTA classification [7–10] (Fig. 4.1, Table 4.1).

4.1.1.4 Clinical Significance of the Tile Classification

The Tile classification is of prognostic relevance as an increase of the mortality rate was observed from 8.8% for type A injuries to 13.8% for type B injuries and to 25% for type C injuries [11].

A recent analysis [12] reported an increase of mortality from B1 to B3. In type C injuries, highest mortality rates were observed after C2 injuries. The mortality rate of B3 injuries was comparable to C-type injuries.

This can be explained, as after open book injuries, a high rate of concomitant intrapelvic vessel injuries is observed due to the increase of the pelvic volume [13].

A further analysis by Rommens et al. for type B and type C injuries [14] reported a threefold higher mortality rate in type C injuries. The rate of anatomic reductions decreased from 93.5% in type B1 to 75% in type B2/B3 and to 62.7% in type C injuries. The functional outcome was worse after type C than type B injuries.

Within the type B group, B1 injuries were associated with less favorable functional results compared to type B2 or B3 injuries. Additionally, the frequency of associated neurological and urological lesions was higher after type B1 injuries than in the B2/B3 group [14, 15].

4.1.2 Young-Burgess Classification

The Young-Burgess classification analyzes the amount of the potential injury force vector and therefore the proposed injury mechanism in detail (Fig. 4.2).

Young and Burgess performed a radiographic analysis of 142 conventional pelvic X-rays (pelvis a.p. view, pelvic inlet view, pelvic outlet view) and identified four principle force vectors [16]:

- Anterior-posterior compression (APC, external rotation of the hemipelvis).

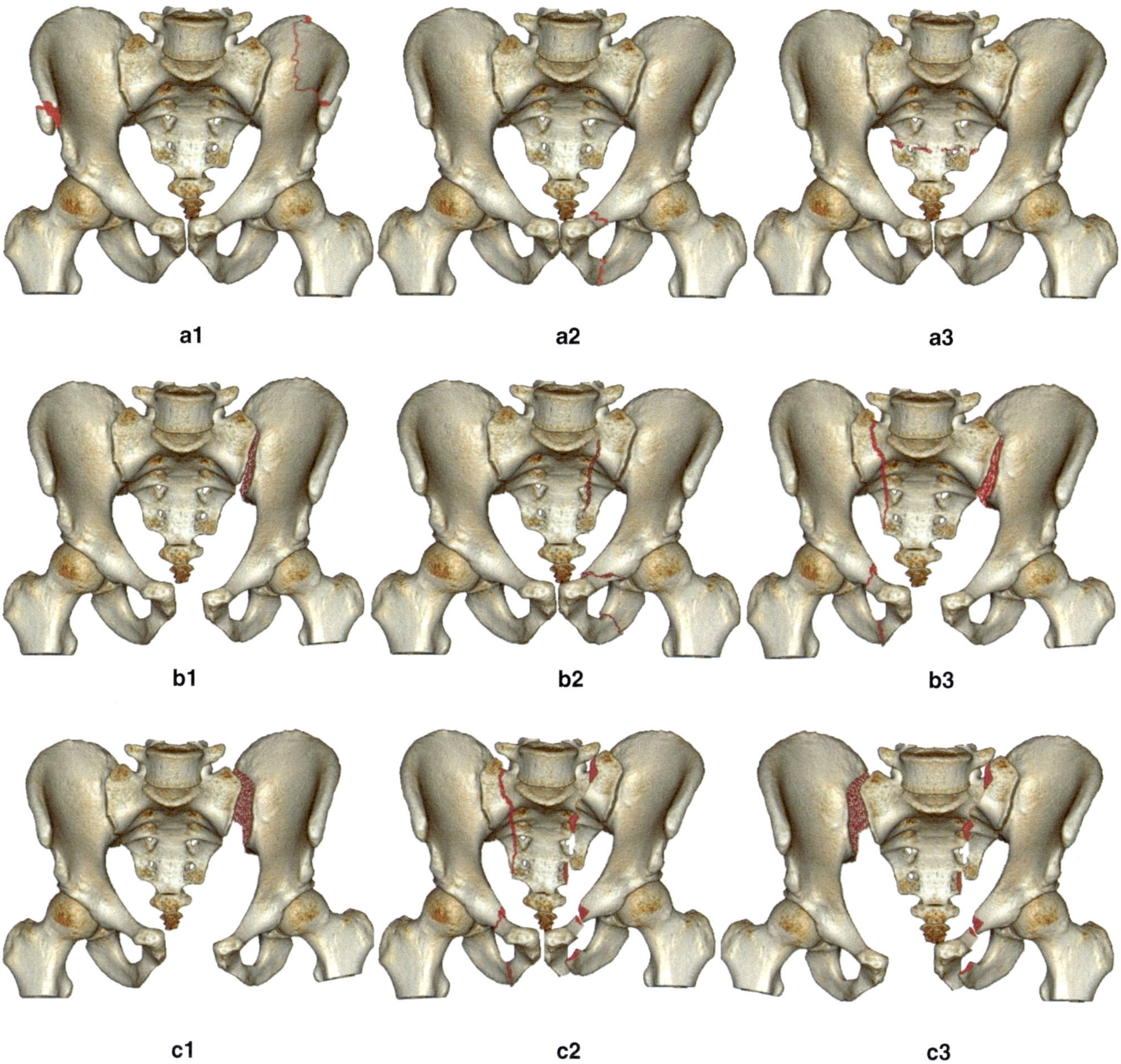

Fig. 4.1 Tile classification (1996) of pelvic ring injuries (see text)

Table 4.1 AO/OTA classification according to Tile's recommendation [4]

Type A: stable pelvic ring	
A1	Avulsion of the innominate bone
A2	Stable iliac wing for stable minimally displaced ring fracture
A3	Transverse fractures of the sacrum and coccyx below the SI joint level
Type B: Partially stable pelvic ring	
B1	Open book injury
B2	Lateral compression injury
B3	Bilateral B injuries
Type C: Complete unstable pelvic ring	
C1	Unilateral
C2	Bilateral, one side B, one side C
C3	Bilateral C lesions

- Lateral compression (LC, internal rotation of the hemipelvis).
- Vertical shear (VS).
- Complex fracture pattern.

4.1.2.1 AP Compression Injuries

AP compression (APC) injuries most frequently result in injuries of the pubic rami ± ligamentous injuries of the pubic symphysis, the SI joint(s), and the pelvic floor ligaments with different severity of the resulting ligamentous injury.

The classical open book deformity consists of a symphyseal separation with a concomitant SI joint injury. Pubic rami fractures always present with a vertical oriented fracture line.

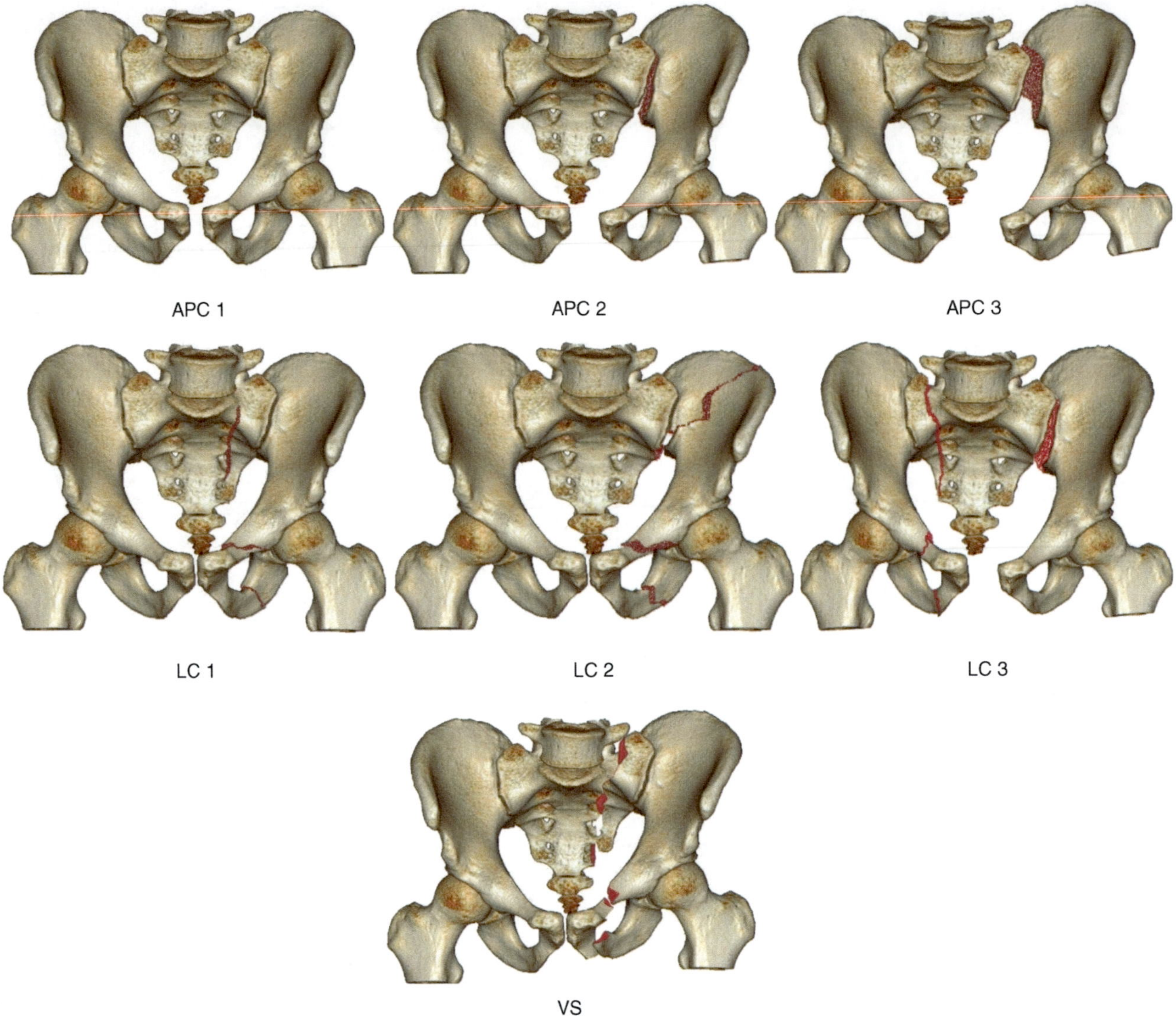

Fig. 4.2 Young-Burgess classification based on the suspected injury mechanism (details: see text)

It was observed that symphyseal separation <2.5 cm was not combined with SI joint instability [16]. Burgess et al. observed no cranio-caudal displacement of the hemipelvis in APC mechanisms [17].

Severity grading of the posterior injury was based on Bucholz' recommendations [18]:

- APC 1 (Fig. 4.3): anterior pelvic ring injury without radiographic or clinical posterior instability (symphyseal widening typically below 2.5 cm) (Fig. 4.3).
- APC 2 (Fig. 4.4a, b): combined symphyseal dislocation (often >2.5 cm) and anterior SI joint injury; an injury to iliac internal artery branches and the lumbosacral plexus should be considered [17].
- APC 3 (Fig. 4.5): complete SI joint disruption (no ligamentous connection between the ilium and the sacrum).

An accompanying acetabular fracture can be present in up to two-thirds of these patients.

Biomechanically, a distinction of APC 1 from APC 2 injuries using the 2.5-cm symphyseal displacement value was not supported. Doro et al. observed that anterior sacroiliac ligament disruption was likely with a symphyseal displacement >4.5 cm, while displacement <1.8 cm was associated with no anterior SI joint ligament injury [19].

4.1.2.2 Lateral Compression Injuries

Lateral compression (LC) injuries present with characteristic horizontal (comminuted) pubic rami fractures in approximately 100%. Sacrum fractures were present in 88%, while additional acetabular fractures (19%) showed medial (central) displaced fracture patterns [16, 17]. Ligamentous injury was rarely observed. Posterior

APC I

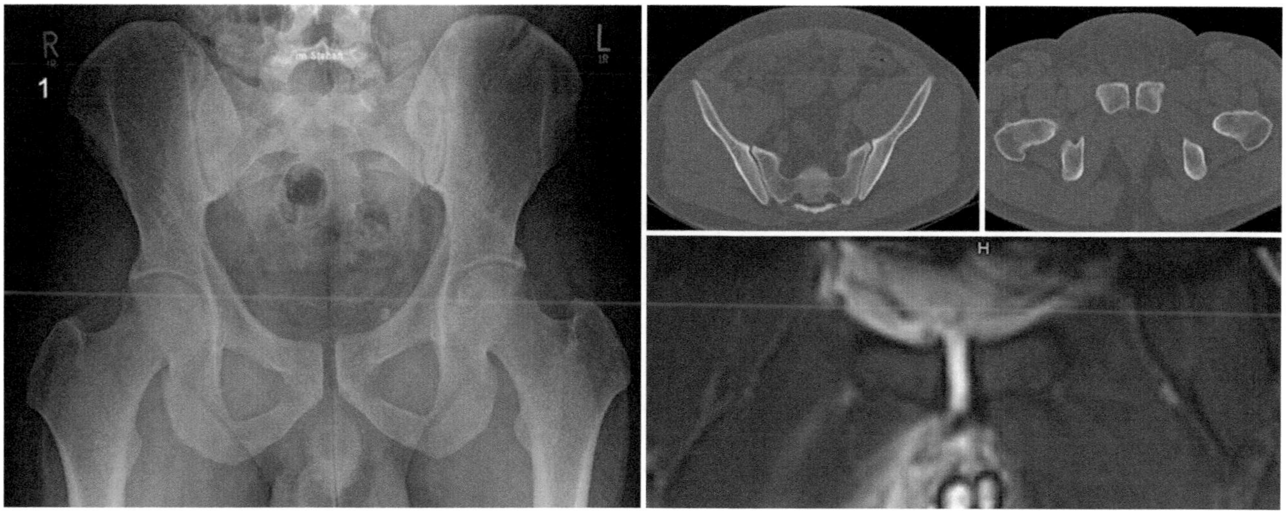

Fig. 4.3 Young-Burgess APC I injury with a symphyseal strain (neglectable instability) and no proven posterior pelvic ring injury

sacroiliac ligament injury can be present. Three subtypes were observed:

- LC 1 (Fig. 4.6): posterior pelvic ring force transmission with minor clinical instability.
- LC 2 (Fig. 4.7): more anterior force transmission with resulting anterior internal (medial) fracture displacement combined with some external rotation of the posterior hemipelvis [16]; crescent fractures were included to this fracture type [17].
- LC 3 (Fig. 4.8): internal rotation of the ipsilateral hemipelvis (LC 1 or LC 2) with (sometimes) external rotation of the contralateral hemipelvis (APC 2 injury) [16, 17].

4.1.2.3 Vertical Shear Injuries

Vertical shear (VS) injuries result from severe vertical force vectors (fall from height), involving one or both sides of the posterior pelvis (Fig. 4.9). A severe posterior pelvic ring instability is present involving the sacrum or the posterior ligamentous complex. Typically, vertically oriented fractures will be observed [16].

Severe VS injuries, especially with caudal hemipelvic displacement, were associated with significant arterial injury, requiring hemipelvectomy [20].

4.1.2.4 Complex Mechanism

Complex fracture patterns (CM) are combinations of at least two of these injury vectors (Fig. 4.10).

Young and Resnik summarized these radiographic findings (Table 4.2) [21].

4.1.2.5 Clinical Significance of the Young-Burgess Classification

Several studies evaluated the clinical relevance of the Young-Burgess classification and its subtypes.

LC injuries are the result of a lateral force vector. The deformity shows a shift of the hemipelvis to the midline [17]. This leads to compression/shortening of the ipsilateral ligaments and neurovascular structures, while tensile or shearing forces are unusual [17]. Vessel injury is therefore supposed to be a result of direct fracture fragment contact.

In contrast, an increased rate of pelvic vascular injury, retroperitoneal hematoma formation, primary hemodynamic shock and 24-h transfusion needs, acute respiratory distress syndrome (ARDS), and sepsis was observed from APC 1 to APC 3 injuries [22].

Problems with using the classical definitions of Young and Burgess were shown in recent analyses.

A computed tomography (CT) analysis of LC 1 fractures indicated that a large proportion of complete sacral fractures were part of this fracture type, indicating more unstable fracture pattern [23]. Risk factors for this injury type were type III sacral fractures according to Denis, significant anterior pelvic ring injury, a higher abdominal abbreviated injury scale (AIS), and a higher injury severity scale (ISS). Complete sacral fractures were integrated into this subgroup [24].

The heterogeneity of LC injuries was confirmed in an analysis of 318 patients. In 4%, no posterior injury was observed, while 51% had an anterior sacral compression fractures and 32% a complete sacral fracture. Thirteen percent presented with a crescent fracture. Overall, 45 complete/unstable posterior pelvic injuries were observed [25].

APC II

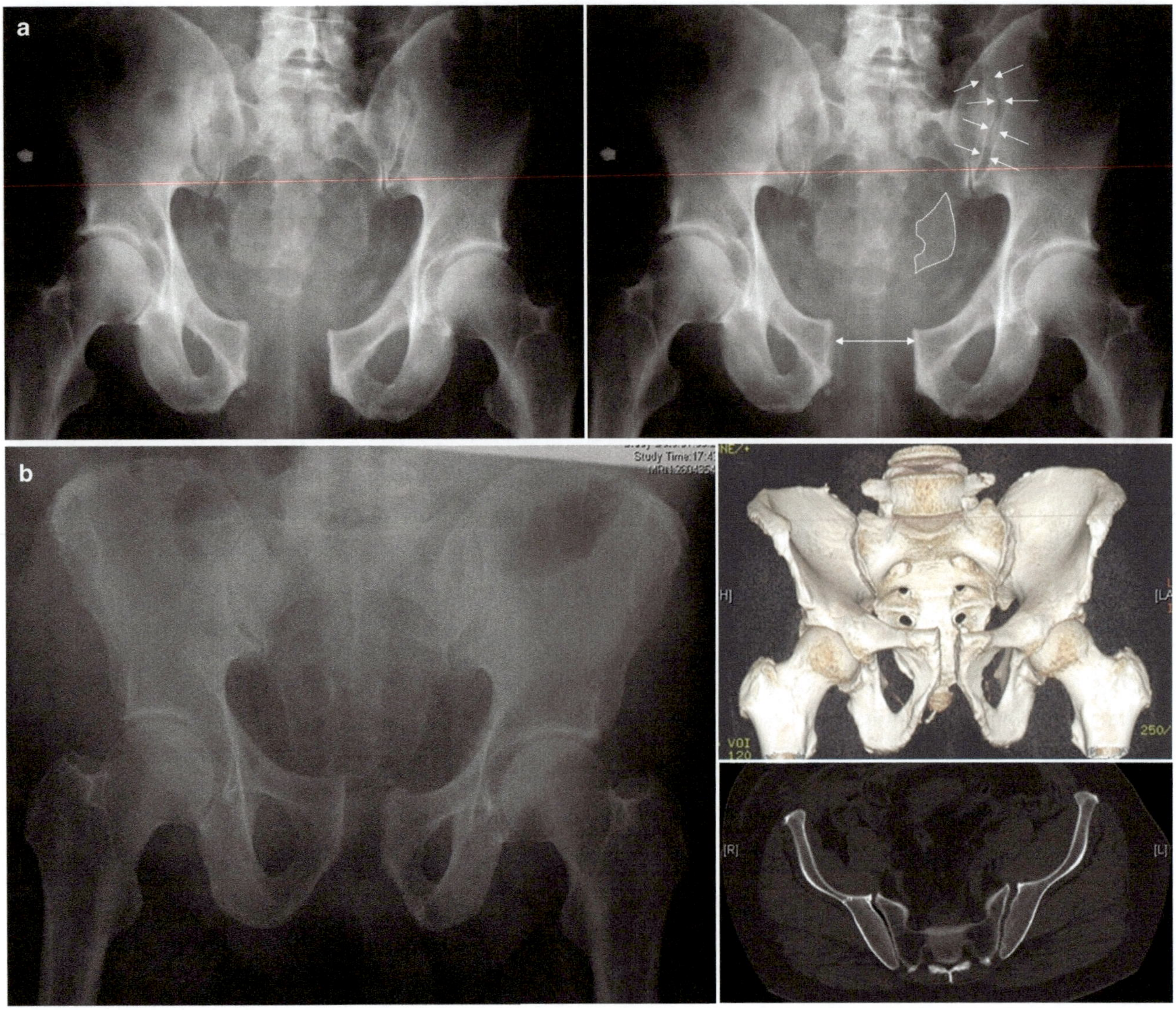

Fig. 4.4 (**a**) Young-Burgess APC II injury with symphyseal and left SI joint dislocation and bony avulsion injury of the sacrospinal ligament. (**b**) Young-Burgess APC II injury with symphyseal and left SI joint dislocation

AP injuries showed an increase of rates of additional spleen, liver, and bowel injuries; pelvic vascular injury with retroperitoneal hematoma formation; primary hemodynamic shock; and 24-h transfusion needs from APC 1 to APC 3 [22].

AP 1 injuries are uncommon [17, 26]. An analysis of AP 1 injuries showed a mean symphyseal diastasis of 1.8 cm on standard a.p. X-rays, while CT evaluation showed 1.4 cm symphyseal widening, which was increased to 2.5 cm using conventional stress radiographs. In one of four patients, symphyseal diastasis was >2.5 cm, which resulted in a change of treatment [27].

As the pelvic a.p. X-ray is only a static radiograph, underestimation of the displacement is common [28].

In an analysis by Sagi et al. using dynamic fluoroscopy, occult instability was observed in 50% of APC 1 injuries (subgroup change to APC 2) and in 39% of APC 2 injuries (subgroup change to APC 3) [29].

In APC 3 injuries, often, the boundaries of the pelvic compartments are completely disrupted leading to large retroperitoneal hemorrhage, and severe local vascular and visceral injuries have to be expected [17]. APC 3 injuries were associated with highest transfusion needs and mortality [22].

APC III

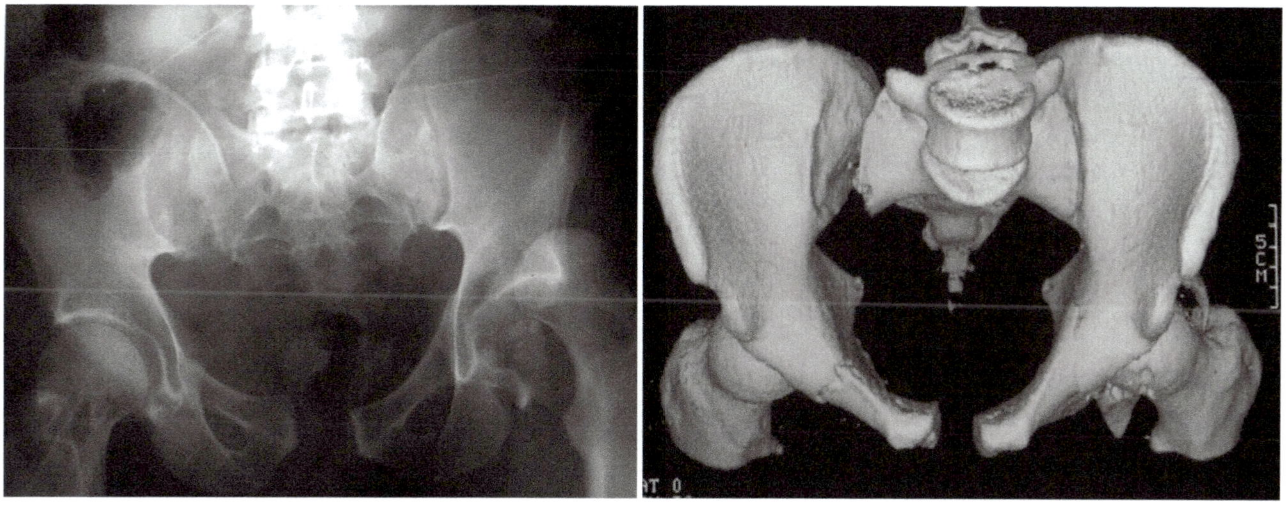

Fig. 4.5 Young-Burgess APC III injury with complete right SI joint dislocation and disruption of the pubic symphysis

LC I

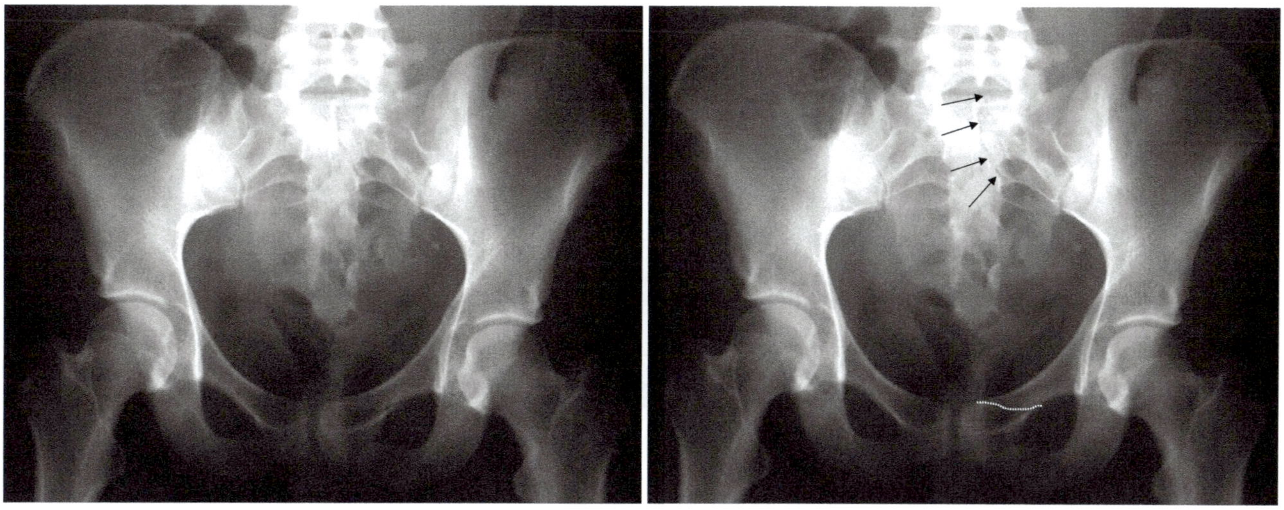

Fig. 4.6 Young-Burgess LC I injury with a central longitudinal sacral fracture, a horizontal superior ramus fracture, and an inferior ramus fracture

Comparing LC 1–3 with APC 2 and APC 3 injury types, an increase of 48-h transfusion needs packed red blood cells (PRBC) from 2.7, 3.1, 7.4, 7.6, and 35.4 was observed, respectively [17]. The corresponding mortality rates were 6.6%, 50%, 4.3%, 20%, and 35.7%, respectively. VS injuries were associated with a 9.4% transfusion rate and a mortality rate of 3.1%. In contrast, Starr et al. found highest mortality rates even in LC 3 and APC 3 injuries [26].

Recently, it was stated that LC 3, APC 2, and APC 3 injuries were associated with higher transfusion requirements than LC 1, APC 1, and VS injuries, while no association to additional injuries of the head, chest, or abdomen was observed [30].

When reducing the Young-Burgess classification into stable (LC 1, APC 1) and unstable (LC 2, LC 3, APC 2, APC 3, VS, CM) fracture types, unstable fracture better predicted mortality rates, concomitant abdominal injury rates, and transfusion requirements [30].

It has to be considered that using dynamic fluoroscopy, occult instability was observed in 37% of LC 1 injuries (subgroup change to LC 2) [29].

LC II

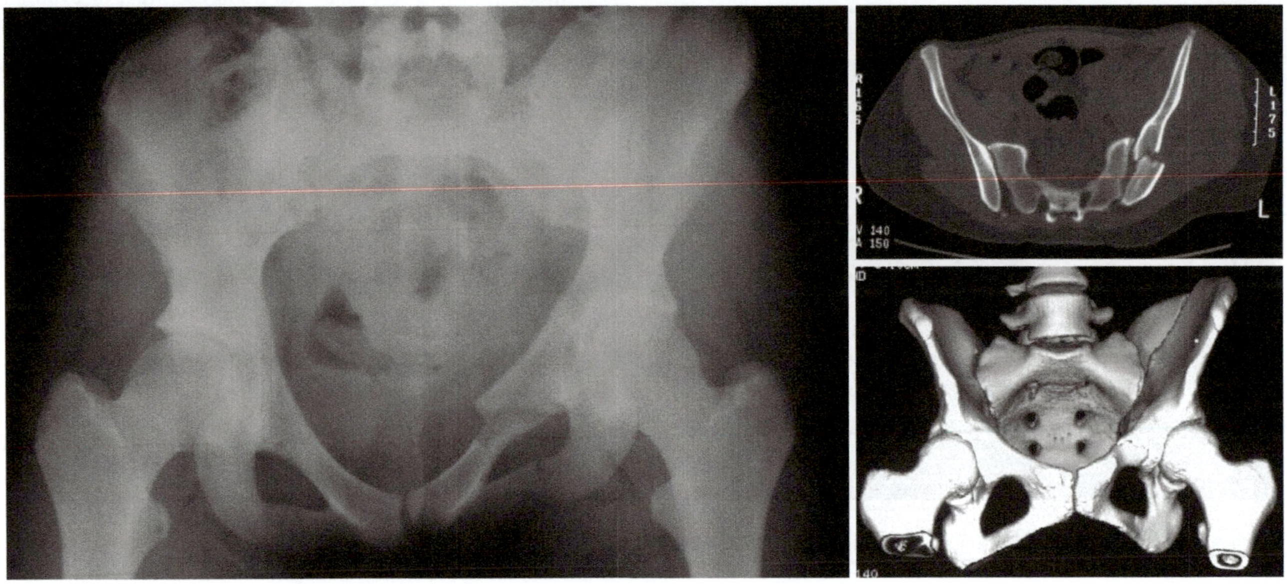

Fig. 4.7 Young-Burgess LC II injury with a fracture dislocation of the left SI joint and left pubic rami fractures

LC III

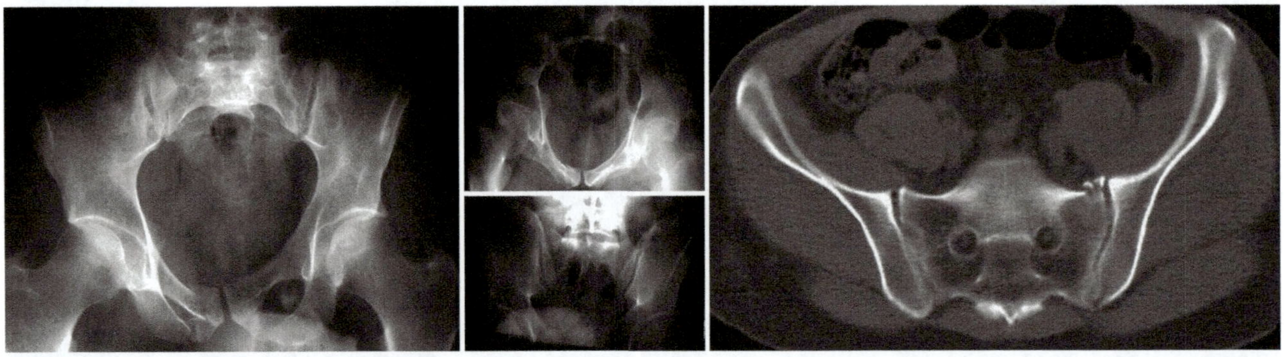

Fig. 4.8 Young-Burgess LC III injury with a combined open book injury of the right SI joint and a lateral compression fracture of the anterior sacrum together with right pubic rami fractures

As dynamic instability testing (Fig. from Sagi) leads to more severe injury subgroups, unstressed imaging may underrepresent the degree of injury and true pelvic instability [31]. Whether stability testing should be performed under general anesthesia is also unknown [29].

The Young-Burgess classification analyzes the injury mechanism, focusing on specific force vectors, especially anterior-posterior mechanisms, lateral compressive forces, and vertical shear mechanisms.

Specific fracture patterns were associated with transfusion requirements and amount of volume replacement [12], while conflicting data exist regarding mortality [12, 17, 26].

Consensus exists that open book APC-type injuries are associated with high risk of fluid requirements and unstable fracture types predicted mortality rate and transfusion requirements [12, 17, 22, 30].

The main disadvantage of the Young-Burgess classification is its limited value regarding guidance of osteoligamentous treatment [31].

4.1.3 AO Classification 2018

The existing Tile AO/OTA classification was recently modified to a 2018 version [32]. Additionally, an attempt was

VS

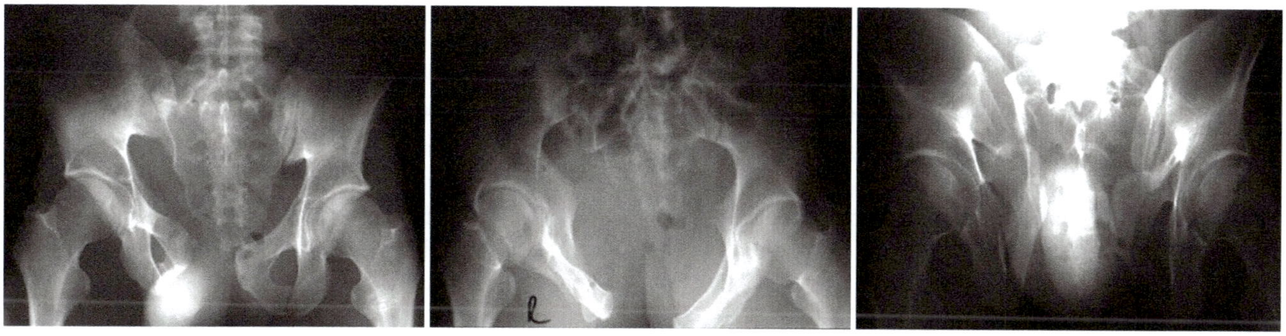

Fig. 4.9 Young-Burgess Vertical Shear (VS) injury with right SI joint dislocation with cranial displacement, symphyseal disruption, right pubic rami fractures, and a left T-type fracture of the acetabulum

CM

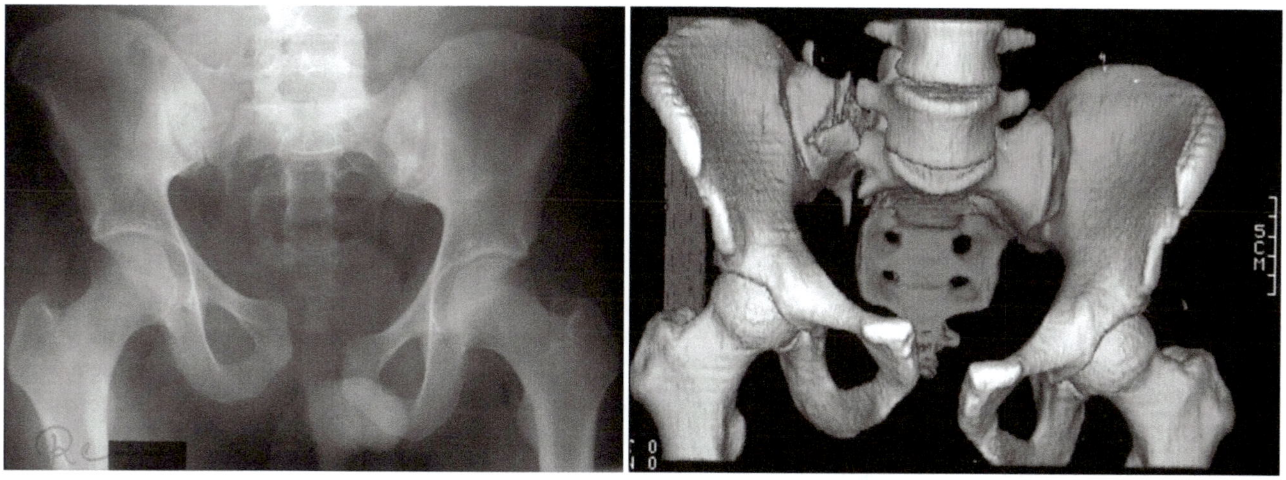

Fig. 4.10 Young-Burgess Complex Mechanism (CM) injury with external rotation injury of the left SI joint, a vertical shear injury of the right sacrum, and a symphyseal disruption

Table 4.2 Typical radiographic findings within the Young-Burgess classification

Fracture type	Pubic #	Sacral #	Acetabular #	Symphysis	SI joint	Iliac wing	Hemipelvic displacement
LC 1	Horizontal	Ipsilateral	Medial wall	No	No	Rare	No
LC 2	Horizontal	Lateral	Medial wall	No	No	Oblique	Minimal medial
LC 3	Horizontal	Lateral	Medial wall	No	AP 2[a]	Oblique/crush	Medio-lateral[b]
AP 1	Vertical	No	A.p. columns	<2.5 cm	No	No	No
AP 2	Vertical	No	A.p. columns	>2.5 cm	Anterior	No	Anterior lateral
AP 3	Vertical	Rare[c]	A.p. columns	Variable	Complete	No	Lateral
VS	Vertical	Vertical	Roof	Variable[d]	Variable[d]	Variable[d]	Vertical

[a]Contralateral SI joint
[b]Ipsilateral medial, contralateral lateral
[c]Sacral avulsion fracture of the pelvic floor ligaments
[d]Vertical displacement

made to correlate the AO classification with the Young-Burgess classification [32].

4.1.3.1 Type A Injuries

61-Type A injuries are defined to have an intact posterior arch. This fracture type is divided into three groups and overall seven subgroups:

61-A1 injuries represent innominate bone avulsion fractures at different locations:

- 61-A1.1: anterior superior iliac spine fracture (Fig. 4.11).
- 61-A1.2: anterior inferior iliac spine fracture (Fig. 4.12).
- 61-A1.3: ischial tuberosity fracture (Fig. 4.13).

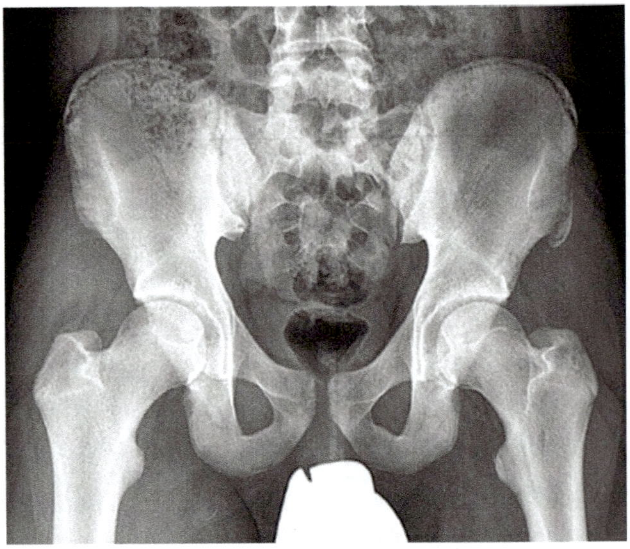

Fig. 4.11 Left anterior superior iliac spine (ASIS) fracture

61-A2 injuries represent innominate bone fractures with an intact posterior arch:

- 61-A2.1: iliac wing fracture (Fig. 4.14).
- 61-A2.2: unilateral fracture of the anterior arch (Fig. 4.15).
- 61-A2.3: bilateral fractures of the anterior arch (Fig. 4.16).

61-A3 injuries represent transverse sacral fractures (S3, S4, S5) below the level of the pelvic brim and the SI joints and coccyx fractures (Fig. 4.17).

4.1.3.2 Type B Injuries

61-Type B injuries are defined as incomplete disruption of posterior arch. This fracture type is divided into three groups and overall eight subgroups:

61-B1 injuries represent with incomplete disruption of the posterior arch without rotational/posterior instability and are subdivided into two subgroups:

- 61-B1.1: lateral compression fracture (LC 1; see Fig. 4.6).
- 61-A1.2: open book fracture (APC 1; see Fig. 4.3).

Modifiers for type B1.1 injuries were added and include an ipsilateral or unilateral pubic ramus fracture, bilateral pubic rami fractures, a contralateral pubic ramus fracture, a parasymphyseal fracture, a tilt fracture, or a locked symphysis.

61-B2 injuries are rotationally unstable and present with a unilateral posterior injury, These injuries are subdivided into three subgroups:

- 61-B2.1: lateral sacral compression fracture with internal rotation instability (LC I04b; see Fig. 4.6).

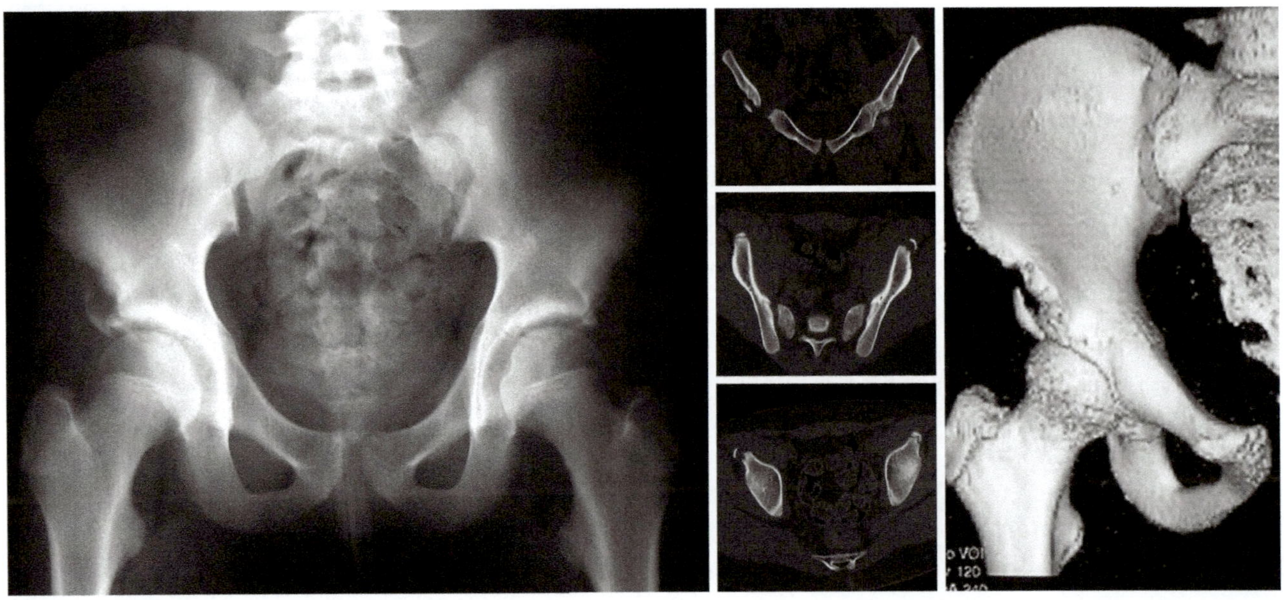

Fig. 4.12 Right anterior inferior iliac spine (AIIS) fracture

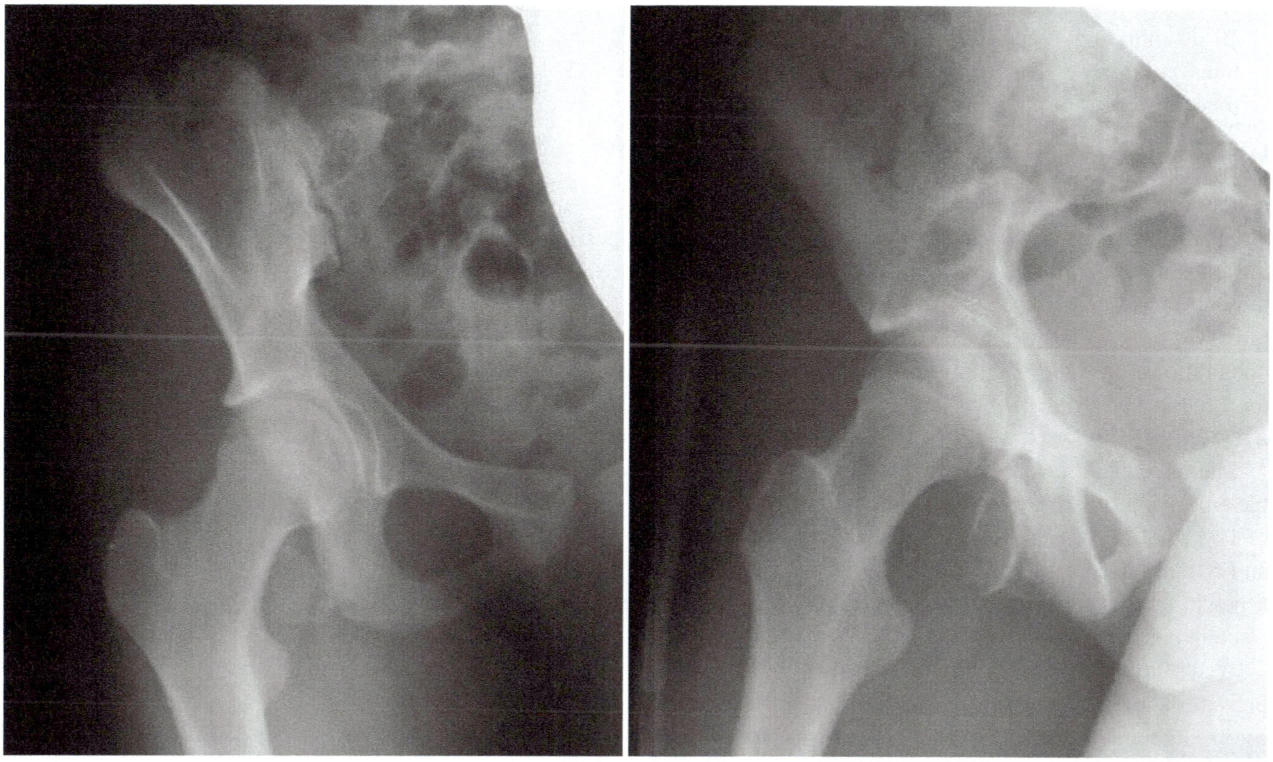

Fig. 4.13 Right avulsion injury of the ischial tuberosity

- 61-B2.2: lateral compression fracture of the ilium (crescent) with internal rotation instability (LC 2; see Fig. 4.7).
- 61-B2.3: open book or external rotation instability (APC 2; see Fig. 4.4b).

Modifiers for type B2 injuries were added and include an ipsilateral or unilateral pubic ramus fracture, bilateral pubic rami fractures, a contralateral pubic ramus fracture, a symphyseal disruption, a parasymphyseal fracture, a tilt fracture, or a locked symphysis.

61-B3 injuries are incomplete posterior arch injuries, which are rotationally unstable, and present with bilateral posterior injury. These injuries are subdivided into three subgroups:

- 61-B3.1: internal rotation instability on one side and external rotation instability on the contralateral side (LC 3; see Fig. 4.8).
- 61-B3.2: bilateral lateral compression (LC) sacral fracture (Fig. 4.18).
- 61-B3.3: open book or external rotation instability (bilateral APC 2, Fig. 4.19).

Modifiers for B3 injuries were added and include an ipsilateral or unilateral pubic ramus fracture, bilateral pubic rami fractures, a symphyseal disruption, a parasymphyseal fracture, a tilt fracture, or a locked symphysis.

4.1.3.3 Type C Injuries

61-Type C injuries are defined as complete disruption of posterior arch. This fracture type is divided into three groups and overall nine subgroups:

61-C1 injuries present with complete unilateral disruption of the posterior arch (APC3, vertical shear) and are subdivided into three subgroups:

- 61-C1.1: posterior complete ilium fracture (Fig. 4.20).
- 61-C1.2: through the sacroiliac joint (Fig. 4.21).
- 61-C1.3: sacrum fracture (Fig. 4.22).

Modifiers of C1 injuries were added and include ipsilateral or unilateral pubic ramus fracture, bilateral pubic rami fracture, contralateral pubic ramus fracture, symphyseal disruption, parasymphyseal fracture, tilt fracture, locked symphysis, and sacroiliac joint fracture dislocation.

61-C2 injuries present with bilateral posterior injury with a complete hemipelvic injury on one side and a contralateral incomplete hemipelvic injury (LC 3) on the other side. These injuries are subdivided into three subgroups:

- 61-C2.1: complete disruption through ilium.
- 61-C2.2: complete disruption through the sacroiliac joint.
- 61-C2.3: sacrum fracture.

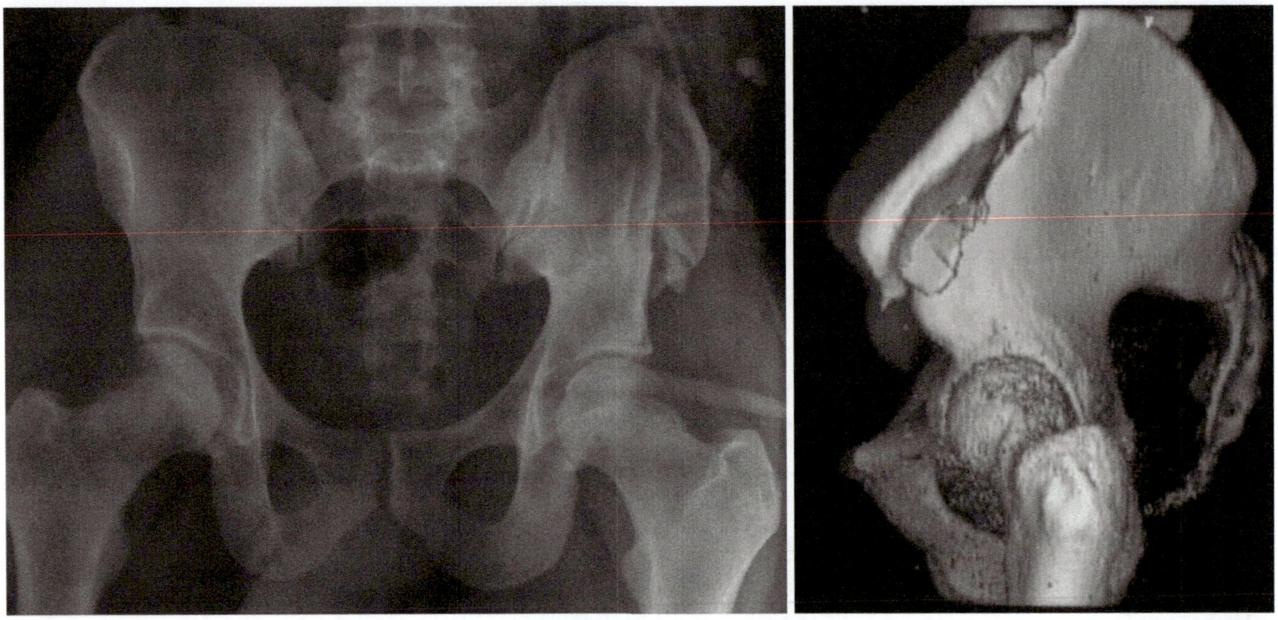

Fig. 4.14 AO/OTA A2.1 left iliac wing fracture without involvement of the pelvic ring

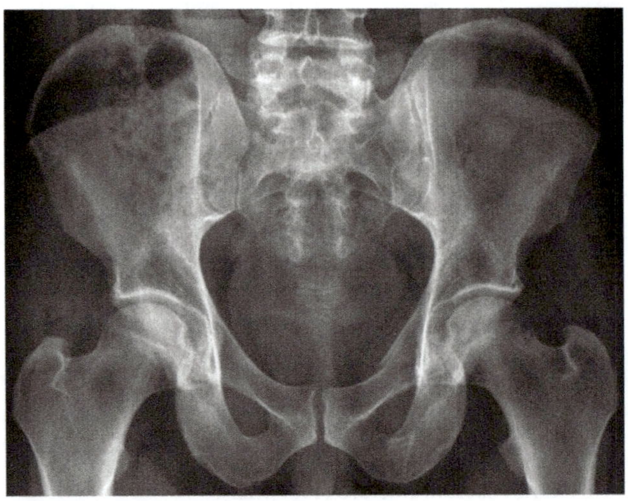

Fig. 4.15 AO/OTA A2.2 isolated unilateral fracture of the left anterior ring without posterior ring injury

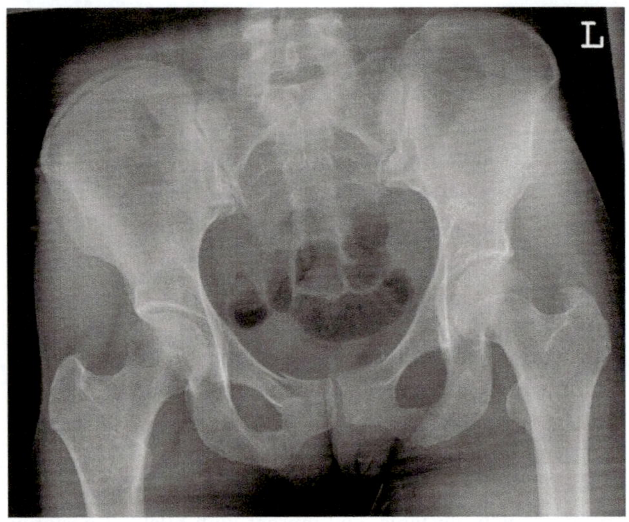

Fig. 4.16 AO/OTA A2.3 isolated bilateral fracture of the anterior ring segment; no signs of posterior pelvic ring involvement

Modifiers of C2 injuries were added and include ipsilateral or unilateral pubic ramus fracture, bilateral pubic rami fracture, contralateral pubic ramus fracture, symphyseal disruption, parasymphyseal fracture, tilt fracture, or locked symphysis. The contralateral posterior injury can consist of a lateral compression sacral fracture, a posterior lateral compression lesion of the ilium (crescent fracture), a posterior external rotation lesion of the SI joint, or a posterior external rotation lesion presenting with a fracture dislocation. No modifiers are added to the type C lesion regarding sacroiliac joint fracture dislocation.

61-C3 injuries present with bilateral complete posterior injury (APC 3, vertical shear) and are subdivided into three subgroups:

- 61-C3.1: extrasacral on both sides.
- 61-C3.2: sacral on one side, extrasacral on the other side.
- 61-C3.3: sacral on both sides.

Modifiers of C3 injuries were added and include ipsilateral or unilateral pubic ramus fracture, bilateral pubic rami fracture, contralateral pubic ramus fracture, symphyseal disruption, parasymphyseal fracture, tilt fracture, locked symphysis, iliac wing fracture, and sacroiliac joint disruption. No modifier is added to the type C lesion regarding sacroiliac joint fracture dislocation.

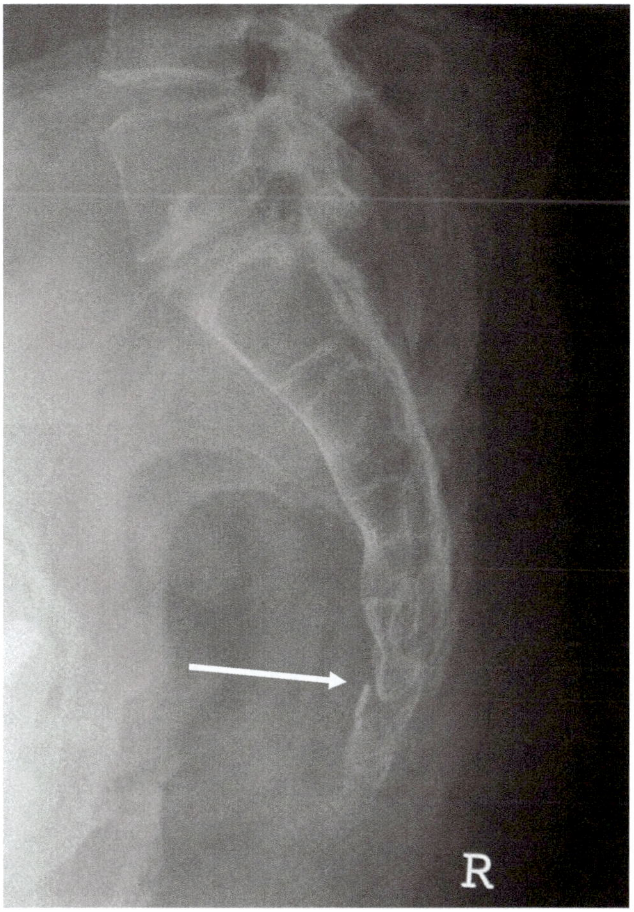

Fig. 4.17 AO/OTA A3 injury: transverse distal sacral fracture below the pelvic ring level

Fractures of the upper sacral segments attached to sacroiliac joints (S1, S2) are classified as part of the pelvic ring injury.

An additional sacral classification as part of the spinal fracture classification was recommended.

4.1.3.4 Authors' Comment

It seems useful to combine the presently most commonly used pelvic ring classification Schemes (AO/OTA and Young-Burgess).

Even the 2018 version of the AO/OTA classification shows some difficult parts.

A classification should be simple and easy to use [33], giving the possibility of logical treatment decisions [6, 34, 35] and thus helping the surgeon to choose a fracture type-based treatment concept. Additionally, for the selected treatment, a prognostic estimation should be possible [7].

The present universal and comprehensive classification still favors prognostic relevance with increasing pelvic ring instability from A1 to C3 injuries.

Especially, B type injuries became more unclear. In contrast to prior versions, the B1 injury is no longer a rotationally unstable injury as before.

B2 and B3 injuries now exclusively represent rotationally unstable injuries with partial persistent posterior stability. B2.1, B2.3, and all B3 injuries are classical type B injuries, which most often only require anterior pelvic ring fixation, while B2.2 injuries are primarily focused on the injury mechanism (lateral compression) resulting in a crescent type fracture. The majority of these injuries lead to complete injury of the posterior arch, and therefore, anterior and posterior fixation is required. For a long time, this is an ongoing problem with the Young-Burgess classification, as the

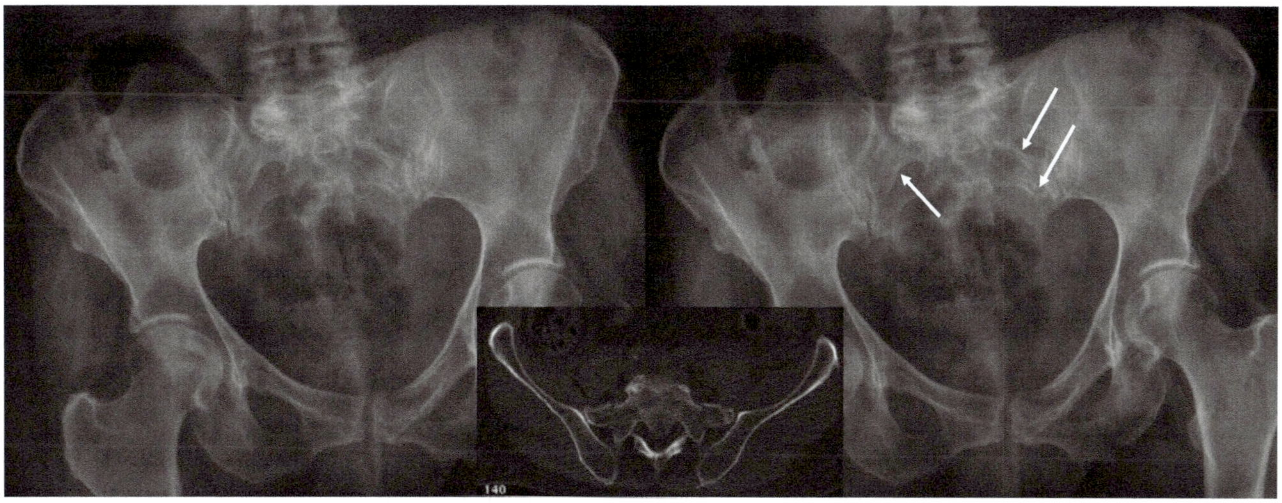

Fig. 4.18 AO/OTA B3.2: bilateral posterior lateral compression injury of the sacrum (arrows) confirmed on CT evaluation, often seen in geriatric (insufficiency) fractures

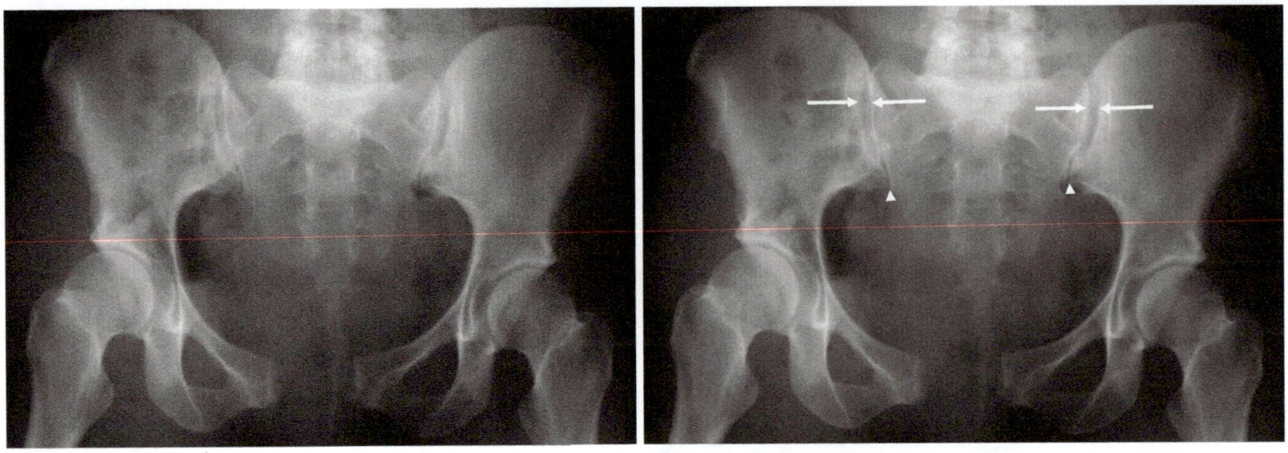

Fig. 4.19 AO/OTA B3.3: bilateral posterior external rotation injury (bilateral APC II). Anterior widening of both SI joints is visible (arrows), while the posterior SI joint ligaments remain intact (arrowhead)

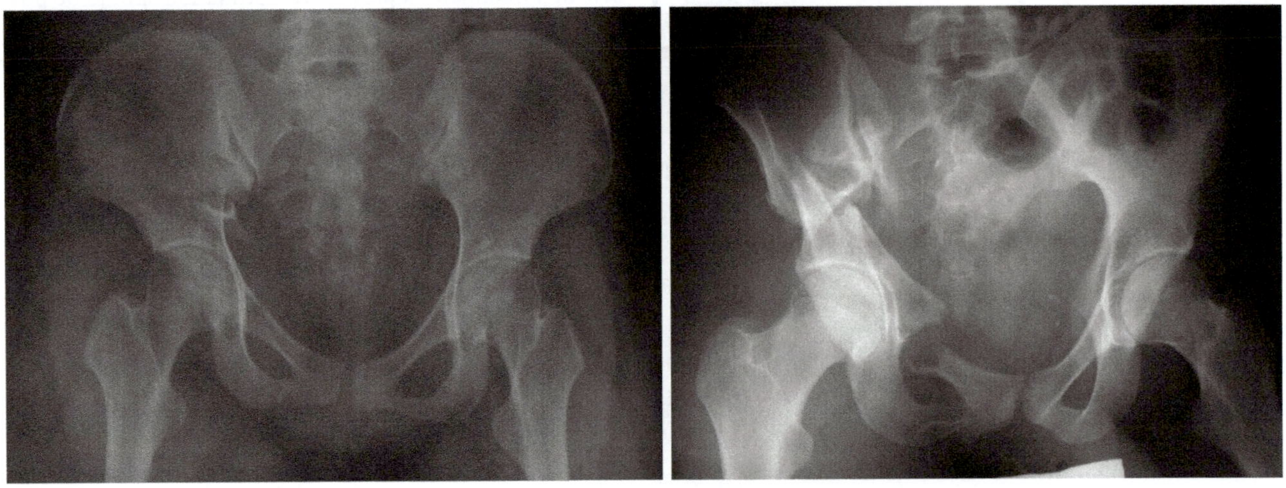

Fig. 4.20 Two cases of an AO/OTA C1.1 injury with a right unilateral complete ilium fracture not extending into the SI joint or acetabulum

morphology of the crescent fracture represents complete posterior disruption.

Another disadvantage of the present classification is the incomplete description of the posterior ring involvement. In C1 injuries, an injury to the SI joint can be modified by description of a sacroiliac joint fracture dislocation, while in C2 and C3 injuries, this option does not exist.

4.1.4 Reliability Analyses

Data on reliability analyses reported conflicting data regarding the classical classification systems.

The relevance of the pelvic a.p. X-ray has been reported by several authors. Accordingly, primary correct diagnoses can be expected in up to 90% of patients [16, 36, 37].

Young et al. reported a rate of primarily correct identifications of pelvic ring injuries in up to 94% [16]. Conventional radiographic results were compared with CT data.

Similar results were stated in the analysis by Edeicken-Monroe et al., who were able to confirm the primary diagnoses compared to a pelvic CT in 88% [36]. Resnik et al. used the pelvic CT as a gold standard and were able to confirm fractures and dislocations of the pelvic ring [37]. Only 9% of the injuries were overlooked without therapeutic consequence.

Koo et al. analyzed the Tile and Young-Burgess classification comparing standard three conventional radiographic views with CT scans in 30 patients [38].

When only analyzing plain radiographs, experienced acetabular/pelvic surgeons were able to adequately classify the injury using the Young-Burgess system as well as the Tile fracture type and subgroup with an excellent level of agreement.

In contrast, the Tile classification was inadequate for orthopedic traumatologists and senior trainees with only slight agreement levels, while orthopedic traumatologists and senior trainees showed substantial and moderate agreement using the Young-Burgess classification, respectively.

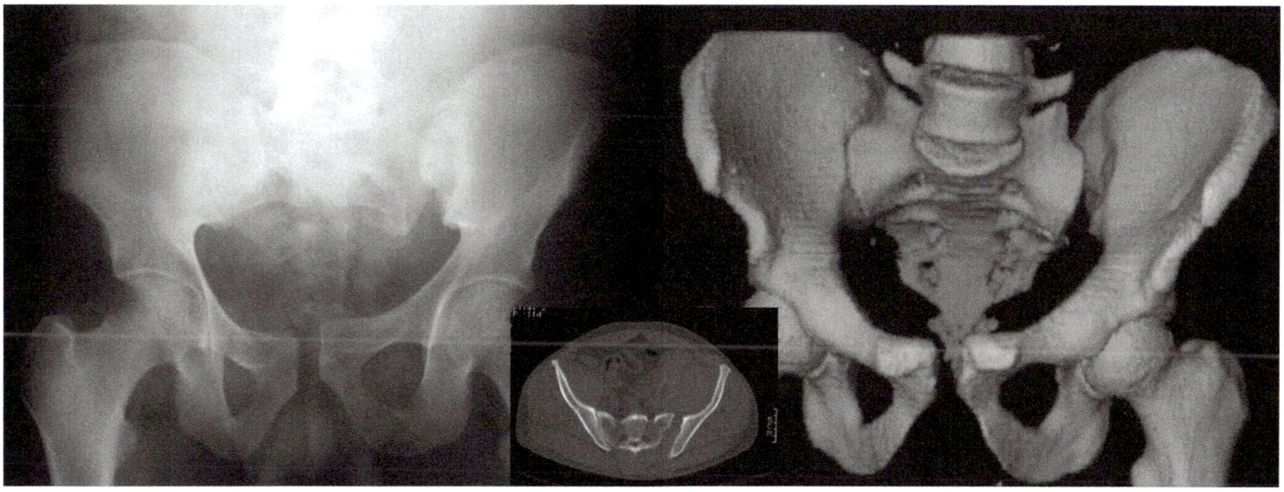

Fig. 4.21 AO/OTA C1.2 injury with left unilateral complete SI joint dislocation and symphyseal disruption

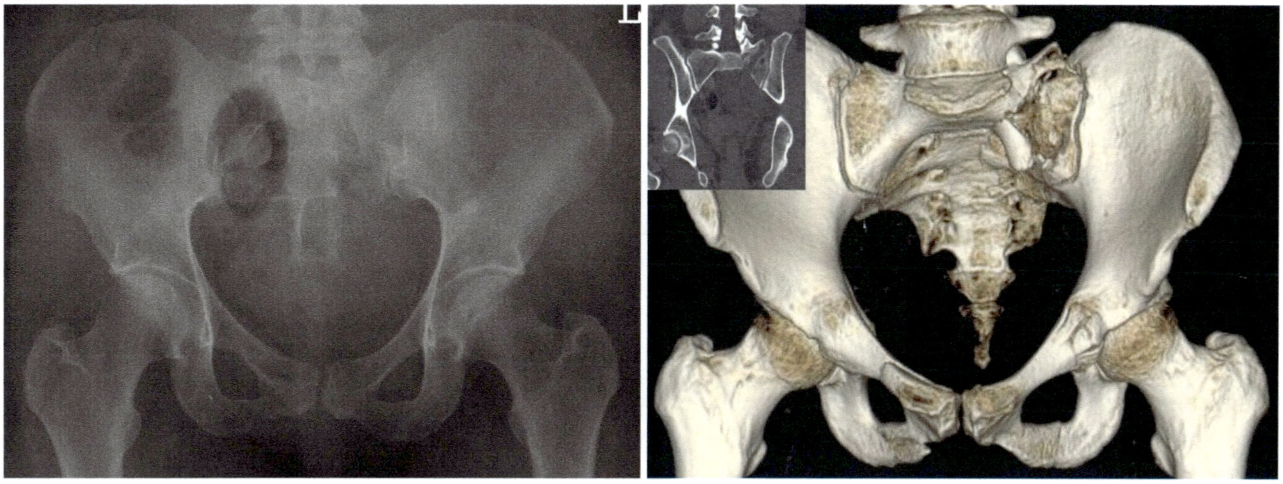

Fig. 4.22 AO/OTA C1.3 injury with left unilateral complete transforaminal sacral fracture and bilateral pubic rami fractures

Adding the CT resulted in only slight better result for less experienced surgeons.

Additionally, some special radiographic features were analyzed. Using plain radiographs alone showed high agreement in detecting posterior displacement >1 cm and symphysis diastasis >2.5 cm, while moderate agreement was found regarding identification of a fracture of the L5 transverse process and stability analysis of the pelvis.

The additional CT evaluation increased the agreement rate for pelvic stability to excellent agreement, while the rate of posterior displacement >1 cm did not change.

It was concluded that:

- CT scan is of value regarding assessment of pelvic stability.
- The Young-Burgess system is ideal for the learning surgeon.
- The Tile classification system may be of benefit for pelvic and acetabular surgeons.

Furey et al. analyzed the conventional radiographs and CT scans in 89 patients by five experienced orthopedic surgeons and reported high agreement for the Young and Burgess classification and moderate agreement for the Tile comprehensive classification [39].

In a recent analysis by Gabbe et al., experienced orthopedic trauma surgeons evaluated the Young-Burgess classification system in 100 patients using plain a.p. radiographs and 3D CT data [40]. The overall agreement rate for both the Young-Burgess and Tile classification systems was low.

4.1.5 Fragility Fractures of the Pelvis (FFP)

With the ongoing demographic change, new pelvic fracture patterns were identified in the elderly population, leading to special treatment considerations.

The present well-accepted comprehensive FFP classification (Fig. 4.23) of these geriatric fractures was proposed by

Rommens et al. and guided by special stabilization techniques [41–43].

FFP type I injuries represent isolated anterior pelvic ring injuries. With increasing use of CT diagnostics in the majority of all suspected pelvic fracture patients, these injuries are expected in low frequency. Two subgroups were distinguished:

- FFP type Ia: unilateral anterior pelvic ring fracture (Fig. 4.23a).
- FFP type Ib: bilateral anterior pelvic ring fracture (Fig. 4.23b).

FFP type II injuries are defined as non-displaced posterior lesions with or without an additional anterior pelvic ring injury. These injuries account for approximately 50% of all FFP [43].

- FFP type IIa: isolated non-displaced posterior injury (most commonly an anterior sacral fracture (Fig. 4.23c)).
- FFP type IIb: sacral crush fracture with a concomitant anterior pelvic ring injury (B2 or LC 1 injury (Fig. 4.23d)).
- FFP type IIc: non-displaced sacral, sacroiliac, or iliac fracture with a concomitant anterior pelvic ring injury (Fig. 4.23e).

FFP type III injuries present with a displaced unilateral posterior injury combined with an anterior pelvic ring lesion, according to a type C injury of the pelvis.

- FFP type IIIa: displaced ilium fracture (Fig. 4.23f).
- FFP type IIIb: displaced SI joint disruption (Fig. 4.23g).
- FFP type IIIc: displaced unilateral sacral fracture (Fig. 4.23h).

FFP type IV injuries are defined as displaced bilateral posterior pelvic ring injuries.

- FFP type IVa: bilateral ilium fractures or bilateral SI joint disruptions (Fig. 4.23i).
- FFP type IVb: spinopelvic dissociation with a bilateral longitudinal Denis zone I injury and an additional transverse fracture component (H- and U-type injuries: Fig. 4.23j).
- FFP type IVc: combination of different posterior instabilities (Fig. 4.23k).

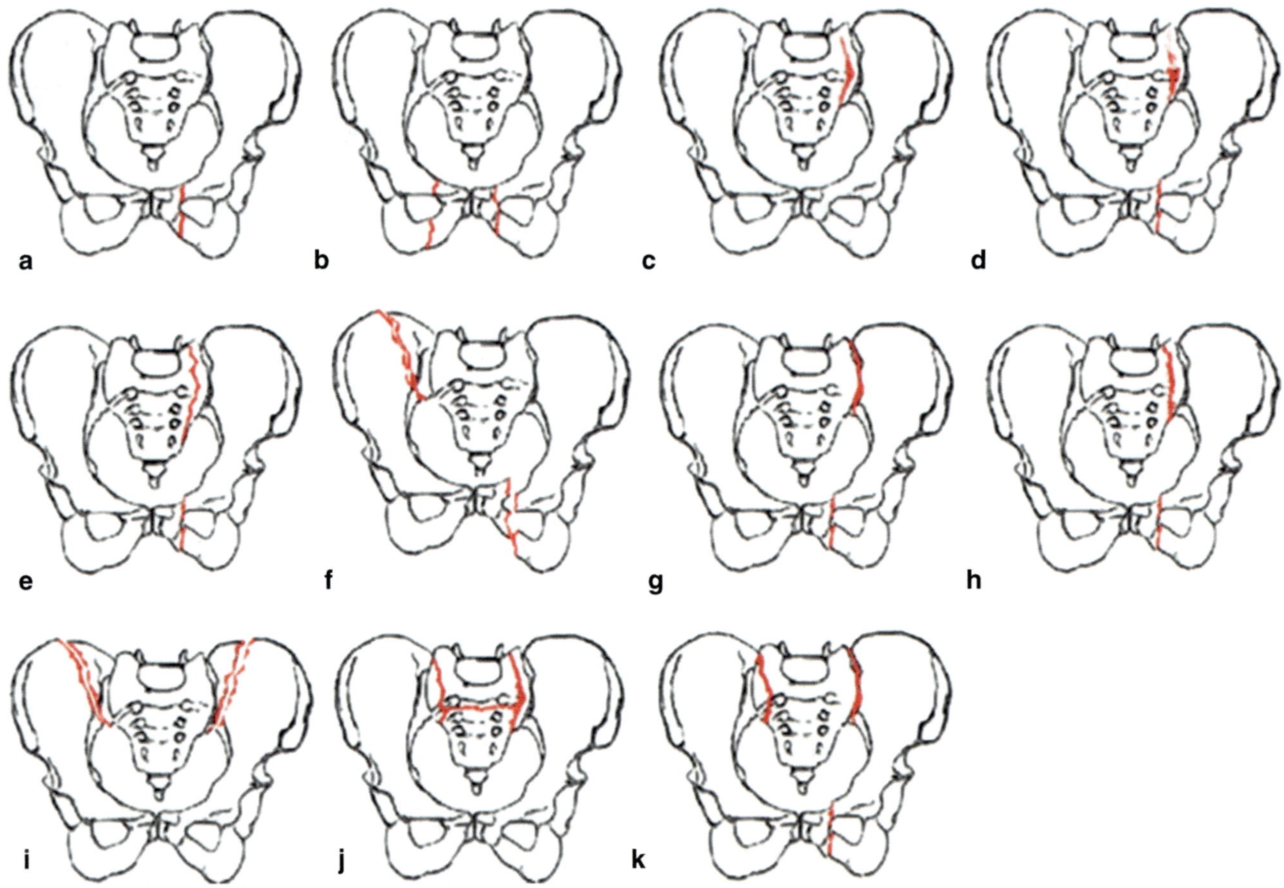

Fig. 4.23 (**a**) FFP type Ia: unilateral anterior pelvic ring fracture. (**b**) FFP type Ib: bilateral anterior pelvic ring fracture. (**c**) FFP type IIa: isolated non-displaced posterior injury (most commonly an anterior sacral fracture). (**d**) FFP type IIb: sacral crush fracture with a concomitant anterior pelvic ring injury (B2 or LC 1 injury). (**e**) FFP type IIc: non-displaced sacral, sacroiliac, or iliac fracture with a concomitant anterior pelvic ring injury. (**f**) FFP type IIIa: displaced ilium fracture. (**g**) FFP type IIIb: displaced SI joint disruption. (**h**) FFP type IIIc: displaced unilateral sacral fracture. (**i**) FFP type IVa: bilateral ilium fractures or bilateral SI joint disruptions. (**j**) FFP type IVb: spinopelvic dissociation with a bilateral longitudinal Denis zone I injury and an additional transverse fracture component (H- and U-type injuries). (**k**) FFP type IVc: combination of different posterior instabilities

4.1.6 Classifications of the Posterior Pelvic Ring Complex

The relevance of the posterior pelvic ring complex in terms of prognostic and therapeutic challenges led to several subclassifications.

These subclassifications include different sacrum classifications and a classification of SI joint injuries.

4.1.6.1 SI Joint Injuries

Tan et al. subdivided SI joint injuries (Fig. 4.24) [44].

- Type I: sacroiliac anterior dislocation (Fig. 4.24).
- Type II: sacroiliac posterior dislocation (Fig. 4.25).
- Type III: crescent fracture dislocation of the SI joint.

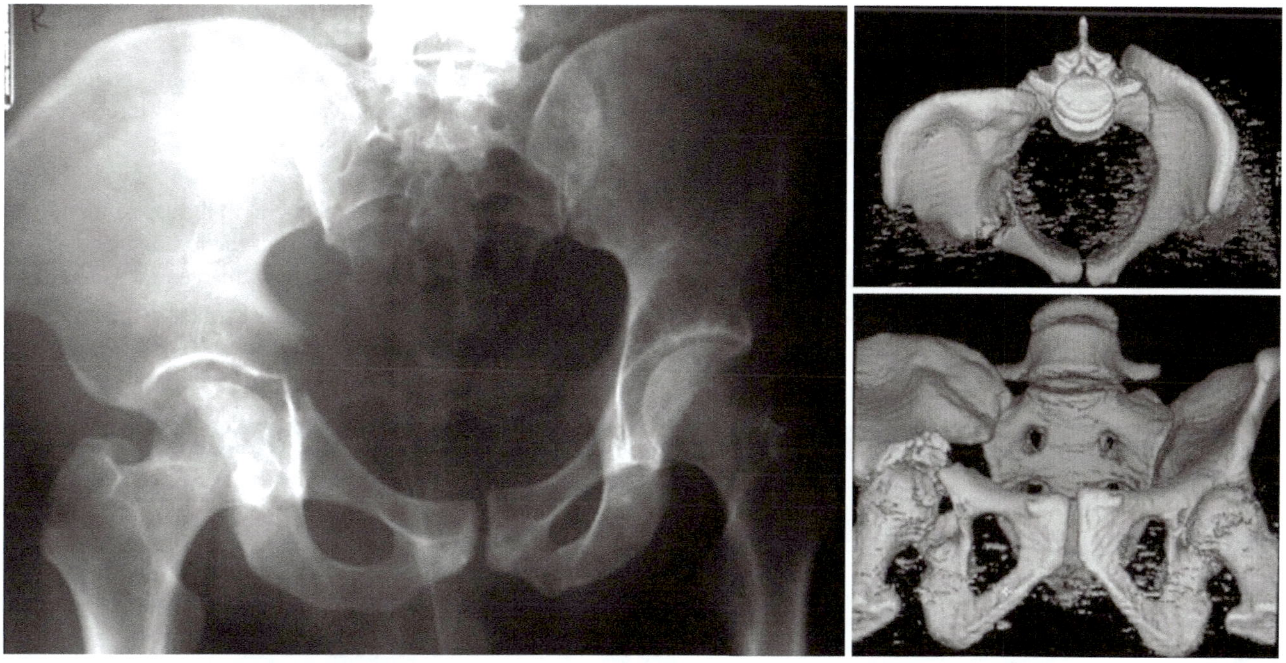

Fig. 4.24 Type I SI joint injury with anterior hemipelvic dislocation

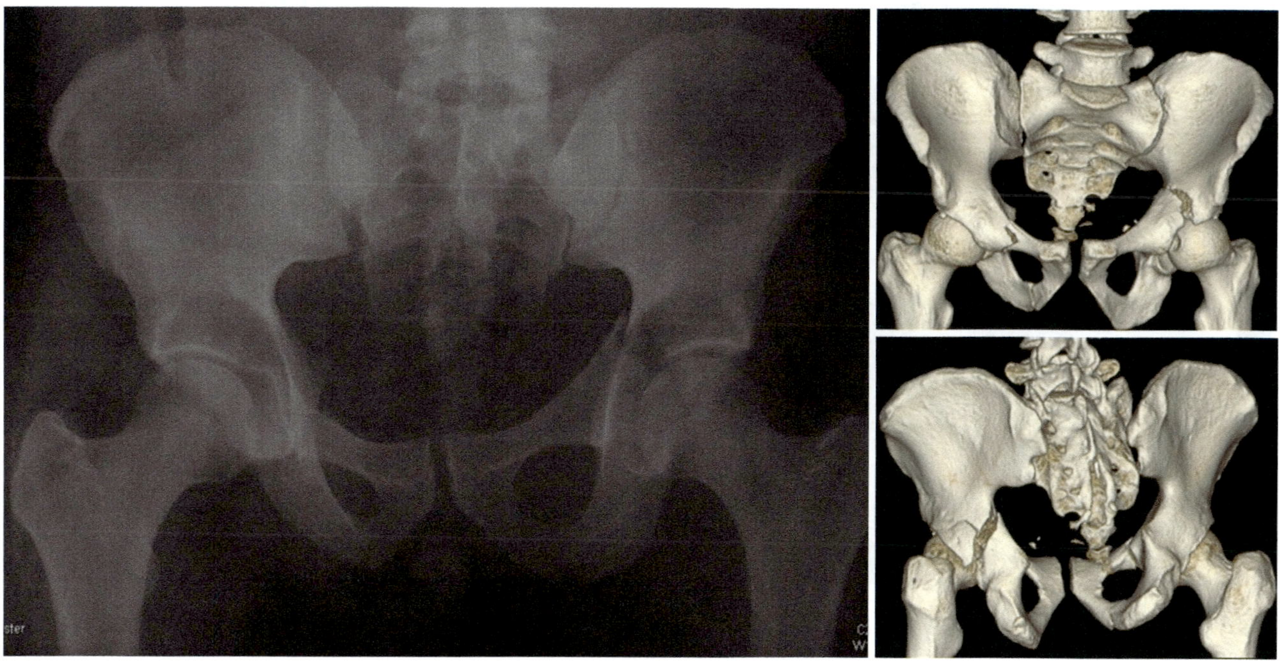

Fig. 4.25 Type II SI joint injury with posterior hemipelvic dislocation

The crescent fracture types are further subdivided into three categories (Fig. 4.26):

- Type IIIa: <1/3 involvement of the SI joint with a large crescent fragment (Fig. 4.27).
- Type IIIb: 1/3–2/3 SI joint involvement with an intermediate crescent fragment (Fig. 4.28).
- Type IIIc: >2/3 SI joint involvement and a small crescent fragment (Fig. 4.29).

4.1.6.2 Sacral Fracture Classifications

Sacral fracture classifications primarily focused on additional nerve injury, posterior stability with involvement of the lumbosacral region, and lumbosacral fractures.

Focus on Nerve Injury

Schmidek et al. proposed a classification of sacral fractures, distinguishing between direct and indirect traumas [45]. Direct trauma resulted in penetrating sacral fractures or in transverse fractures below the level of S2. Indirect fractures can be present isolated as high transverse fractures at the level of S1 or S2 or present as lumbosacral fracture dislocations. Additionally, several sacral fractures were seen in combination with other pelvic ring lesions (lateral sacral mass fracture, juxtaarticular fracture, cleaving fracture (central fracture), avulsion fractures, and combination of these) [45].

With increasing understanding of sacral fractures and upcoming surgical stabilization methods, several new classifications were developed, especially to focus on prognosis and accompanying nerve deficits.

The well-accepted classification of sacral fractures was described by Denis et al., who distinguished three types of sacral fractures (Fig. 4.30) [46]:

- Zone 1 fractures: ala zone, lateral to the sacral foramina.
- Zone 2 fractures: in the region of the foramina.
- Zone 3 fractures: involvement of the central sacral canal region.

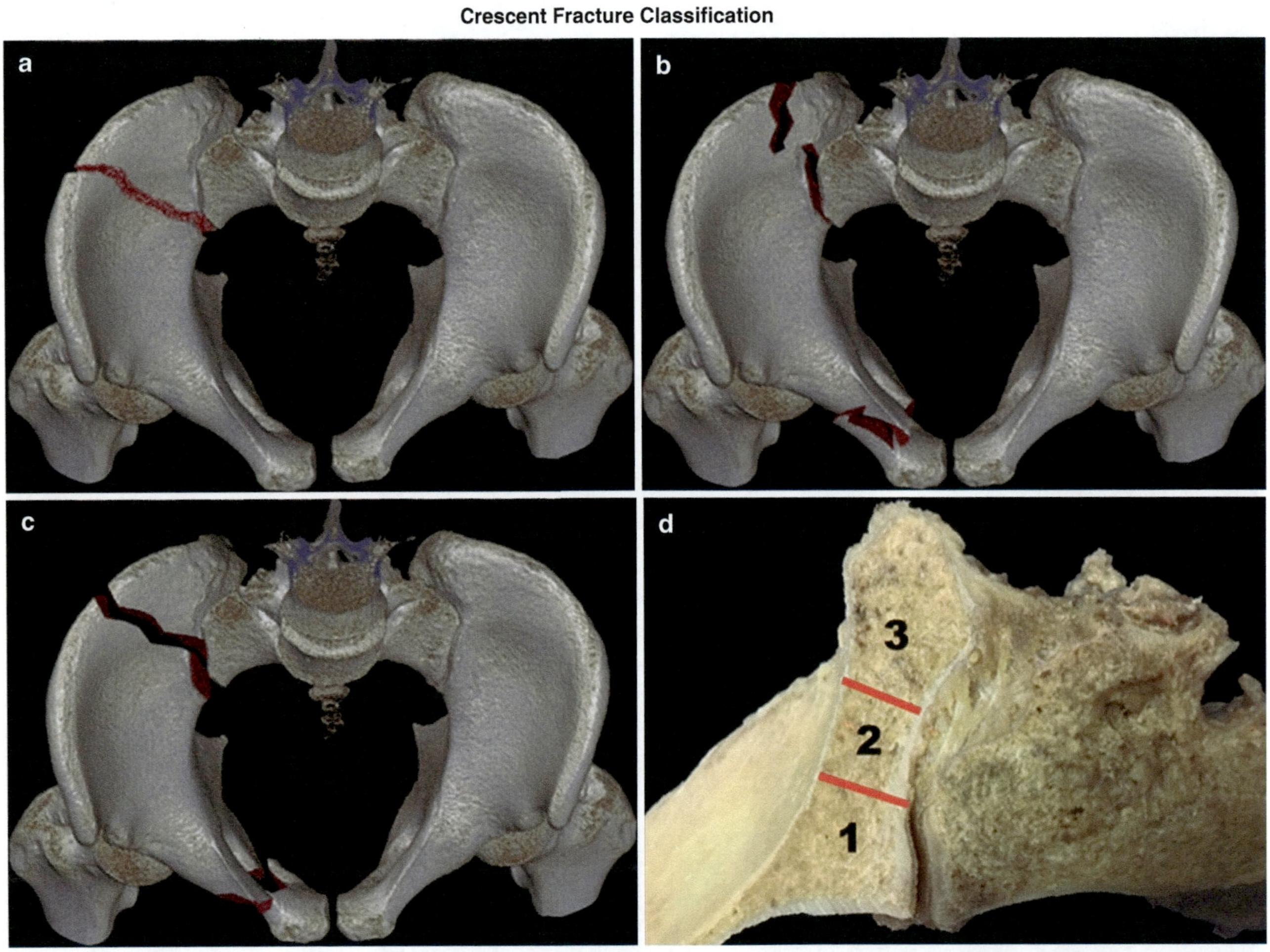

Fig. 4.26 Type III SI joint injury: three types of crescent fracture dislocations (anterior (**a**), intermediate (**b**), and posterior (**c**) SI joint injury) and anatomic definition (**d**)

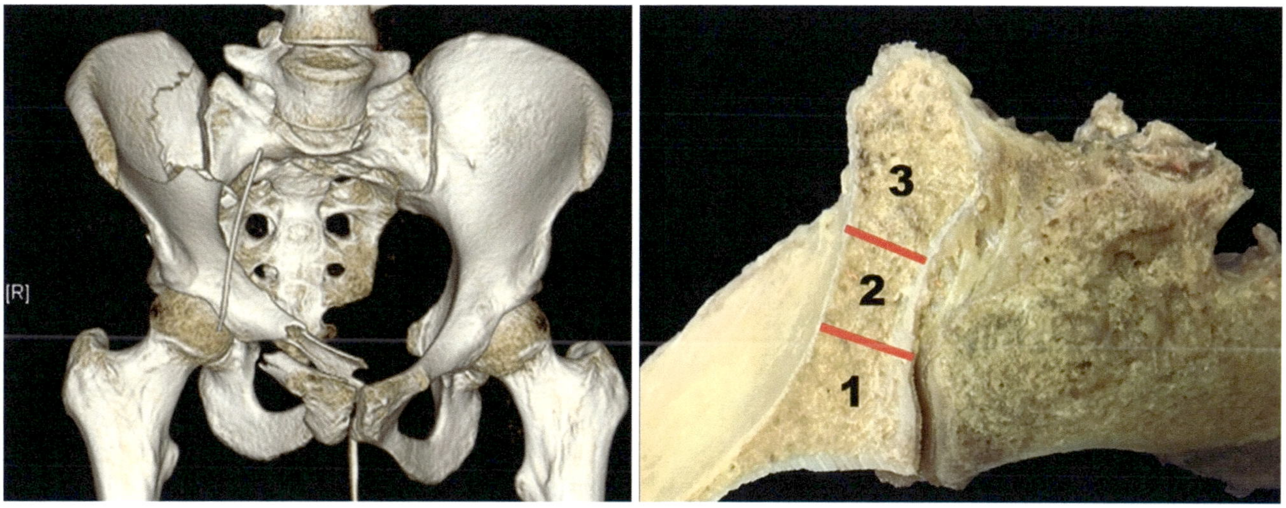

Fig. 4.27 Type I SI joint injury with anterior (1) SI joint injury.

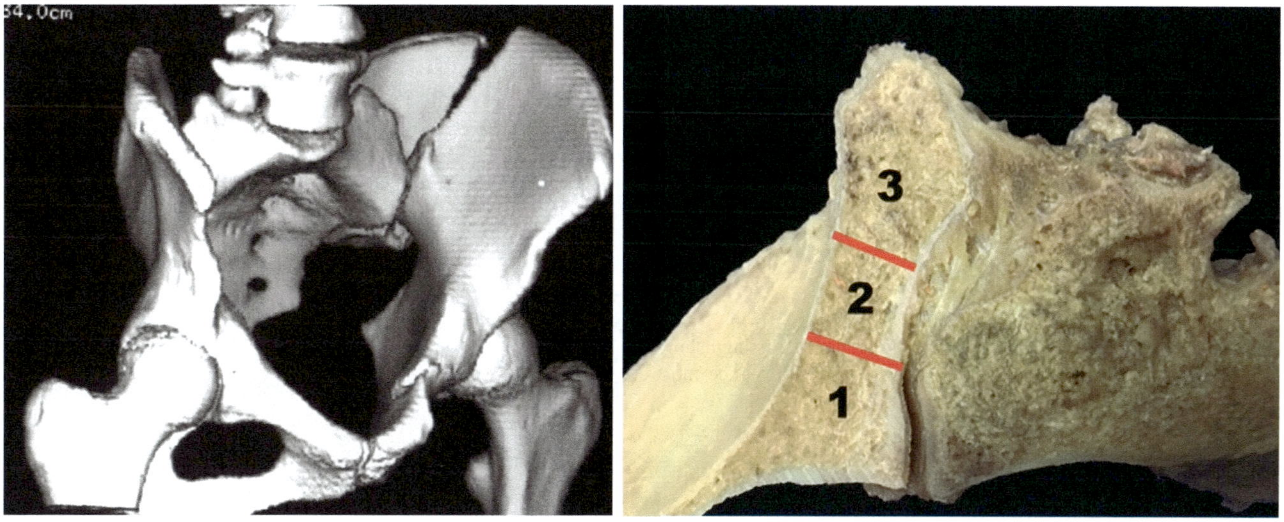

Fig. 4.28 Type II SI joint injury with intermediate (2) SI joint injury

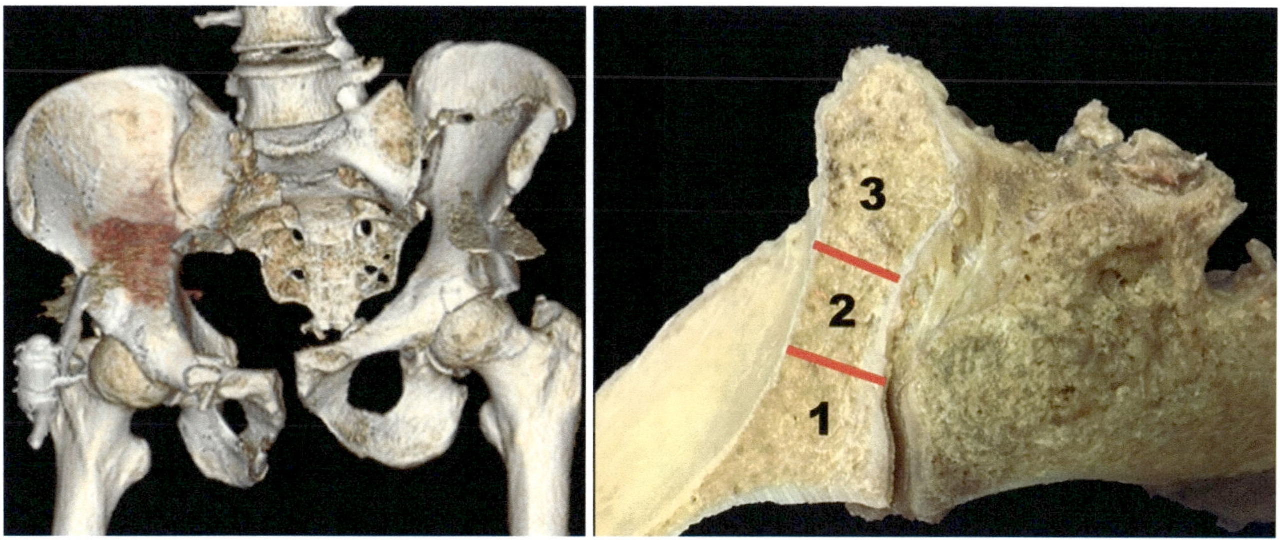

Fig. 4.29 Type III SI joint injury with posterior (3) SI joint injury

This classification is clinically useful, as it showed an increased risk of additional nerve injuries from zone 1 to zone 3 [46–51]. Zone 3 injuries included severely displaced transverse sacral fractures below the level of S2 as well as lumbosacral fracture dislocations [46] and were associated with the highest risk of fracture-related nerve injury [46, 47, 50–52].

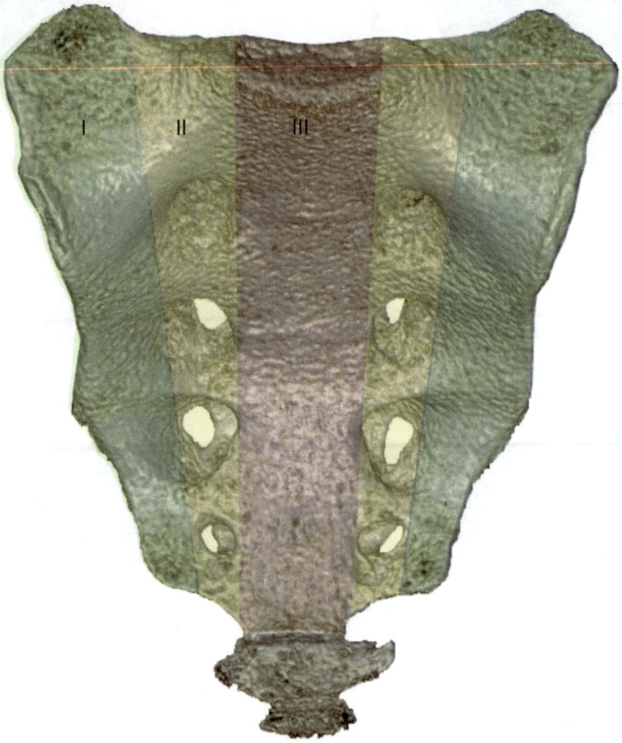

Fig. 4.30 Denis classification of sacral fractures distinguishing between alar (I), foraminal (II), and central (III) fractures. The most medial fracture defines the classification

Focus on Lumbosacral Lesions

Isler identified three types of associated lumbosacral junction lesions (Fig. 4.31) in an analysis of 134 unstable pelvic ring injuries [53]:

- Extraarticular L5/S1 facet joint fractures either involving the L5 articular process or the S1 articular process.
- Articular L5/S1 facet joint fractures presenting with complete fracture dislocations, subluxations, or locked dislocations.
- Complex injuries with fractures of the articular processes, interarticular portions, laminae, and pedicles.

These injuries are clinically relevant, as sacral fracture reduction can be impaired and joint degeneration can lead to persistent and increasing lumbosacral pain [53].

Oransky et al. and Leone et al. added a fourth category with an L5-S1 intervertebral disk injury, lateral bending of the L5 body, and asymmetry of L5/S1 intervertebral space [54, 55].

Lumbosacral Dissociations

Since the first description of lumbopelvic dissociation fractures by Roy-Camille et al. [56], several modifications of these specific injury types were reported in the literature.

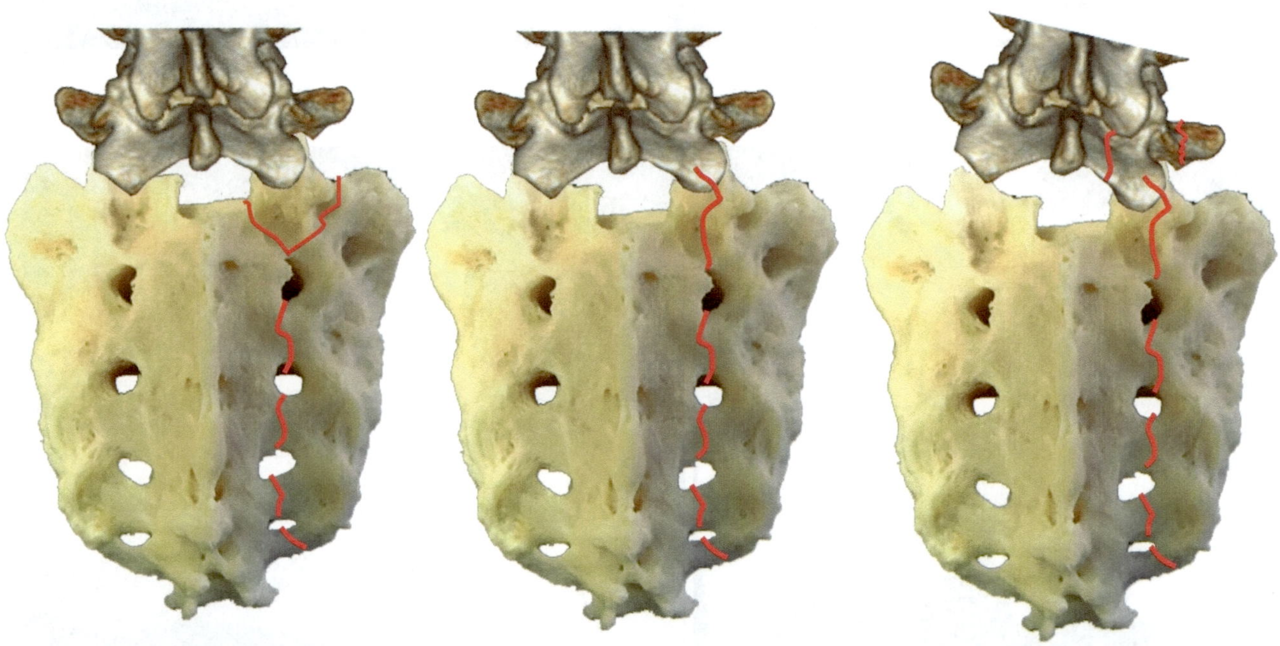

Fig. 4.31 Lumbosacral junction lesions according to Isler (details: see text)

Roy-Camille et al. already described the spinopelvic dissociation injury, but they classified only the transverse sacral fracture, not the bilateral vertical fracture components [57]. Roy-Camille et al. divided these superior transverse sacral fractures into three types:

- Type 1: flexion fracture with anterior simple bending of the upper sacrum without translational displacement.
- Type 2: flexion fracture with posterior displacement of the upper sacrum that becomes more or less horizontal and settles itself on the fractured surface of the lower fragment.
- Type 3: extension fracture with anterior displacement of the upper fragment more or less vertical that slips downward in front of the lower fragment.

Strange-Vongsen and Lebech added a fourth type [58]:

- Type 4: neutral position fracture with total comminution of the upper sacrum without displacement from the lower fragment.

This type 4 fracture is more a burst fracture of S1-S2 with bone retropulsion and not a true transverse sacral fracture [59].

This subclassification is well accepted in the scientific literature [60–64]. The additional, often bilateral vertical sacral fractures associated with a transverse fracture might form the so-called H-, U-, Y-, or lambda-shaped fracture patterns [60–65].

These sacral fracture types, together with the upper sacral burst fracture or complete sacral burst fractures, are clinically observed.

Lehman et al. proposed a lumbosacral injury classification system based on injury morphology, posterior ligamentous complex integrity, and the neurologic status, with a severity analysis of each parameter [65].

Morphological criteria included the presence of:

- Flexion compression: ≤20° kyphosis (1 point), >20° kyphosis (2 points).
- Axial compression (comminution of upper sacrum); with/without (3 points/2 points) sacral canal or neuroforaminal encroachment.
- Translation/rotation (3 points): anterior or posterior translation of upper sacrum, lumbosacral facet injury, or dislocation or vertical translation or instability.
- Blast/shear injury (4 points, severe comminution or segmental bone loss).

Modifiers are the integrity of the posterior ligamentous complex (PLC), which includes the supraspinous ligament, interspinous ligament, ligamentum flavum, iliolumbar ligament, lateral lumbosacral ligament, and the facet joint capsule. These ligamentous structures provide restraint against deforming forces, particularly anterior translation and flexion deformity [65].

The PLC status distinguishes between intact ligamentous structures (0 points) and an indeterminate (1 point) or disrupted status (2 points) [65].

The additional neurological scoring was graded into five categories [65]:

- Neurologically intact (0 points).
- Paresthesias only (1 point).
- Lower extremity motor deficit (2 points).
- Bowel/bladder dysfunction (3 points).
- Progressive neurologic deficit (4 points).

The total score of the resulting "Cumulative Injury Severity Score" (CISS) can range from 1 to 10 points. Patients with a score < 4 points can be treated conservatively, while patients with a score > 4 points should be treated with osteosynthesis. In patients with a score of 4 points, the surgeon can decide for either surgical or nonsurgical treatment [65].

Lindahl et al. analyzed 36 consecutive patients with an H-type sacral fracture and spinopelvic dissociation [66]. Due to their outcome analysis, a modification of type 2 and type 3 injuries according to Roy-Camille was proposed, as specific fracture types led to a higher amount of worse outcomes (Fig. 4.32):

- Type 1: flexion injury without translational displacement.
- Type 2a: flexion injury with partial anterior translational displacement.
- Type 2b: flexion injury with complete anterior displacement of the distal sacral segment.
- Type 3a: extension injury with partial posterior translational displacement.
- Type 3b: extension injury with complete posterior displacement of the distal sacral segment.

It was found that neurological recovery and clinical outcome were associated with the degree of initial translational displacement of the transverse sacral fracture and permanent neurological deficits were more frequent in patients with complete transverse sacral fracture displacement compared with patients with partially displaced sacral fractures [66].

The new AO/OTA classification integrates a sacral fracture classification for fractures without additional pelvic ring injury [67].

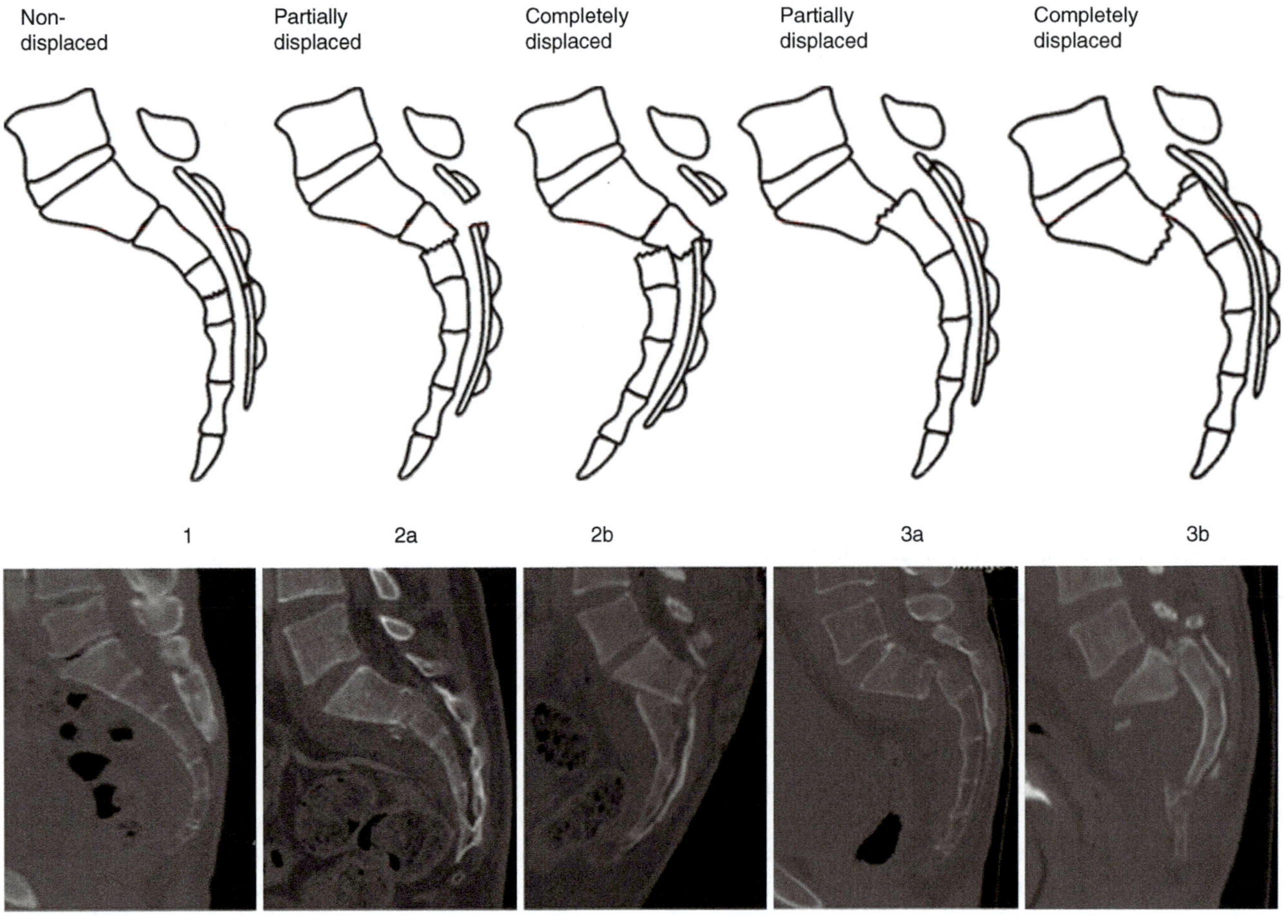

Fig. 4.32 Spinopelvic dissociation injuries according to Lindahl

4.1.6.3 Sacral Fractures According to the AO Spine Classification

Isolated sacral fractures, not part of a pelvic ring instability, were recently integrated in the spinal fracture classification Scheme [67].

Isolated sacral fractures are divided into three categories (Fig. 4.33):

- Type A: fractures of the lower segments not associated with sacroiliac joint.
- Type B: unilateral longitudinal or vertical fractures involving the upper sacral segments associated with sacroiliac joint, which have an impact on pelvic stability.
- Type C: sacral fractures resulting in spinopelvic instability.

Type A Fractures

Three subgroups of lower sacral segment fractures can be distinguished:

- A1 injuries: coccygeal or sacral compression injuries.
- A2 injuries: non-displaced transverse fractures.
- A3 injuries: displaced transverse fractures.

Type B Fractures

Three subgroups of longitudinal fractures can be distinguished according to the Denis classification of sacral fractures:

- B1 injuries: Denis III injuries, medial to the foraminal zone.
- B2 injuries: Denis I injuries, lateral to the foraminal zone.
- B3 injuries: Denis II intraforaminal injuries.

Besides their effect on posterior pelvic stability, additional neurological impairment can be possible.

Type C Fractures

Sacrum fractures resulting in spinopelvic instability present with U-, Y-, H-, and lambda-type variants and can be distinguished into four fracture types:

- C0 injuries: non-displaced, most often low-energy insufficiency fractures.
- C1 injuries: no posterior pelvic instability; any unilateral type B injury with concomitant S1 facet injury attached to the lateral fragment.

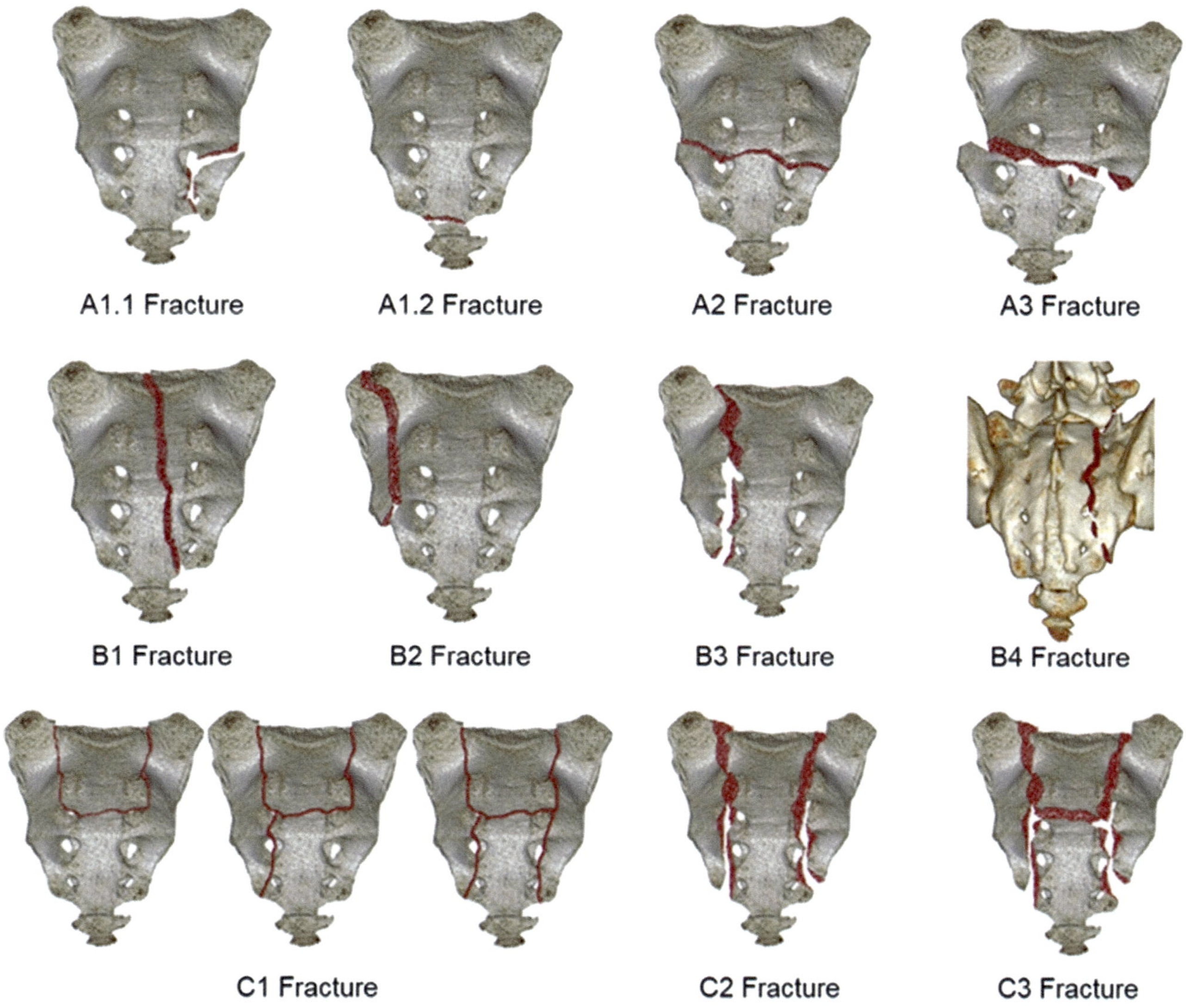

Fig. 4.33 AO spine sacral fracture classification

- C2 injuries: bilateral complete B-type injuries without a transverse fracture.
- C3 injuries: displaced fractures.

Additionally, two modifiers were added, defining an additional neurological deficit and specific patient conditions. Multiple qualifications can be graded.

Neurological Deficit

- NX: cannot be examined.
- N0: neurologically intact.
- N1: transient neurological deficit.
- N2: nerve root injury.
- N3: cauda equina injury or incomplete spinal cord injury.

Patient Specific Conditions

- M1: soft tissue injury.
- M2: metabolic bone disease.
- M3: anterior pelvic ring injury.
- M4: sacroiliac joint injury.

4.2 Complex Pelvic Trauma

The additional peripelvic soft tissue injury, including pelvic organ injury, is of prognostic relevance [68].

Bosch defined the term “complex pelvic trauma” in 1992 as a pelvic fracture accompanied by pelvic soft tissue injuries [68].

Using part of the Hannover Fracture Scale, the pelvic ring stability according to Tile, the amount of soft tissue contusions or laceration including perineal injuries, an additional polytrauma situation, and pelvic organ injuries (bladder, urethra, ureter, vagina, sigma, rectum, large vessel involvement, and lumbosacral plexus involvement) were integrated into a score, which was predictive of mortality.

Complex pelvic trauma is associated with a significant higher mortality, which is as high as 20% and is nearly unchanged for decades [11, 69].

From a practical perspective, Pohlemann et al. further defined two subgroups of complex pelvic trauma with prognostic effects on mortality [70]:

- Combined mechanical and hemodynamically unstable pelvic injuries.
- Traumatic hemipelvectomy.

Patients with these injuries present with significant higher mortality and can be defined most often as "patients in extremis" [71, 72].

4.2.1 WSES Classification

The WSES Classification classifies these hemodynamically unstable patients and combined it with the Young-Burgess classification [73].

Four categories are described:

- WSES grade I: mechanically stable lesions (APC 1, LC 1), hemodynamically stable.
- WSES grade II: hemodynamically stable *and* mechanically unstable (APC 2–3 and LC 2–3).
- WSES grade III: hemodynamically stable *and* mechanically unstable (VS, CM).
- WSES grade IV: all hemodynamically unstable lesions independent of the mechanical stability.

4.2.2 Open Pelvic Fracture Classification

Open pelvic fractures are a subgroup of complex pelvic trauma. There are two open pelvic fracture classifications [74, 75].

In 1997, Jones et al. published an open pelvic fracture classification on the basis of pelvic ring stability and perineal and rectal injury [75]:

- Class 1: stable pelvic ring.
- Class 2: unstable pelvic ring, no rectal or perineal wound.
- Class 3: unstable pelvic ring with rectal or perineal wound.

Bircher and Hargrove in 2004 based their classification on the primary skin lesion, additional soft tissue injury, and the instability of the pelvic ring according to Tile's classification [74].

- Type A1: penetrating trauma resulting in a type A pelvic ring injury with an additional soft tissue injury dependent on the missile and its path.
- Type A2: "outside in" type A iliac crest fracture, with minimal soft tissue damage.
- Type A3: "outside in" type A iliac crest fracture, with extensive soft tissue damage.
- Type B1: "inside out" LC type B2 injury with little external damage but possible genitourinary injury.
- Type B2: "inside out" LC type B2 injury with moderate tissue damage (Morel-Lavallée lesion).
- Type B3: "perineal split" B1 ("open book") fracture.
- Type C1: "perineal split" and/or "sacral shear/split" type C injury with moderate to extensive skin loss, complete genitourinary disruption, and rectal lesions with subsequent fecal contamination.
- Type C2: "hemipelvic destabilization" type C injury with severe tissue damage, complete urogenital and bowel injury combined with extensive contamination of all tissue layers.
- Type C3: "pelvic crush" with bilateral complex type C pelvic instability and massive damage to soft tissues and intrapelvic organs.

4.3 Summary

The 1996 version of the AO/OTA pelvic ring classification seems to be optimal from the authors' standpoint.

In 2018, the "new" AO/OTA classification and the AO Spine Sacrum classification were published. The latter has the following disadvantages compared to the 1996 version:

- In the 2018 version, type B1 was changed to type B2.
- The AO Spine Sacrum classification presents type B injuries, which are predominantly type C injuries of the pelvic ring.
- In the AO Spine Sacrum classification, no pelvic ring type B injuries are integrated.

These changes will potentially lead to confusion, when comparing "old" and future papers dealing with pelvic ring injuries.

References

1. Pennal G, Tile M, Waddell J, Garside H. Pelvic disruption: assessment and classification. Clin Orthop. 1980;151:12–21.
2. Tile M, Pennal G. Pelvic disruptions: principles of management. Clon Orthop. 1980;151:56–64.
3. Tile M. Pelvic ring fractures: should they be fixed ? J Bone Joint Surg. 1988;70-B:1–12.
4. Schatzker J, Tile M. The rationale of operative fracture care. 3rd ed. Berlin, Heidelberg, New York: Springer-Verlag; 2005.
5. Tile M. Fractures of the pelvis and acetabulum. 2nd ed. Baltimore: Williams & Wilkings; 1995.
6. Tile, M., Helfet, D. and Kellam, J., Fractures of the pelvis and acetabulum. 2003.
7. Müller M. CCF Comprehensive Classification of Fractures. Bern: M.E. Müller Foundation; 1996.
8. Müller M. The comprehensive classification of fractures: pelvis. 1996.
9. OTA. Fracture and dislocation compendium. J Orthop Trauma. 1996;10(Suppl. 1):71–5.
10. Pohlemann T. Pelvic ring injuries: assessment and concepts of surgical management. In: Rüedi TP, Murphy WM, editors. AO principles of fracture management. Stuttgart, New York: Thieme-Verlag; 2000. p. 391–414.
11. Gänsslen A, Pohlemann T, Paul C, Lobenhoffer P, Tscherne H. Epidemiology of pelvic ring injuries. Injury. 1996;Suppl. 1(Part 1):13–20.
12. Osterhoff G, Scheyerer M, Fritz Y, Bouaicha S, Wanner G, Simmen H, Werner C. Comparing the predictive value of the pelvic ring injury classification systems by Tile and by Young and Burgess. Injury. 2014;45:742–7.
13. Baqué P, Trojani C, Delotte J, Séjor E, Senni-Buratti M, de Baqué F, Bourgeon A. Anatomical consequences of "open-book" pelvic ring disruption: a cadaver experimental study. Surg Radiol Anat. 2005;27:487–90.
14. Rommens PM, Hessmann MH. Staged reconstruction of pelvic ring disruption: differences in morbidity, mortality, radiologic results, and functional outcomes between B1, B2/B3, and C-type lesions. J Orthop Trauma. 2002;16(2):92–8.
15. Rommens P, Gercek E, Hansen M, Hessmann M. Mortality, morbidity and functional outcome after open book and lateral compression lesions of the pelvic ring. A retrospective analysis of 100 type B pelvic ring lesions according to Tile's classification. [Article in German]. Unfallchirurg. 2003;106:542–9.
16. Young JW, Burgess AR, Brumback RJ, Poka A. Pelvic fractures: value of plain radiography in early assessment and management. Radiology. 1986;160(2):445–51.
17. Burgess A, Eastridge B, Young J, Ellison T, Ellison P, Poka A, Bathon G, Brumback R. Pelvic ring disruption: effective classification systems and treatment protocols. J Trauma. 1990;30(7): 848–56.
18. Bucholz R. The pathological anatomy of malgaigne fracture-dislocations of the pelvis. J Bone Joint Surg. 1981;63-A(3):400–4.
19. Doro C, Forward D, Kim H, Nascone J, Sciadini M, Hsieh A, Osgood G, O'Toole R. Does 2.5 cm of symphyseal widening differentiate anteroposterior compression I from anteroposterior compression II pelvic ring injuries? J Orthop Trauma. 2010;24:610–5.
20. Manson T, Nascone J, O'Toole R. Traction vertical shear pelvic ring fracture: a marker for severe arterial injury? A case report. J Orthop Trauma. 2010;24:e90–4.
21. Young J, Resnik C. Fracture of the pelvis: current concepts in classification. AJR. 1990;155:1169–75.
22. Dalal S, Burgess A, Siegel J, Young J, Brumback R, Poka A, Dunham C, Gens D, Bathon H. Pelvic fracture in multiple trauma: classification by mechanism is key to pattern of organ injury, resuscitative requirements, and outcome. J Trauma. 1989;29(7):981–1000.
23. Lefaivre K, Padalecki J, Starr A. What constitutes a Young and Burgess lateral compression-I (OTA 61-B2) pelvic ring disruption? A description of computed tomography-based fracture anatomy and associated injuries. J Orthop Trauma. 2009;23:16–21.
24. Manson T, Nascone J, Sciadini M, O'Toole R. Does fracture pattern predict death with lateral compression type 1 pelvic fractures? J Trauma. 2010;69:876–9.
25. Weaver M, Bruinsma W, Toney E, Dafford E, Vrahas M. What are the patterns of injury and displacement seen in lateral compression pelvic fractures? Clin Orthop Relat Res. 2012;470:2104–10.
26. Starr A, Griffin D, Reinert C, Frawley W, Walker J, Whitlock S, Borer D, Rao A, Jones A. Pelvic ring disruptions: prediction of associated injuries, transfusion requirement, pelvic arteriography, complications, and mortality. J Orthop Trauma. 2002;16:553–61.
27. Suzuki T, Morgan S, Smith W, Stahel P, Flierl M, Hak D. Stress radiograph to detect true extent of symphyseal disruption in presumed anteroposterior compression type I pelvic injuries. J Trauma. 2010;69:880–5.
28. Gardner M, Krieg J, Simpson T, Bottlang M. Displacement after simulated pelvic ring injuries: a cadaveric model of recoil. J Trauma. 2010;68:159–65.
29. Sagi H, Coniglione F, Stanford J. Examination under anesthetic for occult pelvic ring instability. J Orthop Trauma. 2011;25:529–36.
30. Manson T, O'Toole R, Whitney A, Duggan B, Sciadini M, Nascone J. Young-Burgess classification of pelvic ring fractures: does it predict mortality, transfusion requirements, and non-orthopaedic injuries? J Orthop Trauma. 2010;24:603–9.
31. Alton T, Gee A. Classifications in brief: young and burgess classification of pelvic ring injuries. Clin Orthop Relat Res. 2014;472:2338–42.
32. Kellam J, Meinberg E, Agel J, Karam M, Roberts C. Pelvic ring. In: fracture and dislocation classification compendium-2018: international comprehensive classification of fractures and dislocations committee. J Orthop Trauma. 2018;32:S71–6.
33. Lindsjö U. Classification of ankle fractures: the Lauge-Hansen or AO system? Clin Orthop. 1985;199:12–6.
34. Frandsen P, Andersen E, Madsen F, Skjodt T. Garden's classification of femoral neck fractures: an assessment of inter-observer variation. J Bone Joint Surg. 1988;70-B:588–90.
35. Thomsen N, Overgaard S, Olson L, Hansen H, Nielsen S. Observer variation in the radiographic classification of ankle fractures. J Bone Joint Surg. 1991;73-B:676–8.
36. Edeiken-Monroe B, Browner BD, Jackson H. The role of standard roentgenograms in the evaluation of instability of pelvic ring disruption. Clin Orthop. 1989;240:63–76.
37. Resnik C, Stackhouse D, Shanmuganathan K, Young J. Diagnosis of pelvic fractures in patients with acute pelvic trauma: efficiency of plain radiographs. AJR. 1992;158:109–12.
38. Koo H, Leveridge M, Hompson C, Zdero R, Bhandari M, Kreder H, Stephen D, McKee M, Schemitsch E. Interobserver reliability of the young-burgess and tile classification systems for fractures of the pelvic ring. J Orthop Trauma. 2008;22:379–84.
39. Furey A, O'Toole R, Nascone J, Sciadini M, Copeland C, Turen C. Classification of pelvic fractures: analysis of inter- and intraobserver variability using the Young-Burgess and Tile classification systems. Orthopedics. 2009;32:401. https://doi.org/10.3928/01477447-20090511-05.
40. Gabbe B, Esser M, Bucknill A, Russ M, Hofstee D, Cameron P, Handley C, de Steiger R. The imaging and classification of severe pelvic ring fractures: experiences from two level 1 trauma centres. Bone Joint J. 2013;95-B:1396–401.
41. Oberkircher L, Ruchholtz S, Rommens P, Hofmann A, Bücking B, Krüger A. Osteoporotic pelvic fractures. Dtsch Arztebl Int. 2018;115:70–80.
42. Rommens P, Dietz S, Ossendorf C, Pairon P, Wagner D, Hofmann A. Fragility fractures of the pelvis: should they be fixed? Acta Chir Orthop Traumatol Cechoslov. 2015;82:101–12.

43. Rommens P, Ossendorf C, Pairon P, Dietz S, Wagner D, Hofmann A. Clinical pathways for fragility fractures of the pelvic ring: personal experience and review of the literature. J Orthop Sci. 2015;20:1–11.
44. Tan Z, Huang Z, Li L, Meng W, Liu L, Zhang H, Wang G, Huang F. Classification and treatment of sacroiliac joint dislocation. [Article in Chinese]. Sichuan Da Xue Xue Bao Yi Xue Ban. 2017;48:661–7.
45. Schmidek H, Schmith D, Kristiansen D. Sacral fractures. Neurosurgery. 1984;15:735–46.
46. Denis F, Steven D, Comfort T. Sacral fractures: an important problem, retrospective analysis of 236 cases. Clin Orthop. 1988;227:67–81.
47. Gibbons K, Soloniuk D, Razack N. Neurological injury and patterns of sacral fractures. J Neurosurg. 1990;72:889–93.
48. Pohlemann T, Bosch U, Gänsslen A, Tscherne H. The Hannover experience in management of pelvic fractures. Clin Orthop. 1994;305:69–80.
49. Pohlemann T, Gänsslen A, Hartung S, für die Arbeitsgruppe Becken HT. Beckenverletzungen/Pelvic Injuries, Hefte zu "Der Unfallchirurg", vol. 266. Berlin, Heidelberg: Springer-Verlag; 1998.
50. Pohlemann T, Gänsslen A, Tscherne H. Die Problematik der Sakrumfraktur, klinische Analyse von 377 Fällen. Orthopade. 1992;21:400–12.
51. Pohlemann T, Gänsslen A, Tscherne H. Sacral fractures. In: Tile M, Helfet DL, Kellam JF, editors. Fractures of the pelvis and acetabulum. 3rd ed. Philadelphia: Lippincot Williams & Wilkins; 2003. p. 294–322.
52. Khan J, Marquez-Lara A, Miller A. Relationship of sacral fractures to nerve injury: is the Denis classification still accurate? J Orthop Trauma. 2017;31:181–4.
53. Isler B. Lumbosacral lesions associated with pelvic ring injuries. J Orthop Trauma. 1990;4(1):1–6.
54. Leone A, Cerase A, Priolo F, Marano P. Lumbosacral junction injury associated with unstable pelvic fracture: classification and diagnosis. Radiology. 1997;205:253–9.
55. Oransky M, Gasparini G. Associated lumbosacral junction injuries (LSJi) in Ppelvic fractures. J Orthop Trauma. 1997;11(7):509–12.
56. Roy-Camille R, Saillant G, Gagana G, Mazel C. Transverse fracture of the upper sacrum: suicidal jumper's fracture. Spine. 1985;10(9):838–45.
57. Lindahl J. Management of Pelvic Ring Fractures. Academic Dissertation. Helsinki, Finland: Helsinki University; 2015. ISBN 978-951-51-1414-3 (PDF); ISBN 978-951-51-1413-6 (paperback).
58. Strange-Vognsen H, Lebech A. An unusual type of fracture in the upper sacrum. J Orthop Trauma. 1991;5(2):200–3.
59. Robles L. Transverse sacral fractures. Spine J. 2009;9:60–9.
60. Hunt N, Jennings A, Smith M. Current management of U-shaped sacral fractures or spino-pelvic dissociation. Injury. 2002;33(2):123–6.
61. Nork SE, Jones CB, Harding SP, Mirza SK, Routt ML Jr. Percutaneous stabilization of U-shaped sacral fractures using iliosacral screws: technique and early results. J Orthop Trauma. 2001;15(4):238–46.
62. Schildhauer T, Bellabarba C, Nork S, Barei D, Routt MJ, Chapman J. Decompression and lumbopelvic fixation for sacral fracture-dislocations with spino-pelvic dissociation. J Orthop Trauma. 2006;20:447–57.
63. Tan G, He J, Fu B, Li L, Wang B, Zhou D. Lumbopelvic fixation for multiplanar sacral fractures with spinopelvic instability. Injury. 2012;43:1318–25.
64. Yi C, Hak D. Traumatic spinopelvic dissociation or U-shaped sacral fracture: a review of the literature. Injury. 2012;43:402–8.
65. Lehman RJ, Kang D, Bellabarba C. A new classification for complex lumbosacral injuries. Spine J. 2012;12:612–28.
66. Lindahl J, Mäkinen T, Koskinen S, Söderlund T. Factors associated with outcome of spinopelvic dissociation treated with lumbopelvic fixation. Injury. 2014;45:1914–20.
67. Kellam J, Meinberg E, Agel J, Karam M, Roberts C. Spine. In: fracture and dislocation classification compendium-2018: international comprehensive classification of fractures and dislocations committee. J Orthop Trauma. 2018;32:S145–60.
68. Bosch U, Pohlemann T, Haas N, Tscherne H. Classification and management of complex pelvic trauma. Unfallchirurg. 1992;95:189–96.
69. Hauschild O, Strohm P, Culemann U, Pohlemann T, Suedkamp N, Koestler W, Schmal H. Mortality in patients with pelvic fractures: results from the German pelvic injury register. J Trauma. 2008;64:449–55.
70. Pohlemann T, Gänsslen A and Stief C. Komplexe verletzungen des beckens und acetabulums. Orthopäde. 1998;27:32–44.
71. Gänsslen A, Giannoudis P, Pape H. Hemorrhage in pelvic fracture: who needs angiography? Curr Opin Crit Care. 2003;9:515–23.
72. Gänsslen A, Hildebrand F, Pohlemann T. Management of hemodynamic unstable patients "in extremis" with pelvic ring fractures. Acta Chir Orthop Traumatol Cechoslov. 2012;79:193–202.
73. Coccolino F, Stahel P, Montori G, Biffl W, Horer T, Catena F, Kluger Y, Moore E, PÜeitzman A, Ivatury R, Coimbra R, Pereira Frago G, Pereira B, Risoli S, Kirkpatrick A, Leppaniemi A, Manfredi R, Magnone S, Chiara O, Solaini L, Ceresoli M, Allievi N, Arvieux C, Velmahos G, Balogh Z, Naidoo N, Wber D, Abu-Ziran F, Sartelli M, Ansaloni L. Pelvic trauma: WSES classification and guidelines. World J Emerg Surg. 2017;12:5.
74. Bircher M, Hargrove R. Is it possible to classify open fractures of the pelvis? Eur J Trauma. 2004;30:74–9.
75. Jones A, Powell J, Kellam J, McCormack R, Dust W, Wimmer P. Open pelvic fractures. A multicentern retrospective analysis. Orthop Clin North Am. 1997;28:345–50.

5 Prehospital Treatment of Suspected Pelvic Injuries

Mario Staresinic, Bore Bakota, Stephan Grechenig, and Axel Gänsslen

The immediate treatment of the multiply injured patient with suspected pelvic fracture follows general Advanced Trauma Life Support principles, even in the prehospital setting [1].

The main risk after high-energy injuries of the pelvis is due to hemorrhage. If pelvis-related life-threatening hemorrhage can be controlled in the prehospital environment, survival of these patients can potentially be increased.

During primary resuscitation at the accident scene, the severity of a pelvic injury is often underestimated [2].

In general, prehospital treatment should focus on possible clinical identification of pelvic injuries, mechanical stabilization of the pelvis, and optimization of pelvic-related ongoing hemodynamic instability [3].

The benefits of mechanical stabilization of the pelvis, even in the prehospital setting, allow clot formation and reduction of the pelvic volume (tamponade effect) leading to reduced narcotic needs and facilitate the patient transport [4].

A literature overview gave some clear statements for prehospital management of suspected pelvic fractures [3]:

- Analysis of the mechanism of injury is of major importance as this guides to pelvic injury suspicion.
- In alert patients, reporting of pain in the pelvic back or groin regions indicates possible pelvic injuries.
- In alert patients, routine pelvic immobilization is clearly recommended in positive clinical findings.
- Pelvic manipulation should be avoided as clinical examination is unreliable.
- External compression splinting should be performed in every patient with a suspected pelvic ring fracture.
- Log-rolling the patient should be performed carefully to avoid clot dislodgement.
- Use of a scoop stretcher to move the patient for definitive transport.
- Transport on a spinal board or vacuum mattress.
- Adequate fluid resuscitation.

5.1 Prehospital Identification of Patients with Pelvic Injuries

Based on the recommendations by Lee et al. [3] and newer reports on managing these patients, today, a more clear concept was developed.

5.1.1 Analysis of the Injury Mechanism

The first parameter for suspicion of pelvic injuries is the knowledge of the injury mechanism.

In the majority of cases, a high-energy mechanism is responsible for potential high-risk pelvic fractures. In polytraumatized patients, approximately one-fourth of patients have additional pelvic injuries [5–7].

- Data from the German Pelvic Multicenter Study Group from the early 1990s indicated that the majority of patients sustained their pelvic fracture due to road traffic accidents (59.7%), predominantly involving in car accidents and mechanism against pedestrians (Fig. 5.1); the second most common mechanism was a fall [8].
- Balogh et al. compared the mechanism of injury among low-energy and high-energy injuries; low-energy injuries exclusively occurred after simple falls from less than 1 m, whereas high-energy injuries were the result of motor

M. Staresinic
General and Sports Trauma Department, University Hospital Merkur Zagreb, Zagreb, Croatia

B. Bakota
Department of Orthopaedics and Trauma, Medical University of Graz, Graz, Austria

S. Grechenig
Department of Orthopedics and Trauma Surgery, AUVA Trauma Hospital Klagenfurt, Klagenfurt, Austria

Department of Trauma Surgery, University Hospital Regensburg, Regensburg, Germany

A. Gänsslen (✉)
Department of Trauma Surgery, Orthopedics and Hand Surgery, Hospital Wolfsburg, Wolfsburg, Germany

A. Gänsslen et al. (eds.), *Pelvic Ring Fractures*, https://doi.org/10.1007/978-3-030-54730-1_5

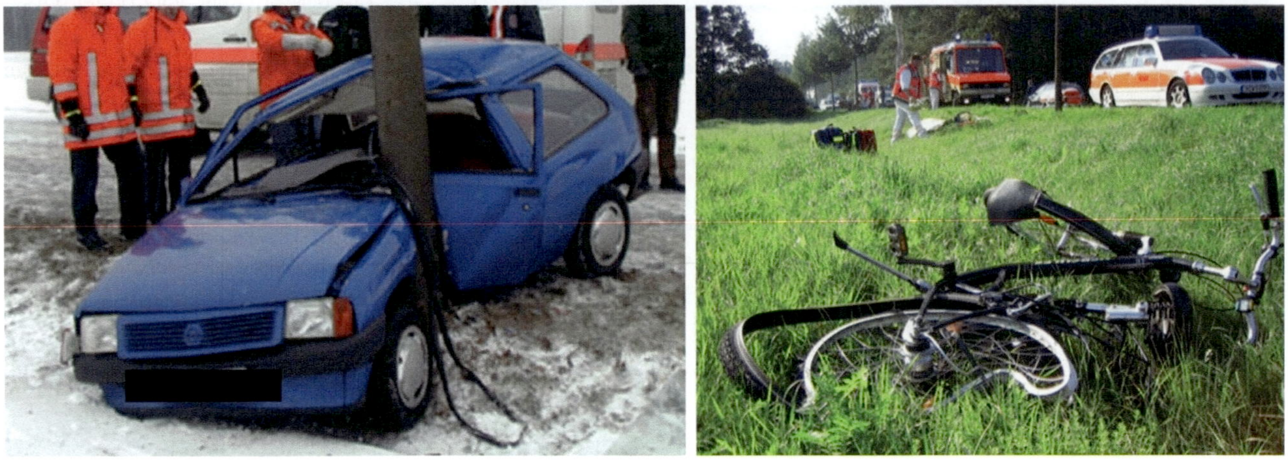

Fig. 5.1 Possible injury mechanisms resulting in pelvic ring injuries: lateral side impact in an MVA (left) or injury to an unrestrained bicycle driver (right)

vehicle accidents (MVA), with 31% motorbike crashes, 27% car crashes, and 22% pedestrians hit by a car [9].

- The injury mechanism in 1012 patients, treated between 1994 and 2005 in Germany, was an MVA in 68.2% and a fall from a height (>3 m) in 16.6%, whereas simple falls were responsible in only 8.5% [10].
- In children, more pedestrian-related injuries occurred, compared to classical MVAs [11].
- Children aged 5–14 years had a six times higher possibility of sustaining a pelvic fracture after being struck by a vehicle and a twice higher likelihood after being occupants in motor vehicle accidents compared to falls [12].

> A high-energy mechanism should always lead to suspicion of an unstable critical pelvic injury [13].

Typical injury mechanisms resulting in pelvic injuries are [2, 14]:

- High-speed road traffic accidents
- Side-impact automobile accidents with the patient on the side of the impact
- Falls from great heights
- Axial forces through the outstretched lower limb
- High-speed trauma in unprotected travelers, such as motorcyclists
- Roll-over accidents

5.1.2 Clinical Signs

Classical clinical signs are often missing in the initial treatment phase. External pelvic hemorrhage, which is rare [15], is more easily identified, whereas internal hemorrhage is hard to identify as obvious clinical signs are normally missing.

Open pelvic injuries can lead to spectacular clinical presentations (see Chap. 17) of external massive bleeding and/or severe pelvic deformities, whereas contour changes after internal hemorrhage are usually even more inconspicuous [16].

Prehospital assessment of traumatic injuries by emergency medical service physicians showed the lowest values for detecting abdominal and pelvic injuries [17]. The sensitivity was only 57% for pelvic injuries, and 43% of relevant pelvic injuries were preclinically missed [17].

At the scene, after initial ABC stabilization according to standard protocols (e.g., advanced trauma life support (ATLS), prehospital trauma life support (PHTLS), etc.), whenever possible, clinical assessment involves the general inspection of the pelvis for hematomas, open wounds, variations of the external contour (see Chap. 17), and deformities of the pelvis and/or lower extremities (shortening, external rotation deformities) [2], as well as an assessment of the gross neurovascular status.

In awake patients, reported pain in the pelvic region can be a sign of a pelvic fracture, but a high rate of misinterpretation is observed [18–25]:

- Salvino et al. observed that 7.7% of 39 radiographically confirmed pelvic fractures were not identified by patient history or clinical examination, whereas 3.6% (28/771) of fractures were clinically suspected but not confirmed on X-rays [23].
- Yugueros et al. observed that 3.4% of 59 radiographically confirmed pelvic fractures were not identified by patient history or clinical examination, whereas 32.1% of fractures were clinically suspected but not confirmed on X-rays [25].
- Kaneriga et al. observed that 52.6% of pelvic fractures were not suspected by clinical examination [21].
- Tien et al. analyzed 763 blunt trauma patients with radiographically confirmed 55 pelvic fractures; approximately 9.1% of patients with a pelvic injury had no clinical signs of pelvic injury or negative history of pain; ethanol abuse did not change these results [24].

- Duane et al. reported on 45 pelvic fractures in a group of 520 blunt trauma patients; all pelvic fractures could be identified on history or clinical examination; in contrast, 73.8% had positive clinical signs without a confirmed pelvic fracture [19].
- Gonzales et al. missed 7.2% of pelvic fractures on clinical examination, whereas 65.1% had clinical pelvic fracture signs without having a fracture [20].
- Pehle et al. reported that patients with clinical instability during pelvic examination had higher injury severity scores, a higher risk of shock-associated problems, and a higher mortality [22]; clinical examination was associated with a sensitivity of 44.1%, a specificity of 99.7%, a positive predictive value of 96%, and a negative predictive value of 93.3%.
- Duane et al. prospectively compared the results of clinical examination with X-rays and computed tomography (CT) diagnosis of pelvic fractures; all pelvic fractures could be clinically confirmed (100% sensitivity, 100% negative predictive value); six patients with CT diagnosis of the pelvic fracture had negative clinical signs [18].

Sauerland et al. performed a meta-analysis of 12 pooled studies with 5454 patients on clinical examination of suspected pelvic fractures [26]. Five hundred forty-nine patients were identified with a pelvic fracture. An overall sensitivity and specificity of 90% and a false negative and a false positive rate of 10% were reported.

In awake patients, the sensitivity was close to 100%, indicating that neurological normal patients were easier to analyze. Overall, 11.1% of pelvic fractures were missed during clinical examination [26].

Typical clinical signs in awake patients indicating suspicion of a pelvic fracture were identified by Duane et al. [18]:

- Subjective hip pain
- Internal rotation of the leg
- Tenderness to palpation over the sacrum
- Tenderness to palpation over the hips
- Diffuse tenderness to palpation throughout the pelvis

Even in patients with reduced consciousness, these factors were still predictive of pelvic fractures [18].

In contrast, Mackersie et al. reported a high incidence of occult major pelvic fractures, when clinical examination was negative [27] and Gonzales et al. reported only one-third of patients reporting pain on lateral compression or palpation of the pubic symphysis [20].

In a recent analysis, Shlamovitz et al. analyzed 81 stable and 34 unstable pelvic injuries [28] and reported on different sensitivities and specificities dependent on several parameters:

- All pelvic fractures: 8% sensitivity, 99% specificity
- Unstable fractures: 26% sensitivity, 99.9% specificity
- Pelvic pain or tenderness (GCS >13), all fractures: 74% sensitivity, 97% specificity
- Pelvic pain or tenderness (GCS >13), unstable fractures: 100% sensitivity, 93% specificity
- Pelvic deformity, all fractures: 30% sensitivity, 99% specificity
- Pelvic deformity, unstable fractures: 55% sensitivity, 97% specificity

When clinical signs are missing during prehospital evaluation, relevant pelvic fractures can normally be excluded, especially in awake patients.

Clinical signs, even in patients with impaired consciousness, alerting for pelvic fractures can be [3, 14]:

- Deformity
- Bruising or swelling over the bony prominences, pubis, perineum, or scrotum
- Leg-length discrepancy
- Rotational deformity of a lower limb (without fracture in that extremity)
- Wounds around the pelvis
- Bleeding from the patient's rectum, vagina, or urethra.
- Neurological abnormalities.

5.1.3 Stability Testing of the Pelvis

Mechanical pelvic instability was suspected to be a marker of severe pelvic fractures.

Pelvic stability can be investigated by manual compression of the pelvic ring in anterior-posterior and lateral-medial directions. It was recommended that stability testing should be performed carefully and gently as these measures can result in additional pelvic bleeding [2]. The presence of a pelvic instability was supposed to be often associated with a high risk of pelvic bleeding [22].

In a recent online survey from German hospitals, 91% of surgeons recommended stability testing in suspected pelvic fractures, whereas 31.2% stated that unnecessary manipulation should be avoided [29]. Additionally, 70.7% indicated pelvic emergency stabilization only after clinically testing pelvic stability [29].

In the hospital setting, in patients with a mechanically unstable pelvis and accompanying hemodynamic instability, the pelvic binder is favored by 88.7% of surgeons [29].

In a prospective analysis of 254 patients with clinically suspected pelvic fractures, only 45.7% had radiologically confirmed pelvic fractures [30]. Clinical stability testing was positive in 25 patients with 72% of these presented with unstable fracture pattern on later CT examination.

Overall, manual stability testing missed 68.4% of radiologically unstable fractures and leads to the following statistical results in detecting unstable pelvic fractures [30]:

- 31.6% sensitivity.
- 92.2% specificity.
- 72% positive predictive value.
- 68% negative predictive value.

A recent analysis stated that "feeling" instability during clinical examination or the presence of pelvic deformity was associated with poor sensitivity in detecting mechanically unstable pelvic fractures, whereas absence of pelvic pain or tenderness in awake patients can normally exclude relevant (unstable) pelvic injury [28].

In unresponsive trauma patients, instability testing should be avoided, even when a pelvic fracture is assumed [3], although stability testing is favored by many surgeons [29].

Additionally, it has to be considered that stability testing is without (therapeutic) relevance and no advantage is observed regarding the choice of the target hospital for these patients.

Clinical examination in unresponsive patients is difficult and cannot confirm every patient with a pelvic fracture.

Log-rolling the patient onto a spinal board should be avoided for the same reasons [3].

5.1.4 Hemodynamic Identification of Patients at Risk

For a long time, science focused on parameters identifying patients at risk for ongoing hemorrhage.

Prehospital hypotension (systolic blood pressure ≤ 90 mmHg) is associated with a higher mortality risk [31–33] and predicts the need for an emergency surgical procedure, even when blood pressure has become normal at admission [34].

In-hospital identification of patients in hemorrhagic shock is based on beside clinical parameters on lactate and base deficit analysis.

Thus, it was logical to integrate these parameters into the prehospital evaluation using point-of-care monitoring.

Overall, prehospital lactate measurement was found to be more sensitive than conventional parameters (systolic blood pressure) in identifying patients at risk for occult hypoperfusion, surgical intervention, or critical care treatment [35–38] with a lactate cut-off of >2 mmol/L [35, 36].

Point-of-care prehospital lactate analysis can identify patients at risk for ongoing hemorrhage with a threshold of 2 mmol/L.

5.2 Mechanical Stabilization of the Pelvis

European guidelines on management of the hemodynamically unstable patient clearly favor immediate pelvic ring closure and stabilization in the clinical setting [39, 40]. Additionally, clear recommendations exist for mechanically stabilizing the pelvis, especially in patients with reduced consciousness, even in the prehospital setting [2, 3, 13, 29, 30].

The primary pathophysiological aim is to control fracture side bleeding and venous bleeding (clotting) by reducing pelvic movements [41].

Historically, prehospital application of military antishock trousers (MAST) has been used to induce a pelvic tamponade effect and a reduction of venous return to the heart, but randomized trials confirmed no evidence regarding reduction in mortality [42], whereas complications, including compartment syndrome, crush syndrome, or electrolyte imbalance, were frequently observed [43–47].

Several options exist to mechanically stabilize the pelvis in the prehospital setting:

- Elastic bindings
- Towels (Fig. 5.2)
- Pelvic binders
- Vacuum mattress (Fig. 5.3)

Elastic stabilization was favored in the Anglo-American area performed by using simple elastic bindings, towel wrapping, or bed sheets.

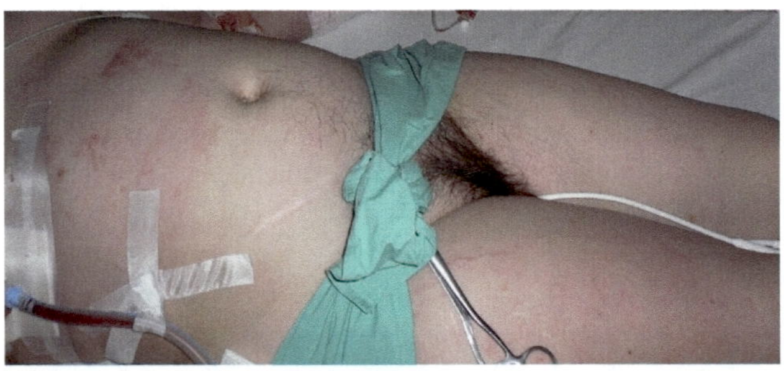

Fig. 5.2 Acute pelvic ring stabilization using a towel

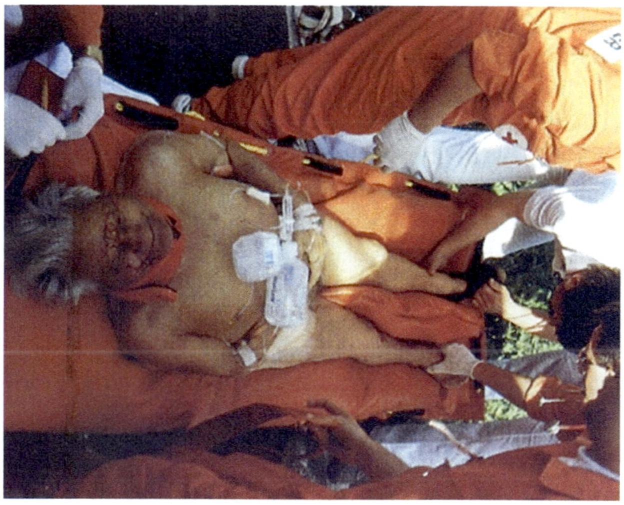

Fig. 5.3 Acute pelvic ring stabilization using the vacuum mattress

- Routt et al. reported a case of an unstable pelvic injury with in-hospital stabilization with a longitudinally folded bed sheet circumferentially placed around the pelvis and secured by anterior clamping [48].
- Simpson reported on two further patients using this technique [49].
- Duxbury et al. modified this technique by twisting the bed sheet anteriorly and fixing it with two cable ties [50].
- Additional internal rotation of the lower limbs was further recommended [16].
- The combination of internal rotation and taping of the lower extremities was favored by Gardner et al. using a 4-in-wide foam tape at the anterior thighs and the feet [51]; no adverse effects were reported, and 15–20% of anatomical reductions were achieved.
- Nun et al. combined pelvic towel sheeting with elastic extremity foam tape sheeting in seven awake patients presenting with severe shock and an unstable pelvis; the shock index improved from 1.89 to 0.71, and transfusion requirements were reduced from 11.3 PRBC/12 to 0.94 PRBC/h [52].

These simple, cheap, and always available techniques can also be used in the prehospital setting.

Baumgärtel introduced a narrow pneumatic belt placed around the injured pelvic ring. By inflating three chambers, a circular compression is achieved. The main advantage is that it can be quickly applied and leads to a targeted pelvic compression without significantly impairing the accessibility to the patient [53].

Vermeulen et al. first introduced a pelvic strap belt to stabilize the pelvis in the prehospital setting in 1999. Their experience in 19 patients showed encouraging results without observing complications related to its use [54].

These mechanical stabilization devices were tested in several studies. Cadaveric analyses have shown that 150–180 N (15–18 kg) was necessary to adequately stabilize and reduce an open book type B or type C pelvic injury [55, 56]. The adequate application site was identified as being the level of the greater trochanter or pubic symphysis, whereas application at the iliac crest leads to insufficient stability and delayed hemodynamic effects [57]. The resulting biomechanical forces were comparable to application of a pelvic C-clamp in the emergency room setting and better than classical external fixation devices [55, 56, 58].

These results were confirmed by later studies [59, 60]. Several binder types resulted in adequate provisional stability of the pelvis [61].

Krieg et al. performed a prospective clinical study on the feasibility of a circumferential pelvic device [62] and reported a significant reduction of the pelvic volume on X-rays and CT examination with no adverse effects even in lateral compression injuries (no over-compression). Mortality could be reduced by prehospital application of such a device [4], and application prior to transfers reduces transfusion requirements [63].

In contrast, there is a high rate of its uncritical use [64]. In a clinical study, 60% of applications were performed without pelvic injury, and in 6.4%, no binder was applied, despite the later diagnosis of an unstable pelvic injury.

Potentially, there is a risk for relevant soft tissue injury, making later frequent soft tissue evaluation necessary [65, 66]. But in the prehospital phase, the benefit of the binders is superior to this reported soft tissue risk.

> Application of a circumferential pelvic binder is the present gold standard for prehospital management of suspected pelvic injuries [67, 68], but not every patient needs a binder.

In summary, the benefits of the pelvic circumferential binders include:

- Providing mechanical pelvic stability.
- Allowing clot formation.
- Preventing ongoing hemorrhage.
- Allowing early application.

Especially in conjunction with internal rotation of the thighs and wrapping of the knees and ankles. But an adequate training must be provided to avoid misplacement.

> Prophylactic application of these devices at the scene appears to be warranted. They are easily and effectively used, readily available, and inexpensive. Potential disadvantages may be related to soft tissue pressure and the risk of visceral injury or sacral nerve root compression, though there were rarely reported complications in small clinical series [1].

Additionally, as a simple measure, the Polytrauma Guideline Update Group of the German Trauma Society recommends leaving leather clothing in place for splinting and compression effects, especially in motorcycle injuries [69–71].

5.2.1 Fluid Resuscitation

In every patients with a suspected pelvic injury or in multiply injured patients, a clinical assessment of the gross cardiovascular status of the patient should be made [1].

Prehospital intravenous access does not delay patient's transfer [72, 73]. The optimal volume for fluid resuscitation remains controversial [1]. The presence or absence of a radial pulse can be used to guide fluid resuscitation [74], although these "hypotensive resuscitation "recommendations are based on studies evaluating penetrating trauma patients [75]. No evidence from randomized controlled trials is available to support early aggressive fluid administration in uncontrolled hemorrhage. In massive trauma patients including patients with hemodynamically unstable pelvic fractures, a massive fluid resuscitation is still performed. A low-volume resuscitation is not the accepted practice in Germany [76].

Fluid resuscitation can lead to a reduced rate of shock in the emergency department (ED) (optimized shock index) if low volumes were infused, whereas volumes >1 L were associated with an increased blood transfusion rate in the ED [77].

> There is still controversy on the adequate fluid management for trauma patients with pelvic fractures.

5.3 Prehospital Control of Life-Threatening Pelvic Hemorrhage

Prehospital options for pelvic hemorrhage control are discussed in the literature. These include the resuscitative endovascular balloon occlusion of the aorta (REBOA) concept [78] and prehospital blood product (PHBP) resuscitation [79].

5.3.1 Resuscitative Endovascular Balloon Occlusion of the Aorta (REBOA)

Pelvic hemorrhage is often noncompressible. During the last decade, resuscitative endovascular balloon occlusion of the aorta (REBOA) was reintroduced into emergency treatment protocols for hemorrhage damage control.

This concept also was considered to be effective in the preclinical setting as uncontrolled pelvic bleeding can lead to death.

The concept of temporary aortic occlusion can result in systolic blood pressure increase and superior perfusion of the heart and brain by temporary control of distal bleeding until permanent hemostasis is achieved. REBOA is performed by using an occlusive balloon catheter, introduced into the aorta via endovascular access of the common femoral artery as a less-invasive procedure [78]. A first case report showed a promising result, even in the prehospital area [80]. Military concepts favor future integration of REBOA for patients in extremis in combat casualties [81, 82].

> In the near future, REBOA can be an option in the prehospital management of patients in extremis with uncontrollable pelvic bleeding.

5.3.2 Prehospital Blood Product Resuscitation

Already in 2004, Soudry et al. extensively discussed the concept of prehospital blood product (PHBP) resuscitation [83].

Based on a literature review, their management strategies could include [83]:

- Low-volume resuscitation to maintain perfusion without worsening further bleeding
- Packed red blood cells to maintain perfusion and oxygen delivery, but associated with logistic problems, e.g., storage, aging, cross-matching
- Perfluorocarbons as artificial solutions with enlarged oxygen-carrying capacities
- Artificial hemoglobin solutions with enlarged oxygen-carrying capacities and oxygen delivery without these logistic problems but a risk of several possible adverse reactions including hypertension
- Recombinant activated factor VII (rFVIIa) which enhances coagulation at injured small blood vessels, at that time without clinical experience

They concluded that early administration of hemoglobin solutions and rFVIIa is the possible future in prehospital control of bleeding [83].

In a recent systematic review on PHBP resuscitation, no association between PHBP and survival was reported [79].

Tranexamic acid was used in the prehospital setting in highly unstable patients and was considered effective and

Table 5.1 Coagulopathy of severe trauma (COAST) score

Variable	Value	Score
Entrapment	Yes	1
Systolic blood pressure	<100 mmHg	1
	<90 mmHg	2
Temperature	<35 °C	1
	<32 °C	2
Chest decompression	Yes	1
Abdominal or pelvic content injury	Yes	1
Highest total possible		7

A score ≥ 3 indicates the need of TXA

safe. A trend of a reduced mortality rate was observed [84–87].

Two scores can guide the prehospital emergency personnel to indication of administration of coagulative medication.

The COAST score (prehospital coagulopathy of severe trauma, Table 5.1) was introduced by Mitra et al. [88], and the Prediction of Acute Coagulopathy of Trauma (PACT) score, which includes the parameters age, injury mechanism, prehospital shock index, Glasgow Coma Score values, prehospital cardiopulmonary resuscitation, and endotracheal intubation, was proposed by Peltan et al. [89]. Peltan et al. reported that the PACT score better discriminated the necessity of coagulative medication.

Indications for PHBP resuscitation were reported if two or more of the following points are present [90]:

- Hypotension (single systolic blood pressure ≤ 90 mmHg)
- Tachycardia (single heart rate ≥ 120/min)
- Penetrating injury
- Lactate ≥5 mg/dL (measurement by portable point-of-care device)
- INR ≥ 1.5 (measurement by portable point-of-care device)
- Base deficit ≤−5 mmol/L (measurement by portable point-of-care device)
- Clinical impression

Data on prehospital blood product transfusion are still conflicting, and indications are dependent on transport times and the local rescue system [85].

> Resuscitation with blood products is possible, but presently not the standard of care. Tranexamic acid can be an interesting future option in bleeding trauma patients with pelvic fractures.

References

1. Gänsslen A, Giannoudis P, Pape H. Hemorrhage in pelvic fracture: who needs angiography? Curr Opin Crit Care. 2003;9:515–23.
2. Gänsslen A, Krettek C, Pape H, Machtens S. Acute management of pelvic fractures: a european perspective. In: Smith WR, Ziran BH, Morgan SJ, editors. Fractures of the pelvis and acetabulum. New York: Informa Healthcare USA, Inc.; 2007; ISBN-13: 978-0-8247-2846-5.
3. Lee C, Porter K. The prehospital management of pelvic fractures. Emerg Med J. 2007;24:130–3.
4. Wayne M. New concepts in the prehospital and ED management of pelvic fractures. Isr J Emerg Med. 2006;6:39–42.
5. Bosch U, Pohlemann T, Haas N, Tscherne H. Klassifikation und Management des komplexen Beckentraumas. Unfallchirurg. 1992;95:189–96.
6. Pohlemann T, Bosch U, Gänsslen A, Tscherne H. The Hannover experience in management of pelvic fractures. Clin Orthop. 1994;305:69–80.
7. Pohlemann T, Gänsslen A, Hartung S. In: Tscherne H, editor. Beckenverletzungen/pelvic injuries, results of the german multicenter study group. Hefte zu der Unfallchirurg. Heidelberg: Springer-Verlag; 1998. p. 1–402.
8. Gänsslen A, Pohlemann T, Paul C, Lobenhoffer P, Tscherne H. Epidemiology of pelvic ring injuries. Injury. 1996;Suppl. 1(Part 1):13–20.
9. Balogh Z, King K, Mackay P, McDougall D, Mackenzie S, Evans J, Lyons T, Julie A, Evans R, Deane S. The epidemiology of pelvic ring fractures: a population-based study. J Trauma. 2007;63: 1066–73.
10. Gänsslen A, Krettek C. Épidémiologie des fractures instables de l'anneau pelvien et des lésions associées. In: Nordin JY, Tonetti J, editors. Fractures et disjonctions de l'anneau pelvien de l'adulte. Masson: Elsevier; 2006. ISBN-10: 2842998146.
11. Shaath M, Koury KL, Gibson PD, Lelkes VM, Hwang JS, Ippolito JA, Adams MR, Sirkin MS, Reilly MC. Analysis of pelvic fracture pattern and overall orthopaedic injury burden in children sustaining pelvic fractures based on skeletal maturity. J Child Orthop. 2017;11:1863–2548.
12. Nabaweesi R, Arnold M, Chang D, Rossberg M, Ziegfeld S, Sawaya D, Bathurst M, Colombani P, Abdullah F. Prehospital predictors of risk for pelvic fractures in pediatric trauma patients. Pediatr Surg Int. 2008;24:1053–6.
13. Coccolini F, Stahel P, Montori G, Biffl W, Horer T, Catena F, Kluger Y, Moore E, Peitzman A, Ivatury R, Coimbra R, Fraga G, Pereira B, Rizoli S, Kirkpatrick A, Leppaniemi A, Manfredi R, Magnone S, Chiara O, Solaini L, Ceresoli M, Allievi N, Arvieux C, Velmahos G, Balogh Z, Naidoo N, Weber D, Abu-Zidan F, Sartelli M, Ansaloni L. Pelvic trauma: WSES classification and guidelines. World J Emerg Surg. 2017;12:5.
14. Pohlemann R. Bosch, Tscherne, Chapter 1.7: Notfallbehandlung und Komplextrauma. In: Tscherne H, Pohlemann T, editors. Tscherne Unfallchirurgie: Becken und Acetabulum. Berlin, Heidelberg, New York: Springer-Verlag; 1998. ISBN-10: 364263754X.
15. Petrisor B, Bhandari M. Injuries to the pelvic ring: incidence, classification, associated injuries and mortality rates. Curr Orthop. 2005;19:327–33.
16. ATLS. Advanced trauma life support for doctors, ATLS, instructor course manual. Chicago: American College of Surgeons; 1997.
17. Esmer E, Derst P, Lefering R, Schulz M, Siekmann H, Delank K, DGU® T. Präklinische Einschätzung der Verletzungsart und—schwere beim Schwerverletzten durch den Notarzt. Unfallchirurg. 2017;120:409–16.

18. Duane T, Dechert T, Wolfe L, Brown H, Aboutanos M, Malhotra A, Ivatury R. Clinical examination is superior to plain films to diagnose pelvic fractures compared to CT. Am Surg. 2008;74: 476–9.
19. Duane T, Tan B, Golay D, Cole F, Weireter L, Britt L. Blunt trauma and the role of routine pelvic radiographs: a prospective analysis. J Trauma. 2002;53:463–8.
20. Gonzalez R, Fried P, Bukhalo M. The utility of clinical examination in screening for pelvic fractures in blunt trauma. J Am Coll Surg. 2002;195:740.
21. Kaneriga P, Schweitzer M, Spettell C, Cohen M, Karasick D. The cost-effectiveness of routine pelvic radiography in the evaluation of blunt trauma patients. Skelet Radiol. 1999;28:271–3.
22. Pehle B, Nast-Kolb D, Oberbeck R, Waydhas C, Ruchholtz S. Wertigkeit der körperlichen und radiologischen Basisdiagnostik des Beckens in der Schockraumbehandlung. Unfallchirurg. 2003;106:642–8.
23. Salvino C, Esposito T, Smith D, Dries D, Marshall W, Flisak M, Gamelli R. Routine pelvic X-ray studies in awake blunt trauma patients: a sensible policy. J Trauma. 1992;33:413–6.
24. Tien I, Dufel S. Does ethanol affect the reliability of pelvic bone examination in blunt trauma? Ann Emerg Med. 2000;36:451–5.
25. Yugueros P, Sarmiento J, Garcia A, Ferrada R. Unnecessary use of pelvic X-ray in blunt trauma. J Trauma. 1995;39:722–5.
26. Sauerland S, Bouillon B, Rixen D, Raum M, Koy T, Neugebauer E. The reliability of clinical examination in detecting pelvic fractures in blunt trauma patients: a meta-analysis. Arch Orthop Trauma Surg. 2004;124:123–8.
27. Mackersie R, Shackford S, Garfin S, Hoyt D. Major skeletal injuries in the obtunded trauma patient: a case for routine radiological survey. J Trauma. 1988;28:1450–4.
28. Shlamovitz G, Mower W, Bergman J, Chuang K, Crisp J, Hardy D, Sargent M, Shroff S, Snyder E, Morgan M. How (un)useful is the pelvic ring stability examination in diagnosing mechanically unstable pelvic fractures in blunt trauma patients? J Trauma. 2009;66:815–20.
29. Wohlrath B, Trentzsch H, Hoffmann R, Kremer M, Schmidt-Horlohè K, Schweigkofler U. Präklinische und klinische Versorgung der instabilen Beckenverletzung. Ergebnisse einer Online-Umfrage Unfallchirurg. 2016;119:755–62.
30. Schweigkofler U, Wohlrath B, Trentsch H, Greipel J, Tamimi N, Hoffmann R, Wincheringer D. Diagnostics and early treatment in prehospital and emergency-room phase in suspicious pelvic ring fractures. Eur J Trauma Emerg Surg. 2017;44:747. https://doi.org/10.1007/s00068-017-0860-0.
31. Bilello J, Davis J, Lemaster D, Townsend R, Parks S, Sue L, Kaups K, Groom T, Egbalieh B. Prehospital hypotension in blunt trauma: identifying the "crump factor". J Trauma. 2011;70:1038–42.
32. Franklin G, Boaz P, Spain D, Lukan J, Carrillo E, Richardson J. Prehospital hypotension as a valid indicator of trauma team activation. J Trauma. 2000;48:1034–7.
33. Lalezarzadeh F, Wisniewski P, Huynh K, Loza M, Gnanadev D. Evaluation of prehospital and emergency department systolic blood pressure as a predictor of in-hospital mortality. Am Surg. 2009;75:1009–14.
34. Lipsky A, Gausche-Hill M, Henneman P, Loffredo A, Eckhardt P, Cryer H, de Virgilio C, Klein S, Bongard F, Lewis R. Prehospital hypotension is a predictor of the need for an emergent, therapeutic operation in trauma patients with normal systolic blood pressure in the emergency department. J Trauma. 2006;61:1228–32.
35. Guyette F, Meier E, Newgard C, McKnight B, Daya M, Bulger E, Powell J, Brasel K, Kerby J, Egan D, Sise M, Coimbra R, Fabian T, Hoyt D, Investigators R. A comparison of prehospital lactate and systolic blood pressure for predicting the need for resuscitative care in trauma transported by ground. J Trauma Acute Care Surg. 2015;78:600–6.
36. Guyette F, Suffoletto B, Castillo J, Quintero J, Callaway C, Puyana J. Prehospital serum lactate as a predictor of outcomes in trauma patients: a retrospective observational study. J Trauma. 2011;70:782–6.
37. Lewis C, Naumann D, Crombie N, Midwinter M. Prehospital point-of-care lactate following trauma: a systematic review. J Trauma Acute Care Surg. 2016;81:748–55.
38. Shah A, Guyette F, Suffoletto B, Schultz B, Quintero J, Predis E, King C. Diagnostic accuracy of a single point-of-care prehospital serum lactate for predicting outcomes in pediatric trauma patients. Pediatr Emerg Care. 2013;29:715–9.
39. Rossaint R, Bouillon B, Cerny V, Coats T, Duranteau J, Fernández-Mondéjar E, Filipescu D, Hunt B, Komadina R, Nardi G, Neugebauer E, Ozier Y, Riddez L, Schultz A, Vincent J, Spahn D. The European guideline on management of major bleeding and coagulopathy following trauma: fourth edition. Crit Care. 2016;20:100. https://doi.org/10.1186/s13054-016-1265-x.
40. Spahn D, Bouillon B, Cerny V, Coats T, Duranteau J, Fernández-Mondéjar E, Filipescu D, Hunt B, Komadina R, Nardi G, Neugebauer E, Ozier Y, Riddez L, Schultz A, Vincent J, Rossaint R. Management of bleeding and coagulopathy following major trauma: an updated European guideline. Crit Care. 2013;17:R76. https://doi.org/10.1186/cc12685.
41. Gänsslen A, Hildebrand F, Pohlemann T. Management of hemodynamic unstable patients "in extremis" with pelvic ring fractures. Acta Chir Orthop Traumatol Cechoslov. 2012;79:193–202.
42. Dickinson K, Roberts I. Medical anti-shock trousers (pneumatic anti-shock garments) for circulatory support in patients with trauma (Cochrane review). The Cochrane library, issue 2. Oxford: Update Software; 2003.
43. Ali J, Qi W. Fluid and electrolyte deficit with prolonged pneumatic antishock garment application. J Trauma. 1995;38:612–5.
44. Christensen K. Pneumatic antishock garments (PASG): do they precipitate lower-extremity compartment syndromes? J Trauma. 1986;26:1102–5.
45. Clarke G, Mardel S. Use of MAST to control massive bleeding from pelvic injuries. Injury. 1993;24:628–9.
46. Frank L. Is MAST in the past? The pros and cons of MAST usage in the field. JEMS. 2000;25:38–41.
47. Vahedi M, Ayuyao A, Parsa M. Pneumatic antishock garmentassociated compartment syndrome in injured lower extremities. J Trauma. 1995;38:616–8.
48. Routt ML Jr, Falicov A, Woodhouse E, Schildhauer TA. Circumferential pelvic antishock sheeting: a temporary resuscitation aid. J Orthop Trauma. 2002;16(1):45–8.
49. Simpson T, Krieg JC, Heuer F, Bottlang M. Stabilization of pelvic ring disruptions with a circumferential sheet. J Trauma. 2002;52(1):158–61.
50. Duxbury M, Rossiter N, Lambert A. Cable ties for pelvic stabilisation. Ann R Coll Surg Engl. 2003;85:130.
51. Gardner M, Parada S, Routt M. Internal rotation and taping of the lower extremities for closed pelvic reduction. J Orthop Trauma. 2009;23:361–4.
52. Nunn T, Cosker T, Bose D, Pallister I. Immediate application of improvised pelvic binder as first step in extended resuscitation from life-threatening hypovolaemic shock in conscious patients with unstable pelvic injuries. Injury. 2007;38:125–8.
53. Baumgaertel F, Wilke M, Gotzen L. Experimentelle Erprobung eines pneumatischen Gürtels zur äußeren Beckenkompression. Swiss Surg. 1996;Suppl. 2:42.
54. Vermeulen B, Peter R, Hoffmeyer P, Unger P. Prehospital stabilization of pelvic dislocations: a new strap belt to provide temporary hemodynamic stabilization. Swiss Surg. 1999;5:43–6.
55. Bottlang M, Krieg J, Mohr M, Simpson T, Madey S. Emergent management of pelvic ring fractures with use of circumferential compression. J Bone Joint Surg Am. 2002;84(Suppl. 2):43–7.

56. Bottlang M, Simpson T, Sigg J, Krieg JC, Madey SM, Long WB. Noninvasive reduction of open-book pelvic fractures by circumferential compression. J Orthop Trauma. 2002;16(6):367–73.
57. Bonner T, Eardley W, Newell N, Masouros S, Matthews J, Gibb I, Clasper J. Accurate placement of a pelvic binder improves reduction of unstable fractures of the pelvic ring. J Bone Joint Surg (Br). 2011;93:1524–8.
58. Pizanis A, Pohlemann T, Burkhardt M, Aghayev E, Holstein J. Emergency stabilization of the pelvic ring: clinical comparison between three different techniques. Injury. 2013;44:1760–4.
59. Prasarn M, Conrad B, Small J, Horodyski M, Rechtine G. Comparison of circumferential pelvic sheeting versus the T-POD on unstable pelvic injuries: a cadaveric study of stability. Injury. 2013;44:1756–9.
60. Prasarn M, Horodyski M, Conrad B, Rubery P, Dubose D, Small J, Rechtine G. Comparison of external fixation versus the trauma pelvic orthotic device on unstable pelvic injuries: a cadaveric study of stability. J Trauma Acute Care Surg. 2012;72:1671–5.
61. DeAngelis N, Wixted J, Drew J, Eskander M, Eskander J, French B. Use of the trauma pelvic orthotic device (T-POD) for provisional stabilisation of anterior-posterior compression type pelvic fractures: a cadaveric study. Injury. 2008;39:903–6.
62. Krieg J, Mohr M, Ellis T, Simpson T, Madey S, Bottlang M. Emergent stabilization of pelvic ring injuries by controlled circumferential compression: a clinical trial. J Trauma. 2005;59:959–664.
63. Fu C, Wu Y, Liao C, Kang S, Wang S, Hsu Y, Lin B, Yuan K, Kuo I, Ouyang C. Pelvic circumferential compression devices benefit patients with pelvic fractures who need transfers. Am J Emerg Med. 2013;31:1432–6.
64. Yong E, Vasireddy A, Davies G, Lockey D. Pre-hospital pelvic girdle injury: improving diagnostic accuracy in a physician-led trauma service. Injury. 2016;47:383–8.
65. Jowett A, Bowyer G. Pressure characteristics of pelvic binders. Injury. 2007;38:118–21.
66. Knops S, Van Lieshout E, Spanjersberg W, Patka P, Schipper I. Randomised clinical trial comparing pressure characteristics of pelvic circumferential compression devices in healthy volunteers. Injury. 2011;42:1020–6.
67. Bakhshayesh P, Boutefnouchet T, Tötterman A. Effectiveness of non invasive external pelvic compression: a systematic review of the literature. Scand J Trauma Resusc Emerg Med. 2016;24:73. https://doi.org/10.1186/s13049-016-0259-7.
68. Spanjersberg W, Knops S, Schep N, van Lieshout E, Patka P, Schipper I. Effectiveness and complications of pelvic circumferential compression devices in patients with unstable pelvic fractures: a systematic review of literature. Injury. 2009;40:1031.
69. DGU PGUG. Level 3 guideline on the treatment of patients with severe/multiple injuries. AWMF Register-Nr. 012/019. Eur J Trauma Emerg Surg. 2018;44(Suppl 1):S3–S271.
70. Hinds J, Allen G, Morris C. Trauma and motorcyclists: born to be wild, bound to be injured? Injury. 2007;38:1131–8.
71. Lee C, Porter K. Prehospital management of lower limb fractures. Emerg Med J. 2005;2005:22.
72. O'Gorman M, Trabulsy P, Pilcher D. Zero time prehospital IV. J Trauma. 1989;29:84–6.
73. Pons P, Moore E, Cusick J. Prehospital venous access in an urban paramedic system: a prospective on-scene analysis. J Trauma. 1988;28:1460–3.
74. NICE. Pre-hospital initiation of fluid replacement therapy in trauma. National Institute for Health and Clinical Excellence (NICE). London: NICE; 2004.
75. Bickell W, Wall M, Pepe P. Immediate versus delayed fluid resuscitation for hypotensive patients with penetrating torso injuries. N Engl Med J. 1994;331:1105–9.
76. Burkhardt M, Kristen A, Culemann U, Koehler D, Histing T, Holstein J, Pizanis A, Pohlemann T, Register GPI. Pelvic fracture in multiple trauma: are we still up-to-date with massive fluid resuscitation? Injury. 2014;45S:S70–5.
77. Geeraedts LJ, Pothof L, Caldwell E, de Lange-de Klerk E, D'Amours S. Prehospital fluid resuscitation in hypotensive trauma patients: do we need a tailored approach? Injury. 2015;46:4–9.
78. Qasim Z, Brenner M, Menaker J, Scalea T. Resuscitative endovascular balloon occlusion of the aorta. Resuscitation. 2015;96:175–279.
79. Smith I, James R, Dretzke J, Midwinter M. Prehospital blood product resuscitation for trauma: a systematic review. Shock. 2016;46:3–16.
80. Sadek S, Lockey D, Lendrum R, Perkins Z, Price J, Davies G. Resuscitative endovascular balloon occlusion of the aorta (REBOA) in the pre-hospital setting: an additional resuscitation option for uncontrolled catastrophic haemorrhage. Resuscitation. 2016;107:135–8.
81. Morrison J, Ross J, Rasmussen T, Midwinter M, Jansen J. Resuscitative endovascular balloon occlusion of the aorta: a gap analysis of severely injured UK combat casualties. Shock. 2014;41:388–93.
82. Reva V, Hörer T, Makhnovskiy A, Sokhranov M, Samokhvalov I, DuBose J. Field and en route resuscitative endovascular occlusion of the aorta: a feasible military reality? J Trauma Acute Care Surg. 2017;83(Suppl. 1):S170–6.
83. Soudry E, Stein M. Prehospital management of uncontrolled bleeding in trauma patients: nearing the light at the end of the tunnel. Isr Med Assoc J. 2004;6:485–9.
84. Ausset S, Glassberg E, Nadler R, Sunde G, Cap A, Hoffmann C, Plang S, Sailliol A. Tranexamic acid as part of remote damage-control resuscitation in the prehospital setting: a critical appraisal of the medical literature and available alternatives. J Trauma Acute Care Surg. 2015;78(Suppl. 1):S70–5.
85. Lier H, Bernhard M, Knapp J, Buschmann C, Bretschneider I, Hossfeld B. Ansätze zur prähospitalen Gerinnungstherapie. Aktuelle Übersicht für die zivile Notfallmedizin Anästhesist. 2017;66:867–78.
86. Neeki M, Dong F, Toy J, Vaezazizi R, Powell J, Jabourian N, Jabourian A, Wong D, Vara R, Seiler K, Pennington T, Powell J, Yoshida-McMath C, Kissel S, Schulz-Costello K, Mistry J, Surrusco M, O'Bosky K, Van Stralen D, Ludi D, Sporer K, Benson P, Kwong E, Pitts R, Culhane J, Borger R. Efficacy and safety of tranexamic acid in prehospital traumatic hemorrhagic shock: outcomes of the Cal-PAT study. West J Emerg Med. 2017;18:673–83.
87. Wafaisade A, Lefering R, Bouillon B, Böhmer A, Gäßler M, Ruppert M, DGU T. Prehospital administration of tranexamic acid in trauma patients. Crit Care. 2016;20:143.
88. Mitra B, Cameron P, Mori A, Maini A, Fitzgerald M, Paul E, Street A. Early prediction of acute traumatic coagulopathy. Resuscitation. 2011;82:1208–13.
89. Peltan I, Rowhani-Rahbar A, Vande Vusse L, Caldwell E, Rea T, Maier R, Watkins T. Development and validation of a prehospital prediction model for acute traumatic coagulopathy. Crit Care. 2016;20:371.
90. Jenkins D, Stubbs J, Williams S, Berns K, Zielinski M, Strandenes G, Zietlow S. Implementation and execution of civilian remote damage control resuscitation programs. Shock. 2014;41(Suppl 1):84–9.

6 Inhospital Clinical Examination

Stephan Grechenig, Christian Pfeifer, and Axel Gänsslen

Early management of trauma patients must include a proper diagnosis of all the injuries. The diagnosis of a pelvic injury requires a high index of suspicion, particularly when the patient is unconscious or uncooperative. Assessment of the degree of pelvic instability must always begin with a careful history and physical examination.

According to the Advanced Trauma Life Support (ATLS) concept, a systematic and organized approach to management of these often critically injured patients is first provided. Initially, stabilization of the C-ABCs is mandatory.

6.1 Patient Handover

The trauma team remains silent during this handover, and a member of the prehospital team communicates information about the patient, usually using the AT-MIST acronym. All members should then commence care with a common understanding of the patient's initial condition.

After admission at the hospital, an immediate effective communication focusing on the prehospital details is performed, and relevant information is given to all team members. The prehospital team delivers a "sterile (silent) handover" [1]. One member of the prehospital team communicates the relevant information about the patient.

S. Grechenig
Department of Orthopedics and Trauma Surgery, AUVA Trauma Hospital Klagenfurt, Klagenfurt, Austria

Department of Trauma Surgery, University Hospital Regensburg, Regensburg, Germany

C. Pfeifer
Department of Trauma Surgery, University Hospital Regensburg, Regensburg, Germany
e-mail: christian.pfeifer@ukr.de

A. Gänsslen (✉)
Department of Trauma Surgery, Orthopedics and Hand Surgery, Hospital Wolfsburg, Wolfsburg, Germany

The handover practice includes typically the MIST acronym details:

- **M**—Mechanism of injury/illness
- **I**—Injuries (sustained or suspected)
- **S**—Signs, including observations and monitoring
- **T**—Treatment given

6.2 Injury Mechanism

Knowing the mechanism of injury provides a better understanding of possible forces acted on the pelvis [2]. A considerable force is usually needed to result in pelvic ring injuries in younger patients. Thus, many patients with pelvic ring fractures are polytraumatized, and they present with multiple associated injuries [3, 4]. Low-energy fractures are typically observed either in older patients that have fallen from a standing position or in younger patients who sustained an avulsion at a tendon-bone complex of the pelvis (e.g., the anterior superior iliac spine (ASIS), the anterior inferior iliac spine (AIIS), or the ischial tuberosity) during sport activity [5].

6.3 Pelvic Inspection

A detailed inspection of the whole pelvic area is crucial, as several clinical signs can be suggestive of pelvic injury.

Primary inspection of the undressed patient should focus on pelvic asymmetry, differences in leg length, pelvic soft tissue injury around the complete pelvis, including the perineum, search for urethral or vaginal bleeding, and search for differences of the color of the feet, probably indicating vascular impairments (Fig. 6.1).

The presence of contusions, abrasions, scrotal swelling, and hematomas can provide additional information about the direction and magnitude of the forces involved and any contiguous structures that may have been injured.

A. Gänsslen et al. (eds.), *Pelvic Ring Fractures*, https://doi.org/10.1007/978-3-030-54730-1_6

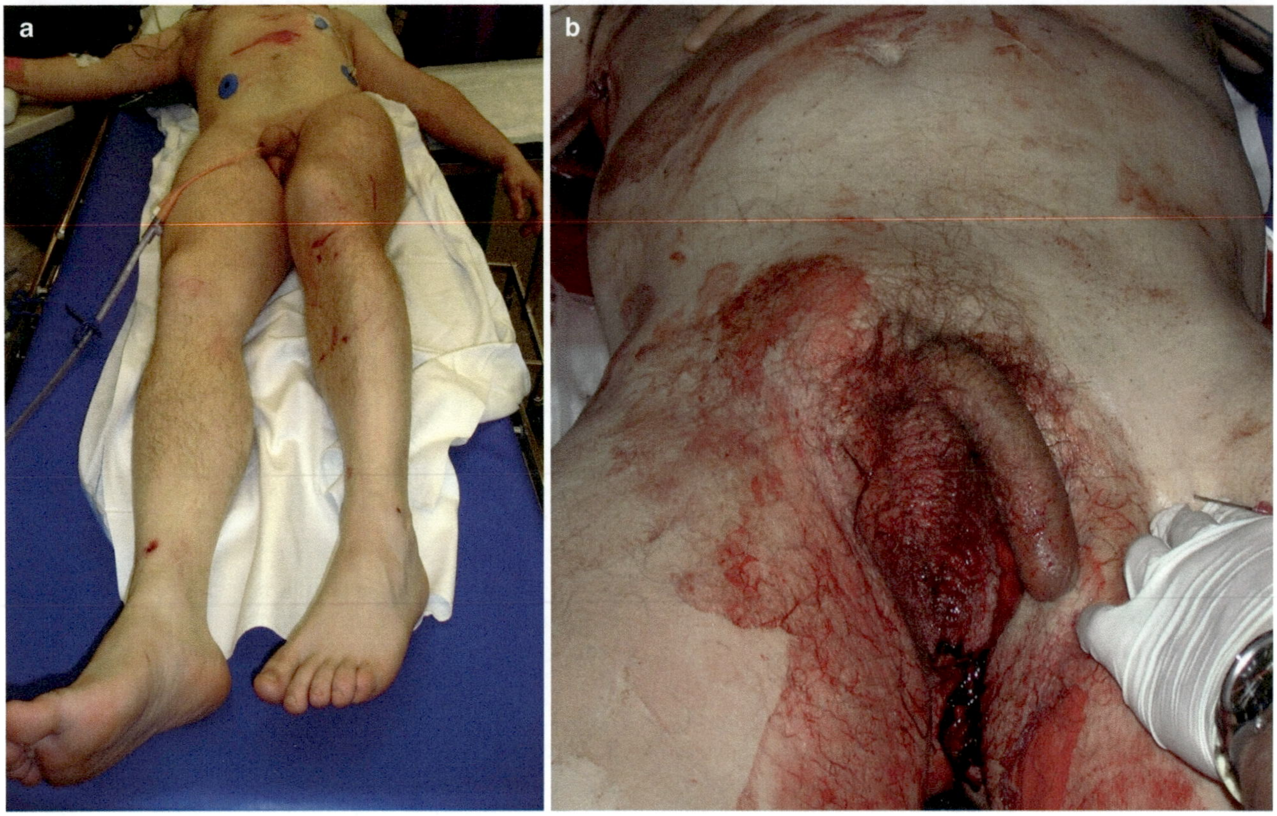

Fig. 6.1 Possible observational signs of a pelvic injury: pelvic and leg asymmetry (**a**), open pelvic wounds (**b**)

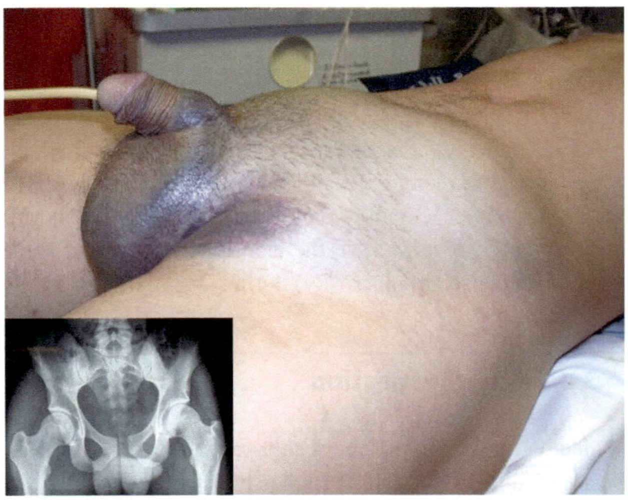

Fig. 6.2 Destot sign: superficial inguinal hematoma: the X-ray confirms symphyseal disruption

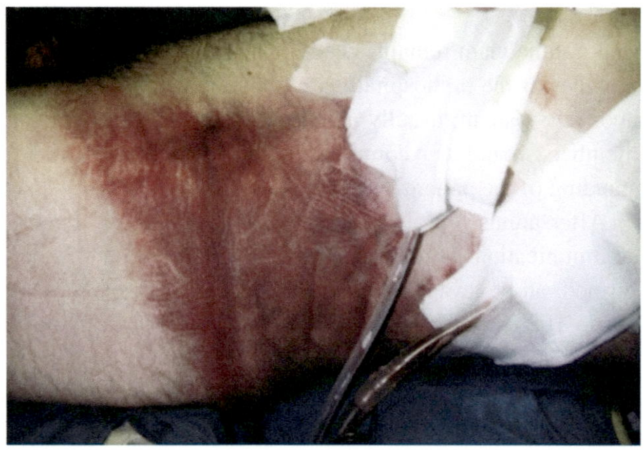

Fig. 6.3 Grey Turner sign: flank ecchymosis, which can indicate retroperitoneal hematoma

The *Destot sign*, a superficial hematoma above the inguinal ligament at the groin (Fig. 6.2), over the scrotum or perineum, or in the upper thigh, may indicate a pelvic fracture [6].

The *Grey Turner sign*, a flank ecchymosis, can indicate retroperitoneal hemorrhage (Fig. 6.3).

Any lacerations, especially in the perineal region, should be examined because they may indicate possible open fractures (Fig. 6.4).

Urogenital injuries can be expected if blood is observed at the rectum or urethra, while vaginal blood is most often due to menses in non-menopausal females.

A rotational deformity of the pelvis or lower extremity and a leg length discrepancy, without an obvious fracture to the long bones, can indicate a displaced pelvic ring injury

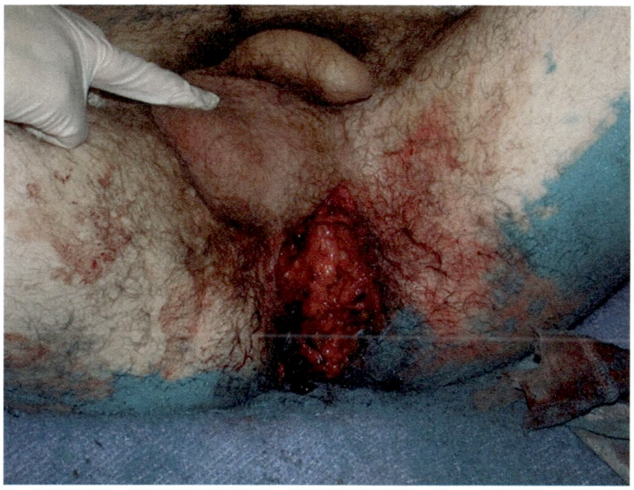

Fig. 6.4 Perineal laceration

[5]. However, according to current literature, the presence of either pelvic deformity or pelvic ring instability on physical examination has a poor sensitivity for detection of mechanically unstable pelvic fractures in blunt trauma patients and is not necessarily recommended. Bimanual compression and distraction of the iliac wings might reveal pain as a first sign of pelvic fracture and is a reliable finding in unstable pelvic injuries [7].

Typical observable clinical signs include:

- Open or closed wounds or abrasions of the groin, buttock, perineum, and flanks
- Blood at the urethral meatus, around the rectum or out of the vagina
- Leg length inequality
- External or internal rotation deformity of the hemipelvis
- Scrotal edema

6.4 Pain Analysis

Pain in the pelvic region is a potential sign of a pelvic fracture, but a high rate of misinterpretation can be present [8–15].

Clinical examination of the pelvis fails to identify later diagnosed pelvic injuries in 3.4–52.6% [8, 9, 11–16]. Approximately 3.6–73.8% pelvic injuries were clinically suspected but later not confirmed on X-rays [8, 13, 15, 16].

In a meta-analysis by Sauerland et al., an overall sensitivity and specificity of 90% and a false negative and a false positive rate of 10% for clinically detecting pelvic injuries were reported. In awake patients, the sensitivity was close to 100%, indicating that neurological normal patients were easier to analyze. Overall, 11.1% of pelvic fractures were missed during clinical examination [17].

In contrast, Mackersie et al. reported a high incidence of occult major pelvic fractures when clinical examination was negative [18], and Gonzales et al. reported only one-third of patients reporting pain on lateral compression or palpation of the pubic symphysis [10].

In a recent analysis, Shlamovitz et al. analyzed 81 stable and 34 unstable pelvic injuries [7] and reported on different sensitivities and specificities dependent on several parameters:

- All pelvic fractures: 8% sensitivity, 99% specificity
- Unstable pelvic fractures: 26% sensitivity, 99.9% specificity
- Pelvic pain or tenderness (GCS >13), all fractures: 74% sensitivity, 97% specificity
- Pelvic pain or tenderness (GCS >13), unstable fractures: 100% sensitivity, 93% specificity
- Pelvic deformity, all fractures: 30% sensitivity, 99% specificity
- Pelvic deformity, unstable fractures: 55% sensitivity, 97% specificity

McCormick et al. could show that pain during posterior palpation was highly sensitive for posterior pelvic ring injuries [19].

Nüchtern et al. could additionally show that in >80% of geriatric patients with positive clinical signs at the posterior pelvic ring (pain, tenderness, positive pelvic stress signs), magnetic resonance imaging (MRI) revealed posterior pelvic ring fractures [20].

6.5 Pelvic Examination

In the conscious cooperative patient, physical examination allows for diagnosis of a pelvic ring injury with a 90% sensitivity [16].

Palpation may reveal localized pain, crepitus, or even an abnormal motion of the hemipelvis, indicative for bony instability.

Palpation of fluctuant areas indicates potential Morel-Lavallée injuries (Fig. 6.5). These are expected in the typical regions around the greater trochanter, the lumbo-gluteal region, and the thigh [21]. Besides local pain, typical clinical signs include [22–29]:

- Presence of a soft fluctuant area with skin hypermobility
- Potentially decreased cutaneous sensation
- Local skin contusion, ecchymosis around the pelvic ring, tire marks, and friction burns

Blood from the rectum or urethra often is indicative of an underlying injury (Fig. 6.6), whereas in the non-menopausal female, bleeding may be indicative of menses.

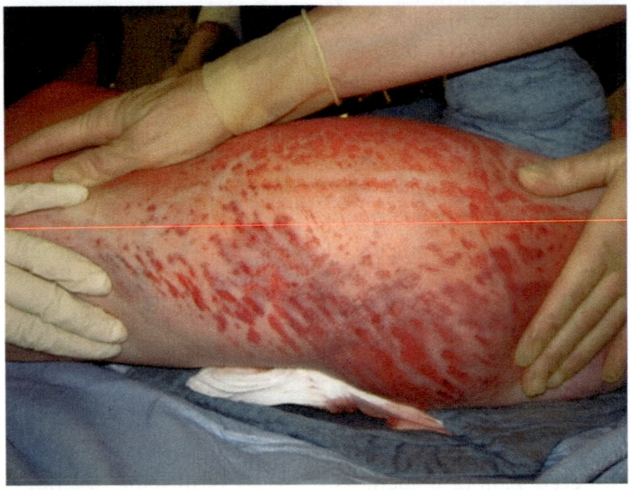

Fig. 6.5 Morel-Levallée lesion of the femoral region in a patient with additional pelvic fracture after a roll-over injury mechanism

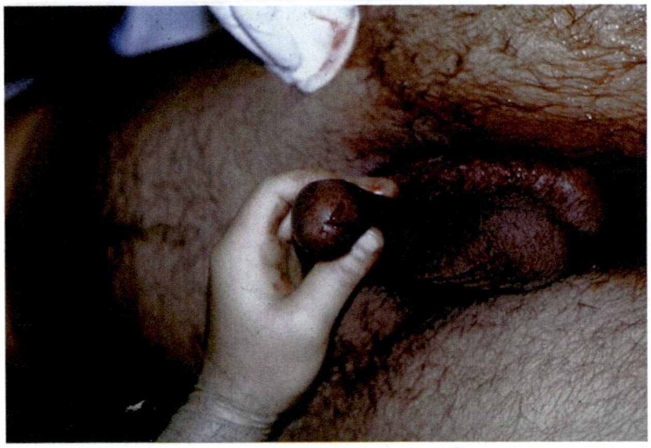

Fig. 6.6 Blood at the urethral meatus, indicating pelvic urological injury

The most common clinical sign of a bladder injury after blunt trauma is a macrohematuria [30, 31]. Further signs include inability to void [30, 32]; abdominal tenderness [31]; suprapubic bruising [30, 32]; abdominal distension [30, 32]; swelling of the scrotum, perineum, abdominal wall, and/or thighs [30]; uremia; and elevated creatinine level [30].

Clinical signs of urethral injuries in male patients include blood at the meatus, inability to void, hematuria, and dysuria. In the case of partial rupture, clinical signs consist of scrotal, perineal, and/or penile swelling, high riding or impalpable prostate on rectal examination and as an indirect sign the difficulty/inability to insert a catheter [33].

In female patients, blood at the urethral meatus and/or vaginal introitus, inability to void, labial swelling, vaginal laceration, and hematuria in the case of partial rupture can be signs of urethral injuries [33].

Detailed examination of all orifices (urethra, rectum) is mandatory to rule out concomitant complex pelvic trauma. Vaginal examination, at least inspection, is warranted in all female patients to rule out mucosal tears. In doubt, urological and gynecological consult can become necessary.

Clinical signs, even in patients with impaired consciousness, alerting for pelvic fractures can include [34, 35]:

- Pelvic deformity
- Bruising or swelling over the bony prominences, pubis, perineum, or scrotum
- Leg length discrepancy
- Rotational deformity of a lower limb (without fracture in that extremity)
- Wounds around the pelvis
- Bleeding from the patient's rectum, vagina, or urethra
- Neurological abnormalities

6.6 Pelvic Instability Testing

For a long time, positive clinical testing of mechanical instability of the pelvis was advised to be a marker of severe pelvic fractures. Careful and gentle manual compression of the pelvic ring in anterior-posterior and lateral-medial directions was recommended [36]. The presence of a pelvic instability was supposed to be often associated with a high risk of pelvic bleeding [12].

In a recent online survey from German hospitals, 91% of surgeons recommended stability testing in suspected pelvic fractures, whereas 31.2% stated that unnecessary manipulation should be avoided. Additionally, 70.7% indicated pelvic emergency stabilization only after clinically testing pelvic stability [37].

In a prospective analysis of 254 patients with clinically suspected pelvic fractures, only 45.7% had radiologically confirmed pelvic fractures. Clinical stability testing was positive in 25 patients with 72% of these presented with unstable fracture pattern on later computed tomography (CT) examination. Overall, manual stability testing missed 68.4% of radiologically unstable fractures, resulting in 31.6% sensitivity, 92.2% specificity, 72% positive predictive value, and 68% negative predictive value [38].

Additionally, it has to be considered that stability testing is without (therapeutic) relevance and no advantage is observed regarding the choice of the target hospital for these patients.

Clinical examination in unresponsive patients is difficult and cannot confirm every patient with a pelvic fracture.

6.7 Identification of Patients at Hemodynamic Risk

In the primary assessment of patients with pelvic ring injuries, the assessment of the accompanying shock state is of major relevance regarding treatment initiation.

The severity of potential hemorrhage, the blood loss, and the extent of the soft tissue injuries remain difficult to assess.

Various parameters such as systolic blood pressure, heart rate, primary base deficit, primary lactate, the course of these parameters, the hemoglobin or hematocrit level at admission, the respiratory rate, the pulse pressure, the mental status, "capillary refill," and the extent of urinary excretion are considered in determining the state of shock state [39–41].

Hypotension in blunt trauma is usually defined as an SBP of ≤90 mmHg [39–48]. In patients with pelvic injuries, Eastridge et al. found that already with an systolic blood pressure (SBP) of 110 mmHg a hypoperfusion of the soft tissues exists [43].

The heart rate value, indicating a pathological shock state, remains unknown. Different cut-off values were reported in the literature [42, 48, 49]. Brasel et al. reported a sufficient specificity of >95% in blunt trauma patients at a heart rate >120/min. In contrast, a heart rate of 80–100/min was associated with a specificity of only 33.2% and a sensitivity of 75.4% [50]. Comparable values were reported by Blackmore et al., who identified an heart rate (HR) of ≥130/min as a risk factor for pelvis-related bleeding [42].

> Isolated analysis of either the heart rate or the systolic blood pressure has no reliable predictive value estimating the pelvis-related shock state.

Victorino et al. tried to correlate both parameters in an analysis of blunt and penetrating injuries [48]. A heart rate ≥90/min was identified as a significant risk factor for hypotension (systolic blood pressure < 90 mmHg).

However, 35% of patients present with a relative bradycardia in combination with hypotension, which corresponds to experiences from other studies [48, 51].

Grimme et al. were able to confirm this relationship, according to a shock index of >1 (HR/SBP). Especially the associated pelvic trauma could be identified as a risk factor of the pathological shock index [52].

Immediate analysis of the primary hemoglobin concentration is performed from capillary, venous, and arterial whole blood by bedside hemoglobinometry (photometry) [53, 54]. The result is available within 40 s. Own observations showed that vital hemorrhage is supposed at a primary hemoglobin concentration of 8 g/dL [55].

It has to be considered that normal admission values cannot exclude significant trauma [56].

> Isolated analysis of the primary hemoglobin concentration has no reliable predictive value estimating the pelvis-related shock state [57].

In contrast, the primary base deficit and lactate levels are considered important parameters for shock monitoring to predict mortality and to estimate shock-related complications [41, 57–62].

Both parameters are important in assessing the "hidden" shock [58, 63].

A primary increased lactate level indicates significant injury severity [59, 64], and persistent increased values are associated with mortality [63, 65, 66].

The value of the primary base excess was extensively analyzed by Rixen et al. [61, 67], who identified a threshold of –6 mmol/L as a prognostic worse indicator.

Recently, a base deficit of −9.35 mmol/L was associated with a 100% specificity and a 70% sensitivity, regarding mortality [68].

> Base deficit and lactate course are useful parameters as worse values are indicative of relevant posttraumatic shock.

Recently, according to extended pathophysiological understanding of posttraumatic induced coagulopathy, a thromboelastography-guided analysis of patients with pelvic ring fractures was initiated [69]. In contrast to established protocols (1:1:1 packed red blood cell (PRBC):fresh frozen plasma (FFP):platelet ratio), a PRBC:FFP:platelet ratio of 2.5:1:2.8 was observed, as >90% of patients had transfusion of at least one PRBC.

> Thromboelastography with adjuvant platelet mapping is a valuable adjunct to guide the acute phase of resuscitation in patients with polytrauma with pelvic injuries [69].

6.8 Rectal Examination

Historically and even today, routine rectal examination in suspected pelvic ring injuries is still recommended in textbooks to confirm or exclude accompanying peripelvic injuries [70].

Already in 2005, Esposito et al. analyzed that digital rectal examination is of minor value, as clinical signs of gastrointestinal bleeding, urethral disruption, or spinal cord injury showed comparable information without changes in management. It was stated that "Elimination of routine digital rectal examination from the secondary survey will presumably conserve time and resources … without any significant negative impact on care and outcome" [71].

Recent further analyses confirmed these recommendations:

The digital rectal examination was found to have a poor sensitivity for diagnosing spinal cord, bowel, rectal, and even bony pelvis and urethral injuries in adult and pediatric patients [72, 73].

Even for detecting urethral injuries ("high riding prostate" during rectal examination), a sensitivity of only 2% was recorded [74].

A recent analysis showed that digital rectal examination missed all urethral and colon injuries. Additionally, 91.7% of spinal cord, 93.1% of small bowel, and 66.7% of rectal injuries were not detected [75].

Digital rectal examination as a screening tool is no longer recommended in blunt trauma patients. However, inspection of the perineum and search for rectal, urethral, or vaginal bleeding are crucial.

6.9 Associated Neurovascular Injuries

Pelvic ring injuries can be associated with neurovascular injuries. Therefore, careful neurovascular examination of the lumbosacral plexus and the lower extremity vessels is mandatory in every suspected pelvic fracture.

Vascular injuries predominantly include venous vessels, while arterial injury is less common.

The vascular status is analyzed by palpation of the pulses of the lower extremities and inspection of capillary refill (normal: <3 s). In suspected cases, Doppler examination of the pulses should be performed.

Neurological screening of the lower extremities is essential and consists of an oriented sensory examination, standard tendon reflex testing, and in awake patients an orientated testing of key muscles.

In pelvic ring injuries, most often the L5 and S1 nerve roots are involved. Sacral fractures can be additionally present with sacral plexus lesions. Thus, testing of the lumbosacral nerve roots is mandatory. A standardized examination is recommended, e.g., the ASIA Scheme [76].

The key myotomes and dermatomes for the lower extremity neurologic testing of the lumbosacral plexus are shown in Table 6.1.

Table 6.1 Key myotomes and dermatomes of the lower extremity for neurologic testing

Root	Functional group	Myotome	Dermatome
L2	Hip flexors	Iliopsoas	Anterior mid-thigh
L3	Knee extensors	Quadriceps	Anterior knee
L4	Ankle dorsiflexors	Tibialis anterior	Medial leg and medial malleolus
L5	Long toe extensors	Extensor hallucis longus	Lateral leg, medial dorsum foot
S1	Ankle plantar flexors	Gastrocsoleus complex	Distal calf, lateral plantar foot

Table 6.2 Muscle function grading

Grade	Description
0	Total paralysis
1	Palpable or visible contraction
2	Active movement, full ROM with gravity eliminated
3	Active movement, full ROM against gravity
4	Active movement, full ROM against gravity and moderate resistance in a muscle specific position
5	(Normal) active movement, full ROM against gravity and full resistance in a functional muscle position expected from an otherwise unimpaired person
5*	(Normal) active movement, full ROM against gravity and sufficient resistance to be considered normal if identified inhibiting factors (i.e., pain, disuse) were not present
NT	Not testable (i.e., attributable to immobilization, severe pain such that the patient cannot be graded, amputation of limb, or contracture greater than 50% of the normal ROM)

Table 6.3 Sensory grading

Grade	Description
0	Absent (or inability to tell sharp from dull)
1	Altered, either decreased or impaired sensation or hypersensitivity
2	Normal
NT	Not testable

The ASIA system additionally includes a standardized muscle strength grading (Table 6.2) and a sensoric grading system (Table 6.3).

Lower sacral nerve root injuries may lead to bowel and bladder disorders and/or sexual dysfunction, which is normally not the primary focus during shock room evaluation.

Minimal examination should consist of testing foot, greater toe and knee flexion and extension, and the typical dermatomes of the lower leg. In doubt, a detailed expert clinical neurological evaluation should be performed.

In unconscious patients, clinical neurological examination is difficult. Here, clues for neurological impairment can include:

- Absence of spontaneous movements
- Missing or weakened response to painful stimuli
- Attenuation/lack of muscle stretching reflexes
- Vegetative dysfunctions (anhidrosis, vasomotor paralysis with temperature side differences)

References

1. Mercer S, Kingston E, Jones C. The trauma call. BMJ. 2018;361:k2272. https://doi.org/10.1136/bmj.k2272.
2. Cryer HM, Miller F, Evers BM, Rouben LR, Seligson DL. Pelvis fracture classification: correlation with hemorrhage. J Trauma. 1988;28:973–80.
3. Giannoudis PV, Grotz M, Tzioupis C, Dino-poulos H, Wells GE, Bouamra O, Lecky F. Prevalence of pelvic fractures, associated injuries, and mortality: the United Kingdom perspective. J Trauma. 2007;63:875–83.
4. Tscherne H, Regel G. Care of the polytrauma-tised patient. J Bone Joint Surg (Br). 1996;78-B:840–52.
5. Pennal GF, Tile M, Waddell JP, Garside H. Pelvic disruption: assessment and classification. Clin Orthop Relat Res. 1980;151:12–21.
6. Failinger MS, McGanity PL. Current concepts review: unstable fractures of the pelvic ring. J Bone Joint Surg Am. 1992;74-A:781–91.
7. Shlamovitz G, Mower W, Bergman J, Chuang K, Crisp J, Hardy D, Sargent M, Shroff S, Snyder E, Morgan M. How (un)useful is the pelvic ring stability examination in diagnosing mechanically unstable pelvic fractures in blunt trauma patients? J Trauma. 2009;66:815–20.
8. Duane T, Dechert T, Wolfe L, Brown H, Aboutanos M, Malhotra A, Ivatury R. Clinical examination is superior to plain films to diagnose pelvic fractures compared to CT. Am Surg. 2008;74:476–9.
9. Duane T, Tan B, Golay D, Cole F, Weireter L, Britt L. Blunt trauma and the role of routine pelvic radiographs: a prospective analysis. J Trauma. 2002;53:463–8.
10. Gonzalez R, Fried P, Bukhalo M. The utility of clinical examination in screening for pelvic fractures in blunt trauma. J Am Coll Surg. 2002;195:740.
11. Kaneriga P, Schweitzer M, Spettell C, Cohen M, Karasick D. The cost-effectiveness of routine pelvic radiography in the evaluation of blunt trauma patients. Skelet Radiol. 1999;28:271–3.
12. Pehle B, Nast-Kolb D, Oberbeck R, Waydhas C, Ruchholtz S. Wertigkeit der körperlichen und radiologischen Basisdiagnostik des Beckens in der Schockraumbehandlung. Unfallchirurg. 2003;106:642–8.
13. Salvino C, Esposito T, Smith D, Dries D, Marshall W, Flisak M, Gamelli R. Routine pelvic X-ray studies in awake blunt trauma patients: a sensible policy. J Trauma. 1992;33:413–6.
14. Tien I, Dufel S. Does ethanol affect the reliability of pelvic bone examination in blunt trauma? Ann Emerg Med. 2000;36:451–5.
15. Yugueros P, Sarmiento J, Garcia A, Ferrada R. Unnecessary use of pelvic X-ray in blunt trauma. J Trauma. 1995;39:722–5.
16. Gonzalez R, Fried P, Bukhalo M. The utility of clinical examination in screening for pelvic fractures in blunt trauma. J Am Coll Surg. 2002;194:121–5.
17. Sauerland S, Bouillon B, Rixen D, Raum M, Koy T, Neugebauer E. The reliability of clinical examination in detecting pelvic fractures in blunt trauma patients: a meta-analysis. Arch Orthop Trauma Surg. 2004;124:123–8.
18. Mackersie R, Shackford S, Garfin S, Hoyt D. Major skeletal injuries in the obtunded trauma patient: a case for routine radiological survey. J Trauma. 1988;28:1450–4.
19. McCormick J, Morgan S, Smith W. Clinical effectiveness of the physical examination in diagnosis of posterior pelvic ring injuries. J Orthop Trauma. 2003;17:257–61.
20. Nüchtern J, Hartel M, Henes F, Groth M, Jauch S, Haegele J, Briem D, Hoffmann M, Lehmann W, Rueger J, Großterlinden L. Significance of clinical examination, CT and MRI scan in the diagnosis of posterior pelvic ring fractures. Injury. 2015;46:315–9.
21. McLean K, Popovic S. Morel-Lavallée lesion: AIRP best cases in radiologic-pathologic correlation. Radiographics. 2017;37:190–6.
22. Collinge C, Tornetta P III. Soft tissue injuries associated with pelvic fractures. Orthop Clin North Am. 2004;35:451–6.
23. Diviti S, Gupta N, Hooda K, Sharma K, Lo L. Morel-Lavallee lesions-review of pathophysiology, clinical findings, imaging findings and management. J Clin Diagn Res. 2017;11:TE01–4.
24. McKenzie G, Niederhauser B, Collins M, Howe B. CT characteristics of Morel-Lavallée lesions: an under-recognized but significant finding in acute trauma imaging. Skelet Radiol. 2016;45:1053–60.
25. Mukherjee K, Perrin S, Hughes P. Morel-Lavallee lesion in an adolescent with ultrasound and MRI correlation. Skelet Radiol. 2007;36(Suppl 1):S43–5.
26. Neal C, Jacobson J, Brandon C, Kalume-Brigido M, Morag Y, Girish G. Sonography of Morel-Lavallée lesions. J Ultrasound Med. 2008;27:1077–81.
27. Robertson N, Anwar I, Nayagam K, Katz R, Farrant J, Holloway B, Marmnery H. Imaging characteristics of the Morel Lavallee Lesion. Poster No. P-0100. ESSR: EPOS; 2014.
28. Tsur A, Galin A, Kogan L, Loberant N. Morel-Lavallee syndrome after crush injury. Harefuah. 2006;145:111–3.
29. Zhong B, Zhang C, Luo C. Percutaneous drainage of Morel-Lavallée lesions when the diagnosis is delayed. Can J Surg. 2014;57:356–7.
30. Gomez R, Ceballos L, Coburn M, Corriere JJ, Dixon C, Lobel B, McAninch J. Consensus statement on bladder injuries. BJU Int. 2004;94:27–32.
31. Wirth G, Peter R, Poletti P, Iselin C. Advances in the management of blunt traumatic bladder rupture: experience with 36 cases. BJU Int. 2010;106:1344–9.
32. Tonkin J, Tisdale B, Jordan G. Assessment and initial management of urologic trauma. Med Clin North Am. 2011;95:245–51.
33. Lumen N, Kuehhas F, Djakovic N, Kitrey N, Serafetinidis E, Sharma D, Summerton D. Review of the current management of lower urinary tract injuries by the EAU trauma guidelines panel. Eur Urol. 2015;67:925–9.
34. Lee C, Porter K. The prehospital management of pelvic fractures. Emerg Med J. 2007;24:130–3.
35. Pohlemann R. Bosch, Tscherne, Chapter 1.7: Notfallbehandlung und Komplextrauma. In: Tscherne H, Pohlemann T, editors. Tscherne Unfallchirurgie: Becken und Acetabulum. Berlin, Heidelberg, New York: Springer-Verlag; 1998. ISBN-10: 364263754X.
36. Gänsslen A, Krettek C, Pape H, Machtens S. Acute management of pelvic fractures: a european perspective. In: Smith WR, Ziran BH, Morgan SJ, editors. Fractures of the pelvis and acetabulum. New York: Informa Healthcare USA, Inc.; 2007; ISBN-13: 978–0–8247-2846-5.
37. Wohlrath B, Trentzsch H, Hoffmann R, Kremer M, Schmidt-Horlohè K, Schweigkofler U. Präklinische und klinische Versorgung der instabilen Beckenverletzung. Ergebnisse einer Online-Umfrage Unfallchirurg. 2016;119:755–62.
38. Schweigkofler U, Wohlrath B, Trentsch H, Greipel J, Tamimi N, Hoffmann R, Wincheringer D. Diagnostics and early treatment in prehospital and emergency-room phase in suspicious pelvic ring fractures. Eur J Trauma Emerg Surg. 2017;44:747. https://doi.org/10.1007/s00068-017-0860-0.
39. ATLS. Advanced trauma life support program for doctors. 8th ed. Chicago: American College of Surgeons; 2008.
40. Rossaint R, Bouillon B, Cerny V, Coats TJ, Duranteau J, Fernandez-Mondejar E, Hunt BJ, Komadina R, Nardi G, Neugebauer E, Ozier Y, Riddez L, Schultz A, Stahel PF, Vincent JL, Spahn DR. Management of bleeding following major trauma: an updated European guideline. Crit Care. 2010;14(2):R52.
41. Siegel J, Rivkind A, Dalal S, Goodarzi S. Early physiologic predictors of injury severity and death in blunt multiple trauma. Arch Surg. 1990;125:498–508.
42. Blackmore CC, Cummings P, Jurkovich GJ, Linnau KF, Hoffer EK, Rivara FP. Predicting major hemorrhage in patients with pelvic fracture. J Trauma. 2006;61(2):346–52.
43. Eastridge B, Salinas J, McManus J, Blackburn L, Bugler E, Cooke W, Concertino V, Wade C, Holomb J. Hypotension beginns at 110 mm hg: redefining "hypotension" with data. J Trauma. 2007;63(2):291–9.

44. Eastridge B, Starr A, Minei J, O'Keefe G, Scalea T. The importance of fracture pattern in guiding therapeutic decision-making in patients with hemorrhagic shock and pelvic ring disruptions. J Trauma. 2002;53(3):446–50.
45. Guzzo J, Bochicchio G, Napolitano L, Malone D, Meyer W, Scalea T. Prediction of outcomes in trauma: anatomic or physiologic parameters? J Am Coll Surg. 2005;201:891–7.
46. Miller PR, Moore PS, Mansell E, Meredith JW, Chang MC. External fixation or arteriogram in bleeding pelvic fracture: initial therapy guided by markers of arterial hemorrhage. J Trauma. 2003;54(3):437–43.
47. Starr A, Griffin D, Reinert C. Pelvic ring disruption: prediction of associated injuries, transfusion requirement, pelvic arteriography, complications, and mortality. J Orthop Trauma. 2002;16:553–61.
48. Victorino G, Battistella F, Wisner D. Does Tachycradia correlate with hypotension after trauma? J Am Coll Surg. 2003;196:679–84.
49. Cook RE, Keating JF, Gillespie I. The role of angiography in the management of haemorrhage from major fractures of the pelvis. J Bone Joint Surg (Br). 2002;84(2):178–82.
50. Brasel K, Guse C, Gentinello L, Nirula R. Heart rate: is it truly a vital sign? J Trauma. 2007;62:812–7.
51. Demetriades D, Chan L, Bhasin P, Berne T, Ramicone E, Huichocea F, Velmahos G, Cornwell E, Belzberg H, Murrey J, Asensio J. Relative bradycardia in patients with traumatic hypotension. J Trauma. 1998;45(3):534–9.
52. Grimme K, Pape H, Probst C, Seelis M, Sott A, Harwood P, Zelle B, Krettek C, Allgöwer M. Calculation of different triage scores based on the German trauma registry. Eur J Trauma. 2005;31(5):480–7.
53. Morris LD, Pont A, Lewis SM. Use of a new HemoCue system for measuring haemoglobin at low concentrations. Clin Lab Haematol. 2001;23(2):91–6.
54. Rippmann CE, Nett PC, Popovic D, Seifert B, Pasch T, Spahn DR. Hemocue, an accurate bedside method of hemoglobin measurement? J Clin Monit. 1997;13(6):373–7.
55. Pohlemann T, Culemann U, Gänsslen A, Tscherne H. Die schwere Beckenverletzung mit pelviner Massenblutung: Ermittlung der Blutungsschwere und klinische Erfahrung mit der Notfallstabilisierung. Unfallchirurg. 1996;99(10):734–43.
56. Paradies N, Balter S, Davison C, Simon G, Rose M. Hematocrit as a predictor of significant injury after penetrating trauma. Am J Emeg Med. 1997;15:224–8.
57. Spahn DR, Cerny V, Coats TJ, Duranteau J, Fernandez-Mondejar E, Gordini G, Stahel PF, Hunt BJ, Komadina R, Neugebauer E, Ozier Y, Riddez L, Schultz A, Vincent JL, Rossaint R. Management of bleeding following major trauma: a European guideline. Crit Care. 2007;11(1):R17.
58. Davis J, Parks S, Kaups K, Gladen H, O'Donnel-Nico S. Admission base deficit predicts transfusion requirements and risk of complications. J Trauma. 1996;41(5):769–74.
59. Ertel W, Keel M, Eid K, Platz A, Trentz O. Control of severe hemorrhage using C-clamp and pelvic packing in multiply injured patients with pelvic ring disruption. J Orthop Trauma. 2001;15(7):468–74.
60. Martin J, FitzSullivan E, Salim A, Brown C, Demetriades D, Long WB. Disordance between lactate and base deficit in the surgical intensive care unit: which one do you trust? Am J Surg. 2006;191:625–30.
61. Rixen D, Raum M, Bouillon B, Neugebauer E, DGU APD. Der base exzess als prognose-indikator bei polytrauma-patienten. Anästhesiol Intensivmed Motfallmed Schmerzther. 2002;37:347–9.
62. Rutherford E, Morris A, Reed G, Hall K. Base deficit stratifies mortality and determines therapy. J Trauma. 1992;33(3):417–23.
63. Abramson D, Scalea T, Hitchcock R, Trooskin S, Henry S, Greenspan J. Lactate clearence and survival following injury. J Trauma. 1993;35:584–9.
64. Manikis P, Jankowski S, Zhang H, Kahn R, Vinect J. Correlation of serial blood lactate levels to organ failure and mortality after trauma. Am J Emeg Med. 1995;13:619–22.
65. Husain F, Martin M, Mullenix P, Steele S, Elliott D. Serum lactate and base deficit as predictors of mortality and morbidity. Am J Surg. 2003;185:485–91.
66. Rixen D, Siegel J. Metablic correlates of oxygen dept predict posttrauma early acute respiratory distress syndrome and the related cytokine response. J Trauma. 2000;49:392–403.
67. Rixen D, Siegel J. Bench-to-bedside review: oxygen dept and its metabolic correlates as quantifiers of the severity of hemorrhagic and posttraumatic shock. Crit Care. 2005;9:441–53.
68. Abt R, Lustenberger T, Stover J, Benninger E, Lenzlinger P, Stocker R, Keel M. Base excess determined within one hour of admission predicts mortality in patients with severe pelvic fractures and severe hemorrhagic shock. Eur J Trauma Emerg Surg. 2009;35(5):429. https://doi.org/10.1007/s00068-009-8245-7. Epub 2009 Jun 19
69. Mamczak C, Maloney M, Fritz B, Boyer B, Thomas S, Evans E, Ploplis V, Castellino F, McCollester J, Walsh M. Thromboelastography in orthopaedic trauma acute pelvic fracture resuscitation: a descriptive pilot study. J Orthop Trauma. 2016;30:299–305.
70. Agarwal A. Chapter 46: Pelvic ring fractures. In: Court-Brown CM, Heckman JD, McQueen MM, Ricci W, Tornetta III P, editors. Rockwood and Green's fractures in adults. Philadelphia, PA: LWW; 2015. ISBN 978-1-4511-7531-8.
71. Esposito T, Ingraham A, Luchette F, Sears B, Santaniello J, Davis K, Poulakidas S, Gamelli R. Reasons to omit digital rectal exam in trauma patients: no fingers, no rectum, no useful additional information. J Trauma. 2005;59:1314–9.
72. Shlamovitz G, Mower W, Bergman J, Crisp J, DeVore H, Hardy D, Sargent M, Shroff S, Snyder E, Morgan M. Lack of evidence to support routine digital rectal examination in pediatric trauma patients. Pediatr Emerg Care. 2007;23:537–43.
73. Shlamovitz G, Mower W, Bergman J, Crisp J, DeVore H, Hardy D, Sargent M, Shroff S, Snyder E, Morgan M. Poor test characteristics for the digital rectal examination in trauma patients. Ann Emerg Med. 2007;50:25–33.
74. Ball C, Jafri S, Kirkpatrick A, Rajani R, Rozycki G, Feliciano D, Wyrzykowski A. Traumatic urethral injuries: does the digital rectal examination really help us? Injury. 2009;40:984–6.
75. Docimo SJ, Diggs L, Crankshaw L, Lee Y, Vinces F. No evidence supporting the routine use of digital rectal Examinations in Trauma Patients. Indian J Surg. 2015;77:265–9.
76. Roberts T, Leonard G, Cepela D. Classifications in brief: American spinal injury association (ASIA) impairment scale. Clin Orthop Relat Res. 2017;475:1499–504.

Radiological Diagnostics

7

Peter Grechenig, Stephan Grechenig, Bore Bakota, and Axel Gänsslen

Many published trauma algorithms have integrated three basic radiographic examinations as a standard in the early emergency treatment phase, including the a.p. chest X-ray, the FAST or eFAST examination, and the pelvic a.p. X-ray, to rule out intrathoracic massive hemorrhage and pneumothorax, massive free intra-abdominal fluid, and pelvic ring instability [1–3].

Despite the ongoing debate, whether to perform a pelvic a.p. X-ray or a computed tomography (CT) during the primary phase of trauma management, many trauma centers still use the pelvic X-ray to exclude significant injury of the pelvis as one source of relevant bleeding after high-energy trauma.

Analysis of the pelvic X-ray should identify or exclude pelvic instability and potential bleeding during the first few minutes of care. Additionally, emergency treatment decisions should be estimated from the result of this analysis.

7.1 Debate on Pelvic X-Ray Versus CT

The anterior-posterior X-ray represents the gold standard in all pelvic injuries and in all polytraumatized patients [1, 4–6].

P. Grechenig
Division of Macroscopic and Clinical Anatomy, Medical University of Graz, Graz, Austria
e-mail: peter.grechenig@stud.medunigraz.at

S. Grechenig
Department of Orthopedics and Trauma Surgery, AUVA Trauma Hospital Klagenfurt, Klagenfurt, Austria

Department of Trauma Surgery, University Hospital Regensburg, Regensburg, Germany

B. Bakota
Department of Orthopaedics and Trauma, Medical University of Graz, Graz, Austria

A. Gänsslen (✉)
Department of Trauma Surgery, Orthopedics and Hand Surgery, Hospital Wolfsburg, Wolfsburg, Germany

The clinical relevance of the pelvic a.p. X-ray has been reported by several authors. Accordingly, primary correct diagnoses can be expected in up to 90% of patients [5, 7, 8].

Young et al. reported a rate of primarily correct identifications of pelvic ring injuries in up to 94% [8]. Similar results were stated in the analysis by Edeicken-Monroe et al., who were able to confirm the primary diagnoses compared to a pelvic CT in 88% [7]. Resnik et al. used the pelvic CT as a gold standard and were able to confirm fractures and dislocations of the pelvic ring. Only 9% of the injuries were overlooked without therapeutic consequence [5].

In the meantime, a discussion on routine use of pelvic X-rays started during the last decade, as in awake and alert patients, no routine need for a pelvic radiograph was recommended, as clinical examination can confirm or exclude pelvic injury. Additionally, elimination from standard trauma protocols can lead to financial savings, and therefore, the main indication was limited to severely injured patients [9].

Computed tomography (CT) is the standard procedure for the detailed diagnosis of pelvic fractures. It allows a more detailed analysis of the posterior pelvic ring and of acetabular fractures. It is helpful in stable patients for detailed surgical planning [10, 11]. In hemodynamically unstable patients with a mechanically unstable pelvis ("patients in extremis"), CT should be avoided, as bleeding control may be delayed.

This was confirmed in a German analysis, comparing clinical and radiological examination. It was stated that all patients with an indication for emergency stabilization of the pelvis should have a pelvic radiograph, already in the emergency room, for surgical planning. Even in patients without clinical signs of pelvic injury, the pelvic X-ray was recommended, as clinical examination cannot reliably rule out surgically significant pelvic fractures, especially in severely injured patients [12].

Newer data indicate that the pelvic a.p. X-ray has limited sensitivity for detecting pelvic fractures, especially at the posterior pelvic ring, and to distinguish between stable and unstable pelvic injuries, compared with CT scanning [13–17].

A. Gänsslen et al. (eds.), *Pelvic Ring Fractures*, https://doi.org/10.1007/978-3-030-54730-1_7

In hemodynamically stable patients, no routine pelvic X-ray was recommended, while the exclusive indication for conventional pelvic radiographs was seen in hemodynamically unstable patients, in patients with relevant clinical findings at the pelvic region, and in patients "in extremis," requiring immediate surgical procedures [13–16].

In contrast, in geriatric patients with low energy injuries of the pelvis, after clinical examination, a pelvic a.p. X-ray is still recommended. In every case with an anterior ring injury, an additional CT is considered mandatory to rule out or confirm posterior injury, as especially sacral fractures were frequently overlooked in up to 91%, representing a low sensitivity of 10.5% [15].

In contrast, Verbeek et al. clearly stated that the pelvic a.p. X-ray still represents an adequate screening tool to rapidly determine the need for immediate interventions [6]. In their analysis, it took 48 min in average until a CT of the pelvis was performed. Interestingly, patients requiring angioembolization had a significant 2-h time delay if only CT evaluation was performed. CT is required in every patient, as especially hip dislocations were observed only with CT in a significant rate [6].

These data are in concordance with German Trauma Registry data. The standard pelvic X-ray is usually available for interpretation within 5–7 min after admission to the hospital, while the trauma whole-body CT scan, including the pelvic area, is performed in average after 22 min [18].

7.2 Pelvic X-Ray Analysis

With only the pelvic a.p. X-ray, the definitive diagnosis regarding stability analysis and therefore fracture type classification of the pelvic ring injury can generally be made.

The classification is based on the injury mechanism according to Pennal and Tile and the resultant AO/OTA classification [19]. Three degrees of pelvic instability are distinguished: stable, rotationally unstable, and translationally unstable.

- Type A: the osteoligamentous integrity of the posterior pelvic ring is preserved; it is a stable pelvic lesion, the pelvic floor is intact, and the pelvis withstands physiological loading without displacement.
- Type B: the posterior pelvic ring is incompletely disrupted, leading to rotational instability around a vertical or transverse axis; the injury is partially unstable, with partially preserved osteoligamentous integrity of the posterior pelvic ring and in some cases also of the pelvic floor.
- Type C: the posterior pelvic ring is completely disrupted; the continuity between all osteoligamentous elements of the posterior pelvic ring is lost, and thus, a three-dimensional translational and rotational instability is present; the pelvic ring injury is unstable.

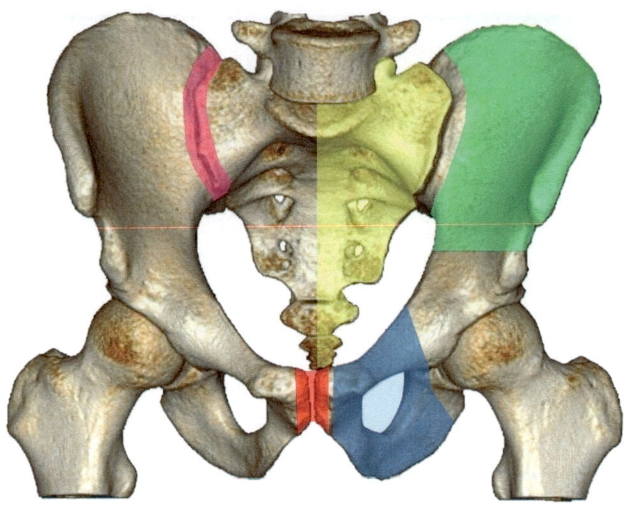

Fig. 7.1 Pelvic regions according to Letournel: symphyseal (red), pubic (blue), iliac (green), iliosacral (pink), and sacral (yellow)

Additionally, an anatomical description of the different pelvic (injury) regions (modified according to Letournel [20], Fig. 7.1) is useful.

Here, the pelvic ring is divided into several anatomical regions:

- Symphyseal
- Pubic
- Acetabular
- Iliac
- Iliosacral
- Sacral

Sacral instabilities are further subdivided into transalar, transforaminal, and central fractures according to Denis [21]. Iliosacral injuries are subdivided into pure sacroiliac (SI) joint dislocations and fracture dislocations including transsacral or transiliac fracture dislocations (crescent fractures).

A standardized analysis of these injury regions (excluding acetabular fractures) is therefore highly recommended.

7.3 Symphyseal Region

Symphyseal injuries are referred to as pure disruptions representing typically as external rotation injuries (Fig. 7.2) or rarely as a locked pubic symphysis due to internal rotation injury of the hemipelvis (Fig. 7.2). These large disruptions are easily identified.

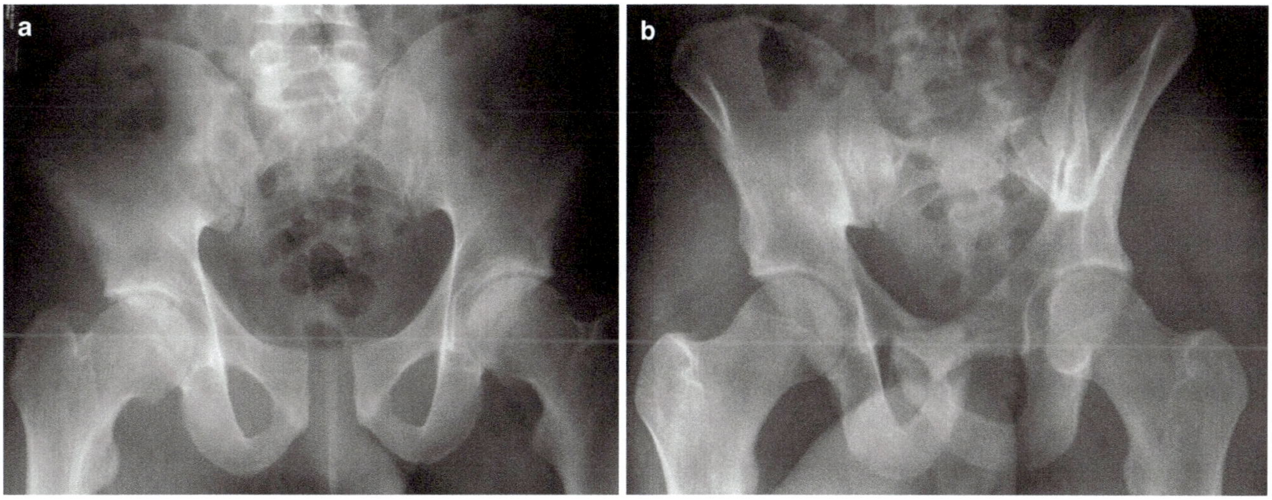

Fig. 7.2 Mechanism-related symphyseal injury: external rotation injury results in symphyseal widening (symphyseal disruption) (**a**) or internal rotation injury resulting in a locked pubic symphysis (**b**)

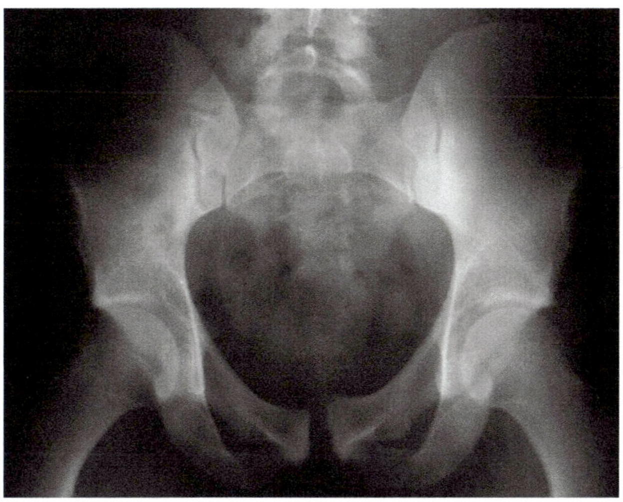

Fig. 7.3 Subtle injury to the pubic symphysis, with asymmetric widening and a nonparallel joint space

Diagnosis of subtle injuries can be difficult (Fig. 7.3). Knowledge of the normal, age-dependent width of the pubic symphysis is important. Consensus exists that the symphysis is wider anteriorly than posteriorly [22–25]. An age and sex dependency of the pubic symphysis width is known. Kraus already in 1930 reported that the width decreases continuously from approximately 10 mm in the toddler age to 2 mm in the older age of 50 years [26]. Patel and Chapman observed a width of 7.4 mm in the first months of life, which decreases to 5.4 mm at the age of 16 [27].

During the last decade, several investigations analyzed especially CT data in patients of different age for standard measurements of the symphysis width (see Chap. 1):

- Alicioglu et al. performed a CT analysis on adult patients >16 years of age in 278 women and 264 men [28]. They reported a constant narrowing of the anterior and posterior part of the symphyseal width, while the middle part showed no significant changes, independent from the number of birth and the body mass index. Female patients were associated with larger values anterior and in the middle.
- McAlister et al. measured the symphyseal width using standard radiographs in 316 consecutive pediatric patients (165 boys, 151 girls), who were separated by gender and divided into three age groups: 2–6 years, 7–10 years, and 11–14 years [29]. Normal values between 5.2–8.4 mm were observed with an average width of 6.8 mm. Interestingly, a subsequent widening was observed within the three age groups: 6.6 mm, 6.8 mm, and 7.2 mm, respectively. It was concluded that a width > 8.4 mm should lead to further evaluation for pathology.
- Bayer et al. analyzed 350 CT scans of children in different age groups: 0–6 years, 7–11 years, 12–15 years, and 16–17 years. The mean width in these age groups was 5.4 mm, 5.3 mm, 4.1 mm, and 3.5 mm in girls and 5.9 mm, 5.4 mm, 5.2 mm, and 4.0 mm in boys, respectively [30].
- A further CT analysis of 1020 CT axial scans in pediatric patients (2–18 years) revealed an average pubic symphyseal width at 2-year-old boys of 6.35 mm and of 5.85 mm in girls. A decrease to 3.68 mm in boys and 3.92 mm in girls at an age of 18 years was observed [31].
- Recently, data on 811 CT measurements of the pubic symphysis were analyzed, stating that from age 2–16 years, the average pubic symphysis width decreased from 5.55 to 3.69 mm [32].

Clinical Relevance

The width of the pubic symphysis decreases from 5–6 mm 2 years after birth to 3–4 mm in early adulthood using CT analyses.

In pediatric trauma patients <10 years of age, a symphyseal width of the SI joint >10 mm should lead to suspicion of injury [31].

Minor injuries can result in interpretational difficulties (Fig. 7.4). The following lines should be analyzed:

- *Iliopectineal line*: the line along the upper pubic ramus is analyzed bilaterally for vertical displacement or asymmetry; vertical displacement can be minimal, as the plane of the pubic symphysis is oblique to the X-ray beam (Fig. 7.5); minor asymmetries can be observed in incomplete injuries which can be present in concomitant acetabular fractures with a transverse fracture component, as the obturator segment shows internal rotation around a longitudinal axis through the symphysis and/or rotation around a sagittal axis (Fig. 7.6).
- *Pubic arch line*: the pubic arch is analyzed regarding asymmetry (Fig. 7.7); however, incorrect positioning of the patient can lead to misalignments (oblique anterior-posterior X-ray).
- *Medial pubic line*: the lateral symphyseal border and thus the medial border of the pubic bones are analyzed for parallelism; asymmetry may indicate an injury to the pubic symphysis (Fig. 7.8).

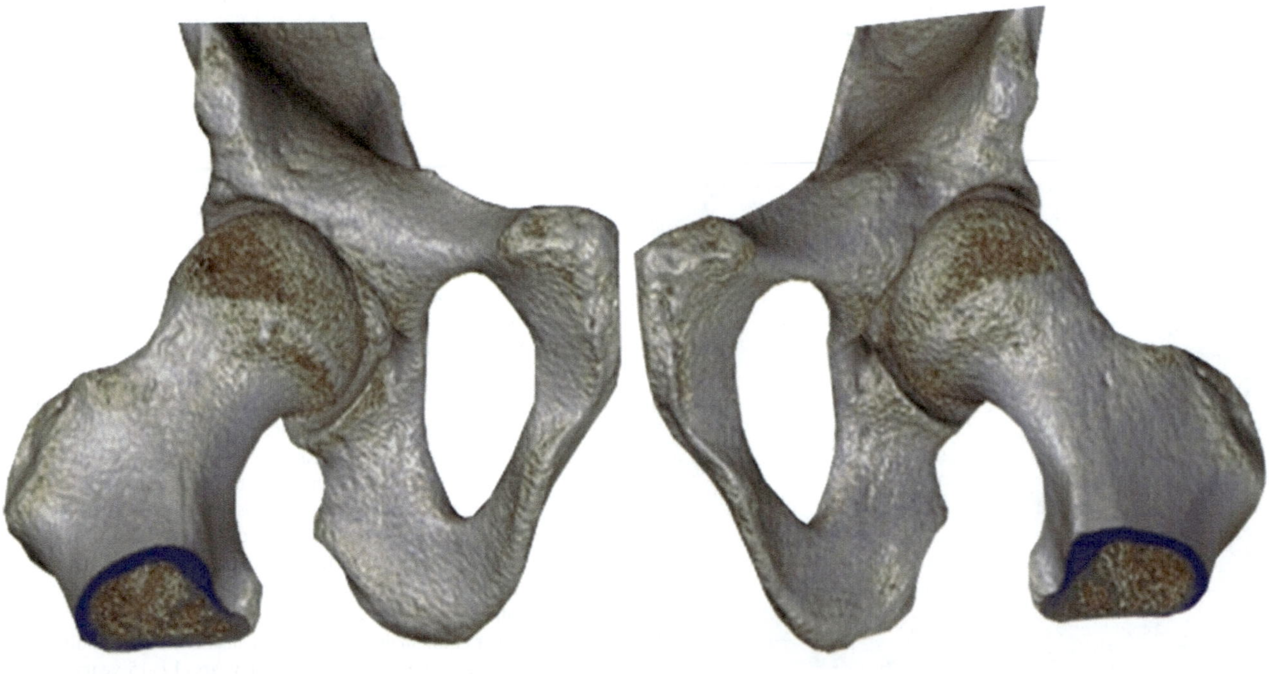

Fig. 7.4 Analysis of symphyseal malposition: the iliopectineal line (line of the upper pubic rami) shows asymmetry, the symphyseal cleft presents without parallelism and a side difference of the inferior pubic rami line is visible

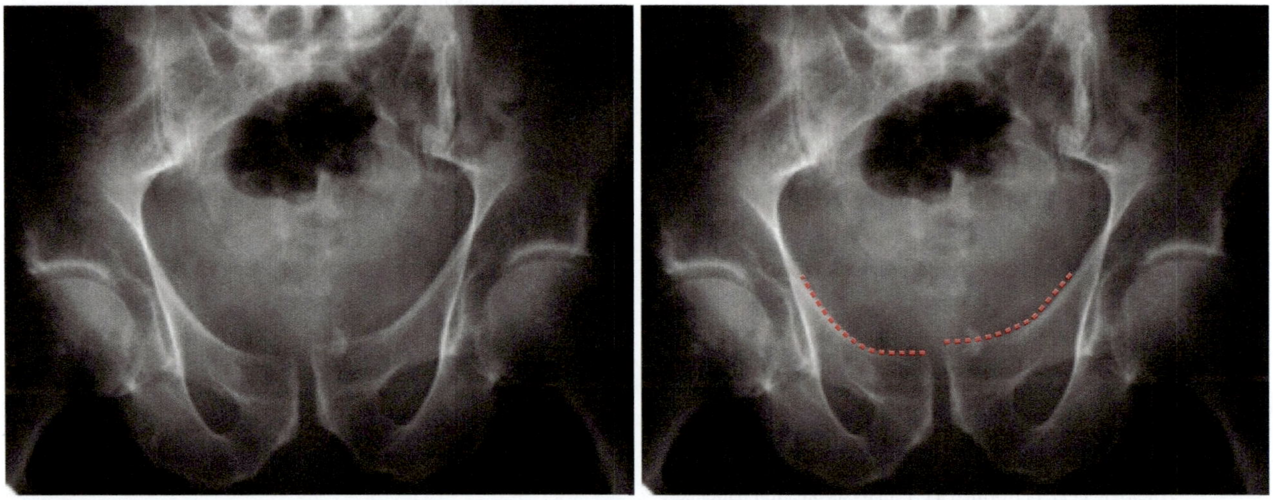

Fig. 7.5 Analysis of the iliopectineal line (upper pubic rami line), showing a side difference in line height

In particular, in transverse fractures of the acetabulum, the rotation of the obturator segment can lead to asymmetry of the symphyseal cleft. It should be noted that in these injuries, the symphysis is not always completely injured (Fig. 7.6).

In inconspicuous analysis of the symphysis using the mentioned lines and still existing clinical impairments, magnetic resonance tomography or bilateral single-leg-stance (flamingo) radiographs can be considered. The latter can show some "step-up" of the pubic bone (Fig. 7.9).

Recently, two analyses dealt with single-leg-stance X-rays [33, 34].

Garras et al. analyzed 45 asymptomatic adult volunteers to determine physiological movement of the symphysis using single-leg-stance X-rays. Male patients showed an average translation of 1.4 mm, nulliparous women showed an average translation of 1.6 mm, and multiparous women showed an average translation of 3.1 mm [33]. It was concluded that up to 5 mm of physiologic motion can be normal.

Siegel et al. analyzed 38 consecutive patients with the presence of pelvic pain for an average of 41 months after trauma, childbirth, or osteopenia. Sixty-five percent showed a mean symphyseal instability of 2 cm [34]. Additionally, symphyseal widening occurs under labor [35].

Single-leg-stance X-rays can be used to detect symphyseal instability. Normal values of translation under load are available. These data and the history of pregnancy should be considered.

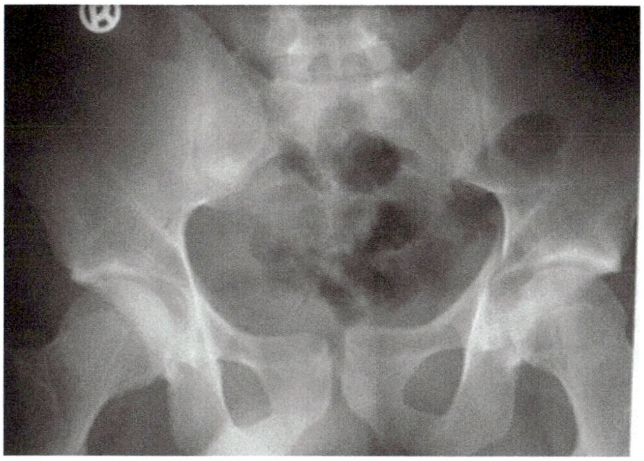

Fig. 7.6 Left transverse acetabular fracture. An internal rotation deformity of the obturator segment results in a symphyseal asymmetry, without symphyseal instability

In rare cases, a bony avulsion injury of the rectus abdominis muscle, which is usually seen on the side of the posterior pelvic lesion (external rotation injury), may be the only indirect sign of a symphyseal injury (Fig. 7.10).

In "open book" injuries of the pelvis with symphyseal disruption and partial or complete posterior injury to the SI joint, a typical radiographic triad can often be observed [36] (Fig. 7.11):

- The injured hemipelvis shows inferior upper pubic rami localization compared to the opposite side.
- External rotation of the affected hemipelvis, visible by a widened iliac fossa.
- Asymmetry of the obturator foramen due to the altered hemipelvic rotation.

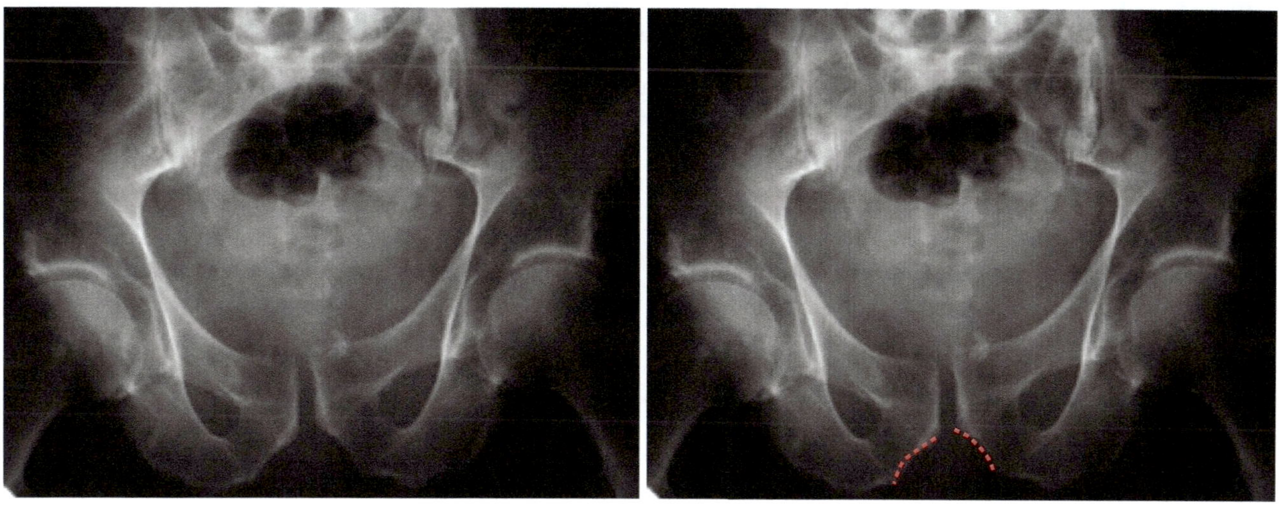

Fig. 7.7 Analysis of the symphyseal arch line (inferior ramus line), showing a step-off

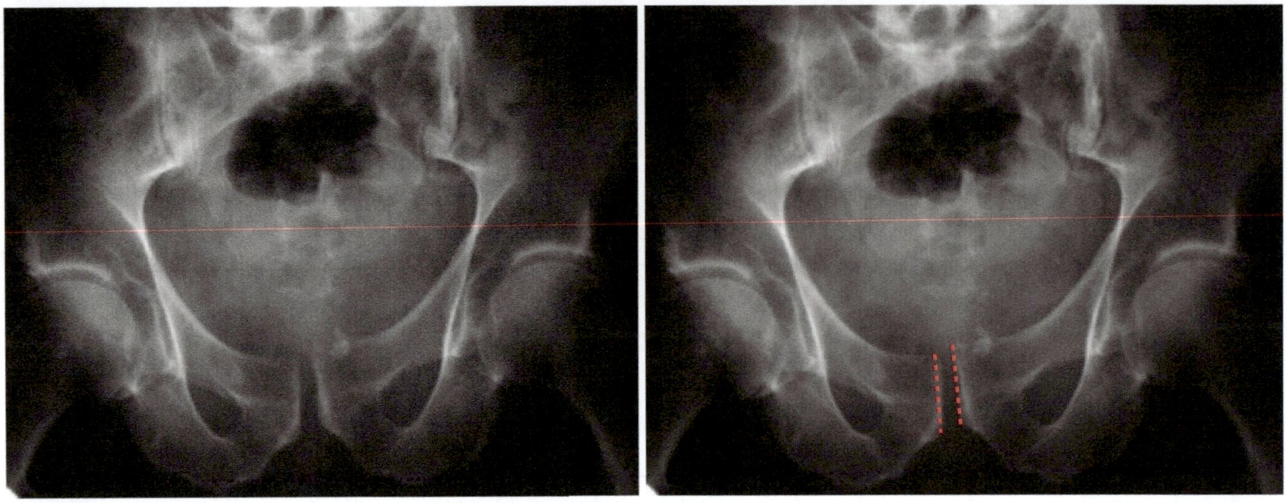

Fig. 7.8 Analysis of the lateral symphyseal border: the symphysis usually shows parallelism

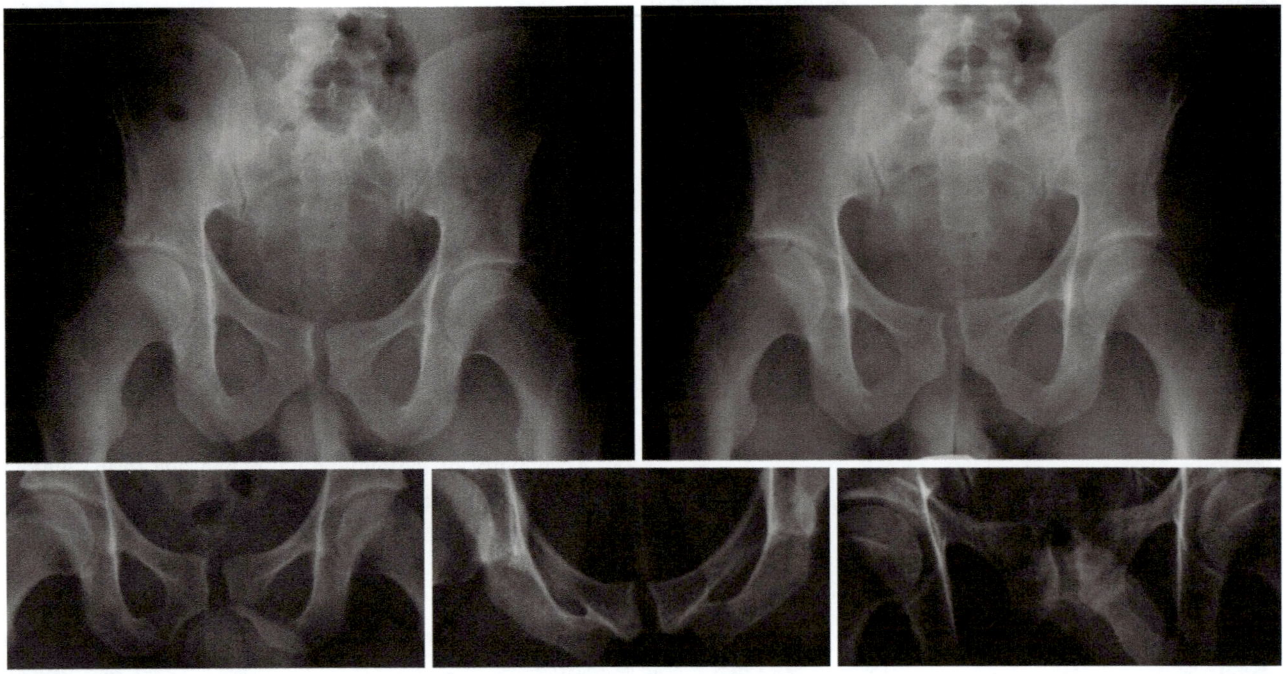

Fig. 7.9 Bilateral single-leg-stance (flamingo) radiographs reveal symphyseal instability. The bottom views show the standard a.p., Inlet and Outlet projections of the symphysis

7.4 Pubic Region

Injuries of the upper and lower pubic rami are the most common injuries of the anterior pelvic ring. While in displaced fractures, usually no diagnostic problems exist, mild or minimal displaced fractures can be difficult to detect, or in fractures close to the acetabulum, a low acetabular anterior column injury can be suspected.

Assessment of the course of the iliopectineal line distal to the acetabulum is analyzed for interruption or diastases and leads to the diagnosis of an upper pubic rami fracture (Fig. 7.12).

Differentiation of "high" fractures of the upper pubic rami from low anterior column fractures is often only possible using CT (Fig. 7.13).

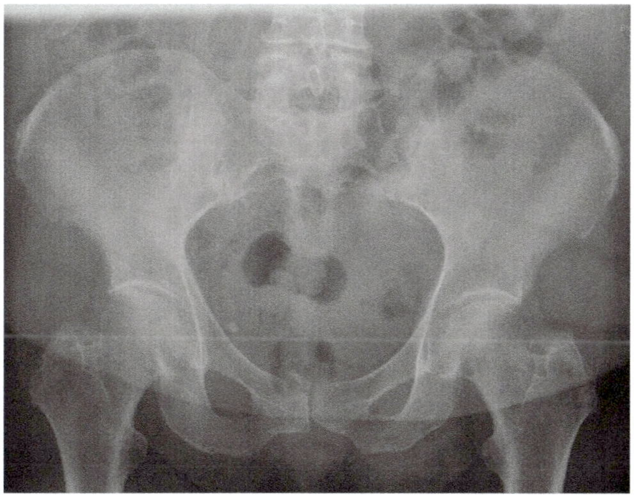

Fig. 7.10 Rectus avulsion injury as a rare radiological sign of a symphyseal disruption

Rarely, fractures of the lower pubic rami may be difficult to assess due to rotational deformity (Fig. 7.14). However, side comparison usually allows final detection. Frequently, superimposing of the fractured fragments leads to clear detection of these fractures (Fig. 7.14).

7.5 Iliac Region

Isolated complete ilium fractures are rare. Diagnostic difficulties exist, as these fractures are often only minimally displaced due to the intrinsic stabilization by the surrounding muscle sling consisting of the iliopsoas and gluteal muscle mass.

The fracture plane is often poorly visualized due to overprojection of different iliac parts. Typically, these fractures are characterized by "fine" fracture lines (<3 mm) (Fig. 7.15).

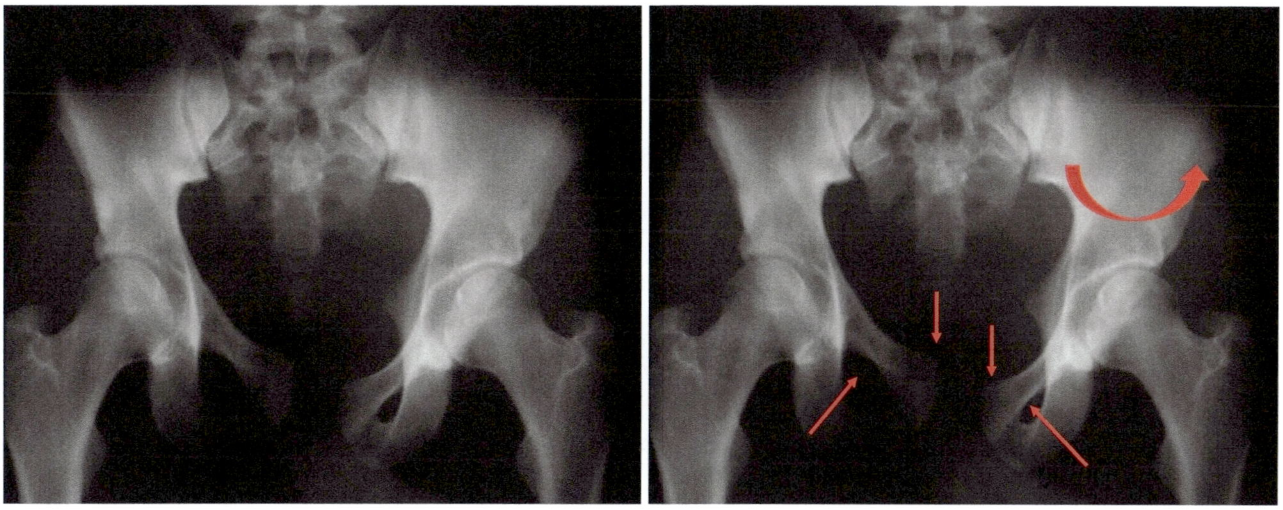

Fig. 7.11 Radiological triad of an open book injury: the affected hemipelvis shows inferior displacement of the upper pubic rami relative to the opposite side, an external rotation deformity with a widened iliac fossa, and asymmetry of the obturator foramen

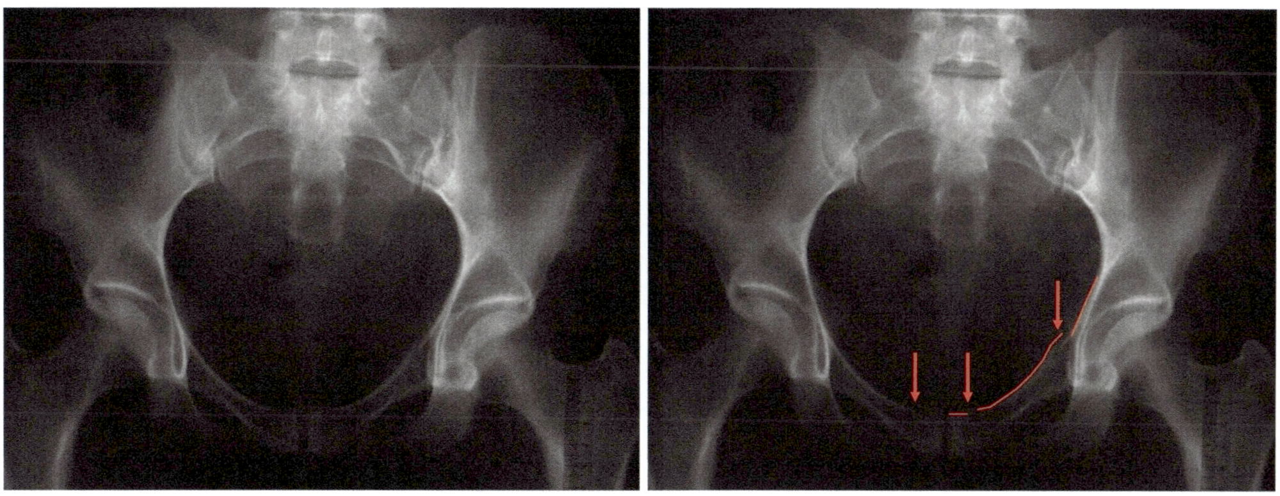

Fig. 7.12 Analysis of the iliopectineal line distal to the acetabulum leads to the diagnosis of an upper pubic rami fracture

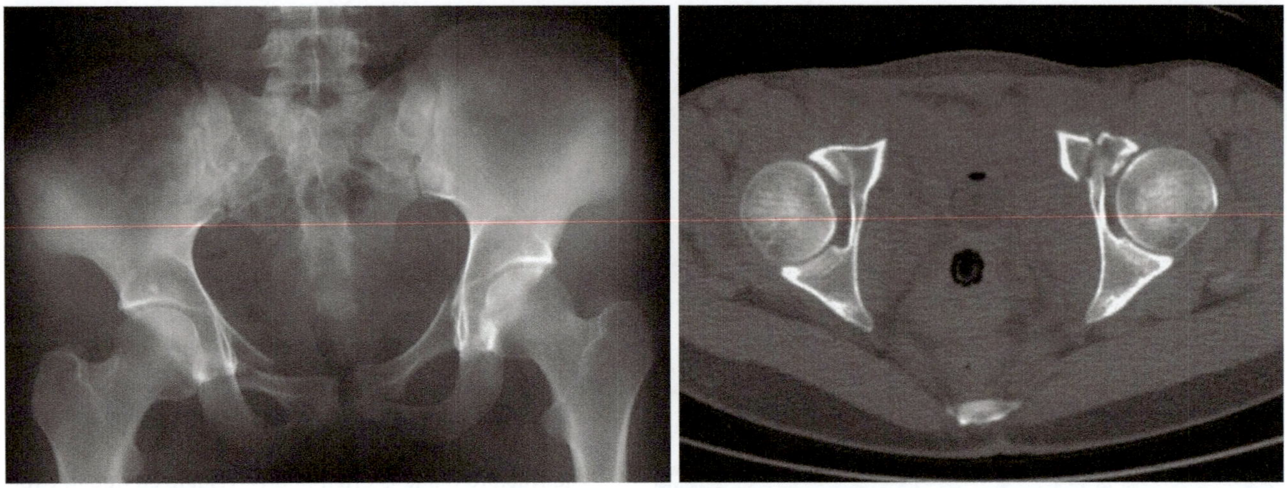

Fig. 7.13 Upper pubic rami fractures (right side) can be distinguished from low anterior column acetabular fractures (left side) often only by CT analysis

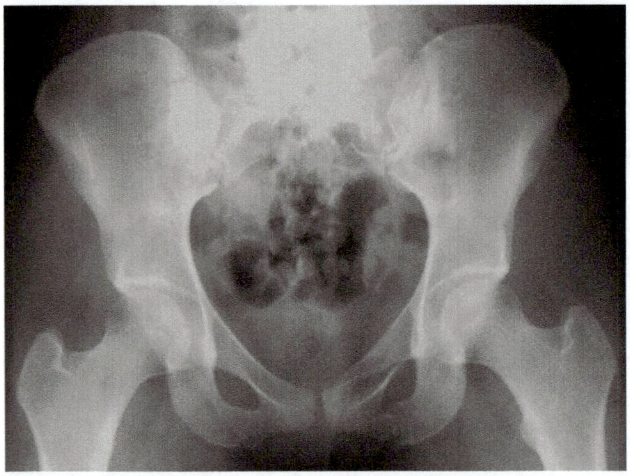

Fig. 7.14 Lower pubic rami fractures can often be sufficiently analyzed by side comparison or by detection of superimposition

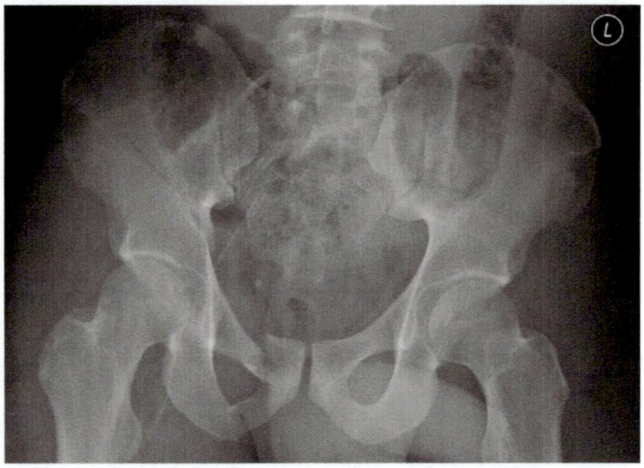

Fig. 7.15 Right complete ilium fracture

Fractures extending into the SI joint region may have to be distinguished from true crescent fractures (iliac fracture dislocations).

More common are isolated iliac wing fractures, not involving the pelvic ring, following direct trauma, with a high rate of fracture comminution (Fig. 7.16) and iliac fractures as part of an acetabular fracture. An accompanying fracture line in the acetabulum is always suspicious of a "pure" acetabular fracture.

The following lines are analyzed:

- *Iliac crest line*: the lateral margin of the superior hemipelvis is checked for interruptions starting between the anterior inferior iliac spine and the posterior sacrum; an additional focus is placed on avulsion injuries (Figs. 7.15 and 7.17).
- *Proximal iliopectineal line*: the medial border of the ilium is analyzed for fractures starting at the iliac crest; fractures involving the iliopectineal line are highly suspicious of a complete iliac fracture (Fig. 7.17).
- *Posterior ilium*: injuries to the posterior part of the ilium, posterior to the sacrum, are difficult to detect due to the overlying sacrum; only high-quality X-rays and lack of intestinal gas superimposition can reliably detect fractures in this region (Fig. 7.18).

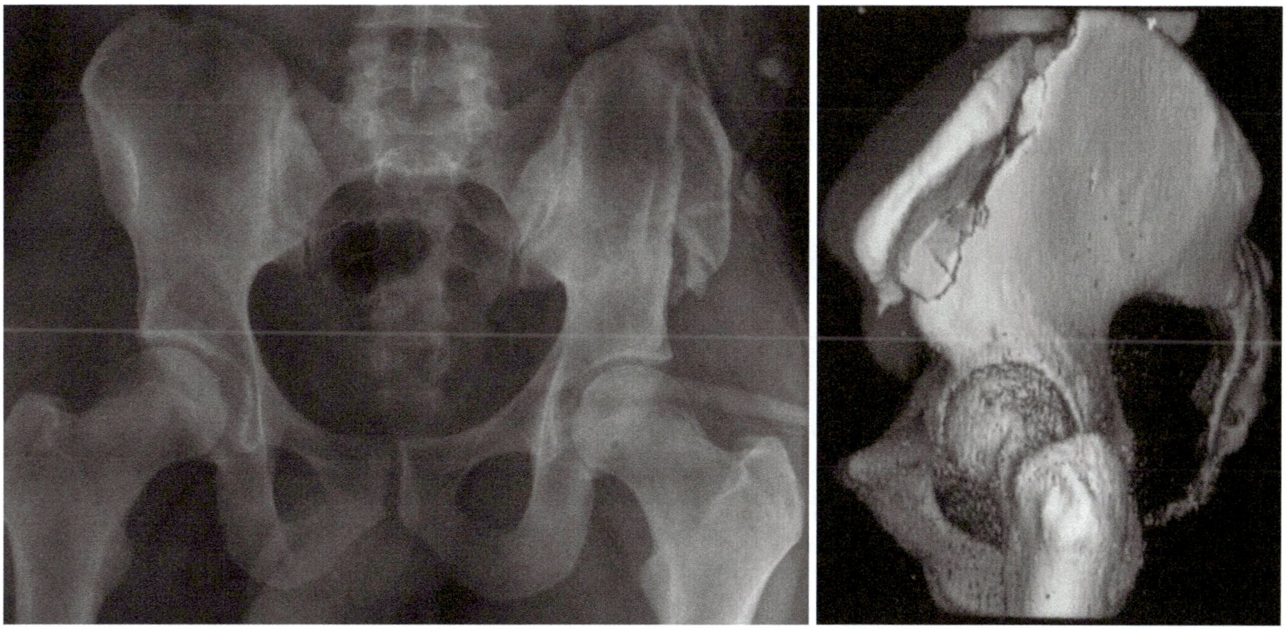

Fig. 7.16 Left iliac wing fracture, not influencing pelvic ring stability (also called Duverney's fracture)

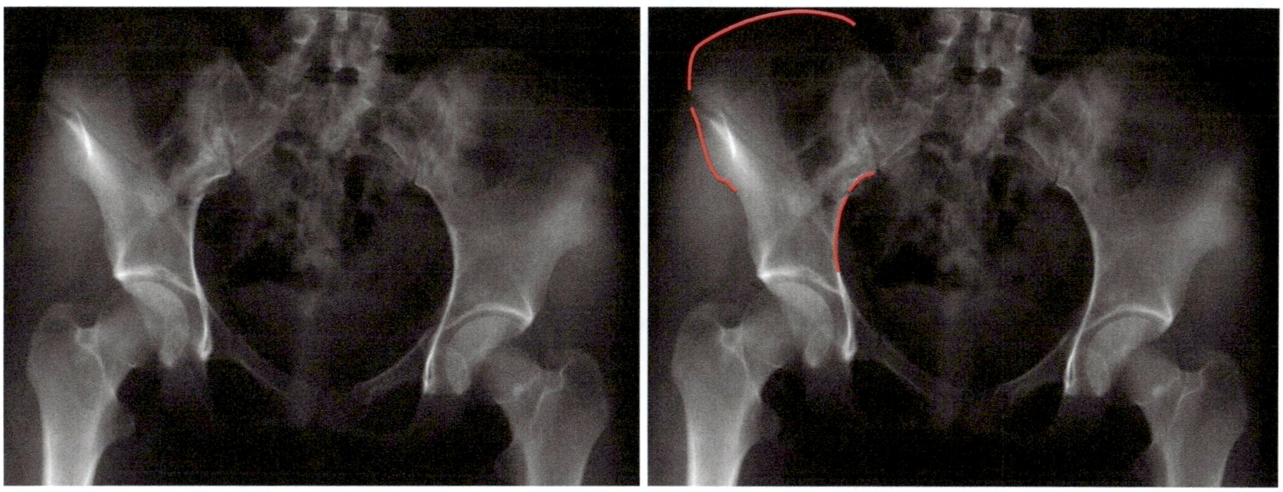

Fig. 7.17 Complete ilium fracture (type C) with disruption of the iliac crest line and the proximal iliopectineal line

7.6 Iliosacral Region

The SI joint presents in an anterior-lateral to posterior-medial orientation on the pelvic a.p. view, which can be usually analyzed by two characteristic lines.

At the junction between the iliopectineal line and the sacrum, the visible gap corresponds to the anterior part of the SI joint. Slightly medially, usually a second gap is present, corresponding to the posterior part of the SI joint (Fig. 7.19). These lines are primarily examined for parallelism.

Lesions of the SI joint are subdivided into pure partial or complete SI joint dislocations and sacral or iliac fracture dislocations.

In pure SI joint dislocations, three injury types can be distinguished:

- *Type B SI joint dislocations* are characterized by intact posterior iliosacral ligaments; the anterior SI joint parts are radiographically widened, while the posterior lines remain intact (Fig. 7.11); the vertical axis of rotation leads to a hemipelvic external rotation with the

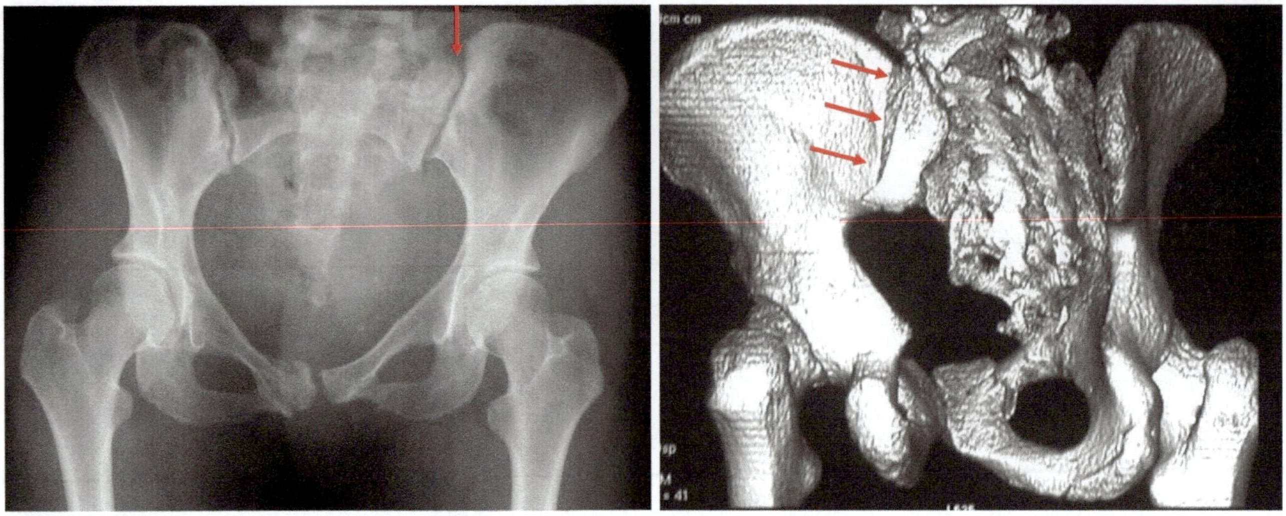

Fig. 7.18 Posterior ilium fracture (posterior to the SI joint)

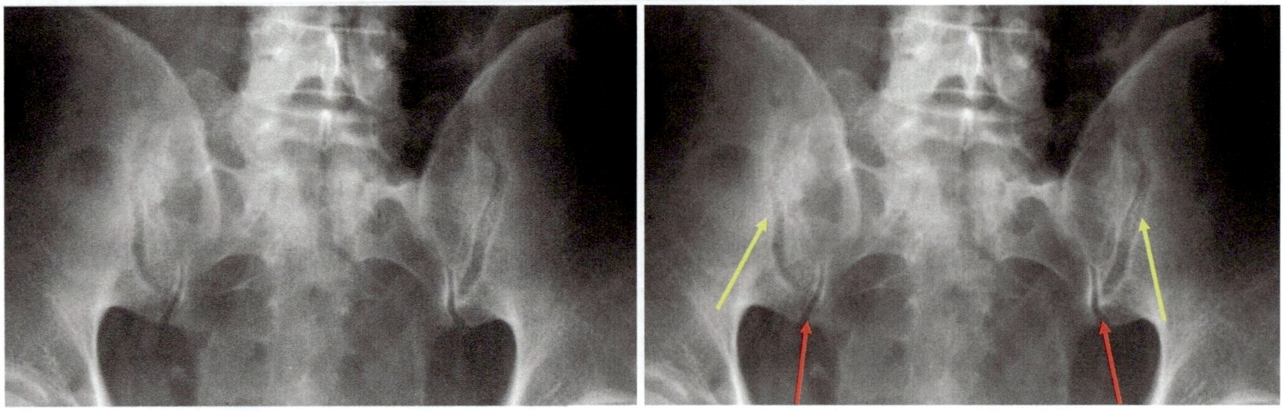

Fig. 7.19 Radiographic features of the SI joint: posterior part of the SI joint (red arrows): identical on both sides; anterior part of the SI joint (yellow arrows): slight widening on the left side

typical radiographic triad; the anterior ring injury most often shows symphyseal disruption ("open book" injury).

- *Type C SI joint dislocations* are characterized by complete disruption of the sacroiliac ligamentous structures; the anterior joint shows wide diastasis, usually >10 mm; the posterior gap is no longer detectable (Fig. 7.20); lateral, superior (vertical shear), and anterior-posterior displacement can be present due to rotations around all three possible axes; the craniocaudal or anterior-posterior displacement can be detected by analysis of the iliopectineal line in relation to the sacrum.

The iliopectineal line nearly always ends at the level of the second arcuate line of the sacrum: malalignment indicates a type C injury (Fig. 7.21).

- *Bucket-handle-type SI joint dislocations* represent a transition between type B and type C injuries; the anterior part of the SI joint usually shows a wide diastasis, while the posterior part is at least partially intact; rotation around a sagittal axis can be expected (Fig. 7.22).

The transition between these three types can be difficult to detect.

In SI joint fracture dislocations, part of the SI joint remains intact. Sacral and iliac fracture dislocations are distinguished:

- Iliac fracture dislocations are also referred to as "crescent fractures" because of the similarity of the remaining intact iliac part to a crescent; the primary fracture line starts variably at the iliac crest and runs to the SI joint (Fig. 7.23); three subtypes can be distinguished, depending on the localization of SI joint involvement (see Chap. 1).

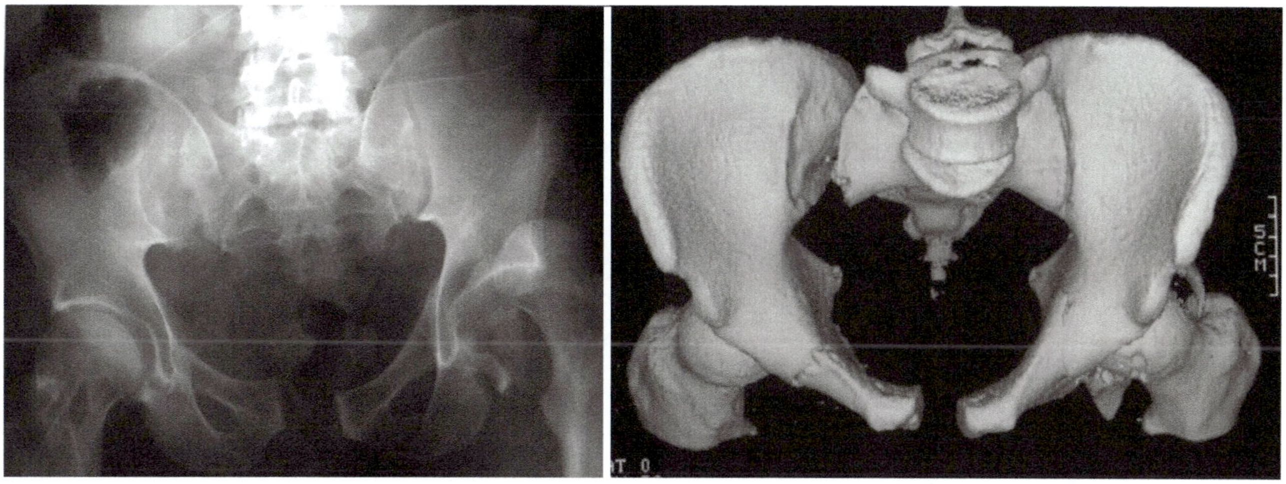

Fig. 7.20 Radiographic features of a complete right SI joint dislocation without detectable anterior and posterior joint space

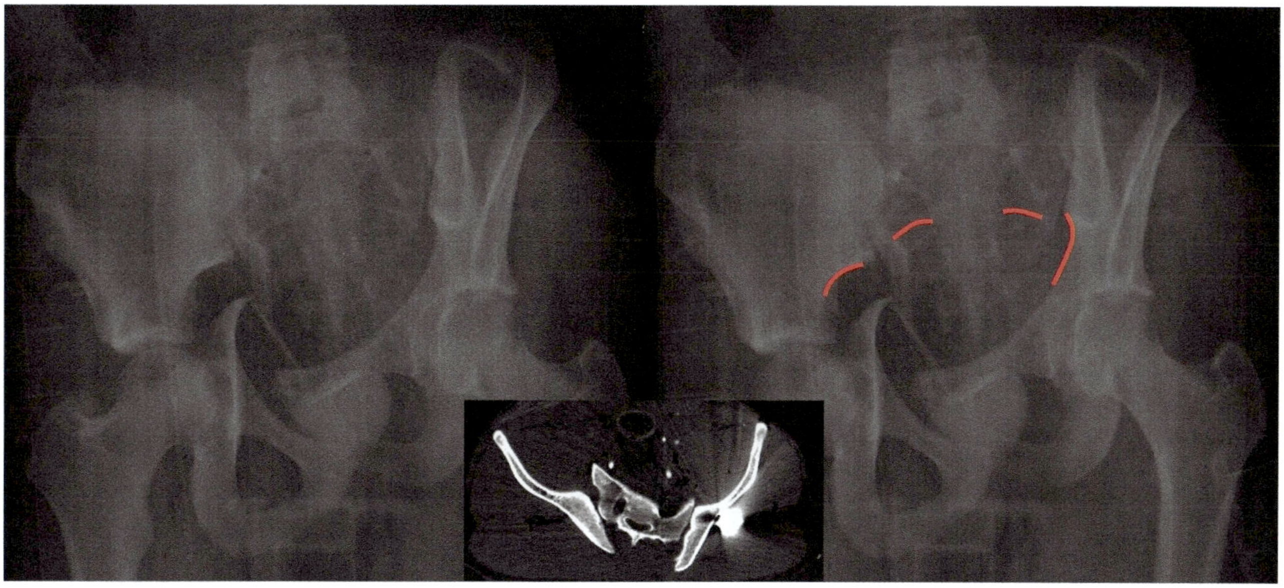

Fig. 7.21 Radiological sign of hemipelvic displacement: the iliopectineal line does not end at the second sacral foramen

- Sacral fracture dislocations present with a proximal sacral fragment attached to an intact part of the SI joint (Fig. 7.24).

Diagnosis of subtle injuries can be difficult. Recent data determine physiological width. The radiological age-dependent physiological width of the joint was analyzed using CT data (see Chap. 1).

A CT analysis by Oetgen et al. in 821 pediatric patients without bony or ligamentous injury aged 2–16 years observed an average SI joint width which decreased from 3.11 to 1.80 mm [32].

A further CT analysis on 1020 CT data observed an average width of 4.4–4.5 mm in 2-year-old children to decrease to 2.0–2.3 mm in 18-year-olds [31]. Girls presented with slightly larger widths with increasing age.

No clear data are available for older adults.

Ligamentous injuries in coincidence with SI joint dislocations can be analyzed using magnetic resonance imaging (MRI) [37]. The sacrospinous, sacrotuberous, anterior sacroiliac, and posterior sacroiliac ligaments could be visualized in 91%, 100%, 98%, and 91%, respectively.

7.7 Sacral Region

Historically, the rate of overlooked sacral fractures was reported to be 30–50% [21, 38]. Still recently, an analysis of geriatric patients reported a low sensitivity (10.5%) of the a.p. pelvic X-ray to detect a sacral fracture [15].

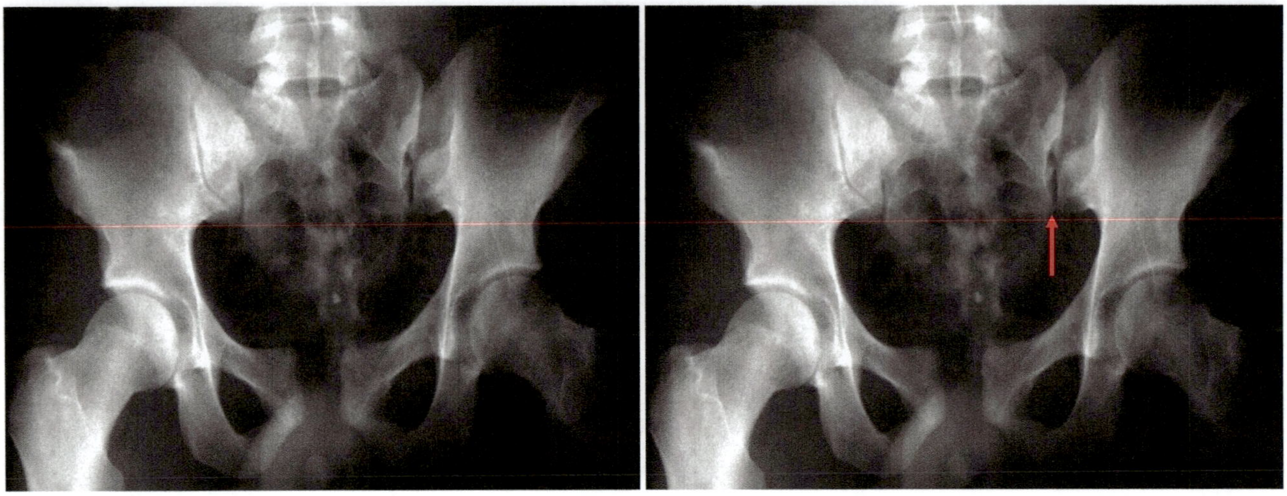

Fig. 7.22 Bucket-handle-type injury of the SI joint with near complete widening but with a persisting partial (inferior) intact part (arrow)

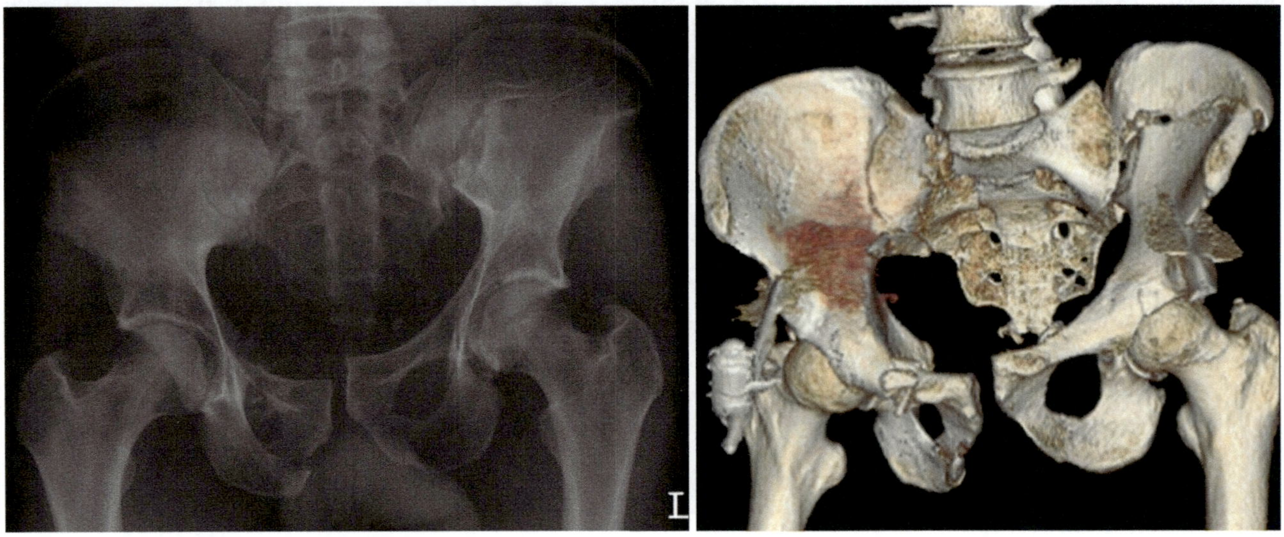

Fig. 7.23 Crescent fracture (iliac fracture dislocation of the SI joint)

The primary analysis should focus on the presence or absence of a sacrum fracture by assessing the arcuate lines of the sacral foramina (Fig. 7.25). Even small breaks of these lines almost always indicate sacral fracture (Fig. 7.26) as CT analysis at least confirms anterior cortical compression fracture. Difficulties can exist due to frequently observed bowel gas overlay.

Additionally, the upper sacral margin (sacrum shoulder, sacral ala) is analyzed. The course from the SI joint to the L5/S1 facet joint is analyzed for interruptions (Fig. 7.27). Further, the distance from the sacral midline to the tip of the sacrum shoulder is analyzed. Different distances are usually associated with type C injuries of the sacrum as part of a pelvic ring injury (Fig. 7.27). Shortened distances can be present in lateral compression fractures.

A rare injury is the so-called suicidal jumper's fracture or lumbo-pelvic dissociation injury [39]. A flexion/compression mechanism can result in bilateral longitudinal sacral fractures with an additional transverse or oblique fracture component. In minor displaced fractures, these injuries are often overlooked on the pelvic a.p. view, as the direction of displacement is situated in the sagittal plane. As sometimes no injury to the anterior pelvic ring is present, an indicative sign can be a prominent promontory, which can be visualized as an oval structure at the proximal sacrum (Fig. 7.28). Only the lateral view or sagittal reformation on CT proves this fracture.

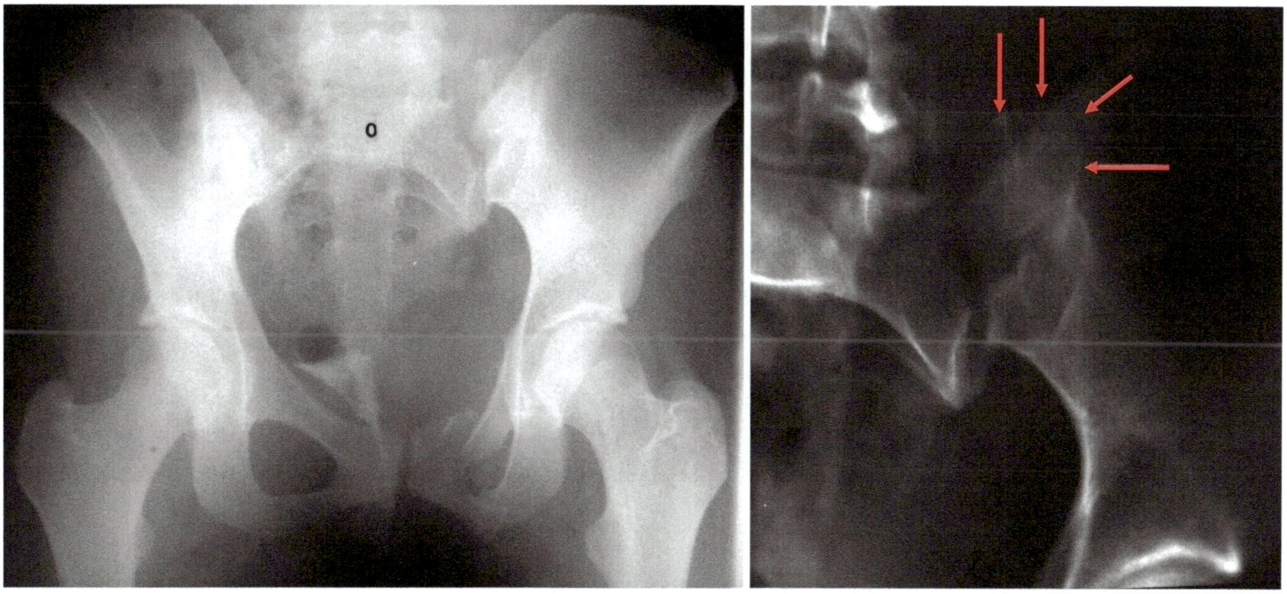

Fig. 7.24 Sacral fracture dislocation of the SI joint with a sacral fragment attached to the left hemipelvis

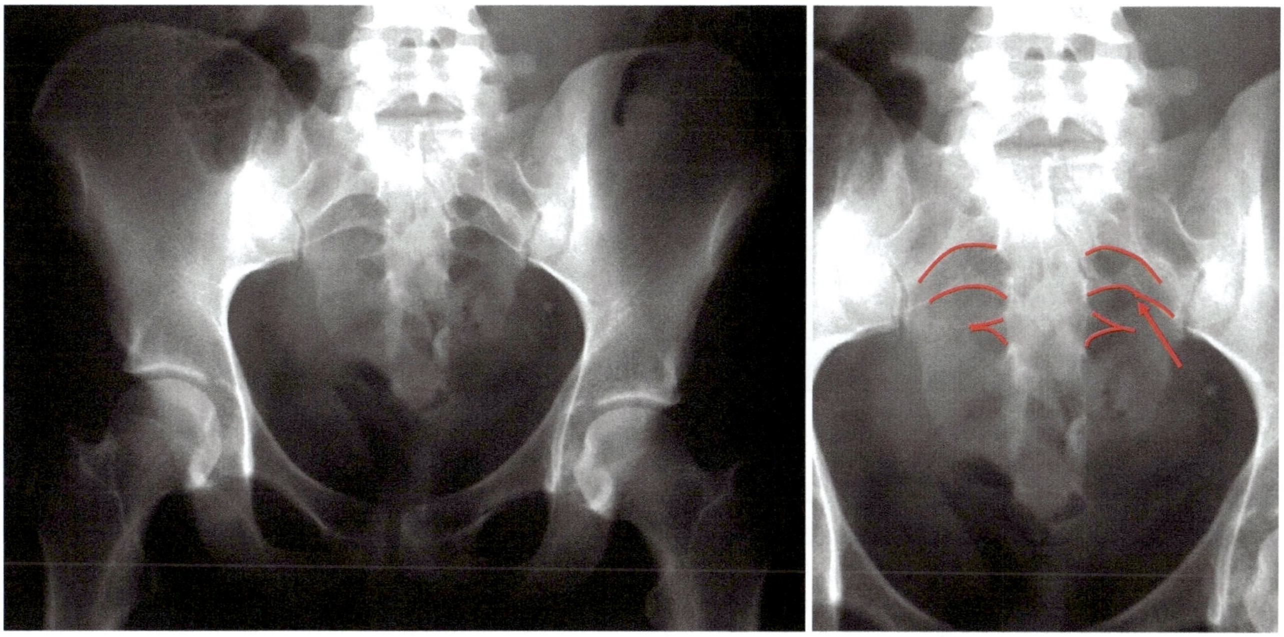

Fig. 7.25 Analysis of sacral arcuate lines on possible interruptions (arrow), indicative for an anterior sacral cortex disruption

7.8 Special Considerations

In addition to the aforementioned injury regions and their fractures or injuries, other important fracture features may occasionally be visible on the pelvic a.p. X-ray.

7.8.1 Injury to the Pelvic Floor Ligaments

In rare cases, osteoligamentous avulsion injuries of the pelvic floor ligaments (sacrotuberous or sacrospinal ligaments) can be observed (Fig. 7.29). Avulsions of the ischial spine

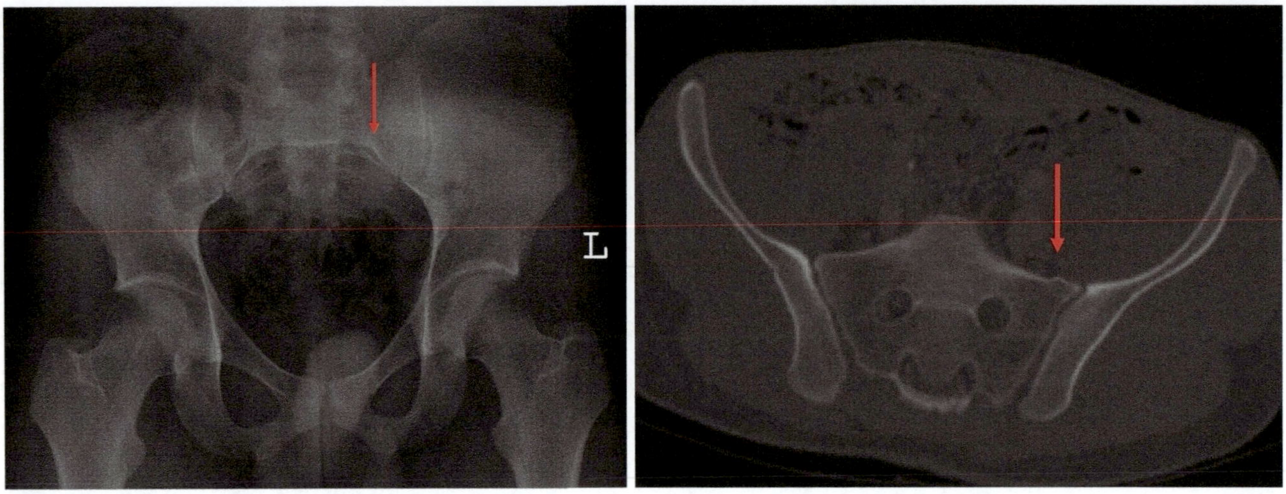

Fig. 7.26 Slight disruption of the first left arcuate line on the a.p. view, confirmed as a break of the anterior cortex on axial CT

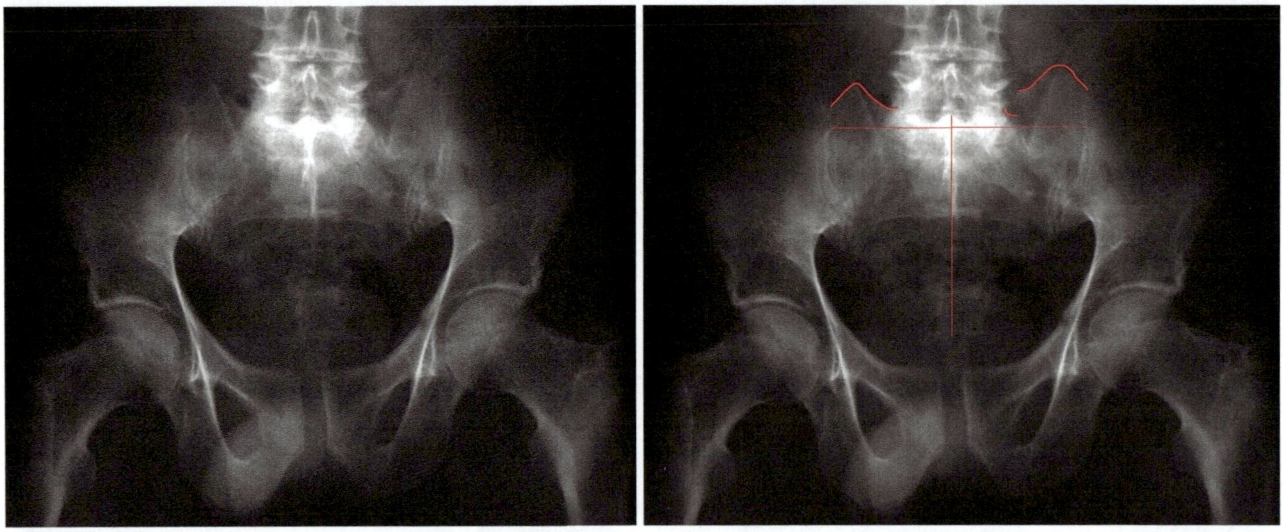

Fig. 7.27 Analysis of the upper sacral margin for interruption and analysis of the hemisacral width

(sacrospinous ligament) or at the ischial tuberosity (sacrotuberous ligament) were not observed and are extremely rare. These injuries can be a sign of significant pelvic instability. Accordingly, they are predominantly seen in type C injuries of the pelvis but can also be observed in considerable rotational instabilities of type B (Fig. 7.29).

7.8.2 L5 Transverse Process Fractures

The iliolumbar ligament complex originates from the lateral and inferior parts of the L5 transverse process to insert on the posterior iliac crest and the sacral ala, respectively. Shearing of hemipelvis in type C injuries may result in a bony avulsion of the transverse process (Fig. 7.30). Thus, these injuries represent an indicator of significant pelvic instability [40–43].

7.8.3 Evaluation After Primary Pelvic Binder Application

There is a potential risk that a pelvic binder can "mask" the amount of initial displacement at the time of injury as sometimes a near anatomic reduction of pelvic instability is observed (for details, see Chap. 9).

Initial CT diagnostics of the pelvic instead of routine pelvic X-ray can result in a significant time delay in diagnosing relevant pelvic ring injuries, requiring immediate pelvic interventions [6]. Thus, the conventional X-ray is still the gold standard in the initial treatment phase.

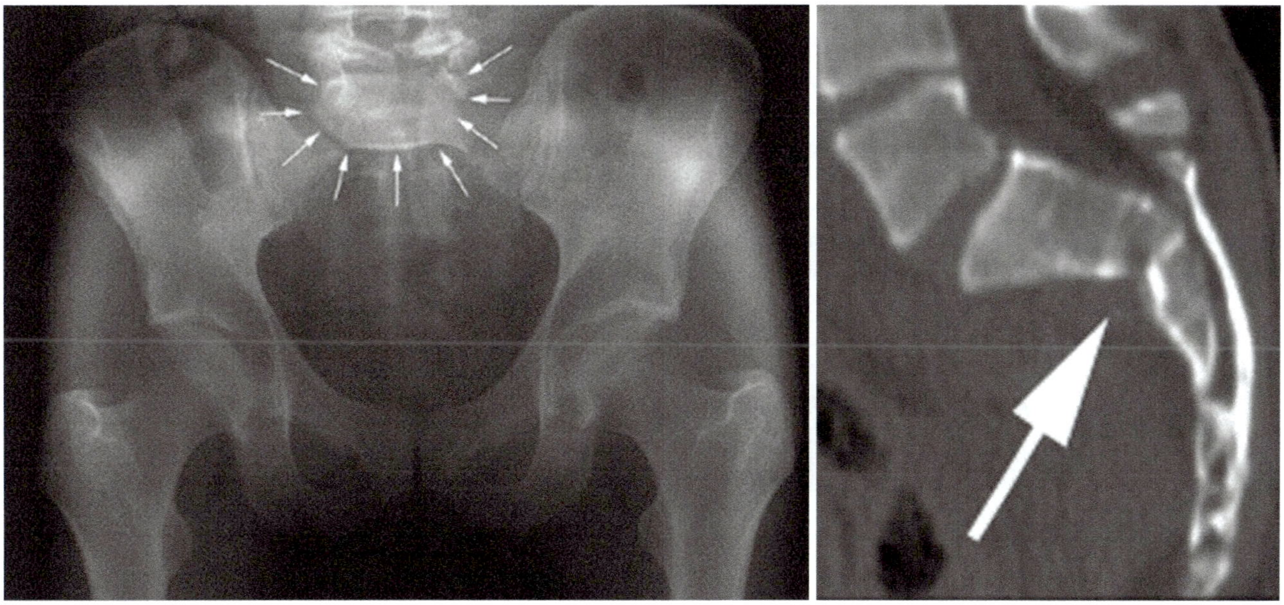

Fig. 7.28 Prominence of the sacral promontory can be indicative for lumbo-pelvic dissociation injury (suicidal jumper's fracture), which is confirmed on sagittal CT

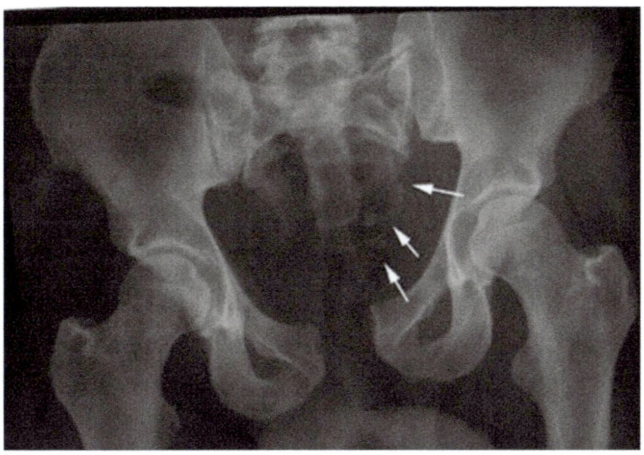

Fig. 7.29 Pelvic floor ligamentous avulsion fracture in a type C injury

7.9 Dynamic Fluoroscopy

Pelvic injury diagnosis using dynamic fluoroscopy was proposed for minor displaced injuries to analyze the degree of instability.

In the supine position, stress examination was recommended under anesthesia. This includes (Fig. 7.31) [44]:

- Adduction and internal rotation of the lower extremities with compression through the greater trochanters
- Abduction force to the knees applied in external rotation (frog-leg position) in a push-and-pull technique to both lower extremities with longitudinal traction on one limb and a simultaneous vertical loading on the contralateral limb and vice versa

Analyzing the pelvis in the standard X-ray planes (anterior-posterior, inlet, outlet) leads to a change of the Young-Burgess classification in 50% of presumed APC 1 injuries, 39% of APC 2 injuries, and 37% of LC 1 injuries, with resulting higher grades of instability [44].

7.10 Inlet and Outlet Views

For a long time, additional oblique views for analysis of pelvic deformity in different planes were considered mandatory.

Inlet and outlet radiographs were classically performed with the X-ray beam directed 45° caudal and 45° cranial, respectively (Fig. 7.32) [45]. The inlet and outlet views according to Pennal and Tile were recommended for several decades. Recent results show that virtual views are sufficient (Fig. 7.33) [46].

Recently, these values were redefined [47, 48]. Pohlemann already described different angulations: 40–60° for the inlet view and 30–45° for the outlet view [49].

Recently, Ricci et al. found a 21° angulation optimal for the inlet view and 63° for the outlet view perpendicular to the S1 body and 57° perpendicular to the S2 body [47]. In a Korean analysis, the optimal inlet angles were 24.2° at S1 and 27.9° at S2, while the outlet angles were 54.8° at S1 and 52.3° at S2 [50].

A further CT analysis revealed an optimal inlet angle of approximately 25° and an outlet angle of 43.8° [46].

Inlct and outlet views were used to analyze the amount of anterior-posterior and vertical displacement, respectively (Fig. 7.34).

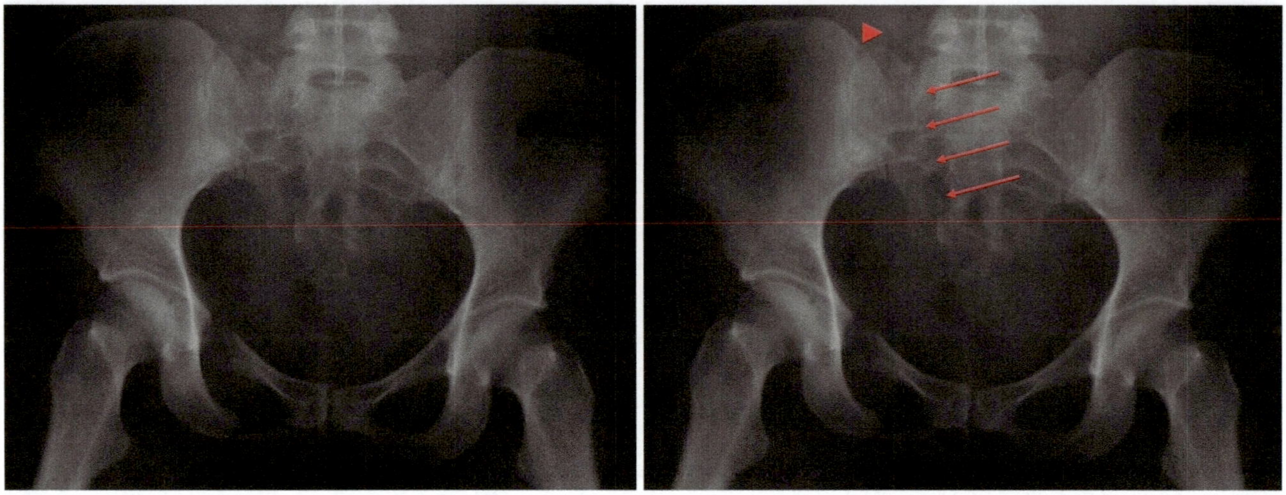

Fig. 7.30 L5 transverse process avulsion fracture (arrowhead) as an indicator of posterior instability (complete right transforaminal sacral fracture (arrows))

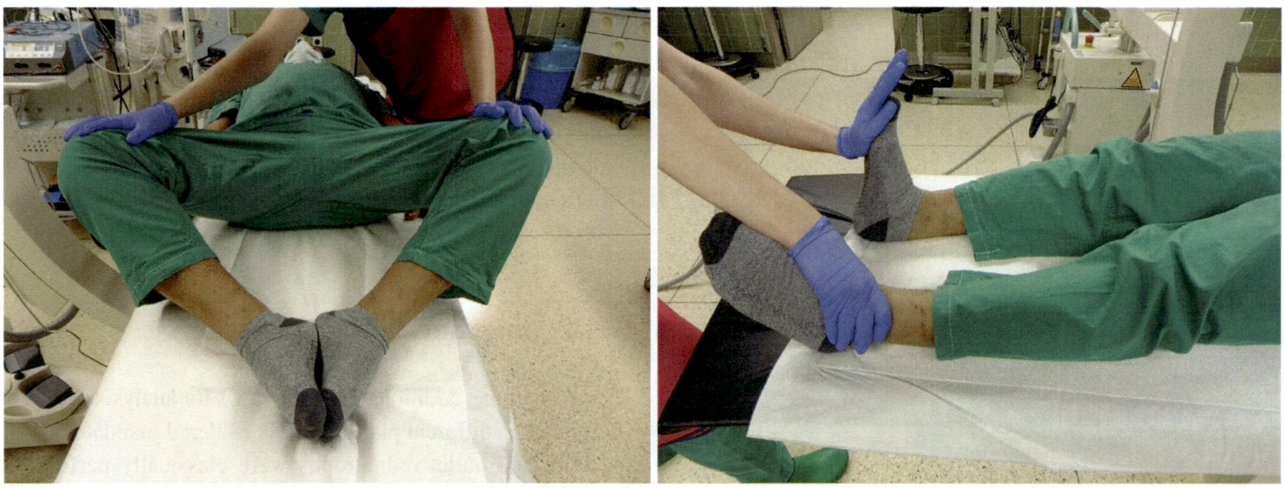

Fig. 7.31 Dynamic stress evaluation of the pelvis in the supine position to detect subtle instabilities or confirm relevant instabilities

Recent analyses stated that the Sagi, Keshishyan, and Lefaivre methods (Figs. 7.34 and 7.35) for analyzing pelvic deformity were associated with only poor reliability. The Sagi method only allows for relevant information in displaced deformities, while the best method was that by Keshishyan, which is difficult to interpret [51].

Nystrom et al. stated that vertical translation of the a.p. view, by measuring the difference in height of the iliac wings in relation to perpendicular lines to the sacral midline and even CT measurement of the anterior SI joint displacement, was unreliable [52]. In contrast, Boontanapibul et al. could show an adequate correlation between cadaver displacement and actual radiographic displacement on the pelvic outlet radiograph with two times of actual displacement [53].

7.11 CT Scanning

Pelvic CT scanning of the pelvis as a contrast-enhanced CT is the imaging modality of choice and therefore the gold standard in evaluating pelvic ring injuries, most commonly performed during the initial whole-body CT examination. In isolated injuries, every conventional diagnosed pelvic ring injury should be additionally analyzed by a pelvic CT scan.

CT of the pelvis allows for a detailed evaluation, especially of the posterior pelvic ring structures to focus on stability analysis of the posterior pelvis.

Overall, the pelvic CT is helpful for analysis of the:

- Mechanism of injury

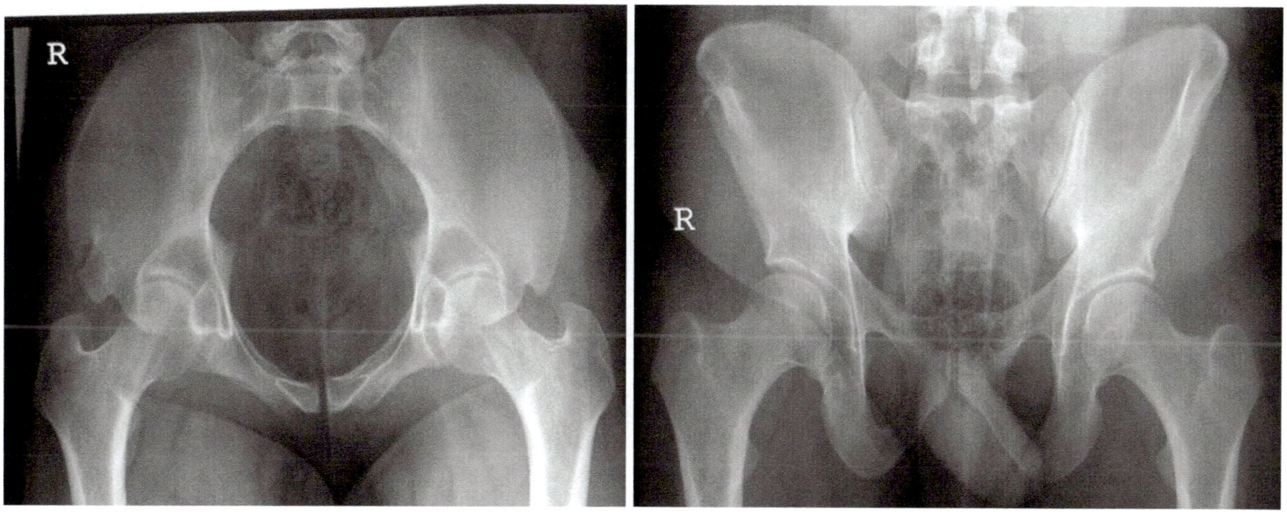

Fig. 7.32 Classical Inlet and Outlet views

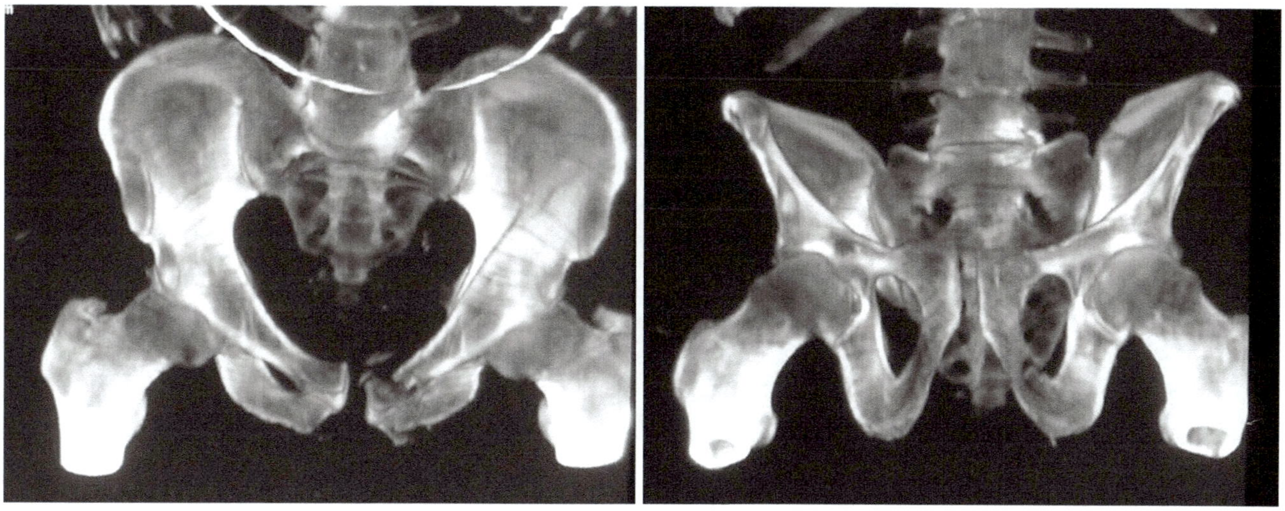

Fig. 7.33 Virtual Inlet and Outlet views derived from CT data

- Degree of stability
- Degree of fracture/injury displacement
- Additional pelvic organ and neurovascular injuries
- Suspected treatment possibilities

Besides images acquired in the axial plane, additional coronal, sagittal multiplanar reconstructions (MPR) (Fig. 7.36) and three-dimensional (3D) volume reconstructions are usually performed to add further understanding of the bony injury.

Postsurgical CT evaluation of the pelvis was recently recommended to allow a safer detection of implant position, especially for evaluation of iliosacral screws [54].

7.11.1 Vascular Injury CT Analysis

Besides analysis of the bony structures, contrast-enhanced CT provides information on pelvic soft tissue injury and the arterial status (Fig. 7.37). Contrast media active extravasation indicates pelvic hematoma formation using an arterial and portal venous phase. These different phases allow for distinguishing arterial and venous hemorrhage [55].

Arterial injuries can be detected during the arterial phase of the CT imaging. The classical sign of arterial injury presents with active bleeding (active contrast extravasation) with an area of hyper-attenuation within a hematoma or hematoma enlargement during further examinations [56]. Vascular

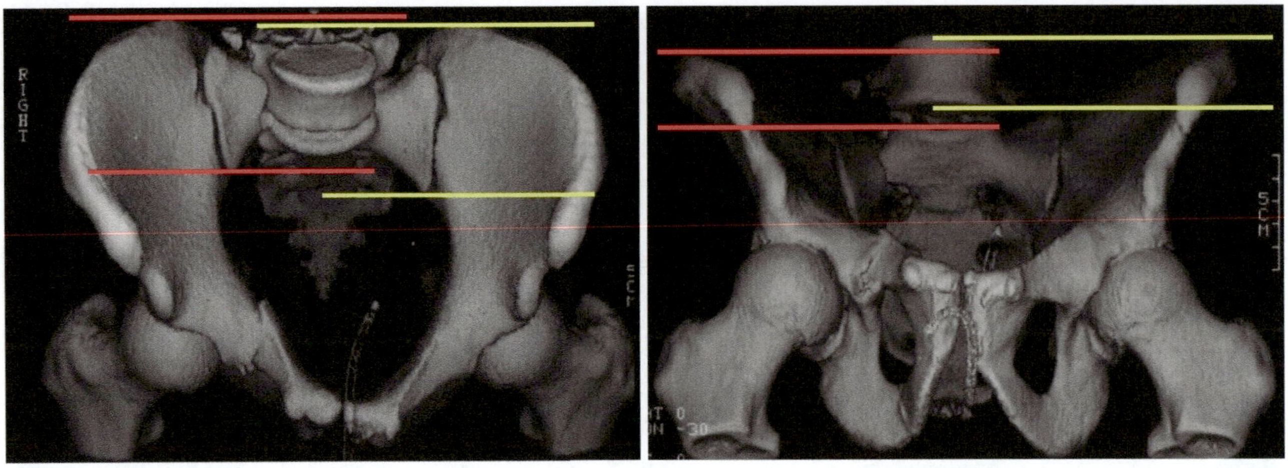

Fig. 7.34 Measurement of anterior-posterior (Inlet) and craniocaudal (Outlet) displacements of pelvic injuries, modified acc. to Lefaivre and Sagi

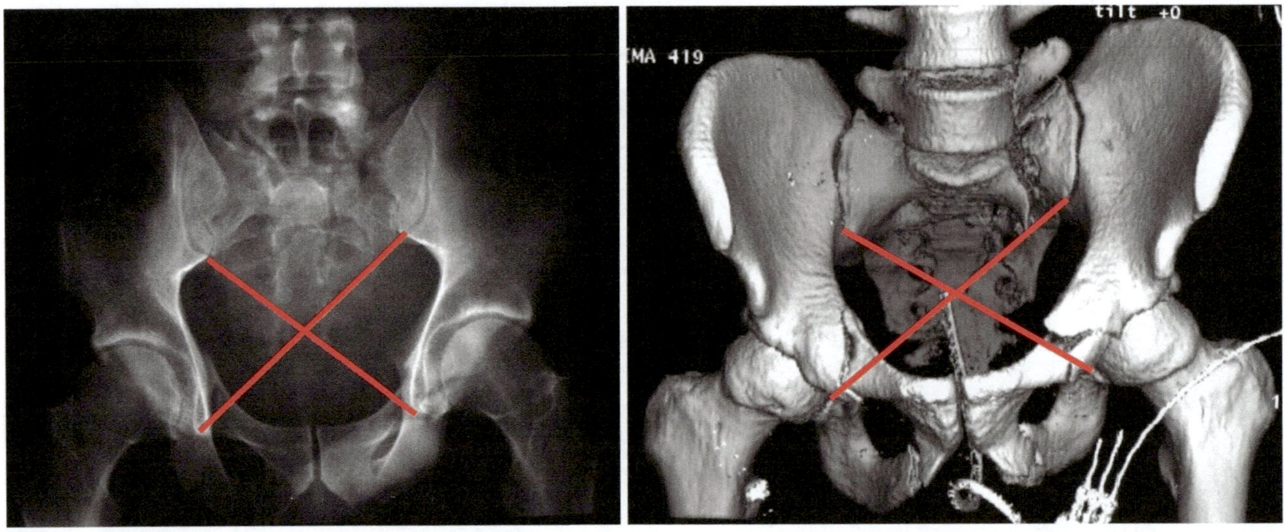

Fig. 7.35 Keshishyan method to measure pelvic obliquity

thrombosis or occlusion is suspected if no vascular enhancement is observed (side comparison).

The sensitivity, specificity, positive predictive value, negative predictive value, and overall accuracy of diagnosing arterial hemorrhage using CT evaluation were found to be 82%, 95%, 60%, 98%, and 94%, respectively [57].

Direct signs of vascular injury include (Fig. 7.38) [58, 59]:

- Arterial thrombosis/occlusion
- Vascular avulsion/complete tear
- Rupture with active extravasation: focal area of hyper-attenuation within a hematoma during the arterial CT phase which can result in an enlarged, enhancing hematoma in the delayed phase
- Arterial pseudoaneurysm: focal area of hyper-attenuation in the arterial phase, stable in size which presents with a "wash-out" in the delayed phase

Indirect signs of venous injuries include:

- Perivascular hematoma: focal area of hyper-attenuation within a hematoma during the venous CT phase which can result in an enlarged, enhancing hematoma in the delayed phase
- Fat stranding
- Vessel wall irregularities

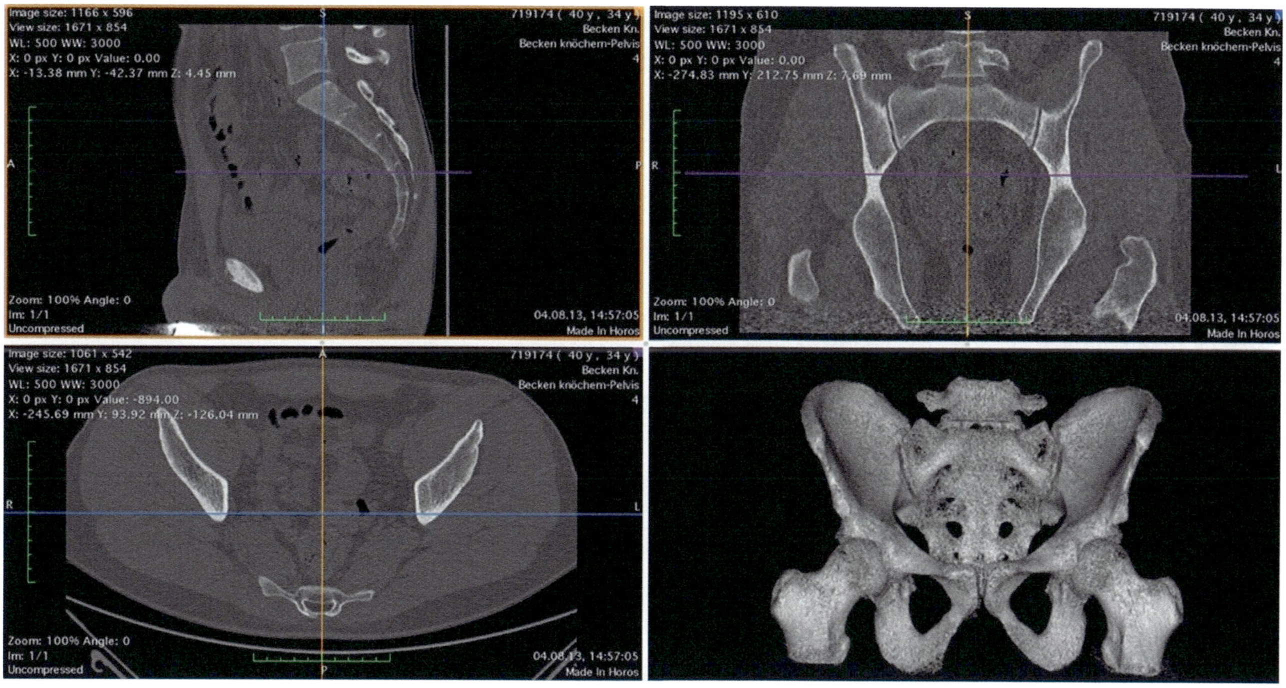

Fig. 7.36 Standard pelvic CT scan with multiplanar reconstructions in the three standard planes and 3D-volume rendering of the pelvis

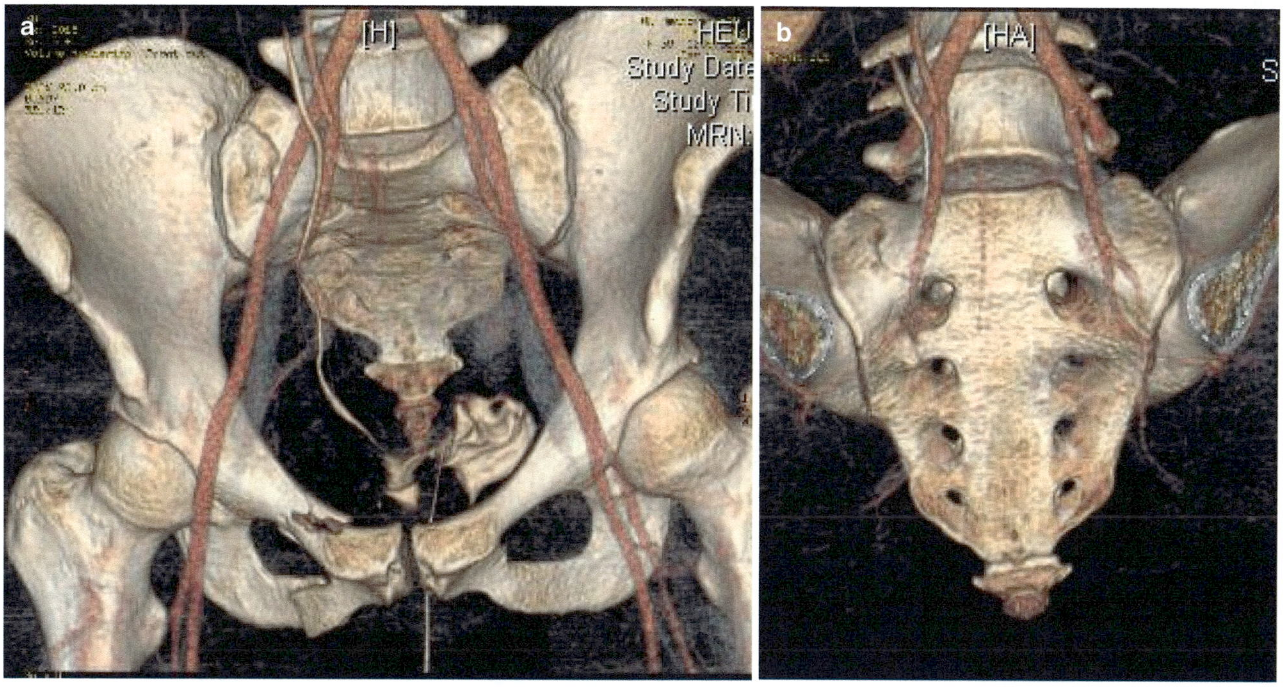

Fig. 7.37 Normal pelvic arterial anatomy (**a**) and anterior to the sacrum (**b**) in a case with a lateral compression injury

The presence of external iliac artery injuries was more often associated with hemodynamic instability than internal iliac artery injuries [60].

Delayed phase imaging has the advantage of easier confirmation of slower active arterial extravasation and of urologic injury [61].

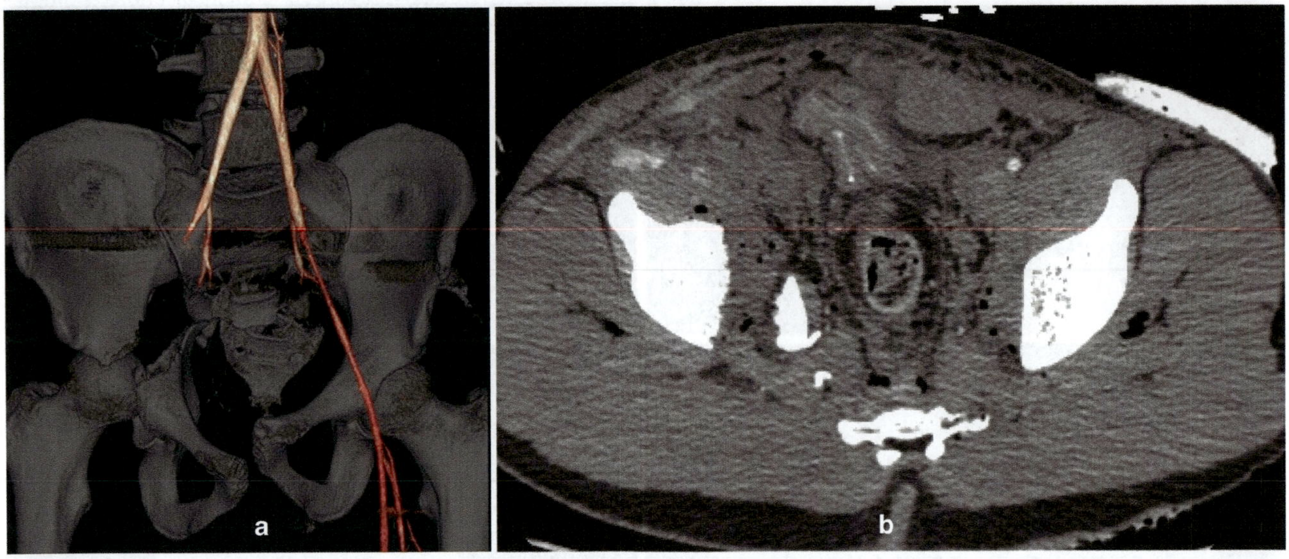

Fig. 7.38 Iliac external artery occlusion with arterial constriction prior to artery disruption (**a**) and active contrast media extravasation distal to the constricted area (**b**)

Table 7.1 Vascular territories on axial CT images and possible injury locations

Artery	Territory	Possible injury site
Iliolumbar	Iliopsoas, quadratus lumborum, ilium	Ilium fracture, SI joint
Lateral sacral	Piriformis, sacrum, erector spinae	Sacrum
Median sacral	Lower lumbar vertebra/Denis zone I + II sacrum	Sacrum
Superior gluteal	Piriformis, gluteal muscles	Ilium, posterior pelvis
Inferior gluteal	Piriformis, gluteal muscles, hamstrings	Ilium, posterior pelvis
Obturator	Obturator internus, adductors	Acetabulum, pubic rami
Internal pudendal	Perineum, urogenital triangle	Pubic rami, posterior pelvis
Inferior epigastric	Rectus abdominis	Pubic symphysis
Visceral branches	Pelvic viscera	Pubic rami

Standard multidetector computed tomography (MDCT) evaluation of arterial hemorrhage was found to show comparable diagnostic value than digital subtraction angiography (DSA) [62, 63].

Hallinan et al. first defined nine major pelvic vascular territories on axial CT images to allow rapid assessment of potential injury locations (Table 7.1, Figs. 7.39, 7.40, and 7.41), based on the arterial hemipelvic anatomy [58].

> It is recommended to perform the CT of the pelvis prior to any urological contrast media filling (e.g., retrograde urethrography, cystography) as the contrast medium can obscure potential arterial extravasation [64].

Uludag et al. performed a comparable analysis and defined the anatomic pelvic hemorrhage distribution after pelvic ring fractures [65].

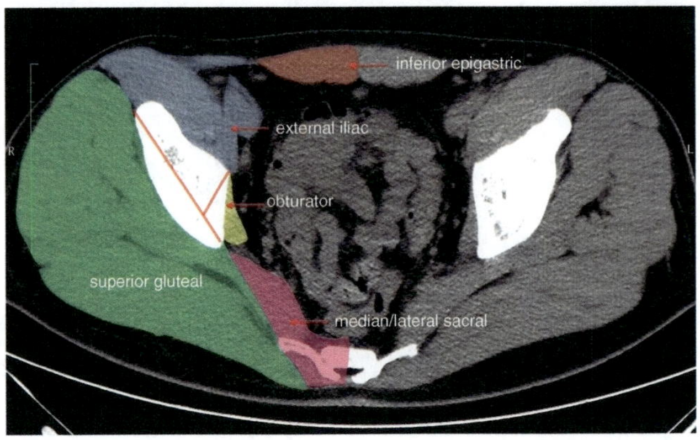

Fig. 7.39 Vascular territories of the intrapelvic muscles, modified according to Hallinan on axial CT images at the mid pelvic level

In an analysis of 60 patients with pelvic ring injuries and hemodynamic instability and pelvic-related hemorrhage, it was found that 47% showed signs of extrapelvic hemorrhage, especially in the gluteal areas. Hemorrhage was

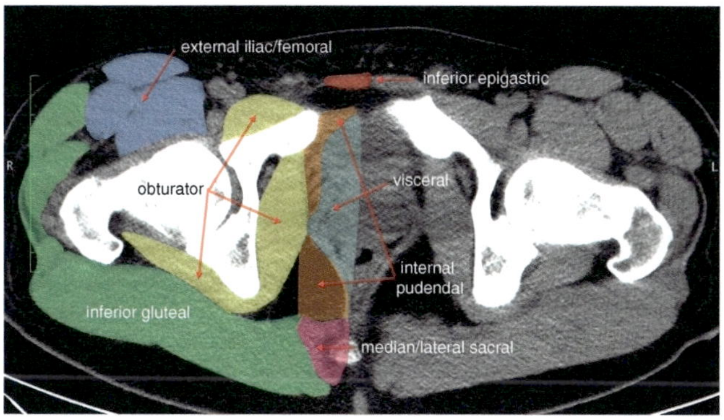

Fig. 7.40 Vascular territories of the intrapelvic muscles, modified according to Hallinan on axial CT images at the hip joint level

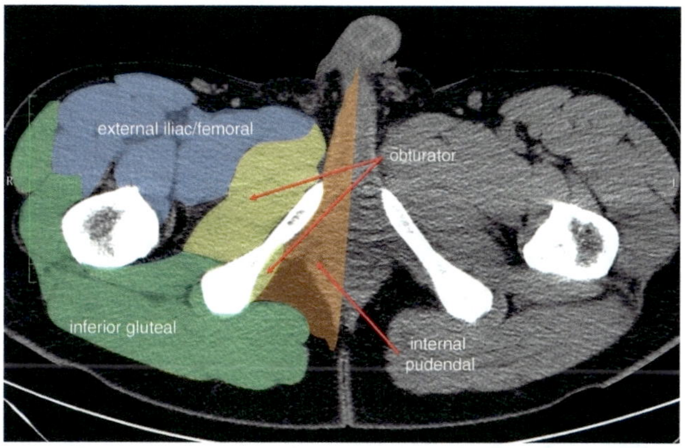

Fig. 7.41 Vascular territories of the intrapelvic muscles, modified according to Hallinan on axial CT images at the ischial tuberosity level

correlated with transfusion requirements, necessity of angiography, and 30-day mortality.

CT analysis consisted of three main regions (zones A–C), with further subdivision on axial CT images into overall 24 true pelvic and five extrapelvic regions. Zones A, B, and C were subdivided into right and left anterior and posterior compartments within and outside the true pelvis:

- Zone A: ischial tuberosity to ischial spine (subdivisions 1–8)
- Zone B: caudal SI joint to the ischial spine (subdivisions 1–8)
- Zone C: caudal SI joint to the iliac crest (subdivisions 1–8)
- Zone D: central extrapelvic paravertebral area from the diaphragm to the sacral promontory with its lateral border being the lateral psoas muscle
- Zone E: lateral extrapelvic flank area from the diaphragm to the iliac crest, lateral to the psoas muscle (2 Zones)
- Zone F: right and left thigh region (2 Zones)

Recently, Dreizin et al. developed a prediction model of major arterial pelvic injury based on radiographic parameters, resulting in angiographic bleeding control [66]. Hematoma volume, contrast media extravasation, atherosclerosis, rotational instability of the pelvis, and an obturator ring fracture were identified to be associated with arterial injury.

A hematoma volume of >433 mL was associated with a positive predictive value of 87–100% for major arterial injury requiring angio-embolization (AE) and transfusion requirements.

A probability equation was calculated:

$$\text{Probability} = \frac{e^{(1.134"OB)+(0.82"AT)+(0.007"HV)+(1.099"ICE)+(-1.237"RT)-2.143}}{1+\left(e^{(1.134"OB)+(0.82"AT)+(0.007"HV)+(1.099"ICE)+(-1.237"RT)-2.413}\right)}"100\%$$

OB obturator ring injury, *AT* atherosclerosis, *HV* hematoma volume, *ICE* intravenous contrast media extravasation, *RT* rotational pelvic instability.

7.12 CT Analysis of Pelvic Urological Trauma

See Chap. 21.

7.13 MRI

During primary evaluation of pelvic ring injuries, the MRI is of minor importance. Primary indications for MRI diagnostics include:

- Detection of subtle injuries, e.g., geriatric fractures [67].
- Evaluation of pelvic thrombosis (Fig. 7.42) [68, 69].
- Analysis of injury-related nerve injuries [70].

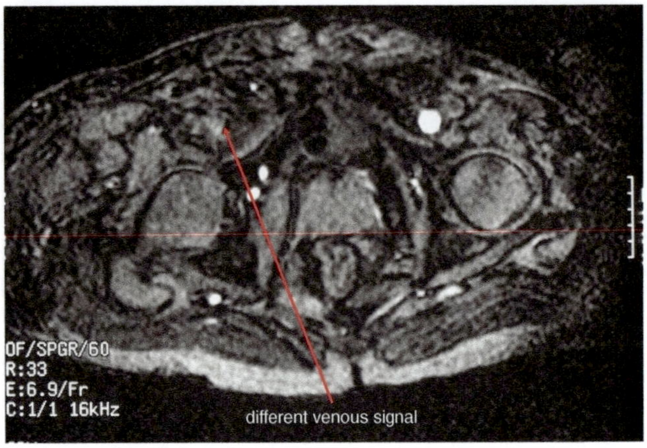

Fig. 7.42 MRI of the pelvic region to detect venous thrombosis

Only one study analyzes the value of MRI during primary evaluation of patients with pelvic injuries. Patients with detected anterior pelvic ring injuries without visible injuries of the posterior ring on a.p. X-rays were clinically examined for posterior pelvic complaints. The resulting CT evaluation confirmed posterior injuries with a sensitivity and specificity of 0.83 and 0.92, respectively. MRI detected posterior injuries, even when not visualized on CT evaluation [71].

The rate of pelvic thrombosis was recorded in up to 63% [72]. As the pelvic region is usually not detectable by ultrasonography, screening for deep vein thrombosis (DVT) was also accomplished by magnetic resonance venography (MRV).

Additionally, MRI was used to detect pelvic floor and iliosacral ligament injuries in detail [37]. The sacrospinous, sacrotuberous, anterior, and posterior sacroiliac ligaments could be analyzed in 91%, 100%, 98%, and 91%, respectively. In all patients with a pelvic ring injury, a ligament injury was detected. Interestingly, the Young-Burgess type APC II injury was associated with a pelvic floor ligament disruption in only 50%.

7.14 Angiography

See Chap. 15.

7.15 Radiation Dose

The effective dose of a pelvic a.p. X-ray is expected to be between 0.3 and 0.7 mSv (http://www.bfs.de).

The radiation exposure of a whole-body CT scan is not negligible. Davies et al. reported a mean dose of 31 mSv with no difference between a 16-line CT scanner and a 128-line CT scanner. The calculated risk development of malignant disease was 1:683 on average [73].

A CT of the pelvis, which is often performed in conjunction with an abdominal CT, leads to a combined effective dose of 6.7 mSv, equivalent to nearly 450 chest radiographs (cited in [59]).

References

1. Advanced trauma life support (ATLS), 9th Edition 2012.
2. Tscherne H, Pohlemann T. Tscherne unfallchirurgie: becken und acetabulum. Berlin, Heidelberg, New York: Springer-Verlag; 1998.
3. Tscherne H, Regel G. Tscherne unfallchirurgie: trauma-management. Berlin, Heidelberg, New York: Springer-Verlag; 1997. p. 257–97.
4. Gercek E, Hessmann M, Rommen P. Bildgebende Diagnostik bei Beckenverletzungen. Akt Traumatol. 2002;32:163–70.
5. Resnik C, Stackhouse D, Shanmuganathan K, Young J. Diagnosis of pelvic fractures in patients with acute pelvic trauma: efficiency of plain radiographs. AJR. 1992;158:109–12.
6. Verbeek D, Burgess A. Importance of pelvic radiography for initial trauma assessment: an orthopedic perspective. J Emerg Med. 2016;50:852–8.
7. Edeiken-Monroe B, Browner BD, Jackson H. The role of standard roentgenograms in the evaluation of instability of pelvic ring disruption. Clin Orthop. 1989;240:63–76.
8. Young JW, Burgess AR, Brumback RJ, Poka A. Pelvic fractures: value of plain radiography in early assessment and management. Radiology. 1986;160(2):445–51.
9. Duane TM, Tan BB, Golay D, Cole FJ Jr, Weireter LJ Jr, Britt LD. Blunt trauma and the role of routine pelvic radiographs: a prospective analysis. J Trauma. 2002;53(3):463–8.
10. Borrelli J Jr, Goldfarb C, Catalano L, Evanoff BA. Assessment of articular fragment displacement in acetabular fractures: a comparison of computerized tomography and plain radiographs. J Orthop Trauma. 2002;16(7):449–56. discussion 456–7
11. Kreitner KF, Mildenberger P, Rommens PM, Thelen M. Rational diagnostic imaging of pelvic and acetabulum injuries. Rofo Fortschr Geb Rontgenstr Neuen Bildgeb Verfahr. 2000;172(1):5–11.
12. Pehle B, Nast-Kolb D, Oberbeck R, Waydhas C, Ruchholtz S. Wertigkeit der körperlichen und radiologischen Basisdiagnostik des Beckens in der Schockraumbehandlung. Unfallchirurg. 2003;106:642–8.
13. Guillamondegui OD, Pryor JP, Gracias VH, Gupta R, Reilly PM, Schwab CW. Pelvic radiography in blunt trauma resuscitation: a diminishing role. J Trauma. 2002;53(6):1043–7.
14. Hilty M, Behrendt I, Benneker L, Martinolli L, Stoupis C, Buggy D, Zimmermann H, Exadaktylos A. Pelvic radiography in ATLS algorithms: a diminishing role? World J Emerg Surg. 2008;3:11. https://doi.org/10.1186/1749-7922-3-11.
15. Schicho A, Schmidt S, Seeber K, Olivier A, Richter P, Gebhard F. Pelvic X-ray misses out on detecting sacral fractures in the elderly - importance of CT imaging in blunt pelvic trauma. Injury. 2016;47:707–10.
16. Soto J, Zhou C, Hu D, Arazoza A, Dunn E, Sladek P. Skip and save: utility of pelvic x-rays in the initial evaluation of blunt trauma patients. Am J Surg. 2015;210:1076–9.
17. Their M, Bensch F, Koskinen S, Handolin L, Kiuru M. Diagnostic value of pelvic radiography in the initial trauma series in blunt trauma. Eur Radiol. 2005;15:1533–7.
18. Traumaregister, Jahresbericht, www.traumaregister.de. 2018.
19. OTA. Fracture and dislocation compendium. J Orthop Trauma. 1996;10(Suppl. 1):71–5.
20. Letournel E. Annotation to pelvic fractures. Injury. 1978;10:145–8.

21. Denis F, Steven D, Comfort T. Sacral fractures: an important problem, retrospective analysis of 236 cases. Clin Orthop. 1988;227:67–81.
22. Björklund K, Bergström S, Lindgren P, Ulmsten U. Ultrasonographic measurement of the symphysis pubis: a potential method of studying symphyseolysis in pregnancy. Gynecol Obstet Investig. 1996;42:151–3.
23. Gamble JG, Simmons SC, Freedman M. The symphysis pubis. Anatomic and pathologic considerations. Clin Orthop Relat Res. 1986;203:261–72.
24. Loeschcke H. Untersuchungen über die Entstehung und Bedeutung der Spaltbildungen in der Symphyse, sowie über physiologische Erweiterungsvorgaenge am Becken Schwangerer und Gebärender. Archiv Gynaek. 1912;96:525–60.
25. Vix V, Ryu C. The adult symphysis pubis: normal and abnormal. Am J Roentgenol Radium Therapy, Nucl Med. 1971;112:517–25.
26. Krauss F. Über Symphysensprengung. Zentbl Chir. 1930;3:134–5.
27. Patel K, Chapman S. Normal symphysis width in children. Clin Radiol. 1993;47:56–7.
28. Alicioglu B, Kartal O, Gurbuz H, Sut N. Symphysis pubis distance in adults: a retrospective computed tomography study. Surg Radiol Anat. 2008;30:153–7.
29. McAlister D, Webb H, Wheeler P, Shinault K, Teague D, Fish J, Beall D. Pubic symphyseal width in pediatric patients. J Pediatr Orthop. 2005;25:725–7.
30. Bayer J, Neubauer J, Saueressig U, Südkamp N, Reising K. Age- and gender-related characteristics of the pubic symphysis and triradiate cartilage in pediatric computed tomography. Pediatr Radiol. 2016;46:1705–12.
31. Kalenderer Ö, Turgut A, Bacaksız T, Bilgin E, Kumbaracı M, Akkan H. Evaluation of symphysis pubis and sacroiliac joint distances in skeletally immature patients: a computerized tomography study of 1020 individuals. Acta Orthop Traumatol Turc. 2017;51:150–4.
32. Oetgen M, Andelman S, Martin B. Age-based normative measurements of the pediatric pelvis. J Orthop Trauma. 2017;31:e205–9.
33. Garras D, Carothers J, Olson S. Single-leg-stance (flamingo) radiographs to assess pelvic instability: how much motion is normal? J Bone Joint Surg Am. 2008;90:2114–8.
34. Siegel J, Templeman D, Tornetta PR. Single-leg-stance radiographs in the diagnosis of pelvic instability. J Bone Joint Surg Am. 2008;90:2119–25.
35. Rustamova S, Predanic M, Sumersille M, Cohen W. Changes in symphysis pubis width during labor. J Perinat Med. 2009;37:370–3.
36. Hefzy MS, Ebraheim N, Mekhail A, Caruntu D, Lin H, Yeasting R. Kinematics of the human pelvis following open book injury. Med Eng Phys. 2003;25(4):259–74.
37. Gary J, Mulligan M, Banagan K, Sciadini M, Nascone J, O'Toole R. Magnetic resonance imaging for the evaluation of ligamentous injury in the pelvis: a prospective case-controlled study. J Orthop Trauma. 2014;28:41–7.
38. Northrop C, Eto R, Loop J. Vertical fracture of the sacral ala: significance of non-continuity of the anterior superior sacral foraminal line. AJR. 1975;124:102–6.
39. Roy-Camille R, Saillant G, Gagana G, Mazel C. Transverse fracture of the upper sacrum: suicidal jumper's fracture. Spine. 1985;10(9):838–45.
40. Maqungo S, Kimani M, Chhiba D, McCollum G, Roche S. The L5 transverse process fracture revisited. Does its presence predict the pelvis fracture instability? Injury. 2015;46:1629–30.
41. Nasef H, Elhessy A, Abushaban F, Alhammoud A. Pelvic fracture instability-associated L5 transverse process fracture, fact or myth? A systematic review and meta-analysis. Eur J Orthop Surg Traumatol. 2018;28:885–91.
42. Starks I, Frost A, Wall P, Lim J. Is a fracture of the transverse process of L5 a predictor of pelvic fracture instability? J Bone Joint Surg (Br). 2011;93:967–9.
43. Winkelmann M, Lopez Izquierdo M, Clausen J, Liodakis E, Mommsen P, Blossey R, Krettek C, Zeckey C. Fractures of the transverse processes of the fourth and fifth lumbar vertebrae in patients with pelvic ring injuries: indicator of biomechanical instability but not shock.´. Bone Joint J. 2018;100:1214–9.
44. Sagi H, Coniglione F, Stanford J. Examination under anesthetic for occult pelvic ring instability. J Orthop Trauma. 2011;25:529–36.
45. Pennal G, Tile M, Waddell J, Garside H. Pelvic disruption: assessment and classification. Clin Orthop. 1980;151:12–21.
46. Pekmezci M, Rotter P, Toogood P, Morshed S, Kandemir U. Reexamination of pelvic inlet and outlet images using 3-dimensional computed tomography reconstructions. J Orthop Trauma. 2014;28:324–9.
47. Ricci W, Mamczak C, Tynan M, Streubel P, Gardner M. Pelvic inlet and outlet radiographs redefined. J Bone Joint Surg. 2010;92-A:1947–53.
48. Ziran B, Wasan A, Marks D, Olson S, Chapman M. Fluoroscopic imaging guides of the posterior pelvis pertaining to iliosacral screw placement. J Trauma. 2007;62:347–56.
49. Pohlemann T, Gänsslen A, Hartung S, Arbeitsgruppe Becken HT, Tscherne H. Beckenverletzungen/Pelvic Injuries. Hefte zu "Der Unfallchirurg". Berlin: Springer; 1998. p. 266.
50. Young P, Ho K, Nair S, Yeon W. Optimal pelvic inlet and outlet radiograph angles in Korean patients. J Korean Orthop Assoc. 2012;47:9–14.
51. Lefaivre K, Blachut P, Starr A, Slobogean G, O'Brien P. Radiographic displacement in pelvic ring disruption: reliability of 3 previously described measurement techniques. J Orthop Trauma. 2014;28:160–6.
52. Nystrom L, McKinley T, Marsh J. Radiographic measurement of rotational deformity in pelvic fractures: a novel method with validity and reliability testing. J Orthop Trauma. 2015;29:365–9.
53. Boontanapibul K, Harnroongroj T, Sudjai N, Harnroongroj T. Vertical pelvic ring displacement in pelvic ring injury: measurements in pelvic outlet radiograph and in cadavers. Ind J Orthop. 2015;49:425–8.
54. Elnahal W, Vetharajan N, Mohamed B, Acharya M, Chesser T, Ward A. Routine postoperative computed tomography scans after pelvic fracture fixation: a necessity or a luxury? J Orthop Trauma. 2018;32:S66–71.
55. Anderson S, Soto J, Lucey B, Burke P, Hirsch E, Rhea J. Blunt trauma: feasibility and clinical utility of pelvic CT angiography performed with 64-detector row CT. Radiology. 2008;246:410–9.
56. Hamilton J, Kumaravel M, Censullo M, Cohen A, Kievlan D, West O. Multidetector CT evaluation of active extravasation in blunt abdominal and pelvic trauma patients. Radiographics. 2008;28:1603–16.
57. Mohseni S, Talving P, Kobayashi L, Lam L, Inaba K, Branco B, Oliver M, Demetriades D. The diagnostic accuracy of 64-slice computed tomography in detecting clinically significant arterial bleeding after pelvic fractures. Am Surg. 2011;77:1176–82.
58. Hallinan J, Tan C, Pua U. Emergency computed tomography for acute pelvic trauma: where is the bleeder? Clin Radiol. 2014;69:529–37.
59. Shenton A, Choudhary S. The emergency radiology of pelvicb-trauma. Trauma. 2014;16:279–91.
60. Tanizaki S, Maeda S, Ishida H, Yamamoto T, Yoshikawa J. Clinical characteristics of external iliac artery branch injury in pelvic trauma. Am J Emerg Med. 2017;35:1636–8.
61. Vasanawala S, Desser T. Value of delayed imaging in MDCT of the abdomen and pelvis. AJR. 2006;187:154–63.
62. Anderson S, Lucey B, Rhea J, Soto J. 64 MDCT in multiple trauma patients: imaging manifestations and clinical implications of active extravasation. Emerg Radiol. 2007;14:151–9.
63. Maturen K, Adusumilli S, Blane C, Arbabi S, Williams D, Fitzgerald J, Vine A. Contrast-enhanced CT accurately detects hemorrhage

in torso trauma: direct comparison with angiography. J Trauma. 2007;62:740–5.
64. Yoon W, Kim J, Jeong Y, Seo J, Park J, Kang H. Pelvic arterial hemorrhage in patients with pelvic fractures: detection with contrast-enhanced CT. Radiographics. 2004;24:1591–605.
65. Uludag N, Tötterman A, Beckman M, Sundin A. Anatomic distribution of hematoma following pelvic fracture. Br J Radiol. 2018;91(1085):20170840. https://doi.org/10.1259/bjr.20170840.
66. Dreizin D, Bodanapally U, Boscak A, Tirada N, Issa G, Nascone J, Bivona L, Mascarenhas D, O'Toole R, Nixon E, Chen R, Siegel E. CT prediction model for major arterial injury after blunt pelvic ring disruption. Radiology. 2018;287:1061–9.
67. Rommens P, Hofmann A. Comprehensive classification of fragility fractures of the pelvic ring: recommendations for surgical treatment. Injury. 2013;44:1733–44.
68. Potter H, Montgomery K, Padgett D, Salvati E, Helfet D. Magnetic resonance imaging of the pelvis. Clin Orthop. 1995;319:223–31.
69. Rubel IF, Potter H, Barie P, Kloen P, Helfet DL. Magnetic resonance venography to evaluate deep venous thrombosis in patients with pelvic and acetabular trauma. J Trauma. 2001;51(3):622.
70. Potter H, Montgomery K, Heise C, Helfet D. MR imaging of acetabular fractures: value in detecting femoral head injury, intraarticular fragments and sciatic nerve injury. AJR. 1994;163:881–6.
71. Nüchtern J, Hartel M, Henes F, Groth M, Jauch S, Haegele J, Briem D, Hoffmann M, Lehmann W, Rueger J, Großterlinden L. Significance of clinical examination, CT and MRI scan in the diagnosis of posterior pelvic ring fractures. Injury. 2015;46:315–9.
72. Geerts W, Coren K, Jay R, Chen E, Szalai J. A prospective study of venous thromboembolism after major trauma. New Engl J Med. 1994;331(24):1601–6.
73. Davies R, Scrimshire A, Sweetman L, Anderton M, Holt E. A decision tool for whole-body CT in major trauma that safely reduces unnecessary scanning and associated radiation risks: an initial exploratory analysis. Injury. 2016;47:43–9.

Part II

Emergency Management

8 Introduction: Emergency Management

Axel Gänsslen and Jan Lindahl

Patients with pelvic ring injuries and accompanying hemodynamic instability represent a special subgroup of complex pelvic trauma patients. Complex pelvic trauma, defined as a pelvic injury with an a significant concomitant peripelvic soft tissue or organ trauma, is potentially life-threatening with a persistent mortality rate of 20% [1].

As a subgroup of these injuries, hemodynamically and mechanically unstable pelvic ring injuries are often called "patients in extremis" and therefore require a demanding primary management concept as exsanguinating hemorrhage is associated with a high mortality rate within the first 24 h after trauma [2].

Since 2007, several European landmark papers were dealing with management recommendations in hemodynamic unstable trauma patients.

Rossaint et al. and Spahn et al. recommend immediate pelvic ring closure and stabilization in hemodynamically unstable patients with pelvic ring injuries followed by early preperitoneal pelvic packing, angiography embolization, and/or surgical bleeding control when hemodynamic instability persists [3, 4].

The Scandinavian guidelines for massive bleeding patients recommend a damage control pelvic approach, where extraperitoneal pelvic packing is favored in patients in extremis and angiography for stable patients requiring ≥4 PRBCs/24 h after exclusion of thoracic and/or abdominal bleeding sources after initial pelvic binder fixation [5].

Geeraerts et al. primarily proposed angiography with arterial embolization as the treatment of choice complemented by pelvic external fixation devices to additionally facilitate venous hemostasis, whereas in major retroperitoneal hematoma, damage control pelvic surgery by pelvic packing and pelvic C-clamps is an effective option [6].

The recent European guideline clearly gave the following statements [7]:

- A pelvic binder should be applied to limit life-threatening bleeding in the presence of a suspected pelvic fracture in the presurgical setting (Grade 1B).
- Patients with pelvic ring disruption and hemorrhagic shock require immediate pelvic ring closure and stabilization (Grade 1B).
- Early surgical bleeding control and/or preperitoneal packing and/or angiographic embolization is recommended in patients with ongoing hemodynamic instability, despite adequate pelvic ring stabilization (Grade 1B).
- Resuscitative endovascular balloon occlusion of the aorta (REBOA) is considered only under extreme circumstances to gain time until appropriate bleeding control measures can be implemented (Grade 2C).

Three principal methods for mechanical stabilization of the pelvis are available [7, 8]:

- Pelvic external fixation
- Pelvic binders/sheets (Chap. 9)
- Pelvic C-clamp (Chap. 10)

A possible option for immediate posterior pelvic ring stabilization as a prerequisite for pelvic packing is the damage control screw/wire stabilization of the posterior pelvic ring (Chap. 11).

Direct surgical bleeding control includes retroperitoneal pelvic packing (Chap. 12) and damage control vascular surgery (Subchapter 7.5).

Indirect vascular control is performed by angiography and selective embolization (Chap. 15) or, in special situations, resuscitative endovascular balloon occlusion of the aorta (REBOA, Chap. 14).

A. Gänsslen (✉)
Department of Trauma Surgery, Orthopedics and Hand Surgery, Hospital Wolfsburg, Wolfsburg, Germany

J. Lindahl
Orthopaedics and Trauma Surgery, Helsinki University Hospital, Helsinki, Finland

A. Gänsslen et al. (eds.), *Pelvic Ring Fractures*, https://doi.org/10.1007/978-3-030-54730-1_8

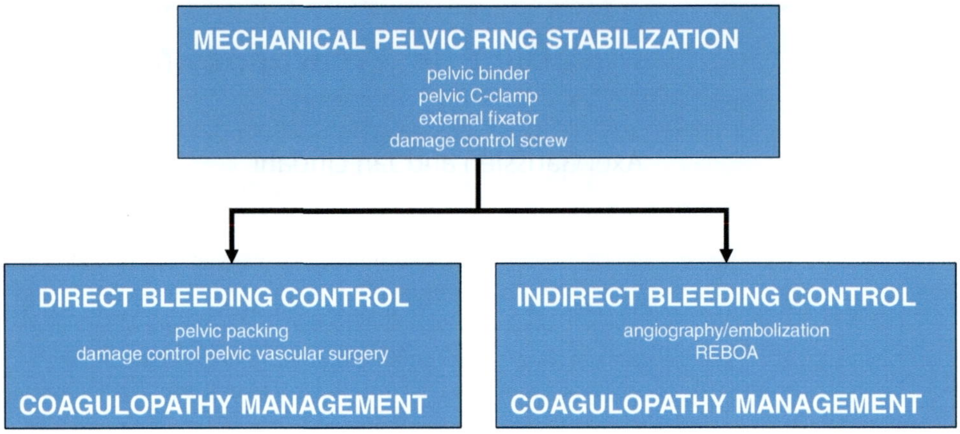

Fig. 8.1 Staged Concept for the treatment of combined hemodynamic and mechanically unstable pelvic ring injuries

Parallel to the concept of mechanical pelvic ring stabilization first, followed by direct surgical or indirect bleeding control, trauma-induced coagulopathy (Chap. 16) has to be addressed (Fig. 8.1).

References

1. Hauschild O, Strohm P, Culemann U, Pohlemann T, Suedkamp N, Koestler W, Schmal H. Mortality in patients with pelvic fractures: results from the German pelvic injury register. J Trauma. 2008;64:449–55.
2. Ertel W, Keel M, Eid K, Platz A, Trentz O. Control of severe hemorrhage using C-clamp and pelvic packing in multiply injured patients with pelvic ring disruption. J Orthop Trauma. 2001;15(7):468–74.
3. Rossaint R, Bouillon B, Cerny V, Coats T, Duranteau J, Fernández-Mondéjar E, Filipescu D, Hunt B, Komadina R, Nardi G, Neugebauer E, Ozier Y, Riddez L, Schultz A, Vincent J, Spahn D. The European guideline on management of major bleeding and coagulopathy following trauma: fourth edition. Crit Care. 2016;20:100.
4. Spahn DR, Cerny V, Coats TJ, Duranteau J, Fernandez-Mondejar E, Gordini G, Stahel PF, Hunt BJ, Komadina R, Neugebauer E, Ozier Y, Riddez L, Schultz A, Vincent JL, Rossaint R. Management of bleeding following major trauma: a European guideline. Crit Care. 2007;11(1):R17.
5. Gaarder C, Naess P, Frischknecht Christensen E, Hakala P, Handolin L, Heier H, Ivancev K, Johansson P, Leppäniemi A, Lippert F, Lossius H, Opdahl H, Pillgram-Larsen J, Røise O, Skaga N, Søreide E, Stensballe J, Tønnessen E, Töttermann A, Ortenwall P, Ostlund A. Scandinavian Guidelines—"The massively bleeding patient". J Surg. 2008;97:15–36.
6. Geeraerts T, Chhor V, Cheisson G, Martin L, Bessoud B, Ozanne A, Duranteau J. Clinical review: initial management of blunt pelvic trauma patients with haemodynamic instability. Crit Care. 2007;11:204.
7. Spahn D, Bouillon B, Cerny V, Duranteau J, Filipescu D, Hunt B, Komadina R, Maegele M, Nardi G, Riddez L, Samama C, Vincent J, Rossaint R. The European guideline on management of major bleeding and coagulopathy following trauma: fifth edition. Crit Care. 2019;23(1):98. https://doi.org/10.1186/s13054-019-2347-3.
8. Gänsslen A, Hildebrand F, Pohlemann T. Management of hemodynamic unstable patients "in extremis" with pelvic ring fractures. Acta Chir Orthop Traumatol Cechoslov. 2012;79:193–202.

Emergency Stabilization: Pelvic Binder

9

Axel Gänsslen, Jan Lindahl, and Bernd Füchtmeier

Historically, military anti-shock trousers (MAST) were used for pelvic emergency stabilization by achieving direct compression and immobilization of the pelvic ring and the lower extremities via pneumatic pressure [1, 2].

However, access to the traumatized region was limited, and assessment and treatment of concomitant injuries were impaired. Major complications, including compartment syndromes and impaired peripheral perfusion necessitating amputation, were reported, particularly after long-term application [1, 3–5].

A Cochrane review of 1075 patients in two randomized trials of MAST found no evidence for reduction of mortality, length of hospitalization, or length of intensive care unit (ICU) stay [6].

In 1996, Baumgärtel introduced a pneumatic "emergency pelvic belt," which acts by local pelvic compression and was easier to apply [7, 8]. This device is placed around the pelvis, and by inflating a pre-symphyseal chamber and two gluteal chambers, circular compression was achieved (Fig. 9.1).

This idea led to the development of different circumferential stabilization techniques, including use of bed sheets, pelvic slings, or pelvic belts for emergency stabilization of pelvic fractures. The main advantage is satisfactory pelvic compression without seriously limiting access to the patient [7–13].

9.1 Elastic Pelvic Sheeting

Routt et al. introduced the concept of pelvic circumferential sheeting using a bed sheet [11]. Advantages include patient comfort, non-invasivity, rapid and temporary pelvic ring stabilization, being readily available, inexpensive, and simple to apply (Fig. 9.2).

A longitudinally folded bed sheet was circumferentially applied around the pelvis and held by two physicians. It was secured by two anterior clamps. Application was performed to allow abdominal and lower extremity assessment. In a hemodynamic unstable patient, after application, hemodynamic stabilization occurred.

Clinical analysis of two patients by Simpson et al. revealed adequate reduction of open book injuries in a safe and time-effective manner [12].

Duxbury et al. modified this technique, fixing the bed sheet by anterior knotting. The ends of the bed sheet were brought out and crossed anteriorly (Fig. 9.2). Fixation was performed with a single twist and secured with two cable ties [10].

Nunn et al. analyzed seven conscious patients with profound hypovolemic shock with anterior posterior compression (APC), lateral compression (LC), and combined mechabnism (CM) injuries treated with a circumferential sheet around the pelvis, the mid-thigh, and the superior ankle region to result in internal rotation of both legs, before definitive emergency fixation with an external fixator [14]. The shock index could be reduced from 1.89 to 0.71. Transfusion requirements were 11.3 packed red blood cells (PRBC)/12 h before application versus 0.94 PRBC/h after application.

Gardner et al. could show that with simple "internal rotation and taping of the lower extremities for closed pelvic reduction" (Fig. 9.2), 15–20% of anatomic reductions could be achieved [15]. Even with the sheet in place around the pelvis, adding "working portals" allows for percutaneous application of implants. These portals are located for percutaneous iliosacral screw fixation, anterior femoral vascular approach, anterior external fixation, and antegrade ramus screw fixation [16].

A. Gänsslen (✉)
Department of Trauma Surgery, Orthopedics and Hand Surgery, Hospital Wolfsburg, Wolfsburg, Germany

J. Lindahl
Orthopaedics and Trauma Surgery, Helsinki University Hospital, Helsinki, Finland

B. Füchtmeier
Department of Trauma Surgery, Hospital Barmherzige Brüder, Regensburg, Germany
e-mail: Bernd.Fuechtmeier@barmherzige-regensburg.de

A. Gänsslen et al. (eds.), *Pelvic Ring Fractures*, https://doi.org/10.1007/978-3-030-54730-1_9

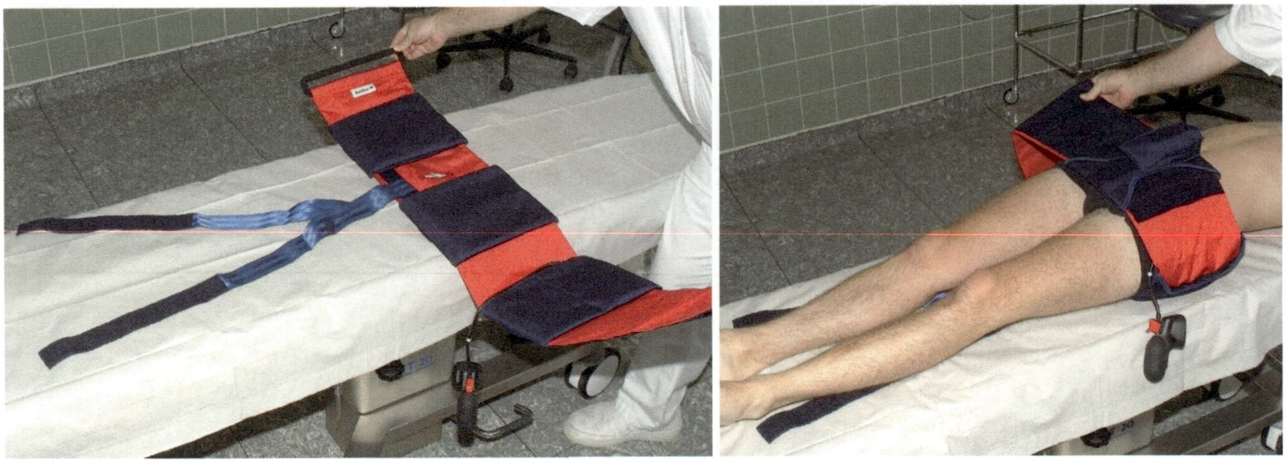

Fig. 9.1 Pelvic binder according to Baumgärtel with three inflatable chambers supporting both gluteal and the pre-symphyseal regions

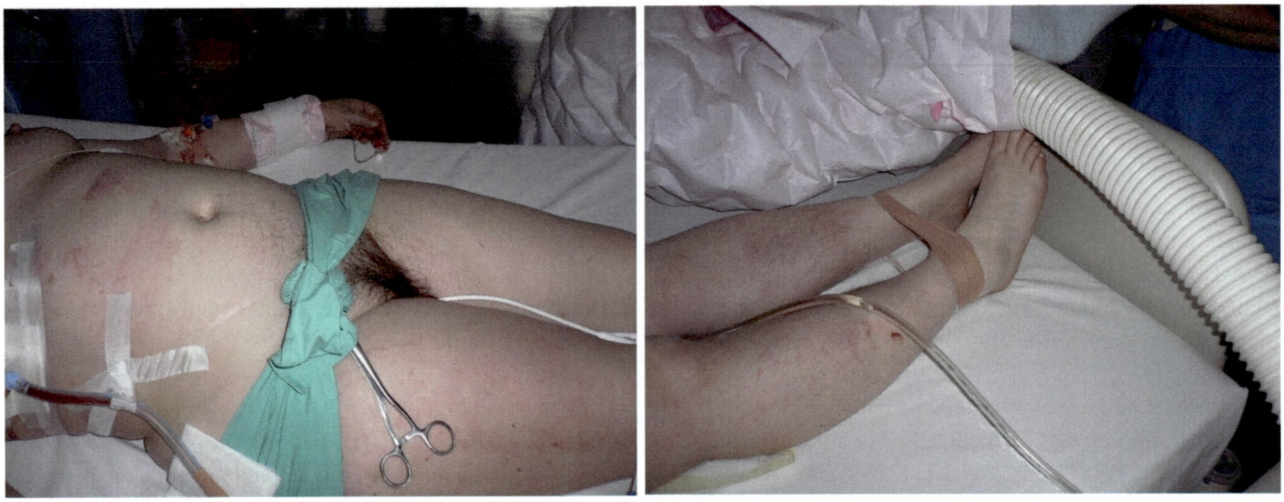

Fig. 9.2 Pelvic sheeting, additionally supported by internal rotation and taping of the lower legs by

Pizanis et al. compared three different emergency stabilization techniques: circumferential sheets, pelvic binders, and pelvic C-clamp. Application was performed in 3.4% of patients with pelvic ring injuries. Circumferential sheeting was the second most common emergency stabilization method with a rate of 16% in type B and C fractures. The mean application time was approximately 10 min after admission [17].

Prasarn et al. experimentally could show that a circumferential sheet was as effective as a classical pelvic binder regarding stability and displacements of the pelvic ring [18].

> Pelvic circumferential sheeting is a cost-effective and simple emergency stabilization method, which allows additional emergency fixation and adequate stability compared to pelvic binders.

9.2 Pelvic Binders

After introduction of Baumgärtel's pelvic belt, several new and well-accepted pelvic binders were introduced (Fig. 9.3).

Pelvic binder application provides stability and allows for clot formation to prevent ongoing hemorrhage [19].

Vermeulen et al. first introduced a pelvic strap belt to stabilize the pelvis in the prehospital setting in 1999. Their experience in 19 patients with suspected pelvic injury before admission showed encouraging results [13]. Thirteen patients had a pelvic fracture. Three polytraumatized patients died of multifactorial causes immediately after admission, and five hemodynamically unstable patients were not believed to have benefited from the prehospital application of the pelvic strap belt. Application times were short (mean: 30 s), and no belt-related complications were recorded.

Besides the potential beneficial effect on hemodynamic stabilization, presently, no pelvic binder device can be

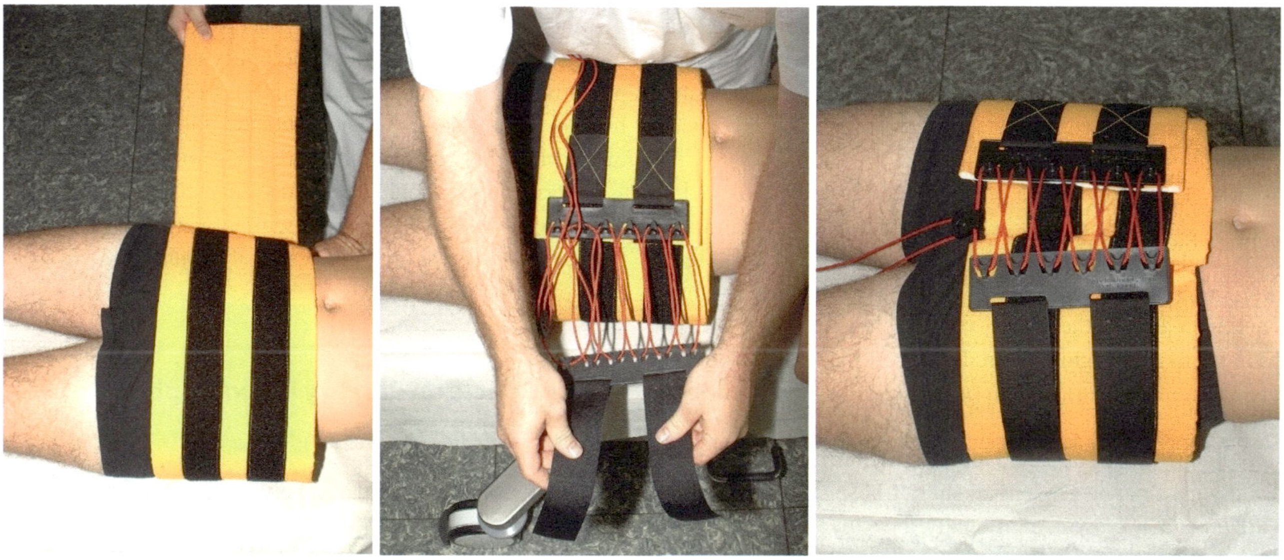

Fig. 9.3 Pelvic binder example

recommended over another, and adequate training must be provided to avoid misplacement [19].

9.2.1 Experimental Results

Bottlang et al. analyzed the efficiency of a pelvic binder to reduce B-type and C-type external rotation injuries of the pelvis in a cadaveric analysis [9, 20]. Adequate reduction of the pubic symphysis was achieved in both injury types [9]. The optimal strap application site was found to be located at the greater trochanteric area, while more superior application sites were associated with a significant increase of intra-abdominal pressure. The minimum strap tension for complete symphyseal reduction was 177–180 N.

In APC III and LC II simulated injuries, the pelvic binder showed comparable stability to the pelvic C-clamp, while an anterior external fixator showed insufficient stability in APC III injuries [20].

Jowett et al. applied a pelvic binder to ten volunteers and measured local pressures at pelvic bony prominences using pressure-sensitive sensors and reported pressures indicating a risk for pressure sore development [21]. These results were confirmed in another analysis [22]. Thus, a frequent soft tissue evaluation is mandatory in prolonged applied binders.

In a B1-type/APC II injury simulation in non-embalmed human cadavers comparing the T-POD and a classical circumferential sheet, AP radiographs revealed a reduction of the created symphyseal diastasis from 39.3 to 17.4 mm with the bed sheet and to 7.1 mm with the T-POD, indicating a more effective reduction using the T-POD [23].

In a comparable biomechanical experimental analysis of available pelvic binders (The Pelvic Binder, SAM Sling, and T-POD), all three were associated with sufficient reduction in simulated type B1 and C injuries. The T-POD was associated with the lowest pulling force for complete reduction [24].

Prasarn et al. could show that the T-POD pelvic binder was as effective as a classical bed sheet but more stable than an external fixator regarding stability and displacements of the pelvic ring [18, 25].

9.2.2 Clinical Results

Krieg et al. performed a prospective clinical study on the feasibility of a circumferential pelvic device and reported a significant reduction of the pelvic volume on X-rays and computed tomography (CT) examination with no adverse effects even in lateral compression injuries (no overcompression) [26]. Sixteen patients with pelvic ring injuries were temporarily stabilized with the pelvic binder, experimentally tested by Bottlang. Displacement of external rotation injuries could be reduced on the a.p. X-ray by 10%. In lateral compression-type injuries, no relevant overcompression was observed.

Ghaemmaghami et al. retrospectively analyzed 118 patients with pelvic fractures and emergency circumferential pelvic binder application and compared the results with a control group without binder treatment [27]. Both groups were comparable regarding fracture patterns, age, and injury severity. The binder group had more LC II and vertical shear (VS) injuries, indicating a higher rate of unstable fracture pattern. Overall, pelvic binder application was not associated with reduced mortality, transfusion requirements, and rate of angioembolization.

In a comparable clinical analysis of external pelvic fixation vs. a pelvic orthotic device (POD), the latter was associated with reduced 24- and 48-h transfusion requirement and a shorter hospital length of stay and especially with a reduced mortality rate (26% vs. 33%) [28].

Tan et al. analyzed 15 patients with unstable pelvic ring injuries and presence of hemodynamic instability, initially stabilized using the T-POD [29]. The main observed effects were a reduction of symphyseal diastasis of 60%, a significant increase of the mean arterial blood pressure (65.3–81.2 mmHg), a significant reduction of the heart frequency (107/min to 94/min), and an overall clinical effectiveness of 70%.

Patients with suspected pelvic fractures initially stabilized with a pelvic binder had shorter hospital and intensive care unit (ICU) stays. Additionally, a positive effect on transfusion requirements and survival was found [30].

In a systematic literature review in 2009, it was stated that a significant reduction of the true pelvic volume was observed after binder application, while no prognostic effect was found [31].

Toth et al. analyzed the effect of pelvic binders on injury types [32]. Especially, patients with type B1, C1, and C2 injuries ± hemodynamic instability were initially stabilized with a pelvic binder. Overall, an improved reduction was observed in 68%, while 21% showed no difference and 11% (type B2 and B3 injuries) were associated with increased deformity.

The optimal position, the greater trochanteric area, was clinically confirmed in an analysis by Bonner et al. [33]. Analyzing 167 patients, only in 50% an optimal binder position was confirmed. A higher position was observed in 39%, which was associated with a 2.8-time greater symphyseal diastasis, which can lead to a delayed bleeding control.

Recently, comparable data were reported. A CT analysis confirmed only 49.1% adequate placements, while 50.9% had unsatisfactory placement. Approximately 44.8% of patients with a pelvic ring injury had no binder applied, of whom 20% had an unstable injury [34].

Fu et al. found that application of a pelvic binder prior to patient transfer was associated with fewer blood transfusions, shorter ICU length of stay, and shorter hospital length of stay (LOS) [35].

Pizanis et al. compared three different emergency stabilization techniques: circumferential sheets, pelvic binders, and pelvic C-clamp. Application was performed in 3.4% of patients with pelvic ring injuries. Pelvic binders were less commonly used in Germany in only 15% in type B and C fractures. The majority of patients was stabilized using the pelvic C-clamp and pelvic sheeting. The mean application time was short, with approximately 10 min after admission [17]. In the UK, pelvic binders are available in approximately three quarters of the trauma units [36].

Mason reported a case of myonecrosis in a pelvic crush injury with significant soft tissue injury and pointed out the potential risk of soft tissue damage associated with pelvic binders [37]. Whether the necrotic complication is the result of the binder or due to the injury itself remains debatable.

Uncritical use should be avoided. In a clinical study, 60% of applications were performed without pelvic injury, and in 6.4%, no binder was applied, despite the later diagnosis of an unstable pelvic injury [38].

9.2.3 Effects on Primary Radiographic Evaluation

There is a potential risk that a pelvic binder can "mask" the amount of initial displacement at the time of injury [39] as adequate reduction of pelvic instability is regular observed [9, 12, 20, 23, 24, 26, 29, 31, 32].

Thus, not to overlook relevant pelvic injuries, a debate started, whether to remove the pelvic binder or not. Recently, Fletcher et al. reported two cases of anatomic reduction after pelvic binder application, who had relevant pelvic injuries [40].

In OTA 61-B1, 61-B3.1, 61-C external rotation injuries, approximately 70% of injuries were diagnosed on standard pelvic X-rays, while after binder application and CT analysis, only 50% could be confirmed [41]. In lateral compression injuries, this effect was not observed.

In a national survey from the UK, 87.5% of emergency department physicians and 78.5% of orthopedic registrars would not release the binder during radiological assessment of the pelvis in a hemodynamically stable patient [36].

Schweigkofler et al. proposed a "clear the pelvis algorithm" defining criteria to open a pelvic binder in polytraumatized patients [42]. The binder should not be opened until X-rays or CT scans are available:

- In patients without clinically suspected pelvic injuries, when no groin access for arterial lines is necessary, the binder is left in place until radiographic exclusion of pelvic injuries.
- In patients without clinically suspected pelvic injuries, when urgent groin access for arterial lines is necessary, opening of the binder should be performed, followed by radiographic diagnostics.
- In clinically suspected pelvic injuries and stable hemodynamics, when no groin access for arterial lines is necessary, the binder is left in place until radiographic exclusion of pelvic injuries.
- In clinically suspected pelvic injuries and stable hemodynamics, when urgent groin access for arterial lines is necessary, opening of the binder should be performed, followed by radiographic diagnostics.

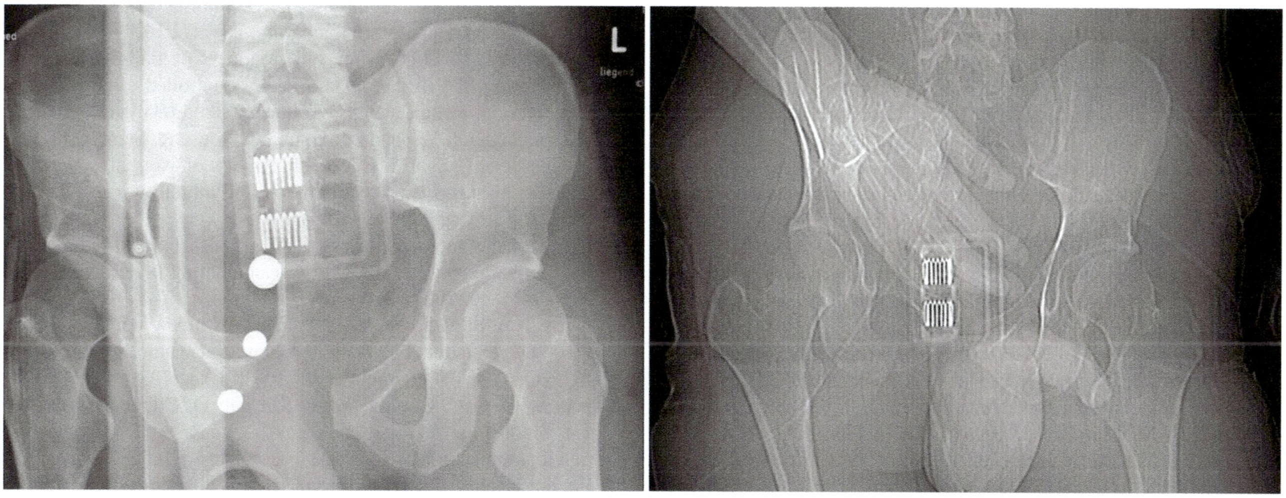

Fig. 9.4 Too superior application of the binder near the iliac crests. After correction, a more anatomic reduction was observed

- In clinically suspected pelvic injuries and unstable hemodynamics, the binder is left in place, binder position is checked, and surgical pelvic stabilization is recommended after radiographic diagnostics.

If radiographic diagnostics could exclude signs of relevant pelvic trauma, e.g., pelvic hematoma, arterial blush, type B or C injuries, and/or intra-abdominal injury, the binder can be opened followed by a detailed clinical examination. If one of the mentioned parameters were identified, opening of the binder should be performed under surgical preparedness [42].

Swartz et al. proposed fluoroscopic manual pelvic stress examination under anesthesia as an essential adjunct [41].

A recent analysis compared primary pelvic X-rays with and without pelvic binder [43]. "Binder-off" imaging resulted in diagnosis of unexpected unstable pelvic ring injuries in 7% that were not identified on CT imaging in binder [43].

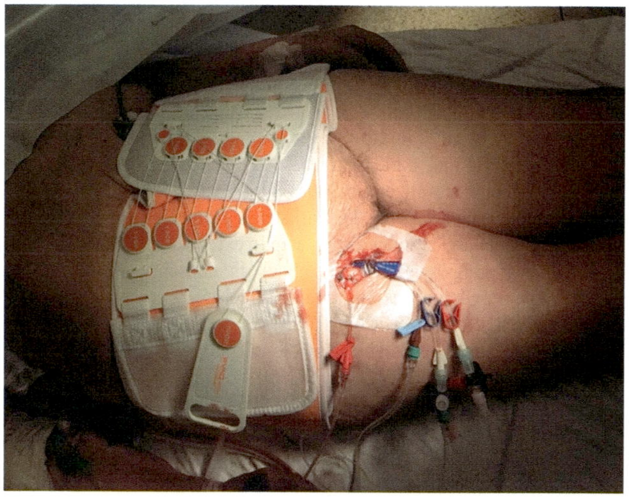

Fig. 9.5 Clinical example of a patient, stabilized with a pelvic binder

9.3 Summary

- The optimal position of pelvic binder application is the greater trochanteric area (Figs. 9.4 and 9.5) [9, 20, 33, 44].
- Pelvic binders and classical bed sheet stabilization are clinically effective for reduction of pelvic displacements [9, 12, 20, 23, 24, 26, 29, 31, 32].
- Potential disadvantages may be related to soft tissue pressure and the risk of visceral injury or sacral nerve root compression [21, 24, 37].
- There is still a high rate, approximately 50%, of inadequate pelvic binder positions [33, 34]. Thus, there is a need for continuing education for pelvic binder application.
- Pelvic binders can mask the severity of pelvic injury found in pelvic X-rays [39–41].
- There is a (theoretical) potential risk of development of hemodynamic instability after binder removal; no clear data are presently available.

References

1. Clarke G, Mardel S. Use of MAST to control massive bleeding from pelvic injuries. Injury. 1993;24(9):628–9.
2. Frank LR. Is MAST in the past? The pros and cons of MAST usage in the field. J Emerg Med Serv JEMS. 2000;25(2):38–41, 44–5
3. Christensen KS. Pneumatic antishock garments (PASG): do they precipitate lower-extremity compartment syndromes? J Trauma. 1986;26(12):1102–5.

4. Vahedi M, Ayuyao A, Parsa M. Pneumatic antishock garmentassociated compartment syndrome in injured lower extremities. J Trauma. 1995;38:616–8.
5. Williams T, Knopp R, Ellyson J. Compartment syndrome after anti-shock trouser use without lower-extremity trauma. J Trauma. 1982;22:595–7.
6. Dickinson K, Roberts I. Medical anti-shock trousers (pneumatic anti-shock garments) for circulatory support in patients with trauma (Cochrane Review). In: The Cochrane Library, Issue 2. Oxford: Update Software; 2003. p. 2003.
7. Baumgaertel F, Wilke M, Gotzen L. Experimentelle Erprobung eines pneumatischen Gürtels zur äußeren Beckenkompression. Swiss Surg. 1996;Suppl. 2:42.
8. Baumgärtel F, Wilke M, Gotzen L. Experimentelle Erprobung eines pneumatischen Gürtels zur äußeren Beckenkompression. Hefte zu "Der Unfallchirurg". 1996;Heft 257:386–7.
9. Bottlang M, Simpson T, Sigg J, Krieg JC, Madey SM, Long WB. Noninvasive reduction of open-book pelvic fractures by circumferential compression. J Orthop Trauma. 2002;16(6):367–73.
10. Duxbury M, Rossiter N, Lambert A. Cable ties for pelvic stabilisation. Ann R Coll Surg Engl. 2003;85:130.
11. Routt ML Jr, Falicov A, Woodhouse E, Schildhauer TA. Circumferential pelvic antishock sheeting: a temporary resuscitation aid. J Orthop Trauma. 2002;16(1):45–8.
12. Simpson T, Krieg JC, Heuer F, Bottlang M. Stabilization of pelvic ring disruptions with a circumferential sheet. J Trauma. 2002;52(1):158–61.
13. Vermeulen B, Peter R, Hoffmeyer P, Unger P. Prehospital stabilization of pelvic dislocations: a new strap belt to provide temporary hemodynamic stabilization. Swiss Surg. 1999;5:43–6.
14. Nunn T, Cosker T, Bose D, Pallister I. Immediate application of improvised pelvic binder as first step in extended resuscitation from life-threatening hypovolaemic shock in conscious patients with unstable pelvic injuries. Injury. 2007;38:125–8.
15. Gardner M, Parada S, Chip Routt MJ. Internal rotation and taping of the lower extremities for closed pelvic reduction. J Orthop Trauma. 2009;23:361–4.
16. Gardner M, Osgood G, Molnar R, Chip Routt MJ. Percutaneous pelvic fixation using working portals in a circumferential pelvic antishock sheet. J Orthop Trauma. 2009;23:668–74.
17. Pizanis A, Pohlemann T, Burkhardt M, Aghayev E, Holstein J. Emergency stabilization of the pelvic ring: clinical comparison between three different techniques. Injury. 2013;44:1760–4.
18. Prasarn M, Conrad B, Small J, Horodyski M, Rechtine G. Comparison of circumferential pelvic sheeting versus the T-POD on unstable pelvic injuries: a cadaveric study of stability. Injury. 2013;44:1756–9.
19. Scott I, Porter K, Laird C, Greaves I, Bloch M. The prehospital management of pelvic fractures: initial consensus statement. Emerg Med J. 2013;30:1070–2.
20. Bottlang M, Krieg J, Mohr M, Simpson T, Madey S. Emergent management of pelvic ring fractures with use of circumferential compression. J Bone Joint Surg. 2002;84-A:43–7.
21. Jowett A, Bowyer G. Pressure characteristics of pelvic binders. Injury. 2007;38:118–21.
22. Knops S, van Riel M, Goossens R, van Lieshout E, Patka P, Schipper I. Measurements of the exerted pressure by pelvic circumferential compression devices. Open Orthop J. 2010;4:101–6.
23. DeAngelis N, Wixted J, Drew J, Eskander M, Eskander J, French B. Use of the trauma pelvic orthotic device (T-POD) for provisional stabilisation of anterior-posterior compression type pelvic fractures: a cadaveric study. Injury. 2008;39:903–6.
24. Knops S, Schep N, Spoor C, van Riel M, Spanjersberg W, Kleinrensink G, van Lieshout E, Patka P, Schipper I. Comparison of three different pelvic circumferential compression devices: a biomechanical cadaver study. J Bone Joint Surg. 2011;93-A:230–40.
25. Prasarn M, Horodyski M, Conrad B, Rubery P, Dubose D, Small J, Rechtine G. Comparison of external fixation versus the trauma pelvic orthotic device on unstable pelvic injuries: a cadaveric study of stability. J Trauma Acute Care Surg. 2012;72:1671–5.
26. Krieg J, Mohr M, Ellis T, Simpson T, Madey S, Bottlang M. Emergent stabilization of pelvic ring injuries by controlled circumferential compression: a clinical trial. J Trauma. 2005;59:959–664.
27. Ghaemmaghami V, Sperry J, Gunst M, Friese R, Starr A, Frankel H, Gentilello L, Shafi S. Effects of early use of external pelvic compression on transfusion requirements and mortality in pelvic fractures. Am J Surg. 2007;194:720–3.
28. Croce M, Magnotti L, Savage S, Wood GN, Fabian T. Emergent pelvic fixation in patients with exsanguinating pelvic fractures. J Am Coll Surg. 2007;204:935–9.
29. Tan E, van Stigt S, van Vugt A. Effect of a new pelvic stabilizer (T-POD®) on reduction of pelvic volume and haemodynamic stability in unstable pelvic fractures. Injury. 2010;41:1239–43.
30. Hsu S, Chen C, Chou Y, Wang S, Chan D. Effect of early pelvic binder use in the emergency management of suspected pelvic trauma: a retrospective cohort study. Int J Environ Res Public Health. 2017;14(10):pii: E1217. https://doi.org/10.3390/ijerph14101217.
31. Spanjersberg W, Knops S, Schep N, van Lieshout E, Patka P, Schipper I. Effectiveness and complications of pelvic circumferential compression devices in patients with unstable pelvic fractures: a systematic review of literature. Injury. 2009;40:1031.
32. Toth L, King K, McGrath B, Balogh Z. Efficacy and safety of emergency non-invasive pelvic ring stabilisation. Injury. 2012;43:1330–4.
33. Bonner T, Eardley W, Newell N, Masouros S, Matthews J, Gibb I, Clasper J. Accurate placement of a pelvic binder improves reduction of unstable fractures of the pelvic ring. J Bone Joint Surg. 2011;93-B:1524–8.
34. Naseem H, Nesbitt P, Sprott D, Clayson A. An assessment of pelvic binder placement at a UK major trauma Centre. Ann R Coll Surg Engl. 2018;100:101–5.
35. Fu C, Wu Y, Liao C, Kang S, Wang S, Hsu Y, Lin B, Yuan K, Kuo I, Ouyang C. Pelvic circumferential compression devices benefit patients with pelvic fractures who need transfers. Am J Emerg Med. 2013;31:1432–6.
36. Jain S, Bleibleh S, Marciniak J, Pace A. A national survey of United Kingdom trauma units on the use of pelvic binders. Int Orthop. 2013;37:1335–9.
37. Mason L, Boyce D, Pallister I. Catastrophic myonecrosis following circumferential pelvic binding after massive crush injury: a case report. Injury Extra. 2009;40:84–6.
38. Yong E, Vasireddy A, Davies G, Lockey D. Pre-hospital pelvic girdle injury: improving diagnostic accuracy in a physician-led trauma service. Injury. 2016;47:383–8.
39. Stahel P, Mauffrey C, Smith W, McKean J, Hao J, Burlew C, Moore E. External fixation for acute pelvic ring injuries: decision making and technical options. J Trauma Acute Care Surg. 2013;75:882–7.
40. Fletcher J, Yerimah G, Datta G. The false security of pelvic binders: 2 cases of missed injuries due to anatomical reduction. J Orthop Case Rep. 2016;6:44–7.
41. Swartz J, Vaidya R, Hudson I, Oliphant B, Tonnos F. Effect of pelvic binder placement on OTA classification of pelvic ring injuries using computed tomography. Does it mask the injury? J Orthop Trauma. 2016;30:325–30.
42. Schweigkofler U, Wohlrath B, Paffrath T, Flohé S, Wincheringer D, Hoffmann R, Trentzsch H. "Clear-the-Pelvis-Algorithmus": Handlungsempfehlung zur Freigabe des Beckens nach nicht invasiver Stabilisierung mittels Beckengurt im Rahmen der Schockraumversorgung. Z Orthop Unfall. 2016;154:470–6.
43. Fagg J, Acharya M, Chesser T, Ward A. The value of 'binder-off' imaging to identify occult and unexpected pelvic ring injuries. Injury. 2018;49:284–9.
44. Prasarn M, Small J, Conrad B, Horodyski N, Horodyski M, Rechtine G. Does application position of the T-POD affect stability of pelvic fractures? J Orthop Trauma. 2013;27:262–6.

10 Emergency Management: Pelvic C-Clamp

Axel Gänsslen and Jan Lindahl

External fixation of unstable pelvic ring injuries using a clamp-type system was introduced in 1937 by Vorschütz [1]. He reported a symphyseal reduction using a special clamp ("Schraubzwinge"), which was applied at the greater trochanter area together with a pelvic cast.

Richter, in 1964, described a strap-type clamp primary used for acetabular dashboard injuries with additional open book injuries of the posterior pelvis to address these posterior ring injuries (Fig. 10.1) [2].

In 1991, Ganz introduced a rectangular pelvic C-clamp (Ganz-clamp), consisting of two long sidearms, which are connected by a crossbar and on the open and, of these sidearms, two percutaneously inserted bolts for lateral insertion opposite to the SI-joints or sacrum, respectively (Fig. 10.2) [3]. He used the term "antishock pelvic clamp" already focusing on its use in hemodynamically unstable patients.

Browner modified this clamp to a more curved clamp (ACE-clamp), which was introduced in 1994 (Fig. 10.2) [4, 5].

Since the early 1990s, these pelvic C-clamps have been in routine use for emergency fixation of the pelvic ring [5–12], especially in European centers.

In a recent online survey of the current management of unstable pelvic injuries, performed by the German Society of Trauma Surgery (DGU), 47.7% recommended pelvic C-clamp stabilization in mechanical and hemodynamic unstable pelvic fracture patients [13]. In 55.6%, a primary X-ray/CT was a prerequisite for C-clamp application.

In 2017, the World Society of Emergency Surgery (WSES) proposed a classification of pelvic trauma, considering the hemodynamic status of the patient and the mechanical stability of the pelvic ring [14]. According to the Young-Burgess classification, for Vertical Shear (VS) injuries, CM-injuries (combined mechanism), and sacroiliac joint disruptions with hemodynamic stability and all patients with any pelvic injury and hemodynamic instability, the pelvic C-clamp was recommended as an option for emergency fixation and a prerequisite for additional pelvic packing.

Contraindications for the use of the pelvic C-clamp were comminuted and transforaminal sacral fractures, iliac wing fractures, and lateral compression (LC)-type pelvic ring disruptions.

There is a clear recommendation for emergency pelvic stabilization, including use of the pelvic C-Clamp to reduce mortality rates in hemodynamically unstable patients [15].

10.1 Indications

From the European perspective, classical indications for application of the pelvic C-clamp include [16, 17]:

- Type C-injuries (acc. to the AO/OTA classification) with complete SI-joint dislocations ± associated hemodynamic instability
- Type C-injuries (acc. to the AO/OTA classification) with unstable sacral fractures ± associated hemodynamic instability
- Some type B-injuries (rotational instability) with associated hemodynamic instability
- Additionally, the C-clamp can be used as a posterior pelvic reduction aid [18–20].

Contraindications are type A pelvic fractures, type B-injuries without hemodynamic instability, longitudinal fractures at the iliac fossa, the majority of "crescent frac-

A. Gänsslen (✉)
Department of Trauma Surgery, Orthopedics and Hand Surgery, Hospital Wolfsburg, Wolfsburg, Germany

J. Lindahl
Orthopaedics and Trauma Surgery, Helsinki University Hospital, Helsinki, Finland

A. Gänsslen et al. (eds.), *Pelvic Ring Fractures*, https://doi.org/10.1007/978-3-030-54730-1_10

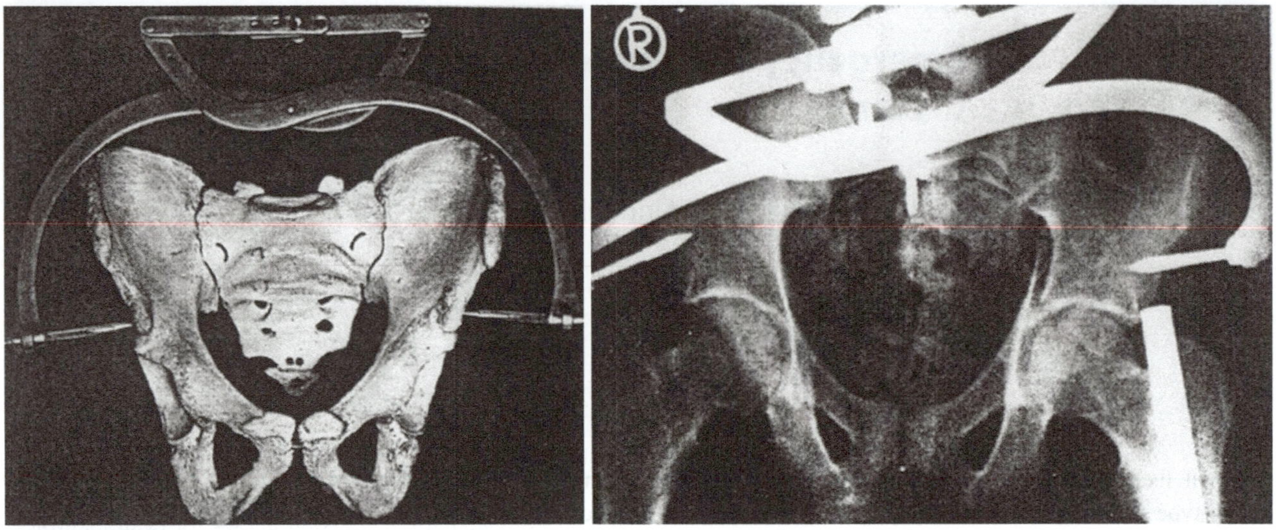

Fig. 10.1 Picture of the pelvic clamp introduced by Richter in 1964 with a clinical application example

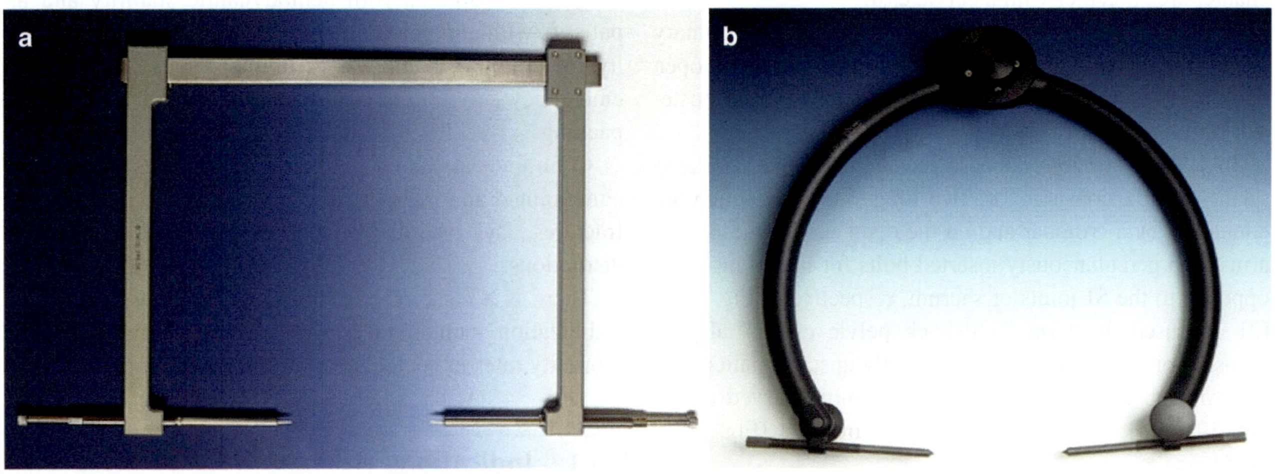

Fig. 10.2 The Ganz pelvic C-clamp (**a**) and the C-clamp introduced by Browner (**b**)

tures", with a large fragment involving the iliac fossa opposite to the SI-joint and acetabular both column fractures [16, 17].

The main advantage of the pelvic C-clamp is direct force transmission to the posterior pelvis leading to a reduction of blood loss from fracture/injury sites and allowing clot formation of the presacral and other posterior venous plexus.

Additionally, after application in the ED, there is no impediment for patient placement into the CT gantry and for further surgery, including laparotomy or femoral osteosynthesis.

Potential disadvantages are a detailed knowledge of the pelvic anatomy, especially in the injured situation, as there is a risk of iliac wing and pelvic organ perforation and a risk of fracture over-compression.

Routinely, an anterior-posterior (AP) plain pelvic X-ray is mandatory.

10.2 Technique of C-Clamp Application

The technique of pelvic C-clamp application follows a step-by-step performance:

- *Patient positioning:* application of the pelvic C-clamp is performed in supine position (Fig. 10.3), ideally on a radiolucent table allowing anterior-posterior (AP) plain pelvic radiographs and, if necessary, oblique views (inlet and outlet views); an image intensifier can be helpful to identify misplacement of the sidearms.
- *Preparation:* desinfection and, whenever possible, depending on the hemodynamic status, draping of both proximal thighs, the anterior pelvis, including the genital region and the buttocks is performed (Fig. 10.3); ideally, the affected leg is disinfected for further manipulation.

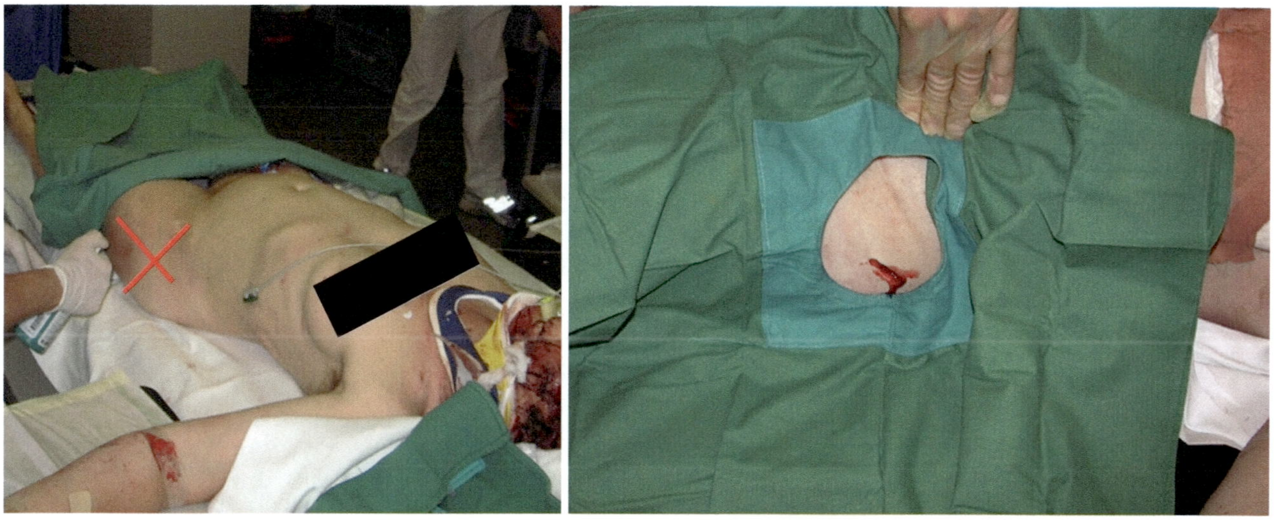

Fig. 10.3 Application of the pelvic C-clamp: supine position, identification of the entry point and step incision

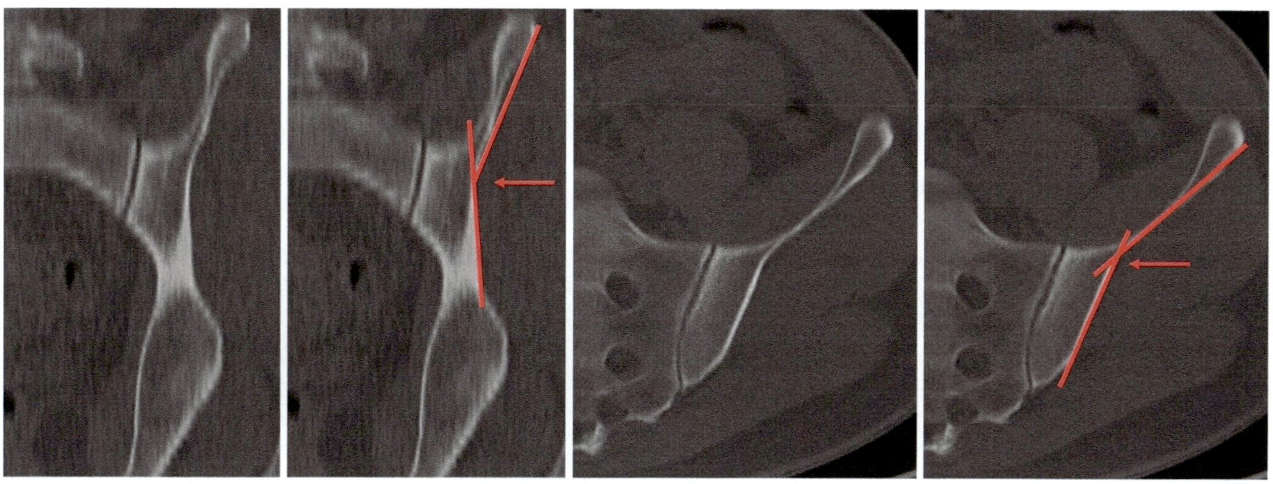

Fig. 10.4 Change of surface orientation on the outer iliac bone in two different planes creating a groove, which can be palpated using a blunt instrument

- *Reduction:* in highly displaced injuries, displacement can be optimized or even corrected by manual traction to the affected leg, together with some internal rotation of the leg and lateral compression to the pelvis; an assistant should hold the reduction until definitive fixation of the C-clamp.
- *Entry point:* due to displacement and hematoma formation, the soft-tissue contours can be altered; thus, it can be difficult to recognize anatomic pelvic landmarks; the classical entry point is located at the intersection between the line of the proximal extension of the femoral axis over the tip of the greater trochanter and a vertical line from the anterior superior iliac spine perpendicular to the table (Fig. 10.3); in markedly displaced injuries or unclear anatomic situations, use of the image intensifier can help to identify the correct entry point.
- *Incision:* a step incision is made at this crossing point and a cannulated blunt instrument is inserted (guide handle for Kirschner wire) to "feel" the outer surface of the ilium (Fig. 10.3); a change of orientation can be indirectly palpated with this instrument as, at the level of the sacroiliac joints, the ilium changes its spatial plane, forming a concavity ("groove") (Fig. 10.4), which can be identified even in displaced injuries or severe soft-tissue swelling [21]; this procedure is started on the healthy side.
- *Contralateral K-wire insertion:* the first K-wire is inserted into the lateral ilium (approximately 1–1.5 cm) through the blunt, cannulated guide handle (if necessary: image intensifier control) by hammering.
- *Contralateral C-clamp insertion:* the pelvic C-clamp is then inserted on the contralateral side with the cannulated nail of the clamp attached to the lower part of the sidearm

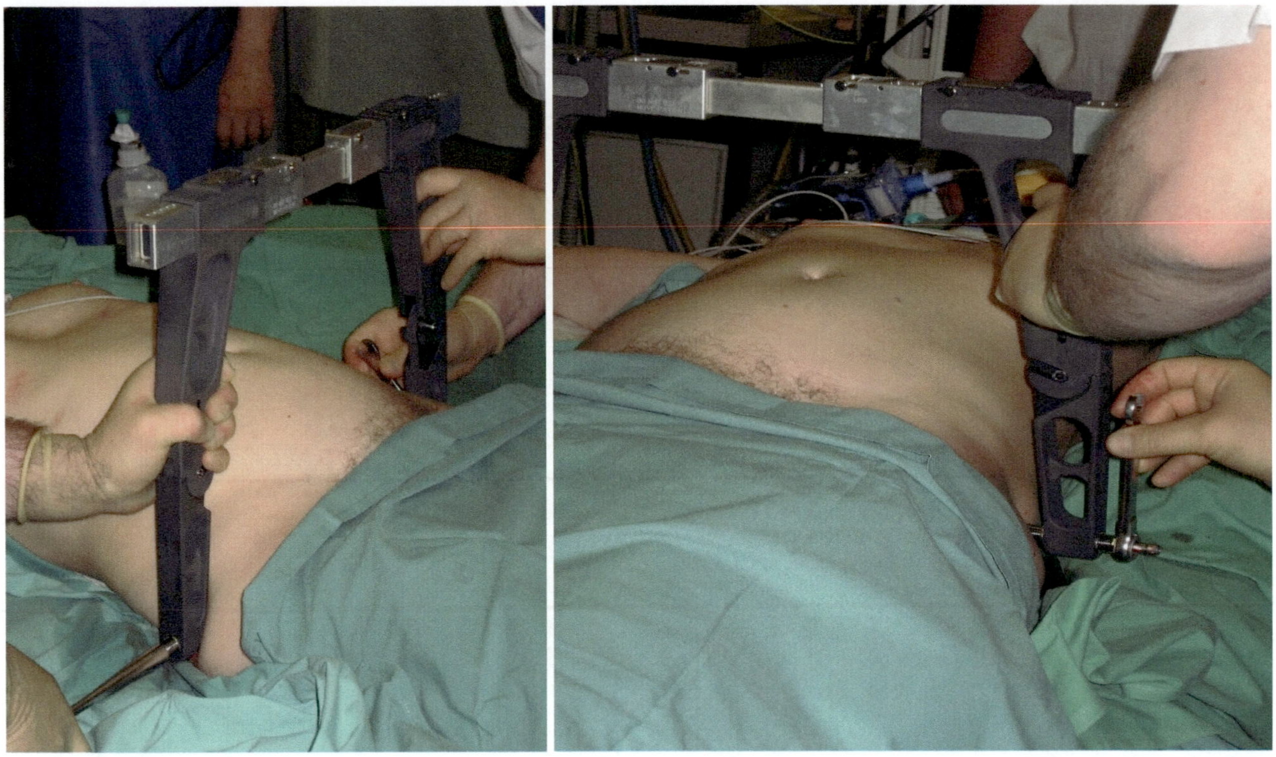

Fig. 10.5 Insertion and tightening of the sidearms

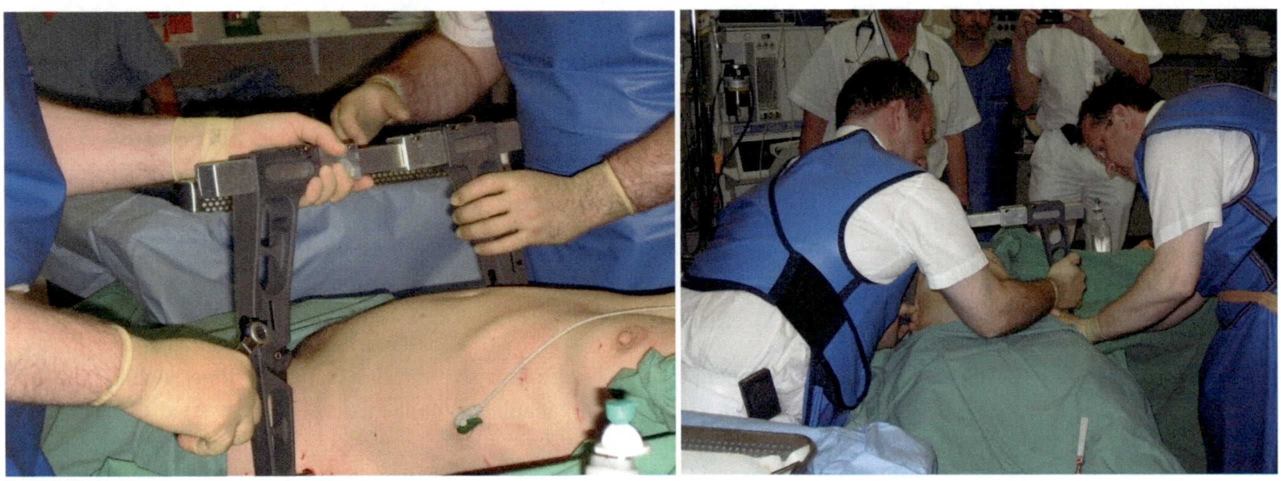

Fig. 10.6 C-clamp compression

over the K-wire (Fig. 10.5); the tip of the nail should safely penetrate into the outer iliac bone.

- *Ipsilateral C-clamp insertion:* the second nail is then inserted on the injured side via additional step incision; normally, no K-wire is necessary; at this point, the reduction should be optimized to be near anatomic; if necessary, or, in mild displacement, a K-wire can be inserted, using the above described technique.
- *C-clamp compression:* manual compression to the upper sidearms is performed, and final nail fixation is performed by tightening the threaded tubes with the ratchet wrench (Fig. 10.6).
- *C-clamp locking:* by using the locking mechanism at the upper buttons, unintended loss of compression during clamp movement is prevented.
- *K-wire management:* removal of the K-wire(s) or K-wire shortening.
- *X-ray control:* after finishing C-clamp application, the a.p. X-ray confirms correct placement of the nails and exclude over-compression of the pelvis (Figs. 10.7 and 10.8).

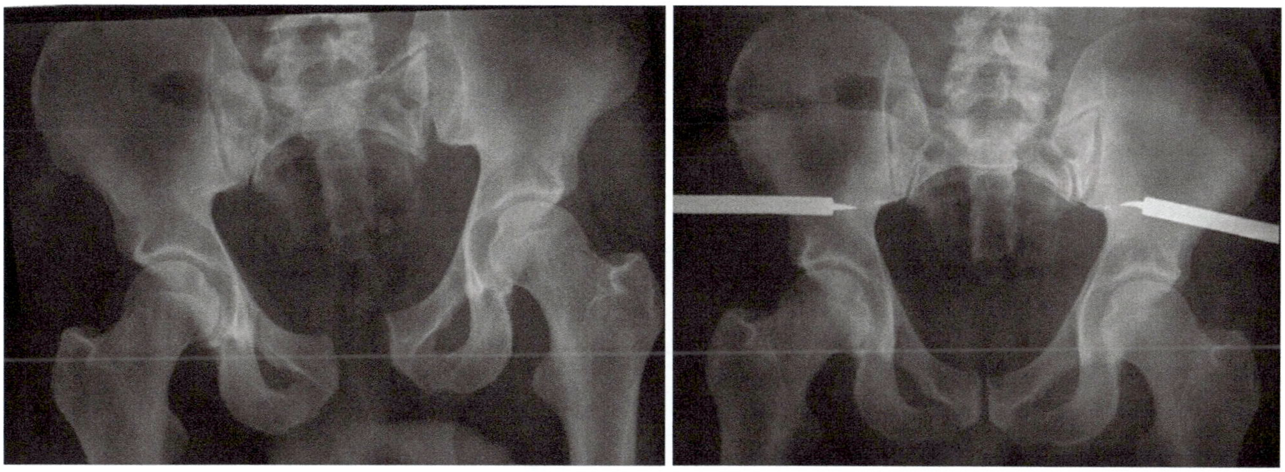

Fig. 10.7 Example of a C-clamp application in a C1.2 c5 injury (left SI-joint dislocation + pubic symphyseal disruption): anatomic reduction, despite nonoptimal side-bar placement

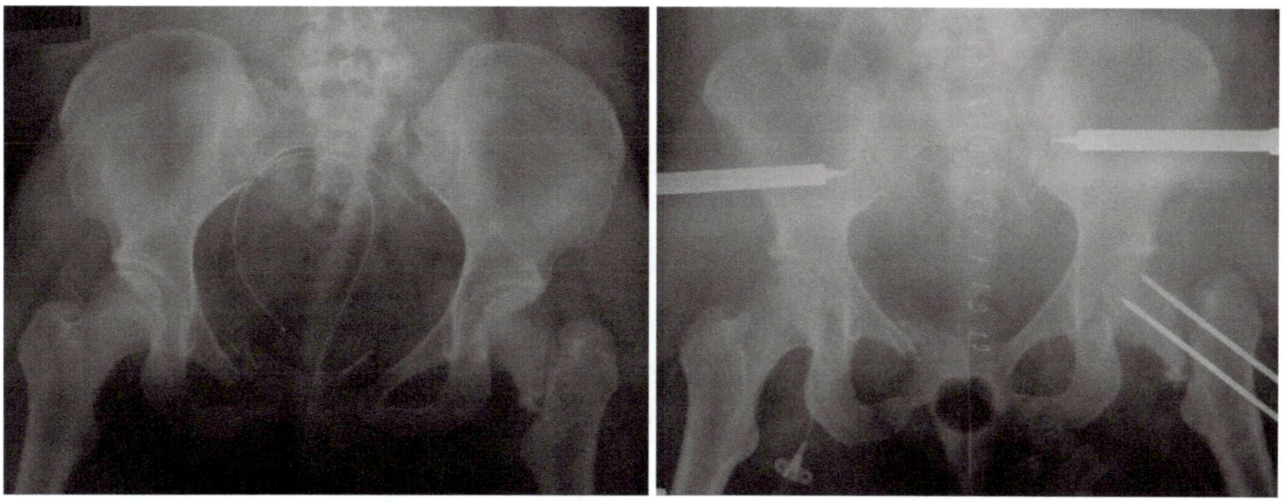

Fig. 10.8 Example of a C-clamp application in a C1.3 injury (left sacral fracture, right type B SI-joint injury + bilateral pubic rami fractures): near anatomic reduction, + damage control fixation of the femoral neck fracture with K-wires

- *Wound closure:* the entry wounds are dressed and padded or, depending on their size, sutured.

After complete and correct application of the pelvic C-clamp, the clamp can be swung caudally and cranially, to allow for a laparotomy or an angiography or femoral fixation (Fig. 10.9), respectively.

10.3 Errors, Hazards, Complications

In the emergency situation, the risk of complications is far behind the benefit of the procedure. Several complications are possible:

- Too anterior placement of the cannulated nails can lead to iliac wing perforation (Figs. 10.10 and 10.11), increasing the risk of hemorrhage and pelvic organ injury.
- Too anterior placement of the cannulated nails can lead to injury of the gluteal neurovascular bundle [17, 22].
- Pelvic over-compression (Fig. 10.12) leads to a risk of iatrogenic sacral nerve root compression.
- Secondary clamp loosening is possible due to frequent patient positioning maneuvers.
- Anterior hemipelvic dislocation due to inadequate nail positioning (Fig. 10.13) [23].

These risks, however, lose relevance in consideration of the critical general condition of the patient [24].

10.4 Pelvic C-Clamp Removal

The pelvic C-clamp is removed when the patient's condition allows definitive treatment of the posterior pelvic ring injury.

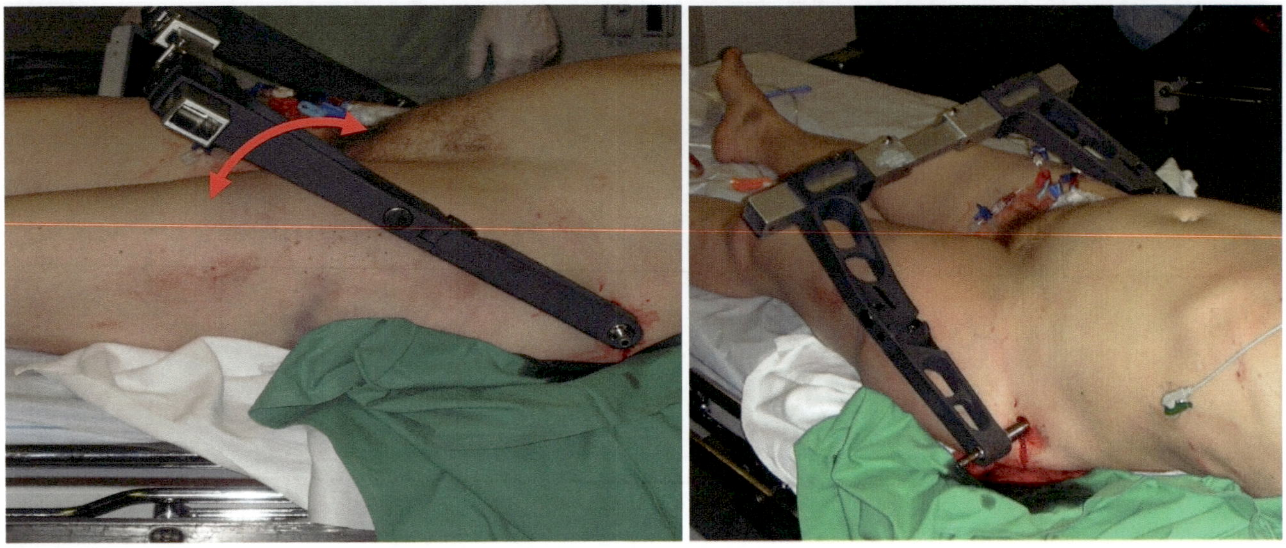

Fig. 10.9 Position of the C-clamp allows for laparotomy and femoral shaft fixation

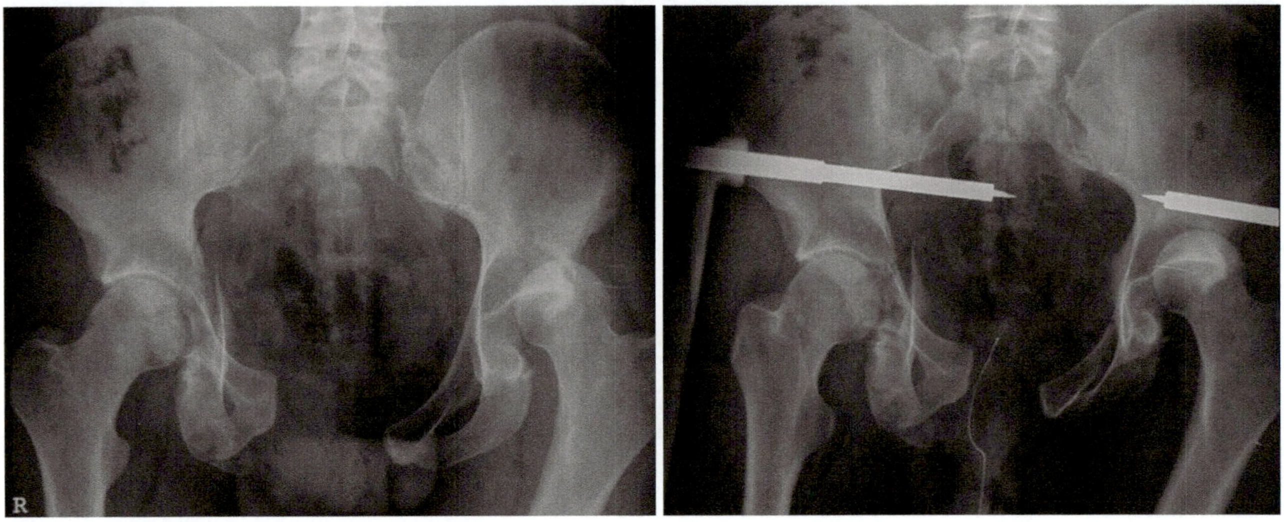

Fig. 10.10 Nail penetration into the true pelvis in a case with too anterior sidearm placement (type C-injury with bilateral transforaminal sacral fracture, symphyseal disruption + bilateral acetabular fractures)

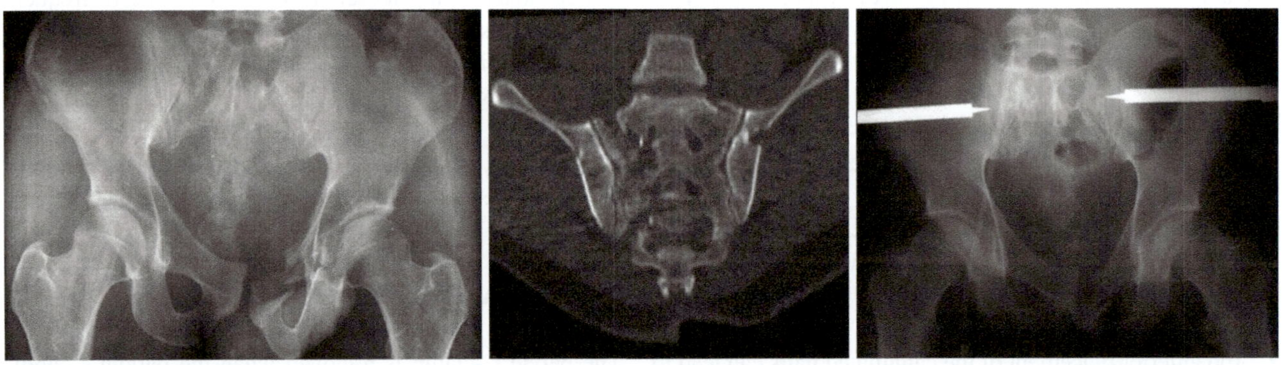

Fig. 10.11 Perforation of the left outer iliac cortex

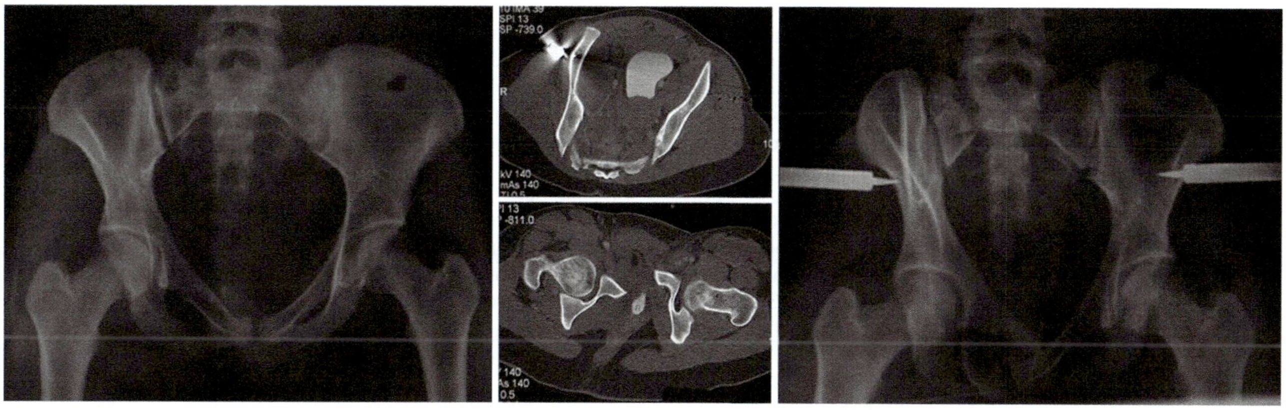

Fig. 10.12 Right hemipelvic over-compression due to too anterior sidearm application with symphyseal overlapping and reduction of the true pelvic volume

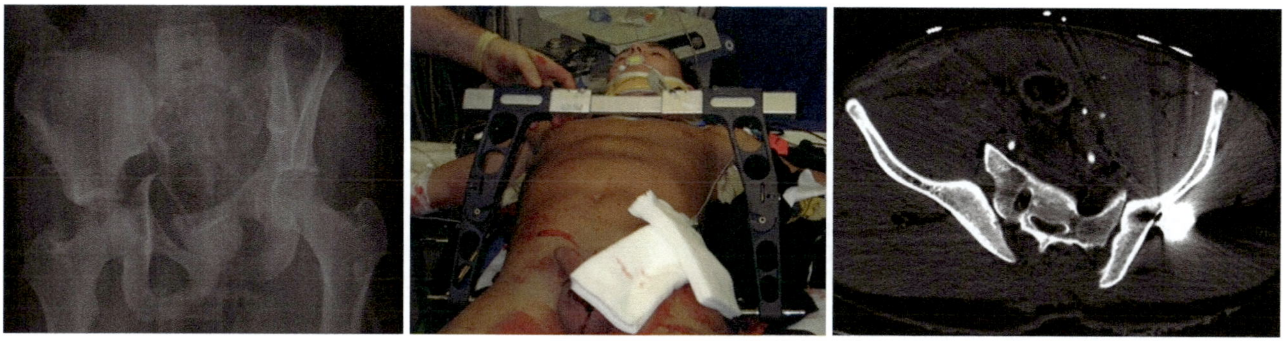

Fig. 10.13 Right posterior hemipelvic dislocation in a highly unstable type C3-injury with bilateral SI-joint dislocations

Depending on the general status, in a few cases, definitive treatment can be performed using the clamp (multiple trauma, acute respiratory distress syndrome, multiple organ failure). Then, the clamp should be removed after 3–4 weeks. Pediculous pin/nail treatment of the entry wounds with antiseptic and sterile dressings is mandatory.

10.5 Results of Treatment

Pelvic C-clamp application is a rare condition, as 1–4% of all patients with pelvic fractures are supposed to be highly unstable patients "in extremis" [25].

In a study of 88 blunt trauma patients with major pelvic fractures (AIS pelvis ≥3), hemodynamic instability, defined as an admission systolic blood pressure ≤ 90 mmHg or 6PRBCs/24 h, and pelvic fixation within 24 h, a pelvic C-clamp was used for emergency stabilization of the pelvis in 3.4% [26].

First results were published from Switzerland and Germany, using the Ganz-clamp [3, 7, 9–12, 17, 27–29].

- Ganz et al., reported on one detailed case and on the acute management in further four patients with type C pelvic injuries. The posterior displacement was adequately reduced [3]. Overall, mortality was 40% (2/5). Two patients (40%) had immediate hemodynamic stabilization. In an on-going analysis by the Bernese group, Witschger et al. analyzed 17 patients with two type B- and 15 type C-injuries [12].
- Heini et al. reported on overall 30 patients [9]. In this series, 25 patients were classified as type C-injuries, three as type B-injuries, and in further two the posterior pelvic injury could not be classified. The mean ISS was 29 points. Indication for c-clamp application was an unstable fracture in 12 cases and a combined mechanical and hemodynamic instability in 18 patients (60%). Hemodynamic instability was defined as a shock index >1. Of the 12 patients with mechanical posterior instability (= prophylactic stabilization), only two patients died (16.7%), whereas of the 18 patients with additional hemodynamic instability, mortality rate was 44.4%. If there was a hemodynamic effect after C-clamp application, mortality was only 20% versus 75% for patients without hemodynamic effect.

  Overall, this specific patient collective had a transfusion requirement within the first 24 h of 24 units of blood in average.

  Application of the C-clamp was performed after a mean of 110 min after admission and a prehospital time of 130 min.

  Heini et al. already stated that this specific group of patients was not comparable to former reports on hemodynamic unstable pelvic fracture patients.

- Schütz et al. reported on nine patients with type C pelvic injuries [11]. Two different C-clamps were used. The indication for C-clamp application was pelvic mechanical instability in four patients and additional hemodynamic instability in five. Two patients had secondary clamp loss of reduction due to inadequate pin alignment. Overall, three patients died (33.3%) due to non-pelvic causes.
- Pohlemann et al. analyzed 19 patients with type C-injuries and an applied pelvic C-clamp and a mean Hannover Polytrauma Score of 47.4 points [10]. The mean prehospital time in primary admitted patients was 72.3 min; the pelvic C-clamp was applied after an average of 14 min after admission in this group.

  Transfusion requirements within the first 3 h after admission were 12.3 PRBC for survivors and 18.5 PRBC in non-survivors. The 24 h transfusion rate was 23.3 PRBC versus 33.6 PRBC, respectively. The overall mortality rate was 57.8%.

  In 13 cases, hemodynamic stabilization could be achieved after C-clamp application (46% survivors), whereas, in six cases, persistent hemodynamic instability was observed (66.6% mortality rate). Four patients had C-clamp related complications: 1 gluteal bleeding from a Morel-Levallé lesion, 1 bleeding from pin placement near the gluteal artery, 1 pin tract infection, and one secondary loss of reduction.

  It was recommended that the indication for the C-clamp was the combined bony and suspected hemodynamic instability of the pelvis and, therefore, optimal for patients "in extremis".
- Ertel et al. from Zürich confirmed this approach. Only patients "in extremis" or patients with severe hemodynamic instability were treated with a pelvic C-clamp [30].
- In a further detailed analysis of 20 consecutive patients with four type B and 16 type C-injuries, the pelvic C-clamp was used together with pelvic packing to control pelvic hemorrhage [7]. The mean ISS of the type C patient group was 38.5 points. The C-clamp was applied in all patients within 57.4 min after admission. The overall mortality rate was 25%.
- Gänsslen et al. analyzed the use of the pelvic C-clamp in 39 patients with type C-injuries and unstable hemodynamics [17]. The patients' average age was 36 years. The mean Hannover Polytrauma Score (PTS) was 39.9 points. The mean admission hemoglobin concentration was 6.7 g/dL, the mean base deficit was −8.7 mmol/L, and the average systolic blood pressure was 82 mmHg. The C-clamp was applied after an average of 4 h after admission.

  Pelvic instability was the primary indication for the C-clamp in 13 patients and, in 26 cases, the combination of mechanical and hemodynamic instability was the main indication. In 15 of these 26 patients, early circulatory stabilization was observed (57.7%), five showed no change and, in six patients, hemodynamics deteriorated.

  Complications occurred in seven patients (17.9%): three over-compressions of sacral fractures without iatrogenic nerve injury, one pin malposition, one ilium perforation, and two with pin tract hemorrhage due to coagulopathy.
- Thiemann et al., reported on 28 polytraumatized patients with a mean age of 38 years with 27 type C- and one type B- injury of the pelvis [29, 31, 32]. The C-clamp was applied after a mean of 64.7 min after trauma and 17 min after admission. Primary hemoglobin concentration was 10.1 g/dL and a mean ISS of 47.1 points was recorded. Nine PRBC had to be transfused within the first hour after admission. The 6-h rate was 15.2 PRBC and the 24-h rate was 19.2 PRBC. Mortality rate was 25%.
- Sadri et al. reported on 14 patients with hemorrhagic shock (definition: systolic blood pressure < 90 mmHg after receiving 2 L crystalloids), where emergency stabilization of the pelvis was performed using the pelvic C-clamp within 2 h after admission and secondary angiography and embolization was performed to control hemorrhage [28]. The mean ISS was 30.1 points. A positive effect after clamp application was recorded. No clamp-related complications occurred. Overall mortality was 14%.
- Lustenberger et al. reported on 50 patients, with 8 type B- and 42 type C-injuries and hemorrhagic shock [27]; emergency stabilization consisted of fixation using the C-clamp and additional laparotomy and extra- and/or intraperitoneal pelvic packing in on-going hemodynamic instability; mean patient's age was 44.7 years, the mean ISS was 41.7 points; 58% of these patients had a systolic blood pressure at admission <90 mmHg; within the first hour, 4.3 PRBC had to be transfused, transfusion requirements within the first 4 h were 12.7 PRBC in average; application of the C-clamp was performed within 39.5 ± 2.2 min of admission and the overall mortality rate was 40%; no C-clamp-related complications were reported.

In the mean-time, modifications of the existing clamp were introduced and a more trochanteric and a supraacetabular application point of the clamp nails was proposed [33–35].

Archdeacon et al. presented a case with percutaneous application of the ACE-clamp at the trochanteric level followed by a cadaveric analysis. The latter could reliably reduce anterior-posterior compression injuries type B and C at the level of the pubic symphysis and at the SI-joints, respectively [33, 34].

Frosch et al. proposed a more supraacetabular insertion point. Results using this approach were reported in 15 patients [35]. Their mean age was 46 years with a mean ISS of 40 points. The mean admission hemoglobin concentration was 7.4 g/dL and the average systolic blood pressure was 69 mmHg. The C-clamp was applied after an average of 54 min after admission. In average, 36.7 PRBC were transfused within 6 h after admission. In 60%, a positive hemodynamic effect was observed within 6 h. Thirty-three point three percent of these patients died. Fourteen of fifteen patients had adequate reduction of their pelvic injury.

Literature analysis showed that there is a learning curve for correct pelvic C-clamp application to avoid C-clamp related complications [17].

Koller et al. found that application training can lead to a positive effect with less rates of mal-positioning of the clamp, as in clinical practice, the clamp is infrequently used due to the less common patient collectives and thus a rare indication. More than 80% of the pins were placed at the correct level within 2.5 min [36, 37].

Conclusion

The Pelvic C-clamp is still an option to provide adequate posterior pelvic ring stability and pelvic bleeding control in the emergency department and thus the basis for further procedures dealing with hemorrhage control, for example, pelvic packing.

Experience and frequent training is necessary to reduce the rates of complications.

References

1. Vorschütz. Schraubenzwingenbehandlung bei Symphysenspaltung. Zentbl Chir. 1937;48:2755–66.
2. Richter H. Die transacetabuläre Beckensprengung und ihre Behandlung mittels percutaner Schraubenzugkompression. Monatsschr Unfallheilkd. 1964;3:109–15.
3. Ganz R, Krushell R, Jakob R, Küffer J. The antishock pelvic clamp. Clin Orthop. 1991;267:71–8.
4. Browner B. The use of the pelvic stabilizer in the emergency management of pelvic ring disruption for the controll of associated hemorrhage. Surgery of the Pelvis and Acetabulum: The second International Consensus. Pittsburgh, October 21–27, 1994, 1994.
5. Buckle R, Browner B, Morandi M. Emergency reduction for pelvic ring disruptions and control of associated hemorrhage using the pelvic stabilizer. Tech Orthop. 1995;9:258–66.
6. Biffl WL, Smith WR, Moore EE, Gonzalez RJ, Morgan SJ, Hennessey T, Offner PJ, Ray CE Jr, Franciose RJ, Burch JM. Evolution of a multidisciplinary clinical pathway for the management of unstable patients with pelvic fractures. Ann Surg. 2001;233(6):843–50.
7. Ertel W, Keel M, Eid K, Platz A, Trentz O. Control of severe hemorrhage using C-clamp and pelvic packing in multiply injured patients with pelvic ring disruption. J Orthop Trauma. 2001;15(7):468–74.
8. Gänsslen A, Giannoudis P, Pape H. Hemorrhage in pelvic fracture: who needs angiography? Curr Opin Crit Care. 2003;9:515–23.
9. Heini P, Witt J, Ganz R. The pelvic C-clamp for the emergency treatment of unstable pelvic ring injuries. A report on clinical experience of 30 cases. Injury. 1996;Suppl. 1(Part 1):38–45.
10. Pohlemann T, Culemann U, Gänsslen A, Tscherne H. Die schwere Beckenverletzung mit pelviner Massenblutung: Ermittlung der Blutungsschwere und klinische Erfahrung mit der Notfallstabilisierung. Unfallchirurg. 1996;99(10):734–43.
11. Schütz M, Stöckle U, Hoffmann R, Südkamp N, Haas N. Clinical experience with two types of pelvic C-clamps for unstable pelvic ring injuries. Injury. 1996;Suppl. 1(Part 1):46–50.
12. Witschger P, Heini P, Ganz R. Beckenzwinge zur Schockbekämpfung bei hinteren Beckenringverletzungen. Orthopade. 1992;21:393–9.
13. Wohlrath B, Trentzsch H, Hoffmann R, Kremer M, Schmidt-Horlohè K, Schweigkofler U. Präklinische und klinische Versorgung der instabilen Beckenverletzung. Ergebnisse einer Online-Umfrage Unfallchirurg. 2016;119:755–62.
14. Coccolini F, Stahel P, Montori G, Biffl W, Horer T, Catena F, Kluger Y, Moore E, Peitzman A, Ivatury R, Coimbra R, Fraga G, Pereira B, Rizoli S, Kirkpatrick A, Leppaniemi A, Manfredi R, Magnone S, Chiara O, Solaini L, Ceresoli M, Allievi N, Arvieux C, Velmahos G, Balogh Z, Naidoo N, Weber D, Abu-Zidan F, Sartelli M, Ansaloni L. Pelvic trauma: WSES classification and guidelines. World J Emerg Surg. 2017;12:5. https://doi.org/10.1186/s13017-017-0117-6.
15. Pizanis A, Pohlemann T, Burkhardt M, Aghayev E, Holstein J. Emergency stabilization of the pelvic ring: clinical comparison between three different techniques. Injury. 2013;44:1760–4.
16. Gänsslen A, Krettek C, Pohlemann T. Emergency stabilization of pelvic instabilities with the pelvic C-clamp. Eur J Trauma. 2004;30:412–9.
17. Gänsslen A, Krettek C, Pohlemann T. Emergency stabilization of pelvic instabilities with the pelvic C-clamp. Oper Orthop Traumatol. 2004;16:192–204.
18. Quintero A, Tarkin I, Pape H. The prone reduction of a sacroiliac disruption with a pelvic C-clamp. Clin Orthop. 2008;467:1103. https://doi.org/10.1007/s11999-008-0508-9.
19. Wiznia D, Swami N, Kim C, Leslie M. A method of using a pelvic C-clamp for intraoperative reduction of a zone 3 sacral fracture. Case Rep Orthop. 2016;2016:1. https://doi.org/10.1155/2016/8586517.
20. Wright R, Glueck D, Selby J, Rosenblum W. Intraoperative use of the pelvic c-clamp as an aid in reduction for posterior sacroiliac fixation. J Orthop Trauma. 2006;20:576–9.
21. Pohlemann T, Braune C, Gänsslen A, Hüfner T, Partenheimer A. Pelvic emergency clamps: anatomic landmarks for a safe primary application. J Orthop Trauma. 2004;18:102–5.
22. Kim W, Lee S, Kim K, Lee J. Superior gluteal artery pseudoaneurysm caused by pelvic C-clamp blind application: a case report. Hip Pelvis. 2017;29:145–9.
23. Bartlett C, Asprinio D, Louis S, Helfet D. Intrapelvic dislocation of the left hemipelvis as a complication of the pelvic "C" clamp: a case report and review. J Orthop Trauma. 1997;11(7):540–2.
24. Gänsslen A, Krettek C, Pape H, Machtens S. Acute management of pelvic fractures: a european perspective. In: Smith WR, Ziran BH, Morgan SJ, editors. Fractures of the pelvis and acetabulum. New York: Informa Healthcare USA, Inc.; 2007, ISBN-13: 978–0–8247-2846-5.
25. Gänsslen A, Hildebrand F, Pohlemann T. Management of hemodynamic unstable patients "in extremis" with pelvic ring fractures. Acta Chir Orthop Traumatol Cechoslov. 2012;79:193–202.
26. Verbeek D, Sugrue M, Balogh Z, Cass D, Civil I, Harris I, Kossmann T, Leibman S, Malka V, Pohl A, Rao S, Richardson M, Schuetz M, Ursic C, Wills V. Acute management of hemodynamically unstable pelvic trauma patients: time for a change? Multicenter review of recent practice. World J Surg. 2008;32:1874–82.
27. Lustenberger T, Meier C, Benninger E, Lenzlinger P, Keel M. C-clamp and pelvic packing for control of hemorrhage in patients with pelvic ring disruption. J Emerg Trauma Shock. 2011;4:477–82.
28. Sadri H, Nguyen-Tang T, Stern R, Hoffmeyer P, PÜeter R. Control of severe hemorrhage using C-clamp and arterial embolization in hemodynamically unstable patients with pelvic ring disruption. Arch Orthop Trauma Surg. 2005;125:443–7.
29. Thiemann A, Böhme J, Josten C. Emergency treatment of multiply injured patients with unstable disruption of the posterior pelvic ring by using the "C-clamp". Eur J Trauma. 2005;31:244–51.
30. Ertel W, Eid K, Keel M, Trentz O. Therapeutical strategies and outcome of polytraumatized patients with pelvic injuries—a six-year experience. Eur J Trauma. 2000;6:278–86.
31. Thiemann A, Böhme J, Josten C. Anwendung der Beckenzwinge beim polytraumatisierten Patienten mit instabilem Becken. Orthopade. 2006;35:1225–36.

32. Thiemann A, Schmidt C, Gonschorek O, Josten C. Notfallbehandlung instabiler Beckenfrakturen - Stellenweret der "Beckenzwinge". Zentralbl Chir. 2004;129:245–51.
33. Archdeacon M, Hiratzka J. The trochanteric C-clamp for provisional pelvic stability. J Orthop Trauma. 2006;20:47–51.
34. Archdeacon M, Safian C, Le T. A cadaver study of the trochanteric pelvic clamp for pelvic reduction. J Orthop Trauma. 2007;21:38–42.
35. Frosch K, Hingelbaum S, Dresing K, Roessler M, Stürmer K. Die supraazetabuläre Beckenzwinge. Unfallchirurg. 2007;110:521–7.
36. Koller H, Balogh Z. Single training session for first time pelvic C-clamp users: correct pin placement and frame assembly. Injury. 2012;43:436–9.
37. Koller H, Keil P, Seibert F. Individual and team training with first time users of the pelvic C-clamp: do they remember or will we need refresher trainings? Arch Orthop Trauma Surg. 2013;133:343–9.

11 Mechanical Stabilization: DC-Osteosynthesis

Axel Gänsslen, Bore Bakota, Mario Staresinic, and Gloria Hohenberger

Standard management concepts in hemodynamically unstable patients with pelvic ring injuries include mechanical stabilization of the pelvic ring first, followed by measures for pelvic hemorrhage control [1, 2].

Established options for mechanical stabilization include pelvic binders and external fixation techniques, for example, simple anterior external fixation frames and the pelvic C-clamp [2] (see Chaps. 9 and 10).

Binders and external fixators have their individual advantages and disadvantages regarding further treatment (Table 11.1). Further, direct pelvic bleeding control, trauma laparotomy and femoral shaft fracture fixation has to be considered.

The pelvic binder and the pelvic C-clamp allow for sufficient posterior pelvic stability. While the pelvic binder is frequently available today, only few hospitals use the pelvic C-clamp. With the binder, depending on its type, the approach to the pelvic area for direct pelvic bleeding control or to the lower abdomen can be restricted to allow adequate surgical treatment of concomitant abdominal-pelvic injuries.

Thus, internal stabilization of the posterior pelvic ring using a simple screw is a further option to get sufficient posterior ring stability, to act as a prerequisite for pelvic packing, which is often necessary in patients in extremis [2].

Table 11.1 Advantages and disadvantages of common emergency mechanical stabilization devices

Device	Advantages	Disadvantages
Pelvic binder	Adequate mechanical stability Simple procedure Application time: <2 min Frequently available	Restricted approach to the true/false pelvis
Anterior external fixator	Simple, applicable Image intensifier not necessary Application time: 15–20 min	Reduced mechanical stability
Pelvic C-clamp	Adequate posterior stability Application time: 15–20 min Adequate approach to abdomen, pelvis and thigh	Learning curve Demanding technique

Gardner et al. introduced the concept of the emergency stabilization using **The Antishock Iliosacral Screw** for posterior pelvic instability in 2010 [3].

It was noted, that this type of screw can be difficult to apply effectively and safely in the acute situation and, therefore, is indicated especially in patients under intensive resuscitation with primary or on-going hemodynamic instability and an unstable pelvic fracture pattern, especially a volume-expanding pelvic ring injury after failure or standard mechanical stabilization methods, for example, pelvic binder application.

The treatment sequence in the presented case can be summarized as:

- Prehospital volume management
- Pelvic binder application in the ER
- CT scan indicating pelvic displacement
- Pelvic angiography, followed by embolization
- Anterior pelvic external fixation (femoral distractor), Synthes, Paoli, PA,
- Percutaneous antishock screw insertion

A. Gänsslen (✉)
Department of Trauma Surgery, Orthopedics and Hand Surgery, Hospital Wolfsburg, Wolfsburg, Germany

B. Bakota
Department of Orthopaedics and Trauma, Medical University of Graz, Graz, Austria

M. Staresinic
General and Sports Trauma Department, University Hospital Merkur Zagreb, Zagreb, Croatia

G. Hohenberger
Department of Orthopaedics and Trauma, Medical University of Graz, Graz, Austria
e-mail: gloria.hohenberger@medunigraz.at

A. Gänsslen et al. (eds.), *Pelvic Ring Fractures*, https://doi.org/10.1007/978-3-030-54730-1_11

11.1 Surgical Technique [3]

The described steps of the proposed surgical technique are summarized:

- Adequate procedure planning using pelvic AP, Inlet and Outlet views and an axial pelvic CT scan
- Planning for screw length and orientation
- Supine position
- Anterior external fixator application (two pins at each iliac crest)
- Limited reduction maneuvers (acceptance of minor malreductions)
- Standard steps of classical iliosacral screw fixation (including serial fluoroscopic views), depending on involvement of the SI-joint or presence of a sacral fracture using two screws.

Application of the Antishock Iliosacral Screw (ASISS) in the presented case report was delayed due to several imaging modalities and on-going hemodynamic stabilization. No data on time requirements of the different procedures were stated.

Taking in consideration, that the typical ER phase in a moderately unstable patient needs 30–40 min, and angio-embolization further requires minimum 60 min [4] (longer times are more likely: up to 3–4 h [5, 6]), transport to the OR needs 15 min and application of the external fixator requires a time of 15–20 min, application of the first iliosacral screw was performed after a minimum of 2–4 h after admission.

Therefore the term "Antishock" is misleading. With a time window of 3–4 h, the standard surgical technique for iliosacral screw application can be performed without harming the patient.

In contrast, European guidelines propose mechanical stabilization of patients in extremis within the first hour of arrival ("golden pelvic hour").

Here, even a damage control percutaneous stabilization method is possible in special situations. In patients, with unresponsive hemodynamics despite adequate volume and coagulation replacement, surgical bleeding control is recommended [1, 2, 7, 8].

In these patients, pelvic packing is favored, which needs some mechanical stability, especially at the posterior pelvis, as a prerequisite for pelvic packing [2].

In these special situations, percutaneous application of an iliosacral screw or a thick Kirschner wire (2.0–3.0 mm) can be an option. Both can be applied without image intensification.

The risk of mal-positioning of such a screw or a K-wire, with a potential risk of sacral nerve root injury, due to inadequate positioning or mal-reduction has to be weighed against the potential life-saving benefit of posterior pelvic ring stabilization [3].

11.2 Surgical Technique Damage-Control-Screw/Wire (DCSW)

The patient is lying in the supine position on the ER table. Usually, the spine board was already removed.

Parallel to anesthesiologic treatment of shock and coagulopathy, the standard concept of evaluating these patients includes, beside clinical examination according to C-ABC-principles [7], diagnostic imaging of the chest, the pelvis and performing the eFAST. Depending on its availability, in some hospitals, a direct CT-evaluation is performed.

After identification of a mechanical unstable pelvic injury pattern (Tile type C injury, APC II/III, VS injuries) with ongoing hemodynamic instability despite initiation of adequate volume replacement, blood product transfusion and optimization of potential trauma-induced coagulopathy, an indication to apply a DCSW is considered.

As hemipelvic deformity avoids adequate palpation of the correct pelvic anatomy, first, closed reduction maneuvers, depending on the analysis of the pelvic a.p. X-ray are performed, which can include [9]:

- Leg traction
- Manual lateral hemipelvic compression
- Internal rotation of the ipsilateral lower extremity

The entry-point for the screw or wire is well-defined and is corresponding to the classical entry-point of the pelvic C-clamp [9–11] or iliosacral screw [12–16].

Due to displacement and hematoma formation, the soft-tissue contours can be altered. Thus, it can be difficult to recognize anatomic pelvic landmarks.

The classical entry-point is located at the intersection between the line of the proximal extension of the femoral axis over the tip of the greater trochanter and a vertical line from the anterior superior iliac spine perpendicular to the Table.

A step incision is made at this crossing point and the K-wire or the drill-bit of the cannulated 7.3 mm screw is inserted until reaching the outer iliac bony surface. Blunt palpation using these instruments to detect the change of orientation is performed, as at the level of the SI-joint, the ilium changes its spatial plane, forming a concavity ("groove"), which can be identified even in displaced injuries or severe soft-tissue swelling [11].

Only a hammer is necessary to intrude the K-wire or the drill-bit through both cortex of the ilium into the sacrum.

As the size of the K-wire does not exceed 3.0 mm and the drill-bit has a diameter of 2.8 mm, the risk of damaging relevant structures is reduced (Fig. 11.1).

The risk of damaging relevant anatomical structures has to be balanced against the potential benefit of posterior pelvic stability.

Depending on the available instruments, overdrilling can be performed and a screw can be inserted. Leaving only the wire in place already allows for sufficient posterior stability. Pelvic packing can then be directly performed in the ER or in the OR.

DCSW application is a simple an easy procedure to get posterior pelvic ring stability. It is rarely necessary, but can support hemodynamic stabilization of the patient (Figs. 11.2, 11.3, and 11.4).

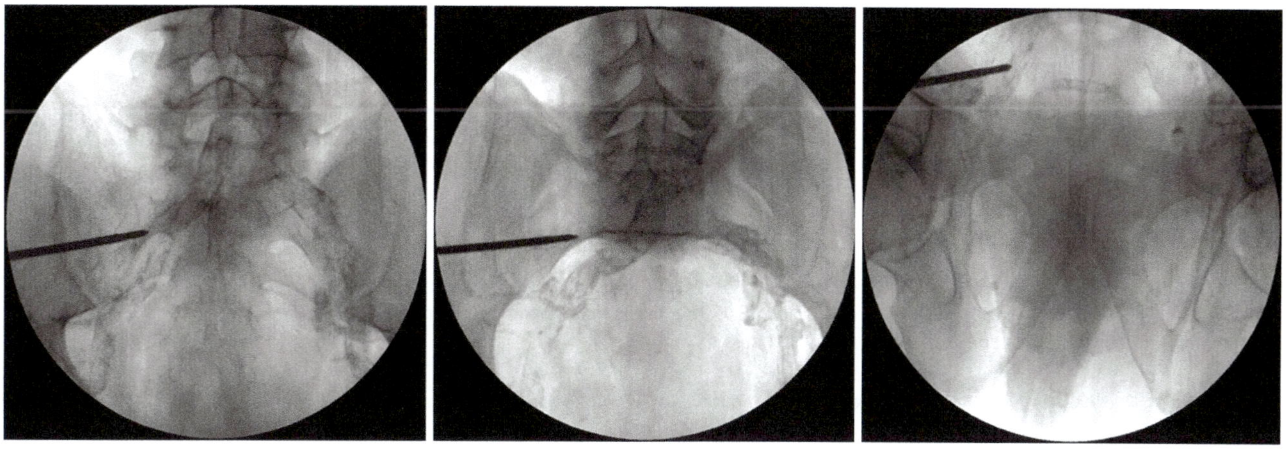

Fig. 11.1 Radiographic control in the three standard planes after percutaneous 2.8 mm K-wire application without X-ray support in a cadaver analysis

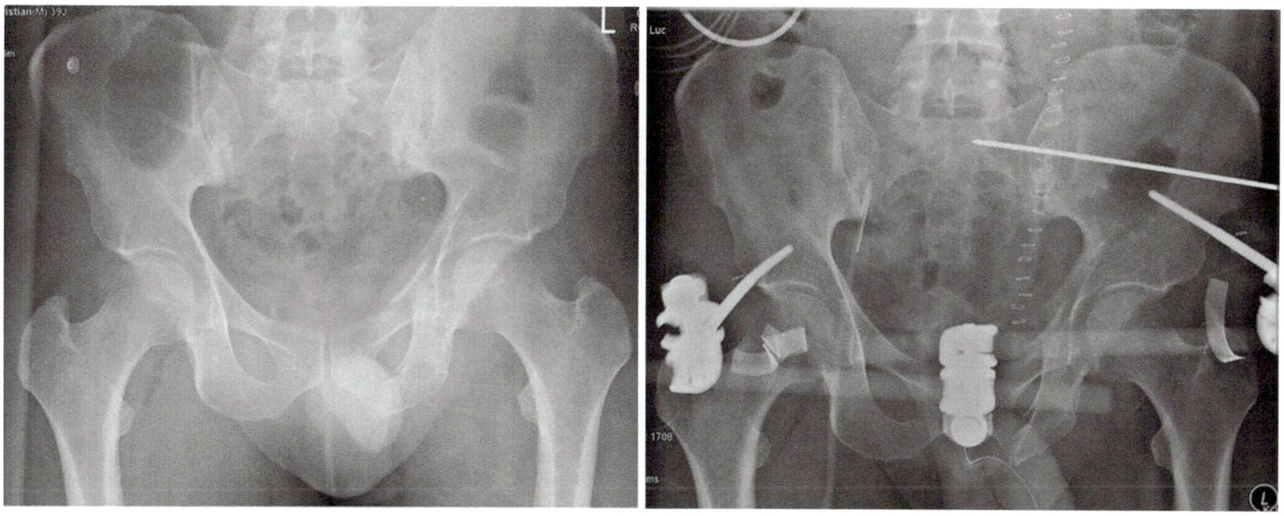

Fig. 11.2 Clinical example of a DC-K-wire application in a hemodynamic unstable patient with a type C injury of the pelvic ring (unstable left SI-joint dislocation + left pubic rami fractures)

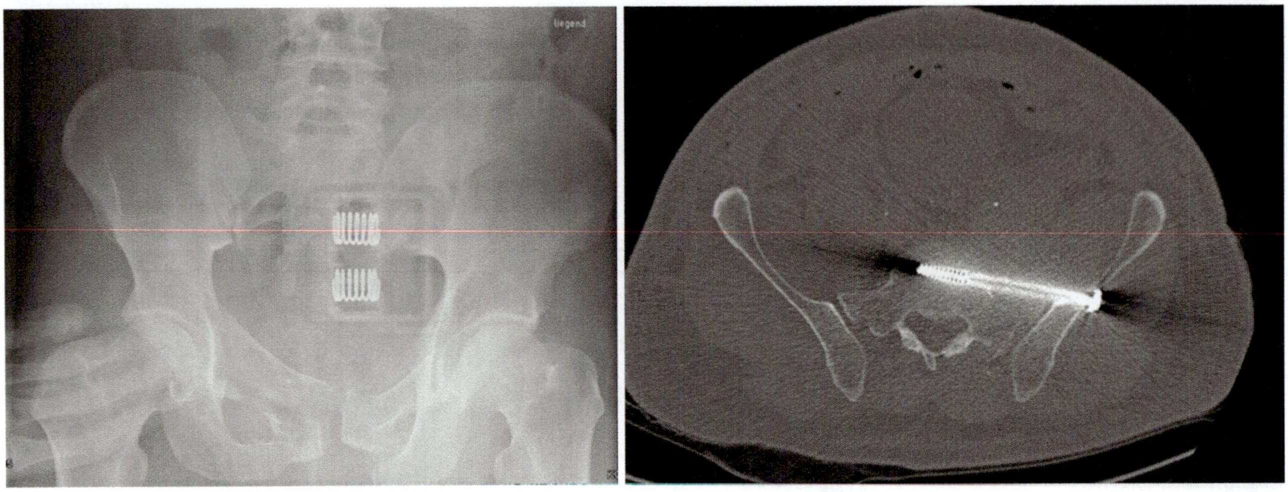

Fig. 11.3 Clinical example of a DC-screw application in a hemodynamic unstable patient with a type C injury of the pelvic ring (left transforaminal sacral fracture + bilateral pubic rami fractures); slightly too anterior screw position stabilizing the posterior pelvis, without neurological impairment during further course

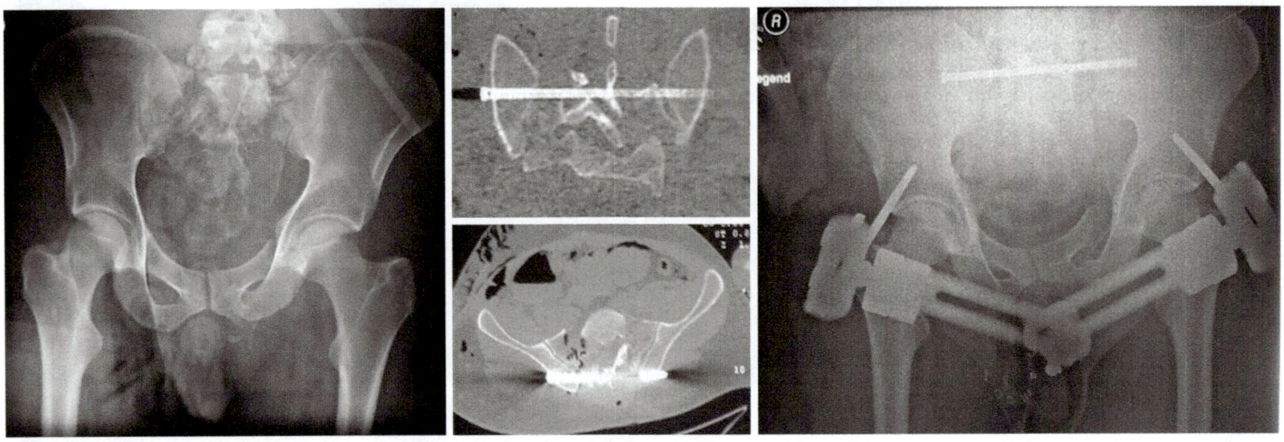

Fig. 11.4 Clinical example of a DC-screw application in a hemodynamic unstable patient with a bilateral type C injury of the pelvic ring (bilateral sacral fracture + left pubic rami fractures); due to the severe sacral comminution, a more posterior screw insertion was used (comparable to sacral bar position)

References

1. Coccolini F, Stahel P, Montori G, Biffl W, Horer T, Catena F, Kluger Y, Moore E, Peitzman A, Ivatury R, Coimbra R, Fraga G, Pereira B, Rizoli S, Kirkpatrick A, Leppaniemi A, Manfredi R, Magnone S, Chiara O, Solaini L, Ceresoli M, Allievi N, Arvieux C, Velmahos G, Balogh Z, Naidoo N, Weber D, Abu-Zidan F, Sartelli M, Ansaloni L. Pelvic trauma: WSES classification and guidelines. World J Emerg Surg. 2017;12:5. https://doi.org/10.1186/s13017-017-0117-6.
2. Gänsslen A, Hildebrand F, Pohlemann T. Management of hemodynamic unstable patients "in extremis" with pelvic ring fractures. Acta Chir Orthop Traumatol Cechoslov. 2012;79:193–202.
3. Gardner M, Chip Routt MJ. The antishock iliosacral screw. J Orthop Trauma. 2010;24:e86–9.
4. Tanizaki S, Maeda S, Matano H, Sera M, Nagai H, Ishida H. Time to pelvic embolization for hemodynamically unstable pelvic fractures may affect the survival for delays up to 60 min. Injury. 2014;45:738–41.
5. Schwartz D, Medina M, Cotton B, Rahbar E, Wade C, Cohen A, Beeler A, Burgess A, Holcomb J. Are we delivering two standards of care for pelvic trauma? Availability of angioembolization after hours and on weekends increases time to therapeutic intervention. J Trauma Acute Care Surg. 2014;76:134–9.
6. Tesoriero R, Bruns B, Narayan M, Dubose J, Guliani S, Brenner M, Boswell S, Stein D, Scalea T. Angiographic embolization for hemorrhage following pelvic fracture: is it "time" for a paradigm shift? J Trauma Acute Care Surg. 2017;82:18–26.
7. ATLS, S.C.M., 9th edition, 2012.
8. Rossaint R, Bouillon B, Cerny V, Coats T, Duranteau J, Fernández-Mondéjar E, Filipescu D, Hunt B, Komadina R, Nardi G, Neugebauer

E, Ozier Y, Riddez L, Schultz A, Vincent J, Spahn D. The European guideline on management of major bleeding and coagulopathy following trauma: fourth edition. Crit Care. 2016;20:100.
9. Gänsslen A, Krettek C, Pohlemann T. Emergency stabilization of pelvic instabilities with the pelvic C-clamp. Oper Orthop Traumatol. 2004;16:192–204.
10. Gänsslen A, Krettek C, Pohlemann T. Emergency stabilization of pelvic instabilities with the pelvic C-clamp. Eur J Trauma. 2004;30:412–9.
11. Pohlemann T, Braune C, Gänsslen A, Hüfner T, Partenheimer A. Pelvic emergency clamps: anatomic landmarks for a safe primary application. J Orthop Trauma. 2004;18:102–5.
12. Routt M, Kregor P, Simonian P, Mayo K. Early results of percutaneous iliosacral screws placed with the patient in the supine position. J Orthop Trauma. 1995;9(3):207–14.
13. Routt M, Simonian P. Closed reduction and percutaneous skeletal fixation of sacral fractures. Clin Orthop. 1996;329:121–8.
14. Routt M, Simonian P. Posterior pelvic ring disruptions: iliosacral screws. In: Wiss DA, editor. Master techniqes in orthopaedics: fractures. Philadelphia, PA: Wolters Kluwers; 1998. p. 595–612.
15. Routt M, Simonian P, Inaba J. Iliosacral screw fixation of the disrupted sacroiliac joint. Tech Orthop. 1995;9(4):300–14.
16. Routt ML Jr, Nork SE, Mills WJ. Percutaneous fixation of pelvic ring disruptions. Clin Orthop. 2000;375:15–29.

Pelvic Packing

12

Axel Gänsslen and Jan Lindahl

Presacral pelvic packing is a well-known procedure in different surgical circumstances [1].

In 1979, Riska et al. first reported on operative bleeding control by local pelvic tamponade or temporary compression of the abdominal aorta in extreme situations in 42 patients with unstable pelvic ring fractures and massive pelvic hemorrhage [2]. Several approaches were used (Fig. 12.1), depending on the source of bleeding, including a midline, a Pfannenstiel approach, an anterior iliac crest-femoral or posterolateral approach, or a combination of different approaches. The source of bleeding was predominantly major arterial injury, whereas bleeding from the pelvic bones was of minor importance.

Pohlemann et al. re-introduced the technique of pelvic packing in 1995, including a detailed description of the technique [3]. This extraperitoneal technique was part of an emergency treatment protocol regarding mechanical and hemodynamic unstable pelvic ring injuries. The packing sites were the anterior presacral venous plexus, the paravesical, and the prevesical areas, respectively.

In these severe injuries, it was proposed that, as the compartmental borders of the pelvic regions were disrupted, temporary (external) fixation of the pelvic ring was the prerequisite for packing.

Ghanayem et al. could show that external fixation sufficiently decreased the true pelvic volume in an unstable pelvic type C fracture model. The abdominal wall showed an additional tension band effect on the iliac wings, as a laparotomy further destabilized an open-book pelvic injury and subsequently increased the pelvic volume and pubic diastasis, which, therefore, can lead to increased blood loss from the pelvic injury and delay a potential tamponade effect [4].

It was recommended to mechanically stabilize the pelvic ring before performing a trauma laparotomy for additional intra-abdominal injuries in patients with unstable pelvic injuries (Fig. 12.2).

During the last decade, several European landmark papers dealt with management recommendations in hemodynamic unstable trauma patients, also focusing on pelvic injuries.

- Rossaint et al. recommended immediate pelvic ring closure and stabilization in hemodynamically unstable patients with pelvic ring injuries, followed by early preperitoneal pelvic packing, angioembolization, and/or surgical bleeding control when hemodynamic instability persists [5].
- The Scandinavian guidelines for massive bleeding patients recommended a damage control pelvic approach, where extraperitoneal pelvic packing is favored in patients in extremis and angiography for stable patients requiring ≥4 PRBCs/24 h after exclusion of thoracic and/or abdominal bleeding sources after initial pelvic binder fixation [6].
- Geeraerts et al. primarily proposed angiography with arterial embolization as the treatment of choice complemented by pelvic external fixation devices to additionally facilitate venous hemostasis, whereas in major retroperitoneal hematoma, damage control pelvic surgery by pelvic packing and pelvic C-clamps were considered effective options [7].
- The recent European guideline recommended early surgical bleeding control and/or preperitoneal packing and/or angiographic embolization for patients with ongoing hemodynamic instability despite adequate pelvic ring stabilization [8].

Recommendations of European landmark papers on hemodynamically and mechanically unstable pelvic injuries proposed mechanical stabilization and surgical/radiographic bleeding control.

A. Gänsslen (✉)
Department of Trauma Surgery, Orthopedics and Hand Surgery, Hospital Wolfsburg, Wolfsburg, Germany

J. Lindahl
Orthopaedics and Trauma Surgery, Helsinki University Hospital, Helsinki, Finland

A. Gänsslen et al. (eds.), *Pelvic Ring Fractures*, https://doi.org/10.1007/978-3-030-54730-1_12

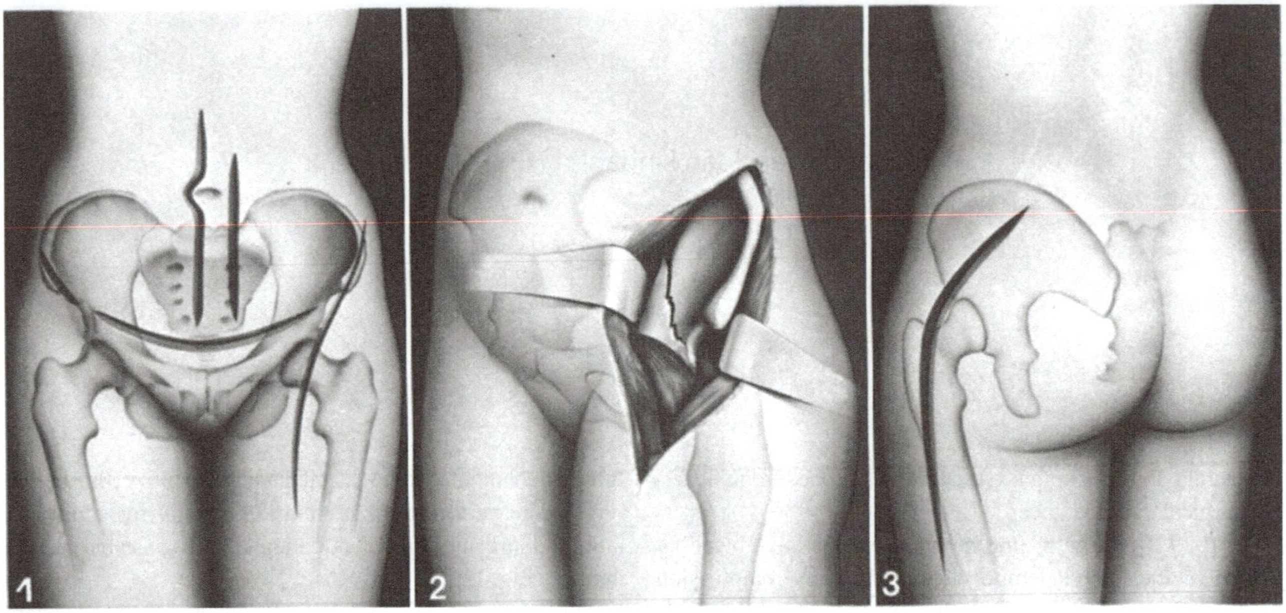

Fig. 12.1 Possible approaches for pelvic bleeding control using tamponades

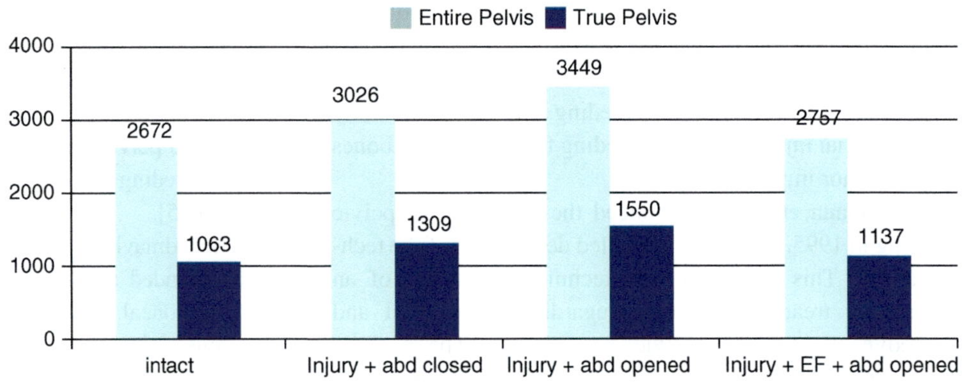

Fig. 12.2 CT measurement of pelvic volume in different injury situations: the abdominal wall provides stability to an unstable pelvic ring injury via a tension band effect on the iliac wings, an external fixation results in a decrease of the pelvic volume by adequate reduction

There are still several controversies regarding treatment of these patients. The source of pelvic bleeding in unstable pelvic ring injuries and, therefore, the optimal treatment method remains unclear.

A recent review on hemodynamically unstable patients with pelvic fractures gave the following evidence-based recommendations regarding the value of pelvic packing [9]:

- Patients with pelvic fracture-related hemodynamic instability should always be considered for preperitoneal pelvic packing, especially in hospitals with no angiography service.
- Direct preperitoneal pelvic packing represents an effective surgical measure of early hemorrhage control in hypotensive patients with bleeding pelvic ring disruptions.
- Pelvic packing should be performed in conjunction with pelvic stabilization to maximize the effectiveness of bleeding.
- Patients with pelvic fracture-related hemodynamic instability with persistent bleeding after angiography should always be considered for preperitoneal pelvic packing.
- Preperitoneal pelvic packing is an effective technique in controlling hemorrhage in patients with pelvic fracture-related hemodynamic instability that have undergone prior anterior/C-clamp fixation.

12.1 Epidemiology

Pelvic packing is a rarely performed procedure. Correspondingly, only few data are available in the literature [2, 9–30].

Table 12.1 Frequency of PPP (*ISS > 15)

Author	Year	Frequency	%	Author	Year	Frequency	%
Pohlemann	1995	11/497	2.2	Li	2016	29/973	3
Tötterman	2006	18/661	2.7	Tesoriero	2016	46/4712	1
Tai	2009	11/632*	1.7	Jang	2016	14/1164*	1.2
Froberg	2016	35/2173	1.6	Burlew	2017	138/2293	6

Pohlemann et al. performed preperitoneal pelvic packing (PPP) in 11 of 497 patients (2.2%) [25]. Several other data confirmed that PPP is only rarely performed (Table 12.1).

Preperitoneal Pelvic Packing is performed in approximately 2.2% of patients with major pelvic fractures.

12.2 Bleeding Sources

Riska already stated that the major bleeding sources were from pelvic arteries and veins [2].

Huitinen et al. performed a postmortem study on fatal pelvic fracture patients and found significant hematoma at the SI joint area (joint, ligaments, fracture) together with disruption of all pelvic compartments in 66.6%, 29.6% osseous bleeding (sacral fractures), 22.2% pelvic floor bleeding (ligaments) and 11.1% bleeding from large branches of the iliac internal artery [31].

Three major sources of bleeding were identified from clinical experience [9, 24, 32, 33]:

- Cancellous bone at the fracture site
- Laceration of retroperitoneal veins in the pelvis
- Venous bleeding (presacral plexus and prevesical veins)
- Arterial bleeding (anterior branches of the internal iliac artery, the pudendal and the obturator artery anteriorly, and superior gluteal artery and lateral sacral artery posteriorly).

From an anatomic standpoint, the venous system follows the arterial system, but is located more posterior (closer to the bones) (Fig. 12.3). Therefore, retroperitoneal venous bleeding can be associated with (posterior) pelvic fractures [7] and venous bleeding is expected to be more common.

Consequently, fatal venous bleeding is more frequent than acknowledged [34, 35] and the significance of arterial bleeding is often over-estimated [35]:

- Rothenberger et al. already reported, that 11 of 12 patients with major vascular injuries with unstable pelvic fractures presented with relevant venous injuries, while five had arterial injuries [36].
- Ertel et al. analyzed 14 polytraumatized patients with an unstable pelvic fracture treated with the pelvic C-Clamp and pelvic packing and observed significant venous bleeding in 13 patients, while no arterial injuries were observed [17].
- An experimental analysis of open-book injuries revealed that, with opening of the pubic symphysis up to 5 cm, in 60% iliolumbar vein injuries, but no arterial injuries were observed [37].
- Kataoka et al. analyzed 72 patients with unstable hemodynamics (systolic blood pressure (sBP) <90 mmHg) and a mean ISS of 34.4; the admission sBP was 76.2 mmHg; angioembolization in 61 patients led to hemodynamic stabilization in 59%, while 25 patients remained hemodynamically unstable; of the latter, 12 patients immediately died; in nine patients, iliac vein injuries were detected (ISS 45.8, mortality 77.8%) [38].

Associated large pelvic vein injuries present with a mortality rate between 11.3% and 31.8% [39].

12.3 Pathophysiology of Pelvic Packing

There is general consensus that an increase of the pelvic volume, especially in type C or massive external rotation injuries (AP II–III according to Burgess) is associated with an increased rate of pelvic bleeding complications.

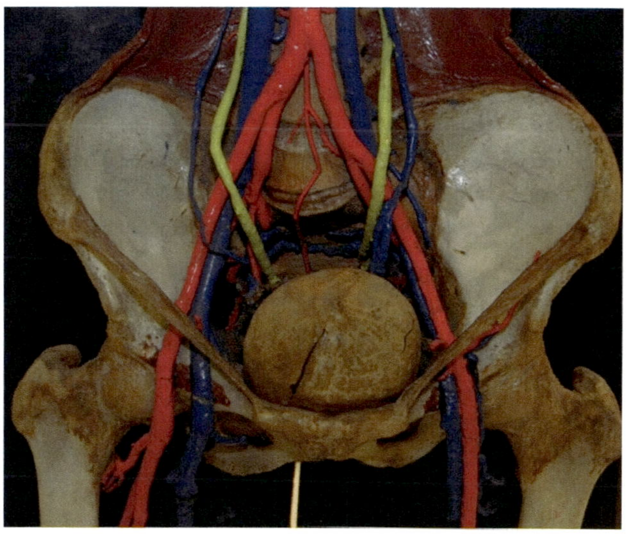

Fig. 12.3 Anatomy of major pelvic vasculature. Note: the venous systems is located closer to the bones

Moss et al. found that with every centimeter symphyseal diastasis, a 4.6% increase in pelvic volume and, with every centimeter SI joint diastasis, an increase of 3.1% of pelvic volume can be expected. Diastases at both regions can be added. A 5 cm symphyseal diastasis was associated with an increase of pelvic volume of approximately 20% [40].

Similar results were reported by Bagué et al., showing a 20.8% increase of pelvic volume with 5 cm of pubic diastasis. In this open-book injury model, 60% venous lacerations of the iliolumbar vein were observed, but no arterial vessel injury or tension on the lumbosacral trunk or the obturator nerve [37].

A self-tamponade effect cannot be expected. Grimm et al. analyzed experimentally, that even 20 L of fluids (blood) infused into the true pelvis and retroperitoneum, lead to an insufficient tamponade effect not reaching values of the intact pelvis. Applying an external fixator led to a temporary immediate-but-reduced effect, while a laparotomy reversed this effect [41]. Similar data were found in a recent analysis [42].

Ghanayem et al. presented similar results and pointed out that the risk of pelvic hemorrhage from a possibly necessary laparotomy is reduced by mechanical stabilization, best by supraacetabular external fixation, as this can reduce the additional instability of the pelvic-abdominal region [4]. Additionally, it was found, that the abdominal wall provides stability to an unstable pelvic ring injury via a tension band effect on the iliac wings.

Therefore, the proposed positive effect of external pelvic ring stabilization alone [43, 44] to control pelvic hemorrhage by "self-tamponade" is only of moderate value, as the potential tamponade effect is lost due to complete disruption of parapelvic fascia (gluteus medius, gluteus minimus, gluteus maximus, iliopsoas compartment). Thus, "haemorrhage from pelvic fracture is essentially bleeding into a free space" [35]. This was proven clinically by Trentz et al. who described this effect as a "chimney effect" in mechanically unstable pelvic ring injuries [45].

Recently, Sato et al. performed a cadaver analysis with pelvic wall pressure measurement after pelvic packing with three sponges [46]. Pelvic packing resulted in an average pressure increase to 12.3 mmHg, a significant pelvic floor and posterior pelvic brim pressure increase, but a non-significant anterior and middle pelvic brim pressure increase.

> Widening of the true pelvis increases the risk of venous bleeding. A self-tamponade effect cannot be expected. Supraacetabular external fixation and laparotomy closure supports and increases intrapelvic pressure, while pelvic packing can sufficiently control venous hemorrhage.

12.4 Prerequisites of PPP

The basis for PPP is mechanical stabilization of the pelvic ring [47]. There is substantial agreement that immediate pelvic ring closure by external stabilization in hemodynamically unstable patients is the first treatment option [3, 5–7, 30, 44, 47].

Three principle methods for mechanical stabilization of the pelvis are available [47]:

- Pelvic binders/sheets allow direct compression and adequate reduction of the pelvic ring, but with the disadvantage of a restricted approach to the true pelvis (the optimal level for a pelvic binder is on the trochanters, not the iliac wings, which allows simultaneous low midline approach).
- Pelvic external fixation is still the most frequently available method, it is quickly applicable, allows bleeding control by compression of fracture sites, but is biomechanically less sufficient; the supraacetabular pin placement is biomechanically superior to the iliac crest placement [48].
- Pelvic C-clamp has a biomechanical advantage of a direct compressive effect on the posterior pelvic ring; the theoretical disadvantages of over-compression of sacral fractures and iliac perforation is of minor importance in the emergency situation [49].

> External mechanical fixation should always be considered in hemodynamic unstable patients with pelvic fractures, especially when laparotomy is indicated [4, 50–52].

12.5 Indications for PPP

Pelvic packing is recommended in patients "in extremis" [47], as it is a fast (within the golden hour of shock) and effective procedure in hemodynamically unstable patients.

Therefore, the following indications are suggested [9, 47, 53, 54]:

- Pelvic fracture-related hemodynamic instability.
- Preperitoneal pelvic packing performed in conjunction with pelvic stabilization (anterior/C-clamp fixation).
- Pelvic fracture-related hemodynamic instability with persistent bleeding after angiography.
- Non-responders.

12.6 Technique of Preperitoneal Pelvic Packing (PPP)

Pohlemann et al. and Tscherne et al. described the technique of PPP in detail [3, 30]. PPP can be performed either in the emergency room [29], in the angio-suite [55] or, most optimally, in the OR [3, 30, 55].

12.6.1 Positioning and Draping

In the supine position, the complete thoraco-abdominal-pelvic area is draped whenever possible. If packing is performed in the emergency room, local abdominal/pelvic draping can be performed.

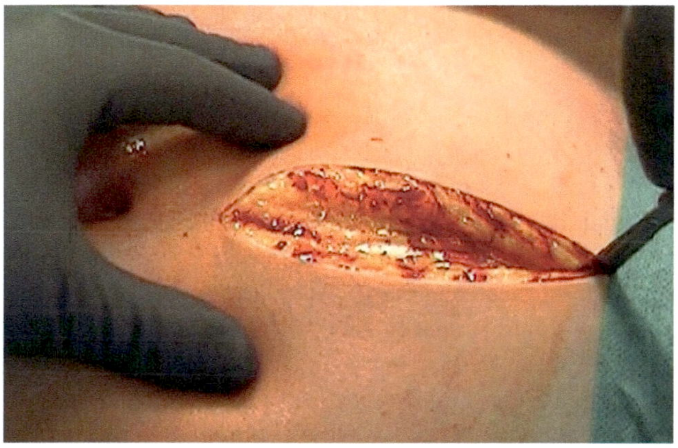

Fig. 12.4 The incision starts from the umbilicus reaching the pubic symphysis. This orientation allows for later complete laparotomy, if necessary

The standard of draping starts from the pubic area to the upper clavicular margins. This allows for pelvic packing, trauma laparotomy and/or emergency thoracotomy.

12.6.2 Incision

Two incisions are possible. The lower midline incision is the gold standard starting at the umbilicus and extending to the pubic symphysis (Fig. 12.4). Alternatively, a Pfannenstiel incision is used, which leaves a potential laparotomy incision without contact to the extraperitoneal packing area to avoid potential contamination, when bowel injuries are present. In the latter, a low horizontal ~10–12 cm incision at the "bikini line" is favored [55].

If a laparotomy is necessary, two separate incisions are favored for optimized effectiveness of the pelvic tamponade [56]. The laparotomy incision starts from the xiphoid to just below the umbilicus. The PPP incision is performed horizontally (Pfannenstiel) or vertically, approximately 6 cm away in the suprapubic area [56].

12.6.3 Retroperitoneal Opening

After skin incision and subcutaneous dissection, the linea alba is identified and incised (Fig. 12.5). The rectus muscle bellies are identified and laterally mobilized, until the posterior layer of the

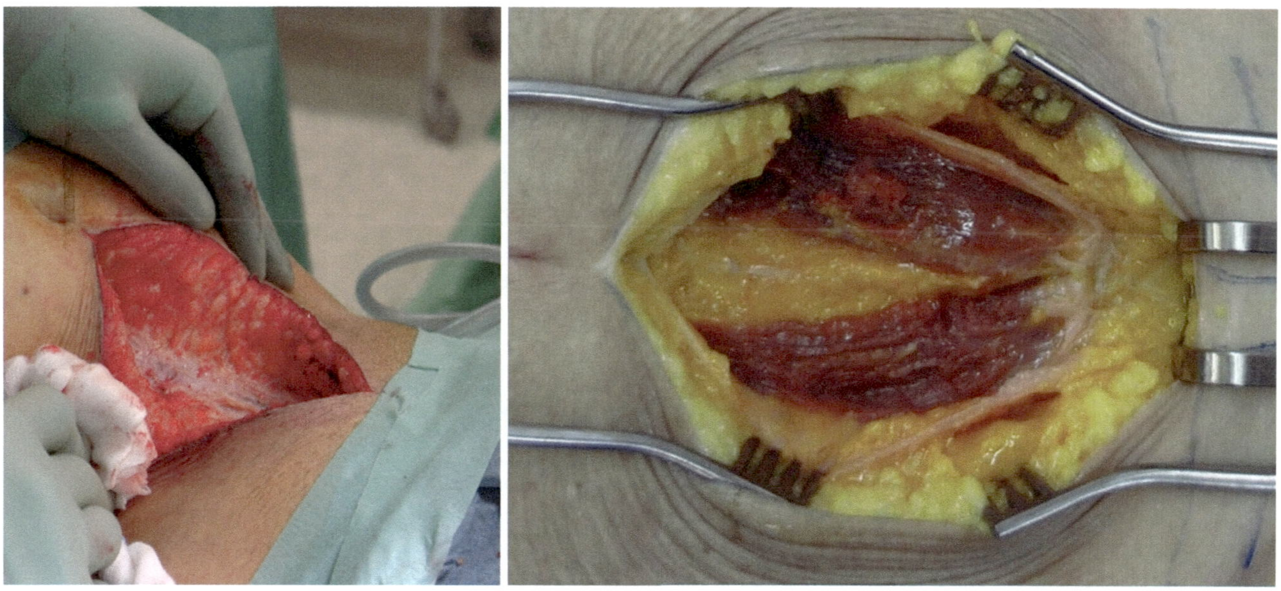

Fig. 12.5 The incision starts from the umbilicus reaching the pubic symphysis. This orientation allows for later complete laparotomy, if necessary

rectus sheath is visible (Fig. 12.5). Near the pubic symphysis, this layer is digitally penetrated to open the space of Retzii (Fig. 12.6). The peritoneum is left intact. On the site of injury, the rectus muscles are left intact and elevated by a hook.

12.6.4 Deep Dissection

On the injured side, the dissection is usually already performed by the injury itself. Thus, direct manual access through the right or left paravesical space down to the presacral region can be achieved without further soft tissue dissection (Fig. 12.7) [30].

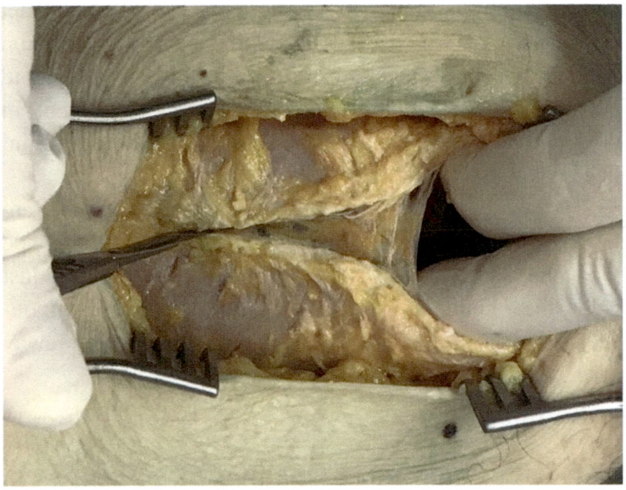

Fig. 12.6 Digital opening of the retrosymphyseal space, without injuring the peritoneum

The urinary bladder is retracted to the contralateral side. The upper pubic ramus is palpated. The obturator neurovascular bundle can become visible, but in patients with significant bleeding, it is not necessary to identify it (Fig. 12.8). Also, the quadrilateral surface site need not be visualized. Further blunt dissection is performed at the inner site of the pelvic brim close to the SI joint.

Bleeding usually originates from the true pelvis and, therefore, pelvic packing should address this area.

In cases where laparotomy is performed prior to pelvic packing, the peritoneum is left intact distally to facilitate packing in the extraperitoneal space [29].

12.6.5 Packing Procedure

In most cases, a specific source of bleeding cannot be identified and the origin of hemorrhage is diffuse either from the venous plexus or the fracture site. In anterior-posterior compression injuries resulting in external rotation, the bleeding source is often primarily seen at the anterior pelvic ring. Closure of the pelvic ring by internal rotation or use of a simple reduction forceps together with paravesical packing is relatively easy and can stop the bleeding. In more unstable fracture pattern (C-type injuries), most commonly the

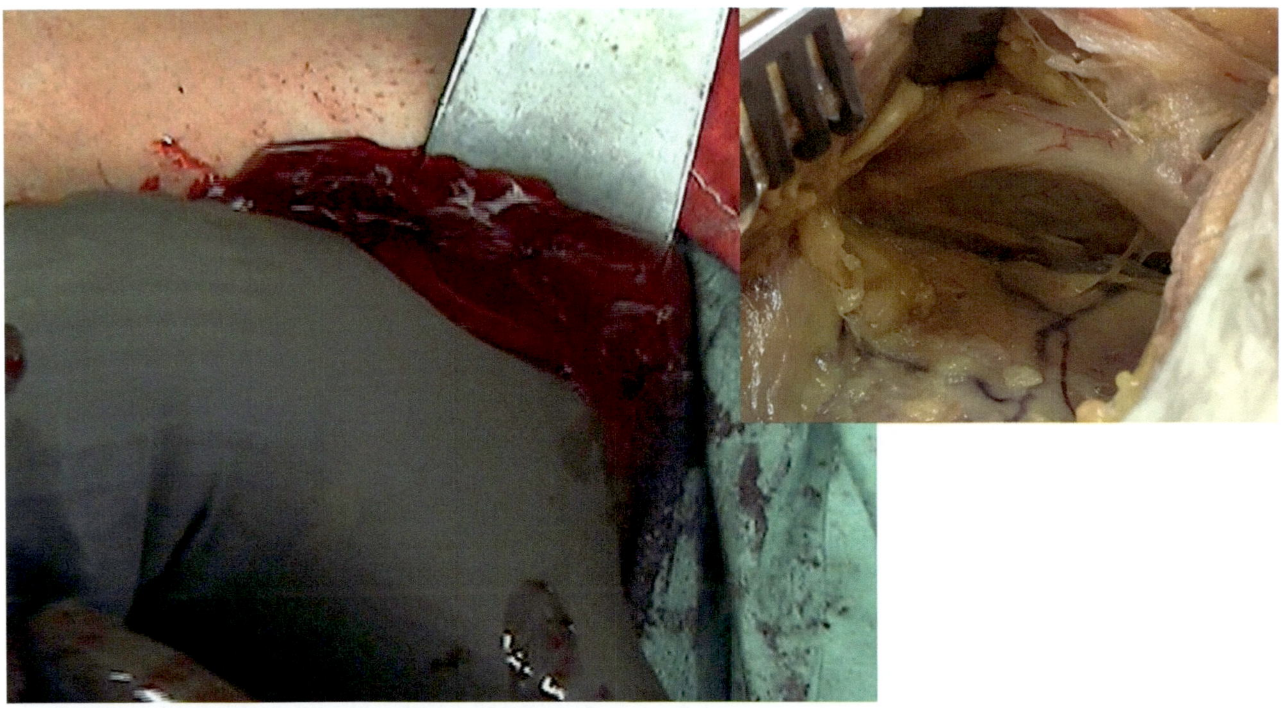

Fig. 12.7 Blunt dissection along the upper pubic rami up to the SI joint

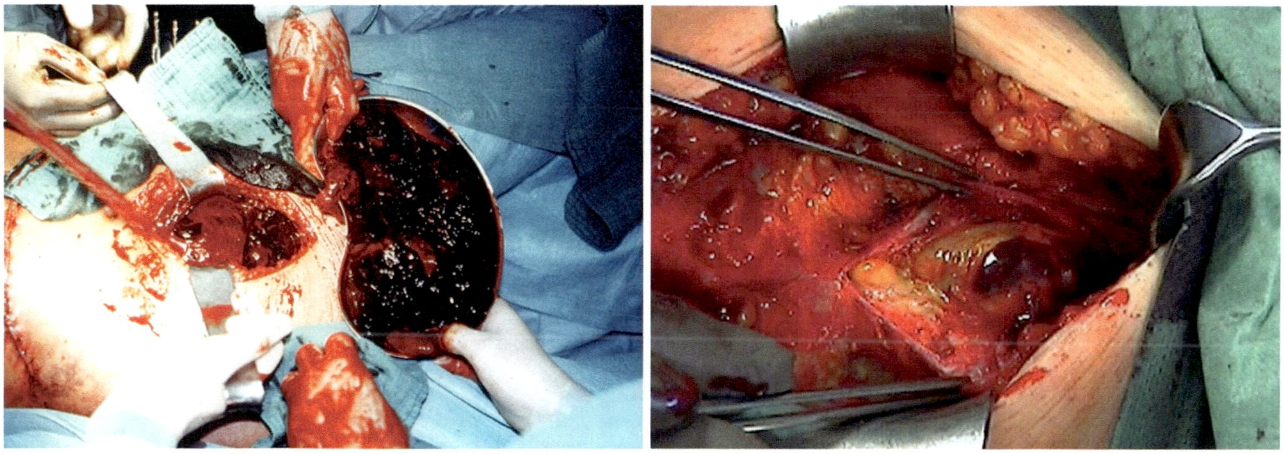

Fig. 12.8 After hematoma evacuation, the contused bladder wall becomes visible. Source: Pohlemann T, Regel G, Bosch U, Stief Ch, Tscherne H. Kapitel 7: Notfallbehandlung und Komplextrauma, p. 99 (Fig. 7.16); in: Tscherne H, Pohlemann T (Ed.). Tscherne Unfallchirurgie – Becken und Acetabulum. Springer Verlag Berlin, Heidelberg, New York, 1998

bleeding source is located at the posterior pelvic (presacral) region [30].

The presacral and paravesical regions are packed using standard surgical tamponades (Fig. 12.9). Due to the amount of blood in the pelvic space, especially in patients in extremis, the pelvic space can usually be inadequately visualized. Thus, rapid packing into the pool of blood has to be performed [56].

Two to three large radio-opaque swabs are placed in the pelvis, starting posteriorly from the SI joint and subsequently reaching the retropubic area [29, 30]. The swabs are placed in the true pelvis to address the internal iliac vessels and the presacral venous plexus, which are in close proximity to the sacrum and pelvic bones (Fig. 12.9b) [29].

> Always, the contralateral site has to be dissected to perform an additional packing here, even when no bleeding is present. From clinical experience, ongoing pelvic bleeding would otherwise result in secondary hematoma and hemodynamic instability.

In open perineal injuries, additional packing of this area is performed.

Superficial and lateral packing should be avoided preventing compression on the femoral vessels [55]. Overall, 6–9 swabs are usually placed into the true pelvis.

If hemodynamic stability is not achieved, swab removal and goal-directed re-packing is performed for optimization of swab localization [3, 55].

If a bladder injury is identified, depending on the hemodynamic status, primary repair can be considered. A suprapubic tube should be inserted through a separate stab incision.

In patients requiring an additional laparotomy due to concomitant intra-abdominal injuries, extraperitoneal packing can even be performed after vascular control (Fig. 12.10).

12.6.6 Wound Closure

Before closure, the effectiveness of the tamponade is re-evaluated. Tamponade localization can be optimized or even identifiable vascular lesions can be controlled by direct surgical means [30].

Whenever possible, the linea alba is closed to support the pelvic tamponade effect. No wound drains are inserted.

In patients with an accompanying laparotomy incision, the abdominal cavity is usually left open to reduce the risk of abdominal compartment syndrome (ACS) [29].

12.6.7 Role of Angioembolization

Tscherne et al. already stated that, in patients with persistent hemodynamic instability, angioembolization should be considered [30].

If the patient is still hemodynamically unstable, and CT evaluation reveals signs of arterial injury, that is, hematoma, contrast extravasation, active hematoma formation, et cetera, the patient is transferred to the angiography suite for angioembolization [9].

Ron et al. proposed to remove the swabs under sterile conditions and directly visualize the iliac vessels, followed by selected angioembolization. The pads are then removed 48–72 h later [55].

In approximately 15% of patients, angioembolization is performed [12]. Indications include >4 units of blood in the 12 h following PPP once coagulopathy is corrected [56].

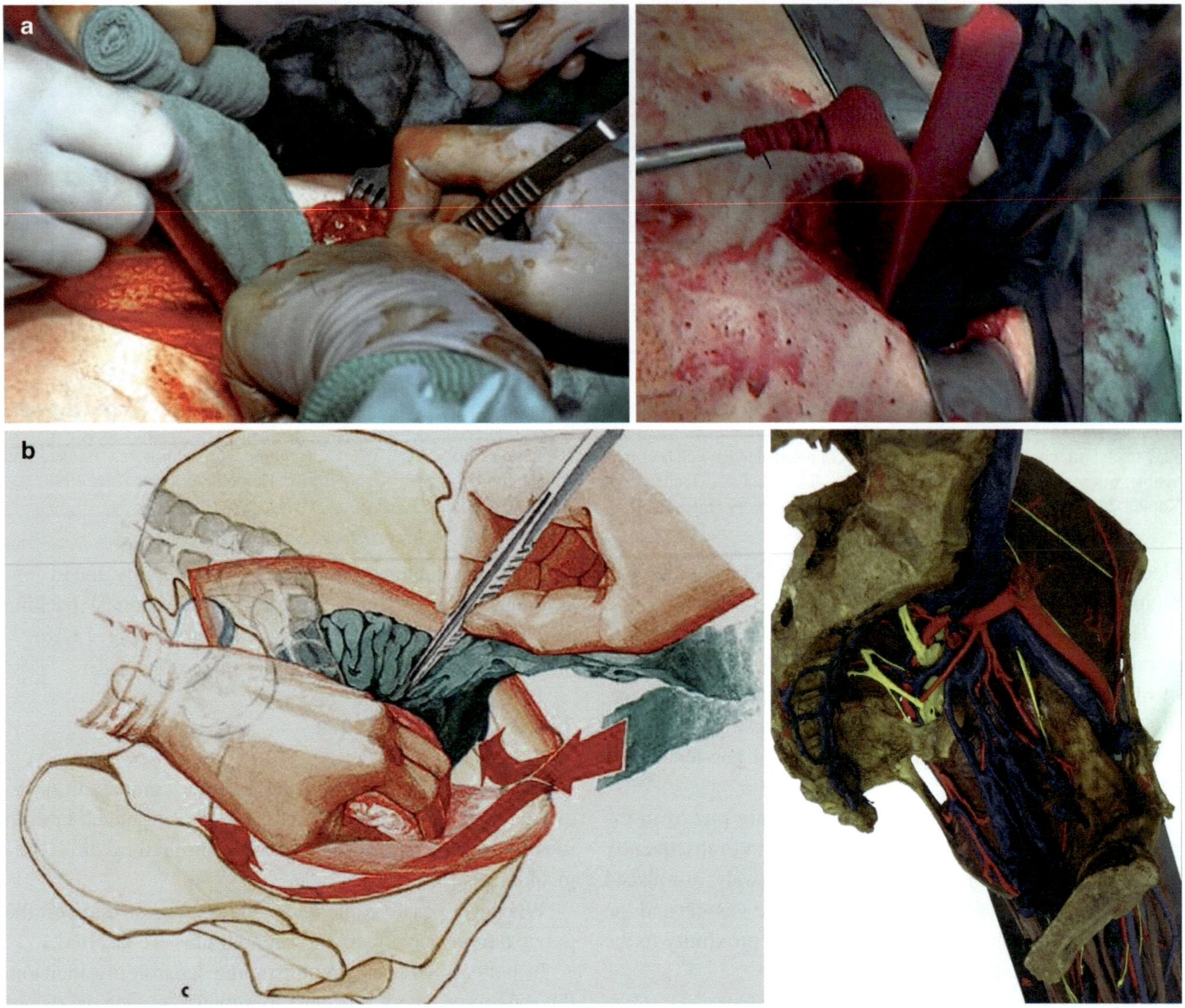

Fig. 12.9 (**a**) Packing is performed using several standard surgical tamponades, starting near the SI joint, then along the pelvic brim, and ending retrosymphyseal. (**b**) Schematic principle of extraperitoneal pelvic packing. Source: Pohlemann T, Regel G, Bosch U, Stief Ch, Tscherne H. Kapitel 7: Notfallbehandlung und Komplextrauma, p. 100 (Fig. 7.17b); in: Tscherne H, Pohlemann T (Ed.). Tscherne Unfallchirurgie – Becken und Acetabulum. Springer Verlag Berlin, Heidelberg, New York, 1998

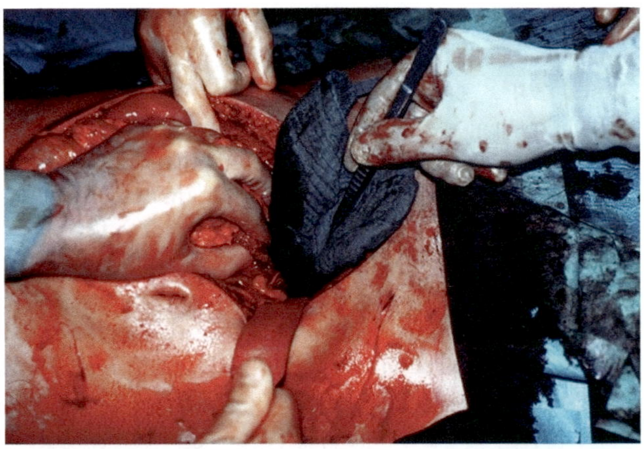

Fig. 12.10 Extraperitoneal pelvic packing during damage control laparotomy. Source: Pohlemann T, Regel G, Bosch U, Stief Ch, Tscherne H. Kapitel 7: Notfallbehandlung und Komplextrauma, p. 100 (Fig. 7.17c); in: Tscherne H, Pohlemann T (Ed.). Tscherne Unfallchirurgie – Becken und Acetabulum. Springer Verlag Berlin, Heidelberg, New York, 1998

12.6.8 Mechanical Stabilization

As a gold standard, pelvic mechanical stabilization is performed prior to PPP to pack against a mechanically stabilized pelvic ring [3, 9, 30, 56]. Others recommend external pelvic fixation secondary to pelvic packing [20, 55].

12.6.9 Second Look

A routine second look is performed after 24–48 h [3, 29, 30, 55, 56].

If there is still relevant bleeding, a re-packing is performed in the same technique. In hemodynamically stable patients without signs of re-bleeding, the swabs are removed and the retroperitoneal true pelvis is closed over one or two drains (without negative pressure).

Dependent on the general status of the patient, definitive anterior ring stabilization or even posterior stabilization can be considered.

Persistent bleeding is treated by re-packing and a "third look" is planned 24–48 h later. Alternatively, angioembolization is performed.

12.7 Data on PPP

Since the first report on Pohlemann et al. in 1995, several case reports [14, 19, 26, 57] and reviews [18, 35, 53, 54, 56, 58–61] were reported.

Pohlemann et al. described the technique of retroperitoneal pelvic packing in detail via an infra-umbilical extraperitoneal approach [3]. The indication performing pelvic packing was first reported in a severely injured group of 19 patients with C-type pelvic injuries. The pelvis was stabilized by pelvic C-clamp. The mean injury severity was 47.4 points (Hannover Polytrauma Scale) and the admission hemoglobin was 7.7 g/dL. Retroperitoneal pelvic packing was performed in 73.7% for controlling venous hemorrhage, which was present in about 70%. Additional abdominal injuries were frequent with a rate of 63%. Overall, in this group of patients, mortality was high with 58%.

Tscherne et al. reported on 15 patients with C-type pelvic injuries and an initial hemoglobin level ≤8 g/dL, where pelvic packing was performed [30]. This patient group additionally was severely injured with an ISS of 37.4 points, a mean systolic blood pressure at admission of 63 mmHg, a mean hemoglobin level of 5.6 g/dL and a mean base deficit of −10.1 mmol/L. During the first hour of treatment, a mean of 7.9 units of blood had to be transfused and, within 12 h after admission, a mean of 37.4 units were necessary. Concomitant abdominal injury was seen in 80%. Overall mortality was high with 66.6%.

Ertel et al. analyzed 41 patients in extremis defined as absent vital signs, severe shock requiring mechanical resuscitation or catecholamines despite transfusion of >12 units within 2 h after admission [16]. The mean ISS was 40.1 points. Nineteen of the forty-one patients had C-type injuries of the pelvis and 12 B-type injuries. Additional abdominal injuries were frequent with a rate of 61%. Stabilization of the pelvis was performed by C-clamp in two patients with C-type injury (10.5%). An external fixator was applied in an additional 26.3% of patients with C-type injuries. The overall rate of pelvic emergency stabilization in C-type injuries in patients in extremis, therefore, was 36.8%. Pelvic packing in the whole group was performed in 29.3%. The overall mortality rate was 90.2%. Two-thirds (62%) of these patients died due to uncontrollable hemorrhage.

A further analysis by the same group on 16 patients with type C-injuries were treated with a pelvic C-clamp for mechanical pelvic stabilization, followed by intraperitoneal pelvic packing in ten cases. The mean ISS in this group was 38.5, with an overall mortality rate of 25%. Of these, 75% died due to uncontrollable hemorrhage [17]. The primary lactate levels were superior to hemoglobin or hematocrit, identifying patients in extremis.

Töttermann et al. analyzed 18 hemodynamically unstable patients with a mean systolic BP of 60 mmHg, a heart rate of 119/min, a base deficit of −6.6 mmol/L and a hemoglobin value of 8.8 g/dL [29]. Seventeen of these were polytraumatized and had additional injuries. The mean ISS was 48% and 28% of these patients died during further course. The mean time from injury to hospital admission was 63 min. After further 41 min, extraperitoneal pelvic packing was performed in 13 patients with manifest shock signs. The overall time to packing was 134 min, indicating an in-hospital treatment window of 2.2 h since injury. The pelvis was stabilized by pelvic sheeting or external fixation. 12 units of blood were transfused on average during this period (5.3 units/h), followed by 0.71 units/h during the following 24 h. Stabilization of systolic blood pressure was observed immediately after the procedure. Despite hemodynamic stabilization after pelvic packing, secondary angiography revealed arterial injury in 80% of these patients.

The complication rate was 11.1%. One patient developed infection as the swabs could not be removed earlier than 3 days post injury and, in another patient, septicemia was due to accidentally left swabs.

As pelvic packing is a procedure which is presently not widespread in use, Bach et al. analyzed teaching of this potentially simple procedure to be easy, and clinical implementation was possible without major problems [62].

The value of this treatment concept has also been identified in the anglo-american area in recent years. Re-discovering this technique led to a paradigm shift.

In a first report, two cases were presented by Smith et al. on two secondarily transferred patients that were treated by pelvic C-clamp and extraperitoneal pelvic packing [26]. Both patients received transfusions prior to packing of approximately 2 units/h. From their hemodynamic status both were moderately hemodynamically unstable. A further case report was presented by Cothren et al. [14]. A secondary transferred 6-year-old child received 5 units of blood before pelvic packing. Angiography after packing showed no arterial extravasation.

Cothren et al. then presented a study on 28 patients with type B- and C-injuries and a systolic blood pressure < 90 mmHg receiving two units of blood. The ISS was 55. The mean primary systolic blood pressure was 77 mmHg, the heart rate was 120/min and the base deficit was 13 mmol/L. Mechanical stabilization of the pelvis was performed by anterior external fixation or posterior pelvic C-clamp prior to pelvic packing. On average, 2.9 units of blood/h were transfused during the initial period. Within 48 h, re-packing was necessary in 32% of these patients. Mortality rate was 25%. Infectious complications due to the procedure were found in one patient. They concluded, that pelvic packing more rapidly and directly addresses the primary source of bleeding with pelvic fractures, the venous and bone hemorrhage and pelvic packing was effective in reducing transfusion requirements [15].

The same group compared angiography/embolization vs. pelvic packing. Osborn et al. reported on 20 patients requiring pelvic packing after resuscitation with 2000 mL of intravenous (IV) crystalloids according to the ATLS protocol. When the systolic blood pressure was <90 mmHg 6 h after admission despite receiving 2 units of blood, packing was performed together with pelvic mechanical stabilization [23].

The mean ISS in the packing group was 54.7, higher than in the angiography group. The mean admission systolic blood pressure and base deficit were comparable in both groups (packing vs. angiography) with 81.5 vs. 75.8 mmHg and 12.7 vs. 13.2 mmol/L, respectively.

Packing was performed in median 45 min after admission. These patients received 11.8 PRBC units before completion of pelvic packing (median: 15.7 units/h) in contrast to 2 units/h in the angiography group (median: 4.2 units/h). There was a trend that patients after pelvic packing had reduced transfusion requirements within 24 h after this procedure compared to the angiography group (6.9 vs. 10.1 PRBC). Overall, the mortality rate was 25% vs. 30%, respectively.

In the Chinese literature, Gao et al. reported on two patients with significant pelvic bleeding, where pelvic packing was performed via a retroperitoneal approach and packing was supported by application of an external fixator. Both patients hemodynamically stabilized after the procedure [19].

Tai et al. analyzed 11 patients receiving pelvic packing after a mean of 78.8 min in patients with a mean systolic blood pressure at admission of 99 mmHg [63]. Two units of blood were transfused prior to packing in average (1.5 units/h). After this procedure, transfusion requirements were 0.37/h within the next 24 h. Overall mortality in this group 36.3%. Comparing these patients to a group where angiography and embolization was performed, showed a higher transfusion requirement prior to intervention (3.1 units/h), a reduced transfusion rate within 24 h after the procedure (0.21 units/h), but a higher mortality rate of 69.2% after primary systolic blood pressure of 61.9 mmHg and a base deficit of −14.8 vs. -10.8 mmol/L. In the packing group, 25% non-survivors died due to persistent hemorrhage compared to 33% in the angiography group.

Older age was found to be a worse prognostic indicator in patients requiring pelvic packing [15, 29].

In a summarized analysis of 364 patients with PPP from the existing literature (Table 12.2), the following results were obtained:

- In the majority of patients, the pelvic ring is highly unstable with 73.6% type C-injuries and 25.2% type B-injuries [13, 17, 21, 22, 29, 30].
- The mean ISS of this patient group is 43 points [13, 17, 20–22, 29, 30, 55, 58, 63, 64].
- The mean sBP at admission was 76 mmHg [20, 29, 30, 55, 58, 63].
- The average lactate at admission was 4.5 mmol/L [13, 17, 20, 64] and the base deficit was −9.4 mmol/L [13, 29, 30, 58, 63, 64].
- The average hemoglobin at admission was 8.2 g/dL [17, 20, 29, 30, 55, 63, 64].
- The time interval between admission and start of PPP was 53.3 min [20, 21, 29, 55, 58, 63].
- During the first hour after admission, an average of 4.7 PRBC's were transfused [29, 30, 55, 58].
- 24-h transfusion requirements were 12.3 PRBC's [13, 29, 58, 63, 64].
- An overall mortality rate of 28% was observed [13, 17, 20–22, 29, 30, 55, 58, 63, 64].

Table 12.2 Patient data on pelvic packing

Author	Year	No.	ISS	sBP	Lactate	BD	Hb	*A*	*B*	*C*	Time to PPP	EK/1st	EK/24 h	Mortality (%)
Tscherne	2000	15	37.4	63		−10.1	5,6	0	0	15		7.9		66.6
Ertel	2001	20	41.2		5.1		7.0	0	4	16				25
Tötterman	2006	18	48.0	80		−7.9	8.0	1	6	8	41.0	4.1	29	27.8
Tai	2011	11	40.0	99		−10.8	11.8				78.8		9	36.4
Ron	2015	14	29.7	63			10.3				83.9	8.6		21.4
Froberg	2016	35	30.0		3.4	−4.3	7.1						9	25.7
Li	2016	29	48.0					0	13	16	77.0			13.9
Burlew	2017	128	48	74		−12.0					44.0	4.0	11	21.1
Jang	2016	14	38.8	95	4.9		10.4				55.0			35.7
Lustenberger	2011	50	41.7					0	8	42				40
Cjiara	2016	30	44.9		5.2	−4.3		1	9	20			13	33.3

Table 12.3 Patient data comparing angioembolization and extraperitoneal pelvic packing

Author	Year	Incidence	Age	ISS	sBP	BD	Lactate	Time/proc	PRBC*	Mortality (%)
EPP										
Osborn	2009	20	37.9	54.7	81.5	12.7	5.3	45	11.8	20
Tai	2011	11/632	51.2	40	99	10.8		78.8	2	36.3
Li	2016	29/973	43	48				77	10.9	13.8
Froberg	2016	35/2173	43	30		4.3	3.4			25.7
Angiography/embolization										
Osborn	2009	20	39.5	45.9	75.8	13.2	4.9	130	9.2	30
Tai	2011	13/632	44.8	42.3	61.2	14.8		139.5	3.2	69.2
Li	2016	27/973	40	43				102	11.2	18.5
Froberg	2016	31/2173	46	30		5.2	3.3			9.7

12.8 Comparable Analyses

The effect of pelvic packing on hemodynamic instability was analyzed by different authors, comparing patients treated with PPP and angioembolization (Table 12.3).

Osborn et al. compared each 20 patients with TAE and PPP [23]. PPP was finished significantly earlier after admission (EPP 45 min vs. TAE 130 min), leading to a significant decrease in 24 h blood transfusions and even mortality was lower than in the TAE group (20% vs. 30%), despite overall ISDS being significantly higher (54.7 points vs. 45.9 points).

Tai et al. compared 13 TAE patients with 11 PPP patients [63]. The mean time from admission to PPP was 78.8 min vs. 139 min for TAE; while the mortality rate was 36.3% for PPP and 69.2% for TAE.

Li et al. compared 27 TAE patients with 29 PPP patients [21]. The ISS in the ANGIO group was lower than in the PACK group (43 vs. 48 points). TAE was performed after 102 min with a procedure time of 84 min (overall: 186 min after admission), while PPP was started 77 min after admission with a procedure time of 60 min (overall: 137 min after admission, 50 min less). The overall mortality rate was higher in the TAE group (mortality (TAE) 18.5%; mortality (PPP) 13.8%).

Several analyses compared pelvic packing against groups without pelvic packing.

Jang et al. analyzed 14 hemodynamically unstable patients treated with PPP. In 69%, type C-injuries were present. The mean ISS was 38.8 pt., the mean hemoglobin at admission was 10.4 g/dL, the lactate was 4.9 and an average of 23.9 units of blood had to be transfused within the first 24 h. Time to procedure start was 55.4 min. The overall mortality was 35.7%. It was concluded, that PPP reduced the mortality rate, when compared to a non-PPP group (14.3% vs. 37.5%) [20].

Chiara et al. reported on 30 hemodynamically unstable patients with PPP, presenting with a mean base deficit of 4.3 mmol/L and a lactate of 5.18. Thirteen PRBC were transfused within the first 24 h after arrival. The mortality rate was 28%. This was significantly less compared to matched non-PPP group (20 vs. 52) [13].

In a literature overview, Hou et al. compared more historical patients with and without pelvic packing [65]. The mortality rate significantly differed, despite a higher ISS: pelvic packing 21.9% vs. non-packing 46.5%.

Pelvic packing is initiated in a faster time interval after hospital admission it might be associated with a lower mortality rate than with TAE, but the direct comparison is difficult, because the study groups and bleeding sources are not comparable and there are also other reasons like head injury and multi-organ failure for mortality.

12.9 Conclusion

In patients "in extremis" the concept of direct extraperitoneal pelvic packing is recommended. In moderately unstable patients or in patients where persistent hemodynamic instability occurs despite shock therapy and mechanical stabilization and pelvic packing, arterial injury is ruled out by angiography, followed by selected embolization of pelvic vessels [47].

References

1. Celentano V, Ausobsky J, Vowden P. Surgical management of presacral bleeding. Ann R Coll Surg Engl. 2014;96:261–5.
2. Riska E, Vin Bonsdorff H, Hakkinen S, Jaroma H, Kiviluato O, Paavilainen T. Operative control of massive haemorrhage in comminuted pelvic fractures. Int Orthop. 1979;3:141–4.
3. Pohlemann T, Gänsslen A, Bosch U, Tscherne H. The technique of packing for control of hemorrhage in complex pelvic fractures. Tech Orthop. 1995;9(4):267–70.
4. Ghanayem A, Wilber J, Lieberman J, Motta A. The effect of laparotomy and external fixator stabilization on pelvic volume in an unstable pelvic injury. J Trauma. 1995;38(3):396–400.
5. Rossaint R, Bouillon B, Cerny V, Coats T, Duranteau J, Fernández-Mondéjar E, Filipescu D, Hunt B, Komadina R, Nardi G, Neugebauer

E, Ozier Y, Riddez L, Schultz A, Vincent J, Spahn D. The European guideline on management of major bleeding and coagulopathy following trauma: fourth edition. Crit Care. 2016;20:100.
6. Gaarder C, Naess P, Frischknecht Christensen E, Hakala P, Handolin L, Heier H, Ivancev K, Johansson P, Leppäniemi A, Lippert F, Lossius H, Opdahl H, Pillgram-Larsen J, Røise O, Skaga N, Søreide E, Stensballe J, Tønnessen E, Töttermann A, Ortenwall P, Ostlund A. Scandinavian Guidelines—"The massively bleeding patient". J Surg. 2008;97:15–36.
7. Geeraerts T, Chhor V, Cheisson G, Martin L, Bessoud B, Ozanne A, Duranteau J. Clinical review: initial management of blunt pelvic trauma patients with haemodynamic instability. Crit Care. 2007;11:204.
8. Spahn D, Bouillon B, Cerny V, Duranteau J, Filipescu D, Hunt B, Komadina R, Maegele M, Nardi G, Riddez L, Samama C, Vincent J, Rossaint R. The European guideline on management of major bleeding and coagulopathy following trauma: fifth edition. Crit Care. 2019;23(1):98. https://doi.org/10.1186/s13054-019-2347-3.
9. Coccolini F, Stahel P, Montori G, Biffl W, Horer T, Catena F, Kluger Y, Moore E, Peitzman A, Ivatury R, Coimbra R, Fraga G, Pereira B, Rizoli S, Kirkpatrick A, Leppaniemi A, Manfredi R, Magnone S, Chiara O, Solaini L, Ceresoli M, Allievi N, Arvieux C, Velmahos G, Balogh Z, Naidoo N, Weber D, Abu-Zidan F, Sartelli M, Ansaloni L. Pelvic trauma: WSES classification and guidelines. World J Emerg Surg. 2017;12:5. https://doi.org/10.1186/s13017-017-0117-6.
10. Abrassart S, Stern R, Peter R. Unstable pelvic ring injury with hemodynamic instability: what seems the best procedure choice and sequence in the initial management? Orthop Traumatol Surg Res. 2013;99:175–82.
11. Alkatary M, Miller J, Fawzi Al-Ayoubi F. Management of hemodynamically unstable patients with fracture pelvis. Int Surg J. 2017;4:1893–2897.
12. Burlew C, Moore E, Smith W, Johnson J, Biffl W, Barnett C, Stahel P. Preperitoneal pelvic packing/external fixation with secondary angioembolization: optimal care for life-threatening hemorrhage from unstable pelvic fractures. J Am Coll Surg. 2011;212:628–35.
13. Chiara O, di Fratta E, Mariani A, Michaela B, Prestini L, Sammartano F, Cimbanassi S. Efficacy of extra-peritoneal pelvic packing in hemodynamically unstable pelvic fractures, a propensity score analysis. World J Emerg Surg. 2016;11:22. https://doi.org/10.1186/s13017-016-0077-2.
14. Cothren C, Moore E, Smith W, Morgan S. Preperitoneal pelvic packing in the child with an unstable pelvis: a novel approach. J Pediatr Surg. 2006;41:E17–9.
15. Cothren C, Osborn P, Moore E, Morgan S, Johnson J, Smith W. Preperitonal pelvic packing for hemodynamically unstable pelvic fractures: a paradigm shift. J Trauma. 2007;62:834–42.
16. Ertel W, Eid K, Keel M, Trentz O. Therapeutical strategies and outcome of polytraumatized patients with pelvic injuries—a six-year experience. Eur J Trauma. 2000;6:278–86.
17. Ertel W, Keel M, Eid K, Platz A, Trentz O. Control of severe hemorrhage using C-clamp and pelvic packing in multiply injured patients with pelvic ring disruption. J Orthop Trauma. 2001;15(7):468–74.
18. Filiberto D, Fox A. Preperitoneal pelvic packing: technique and outcomes. Int J Surg. 2016;33(Pt B):222–4. https://doi.org/10.1016/j.ijsu.2016.05.072.
19. Gao H, Luo C, Chen J, Zhou K, Zeng B. Control of severe pelvic fracture hemorrhage with pelvic packing. Chin J Traumatol. 2008;11:120–2.
20. Jang J, Shim H, Jung P, Kim S, Bae K. Preperitoneal pelvic packing in patients with hemodynamic instability due to severe pelvic fracture: early experience in a Korean trauma center. Scand J Trauma Resusc Emerg Med. 2016;24:3. https://doi.org/10.1186/s13049-016-0196-5.
21. Li Q, Dong J, Yang Y, Wang G, Wang Y, Liu P, Robinson Y, Zhou D. Retroperitoneal packing or angioembolization for haemorrhage control of pelvic fractures—quasi-randomized clinical trial of 56 haemodynamically unstable patients with injury severity score ≥33. Injury. 2016;47:395–401.
22. Lustenberger T, Meier C, Benninger E, Lenzlinger P, Keel M. C-clamp and pelvic packing for control of hemorrhage in patients with pelvic ring disruption. J Emerg Trauma Shock. 2011;4:477–82.
23. Osborn P, Smith W, Moore E, Clothren C, Morgan S, Williams A, Stahel P. Direct retroperitoneal pelvic packing versus pelvic angiography: a comparison of two management protocols for haemodynamically unstable pelvic fractures. Injury. 2009;40:54–60.
24. Papakostidis C, Giannoudis P. Pelvic ring injuries with haemodynamic instability: efficacy of pelvic packing, a systematic review. Injury. 2009;40:53–61.
25. Pohlemann T, Culemann U, Gänsslen A, Tscherne H. Die schwere Beckenverletzung mit pelviner Massenblutung: Ermittlung der Blutungsschwere und klinische Erfahrung mit der Notfallstabilisierung. Unfallchirurg. 1996;99(10):734–43.
26. Smith W, Moore E, Osborn P, Agudelo J, Morgan S, Parekh A, Cothren C. Retroperitoneal packing as a resuscitation technique for hemodynamically unstable patients with pelvic fractures: report of two representative cases and a description of technique. J Trauma. 2005;59:1510–4.
27. Söderlund T, Ketonen T, Handolin L. Bleeding pelvic fracture patients: evolution of resuscitation protocols. Scand J Surg. 2017;106:255–60.
28. Tesoriero R, Bruns B, Narayan M, Dubose J, Guliani S, Brenner M, Boswell S, Stein D, Scalea T. Angiographic embolization for hemorrhage following pelvic fracture: is it "time" for a paradigm shift? J Trauma Acute Care Surg. 2017;82:18–26.
29. Tötterman A, Madsen J, Skaga N, Røise O. Extraperitoneal pelvic packing: a salvage procedure to control massive traumatic pelvic hemorrhage. J Trauma. 2007;62:843–52.
30. Tscherne H, Pohlemann T, Gansslen A, Hufner T, Pape HC. Crush injuries of the pelvis. Eur J Surg. 2000;166(4):276–82.
31. Huittinen V, Slätis P. Postmortem angiography and dissection of the hypogastric artery in pelvic fractures. Surgery. 1973;73:454–62.
32. Blackmore C, Cummings P, Jurkovich G, Linnau K, Hoffer E, Rivara F. Predicting major hemorrhage in patients with pelvic fracture. J Trauma. 2006;61:346–52.
33. Schmal H, Markmiller M, Mehlhorn A, Sudkamp N. Epidemiology and outcome of complex pelvic injury. Acta Orthop Belg. 2005;71:41–7.
34. Hussami M, Grabherr S, Meuli R, Schmidt S. Severe pelvic injury: vascular lesions detected by ante- and post-mortem contrast medium-enhanced CT and associations with pelvic fractures. Int J Legal Med. 2017;131:731–8.
35. Suzuki T, Smith W, Moore E. Pelvic packing or angiography: competitive or complementary? Injury. 2009;40:343–53.
36. Rothenberger D, Fischer R, Perry J. Major vascular injuries secondary to pelvic fractures: an unsolved clinical problem. Am J Surg. 1978;136:660–2.
37. Baqué P, Trojani C, Delotte J, Séjor E, Senni-Buratti M, de Baqué F, Bourgeon A. Anatomical consequences of "open-book" pelvic ring disruption: a cadaver experimental study. Surg Radiol Anat. 2005;27:487–90.
38. Kataoka Y, Maekawa K, Nishimaki H, Yamamoto S, Soma K. Iliac vein injuries in hemodynamically unstable patients with pelvic fracture caused by blunt trauma. J Trauma. 2005;58:704–8.
39. Ksycki M, Ruiz G, Perez-Alonso A, Sciarretta J, Gonzalo R, Iglesias E, Gigena A, Vu T, Asensio J. Iliac vessel injuries: difficult injuries and difficult management problems. Eur J Trauma Emerg Surg. 2012;38:347–57.

40. Moss M, Bircher M. Volume changes within the true pelvis dirung disruption of the pelvic ring—where does the hemorrhage go? Injury. 1996;Suppl. 1(Part 1):21–3.
41. Grimm M, Vrahas M, Thomas K. Pressure-volume characteristics of the intact and disrupted pelvic retroperitoneum. J Trauma. 1998;44(3):454–9.
42. Köhler D, Sellei R, Sop A, Tarkin I, Pfeifer R, Garrison R, Pohlemann T, Pape H. Effects of pelvic volume changes on retroperitoneal and intra-abdominal pressure in the injured pelvic ring: a cadaveric model. J Trauma. 2011;71:585–90.
43. Kellam J. The role of external fixation in pelvic disruptions. Clin Orthop. 1989;241:66–82.
44. Riemer B, Butterfield S, Diamond D, Young J, Raves J, Cottington E, Kislan K. Acute mortality associated with injuries to the pelvic ring: the role of early mobilization and external fixation. J Trauma. 1993;35(5):671–7.
45. Trentz O, Bühren V, Friedl H. Beckenverletzungen. Chirurg. 1989;60:639–48.
46. Sato Y, Sekine K, Shibusawa T, Tajima K, Sasaki J, Imanishi N, Aiso S, Hori S. Effect of retroperitoneal pelvic packing on pelvic cavity pressure: a cadaveric study. Orthopedics. 2017;40:947–51.
47. Gänsslen A, Hildebrand F, Pohlemann T. Management of hemodynamic unstable patients "in extremis" with pelvic ring fractures. Acta Chir Orthop Traumatol Cechoslov. 2012;79:193–202.
48. Gänsslen A, Hildebrand F, Krettek C. Supraacetabular external fixation for pain control in geriatric type B pelvic injuries. Acta Chir Orthop Traumatol Cechoslov. 2013;80:101–5.
49. Gänsslen A, Krettek C, Pohlemann T. Emergency stabilization of pelvic instabilities with the pelvic C-clamp. Oper Orthop Traumatol. 2004;16:192–204.
50. Bottlang M, Simpson T, Sigg J, Krieg JC, Madey SM, Long WB. Noninvasive reduction of open-book pelvic fractures by circumferential compression. J Orthop Trauma. 2002;16(6):367–73.
51. Eastridge B, Starr A, Minei J, O'Keefe G, Scalea T. The importance of fracture pattern in guiding therapeutic decision-making in patients with hemorrhagic shock and pelvic ring disruptions. J Trauma. 2002;53:446–50.
52. Shapiro M, McDonald A, Knight D, Johannigman J, Cuschieri J. The role of repeat angiography in the management of pelvic fractures. J Trauma. 2005;58:227–31.
53. Lustenberger T, Wutzler S, Störmann P, Marzi I. The role of pelvic packing for hemodynamically unstable pelvic ring injuries. Clin Med Insight Trauma Intens Med. 2015;6:1–8. https://doi.org/10.4137/CMTIM.S12257.
54. Marzi I, Lustenberger T. Management of Bleeding Pelvic Fractures. Scand J Surg. 2014;103:104–11.
55. Ron G, Epstein D, Ben-Galim P, Klein Y, Kaban A, Sagiv S. Extraperitoneal pressure packing without external pelvic fixation: a life-saving stand-alone surgical treatment. J Emerg Trauma Shock. 2015;8:181–7.
56. Glass N, Burlew C. Preperitoneal pelvic packing: how and when. Curr Trauma Rep. 2015;1:1–7.
57. Cox S, Westgarth-Taylor C, Dix-Peek S, Millar A. Pre-peritoneal pelvic packing in a paediatric unstable pelvic fracture: an undescribed complication of lower limb compartment syndrome. Injury. 2013;44:258–60.
58. Burlew C. Preperitoneal pelvic packing for exsanguinating pelvic fractures. Int Orthop. 2017;41:1825–9.
59. Cullinane D, Schiller H, Zielinski M, Bilaniuk J, Collier B, Como J, Holevar M, Sabater E, Sems S, Vassy W, Wynne J. Eastern Association for the Surgery of trauma practice management guidelines for hemorrhage in pelvic fracture—update and systematic review. J Trauma. 2011;71:1850–68.
60. Heng M. Acute pelvic packing. Oper Tech Orthop. 2015;25:256–61.
61. Voiglio E, Dubuisson V, Massalou D, Baudoin Y, Caillot J, Létoublon C, Arvieux C. Place et technique de la laparotomie écourtée (LAPEC) ou damage control laparotomy. J Visc Surg. 2016;153:13–24.
62. Bach A, Bendix J, Hougaard K, Frischknecht Christensen E. Retroperitoneal packing as part of damage control surgery in a Danish trauma Centre—fast, effective, and cost-effective. Scand J Trauma Resuscitation Emerg Med. 2008;16(4):1–4.
63. Tai D, Li W, Lee K, Cheng M, Lee K, Tang L, Lai A, Ho H, Cheung M. Retroperitoneal pelvic packing in the management of hemodynamically unstable pelvic fractures: a level I trauma center experience. J Trauma. 2011;71(4):E79–86.
64. Froberg L, Helgstrand F, Clausen C, Steinmetz J, Eckardt H. Mortality in trauma patients with active arterial bleeding managed by embolization or surgical packing: an observational cohort study of 66 patients. J Emerg Trauma Shock. 2016;9:107–14.
65. Hou Z, Smith W, Strohecker K, Bowen T, Irgit K, Baro S, Morgan S. Hemodynamically unstable pelvic fracture management by advanced trauma life support guidelines results in high mortality. Orthopedics. 2012;35:e319–24.

Direct Hemorrhage Control: Vascular DC-Treatment

13

Jan Lindahl and Axel Gänsslen

Bleeding from major vessels inside the false and true pelvis can be dramatic, with the potential risk of whole blood loss.

Therefore, basic knowledge of vascular damage control procedures and vascular access is of major importance in dealing with patients in extremis and pelvic ring instabilities.

The pelvic surgeons should be familiar with the following procedures until a vascular surgeon is available:

- DC approach to the common femoral artery
- DC approach to the iliac external artery and vein
- DC approach to the common and internal iliac artery and vein

13.1 DC Approach to the Common Femoral Artery

The femoral artery is approached in the femoral triangle, which is bordered by the inguinal ligament (superior), the adductor longus muscle (medial) and the sartorius muscle (lateral).

The Damage-Control approach starts with a longitudinal incision lateral to the vessels, which are expected slightly medial to the midline of the inguinal ligament with its palpable origin and insertion points: ASIS and pubic tubercle (Fig. 13.1).

The incision starts slightly above the inguinal ligament and is directed distally approximately 10 cm (Fig. 13.1). After dissecting the subcutaneous fat, near the inguinal ligament, the superficial epigastric vein is usually transsected. After sharp opening of the fascia at the medial border of the sartorius muscle, dissection is performed medial to the vessels until reaching the artery and vein (Fig. 13.2). The lymphatics should be protected, alternatively, they can be ligated to protect against lymphatic fistula. In the emergency situation, this is of minor initial importance.

Typically, even in an arterial injury, the artery can be easily palpated or the injury is directly visualized.

Exposure of the artery near the inguinal ligament allows for proximal vascular control. The femoral circumflex vessels arise lateral to the common branch and inferior epigastric arteries medially.

The common femoral artery bifurcates in direct continuation into the superficial femoral artery (SFA) and further on into 1–2 deep femoral arteries. The SFA runs deep to the sartorius muscle. The profunda femoral arteries exit the common femoral artery lateral into the thigh muscles.

Arterial damage control is performed by direct clamping, followed by direct repair or more often by vascular grafts.

In venous injuries, the extremely fragile vessel wall, the tendency to develop thrombosis and the short time window for relevant blood loss have to be respected. Vein injuries should be primarily treated by digital compression. Clamps should be used with caution, as these can increase the extent of injury.

In the absence of vascular-surgical expertise, under triage conditions, shunting for temporary reperfusion of the limb is considered an alternative [1–7].

Historically, ligation of the common femoral artery results in unacceptable high amputation rates [8]. Recent experience stated that amputation should be an exception [9–11].

This approach can be extended cranially to reach the iliac external artery and vein [12].

The incision is then extended in a hockey-stick-shape to an extraperitoneal approach to these vessels. A lateral curved extension is made reaching the level above the iliac crest.

J. Lindahl
Orthopaedics and Trauma Surgery, Helsinki University Hospital, Helsinki, Finland

A. Gänsslen (✉)
Department of Trauma Surgery, Orthopedics and Hand Surgery, Hospital Wolfsburg, Wolfsburg, Germany

A. Gänsslen et al. (eds.), *Pelvic Ring Fractures*, https://doi.org/10.1007/978-3-030-54730-1_13

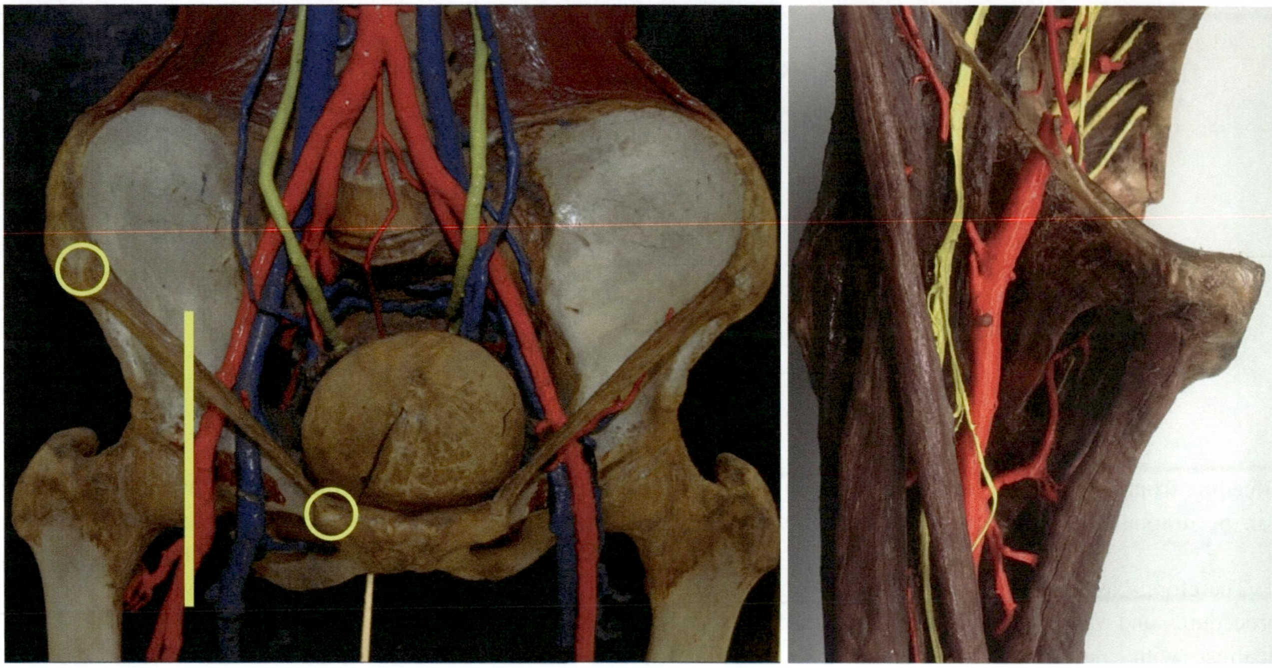

Fig. 13.1 Landmarks an incision for the direct access to the femoral artery

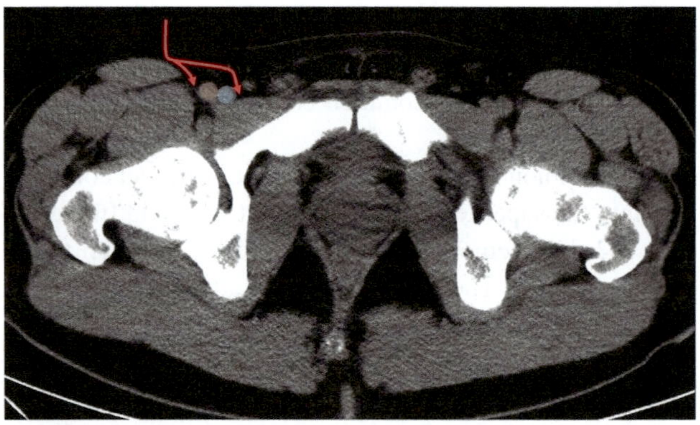

Fig. 13.2 Dissection medial to the sartorius muscle

13.2 DC Approach to the External Iliac Artery and Vein

In patients with injuries of the external iliac artery, ligation can be performed, if the homolateral internal iliac artery is intact [13]. Venous injuries can be either reconstructed or ligated. After reconstruction, venous size narrowing requires direct postoperative anticoagulation therapy.

The approach to the iliac external vessels is the classical extraperitoneal approach, which can be an extension of the vertical approach to the femoral artery.

This extraperitoneal approach is favored [14].

The 10–15 cm long skin incision is made parallel and superior to the inguinal ligament in line with the expected fibers of the external oblique muscle, starting at the ASIS and reaching the lateral border of the rectus abdominis muscle (Fig. 13.3). The superficial epigastric vessels may be ligated [15].

Near the midline, the incision runs lateral to the internal inguinal ring to avoid injury to the spermatic cord structures. After dissection of the subcutaneous fat and tissues, the external oblique aponeurosis is split and the peritoneum is exposed after mobilizing the internal oblique and transversus muscles and lateral opening of the transversalis fascia (Fig. 13.4). The peritoneum is identified and bluntly separated from the extraperitoneal fat and the anterior abdominal wall using a sponge stick [15]. The peritoneum and ureter are reflected medially.

The iliac vessels are then easily exposed (Fig. 13.5). The vein is found posterior and medial to the artery. They are mobilized and controlled using slings by passing a curved (Lahey) forceps around the vessel from medial to lateral [12, 15].

Proximal and distal extension is possible by either retracting the peritoneal sac superior and medially, while caudally retracting the inferior wound margin [15].

Considering the pelvic or acetabular bony injury, the Pararectus approach might be an alternative to address these vessels. This approach allows either primary or secondary treatment of accompanying pelvic ring or acetabular fracture fixation.

The incision is slightly more oblique and starts approximately 3–5 cm medial to the ASIS at the junction of the lateral and the middle third of the connecting line of the umbilicus and the ASIS (Fig. 13.6). The incision runs in a

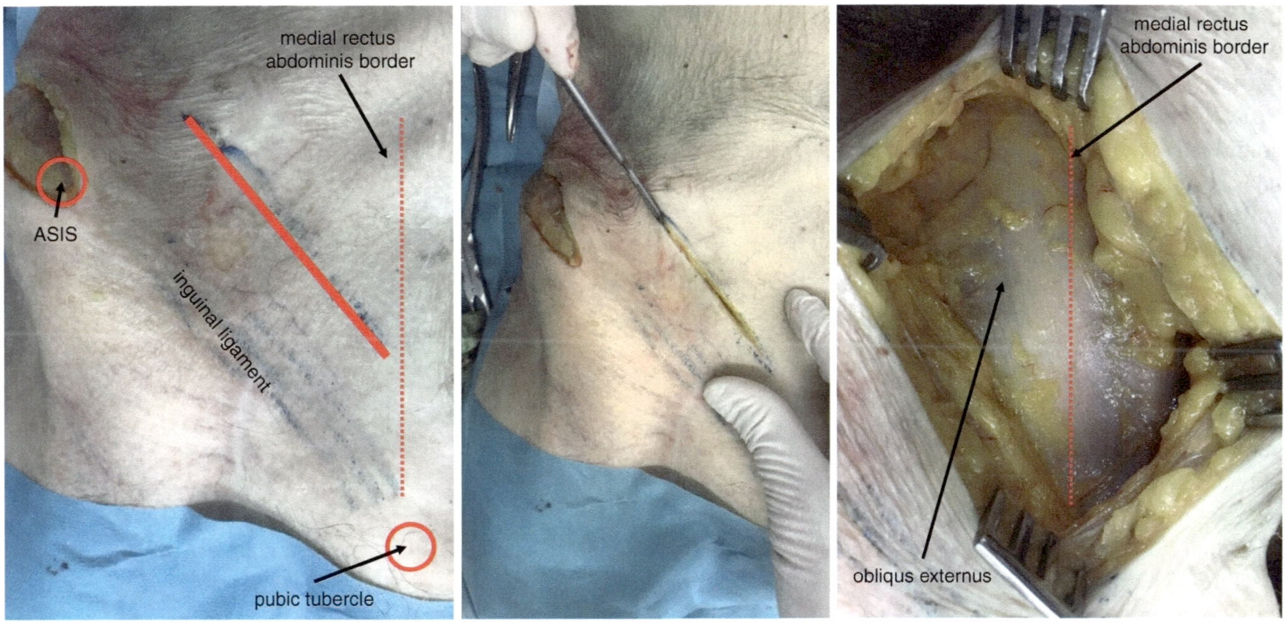

Fig. 13.3 Landmarks, incision and superficial dissection parallel to the inguinal ligament

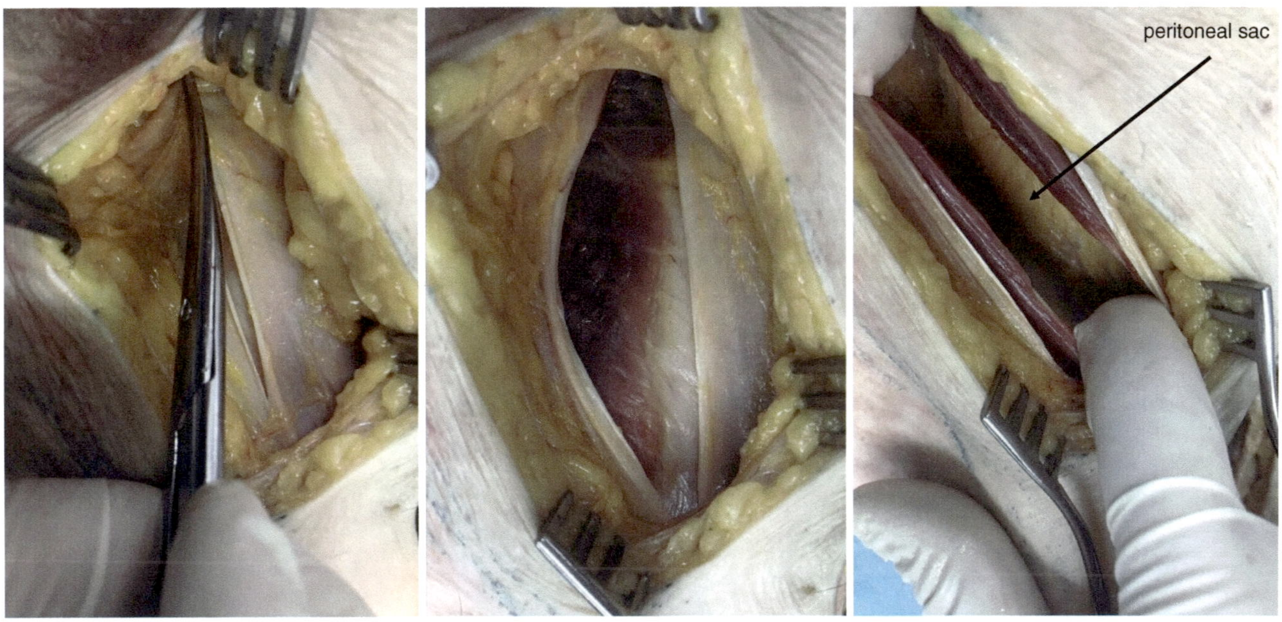

Fig. 13.4 Splitting the external oblique aponeurosis identification and mobilization of the transversus muscle and lateral opening of the transversalis fascia

curve to the junction of the middle and the medial third of a line connecting the ASIS with the symphysis [16].

After subcutaneous dissection, the anterior abdominal fascia is incised in line with the skin incision.

The rectus sheath is incised and the muscle belly is mobilized medially to identify the transversalis fascia, which is incised longitudinally. Perforation of the parietal peritoneum is avoided. With the peritoneum mobilized and retracted craniomedially within the lateral retroperitoneum, the external iliac artery and vein are identified and mobilized as described. This dissection is identical to the described technique (Fig. 13.7). Laterally, the iliopsoas muscle is visualized.

Here, the ilioinguinal, femoral, lateral cutaneous femoral and genitofemoral nerves are protected. Proximal extension of the skin incision allows identification of the SI joint with the lumbosacral trunk (not needed in DC-situation) (Fig. 13.8). Medial mobilization allows for even identification of the common iliac vessels (Fig. 13.9).

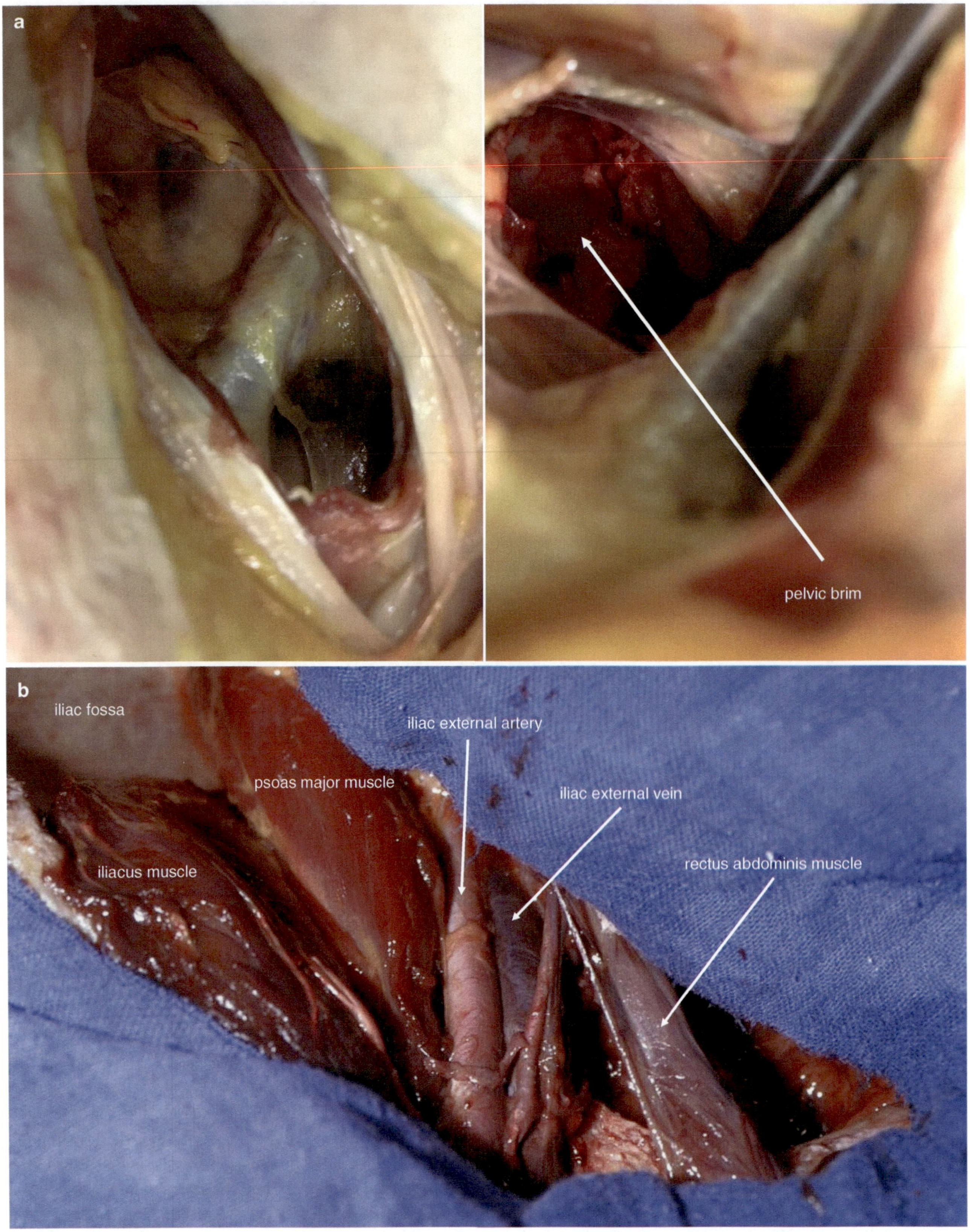

Fig. 13.5 (**a**) After medialization of the peritoneal sac, the iliac vessels are easily identified. By mobilizing the vessels medially, the pelvic brim can be visualized. (**b**) Dissection view of the iliac external vessels

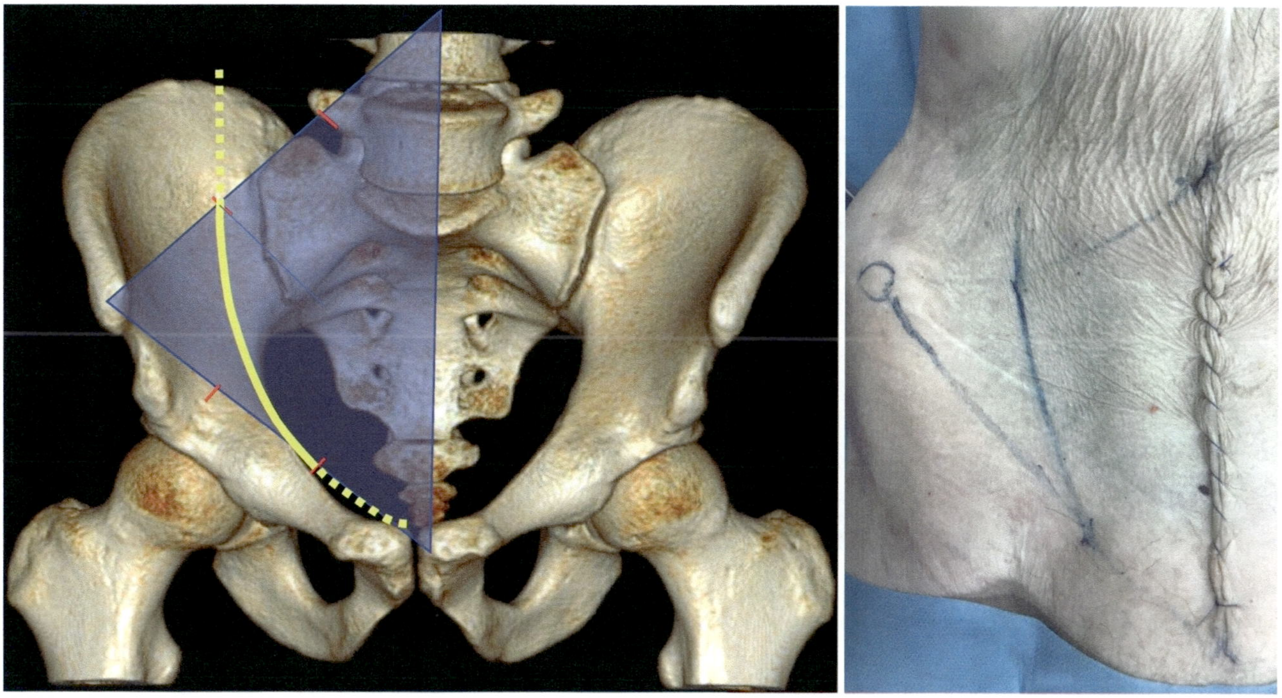

Fig. 13.6 Landmarks and marked skin incision for the Pararectus approach

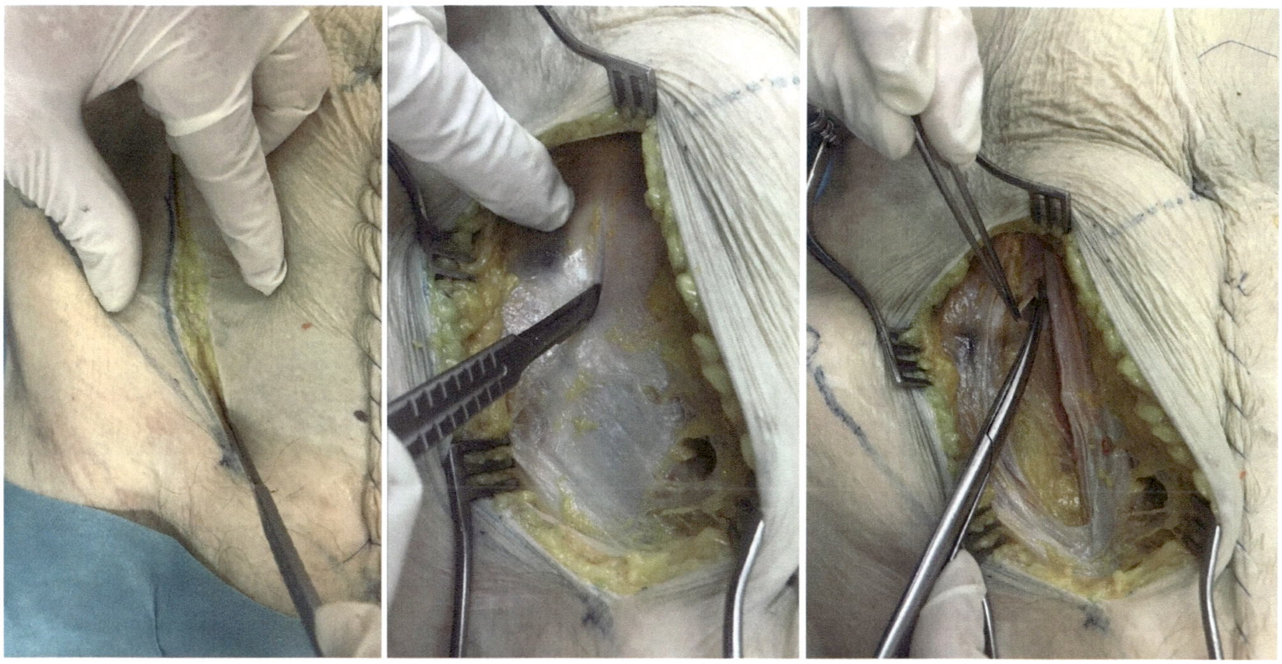

Fig. 13.7 Superficial dissection until reaching the peritoneal sac medially

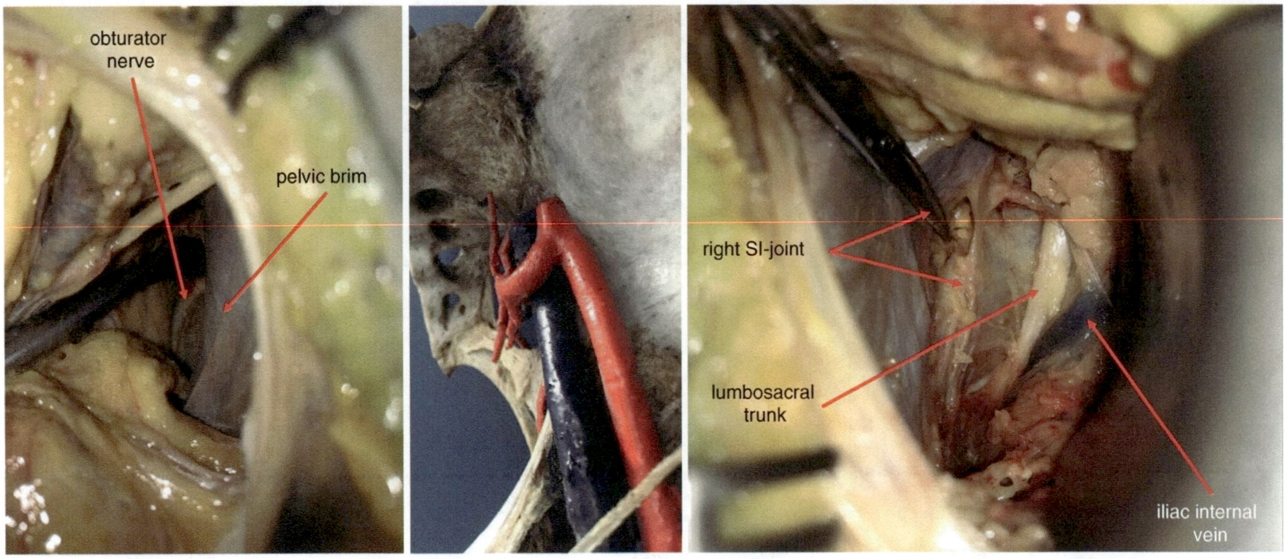

Fig. 13.8 Mobilization of the iliac external vessels medially. Identification of the periacetabular pelvic brim and proximally the SI joint with the anterior neurovascular structures including the iliac internal vessels

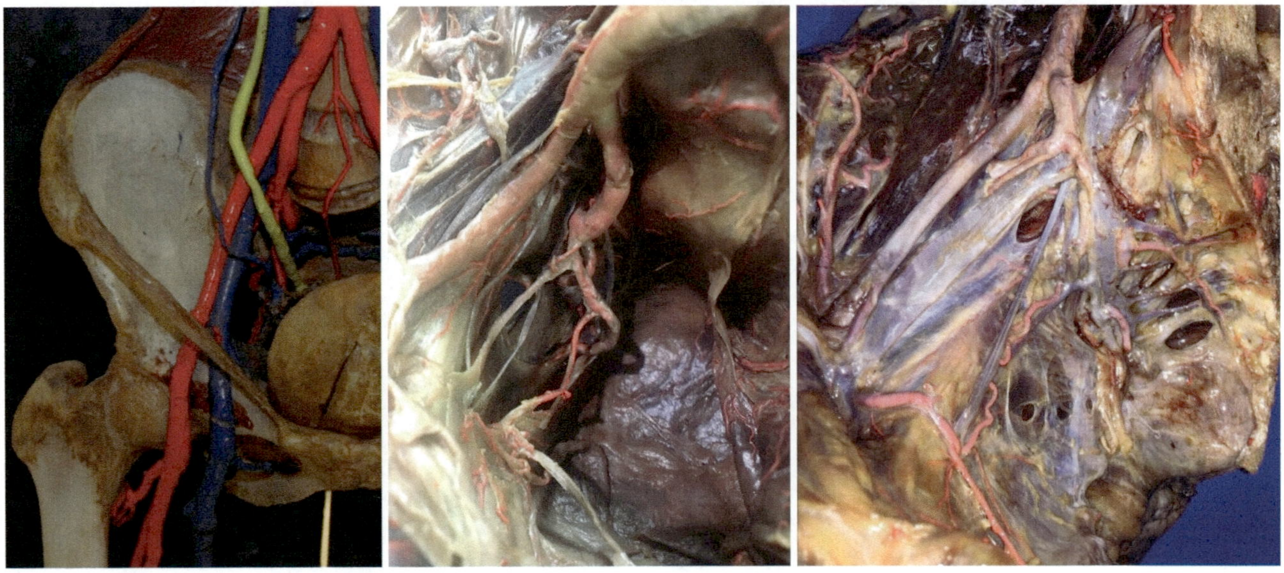

Fig. 13.9 Anatomy of the common, external, and internal iliac vessels in relation to the sacral area. Medial mobilization of the iliac external vessels allows for identification of the iliac internal and common iliac vessels from lateral

13.3 DC Approach to the Common and Internal Iliac Artery and Vein

According to recent guidelines, treatment of common iliac artery injuries consists of emergency shunting or direct suturing with an end-to-end anastomosis or alternatively insertion of a saphenous vein or PTFE graft [13]. Ligation leads to limb ischemia. Venous injuries can be either reconstructed or ligated. After reconstruction, venous size narrowing requires direct postoperative anticoagulation therapy.

A transabdominal approach is favored, as often accompanying intra-abdominal injuries and injuries to major distal abdominal vessels are present.

A classical damage control laparotomy approach is used to reach even the distal aorta and the hypogastric artery. Palpation of the sacral promontory and visualization of an imaginary line between both ASIS led to identify the expected location of the common iliac artery bifurcation.

A longitudinal incision into the posterior parietal peritoneum is performed directly over the bifurcation. The course of the ureter has to be respected, which runs from lateral to medial, crossing the common iliac artery.

The common and internal iliac arteries are in close relationship to the underlying veins, which are in danger to injury, which can result in catastrophic bleeding.

Meticulous dissection with scissors is required to separate the internal iliac vein from the artery if they are adherent [14]. Immediate bleeding control is performed by local compression using fingers or packing.

Temporary shunting should be considered if vascular surgical experience is minor.

13.4 Conclusion

Some basic knowledge on vascular approaches to the intrapelvic major vessels is helpful in treating patients with pelvic ring injuries, which are hemodynamically unstable.

References

1. Abou Ali A, Salem K, Alarcon L, Bauza G, Pikoulis E, Chaer R, Avgerinos E. Vascular shunts in civilian trauma. Front Surg. 2017;4:39. https://doi.org/10.3389/fsurg.2017.00039. eCollection 2017
2. Feliciano D, Subramanian A. Temporary vascular shunts. Eur J Trauma Emerg Surg. 2013;39:553–60.
3. Gifford S, Aidinian G, Clouse W, Fox C, Porras C, Jones W, Zarzabal L, Michalek J, Propper B, Burkhardt G, Rasmussen T. Effect of temporary shunting on extremity vascular injury: an outcome analysis from the Global War on Terror vascular injury initiative. J Vasc Surg. 2009;50:549–55.
4. Hornez E, Boddaert G, Ngabou U, Aguir S, Baudoin Y, Mocellin N, Bonnet S. Temporary vascular shunt for damage control of extremity vascular injury: a toolbox for trauma surgeons. J Visc Surg. 2015;152:363–8.
5. Inaba K, Aksoy H, Seamon M, Marks J, Duchesne J, Schroll R, Fox C, Pieracci F, Moore E, Joseph B, Haider A, Harvin J, Lawless R, Cannon J, Holland S, Demetriades D, M.S.S. Group. Multicenter evaluation of temporary intravascular shunt use in vascular trauma. J Trauma Acute Care Surg. 2016;80:359–64.
6. Oliver J, Gill H, Nicol A, Edu S, Navsaria P. Temporary vascular shunting in vascular trauma: a 10-year review from a civilian trauma centre. S Afr J Surg. 2013;51:6–10.
7. Rasmussen T, Clouse W, Jenkins D, Peck M, Eliason J, Smith D. The use of temporary vascular shunts as a damage control adjunct in the management of wartime vascular injury. J Trauma. 2006;61:8–12.
8. Newton E, Arora S. Chapter 48: Peripheral vascular injury. In: Marx JA, Hockberger RS, Walls RM, editors. Rosen's emergency medicine—concepts and clinical practice. Philadelphia: Saunders; 2013.
9. Fox C, Gillespie D, O'Donnell S, Rasmussen T, Goff J, Johnson C, Galgon R, Sarac T, Rich N. Contemporary management of wartime vascular trauma. J Vasc Surg. 2005;41:638–44.
10. Peck M, Clouse W, Cox M, Bowser A, Eliason J, Jenkins D, Smith D, Rasmussen T. The complete management of extremity vascular injury in a local population: a wartime report from the 332nd Expeditionary Medical Group/AirForce Theater Hospital, balad air base. Iraq J Vasc Surg. 2007;45:1197–205.
11. Taller J, Kamdar J, Greene J, Morgan R, Blankenship C, Dabrowski P, Sharpe R. Temporary vascular shunts as initial treatment of proximal extremity vascular injuries during combat operations: the new standard of care at Echelon II facilities? J Trauma. 2008;65:595–601.
12. Brohi K. Extraperitoneal approach to the iliac vessels. www.trauma.org; 7:12, December 2002. 2002.
13. Pereira B, Chiara O, Ramponi F, Weber D, Cimbanassi S, De Simone B, Musicki K, Meirelles G, Catena F, Ansaloni L, Coccolini F, Sartelli M, Di Saverio S, Bendinelli C, Fraga G. WSES position paper on vascular emergency surgery. World J Emerg Surg. 2015;10:49. https://doi.org/10.1186/s13017-015-0037-2. eCollection 2015
14. B-Lynch C, Keith L, Campbell W. Chapter 52: Internal iliac (hypogastric) artery ligation. In: B-Lynch C, Keith L, Lalonde A, Karoshi M, editors. A textbook of postpartum hemorrhage. Jerusalem: Sapiens Publishing; 2006.
15. Radowsky J, Rodriguez C, Wind G, Elster E. A surgeon's guide to obtaining hemorrhage control in combat-related dismounted lower extremity blast injuries. Mil Med. 2016;181:1300–4.
16. Keel M, Ecker T, Cullmann J, Bergmann M, Bonel H, Büchler L, Siebenrock K, Bastian J. The Pararectus approach for anterior intrapelvic management of acetabular fractures: an anatomical study and clinical evaluation. J Bone Joint Surg (Br). 2012;94:405–11.

14 Emergency Management: Resuscitative Endovascular Balloon Occlusion of the Aorta (REBOA)

Axel Gänsslen and Jan Lindahl

Pelvic bleeding, abdominal and thoracic bleeding are summarized under noncompressible torso hemorrhage (NCTH). These bleeding sources are still leading causes of early deaths among trauma patients and, therefore, preventable trauma deaths in civilian trauma [1].

For a long time, arrest of the arterial inflow into the pelvic area was considered an option for emergency pelvic bleeding control. The principle options described were ligation of the hypogastric artery and occlusion of the aorta by temporary clamping during emergency laparotomy [2, 3].

Clinical experience showed that ligation of the hypogastric artery was not associated with satisfactory reduction of pelvic area bleeding due to the remarkable collateral supply within the [4–8].

Occlusion of the aorta has been described as a temporary measure to control catastrophic hemorrhage. It was often performed by direct, open infrarenal or thoracic cross-clamping [9].

The concept of percutaneous Resuscitative Endovascular Balloon Occlusion of the Aorta (REBOA) was already introduced in the mid-1950s for control of dramatic intra-abdominal hemorrhage [10]. This concept was used to control excessive retroperitoneal hemorrhage or penetrating injuries [11, 12].

Bühren first described this technique for hemodynamically unstable patients with pelvic fractures [13]. Pelvic bleeding belongs to the Zone 3 of noncompressible torso hemorrhage from the lowest renal artery to the aortic bifurcation [14].

Today, REBOA is considered a temporary method for truncal bleeding control within the first 30–60 min, until definitive surgical hemostasis is possible [15].

Even in the prehospital setting, this procedure was already considered an option [16].

Overall, present data support REBOA over DC thoracotomy with open aortic cross-clamping with a positive effect on mortality [17].

14.1 REBOA Principle

Two main principles are the basis for REBOA [18]:

- Assisted resuscitation with temporary restoration of aortic blood pressure in noncompressible truncal hemorrhage of the chest, abdomen, and/or pelvis until damage control resuscitation procedures (DC resuscitation, DC surgery) can be definitively performed.
- Emergent maintenance of cerebral and myocardial organ perfusion to allow temporal correction of physiologic coagulation and blood volume abnormalities until surgical hemostasis is achieved.

14.2 REBOA-Technique

The technique of REBOA is described in detail and can, therefore, be easily performed. It follows a standardized step-by-step concept [14]:

- Arterial access
- Balloon selection and positioning
- Balloon inflation
- Balloon deflation
- Sheath removal

A. Gänsslen (✉)
Department of Trauma Surgery, Orthopedics and Hand Surgery, Hospital Wolfsburg, Wolfsburg, Germany

J. Lindahl
Orthopaedics and Trauma Surgery, Helsinki University Hospital, Helsinki, Finland

A. Gänsslen et al. (eds.), *Pelvic Ring Fractures*, https://doi.org/10.1007/978-3-030-54730-1_14

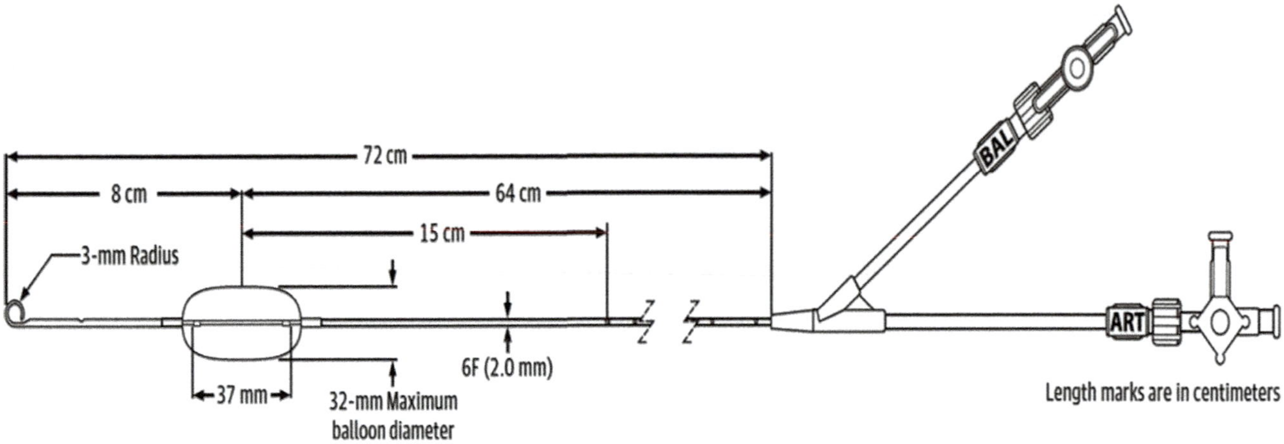

Fig. 14.1 Schematic drawing of the REBOA-catheter (from [19])

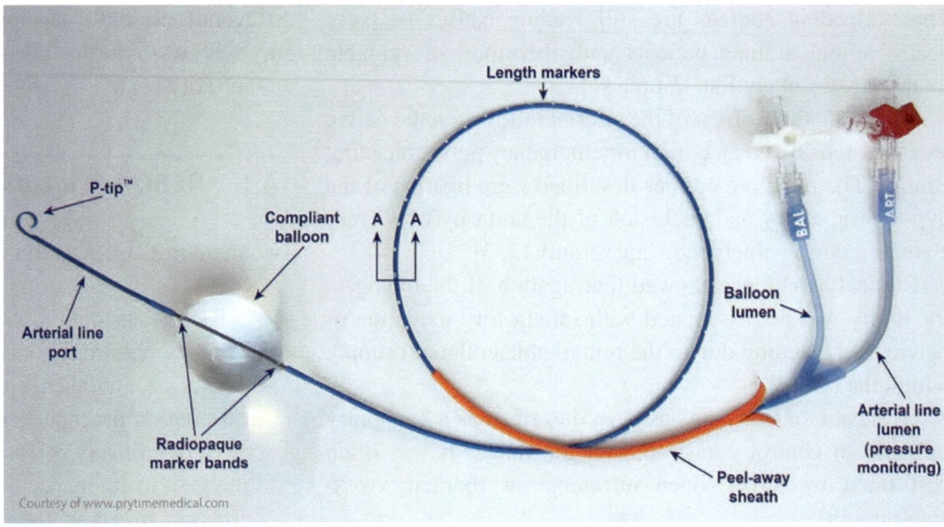

Fig. 14.2 REBOA-catheter (from [20]; courtesy of www.prytimemedical.com)

14.3 Materials

A standardized set (REBOA-Kit) is necessary for application, including an "introducer", special sheaths, Seldinger wires, occlusive balloon catheter and a surgical set for vessel exposure and fixation of the catheter (Figs. 14.1 and 14.2). Additionally, sterile drapes, syringes, and sutures are supplemented.

The present standard is a wire-related REBOA-technique. Recently, even wireless techniques were introduced with acceptable and comparable results [21].

14.4 Prerequisites

A pelvic a.p. X-ray is a prerequisite for REBOA application to analyze relevant fractures in the area of the chosen femoral artery together with clinical analysis of peripheral pulses to exclude relevant pelvic arterial injury at the chosen approach.

In cases where a pelvic binder is already in place, removal depends on the decision of the trauma team leader. Pelvic binders, which allow a local opening without influencing the binder stability, are advantageous [22].

14.5 Indications

In a French analysis, REBOA indications were "patients in extremis" with extreme hemodynamic instability (systolic arterial blood pressure <60 mmHg on admission, persistent systolic arterial blood pressure <90 mmHg despite initial resuscitation, post-traumatic cardiac arrest and a positive pelvic X-ray [23]).

14.6 Vascular Approach

The standard approach for REBOA application in pelvic fracture bleeding is via the femoral artery.

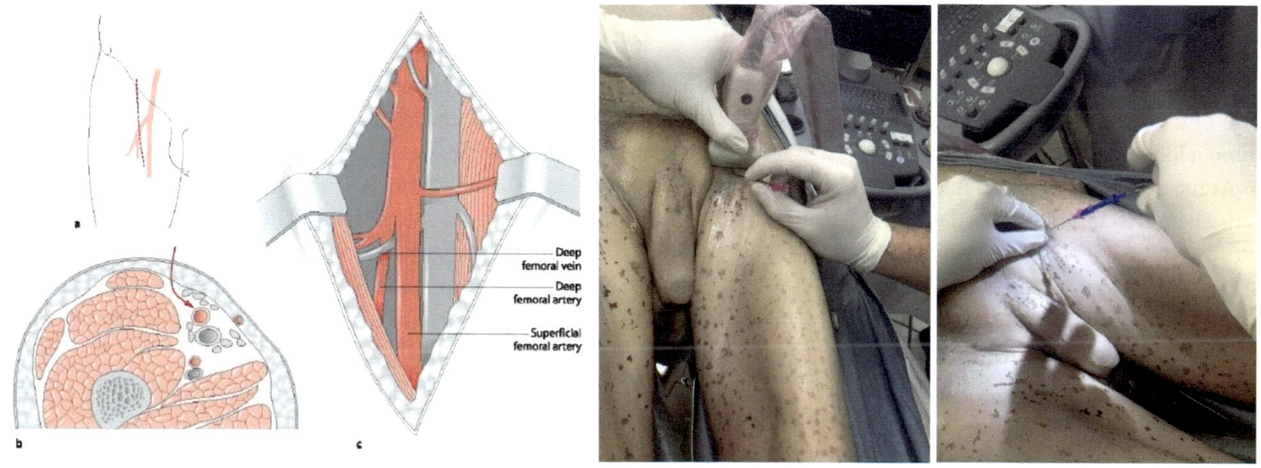

Fig. 14.3 Open (*) and percutaneous vascular access to the femoral artery for REBOA application (*: Fig. from Eric Wahlberg, Pär Olofsson, Jerry Goldstone (Ed.): Emergency Vascular Surgery—A Practical Guide, 2007 Springer, with permission)

Three possible approaches are reported accessing the femoral artery [14, 15]:

- Percutaneous (ultrasound-based) Seldinger technique approach (Fig. 14.3).
- Open arterial cut-down (Fig. 14.3).
- Exchange approach after already inserted arterial catheter (consider compatibility of Guidewires with sheath system).

In the emergency situation, insertion of the needle or guide can be performed without ultrasound support. Depending on the hemodynamic status, ultrasound-guided insertion is helpful, especially in hypotensive patients without palpable pulses.

14.7 Zones of Truncal Hemorrhage

Three zones of truncal hemorrhage are distinguished (Fig. 14.4):

- Zone I: origin of left subclavian artery to celiac artery.
- Zone II celiac artery to lowest renal artery (no-occlusion zone!)
- Zone III: lowest renal artery to aortic bifurcation.

In isolated pelvic injuries, after exclusion of additional intra-abdominal or intrathoracic bleeding sources with FAST examination and a chest X-ray (or even a CT examination, depending on the hemodynamic status) [24], only balloon positioning and aortic occlusion at the aortic bifurcation is sufficient.

In cases with combined pelvic and intra-abdominal bleeding, the balloon should be placed at zone I, whereas zone II positioning is contraindicated due to the risk of consecutive mesenteric ischemia, while occluding the celiac and superior mesenteric artery [14].

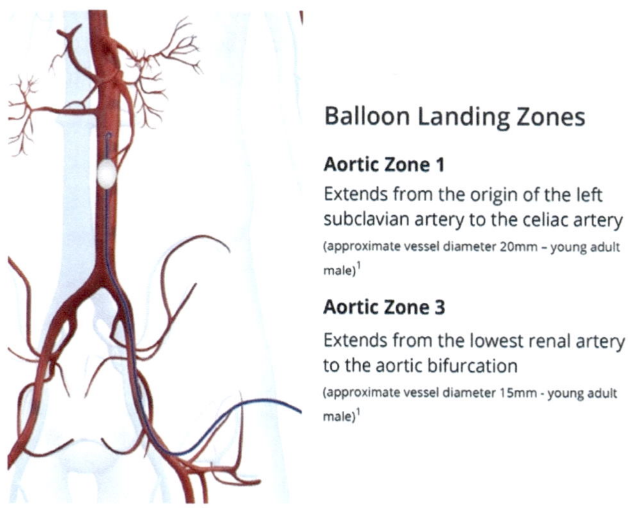

Fig. 14.4 Zones of truncal hemorrhage: zone I and III are relevant for REBOA application, while zone II should be avoided (courtesy of www.prytimemedical.com)

It is of practical relevance to distinguish the indications of these different zones, as in isolated pelvic fracture hemorrhage (zone III), small diameter balloons are sufficient, as the aortic bifurcation secures the balloon against pulsation [14].

In contrast, balloon positioning at zone I needs larger diameter balloons and a longer sheath (45–60 cm), which has to be guided up to the thoracic aorta.

14.8 Vascular Opening

The femoral artery is punctured with an appropriate needle and the starter wire is inserted. The wire should be passed forward without resistance. If a short sheath is chosen, it can be inserted without fluoroscopic guidance, whereas zone I sheaths should be inserted under fluoroscopic control.

If "rewiring" is considered with an existing arterial line, a wire of 2× the length of the existing arterial catheter is recommended [14].

At the completion, in isolated pelvic injuries, a 10–15 cm long sheath is inserted into the femoral and external iliac artery.

14.9 Interventional Landmarks

For optimal placement of the desired sheaths, identification of some anatomical landmarks is helpful for insertion (Fig. 14.5):

- Zone I: the sheath length is expected between the upper margin of the 12th rib and distal to the sterno-clavicular joint [14]; the balloon length can be estimated from the distance between the puncture site and the mid sternum [25] or should be shorter than the distance between the puncture site and the suprasternal notch and longer than the distance between the puncture site and the xiphoid [26]; radiographically, a zone I REBOA should be in place between the level of fourth and eleventh thoracic spine [27].
- Zone III: the balloon length can be estimated from the distance from the puncture site to the umbilicus; radiographic optimal balloon position is below the level of the second lumbar spine [27]; a position at the aortic bifurcation can be seen, as aortic pulsation pushes the balloon to the bifurcation [28].

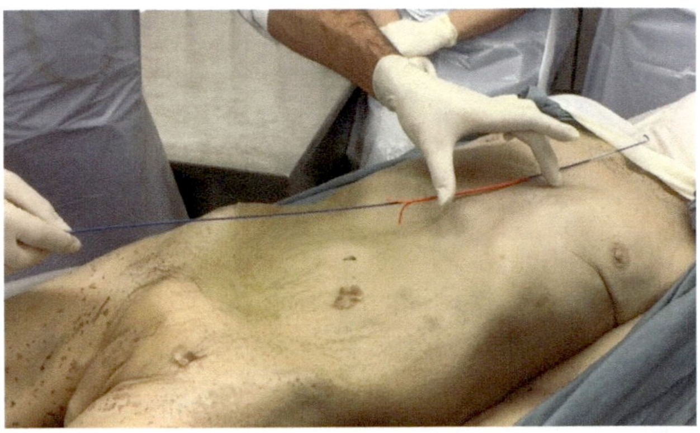

Fig. 14.5 Estimation of the catheter length

14.10 Balloon Insertion

The depth of balloon insertion depends on the hemorrhage zone:

- Zone I: a 260-cm long, 0.035-in. wire is inserted through the initial sheath (Fig. 14.6) and advanced to the chest area under fluoroscopic guidance until the tip is reaching the distal aortic arch; the depth of wire insertion should be controlled to avoid wire dislocation with potential subsequent injury to coronary or cerebral vessels; a sheath change is then performed over the wire (without wire dislocation) to a more larger and longer sheath for balloon insertion guided into the thoracic aorta; fluoroscopic evaluation is mandatory at this part of the procedure; the balloon is then advanced to the target area under fluoroscopic control (Fig. 14.7) [14].
- Zone III: the inserted sheath should be larger and shorter that the balloon reaches the inferior aorta under fluoroscopic visualization.

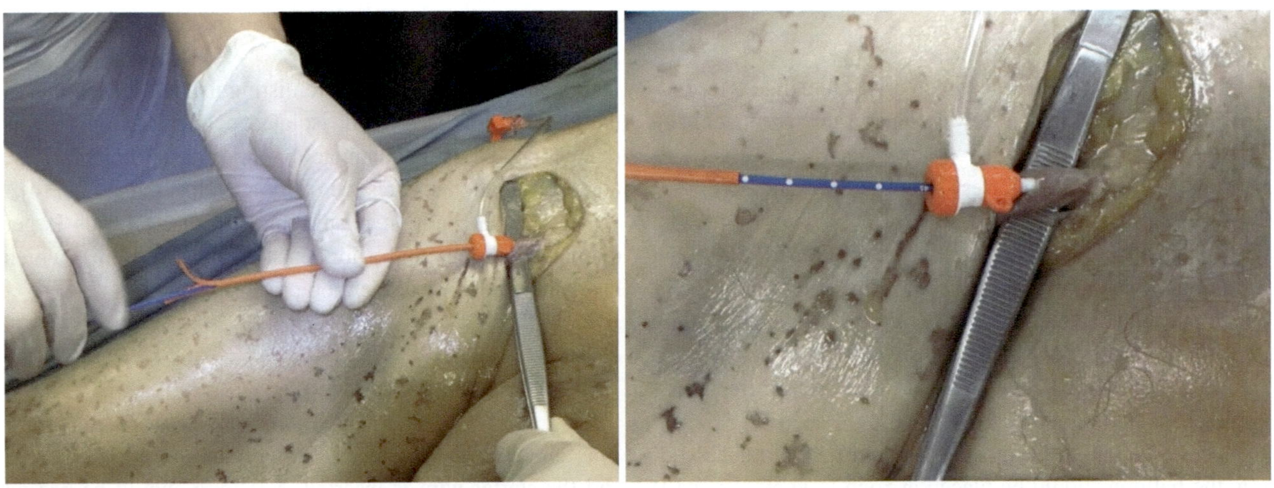

Fig. 14.6 REBOA-catheter insertion: 45 cm insertion for zone I application

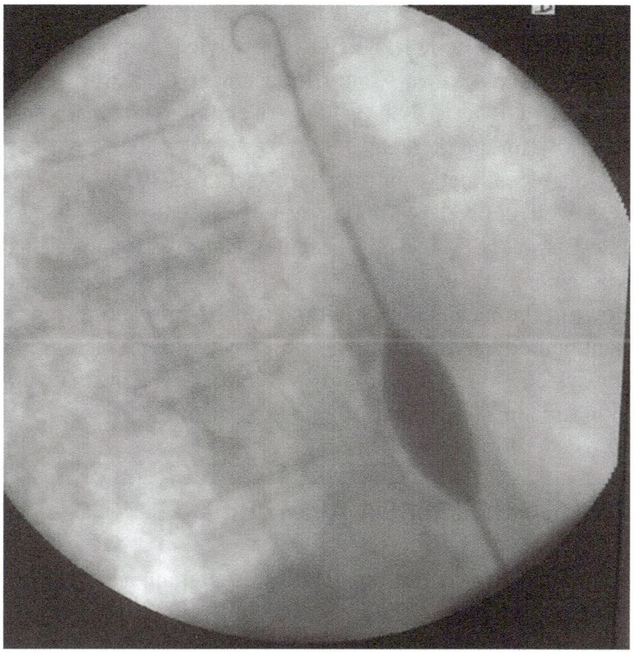

Fig. 14.7 Radiographic control of the balloon position after balloon filling with 4 mL of contrast media fluid

14.11 Balloon Inflation

During balloon inflation, the recommended volumes have to be considered:

- Zone I: the balloon is filled with approximately 8–9 mL sterile saline together with some contrast media, using a large-volume syringe and fluoroscopic control until the outer shape of the balloon changes from a convex orientation to a more parallel contouring; during the systole, a "mushroom cap" shape can be visible [14]; during this procedure, an assistant should hold the balloon, the sheath, and the wire in its adequate position; as with return of adequate blood pressure, there is a risk of caudal balloon migration.
- Zone III: smaller volumes are necessary for balloon filling (approximately 4–5 mL); after inflating the balloon under fluoroscopic guidance, the aortic pulsation often pushes the balloon to the bifurcation [28].

CAUTION: too heavy inflammation must be avoided, as it can result in aortic intima injury or even aortic rupture; clinically, invasively measured blood pressure distal to the balloon should show a loss of the pulsatile pressure curve [15].

14.12 Monitoring

During the whole procedure, the mean arterial pressure, the balloon position, and the maintenance of inflation should continuously be known and reported by an assistant.

Zone I balloons can also be monitored by TEE [15] or by ultrasound [29]; Zone III balloons are monitored by ultrasound [15]. The balloon can be additionally secured by sutures or an occlusive dressing [14].

14.13 Deflation

Deflation should be performed by the surgeon who inserted the balloon, while the assistant holds the balloon, sheath, and wire in its location [14].

CAUTION: deflation after prolonged balloon inflation or during incomplete resuscitation can lead to reperfusion injury due to washout of metabolic products and acidosis; a reperfusion syndrome can be expected when the patient presents with hypotension, hyperkalemia, and metabolic acidosis.

Thus, deflation should be performed in a slow and step-by-step manner. It was recommended to deflate the balloon ml per ml under hemodynamic reaction control or balloon opening over 5 min without increase of systolic blood pressure of more than 50% below the balloon level [15, 30].

Even using this concept, clinical reperfusion problems can be observed over 30 min after aortic opening [31]. Thus, all aspects of extended shock therapy should be available. Frequent periodical blood gas analyses, electrolyte evaluation, and ROTEM control of coagulopathy are recommended every 5–10 min after deflation [15].

Removal of the deflated balloon and the guide should be followed by flushing heparinized saline into the sheath. In large diameter sheaths, open surgical exposure of the femoral artery has to be considered for sheath removal, using a longitudinal or transverse groin incision. The resulting arteriotomy is sutured in a standardized way [14].

14.14 Complications

Local approach-related complications or balloon associated complications are rare and should be related to the positive hemodynamic effects, reported in the literature [20, 32–34]. Local complications included intracranial massive hemorrhage, arterial injury at the access site, renal failure, balloon migration, infections, retroperitoneal hematoma, and balloon rupture, all far below 1% [35].

Systemic complications are potentially a function of the occlusion time, as the potential injury-related consequences of the initial hemodynamic instability have to be considered. The "occlusion window" should be as short as possible.

The maximum occlusion time at zone I should be below 60–90 min, whereas, in Zone III, longer times can potentially be accepted [16, 18, 19, 36, 37].

To reduce the time window for definitive surgical bleeding control, Damage Control procedures should be performed already in the ED after REBOA-associated hemodynamic stabilization [15].

Recently, the concept of partial REBOA [30] (pREBOA) proved to extend occlusion times without negative effects on complications and mortality [34, 38–40].

14.15 Results of Pelvic REBOA

Martinelli et al. were the first to control relevant pelvic fracture bleeding by REBOA [28]. In 13 patients, after sufficient balloon placement, an average systolic blood pressure (SBP) increase of 70 mmHg was observed. The overall survival rate was 46%.

In 24 patients with blunt injury, REBOA was performed in patients with hemoperitoneum and/or pelvic ring fracture. A significant increase of SBP of 46 mmHg was observed. The overall mortality rate was 41.7% [34].

Further Japanese data on 10 patients with pelvic fractures showed a 40% survival rate [41].

In a French analysis of 32 patients, a survival rate of 40.6% was reported. REBOA led to a significant increase of SBP from 60 to 115 mmHg. A 19% rate of vascular complications was reported. Thirty-four percent needed renal replacement therapy and nearly half of the patients suffered from severe rhabdomyolysis [23]. In contrast, Tsurukiri reported a survival rate of only 25% [42].

Moore compared different trauma and non-trauma patients with initial REBOA treatment. The highest survival rate (53.8%) was observed in patients with vital signs at admission and Zone III REBOA for pelvic hemorrhage [43]. Of 17 patients with a Zone III placement, 70% were transferred to OR for pelvic packing or exploratory laparotomy and 30% for angiography.

In a recent meta-analysis, the effect of REBOA in trauma was well defined [44]. The overall mortality rate in 865 patients was 63%. In 97%, the femoral artery was approached via a percutaneous approach in 79.7% (20.3% open cutdown). The mean occlusion time was 52 min and a significant hemodynamic effect was observed, with an increase of the systolic blood pressure of 79.8 mmHg. The mean occlusion time in Zone III was longer with 68 min.

14.16 Pelvic REBOA-Algorithms

REBOA is already integrated into present trauma algorithms. While, during the last decade, polytrauma algorithms often included primary whole-body CT examination and abandoned conventional X-rays, REBOA-algorithms returned to the classical ATLS protocol, which included conventional X-rays of the chest and pelvis and the (extended) FAST examination for immediate detection of possible life-threatening truncal bleeding sources [43, 45, 46].

These three algorithms have NOT integrated a CT evaluation, as the basis for REBOA is the highly unstable patient. This specific patient group belongs to the term "patient in extremis".

Presently, no universal concept is supported by literature. Thus, the presently accepted algorithms are presented:

The basis of the Denver Health Medical Center algorithm for the management of combined hemodynamically and mechanically unstable pelvic fractures is the pelvis a.p. X-ray, according to the ATLS protocol [45]. This algorithm includes an equivalent concept of pelvic packing and REBOA for primary hemodynamic stabilization. If REBOA is chosen, this procedure is performed prior to mechanical pelvic ring stabilization, whereas pelvic packing is combined with an external fixation technique of the pelvis.

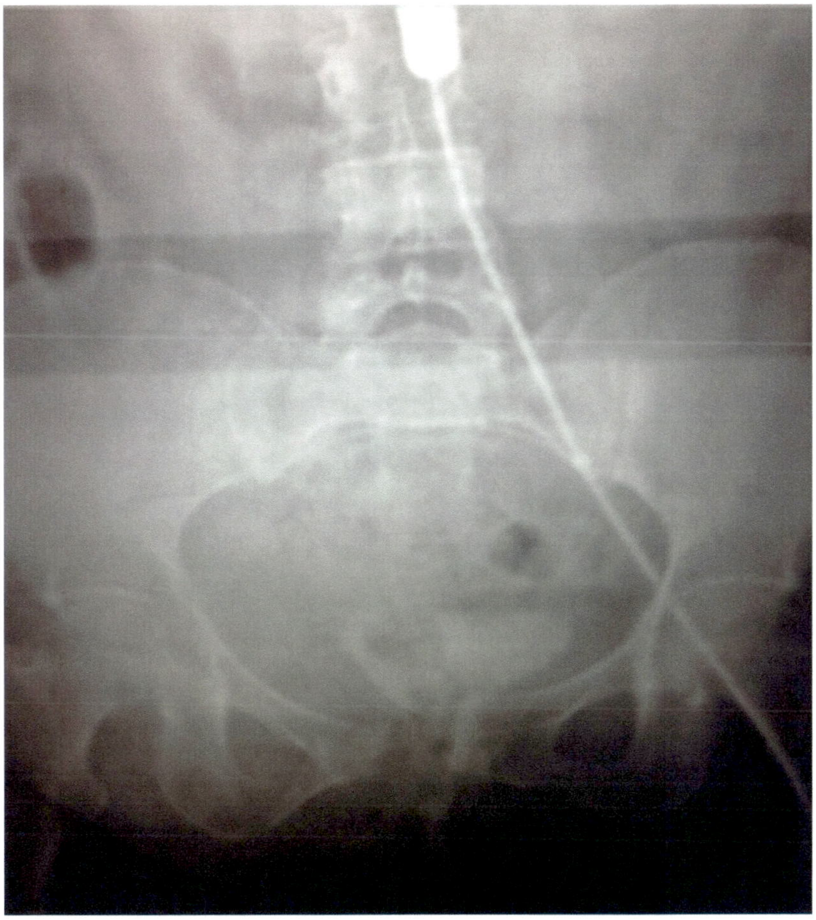

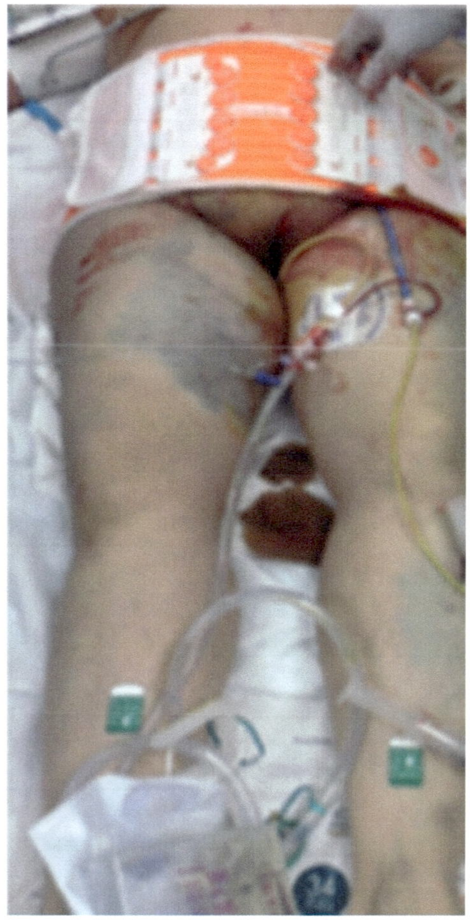

The basis of the Houston algorithm is the identification of potential aortic injury, intra-abdominal or relevant pelvic injury in ATLS partial- or non-responders [43]. In this specific patient group, all patients have femoral artery access in the ED, either for arterial blood pressure management or as an option for rewiring for REBOA. Diagnostics include chest and pelvic X-rays and the FAST evaluation.

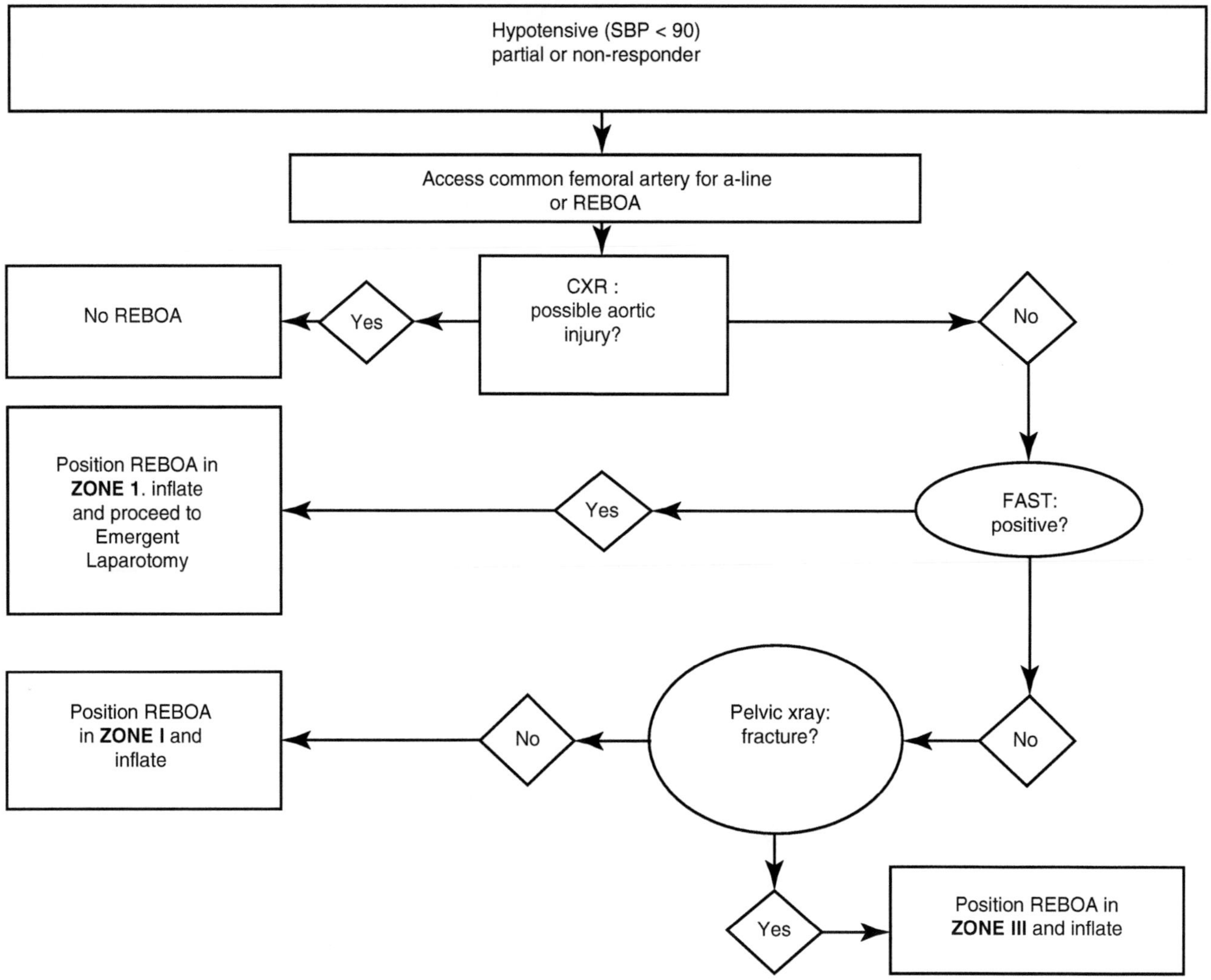

A recent German algorithm for REBOA application distinguished between penetrating and blunt injury mechanisms. All patients get femoral arterial access and are treated according to a massive transfusion protocol and the ATLS protocol. After excluding cardiac or intrathoracic aortic injury with chest X-ray and chest FAST, abdominal FAST evaluation is performed to detect intra-abdominal injuries. The presence of free fluid leads to Zone I REBOA application. This is followed by pelvic a.p. X-ray. If an open-book injury is present or a complex fracture/dislocation of the pelvis, a Zone III REBOA is performed. Interestingly no recommendation is performed regarding pelvic mechanical stabilization [46].

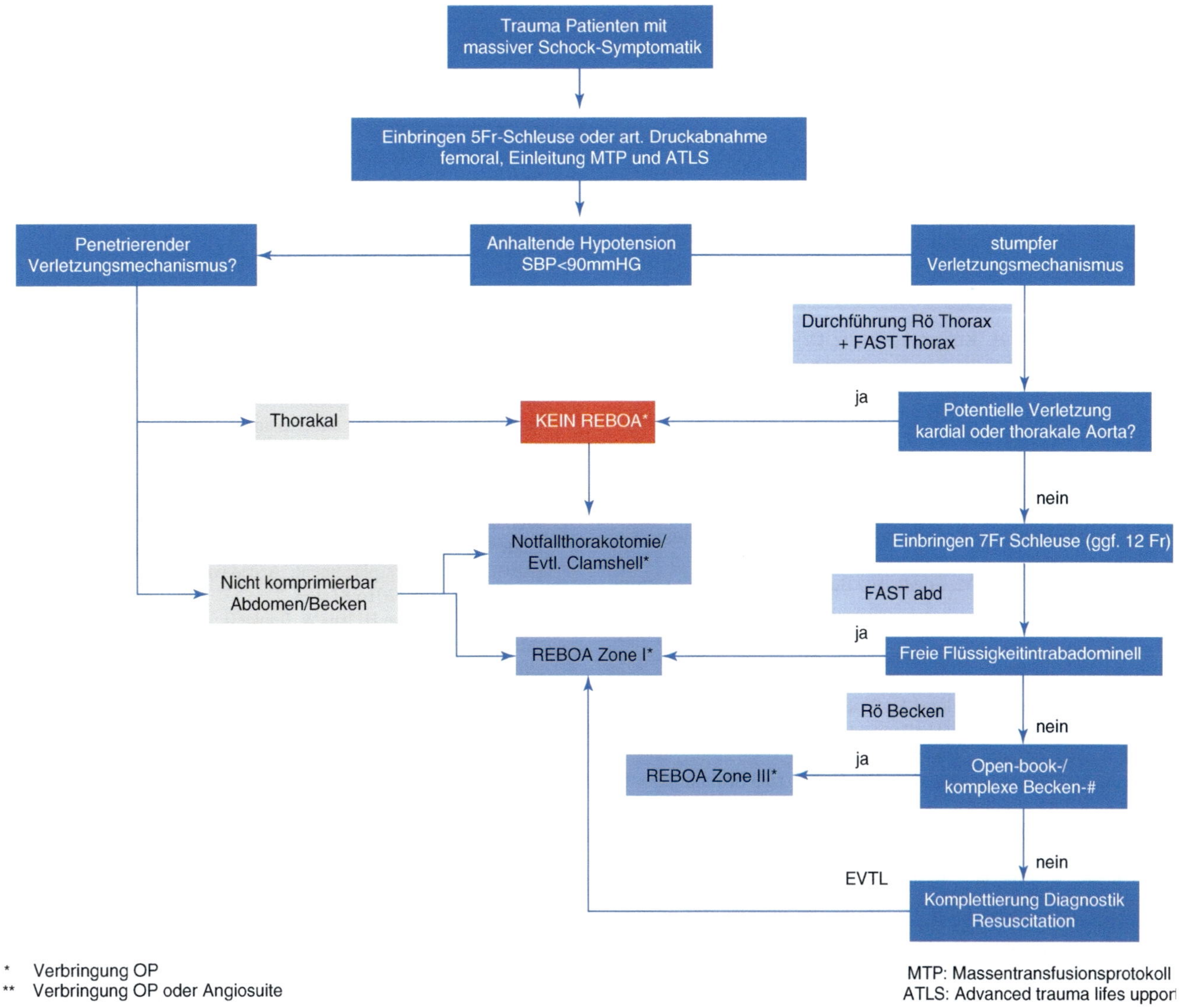

14.17 Conclusion

REBOA is only a temporary measure for cardiocirculatory stabilization and should be followed by definitive surgical bleeding control as part of a Damage Control Surgical Concept [47, 48]. Surgical hemodynamic stabilization should be performed after Zone I REBOA within 45 min (Fig. 14.8), otherwise mortality is unacceptably increased [39]. In Zone III, often longer inflation times can be accepted, especially when partial occlusion or intermittent deflation is performed [49]. It is of crucial mortality-related relevance to immediately start with REBOA for patients "in extremis" [50].

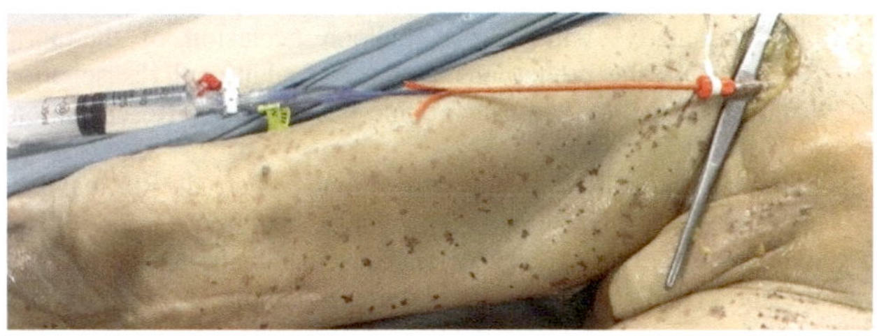

Fig. 14.8 Overview after application

References

1. Morrison J, Rasmussen T. Noncompressible torso hemorrhage: a review with contemporary definitions and management strategies. Surg Clin North Am. 2012;92:843–52.
2. Gänsslen A, Giannoudis P, Pape H. Hemorrhage in pelvic fracture: who needs angiography? Curr Opin Crit Care. 2003;9:515–23.
3. Gänsslen A, Hildebrand F, Pohlemann T. Management of hemodynamic unstable patients "in extremis" with pelvic ring fractures. Acta Chir Orthop Traumatol Cechoslov. 2012;79:193–202.
4. Hauser C, Perry J. Control of massive hemorrhage from pelvic fractures by hypogastric artery ligation. Surg Gynecol Obstet. 1964;121:313.
5. Platz A, Friedl H, Kohler A, Trentz O. Chirurgisches management bei schweren Beckenquetschverletzungen. Helv Chir Acta. 1992;58:925–9.
6. Ravdin I, Ellison E. Hypogastric artery ligation in acute pelvic trauma. Surgery. 1964;56:601–2.
7. Saueracker A, McCroskey B, Moore E, Moore F. Intraoperative hypogastric artery embolization for life-threatening pelvic hemorrhage: a preliminary report. J Trauma. 1987;27:1127–9.
8. Seavers F, Robinson R. Hypogastric artery ligation for uncontrollable hemorrhage in acute pelvic trauma. Surgery. 1964;55:516.
9. Trentz O, Bühren V, Friedl H. Beckenverletzungen. Chirurg. 1989;60:639–48.
10. Hughes C. Use of an intra-aortic balloon catheter tamponade for controlling intraabdominal hemorrhage in man. Surgery. 1954;36:65–8.
11. Gupta B, Khaneja S, Flores L, Eastlick L, Longmore W, Shaftan G. The role of intra-aortic balloon occlusion in penetrating abdominal trauma. J Trauma. 1989;29:861–5.
12. Ledgerwood A, Kazmera M, Lucas C. The role of thoracic aortic occlusion for massive hemoperitoneum. J Trauma. 1976;16:610–5.
13. Bühren V, Trentz O. Intraluminäre Ballonblockade der Aorta bei traumatischer Massivblutung. Unfallchirurg. 1989;92:309–13.
14. Stannard A, Eliason J, Rasmussen T. Resuscitative endovascular balloon occlusion of the aorta (REBOA) as an adjunct for hemorrhagic shock. J Trauma. 2011;71:1869–72.
15. Knapp J, Bernhard M, Haltmeier T, Bieler D, Hossfeld B, Kulla M. Resuscitative endovascular balloon occlusion of the aorta: Option for incompressible trunk bleeding? Anaesthesist. 2018;67:280–92.
16. Sadek S, Lockey D, Lendrum R, Perkins Z, Price J, Davies G. Resuscitative endovascular balloon occlusion of the aorta (REBOA) in the prehospital setting: an additional resuscitation option for uncontrolled catastrophic haemorrhage. Resuscitation. 2016;107:135–8.
17. Manzano Nunez R, Naranjo M, Foianini E, Ferrada P, Rincon E, García-Perdomo H, Burbano P, Herrera J, García A, Ordoñez C. A meta-analysis of resuscitative endovascular balloon occlusion of the aorta (REBOA) or open aortic cross-clamping by resuscitative thoracotomy in non-compressible torso hemorrhage patients. World J Emerg Surg. 2017;12:30. https://doi.org/10.1186/s13017-017-0142-5. eCollection 2017
18. Sridhar S, Gumbert S, Stephens C, Moore L, Pivalizza E. Resuscitative endovascular balloon occlusion of the aorta: principles, initial clinical experience, and considerations for the anesthesiologist. Anesth Analg. 2017;125:884–90.
19. Rich J, Coleman J, Devaux C, Hoffman K. Acute rehabilitation after resuscitative endovascular balloon occlusion of the aorta (REBOA) in major trauma. BMJ Case Rep. 2017;2017:bcr2017220885.
20. Teeter W, Matsumoto J, Idoguchi K, Kon Y, Orita T, Funabiki T, Brenner M, Matsumura Y. Smaller introducer sheaths for REBOA may be associated with fewer complications. J Trauma Acute Care Surg. 2016;81:1039–45.
21. Romagnoli A, Teeter W, Wasicek P, Gamble W, Hu F, Stein D, Scalea T, Brenner M. No wire? No problem: resuscitative endovascular balloon occlusion of the aorta (REBOA) can be performed effectively and more rapidly with a wire-free device. J Trauma Acute Care Surg. 2018;85:894. https://doi.org/10.1097/TA.0000000000002003.
22. Brenner M, Moore L, DuBose J, Tyson G, McNutt M, Albarado R, Holcomb J, Scalea T, Rasmussen T. A clinical series of resuscitative endovascular balloon occlusion of the aorta for hemorrhage control and resuscitation. J Trauma Acute Care Surg. 2013;75:506–11.
23. Pieper A, Thony F, Brun J, Rodière M, Boussat B, Arvieux C, Tonetti J, Payen J, Bouzat P. Resuscitative endovascular balloon occlusion of the aorta for pelvic blunt trauma and life-threatening hemorrhage: a 20-year experience in a level I trauma center. J Trauma Acute Care Surg. 2018;84:449–53.
24. Moore L, Brenner M, Kozar R, Pasley J, Wade C, Baraniuk M, Scalea T, Holcomb J. Implementation of resuscitative endovascular balloon occlusion of the aorta as an alternative to resuscitative thoracotomy for noncompressible truncal hemorrhage. J Trauma Acute Care Surg. 2015;79:523–30.
25. Linnebur M, Inaba K, Haltmeier T, Rasmussen T, Smith J, Mendelsberg R, Grabo D, Demetriades D. Emergent non-image-guided resuscitative endovascular balloon occlusion of the aorta (REBOA) catheter placement: A cadaver-based study. J Trauma Acute Care Surg. 2016;81:453–7.
26. Okada Y, Narumiya H, Ishi W, Iiduka R. Anatomical landmarks for safely implementing resuscitative balloon occlusion of the aorta (REBOA) in zone 1 without fluoroscopy. Scand J Trauma Resusc Emerg Med. 2017;25:63.
27. Perkins Z, Lendrum R, Brohi K. Resuscitative endovascular balloon occlusion of the aorta: promise, practice, and progress? Curr Opin Crit Care. 2016;22:563–71.
28. Martinelli T, Thony F, Decléty P, Sengel C, Broux C, Tonetti J, Payen J, Ferretti G. Intra-aortic balloon occlusion to salvage patients with life-threatening hemorrhagic shocks from pelvic fractures. J Trauma. 2010;68:942–8.
29. Ogura T, Lefor A, Nakamura M, Fujizuka K, Shiroto K, Nakano M. Ultrasound-guided resuscitative endovascular balloon occlusion of the aorta in the resuscitation area. J Emerg Med. 2017;52:715–22.
30. Johnson M, Neff L, Williams T, DuBose J, Group ES. Partial resuscitative balloon occlusion of the aorta (P-REBOA): Clinical technique and rationale. J Trauma Acute Care Surg. 2016;81(5):S133–7. Suppl 2 Proceedings of the 2015 Military Health System Research Symposium
31. Yeung K, Groeneveld M, Lu J, van Diemen P, Jongkind V, Wisselink W. Organ protection during aortic cross-clamping. Best Pract Res Clin Anaesthesiol. 2016;30:305–15.
32. DuBose J, Scalea T, Brenner M, Skiada D, Inaba K, Cannon J, Moore L, Holcomb J, Turay D, Arbabi C, Kirkpatrick A, Xiao J, Skarupa D, Poulin N, Group AAS. The AAST prospective aortic occlusion for resuscitation in trauma and acute care surgery (AORTA) registry: data on contemporary utilization and outcomes of aortic occlusion and resuscitative balloon occlusion of the aorta (REBOA). J Trauma Acute Care Surg. 2016;81:409–19.
33. Napolitano L. Resuscitative endovascular balloon occlusion of the aorta: indications, outcomes, and training. Crit Care Clin. 2017;33:55–70.
34. Saito N, Matsumoto J, Yagi T, Hara Y, Hayashida K, Motomura T, Mashiko K, Iida H, Yokota H, Wagatsuma Y. Evaluation of the safety and feasibility of resuscitative endovascular balloon occlusion of the aorta. J Trauma Acute Care Surg. 2015;78:897–903.
35. Gamberini E, Coccolini F, Tamagnini B, Martino C, Albarello V, Benni M, Bisulli M, Fabbri N, Hörer T, Ansaloni L, Coniglio C, Barozzi M, Agnoletti V. Resuscitative endovascular balloon occlusion of the aorta in trauma: a systematic review of the literature.

World J Emerg Surg. 2017;12:42. https://doi.org/10.1186/s13017-017-0153-2. eCollection 2017
36. Markov N, Percival T, Morrison J, Ross J, Scott D, Spencer J, Rasmussen T. Physiologic tolerance of descending thoracic aortic balloon occlusion in a swine model of hemorrhagic shock. Surgery. 2013;153:848–56.
37. Scott D, Eliason J, Villamaria C, Morrison J, Houston RT, Spencer J, Rasmussen T. A novel fluoroscopy-free, resuscitative endovascular aortic balloon occlusion system in a model of hemorrhagic shock. J Trauma Acute Care Surg. 2013;75:122–8.
38. Matsumura Y, Matsumoto J, Kondo H, Idoguchi K, Ishida T, Kon Y, Tomita K, Ishida K, Hirose T, Umakoshi K, Funabiki T, Investigators D-I. Fewer REBOA complications with smaller devices and partial occlusion: evidence from a multicenter registry in Japan. Emerg Med J. 2017;34:793–9.
39. Norii T, Crandall C, Terasaka Y. Survival of severe blunt trauma patients treated with resuscitative endovascular balloon occlusion of the aorta compared with propensity scoreadjusted untreated patients. J Trauma Acute Care Surg. 2015;78:721–8.
40. Russo R, Neff L, Lamb C, Cannon J, Galante J, Clement N, Grayson J, Williams T. Partial resuscitative endovascular balloon occlusion of the aorta in swine model of hemorrhagic shock. J Am Coll Surg. 2016;223:359–68.
41. Sato R, Kuriyama A, Takaesu R, Miyamae N, Iwanaga W, Tokuda H, Umemura T. Resuscitative endovascular balloon occlusion of the aorta performed by emergency physicians for traumatic hemorrhagic shock: a case series from Japanese emergency rooms. Crit Care. 2018;22:103.
42. Tsurukiri J, Akamine I, Sato T, Sakurai M, Okumura E, Moriya M, Yamanaka H, Ohta S. Resuscitative endovascular balloon occlusion of the aorta for uncontrolled haemorrahgic shock as an adjunct to haemostatic procedures in the acute care setting. Scand J Trauma Resusc Emerg Med. 2016;24:13.
43. Moore L, Martin C, Harvin J, Wade C, Holcomb J. Resuscitative endovascular balloon occlusion of the aorta for control of non-compressible truncal hemorrhage in the abdomen and pelvis. Am J Surg. 2016;212:1222–30.
44. van der Burg B, van Dongen T, Morrison J, Hedeman Joosten P, DuBose J, Hörer T, Hoencamp R. A systematic review and meta-analysis of the use of resuscitative endovascular balloon occlusion of the aorta in the management of major exsanguination. Eur J Trauma Emerg Surg. 2018;44(4):535–50. https://doi.org/10.1007/s00068-018-0959-y.
45. Biffl W, Fox C, Moore E. The role of REBOA in the control of exsanguinating torso hemorrhage. J Trauma Acute Care Surg. 2015;78:1054–8.
46. Elias K, Engelhardt M. Resuscitative endovascular balloon occlusion of the aorta—ÜberbrückendeMaßnahme bis zur operativen Versorgung. Unfallchirurg. 2018;121:537–43.
47. Bouillon B, Rixen D, Maegele M, Steinhausen E, Tjardes T, Paffrath T. Damage control orthopedics. What is the current situation? Unfallchirurg. 2009;112:860.
48. Rotondo M, Zonies D. The damage control sequence and the underlying logic. Surg Clin North Am. 1997;77:761–77.
49. Andres J, Scott J, Giannoudis P. Resuscitative endovascular balloon occlusion of the aorta (REBOA): what have we learned? Injury. 2016;47:2603–5.
50. Matsumura Y, Matsumoto J, Kondo H, Idoguchi K, Ishida T, Okada Y, Kon Y, Oka K, Ishida K, Toyoda Y, Funabiki T, Investigators D-I. Early arterial access for REBOA is related to survival outcome in trauma. J Trauma Acute Care Surg. 2018;85(3):507–11. https://doi.org/10.1097/TA.0000000000002004.

Indirect Hemorrhage Control: Angiography/Embolization (AE)

15

Jan Lindahl and Axel Gänsslen

The rapid assessment and control of massive arterial bleeding, associated with pelvic injuries secondary to blunt trauma, pose a challenge for emergency trauma care. Exsanguinating bleeding has been identified as the major cause of early death during the first 24–48 h after trauma in multiple-trauma patients with pelvic ring injuries [1–7]. Treatment decisions during this time interval have significant influence on patient survival [8]. Patients with arterial bleeding must be identified early to prevent further bleeding-related complications.

Emergency treatment of hemodynamically unstable pelvic ring patients should focus on hemorrhage control and extensive shock therapy. However, upon admission, early detection of the major source of the hemorrhage responsible for shock is difficult [9]. Significant variation of optimal treatment of patients with pelvic fractures that are hemodynamically unstable exists across institutions [10].

Four main options to control massive pelvic bleeding have been suggested by the World Society of Emergency Surgery, including closed reduction and temporary mechanical stabilization of the pelvic ring, preperitoneal pelvic packing (PPP), resuscitative endovascular balloon occlusion of the aorta (REBOA), and transcatheter angiographic embolization (AE) [11]. The recent evolution of these four procedures has significantly decreased the mortality rates of devastating pelvic injuries [12].

Current trauma protocols are based on rapid control of external and internal bleeding; prevention of the lethal triad (acidosis, hypothermia, and coagulopathy); control of emergent laboratory parameters (e.g., blood hemoglobin, platelets, pH, base deficit, lactate, serum calcium); appropriate use of blood components; maintenance of tissue perfusion; and pharmacological treatment [13, 14].

J. Lindahl
Orthopaedics and Trauma Surgery, Helsinki University Hospital, Helsinki, Finland

A. Gänsslen (✉)
Department of Trauma Surgery, Orthopedics and Hand Surgery, Hospital Wolfsburg, Wolfsburg, Germany

Pelvic angiography and embolization was initially used to control arterial sources of intrapelvic bleeding in the 1970s [15].

Angiography can precisely identify the source of hemorrhage, and selective transcatheter angiographic embolization (AE) can definitively treat arterial bleeding [16–22]. However, there is no clear consensus on the appropriate indication, timing, or order for applying angiographic interventions in pelvic fractures accompanied by exsanguinating retroperitoneal bleeding.

15.1 Pelvic Fracture-Related Bleeding

Major pelvic injuries are associated with a high risk of venous and arterial bleeding [23–25]. The presence of hypotension (sBP < 90 mmHg) at the time of arrival was found to significantly increase mortality (Table 15.1). Pelvic fractures, however, may be caused by low- or high- energy trauma, and they may be an isolated injury or associated with additional injuries to other body regions. In patients that sustain polytraumas, the injury distribution and injury severity vary substantially, and hemodynamic instability may be caused by conditions other than hemorrhage. Approximately 10% of pelvic fractures among hospital admissions are characterized by hemodynamic instability [36].

Pelvic hemorrhage can be massive [19, 37]. Pelvic fracture-related hemorrhage typically originates directly from the cancellous bony surfaces and bony edges of the fracture lines [24, 38], from an injured retroperitoneal presacral venous plexus [13, 38], or from the arteries and veins of the internal or external iliac systems [6, 17, 19, 24, 37, 39, 40].

Huittinnen et al. performed an angiographic postmortem analysis of 27 patients after MVA [24]. Soft-tissue bleeding and bleeding from fracture sites were observed in 23 patients, originating from rami of the hypogastric artery. Complete arterial dissection was observed in only three cases. Sacral fracture site bleeding was seen from intraosseous branches of the lateral sacral artery, while injuries of the SI-joint were associated with bleeding sources from the cancellous bone surfaces, torn ligaments, and the SI-joint itself.

A. Gänsslen et al. (eds.), *Pelvic Ring Fractures*, https://doi.org/10.1007/978-3-030-54730-1_15

Table 15.1 Factors predicting hemorrhage and mortality in blunt pelvic trauma patients

Risk factor	References
A. Hemodynamic and laboratory parameters	
Systolic blood pressure (<90/100 mmHg)	[2–4, 19, 26, 27]
Pulse rate (100/130 or greater)	[2, 23]
Low hemoglobin concentration	[3, 4, 27]
Hematokrit (30 or less)	[23]
Base excess	[17, 27]
High blood lactate level	[28]
Transfusion requirements	[3, 4, 7, 26]
B. Patient-related aspects	
Age of the patient	[2, 6, 7, 26, 27, 29]
Gender (male)	[4]
C. Fracture-related aspects	
Pelvic fracture type	[1, 3, 4, 6, 26, 29–31]
Mechanism of pelvic ring injury	[26, 30–32]
Degree of displacement of pelvic fracture	[23, 26]
D. Pattern and severity of injuries	
ISS	[3, 4, 7, 26, 29, 33–35]
Revised trauma score (RTS)	[7, 27]
Head injury	[3]
Glasgow coma scale (GCS)	[7]

With permission from: Jan Lindahl, Management of Pelvic Ring Injuries, Thesis, University of Helsinki, Helsinki, Finland 2015

The presacral venous plexus is located just anterior to the sacrum and SI-joints, and therefore, they are subject to injury in fractures that affect the posterior sacroiliac complex. When a thin-walled, presacral venous plexus is damaged, the escaping venous blood often passes into the retroperitoneum. The retroperitoneum is a closed space; thus, hemorrhage from a venous plexus eventually stops, when the counter-pressure exceeds venous pressure [13], and the patient's coagulation status is maintained within acceptable limits [41]. On the other hand, arterial hemorrhage can overcome a tamponade effect, and this condition can lead to hypovolemic shock. The volume of the retroperitoneal space is large; it extends from the diaphragm to the true pelvis; thus, it can accommodate several liters of blood.

Severe venous bleeding seems to be more frequent than generally acknowledged and most treatment approaches might overestimate the significance and incidence of arterial bleeding, while underestimating the significance of venous bleeding [40]:

- Already, Rothenberger et al. found that 11 of 12 patients with major vascular injuries secondary to pelvic fractures had venous injuries, while 5 of 12 patients presented with arterial injuries [6].
- Ertel et al. analyzed 14 patients with highly hemodynamic unstable pelvic ring injuries and observed venous plexus bleeding in 13 of 14 patients, but no arterial injury was intraoperatively detected [28].
- Kataoka et al. analyzed patients with major venous injuries and observed relevant venous bleeding in 9 of 11 patients after successful embolization [37].

An experimental "open-book" cadaveric pelvic injury model showed, that 5 cm symphyseal diastasis resulted in 60% iliolumbar vein injuries, but in no arterial injuries [42].

The internal iliac artery is the main artery that supplies the intrapelvic structures. This artery, which is about 4 cm long, arises from the common iliac artery above the pelvic brim (linea terminalis), at the same level as the lumbosacral intervertebral disc, and anterior to the lateral sacrum. It then descends to the upper margin of the greater sciatic foramen (Fig. 15.1), where it divides into its main branches in the true

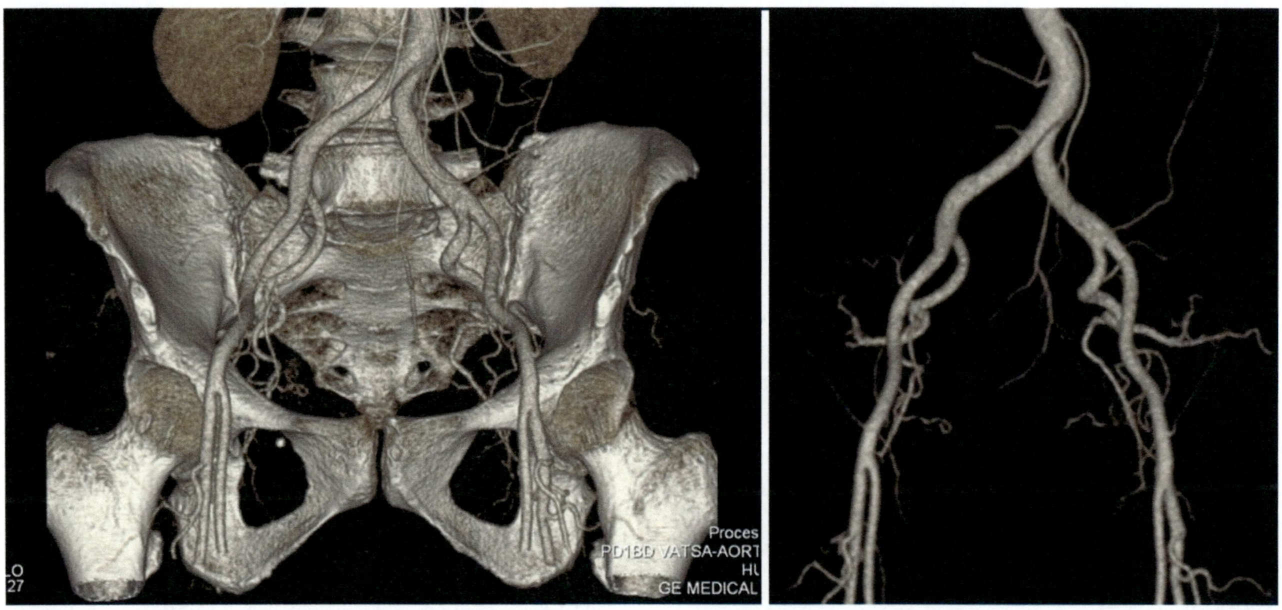

Fig. 15.1 Normal vascular anatomy using angio-CT data

pelvis. Severe trauma to the pelvis may disrupt the main internal iliac artery [17, 19], the common iliac artery, or the external iliac artery [6, 17, 39]. Damage to the superior or inferior gluteal arteries, the largest branches of the internal iliac artery, are a common cause of massive hemorrhage. Because superior gluteal artery courses through the upper part of the greater sciatic foramen, it is prone to damage from traumas that injure the SI-joint (Fig. 15.1). In the true pelvis, important bleeding can originate from the obturator artery, which runs along the lateral wall of the pelvis (the quadrilateral surface of the acetabulum) and enters the obturator foramen. Also, several other branches of the iliac arteries may be a potential source of arterial bleeding associated with pelvic fractures [17, 19].

The study by Huittinen and Slätis showed that death from hemorrhage is rare, but, when it does occur, it most often originates from an arterial source in the pelvic ring [24]. In addition, nearly half of these patients have other sources of bleeding, often from a thoracic or abdominal injury [43].

Rupture of the main iliac vein due to blunt pelvic trauma is rare. These injuries are difficult to diagnose, because bleeding veins do not show up on angiograph [37]. A diagnosis can be made based on pelvic venography, but this technique is seldom used during the initial resuscitation or during emergent laparotomy when continuous venous bleeding is observed from a ruptured retroperitoneum in the pelvis. Bleeding from the internal iliac vein is often controllable with pelvic packing [13] or with an endovascular stent placement [37]. Massive venous bleeding might occur more frequently than generally acknowledged [40].

15.2 Massive Bleeding

The extent of a life-threatening injury is difficult to judge adequately. Spahn et al. defined massive bleeding in trauma patients as the loss of one blood volume within 24 h or the loss of 0.5 blood volumes within 3 h [44]. To facilitate early recognition, Scandinavian guidelines defined massive bleeding due to trauma in the adult patient as a continuing need for pressure-driven intravenous fluid and blood component replacement [45]. Massive bleeding is often caused by a combination of vascular injury and coagulopathy [44].

Patients that are exsanguinating "in extremis" are at the greatest risk of death. This patient group is characterized by absent vital signs or severe shock, with an initial systolic blood pressure <70 mmHg and/or they require mechanical resuscitation or catecholamines despite more than 12 blood transfusions within the first 2 h after admission [46].

Patients that receive massive blood transfusions exceeding 50 U have a low survival rate [47, 48]. In general, the mortality rate for patients that require massive transfusions was reported to be approximately 50% [49–51].

Life-threatening bleeding from pelvic or acetabular fractures in pediatric patients is even more rare (2.8%). Therefore, this population does not substantially contribute to the overall mortality [52].

15.3 Detection of Pelvic Bleeding

Identifying patients with major arterial hemorrhage after a blunt pelvic trauma might be difficult. There is no emergent parameter or single test for detecting hemorrhage. Assessments of bleeding require a complex, combined evaluation of the trauma mechanism, vital signs, and physiological parameters. The detection of external and internal bleeding sources is based on injuries found on the trauma CT scan and other secondary investigations, a need for blood product replacements, and the response to treatment [14].

The source of arterial bleeding is verified with angiography. Contrast-enhanced trauma CT might detect active arterial bleeding, but not all instances require invasive intervention [53] and, conversely, the absence of a contrast blush on a trauma CT scan does not rule out active arterial bleeding [54]. All imaging techniques for detecting the arterial source of bleeding are time-consuming. A precise assessment and control of exsanguinating bleeding from large pelvic arteries requires time.

Pelvic fracture classifications have limited utility in predicting the risk of hemorrhage for individual patients [55]. Common scoring systems for assessing injury severity, such as the Injury Severity Score (ISS) [56], the New Injury Severity Score (NISS) [57], and the Revised Trauma Score (RTS) [58], are not sufficiently specific to be useful for the early diagnosis of bleeding.

The ideal emergency parameter for hemorrhage (a risk factor of mortality) should be available early, within the first 10–15 min. Several general risk factors have been found to predict major hemorrhage and mortality (Table 15.1), but none of the known general parameters is sufficiently specific to identify patients that are at the highest risk of death.

15.3.1 Signs of Arterial Injury on CT Evaluation

Analysis of contrast-enhanced CT (Fig. 15.1) is helpful to predict the potential need of pelvic angiography and further embolization.

Classical CT-based parameters to angiography/embolization can include [59]:

- Contrast media extravasation (CE).
- Pelvic hematoma in hemodynamically unstable pelvic fracture patients.
- Positive blush on CT in hemodynamic unstable patients.

The sensitivity was calculated to 60–90%, with a specificity of CT of 92–100% [60–63].

Additionally, the pelvic hematoma size can guide to AE [64, 65]. Pelvic hematoma formation ≥500 cm^3 increases the risk of the presence of an arterial injury, even in the absence of a visible contrast blush [64].

Recently, it was found that CE was associated with a higher angiography and angioembolization rate (40% and 23%), representing a sensitivity, specificity, positive predictive value, and negative predictive value of CE on CT of 100%, 87.9%, 22.7%, and 100%, respectively. The presence of CE was additionally associated with a doubled mortality rate (13% vs. 6%) [66].

15.3.2 Signs of Arterial Injury on Angiography

After initiation of angiography, the following signs indicate the necessity of embolization [67]:

- Contrast extravasation (Fig. 15.2)
- Pseudoaneurysm
- Arteriovenous fistula
- Abrupt cutoff of flow
- Vessel narrowing

15.3.3 Indications for Pelvic Angiographic Embolization

AE should be considered without delay in patients with pelvic fractures that remain hemodynamically unstable despite adequate resuscitation and provisional stabilization of the pelvic ring. Bleeding can be occluded definitively with embolization.

AE is an effective and safe procedure.

Arterial bleeding usually requires angiographic embolization [15, 21, 49]. Significant arterial bleeding is only seen in 10–20% of cases [27, 57, 68].

In patients in whom bleeding can be identified with angiography, transcatheter embolization definitively treats this bleeding. Usually the bleeding vessels are catheterized selectively and embolized with coils or glue. If this is not possible because of multiple bleeding vessels or uncontrolled bleeding, embolization of internal iliac artery with coils is performed. Because of extensive collateral circulation, even the main internal iliac artery can be occluded bilaterally [69].

The following indications are suggested [11, 46, 64, 67, 70, 71]:

- Pelvic fracture-related hemodynamic instability (SBP < 90 mmHg) and persistent bleeding (with no evidence of intra-abdominal bleeding).
- Pelvic fracture-related hemodynamic instability with persistent bleeding after provisional pelvic stabilization (pelvic binder, anterior external fixator, or C-clamp).
- Pelvic fracture-related hemodynamic instability with persistent pelvic bleeding after preperitoneal pelvic packing (PPP).

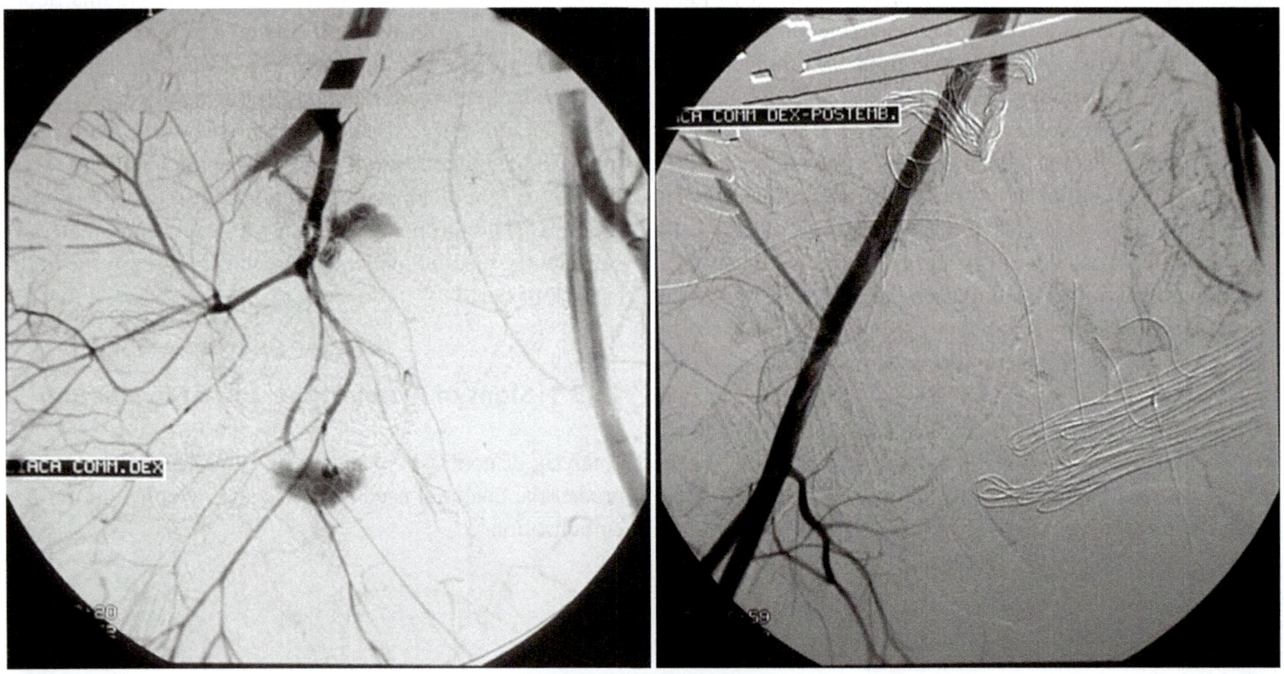

Fig. 15.2 Angiography of the internal iliac artery before and after embolization (nonselective embolization). (**a**) Initial angiogram shows several bleeding vessels; (**b**) the control angiogram shows no bleeding

- Bleeding from the branches of the external iliac artery (detected in angiography).
- Non-responders (after PPP or REBOA).
- Evidence of arterial contrast extravasation by CT may require AE, regardless of hemodynamic status.
- Large hematoma on CT scan or expanding gluteal hematoma.
- Persistent hemorrhage in a stable (or stabilized) pelvis.
- Recurrent hemorrhage after initial angioembolization.

Bleeding from the common iliac artery or the external iliac artery is unique, because it is the only pelvic arterial injury that requires immediate surgical repair (see below). The diagnosis is made with angiography.

The ATLS concepts recommended angiography for pelvic bleeding control [72]. Hou et al. analyzed this concept in 48 consecutive patients with hemodynamically unstable pelvic fractures [73]. Primary angiography was performed based on the trauma surgeon's preference in 14 cases. The mean ISS of these 48 patients was 43.2 points and shock parameters include a mean systolic blood pressure of 74.8 mmHg, a heart rate of 102 bpm, resulting in a shock index of 1.37. The mean transfusion requirements during the first 6 h after admission were 7.06 PRBC +4.2 FFP. The mean time to angiography was 235 min. The overall mortality rate was 41.7%.

Hou et al. concluded, that these ATLS guidelines result in unacceptably high mortality rates compared with more specific approaches using transfusion protocols and interventions, such as pelvic packing [73].

The recent ATLS concept integrated pelvic packing as an alternative [74], when angioembolization is delayed or unavailable.

Angiography followed by embolization is a well-accepted treatment modality in patients with pelvic ring injuries and hemodynamic instability.

Angiography and embolization are both often used in North-American trauma centers. In a multi-institutional trial analysis of 178 patients with pelvic injuries admitted in hemodynamic shock (systolic blood pressure < 90 mmHg or heart rate > 120 beats/min or base deficit < −5), an overall angioembolization rate of 17.5% was observed [10].

The World Society of Emergency Surgery (WSES) recommended AE as an effective measure of hemorrhage control secondary to mechanical pelvic stabilization, especially when CT evaluation presented with signs of potential pelvic bleeding [11].

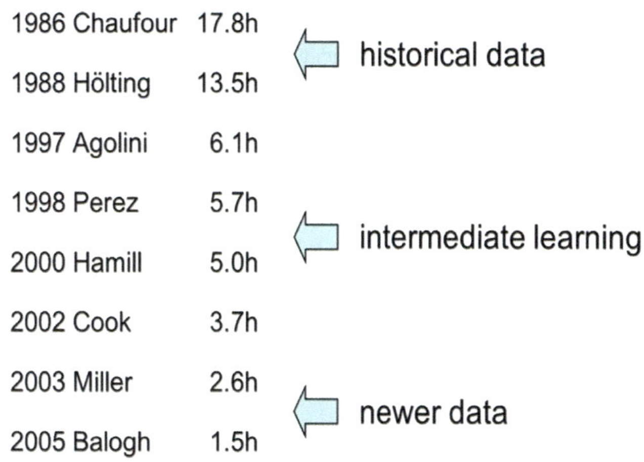
1986 Chaufour 17.8h
1988 Hölting 13.5h
1997 Agolini 6.1h
1998 Perez 5.7h
2000 Hamill 5.0h
2002 Cook 3.7h
2003 Miller 2.6h
2005 Balogh 1.5h
historical data
intermediate learning
newer data

Fig. 15.3 Time from admission to AE based on selected historical data

15.4 Timing of AE

Historical data showed a clear trend to faster AE [16, 61, 75–80] (Fig. 15.3).

Already, in 1997, Agolini et al. demonstrated improved survival if AE was performed within 3 h after admission [75]. Mortality in patients embolized within 3 h was 36.4% and 75% for patients with delayed AE. Based on this study, Hak et al. recommended angiography within 90 min after admission [81].

Recently, Tanizaki et al. reported on a 16% mortality rate, if angioembolization was started within 60 min compared to 64%, if AE was delayed [63].

Angioembolization should be performed as early as possible in the emergency treatment phase of hemodynamically unstable patients with unstable pelvic ring injuries.

In contrast, Gänsslen et al. analyzed the time interval from hospital admission to start of angiography in detail [46], based on 320 embolized patients and reported an average time window of 5.6 h until embolization was finished [22, 82–87].

Recent data could be analyzed regarding pre-procedure times, procedure times, and whole treatment times (Table 15.2):

- Shapiro et al. analyzed 31 patients with angiography and reported a time interval between admission and start of angiography of 187.3 min [88].
- Töttermann et al. reported a mean time from admission to angiography of 240 min [22].
- Westhoff et al. reported a mean time to start of AE of 62 min and a procedure time of 25 min for 21 patients [87].
- Osborn et al. observed a median time from admission to angiography of 130 min and a mean time of 276 min [89].

Table 15.2 Analysis of AE timing

Year	Author	No.	Time admission to angio	AE time	Total time
2005	Shapiro	31	187,3		
2006	Tötterman	31	240		
2008	Westhoff	21	62	25	87
2009	Osborn*	20	276		
2009	Fang	140	584		
2009	Jeroukhimov	29	210		
	SUM I	**272**	**396.8**		
2010	Jeske	45		60.4	
2010	Morozumi	29	87.9	73.3	161.2
2011	Barentsz	19		68.3	
2011	Tai	13	139.5	61.9	201,4
2011	Seif	17		92.8	
2012	Tanizaki	43	76.3		
2012	Hou	48	235		
2014	Tanizaki	68	76	58	134
2014	Brun	27	120	105	225
2017	Tesoriero*	344	286	51	337
	SUM II	**653**	**219.8**	**58.4**	**278.2**

Mean time in minutes; *median time

- Fang et al. reported an interval between admission and start of angiography of 584 min [82].
- Jeroukhimov et al. performed all angiographies within 3.5 ± 2 h after admission [84].
- Jeske et al. reported a procedure time of 60.4 min [85].
- Morozumi et al. analyzed 29 patients with angiography and reported a mean time to intervention of 87.9 min and a mean procedure time of 73.3 min. Thus, AE was completed on average 161.2 min after admission [86].
- Barentsz et al. reported a procedure time of 68.3 min [60].
- Tai et al. analyzed 13 patients with angiography as the primary stabilization method and reported a time to intervention of 139.5 min and a procedure time of 61.9 min. Thus, AE was completed in average 201.4 min after admission [90].
- Seif et al. reported an average procedure time of 92.8 min, including angiographic performance and time loss during patient transport, preparation, and puncture site compression [91].
- Tanizaki et al. reported a fast time until start of angiography of 76.3 min [92].
- Hou et al. analyzed 48 consecutive patients with hemodynamically unstable pelvic fractures [73]. The mean time to angiography was 235 min.
- Tanizaki et al. reported an average time interval between hospital admission and arrival at the angiography suite of 76 min and a mean procedure time of 58 min (30–125 min) [63]. Thus, the whole time, from admission until the end of embolization, was 134 min.
- Brun et al. analyzed 27 patients with unstable pelvic ring injuries requiring angiography. The average time from admission to pelvic angiography was 120 min, and a median procedure time of 105 min was reported. In the hemodynamically unstable, start of angiography was faster, within 80 min after admission [93].

Even today, in experienced centers, a too extended time interval is observed until angioembolization is initiated. Tesoriero et al. analyzed the results of angiography in 344 patients [94]. The median time to angiography was 286 min (264 min in unstable patients and 309 min in stable patients). The procedure time (AE) was 51 min. Interestingly, no learning effect regarding whole AE time after admission was observed, as, during the last 2 years, only 21 min' saving was observed.

> Despite an overall decrease of nearly 50% during the last decade until start of AE, there is still a significant treatment delay for hemodynamic stabilization. AE, on average, starts 3.5 h after admission.

Therapeutic angiography and embolization procedure is time-consuming and needs the 24-h service of an interventional radiologist. The angiography suite should be close to the emergency department. The future trauma center should be equipped with all diagnostic, interventional radiological, and operative facilities to avoid transporting an unstable patient to another location for imaging and management.

In massive hemorrhage with several bleeding arteries uni- or bilaterally, it is reasonable to use nonselective embolization by promptly occluding the main trunk of the internal iliac artery, either uni- or bilaterally [17].

15.5 Technique of AE

15.5.1 Positioning and Draping

The procedure is done with the patient in a supine position. The complete thoraco-abdominal-pelvic-inguinal area is draped (Fig. 15.4). The standard draping starts from the inguinal area to the upper clavicular margins. This allows for pelvic packing, trauma laparotomy and/or emergency thoracotomy, also during the AE procedure if the patient's hemodynamical status gets worse.

15.5.2 Puncture of the Femoral Artery

The puncture of the femoral artery is usually made in the contra-lateral side to the pelvic fracture in unilateral injuries (Fig. 15.4).

15.5.3 Diagnostic Angiography

The source of arterial bleeding is verified with angiography. The procedure is started with diagnostic angiography performed through the femoral artery with 5F catheters and this consists of aortal, bilateral common iliac artery, and internal iliac artery injections [17]. Aortogram gives knowledge of

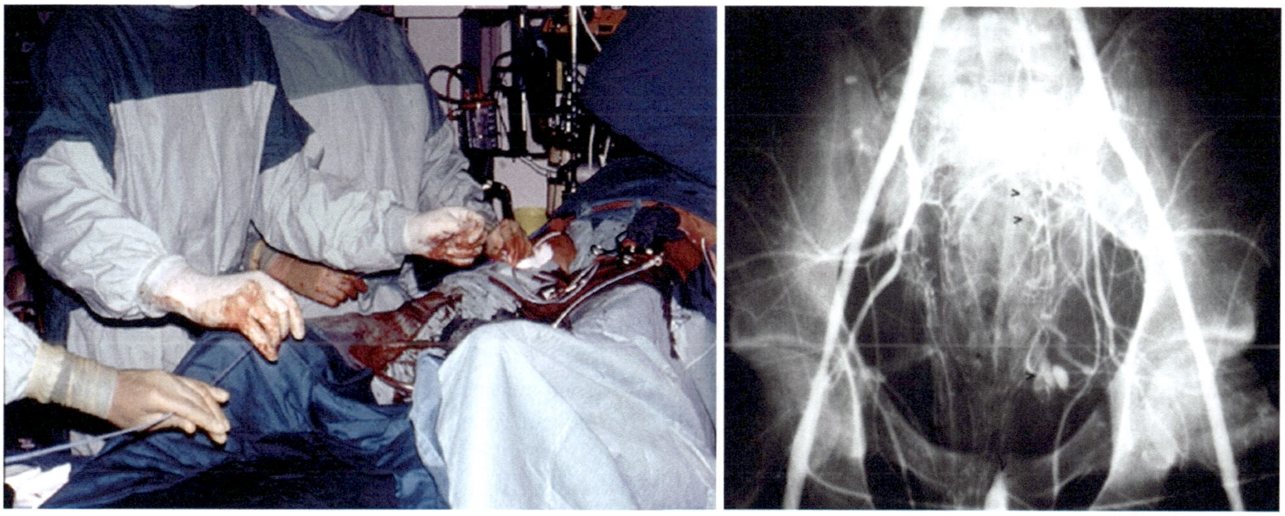

Fig. 15.4 Vascular approach to the femoral artery for angiography: injury of the lateral sacral artery and spasm of the inferior gluteal artery

the major arterial anatomy and may reveal the bleeding site. Selective internal iliac arteriography usually demonstrates clinically significant bleeding. The bleeding artery is identified by extravasation of contrast in the arterial phase, usually persisting well into venous phase. Associated findings may be local arterial spasm, displacement, and compression of arteries owing to hematoma.

15.5.4 Embolization

When the actively bleeding artery is found, a 3F microcatheter with a Guidewire is introduced via the angiographic catheter close to the bleeding point and embolization is performed using various materials, according to the preference of the radiological unit.

15.5.5 Occluding Adjuncts

A variety of hemostatic adjuncts can be used to promote the arrest of hemorrhage using endovascular techniques.

Embolic agents can be distinguished into solid or liquid, mechanical or chemical, and autologous or biosynthetic/synthetic.

Liquid agents can be gelfoam, glue, PVA (polyvinyl alcohol), or Onyx, while mechanical agents include coils and plugs [95].

Additionally, temporary and permanent agents can be distinguished. Temporary agents allow early (autologous blood) or delayed (gelatin sponge) recanalization of the embolized vessels. Permanent agents include nonabsorbable microparticles (PVA, gelatin microspheres), mechanical agents (coils, plugs) or liquid agents [95].

Historically, clotted autologous blood was first used as coagulation agent [15, 96, 97], followed by the use of gelfoam for small arteries [18] and metallic coils with or without gelfoam [98, 99].

Recently, Rehwald et al. reported a higher AE failure rate (higher mortality and higher re-angiography rate) when using too few coils and not using microparticles [100].

- **Autogenous clot.** First, after catheterization of the femoral artery, 25 mL of blood sample is taken and placed in a sterile beaker. Formation of the clot occurs in 15 min. A clot may not form, if the patient has bled massively. An autogenous clot will lyse early (within 12 h), and the risk for rebleeding is high. Therefore, it is not used in author's clinics.
- **Metal coils.** Fibered platinum microcoils provide a good option for definitive occlusion of the bleeding artery. The size of microcoils used should be correct. Therefore, fibered platinum microcoils are our adjunct of choice (with or without glue).
- **Glue.** Glue (mixture of n-bytyl-cyanoacrylate and iophendylate, at a ratio of 1:1 [17] or isobutyl 2-cyanoacrylate) offers a good alternative to metals coils to occlude the bleeding pelvic arteries. It provides a definitive occlusion of a treated artery.
- **Gelfoam.** Gelfoam facilitates more temporary hemorrhage control by promoting clot formation locally. In internal iliac artery lacerations, embolization with Gelfoam might not be effective because the agent merely passes out of the lumen through the injury site. In these rare cases with massive bleeding, metal coils and/or glue is used in the author's clinic.
- **Nitinol plugs.** Nitinol plugs, like metal coils, provide lasting occlusion of a treated vessel.

15.5.6 Nonselective Vs. Selective Embolization

In critical situations, it is reasonable to use nonselective embolization by promptly occluding the main trunk of the internal iliac artery, either uni- or bilaterally. Also, if the patient is in extremis and/or several bleeding points are found in angiography, then proximal nonselective embolization of the internal iliac artery should be carried out (Fig. 15.2). This procedure is considered time-saving and effective compared to selective embolization of more distal, smaller arteries or multiple arteries. On the other hand, selective embolization is preferable in patients that respond to initial shock therapy and exhibit extravasation from a single arterial branch.

15.5.7 Control Angiography

The embolization procedure is stopped when the control angiogram shows no bleeding.

15.6 Special Situations

15.6.1 Bleeding from the Common or External Iliac Artery

Arterial bleeding may occur from any branch of the internal or external iliac system. However, injuries to the main trunk of the common iliac artery and to the external iliac artery are uncommon [6, 19, 39]. In the study by Lindahl et al., 86% of patients exhibited bleeding from the main trunk or main branches of the internal iliac artery, 4% from the main trunk or main branch of the external iliac artery, and 10% from both the internal and external iliac systems [17].

This condition represents an exception to the general principles of managing bleeding from the internal iliac system. In this condition, the clinician should always attempt to repair the injury to the common iliac and external iliac arteries, because the patient is at significant risk of critical ischemia in the lower leg, which can result in limb loss [13, 101]. An endovascular stent placement might be an option for bleeding control.

Angiography is an effective tool for identifying rare bleeding sources, such as the femoral circumflex artery in the external iliac system. Bleeding from the branches of the external iliac artery can be best controlled with selective angiographic embolization. PPP will not tamponade this more lateral, anterior source of hemorrhage, and direct surgical bleeding control is too difficult without angiographic information about the anatomical location of the bleeding artery.

On the other hand, rupture of the main trunk of the external iliac artery is unique, because it is the only pelvic arterial injury that requires immediate surgical repair. This arterial injury might be suspected in connection with a crushed pelvis [24]. A rupture of the common iliac artery is also possible, but rare. It is also an indication for early surgical repair to restore the arterial supply and avoid critical ischemia of the lower leg.

15.6.2 Intra-Abdominal and Pelvic Arterial Bleeding

In combined pelvic ring and abdominal injuries, numerous investigators have recommended that laparotomy, when indicated, should be performed before AE [33, 102, 103]. However, Eastridge et al. reviewed 193 pelvic fractures and found that patients ($n = 4$) that underwent angiography before laparotomy had better outcomes than patients ($n = 10$) that underwent laparotomy first (mortality 25% and 60%, respectively) [36].

In the outcome study by Lindahl et al., 49 patients with pelvic fracture-related arterial bleeding were treated with AE [17]. Nine of these patients had concomitant intra-abdominal bleeding necessitating laparotomy. Six patients had emergency laparotomy before AE, and three after AE. The overall mortality in patients with concomitant intra-abdominal bleeding necessitating laparotomy was 44%, whereas the overall mortality in patients without intra-abdominal bleeding was 25%.

15.6.3 Packing and AE in Patient in Extremis

Direct pelvic packing via a retroperitoneal approach has been proposed as a damage control treatment for patients that are exsanguinating, but are not in an adequate condition for transport to the angiography suite [2, 5, 28, 89, 104]. In these rare cases, when the patient is in extremis, pelvic packing may slow down the bleeding sufficiently to gain time for resuscitating the patient to a status suitable for tolerating the definitive arterial bleeding control provided with TAE [40, 45, 89, 104]. Pelvic packing and AE play complementary roles in the control of massive intrapelvic bleeding [104, 105]. In a systematic review of pelvic packing studies, Papakostidis and Giannoudis concluded that this procedure can facilitate early control of intrapelvic bleeding and provide crucial time for more selective management of hemorrhage with embolization [5].

15.6.4 Temporary Occlusion of the Aorta

A precise assessment and control of massive bleeding from large pelvic arteries requires time. This time can be gained partly by applying PPP, and partly by temporarily occluding the aorta with a left side resuscitative thoracotomy and aortic cross-clamping. This procedure has been incorporated into clinical guidelines, but survival is rare [106].

More recently, resuscitative endovascular balloon occlusion of the aorta (REBOA) has been accepted as the preferred initial maneuver for controlling massive pelvic hemorrhage [106, 107].

Sadeghi et al. first reported an observational multicenter study of results regarding continuous and non-continuous REBOA with favorable outcomes. However, the authors summarized that further prospective studies are needed to be able to draw conclusions on morbidity and mortality [108].

15.6.5 Multiple and Bilateral Arterial Pelvic Bleeding

Arterial bleeding may occur from any branch of the internal or external iliac system. In the study by Lindahl et al., angiography revealed multiple bleeding vessels in two-thirds of the cohort and bilateral arterial bleeding in one-third of the cohort [17]. Similar incidences were reported by O'Neill et al. [19]. A higher incidence of bilateral bleeding (64%) was reported in a postmortem angiography study by Huittinen and Slätis on individuals that sustained pelvic fractures in accidents [24]. The worst prognosis is related to exsanguinating bleeding from the large pelvic arteries or from multiple smaller arteries [17, 19]. All bleeding from the internal iliac arteries and from the smaller branches of the external iliac artery might be occluded successfully with embolization.

15.6.6 Bleeding from the Main Trunk of the Internal Iliac Artery

Massive bleeding and the worst prognosis are often associated with rupture of the internal iliac artery and, in some rare cases, with rupture of the external iliac artery. The prognosis was worse for patients bleeding from the internal or external iliac artery (mortality 57%) compared to patients bleeding from more distal, smaller pelvic arteries (mortality 24%) [17].

Hemorrhage control of a ruptured internal iliac artery might be technically difficult with packing. The internal iliac artery is short, about 4 cm long, and it arises from the common iliac artery, above the pelvic brim (Fig. 15.1), at the level of the lumbosacral intervertebral disc. From there, it descends to the upper margin of the greater sciatic foramen, where it divides into its main branches. Even when retroperitoneal pelvic packing is considered for reducing internal iliac artery bleeding, it is difficult to achieve a tamponade when the compression swabs are only placed into the true pelvis. In theory, the swabs should also be placed above the pelvic brim, against the trunk of internal iliac artery. However, in that location, the swabs may also cause compression of the external iliac artery, which would increase the risk of critical ischemia in the lower leg.

Due to the extensive collateral circulation in the pelvis, even the main internal iliac artery can be occluded [109–111]. The complication rate after emergency uni- or bilateral internal iliac artery embolization is typically low [17, 112].

Table 15.3 Angiography rates in pelvic ring injuries

Year	Author	No. of patients	No. angio	Angio-rate (%)	Location
2016	Costantini	1339	77	5.8	North America
2016	Froberg	2173	31	1.4	Europe
2013	Metsemakers	803	15	1.9	Europe
2012	Hauschild	5040	17	0.3	Europe
2011	Cherry	912	65	7.1	North America
2011	Karadimas	400	34	8.5	Europe
2010	Jeske	1476	42	2.8	Europe
2010	Costantini	819	31	3.8	North America
2009	Fang	964	174	18	Asia
2005	Shapiro	678	31	4.6	North America
	SUM	**14,604**	**517**	**3.5**	

15.7 Epidemiology

Some analyses reported AE frequency rates (Table 15.3):

- Costantini et al. prospectively analyzed 1339 patients with pelvic ring injuries and reported an angiography rate of 5.8% and an embolization rate of 1.6% [10].
- Froberg et al. performed AE in 31 of 2173 patients (AE rate: 1.4%) [113].
- Metsemakers et al. analyzed 803 patients with pelvic ring injuries, of which 15 underwent AE (1.9%) [114].
- Hauschild et al. analyzed data from 5040 patients from the German Pelvic Trauma Registry and identifies 152 patients with pelvic bleeding, of whom 17 underwent angiography and angioembolization (0.3% of all patients, 11.2% of patients with CT diagnosed bleeding) [34].
- Cherry et al. performed angioembolization in 65 patients from a group of 912 pelvic ring fracture patients (angiography rate: 7.1%) [115].
- Karadimas et al. reported an angiography rate of 8.5% (34 of 400 patients with pelvic ring injuries) [116].
- Jeske et al. analyzed 1476 pelvic fracture patients, including 42 with angiographic embolization (2.8%) [85].
- Costantini et al. reported on 819 patients, with only 31 patients (3.8%) undergoing diagnostic pelvic angiography [117].
- In the analysis by Fang et al., pelvic angiography was performed on174 of 964 patients with pelvic fractures (18%) and 140 patients needed embolization (14.5% of all patients, 80.4% embolization rate) [82].
- Shapiro et al. analyzed 678 patients with pelvic fractures and performed angiography in 31 patients (4.6%) [88].

Table 15.4 Analysis of different historical embolization studies

Year	Author	No.	Time	PRBC	PRBC/h	Mortality (%)
1986	Chaufour	9	17.8	13.9	0.78	11.1
1989	Grabenwöger	6	n.e.	24	n.e.	50.0
1992	Hölting	20	13.5	28	2.1	55
1995	Piotin	6	44	11.3	0.25	0
1998	Perez	8	5.7	120.6	1.8	25
2000	Hamill	20	5	14	2.8	45
2002	Cook	23	3.7	n.e.	n.e.	43
	SUM	**92**	**10.6**	**18.3**	**1.65**	**39.1**

A difference was observed comparing angiography rate from North America and Europe.

In North America (USA), a significantly higher amount of patients is treated using angiography and/or embolization to control pelvic ring injury-related hemorrhage [10, 88, 115, 117]. The overall angiography rate was 5.4% (204 angiographies/3748 patients with pelvic injuries). Roudsari et al. observed a reduction of performed angiographies from 31% in 1996 to 9% in 2010 in an analysis of 6315 pelvic ring injury patients [118].

In contrast, in European trauma centers, angiography is performed in only 1.4% of patients (517 angiographies/9892 patients with pelvic injuries) [34, 85, 113, 114, 116].

> Pelvic angiography is performed in 1–4% of patients with (major) pelvic fractures.

15.8 Patient Groups Requiring Angioembolization

The available literature of angioembolization until 2017 was analyzed for specific patient data.

Gänsslen et al. reviewed different embolization studies [16, 21, 68, 77, 78, 80, 119] in 2003 (Table 15.4) and analyzed the number of patients with embolization (no.), time to embolization (hours), transfusion requirements before embolization (PRBC), PRBC/h and mortality [120].

These patient groups represent highly heterogeneous groups, with multiple other injuries. The average time to intervention decreased over time from 17 to 5 h, but the average time is still very long with 10.7 h. During this time, a mean of 18.3 PRBC were transfused, indicating a rate of 1.65 PRBC/h.

15.9 Analysis of Data from Studies 1997–2005

Analysis of studies, published between 1997 and 2005, revealed a rate of 2.9% performed angiographies on 3879 patients with an incidence of arterial bleeding of 65% and a mortality rate of 32% [16, 36, 61, 75, 80, 88, 121–123]. The rate of clinically relevant bleeding could not be confirmed.

A more recent analysis [46] stated that angiographic embolization is necessary in about 3% of cases [61, 75, 80, 88, 123], with a success rate as high as 95% [88, 122–124] despite an overall mortality rate in these patients of 1/3 of cases [3, 16, 20, 29, 33, 75, 80, 88, 102, 122, 123].

A problem of angiographic data analyses are still different definitions of hemodynamic instability, such as 6 PRBCs/24 h to 6 PRBCs/72 h [27, 125] and the clinical definition of hemodynamic instability.

Interestingly, more recent data show a much higher incidence of performed angiography/embolization, up to 31% [22, 82, 83, 126, 127].

15.10 Analysis of Data from Recent Studies 2005–2017

Data from 33 recent studies were analyzed in terms of patient demographics, clinical and laboratory hemodynamic parameters, and mortality [22, 34, 55, 60, 66, 82–90, 92–94, 113, 114, 116, 117, 127–138].

15.10.1 Demographics

The mean or median age was reported in 28 studies [22, 34, 55, 60, 66, 82, 83, 85–90, 92–94, 113, 114, 116, 117, 127, 128, 130, 131, 133, 134, 136, 138].

Analysis of these 1497 patients showed an average age of 45 years (range: 33–58 years).

The rate of male or female patients was reported in 23 studies [34, 55, 60, 66, 82, 85, 87, 88, 92–94, 113, 116, 117, 127, 128, 130, 133–138].

In this group of 1438 patients, 964 were male (67%), representing a male/female ratio of 2:1.

15.10.2 Injury Severity

The mean or median Injury Severity based on the Injury Severity Score (ISS) was reported in 27 studies [22, 34, 55, 82, 83, 85–90, 92–94, 113, 114, 116, 117, 127–129, 131, 133–135, 137, 138].

Analysis of these 1464 patients showed an average ISS of 29 points (range: 16.6–45.9 points).

15.10.3 Shock Parameters

The combined mean or median systolic blood pressure (sBP) and the heart rate (HR) were reported in 10 studies [66, 92–94, 116, 117, 127, 130, 135, 138].

Analysis of these 826 patients showed an average sBP of 113.7 mmHg (range: 92–119.1 mmHg) and an HR of

102.9 bpm (range: 91–109.3 bpm). The calculated shock index (SI) for this group of patients was 0.9.

Additionally, these data were analyzed in relation to age (<45 years, >45 years) and ISS.

No relevant difference was observed comparing these age groups (sBP: 116.9 vs. 112.6 mmHg, HR: 102.1 vs. 103.2 bpm; SI: 0.87 vs. 0.92). Combined data of ISS, sBP, and HR were reported in eight studies [92–94, 116, 117, 127, 135, 138]. The mean ISS in 759 patients was 27.2 points.

Data grouping to ISS groups <30 points and >30 points showed different shock parameters, but the shock index in both groups was below 1 (0.89 vs. 0.97). The HR was identical in both groups with 103 bpm, while the sBP was slightly lower in patients with higher ISS (107.3 vs. 116.7 mmHg).

Laboratory parameters included hemoglobin concentration (Hb (g/dl)), lactate (Lac, mmol/L) and base deficit (BD, mmol/L).

The mean or median Hb was reported in 11 studies [34, 82, 83, 85, 87, 90, 93, 113, 127, 130, 138]. In 492 patients, an average Hb concentration of 9.97 g/dL could be calculated.

The mean or median Lac was reported in five studies [85, 89, 93, 113, 138]. In 139 patients, an average Lac concentration of 4.3 mmol/L could be calculated.

The mean or median BD was reported in six studies [85, 88–90, 113, 117]. In 171 patients, an average BD of −8.1 mmol/L could be calculated.

The mean or median transfusions (packed red blood cells, PRBC) within the first 24 h after admission were reported in eight studies [55, 86, 90, 92, 94, 113, 116, 135]. In 725 patients, a mean of 6.9 PRBC/24 h were transfused.

15.10.4 Mortality

Data on patient mortality were reported in 25 studies [22, 34, 55, 82, 83, 85, 86, 88, 90, 92–94, 113, 114, 116, 117, 127, 128, 130, 131, 133–136, 138].

Analysis of these 1603 patients showed an average mortality rate of 17.5%. A trend to lower mortality rates can be observed, when grouping patients to the years 2005–2010, 2011–2014, and 2015–2017. The corresponding mortality rates were 18.7%, 17.9%, and 16.7%, respectively.

Mortality correlated well with Injury Severity. An ISS <35 was associated with a mortality rate of 16.9%, while patients with a median/mean ISS >35 had a mortality rate of 31.4%.

In the patient group (*n* = 471) with a recorded Hb (9.96 g/dL) [34, 82, 83, 85, 87, 90, 93, 113, 127, 130, 138], the overall mortality rate was 19.3%.

In the patient group (*n* = 471) with a recorded Lac (4.2 mmol/L) [85, 89, 93, 113, 138], the overall mortality rate was 27.7%.

In the patient group (*n* = 171) with a recorded BD (−8.1 mmol/L) [85, 88–90, 113, 117], the overall mortality rate was 21.6%.

> During the last 1.5 decades, the group of patients requiring AE presented with moderate hemodynamic instability with a shock index <1, low transfusion requirements within the first 24 h and, compared to patients with pelvic packing, a relatively lower mortality rate of 17.5%.

15.11 Drawbacks of Angiography

Several drawbacks have been associated with performing AE.

- AE can be time-consuming due to transporting the patient to the angiography suite and, therefore, simultaneous treatment of associated injuries must be delayed [3, 9, 74, 120].
- AE requires a skilled interventional radiologist; thus, this individual must be available 24 h/day, which might be difficult to organize in small trauma units.
- A procedure delay of 1–5.5 h was recorded; thus, only 14.7% of angiographies were performed within 90 min [139].
- Access to the femoral artery might be difficult, due to obesity, hypotension, or soft tissue injuries [19, 20].
- There is a risk of hematoma development and pseudoaneurysm at the arterial puncture site [16].
- AE of the internal iliac arteries can cause ischemia and necrosis of the gluteal muscle, bladder wall, uterus, colon, and femoral head [140–145].
- AE can result in neurological defects, paresis of the lower leg, and impotence [16, 22, 25, 140].
- AE can be accompanied with recurrent bleeding, requiring ongoing blood product administration, and re-embolization [82, 88, 126].
- Historically, 20% of patients required CPR during AE [146].

15.12 Advantages of AE

In contrast to the potential drawbacks, several advantages of AE are clearly stated in the recent literature.

- Auerbach et al. could find, that selective AE of branches of the internal iliac artery was without potential harmful risk for patients with pelvic ring injuries; even nonselective AE was safe when performed unilaterally [128].

- Velmahos et al. [147] reported 30 patients who underwent bilateral internal iliac artery embolization. Thirteen patients had first undergone laparotomy with unsuccessful control of the bleeding. In the remaining 17 patients, embolization was performed as the primary treatment for control of hemorrhage. The overall success rate was 97% for patients with blunt pelvic trauma. The authors concluded that the procedure appears to be useful in selected patients.
- Agolini et al. [75] retrospectively investigated 15 patients who underwent pelvic angiography and embolization. All embolizations were successful; no deaths resulted from ongoing hemorrhage. Embolization was performed between 50 min and 19 h after arrival in the ICU. The average time to perform angiography was 90 min (50–140 min). Patients who underwent embolization within 3 h of arrival had a significantly greater survival rate. No data were given for pelvic ring instability or hemodynamic instability. The authors concluded that embolization is effective, but is indicated in only a small percentage of patients with pelvic fractures.
- Hamill et al. [78] retrospectively analyzed 76 pelvic trauma patients who received more than 6 U of blood within the first 24 h. Twenty patients underwent pelvic embolization, with a primary success rate of 90%.

An adequate clinical success rate after AE is reported.

In 2012, Papakostidis et al. performed a systematic review of the available literature based on 21 articles [16, 18, 20, 22, 27, 29, 33, 55, 75, 82–85, 88, 89, 121, 123, 127, 139, 148, 149]. The main findings included:

- After AE, often a reduction of transfusion requirements can be expected.
- AE was associated with a high success rate (81–100%).
- Repeated angiography was necessary in 0–26%.
- Repeated AE was necessary in 0–19%.
- Patients requiring angiography/embolization presented with a mortality rate of 7—50%.
- In 6.3% of patients, pelvic hemorrhage was responsible for mortality.
- In 5% of patients, concomitant injuries were responsible for mortality.
- In 8% of patients, shock-related complication (ARDS, MOF, sepsis) were responsible for mortality.
- The overall procedure complication rate was 1% (0–9.7%).

A recent review of 26 studies analyzed comparable parameters [59]:

- Aangiography incidence ranged from 0.34% to 48.6%.
- 13.1% to 100% required embolization.
- A 74% to 100% success rate was observed.
- A 2.2% to 34% rate of repeated angiographies was stated.
- An 11.3% to 40.0% embolization rate was stated (re-angiography/embolization was associated often with a new bleeding site [36, 78, 126]. These patients, additionally, presented more often with multiple injuries and more hemodynamic instability [36].).
- High mortality rates were observed for patients requiring pelvic embolization.

15.13 Involved Vessels

No clear statement can be given from analysis of the literature. Several studies analyzed involved vessels for embolization, but were associated with a wide range of different vessels.

Lindahl et al. analyzed 49 patients with AE [69]. The internal iliac artery (IIA) was involved in 42 patients (86%), including main trunk involvement in six patients (12%) and main branches in 36 patients (74%) of all vessels involved. Lesions of the external iliac artery (EIA) were seen in two patients (4%), with one main trunk and one main branch (femoral circumflex artery) involvement (Fig. 15.5). In five patients, a combined injury to the EIA and IIA was observed. Overall, more than one bleeding artery was seen in 59% and bleeding from both sides of the pelvic ring in 30%.

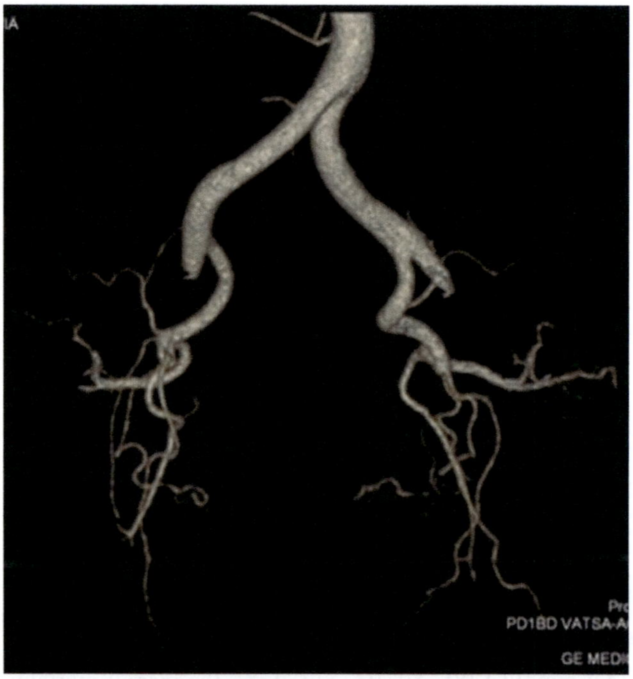

Fig. 15.5 Interruption of the IEA flow

Table 15.5 Analysis of involved vessels

Year	Author	No.	CIA	IEA	IIA	ILA	SGA	IGA	MSA	LSA	OA	PA	FA
2017	Cha	19	0	0	0	4	2	3	1	6	8	3	0
2015	Ierardi	168	0	1	0	19	55	10	0	27	29	44	1
2010	Jeske	45	1		14	1	9		1		4	16	
2008	Westhoff	21	0	0	0	6	5	3	0	2	2	1	0
2006	Tötterman	31	0	0	28	2	11	0	0	4	4	3	1

CIA common iliac artery, *IEA* iliac external artery, *IIA* internal iliac artery, *ILA* iliolumbar artery, *SGA* superior gluteal artery, *IGA* inferior gluteal artery, *MSA* median sacral artery, *LSA* lateral sacral artery, *OA* obturator artery, *PA* internal pudendal artery, *FA* femoral artery

Large arterial disruptions (internal or external iliac artery) were associated with type C pelvic ring injuries, relevant shock (BD14.0 mmol/L) and a mortality rate of 57%.

Other relevant vessels include the superior gluteal artery (SGA), the iliolumbar artery (ILA), the obturator artery (OA), and the internal pudendal artery (PA) (Table 15.5).

15.14 Complications

AE is associated with complications affecting the outcome of survivors. Vaidya et al. analyzed the literature until 2017 and reported complication rates ranging from 0% to 63% [59]. Matityahu et al. focused on complications in 98 patients after pelvic AE [150]. The overall complication rate was 11.2%. Six patients developed gluteal muscle necrosis (6.1%), five patients developed surgical wound breakdown (5.1%), four showed deep infections (4.1%), and one a superficial infection. Urogenital complications included erectile dysfunction in two and bladder necrosis in one patient. Risk factors included the presence of Morel-Levallée lesions and (bilateral) nonselective embolization.

Puncture site complications are rarely observed, but can include local hematoma at the puncture site, and pseudoaneurysm at the arterial puncture site [16].

Overall, complications associated with AE can include:

- Surgical wound breakdown.
- Deep infection.
- Gluteal muscle necrosis, especially after nonselective internal iliac artery embolization [145, 150].
- Nerve injury.
- Bladder or ureteral infarction [151].
- Rebleeding or re-hemorrhage.
- Bowel infarction.
- Thigh or buttock claudication.
- Erectile dysfunction.
- Increased rates of buttock, thigh, or perineal paresthesia [112].
- Contrast nephropathy [152].

Recently, two studies from Taiwan reported results on sexual dysfunction after angioembolization of pelvic hemorrhage:

- Male patients presented with a higher risk of erectile dysfunction [153].
- In female patients, a higher risk of infertility was observed [154].

> When employed to control potentially life-threatening hemorrhage, the frequent benefits surely outweigh the rare risk [67].

Conflicting results were reported regarding the effect of (non-selected) bilateral Internal Iliac Artery (IIA) embolization. Several authors suggested increased complication rates [63, 80, 112, 131, 150]. In contrast, Travis et al. reported no differences regarding skin necrosis, sloughing, pelvic perineal infection, or nerve injury within 30 days after embolization compared to patients without embolization [112].

Embolization of the internal iliac arteries was rarely reported to cause ischemia and necrosis of the gluteal muscle, bladder wall, uterus, colon, or femoral head. In addition, very rare complications include neurological defects, paresis of the lower leg, and impotence [16, 22, 25, 140].

In a recent study, unilateral necrosis of the gluteal muscle was seen in 1 out of 49 patients [17]. The etiology of ischemia of the gluteal muscle in this case was either the embolization of the internal iliac artery or direct impact and compartment syndrome of the buttock.

Even bilateral IIA embolization was not associated with negative effects on urogenital function [155], and other authors reported no complications after bilateral nonselective embolization [60, 63]. Possibly, larger-than-average gelatin sponge use allows some collateral blood flow of smaller vessels, resulting in less tissue ischemia and reduced complication rates [63, 144].

15.15 Re-bleeding and Repeat AE

Some studies have reported recurrent bleeding after TAE; this condition requires ongoing blood product administration and re-embolization [82, 88, 126].

Shapiro et al. reported re-angiographies in three of 16 patients (18.8%) with primary AE due to ongoing hemodynamic instability [88]. Additionally, of 15 patients with initial negative angiography, five patients required re-angiography (33.3%) after secondary diagnosed arterial bleeding. Recurrent hypotension (sBP < 90), absence of intra-abdominal injury, and a persistent base deficit of >10 for >6 h were predictive for re-angiography. However, they did not report the source of rebleeding.

Gourlay et al. analyzed 556 patients with primary angiography and reported a re-angiography rate of 7.5% [126]. New bleeding sites were observed in 82% of these patients and 32% presented with persistent bleeding areas. Risk factors for recurrent angiography were ongoing transfusion requirements (>2 PRBC/h) and >2 arterial bleeding sites on initial angiography. The time between the first and the second angiography was 24.3 h on average.

Fang et al. analyzed 964 patients with different pelvic ring injuries. In 174 patients, an angiography was performed, of which 135 showed active contrast media extravasation. In 133 of these patients, an AE was performed [82].

The rate of re-angiographies was 25.2% ($n = 34$) and the re-embolization rate was 19.5%. The time between the first and the second angiography was 3–58 h, with a mean of 21 h. Re-AE was clinically effective in 100%. Interestingly, 69.2% of patients with re-angiography had stable pelvic injuries (LC I + II; AP I). The sources of bleeding were new sites in 38%, previously embolized sites in 27%, and both of these in 35% of patients.

In the study by Lindahl et al., they used coils and/or glue to occlude the bleeding arteries, and no rebleeding occurred from embolized vessels [17]. On the other hand, one repeated angiography revealed a new bleeding artery, which was treated with selective embolization.

One potential explanation for new bleeding arteries is that they were in vasospasm or had thrombosed during the first TAE, and they started to bleed again later. Alternatively, rebleedings might have resulted from the use of gelatin sponges (gel foam) to occlude the vessels; these sponges absorb quickly, and recanalization can occur between 48 h and a few weeks after the embolization [25, 147].

> Re-angiographies are performed between 2% and 25% after a mean of 24 h. Ongoing hemodynamic instability and shock are the main risk factors to identify new or persistent bleeding sites.

15.15.1 30-Day Mortality

The cause of death in patients with multiple injuries is often multifactorial; therefore, the contribution of major hemorrhage to mortality is difficult to determine [5].

The present mortality rate of patients with performed AE from 25 studies showed an average mortality rate of 17.5% [22, 34, 55, 82, 83, 85, 86, 88, 90, 92–94, 113, 114, 116, 117, 127, 128, 130, 131, 133–136, 138].

In a previous study, head injury was the major cause of death in patients that sustained pelvic fractures, with or without injuries to other body regions [4]. In that study, the most common general reason for death, not related to a specific body region, was major hemorrhage, and the primary source of lethal bleeding was the pelvis.

Lindahl et al. reported that five of 14 non-survivors (36%) died from head injuries [17]. Among non-survivors, none died from ongoing pelvic bleeding, but five died from the bleeding-related, irreversible, lethal triad (acidosis, hypothermia, and coagulopathy) within the first 24 h. In addition, three late deaths were due to prolonged, hypovolemia-related, multiple organ failure (MOF), and one died from cardiac arrest. In their series, bleeding-related mortality was 16%, after excluding deaths from head injuries.

15.16 Predictive Factors for AE

Several studies analyzed predictive factors suggesting necessity of AE.

15.16.1 Fracture Type

Unstable posterior pelvic injuries are associated with an increased need for AE:

- Fractures involving the greater sciatic notch and sacrum fractures were associated with angiography [129].
- A further study reported an association of pelvic blush detected on CT evaluation with complete posterior pelvic injury [134].
- A multicenter study revealed, that especially LC I, LC II and VS injuries, according to Young and Burgess, were associated with the need of different hemorrhage control interventions, including pelvic angioembolization, preperitoneal pelvic packing, pelvic external fixator placement, or REBOA, respectively [156].
- APC pelvic fractures were associated with higher rates of angioembolization and bilateral IIA injuries [133].
- Unstable pelvic fractures are risk factors for need of angioembolization [157].

A recent trauma registry-based study of 5340 patients with pelvic ring disruptions showed that the mortality rate was higher among patients with type C fractures than among patients with types B and A fractures [4]. This result was the same between patients with non-isolated pelvic injuries that had additional injuries in other body regions and patients with isolated pelvic ring injuries.

In a single trauma center study, three-fourths of arterial bleedings (78%) occurred in high-energy type C pelvic ring injuries. The other one-fourth of arterial bleedings was associated with other pelvic ring injuries (type B: 14%; type A: 2%) and with acetabular fractures (6%) [17].

In an analysis of 15 patients with performed angiography, the positive predictive value for embolization using CT evaluated hematoma alone was 39%, while that of isolated pelvic blush was 73% and the presence of an unstable type B or C fracture alone was 47%. The combined positive predictive value of all three parameters was 75% [158].

15.16.2 Hemodynamic Parameters

Further analyses focused on hemodynamic parameters and type of vascular lesions.

In an analysis of 143 patients after high-energy trauma mechanism, a BD <6 mmol/L, systolic blood pressure <104 mmHg, and the need for transfusion in ED were found to be independent predictors of arterial pelvic bleeding during the emergency department phase [159].

15.16.3 Vascular Lesions

Lindahl et al. analyzed 49 patients with AE [17]. Exsanguinating bleeding from the large pelvic arteries (iliac arteries) was associated with extreme mortality compared to bleeding from smaller arteries (57% vs. 24%). Patients with very low initial BD values (<−10.0 mmol/L) were associated with a negative predictive value for survival. In these patients, an aggressive bleeding control protocol with extraperitoneal pelvic packing or REBOA prior to AE was recommended.

15.16.4 Risk Models

Salim et al. developed a risk stratification model for pelvic angiography, including the parameters SI-joint disruption, female gender, and duration of hypotension [127]. The following equation was derived from the multivariable analysis:

> Logarithm odds of therapeutic angiography = −1.408 + (1.361 × gender female) + (1.497 × presence of SIJ disruption) + (0.364 × min of SBP < 100 mmHg during first 2 h: 15).

In the presence of three risk factors, angiography was performed in 99%, while patients with no presented risk factor showed an AE probability of only 20%.

Comparably, Shapiro et al. developed a risk model for recurrent angiography based on recurrent hypotension (sBP <90 mmHg), persistent base deficit of <−10 mmol/L for >6 h following angiography and absence of intra-abdominal injury [88]. The calculated probability of bleeding was estimated by:

> Log odds of rebleeding = −0.667 + (2.0149 × sBP < 90) − (1.6292 × intra-abdominal bleeding) + (2.1282 × BD < −10).

In the presence of all three risk factors, re-angiography was required in 97%, while patients with no presented risk factors showed a recurrent AE probability of 9%.

15.16.5 Patient Age

As the population ages, more elderly people will require acute treatment due to trauma. The number of osteoporotic pelvic fractures in the older population has increased during the past few decades [160, 161]. Patient age was found to be a risk factor for hemorrhage and mortality in patients that sustain pelvic fractures [2, 6, 7, 13, 26, 27, 29]. However, a recent trauma registry-based study of patients with pelvic fractures did not show any differences in mean age or the age distribution between survivors and non-survivors [4]. They explained this with the observation that young patients that sustained high-energy traumas had a higher risk of lethal injures to other body regions than older patients. The elevated risk of hemorrhage in older individuals may be due to the fact that arteriosclerosis is common among older people; this condition may limit the ability of injured vessels to tamponade spontaneously through vasospasm [9]. Thus, older patients frequently require angiographic embolization for vascular control, even with lower grade pelvic fracture patterns [9, 13]. Several comorbidities and the wide use of anticoagulant and antiplatelet medications among older individuals increases the risk of bleeding with a pelvic injury [162]. In the future, we expect a greater need for bleeding control procedures designed for treating older patients.

15.17 Future Aspects of Emergency Treatment

In the resuscitation phase, immediate identification of the major source of pelvic hemorrhage appears to be impossible with the current methods [40]. Contrast blush in a CT scan is the only means for detecting arterial bleeding prior to an angiography, but the CT does not reveal relevant arterial bleeding in all cases [54]. In addition, hemodynamic instability is contraindicative for a trauma CT. The aim of the CT scan is prompt identification of patients with a significant arterial source of bleeding. These patients will benefit most from AE, when it is performed at the appropriate time, with respect to the assessment and management of other associated injuries [9]. This situation highlights the necessity for further advances in diagnostics and medical imaging of massive arterial bleeding.

The use of large vessel balloon occlusion for resuscitation, such as REBOA, has increased during the past decade [163]. Compared to PPP, endovascular techniques are less invasive, and they are associated with reduced morbidity. Open surgical exploration of a retroperitoneal hematoma increases the danger of infection [5, 40, 104, 164]. PPP is a highly invasive approach, and it requires a second procedure for removing the tamponades. In addition, the effectiveness of PPP has not been definitively proven in cases of massive bleeding from the main trunk of the internal iliac artery. Aortic balloon occlusion techniques are likely to appear more frequently in the treatment algorithms for bleeding in patients with pelvic injuries. Before that occurs, it is necessary to treat a large series of patients with pelvic fractures and massive bleeding with REBOA and analyze the results carefully to determine whether the complication rate is lower and patient survival is improved compared to results reported to date from studies that used AE or PPP, followed by AE.

Successful treatment of a patient with a bleeding pelvic trauma requires a multidisciplinary team approach. The future trauma center should be equipped with all diagnostic, interventional radiological, and operative facilities to avoid transporting an unstable patient to another location for imaging and management. This type of integrated CT-angiography unit could optimize the use of current resuscitation resources. The latest interventions in resuscitation are guided by the concept of hypotensive resuscitation. They aim to avoid excess administration of crystalloids and treat traumatic coagulopathy with early use of fresh frozen plasma, fibrinogen concentrate, platelets, and tranexamic acid, guided by viscoelastometric devices (ROTEM, TEG) [165].

It appears that the best chance at survival can be offered with a multidisciplinary approach, prompt pelvic ring stabilization, resuscitation with new strategies, temporary bleeding control with PPP or REBOA, followed by AE, and an integrated CT-angiography trauma unit.

15.18 Summary

One of the landmark papers dealing with angiographic embolization was published by Matalon et al. already 40 years ago [18]. The conclusions of their findings and experiences of angiographic embolization are still valid:

1. Most patients with pelvic fracture and rapid blood loss have pelvic arterial bleeding sites that can be identified by angiography.
2. Transcatheter arteriographic occlusive methods result in prompt reduction or control of pelvic hemorrhage in nearly all attempts.
3. The effect of transcatheter occlusive treatment on the mortality rate cannot be assessed due to lack of suitable controls.
4. Angiography should be performed early in the course of management of pelvic hemorrhage to avoid complications due to massive blood replacement and hypotension.

Based on the available literature, the following conclusions can be made:

- AE is an effective measure of hemorrhage control secondary to mechanical pelvic stabilization.
- AE can definitively treat pelvic arterial bleeding.
- AE should be performed as early as possible.
- Pelvic angiography is performed in 1–4% of patients with (major) pelvic fractures.
- AE is time-consuming.
- Nonselective proximal AE is recommended in critical clinical situations.
- Selective AE should be performed whenever possible.
- AE is mainly related to a high-energy type C pelvic ring fractures.
- Potential drawbacks should be weighed against the benefits to control potentially life-threatening hemorrhage.

References

1. Cryer HM, Miller FB, Evers BM, Rouben LR, Seligson DL. Pelvic fracture classification: correlation with hemorrhage. J Trauma. 1988;28(7):973–80.
2. Ertel W, Eid K, Keel M, Trentz O. Therapeutical strategies and outcome of polytraumatized patients with pelvic injuries—a six-year experience. Eur J Trauma. 2000;6:278–86.
3. Gilliland M, Ward R, Flynn T, Miller P, Ben-Menachem Y, Duke J. Peritoneal lavage and angiography in the management of patients with pelvic fractures. Am J Surg. 1982;144:744–7.
4. Holstein J, Culemann U, Pohlemann T. Mortality in pelvic fracture patients. What are predictors of mortality in patients with pelvic fractures? Clin Orthop Relat Res. 2012;470:2090–7.
5. Papakostidis C, Giannoudis P. Pelvic ring injuries with haemodynamic instability: efficacy of pelvic packing, a systematic review. Injury. 2009;40:53–61.
6. Rothenberger D, Fischer R, Perry J. Major vascular injuries secondary to pelvic fractures: an unsolved clinical problem. Am J Surg. 1978;136:660–2.
7. Smith W, Williams A, Agudelo J, Shannon M, Morgan S, Stahel P, Moore E. Early predictors of mortality in hemodynamically unstable pelvic fractures. J Orthop Trauma. 2007;21:31–3.
8. Kregor PJ, Routt ML Jr. Unstable pelvic ring disruptions in unstable patients. Injury. 1999;30(Suppl 2):B19–28.

9. Hak DJ. The role of pelvic angiography in evaluation and management of pelvic trauma. Orthop Clin North Am. 2004;35(4):439–43. v
10. Costantini T, Coimbra R, Holcomb J, Podbielski J, Catalano R, Blackburn A, Scalea T, Stein D, Williams L, Conflitti J, Keeney S, Suleiman G, Zhou T, Sperry J, Skiada D, Inaba K, Williams B, Minei J, Privette A, Mackersie R, Robinson B, Moore F, Group APFS. Current management of hemorrhage from severe pelvic fractures: results of an American association for the surgery of trauma multi-institutional trial. J Trauma Acute Care Surg. 2016;80:717–23.
11. Coccolini F, Stahel P, Montori G, Biffl W, Horer T, Catena F, Kluger Y, Moore E, Peitzman A, Ivatury R, Coimbra R, Fraga G, Pereira B, Rizoli S, Kirkpatrick A, Leppaniemi A, Manfredi R, Magnone S, Chiara O, Solaini L, Ceresoli M, Allievi N, Arvieux C, Velmahos G, Balogh Z, Naidoo N, Weber D, Abu-Zidan F, Sartelli M, Ansaloni L. Pelvic trauma: WSES classification and guidelines. World J Emerg Surg. 2017;12:5. https://doi.org/10.1186/s13017-017-0117-6.
12. Kim M, Lee J, Lee S. Factors predicting the need for hemorrhage control intervention in patients with blunt pelvic trauma: a retrospective study. BMC Surg. 2018;18(1):101. https://doi.org/10.1186/s12893-018-0438-8.
13. Henry S, Tornetta PI, Scalea T. Damage control for devastating pelvic and extremity injuries. Surg Clin North Am. 1997;77:879–95.
14. Rossaint R, Bouillon B, Cerny V, Coats T, Duranteau J, Fernández-Mondéjar E, Filipescu D, Hunt B, Komadina R, Nardi G, Neugebauer E, Ozier Y, Riddez L, Schultz A, Vincent J, Spahn D. The European guideline on management of major bleeding and coagulopathy following trauma: fourth edition. Crit Care. 2016;20:100.
15. Margolies M, Ring E, Waltman A, Kerr W, Baum S. Arteriography in the management of hemorrhage from pelvic fractures. New Engl J Med. 1972;287:317–3212.
16. Cook RE, Keating JF, Gillespie I. The role of angiography in the management of haemorrhage from major fractures of the pelvis. J Bone Joint Surg (Br). 2002;84(2):178–82.
17. Lindahl J, Handolin L, Söderlund T, Porras M, Hirvensalo E. Angiographic embolization in the treatment of arterial pelvic hemorrhage: evaluation of prognostic mortality-related factors. Eur J Trauma Emerg Surg. 2013;39:57–63.
18. Matalon T, Athanasoulis C, Margolies M, Waltman A, Novelline R, Greenfield A, Miller S. Hemorrhage with pelvic fractures: efficacy of transcatheter embolization. Am J Roentgenol. 1978;133:959–864.
19. O'Neill P, Riina J, Sclafani S, Tornetta PI. Angiographic findings in pelvic fractures. Clin Orthop Relat Res. 1996;329:60–7.
20. Panetta T, Sclafani S, Goldstein A, Phillips T, Shaftan G. Percutaneous transcatheter embolisation for massive bleeding from pelvic fractures. J Trauma. 1985;25:1021–9.
21. Piotin M, Herbreteau D, Guichard J, Houdart E, Reizine D, Aymard A, Payen D, Merland J. Percutaneous transcatheter embolization in multiply injured patients with pelvic ring disruption associated with severe haemorrhage and coagulopathy. Injury. 1995;26(10):677–80.
22. Tötterman A, Dormagen J, Madsen J, Klow N, Skaga N, Roise O. A protocol for angio-graphic embolization in exsanguinating pelvic trauma. A report on 31 patients. Acta Orthop. 2006;77:462–8.
23. Blackmore C, Cummings P, Jurkovich G, Linnau K, Hoffer E, Rivara F. Predicting major hemorrhage in patients with pelvic fracture. J Trauma. 2006;61:346–52.
24. Huittinen V, Slätis P. Postmortem angiography and dissection of the hypogastric artery in pelvic fractures. Surgery. 1973;73:454–62.
25. Mucha PJ, Welch TJ. Hemorrhage in major pelvic fractures. Surg Clin North Am. 1988;68(4):757–73.
26. Sharma O, Oswanski M, Rabbi J, Georgiadis G, Lauer S, Stombaugh H. Pelvic fracture risk assessment on admission. Am Surg. 2008;74:761–6.
27. Starr A, Griffin D, Reinert C. Pelvic ring disruption: prediction of associated injuries, transfusion requirement, pelvic arteriography, complications, and mortality. J Orthop Trauma. 2002;16:553–61.
28. Ertel W, Keel M, Eid K, Platz A, Trentz O. Control of severe hemorrhage using C-clamp and pelvic packing in multiply injured patients with pelvic ring disruption. J Orthop Trauma. 2001;15(7):468–74.
29. Mucha P, Farnell M. Analysis of pelvic fracture management. J Trauma. 1984;24(5):379–86.
30. Burgess A, Eastridge B, Young J, Ellison T, Ellison P, Poka A, Bathon G, Brumback R. Pelvic ring disruption: effective classification systems and treatment protocols. J Trauma. 1990;30(7):848–56.
31. Magnussen R, Tressler M, Obremskey W, Kregor P. Predicting blood loss in isolated pelvic and acetabular high-energy trauma. J Orthop Trauma. 2007;21:603–7.
32. Dalal S, Burgess A, Siegel J, Young J, Brumback R, Poka A, Dunham C, Gens D, Bathon H. Pelvic fracture in multiple trauma: classification by mechanism is key to pattern of organ injury, resuscitative requirements, and outcome. J Trauma. 1989;29(7):981–1000.
33. Evers BM, Cryer HM, Miller FB. Pelvic fracture hemorrhage: priorities in management. Arch Surg. 1989;124(4):422–4.
34. Hauschild O, Aghayev E, von Heyden J, Strohm P, Culemann U, Pohlemann T, Suedkamp N, Schmal H. Angioembolization for pelvic hemorrhage control: results from the German pelvic injury register. J Trauma Acute Care Surg. 2012;73:679–84.
35. Lunsjo K, Tadros A, Hauggaard A, Blomgren R, Kopke J, Abu-Zidan F. Associated injuries and not fracture instability predict mortality in pelvic fractures: a prospective study of 100 patients. J Trauma. 2007;62:687–91.
36. Eastridge B, Starr A, Minei J, O'Keefe G, Scalea T. The importance of fracture pattern in guiding therapeutic decision-making in patients with hemorrhagic shock and pelvic ring disruptions. J Trauma. 2002;53(3):446–50.
37. Kataoka Y, Maekawa K, Nishimaki H, Yamamoto S, Soma K. Iliac vein injuries in hemodynamically unstable patients with pelvic fracture caused by blunt trauma. J Trauma. 2005;58:704–10.
38. Sadri H, Nguyen-Tang T, Stern R, Hoffmeyer P, Peter R. Control of severe hemorrhage using C-clamp and arterial embolization in hemodynamically unstable patients with pelvic ring disruption. Arch Orthop Trauma Surg. 2005;125(7):443–7.
39. Carrillo E, Wohltmann C, Spain D, Schmieg RJ, Miller F, Richardson J. Common and external iliac artery injuries associated with pelvic fractures. J Orthop Trauma. 1999;13:351–5.
40. Suzuki T, Smith W, Moore E. Pelvic packing or angiography: competitive or complementary? Injury. 2009;40:343–53.
41. Durkin A, Sagi H, Durham R, Flint L. Contemporary management of pelvic fractures. Am J Surg. 2006;192:211–23.
42. Baqué P, Trojani C, Delotte J, Séjor E, Senni-Buratti M, de Baqué F, Bourgeon A. Anatomical consequences of "open-book" pelvic ring disruption: a cadaver experimental study. Surg Radiol Anat. 2005;27(6):487–90.
43. Papadopoulos I, Kanakaris N, Bonovas S, Triantafillidis A, Garnavos C, Voros D. Auditing 655 fatalities with pelvic fractures by autopsy as a basis to evaluate trauma care. J Am Coll Surg. 2006;203:30–43.
44. Spahn DR, Cerny V, Coats TJ, Duranteau J, Fernandez-Mondejar E, Gordini G, Stahel PF, Hunt BJ, Komadina R, Neugebauer E, Ozier Y, Riddez L, Schultz A, Vincent JL, Rossaint R. Management of bleeding following major trauma: a European guideline. Crit Care. 2007;11(1):R17.

45. Gaarder C, Naess PA, Frischknecht Christensen E, Hakala P, Handolin L, Heier HE, Ivancev K, Johansson P, Leppaniemi A, Lippert F, Lossius HM, Opdahl H, Pillgram-Larsen J, Roise O, Skaga NO, Soreide E, Stensballe J, Tonnessen E, Tottermann A, Ortenwall P, Ostlund A. Scandinavian guidelines—"the massively bleeding patient". Scand J Surg. 2008;97(1):15–36.
46. Gänsslen A, Hildebrand F, Pohlemann T. Management of hemodynamic unstable patients "in extremis" with pelvic ring fractures. Acta Chir Orthop Traumatol Cechoslov. 2012;79:193–202.
47. Kivioja A, Myllynen P, Rokkanen P. Survival after massive transfusions exceeding four blood volumes in patients with blunt injuries. Am Surg. 1991;57:398–401.
48. Michelsen T, Salmela L, Tigerstedt I, Mäkeläinen A, Linko K. Massive blood transfusion: is there a limit? Crit Care Med. 1989;17:699–700.
49. Hakala P, Lindahl J, Alberty A, Tanskanen P, Nieminen H, Porras M. Massive transfusion exceeding 150 units of packed red cells during the first 15 hours after injury. J Trauma. 1998;44:410–2.
50. Phillips T, Soulier G, Wilson R. Outcome of massive transfusion exceeding two blood volumes in trauma and emergency surgery. J Trauma. 1987;27:903–10.
51. Wudel J, Morris J, Yates K, Wilson A, Bass S. Massive transfusion: outcome in blunt trauma patients. J Trauma. 1991;31:1–7.
52. Tuovinen H, Söderlund T, Lindahl J, Laine T, Åström P, Handolin L. Severe pelvic fracture-related bleeding in pediatric patients: does it occur? Eur J Trauma Emerg Surg. 2012;38:163–9.
53. Diamond I, Hamilton P, Garber A, Tien H, Chughtai T, Rizoli S, Tremblay L, Brenneman F. Extravasation of intravenous computed tomography scan contrast in blunt abdominal and pelvic trauma. J Trauma. 2009;66:1102–7.
54. Brown C, Kasotakis G, Wilcox A, Rhee P, Salim A, Demetriades D. Does pelvic hematoma on admission computed tomography predict active bleeding at angiography for pelvic fracture? Am Surg. 2005;71:759–62.
55. Sarin E, Moore J, Moore E, Shannon M, Ray C, Morgan S, Smith W. Pelvic fracture pattern does not always predict the need for urgent embolization. J Trauma. 2005;58:973–7.
56. Baker S, O'Neill B, Haddon W, Long W. The injury severity score: a method for describing patients with multiple injuries and evaluating emergency care. J Trauma. 1974;14(3):187–96.
57. Osler T, Baker S, Long W. A modification of the injury severity score that both improves accuracy and simplifies scoring. J Trauma. 1997;43:922–5.
58. Champion H, Sacco W, Copes W, Gann D, Gennarelli T, Flanagan M. A revision of the trauma score. J Trauma. 1989;29:623–9.
59. Vaidya R, Waldron J, Scott A, Nasr K. Angiography and embolization in the management of bleeding pelvic fractures. J Am Acad Orthop Surg. 2018;26:68–76.
60. Barentsz M, Vonken E, van Herwaarden J, Leenen L, Mali W, van den Bosch M. Clinical outcome of intra-arterial embolization for treatment of patients with pelvic trauma. Radiol Res Pract. 2011;2011:935484.
61. Miller PR, Moore PS, Mansell E, Meredith JW, Chang MC. External fixation or arteriogram in bleeding pelvic fracture: initial therapy guided by markers of arterial hemorrhage. J Trauma. 2003;54(3):437–43.
62. Pereira SJ, O'Brien DP, Luchette FA, Choe KA, Lim E, Davis K Jr, Hurst JM, Johannigman JA, Frame SB. Dynamic helical computed tomography scan accurately detects hemorrhage in patients with pelvic fracture. Surgery. 2000;128(4):678–85.
63. Tanizaki S, Maeda S, Matano H, Sera M, Nagai H, Ishida H. Time to pelvic embolization for hemodynamically unstable pelvic fractures may affect the survival for delays up to 60 min. Injury. 2014;45:738–41.
64. Cullinane D, Schiller H, Zielinski M, Bilaniuk J, Collier B, Como J, Holevar M, Sabater E, Sems S, Vassy W, Wynne J. Eastern Association for the Surgery of trauma practice management guidelines for hemorrhage in pelvic fracture--update and systematic review. J Trauma. 2011;71:1850–68.
65. Hallinan J, Tan C, Pua U. Emergency computed tomography for acute pelvic trauma: where is the bleeder? Clin Radiol. 2014;69:529–37.
66. Juern J, Milia D, Codner P, Beckman M, Somberg L, Webb T, Weigelt J. Clinical significance of computed tomography contrast extravasation in blunt trauma patients with a pelvic fracture. J Trauma Acute Care Surg. 2017;82:138–40.
67. Klein E, Kirton O. Angioembolization: indications, approach and optimal use. Curr Trauma Rep. 2015;1:26–34.
68. Hölting T, Buhr H, Richter G, Roeren T, Friedl W, Herfarth C. Diagnosis and treatment of retroperitoneal hematoma in multiple trauma patients. Arch Orthop Trauma Surg. 1992;111(6):323–6.
69. Lindahl J. Management of pelvic ring injuries. Thesis. Finland: University of Helsinki; 2015.
70. Lustenberger T, Wutzler S, Störmann P, Marzi I. The role of pelvic packing for hemodynamically unstable pelvic ring injuries. Clinical Medicine Insights: Trauma and Intensive Medicine. 2015;6:1–8. https://doi.org/10.4137/CMTIM.S12257.
71. Marzi I, Lustenberger T. Management of Bleeding Pelvic Fractures. Scand J Surg. 2014;103:104–11.
72. ATLS. Advanced trauma life support program for doctors, 8th edn. Chicago: American College of Surgeons. 9th Edition; 2012.
73. Hou Z, Smith W, Strohecker K, Bowen T, Irgit K, Baro S, Morgan S. Hemodynamically unstable pelvic fracture management by advanced trauma life support guidelines results in high mortality. Orthopedics. 2012;35:e319–24.
74. ATLS. Advanced trauma life support program for doctors, 8th edn. Chicago: American College of Surgeons. 10th Edition; 2016.
75. Agolini S, Shah K, Jaffe J, Newcomb J, Rhodes M, Reed J. Arterial embolization is a rapid and effective technique for controlling pelvic fracture hemorrhage. J Trauma. 1997;43(3):395–9.
76. Balogh Z, Caldwell E, Heetveld M, D'Amours S, Schlaphoff G, Harris I, Sugrue M. Institutional practice guidelines on management of pelvic fracture-related hemodynamic instability: do they make a difference? J Trauma. 2005;58:778–82.
77. Chaufour J, Melki JP, Riche MC, Fernand M, Cormier JM, Laurian C, Fichelle JM, Gigou F. Complications vasculaires hémorragiques des fractures du bassin. Presse Med. 1986;15(42):2097–100.
78. Hamill J, Holden A, Paice R, Civil I. Pelvic fracture pattern predicts pelvic arterial haemorrhage. Aust N Z J Surg. 2000;70(5):338–43.
79. Holting T, Ruf W, Buhr H, Teller P, Kretzschmar U. Life-threatening hemorrhage in pelvic fractures of polytraumatized patients. Diagnostic issues and embolization treatment. Chirurg. 1988;59(8):547–51.
80. Perez JV, Hughes TM, Bowers K. Angiographic embolisation in pelvic fracture. Injury. 1998;29(3):187–91.
81. Hak DJ, Smith WR, Suzuki T. Management of hemorrhage in life-threatening pelvic fracture. J Am Acad Orthop Surg. 2009;17(7):447–57.
82. Fang J, Shih L, Wong Y, Lin B, Hsu Y. Repeat transcatheter arterial embolization for the management of pelvic arterial hemorrhage. J Trauma. 2009;66:429–35.
83. Fangio P, Asehnoune K, Edouard A, Smail N, Benhamou D. Early embolization and vasopressor administration for management of life-threatening hemorrhage from pelvic fracture. J Trauma. 2005;58(5):978–84. discussion 984
84. Jeroukhimov I, Ashkenazi I, Kessel B, Gaziants V, Peer A, Altshuler A, Nesterenko V, Alfici R, Halevy A. Selection of patients with severe pelvic fracture for early angiography remains controversial. Scand J Trauma Resuscitation Emerg Med. 2009;17:62–8.
85. Jeske H, Larndorfer R, Krappinger D, Attal R, Klingensmith M, Lottersberger C, Dunser M, Blauth M, Falle S, Dallapozza

C. Management of hemorrhage in severe pelvic injuries. J Trauma. 2010;68:415–20.
86. Morozumi J, Homma H, Ohta S, Noda M, Oda J, Mishima S, Yukioka T. Impact of mobile angiography in the emergency Department for Controlling Pelvic Fracture Hemorrhage with Hemodynamic Instability. J Trauma. 2010;68:90–5.
87. Westhoff J, Laurer H, Wutzler S, Wyen H, Mack M, Maier B, Marzi I. Interventionelle Notfallembolisation bei schweren Beckenfrakturen mit arterieller Blutung. Unfallchirurg. 2008;111:821–8.
88. Shapiro M, McDonald AA, Knight D, Johannigman JA, Cuschieri J. The role of repeat angiography in the management of pelvic fractures. J Trauma. 2005;58(2):227–31.
89. Osborn P, Smith W, Moore E, Clothren C, Morgan S, Williams A, Stahel P. Direct retroperitoneal pelvic packing versus pelvic angiography: a comparison of two management protocols for haemodynamically unstable pelvic fractures. Injury. 2009;40:54–60.
90. Tai D, Li W, Lee K, Cheng M, Lee K, Tang L, Lai A, Ho H, Cheung M. Retroperitoneal pelvic packing in the management of hemodynamically unstable pelvic fractures: a level I trauma center experience. J Trauma. 2011;71:E79–86.
91. Seif M, Emam Y. Efficacy and procedural time of angioembolization in ongoing pelvic fracture hemorrhage. Egypt J Radiol Nucl Med. 2011;42:185–91.
92. Tanizaki S, Maeda S, Hayashi H, Matano H, Ishida H, Yoshikawa J, Yamamoto T. Early embolization without external fixation in pelvic trauma. Am J Emerg Med. 2012;30:342–6.
93. Brun J, Guillot S, Bouzat P, Broux C, Thony F, Genty C, Heylbroeck C, Albaladejo P, Arvieux C, Tonetti J, Payen J. Detecting active pelvic arterial haemorrhage on admission following serious pelvic fracture in multiple trauma patients. Injury. 2014;45:1201–106.
94. Tesoriero R, Bruns B, Narayan M, Dubose J, Guliani S, Brenner M, Boswell S, Stein D, Scalea T. Angiographic embolization for hemorrhage following pelvic fracture: is it "time" for a paradigm shift? J Trauma Acute Care Surg. 2017;82:18–26.
95. Medsinge A, Zajko A, Orons P, Amesur N, Santos E. A case-based approach to common embolization agents used in vascular interventional radiology. AJR Am J Roentgenol. 2014;203:699–708.
96. Ayella R, DuPriest R, Khaneja S, Maekawa K, Soderstrom C, Rodriguez A, Cowley R. Transcatheter embolization of autologous clot in the management of bleeding associated with fractures of the pelvis. Surg Gynecol Obstet. 1978;147:849–52.
97. Ring E, Athanasoulis C, Waltman A. Arteriographic management of hemorrhage following pelvic fracture. Radiology. 1973;109:65.
98. Lang E. Transcatheter embolization of pelvic vessels for control of intractable hemorrhage. Radiology. 1981;140:331–9.
99. Yellin A, Lundell C, Finck E. Diagnosis and control of posttraumatic pelvic hemorrhage. Arch Surg. 1983;118:1378–83.
100. Rehwald R, Schönherr E, Petersen J, Jeske H, Fialkovska A, Luger A, Grams A, Loizides A, Jaschke W, Glodny B. Prognostic factors in endovascular treated pelvic haemorrhage after blunt trauma. BMC Surg. 2017;17(1):89. https://doi.org/10.1186/s12893-017-0283-1.
101. Green N, Allen B. Vascular injuries associated with dislocation of the knee. J Bone Joint Surg. 1977;59-A:236–9.
102. Moreno C, Moore EE, Rosenberger A, Cleveland HC. Hemorrhage associated with major pelvic fracture: a multispecialty challenge. J Trauma. 1986;26(11):987–94.
103. Yang A, Iannacone W. External fixation for pelvic ring disruptions. Orthop Clin North Am. 1997;28(3):331–44.
104. Tötterman A, Madsen J, Skaga N, Røise O. Extraperitoneal pelvic packing: a salvage procedure to control massive traumatic pelvic hemorrhage. J Trauma. 2007;62:843–52.
105. Cothren C, Osborn P, Moore E, Morgan S, Johnson J, Smith W. Preperitonal pelvic packing for hemodynamically unstable pelvic fractures: a paradigm shift. J Trauma. 2007;62:834–42.
106. White J, Cannon J, Stannard A, Markov N, Spencer J, Rasmussen T. Endovascular balloon occlusion of the aorta is superior to resuscitative thoracotomy with aortic clamping in a porcine model of hemorrhagic shock. Surgery. 2011;150:400–9.
107. Stannard A, Eliason J, Rasmussen T. Resuscitative endovascular balloon occlusion of the aorta (REBOA) as an adjunct for hemorrhagic shock. J Trauma. 2011;71:1869–72.
108. Sadeghi M, Nilsson K, Larzon T, Pirouzram A, Toivola A, Skoog P. The use of aortic balloon occlusion in traumatic shock: first report from the ABO trauma registry. Eur J Trauma Emerg Surg. 2017;44:491. https://doi.org/10.1007/s00068-017-0813-7.
109. Chait A, Moltz A, Nelson J. The collateral arterial circulation in the pelvis. An angiographic study. Am J Roentgenol. 1967;102:392–400.
110. Ravitch M. Hypogastric artery ligation in acute pelvic trauma. Surgery. 1964;56:601–2.
111. Seavers F, Robinson R. Hypogastric artery ligation for uncontrollable hemorrhage in acute pelvic trauma. Surgery. 1964;55:516.
112. Travis T, Monsky W, London J, Danielson M, Brock J, Wegelin J, Link D. Evaluation of short-term and long-term complications after emergent internal iliac artery embolization in patients with pelvic trauma. J Vasc Interv Radiol. 2008;19:840–7.
113. Froberg L, Helgstrand F, Clausen C, Steinmetz J, Eckardt H. Mortality in trauma patients with active arterial bleeding managed by embolization or surgical packing: an observational cohort study of 66 patients. J Emerg Trauma Shock. 2016;9:107–14.
114. Metsemakers W, Vanderschot P, Jennes E, Nijs S, Heye S, Maleux G. Transcatheter embolotherapy after external surgical stabilization is a valuable treatment algorithm for patients with persistent haemorrhage from unstable pelvic fractures: outcomes of a single centre experience. Injury. 2013;44:964–8.
115. Cherry R, Goodspeed D, Lynch F, Delgado J, Reid S. Intraoperative angioembolization in the management of pelvic-fracture related hemodynamic instability. J Trauma Manag Outcomes. 2011;5:6. https://doi.org/10.1186/1752-2897-5-6.
116. Karadimas E, Nicolson T, Kakagia D, Matthews S, Richards P, Giannoudis P. Angiographic embolisation of pelvic ring injuries. Treatment algorithm and review of the literature. Int Orthop. 2011;35:1381–90.
117. Costantini T, Bosarge P, Fortlage D, Bansal V, Coimbra R. Arterial embolization for pelvic fractures after blunt trauma: are we all talk? Am J Surg. 2010;200:752–7.
118. Roudsari B, Psoter K, Padia S, Kogut M, Kwan S. Utilization of angiography and embolization for abdominopelvic trauma: 14 years' experience at a level I trauma center. AJR Am J Roentgenol. 2014;202:580–5.
119. Grabenwöger F, Dock W, Ittner G. Perkutane Embolisation von retroperitonealen Blutungen bei Beckenfrakturen. RöFo. 1989;150(3):335–8.
120. Gänsslen A, Giannoudis P, Pape H. Hemorrhage in pelvic fracture: who needs angiography? Curr Opin Crit Care. 2003;9:515–23.
121. Kimbrell B, Velmahos G, Chan L, Demetriades D. Angiographic embolization for pelvic fractures in older patients. Arch Surg. 2004;139:728–33.
122. Sugahara T, Saito R, Murakami R, Miyazaki T. Clinical evaluation of transcatheter arterial embolization for the management of retroperitoneal bleeding in cases of pelvic fracture. Nihon Igaku Hoshasen Gakkai Zasshi. 2004;64:197–203.
123. Wong YC, Wang LJ, Ng CJ, Tseng IC, See LC. Mortality after successful transcatheter arterial embolization in patients with unstable pelvic fractures: rate of blood transfusion as a predictive factor. J Trauma. 2000;49(1):71–5.
124. Velmahos GC, Toutouzas KG, Vassiliu P, Sarkisyan G, Chan LS, Hanks SH, Berne TV, Demetriades D. A prospective study on the safety and efficacy of angiographic embolization for pelvic and visceral injuries. J Trauma. 2002;53(2):303–8. discussion 308

125. O'Sullivan R, White T, Keating J. Major pelvic fractures: identification of patients at high risk. J Bone Joint Surg. 2005;87-B(4):530–3.
126. Gourlay D, Hoffer E, Routt M, Bulger E. Pelvic angiography for recurrent traumatic pelvic arterial hemorrhage. J Trauma. 2005;59(5):1168–74.
127. Salim A, Teixeira P, DuBose J, Ottochian M, Inaba K, Margulies D, Demetriades D. Salim predictors of positive angiography in pelvic fractures. A prospective study. J Am Coll Surg. 2008;207:656–62.
128. Auerbach A, Rehman S, Kleiner M. Selective transcatheter arterial embolization of the internal iliac artery does not cause gluteal necrosis in pelvic trauma patients. J Orthop Trauma. 2012;26:290–5.
129. Cha Y, Kim J, Kim Y, Sul Y, Kim H, Choy W. Correlation between pelvic bone fracture site and arterial embolization in severe trauma patients: a retrospective study in a single Korean institute. Trauma Mon. 2017;22(3):e33461.
130. Comai A, Zatelli M, Haglmuller T, Bonatti G. The role of Transcatheter arterial embolization in traumatic pelvic hemorrhage: not only pelvic fracture. Cureus. 2016;8(8):e722. https://doi.org/10.7759/cureus.722.
131. El-Haj M, Bloom A, Mosheiff R, Liebergall M, Weil Y. Outcome of angiographic embolisation for unstable pelvic ring injuries: factors predicting success. Injury. 2013;44:1750–5.
132. Fang J, Shih L, Wong Y, Lin B, Hsu Y. Angioembolization and laparotomy for patients with concomitant pelvic arterial hemorrhage and blunt abdominal trauma. Langenbeck's Arch Surg. 2011;396:243–50.
133. Fu C, Hsieh C, Wu S, Chen R, Wang Y, Shih C, Huang H, Huang J, Tsuo H, Tung H. Anterior-posterior compression pelvic fracture increases the probability of requirement of bilateral embolization. Am J Emerg Med. 2013;31:42–9.
134. Gwak J, Yoon Y, Lee M, Yu B, Jang M, Choi K. Blush on computed tomography and transcatheter arterial embolization in pelvic fracture. J Trauma Injury. 2016;29(4):161–6. https://doi.org/10.20408/jti.2016.29.4.161.
135. Hymel A, Asturias S, Zhao F, Bliss R, Moran T, Marshall R, Benjamin E, Phelan H, Krause P, Marecek G, Leonardi C, Stuke L, Hunt J, Mooney J. Selective versus nonselective embolization versus no embolization in pelvic trauma: a multicenter retrospective cohort study. J Trauma Acute Care Surg. 2017;83:361–7.
136. Ierardi A, Piacentino F, Fontana F, Petrillo M, Floridi C, Bacuzzi A, Cuffari S, Elabbassi W, Novario R, Carrafiello G. The role of endovascular treatment of pelvic fracture bleeding in emergency settings. Eur Radiol. 2015;25:1854–64.
137. Kuo L, Yang S, Fu C, Liao C, Wang S, Wu S. Relative hypotension increases the probability of the need for angioembolisation in pelvic fracture patients without contrast extravasation on computed tomography scan. Injury. 2016;47:37–42.
138. Ruatti S, Guillot S, Brun J, Thony F, Bouzat P, Payen J, Tonetti J. Which pelvic ring fractures are potentially lethal? Injury. 2015;46:1059–63.
139. Verbeek D, Sugrue M, Balogh Z, Cass D, Civil I, Harris I, Kossmann T, Leibman S, Malka V, Pohl A, Rao S, Richardson M, Schuetz M, Ursic C, Wills V. Acute management of hemodynamically unstable pelvic trauma patients: time for a change? Multicenter review of recent practice. World J Surg. 2008;32:1874–82.
140. Hietala S. Urinary bladder necrosis following selective embolization of the internal iliac artery. Acta Radiol Diagn. 1978;19:316–20.
141. Shimizu T, Matsuda S, Sakuragi A, Tsukie T, Kawanabe K. Simultaneous occurrence of a severe Morel-Lavallée lesion and gluteal muscle necrosis as a sequela of transcatheter angiographic embolization following pelvic fracture: a case report. J Med Case Rep. 2015;9:69. https://doi.org/10.1186/s13256-015-0550-7.
142. Sieber P. Bladder necrosis secondary to pelvic artery embolization: case report and literature review. J Urol. 1994;151:422.
143. Suzuki T, Shindo M, Kataoka Y, Kobayashi I, Nishimaki H, Yamamoto S, Uchino M, Takahira N, Yokoyama K, Soma K. Clinical characteristics of pelvic fracture patients with gluteal necrosis resulting from transcatheter arterial embolization. Arch Orthop Trauma Surg. 2005;125:448–52.
144. Takahira N, Shindo M, Tanaka K, Nishimaki H, Ohwada T, Itoman M. Gluteal muscle necrosis following transcatheter angiographic embolisation for retroperitoneal haemorrhage associated with pelvic fracture. Injury. 2001;32(1):27–32.
145. Yasumura K, Ikegami K, Kamohara T, Nohara Y. High incidence of ischemic necrosis of the gluteal muscle after transcatheter angiographic embolization for severe pelvic fracture. J Trauma. 2005;58:985–90.
146. Niwa T, Takebayashi S, Igari H, Morimura N, Uchida K, Sugiyama M, Matsubara S. The value of plain radiographs in the prediction of outcome in pelvic fractures treated with embolisation therapy. Br J Radiol. 2000;73:945–50.
147. Velmahos GC, Chahwan S, Hanks SE, Murray JA, Berne TV, Asensio J, Demetriades D. Angiographic embolization of bilateral internal iliac arteries to control life-threatening hemorrhage after blunt trauma to the pelvis. Am Surg. 2000;66(9):858–62.
148. Hagiwara A, Minakawa K, Fukushima H, Murata A, Masuda H, Shimazaki S. Predictors of death in patients with life-threatening pelvic hemorrhage after successful transcatheter arterial embolization. J Trauma. 2003;55:696–703.
149. Stephen D, Kreder H, Day A, McKee M, Schemitsch E, El Maraghy A, Hamilton P, McLellan B. Early detection of arterial bleeding in acute pelvic trauma. J Trauma. 1999;47:638–42.
150. Matityahu A, Marmor M, Elson J, Lieber C, Rogalski G, Lin C, Belaye T, Miclau TR, Kandemir U. Acute complications of patients with pelvic fractures after pelvic angiographic embolization. Clin Orthop Relat Res. 2013;471:2906–11.
151. Ali A, Nabi G, Swami S, Somani B. Bladder necrosis secondary to internal iliac artery embolization following pelvic fracture. Urol Ann. 2014;6:166–8.
152. Vassiliu P, Sava J, Toutouzas K, Velmahos G. Is contrast as bad as we think? Renal function after angiographic embolization of injured patients. J Am Coll Surg. 2002;194:142–6.
153. Hsu S, Chen C, Wang I, Lin K, Wang C, Chien W, Chung C, Chang W. The risk of erectile dysfunction following pelvic angiographic embolization in pelvic fracture patients: a Nationwide population-based cohort study in Taiwan. World J Surg. 2019;43:476–85.
154. Hsu S, Lee S, Lin K, Lin C, Chien W, Chen C, Chung C, Chang W. Risk of infertility following pelvic angiographic embolization in female patients with pelvic fractures: a nationwide population-based cohort study in Taiwan. PLoS One. 2017;12(12):e0174733. https://doi.org/10.1371/journal.pone.0174733. eCollection 2017
155. Ramirez J, Velmahos G, Best C, Chan L, Demetriades D. Male sexual function after bilateral internal iliac artery embolization for pelvic fracture. J Trauma. 2004;56:734–9.
156. Costantini T, Coimbra R, Holcomb J, Podbielski J, Catalano R, Blackburn A, Scalea T, Stein D, Williams L, Conflitti J, Keeney S, Hoey C, Zhou T, Sperry J, Skiada D, Inaba K, Williams B, Minei J, Privette A, Mackersie R, Robinson B, Moore F, Group APFS. Pelvic fracture pattern predicts the need for hemorrhage control intervention-results of an AAST multi-institutional study. J Trauma Acute Care Surg. 2017;82:1030–8.
157. Fu C, Wu S, Chen R, Wang Y, Chung P, Yeh C, Huang H. Evaluation of pelvic fracture stability and the need for angioembolization: pelvic instabilities on plain film have an increased probability of requiring angioembolization. Am J Emerg Med. 2009;27:792–6.
158. Anandakumar V, Hussein F, Varuun B, Zhu R. Predictive parameters for angiography and embolization in the bleeding pelvic fracture. J Clin Orthop Trauma. 2013;4:70–4.

159. Toth L, King K, McGrath B, Balogh Z. Factors associated with pelvic fracture-related arterial bleeding during trauma resuscitation: a prospective clinical study. J Orthop Trauma. 2014;28:489–95.
160. Kannus P, Palvanen M, Niemi S, Parkkari J, Jarvinen M. Epidemiology of osteoporotic pelvic fractures in elderly people in Finland: sharp increase in 1970–1997 and alarming projections for the new millennium. Osteoporos Int. 2000;11(5):443–8.
161. Tosounidis G, Holstein J, Culemann U, Holmenschlager F, Stuby F, Pohlemann T. Changes in epidemiology and treatment of pelvic ring fractures in Germany: an analysis on data of German pelvic multicenter study groups I and III (DGU/AO). Acta Chir Orthop Traumatol Cechoslov. 2010;77:450–6.
162. Berndtson A, Coimbra R. The epidemic of pre-injury oral antiplatelet and anticoagulant use. J Trauma Emerg Surg. 2014;40:657–69.
163. Brenner M, Hoehn M, Rasmussen T. Endovascular therapy in trauma. Eur J Trauma Emerg Surg. 2014;40:671–8.
164. Stock J, Harris W, Athanasoulis A. The role of diagnostic and therapeutic angiography in trauma to the pelvis. Clin Orthop. 1980;151:31–40.
165. Spahn D, Bouillon B, Cerny V, Duranteau J, Filipescu D, Hunt B, Komadina R, Maegele M, Nardi G, Riddez L, Samama C, Vincent J, Rossaint R. The European guideline on management of major bleeding and coagulopathy following trauma: fifth edition. Crit Care. 2019;23(1):98. https://doi.org/10.1186/s13054-019-2347-3.

Coagulation Management

16

Jan Lindahl and Axel Gänsslen

Trauma-Induced Coagulopathy (TIC) can be of major relevance, when treating hemodynamically unstable patients with pelvic ring injuries.

Unstable pelvic ring injuries were historically associated with TIC incidence between 25% and 40% [1, 2].

Recent unpublished data from the German Pelvic Injury Register reported a TIC incidence of 36.1% in type A, 50.4% in type B, and 53.1% in type C injuries, with a parallel increase of massive transfusion requirements (>10 units of PRBCs/24 h) of 8.3% in type A, 13.3% in type B, and 18.5% in type C injuries, respectively [3]. The relevance of the mechanical stability of the pelvic ring is clearly shown.

> It is of crucial importance to address potential TIC in all patients with pelvic ring injuries.

During the last two decades, a tremendous scientific work was done on pathophysiological understanding, immediate diagnostics, and development of guided treatment protocols to avoid drawbacks of TIC.

It is beyond the scope of this book to discuss pathophysiology, coagulation assessment, and management of Trauma-Induced Coagulopathy in detail. This is referred to review articles and textbooks [4–10].

The recent European guideline on management of major bleeding and coagulopathy following trauma presents recommendations, which are also suitable for the bleeding pelvic ring injury patient [9]. In summary, the following recommendations were stated for the bleeding trauma patient:

- Early and repeated coagulation monitoring, using traditional laboratory and/or point-of-care (POC) methods should be initiated in the immediate treatment phase.
- POC platelet function devices should assist management in patients with suspected platelet dysfunction.
- Normothermia should be achieved as early as possible to optimise coagulation (administration of tranexamic acid (TXA) within 3 h after trauma).
- One of the two following strategies should be initiated: FFP or pathogen-inactivated FFP in a FFP:RBC ratio of at least 1:2 as needed and/or Fibrinogen concentrate and RBC.
- A goal-directed strategy, guided by standard laboratory coagulation values and/or viscoelastic measures, should be continued.
- FXIII should be monitored and be supplemented in deficient patients, in patients with hypofibrinogenaemia, fibrinogen concentrate, or cryoprecipitate is advised.
- Platelets should be administered to maintain a platelet count above 50 × 109/L.
- Monitoring of ionised calcium levels and correction of hypocalcaemia during massive transfusion.
- Administration of recombinant-activated coagulation factor VII (rFVIIa) is not indicated as a first-line treatment; off-label use should be considered in specific situations.
- Antithrombotic agent reversal is indicated.

> Coagulation monitoring, including POC systems, and a goal-directed treatment protocol, including a massive transfusion protocol should be part of the management of bleeding trauma patients with pelvic ring injuries [9].

J. Lindahl
Orthopaedics and Trauma Surgery, Helsinki University Hospital, Helsinki, Finland

A. Gänsslen (✉)
Department of Trauma Surgery, Orthopedics and Hand Surgery, Hospital Wolfsburg, Wolfsburg, Germany

A. Gänsslen et al. (eds.), *Pelvic Ring Fractures*, https://doi.org/10.1007/978-3-030-54730-1_16

References

1. Brohi K, Singh J, Heron M, Coats T. Acute traumatic coagulopathy. J Trauma Acute Care Surg. 2003;54:1127–30.
2. Cosgriff N, Moore E, Sauaia A, Kenny-Moynihan M, Burch J, Galloway B. Predicting life-threatening coagulopathy in the massively transfused trauma patient: hypothermia and acidoses revisited. J Trauma. 1997;42:857–61.
3. Burkhardt M, Kristen A, Culemann U, Koehler D, Histing T, Holstein J, Pizanis A, Pohlemann T, Register TDGPI. Pelvic fracture in multiple trauma: are we still up-to-date with massive fluid resuscitation? Injury. 2014;45:S70–5.
4. Fröhlich M, Mutschler M, Caspers M, Nienaber U, Jäcker V, Driessen A, Bouillon B, Maegele M, DGU T. Trauma-induced coagulopathy upon emergency room arrival: still a significant problem despite increased awareness and management? Eur J Trauma Emerg Surg. 2019;45:115–24.
5. Gonzalez E, Moore H, Moore E, editors. Trauma induced coagulopathy. Berlin: Springer-Verlag; 2016. ISBN 978-3-319-28306-7, ISBN 978-3-319-28308-1 (eBook); https://doi.org/10.1007/978-3-319-28308-1.
6. Inaba K, Rizoli S, Veigas P, Callum J, Davenport R, Hess J, Maegele M, Panel VTiTC. 2014 consensus conference on viscoelastic test-based transfusion guidelines for early trauma resuscitation: report of the panel. J Trauma Acute Care Surg. 2015;78:1220–9.
7. Maegele M, Nardi G, Schöchl H. Hemotherapy algorithm for the management of trauma-induced coagulopathy: the German and European perspective. Curr Opin Anaesthesiol. 2017;30:257–64.
8. Mauffrey C, Cuellar DR, Pieracci F, Hak D, Hammerberg E, Stahel P, Burlew C, Moore E. Strategies for the management of haemorrhage following pelvic fractures and associated trauma-induced coagulopathy. Bone Joint J. 2014;96-B:1143–54.
9. Spahn D, Bouillon B, Cerny V, Duranteau J, Filipescu D, Hunt B, Komadina R, Maegele M, Nardi G, Riddez L, Samama C, Vincent J, Rossaint R. The European guideline on management of major bleeding and coagulopathy following trauma: fifth edition. Crit Care. 2019;23(1):98. https://doi.org/10.1186/s13054-019-2347-3.
10. Thorn S, Lefering R, Maegele M, Gruen R, Mitra B. Early prediction of acute traumatic coagulopathy: a validation of the COAST score using the German Trauma Registry. Eur J Trauma Emerg Surg. 2019; https://doi.org/10.1007/s00068-019-01142-0.

Open Pelvic Fractures

17

Jan Dauwe and Axel Gänsslen

Open pelvic fractures constitute one of the most devastating injuries in musculoskeletal trauma [1], with an accompanying high risk for injury-related mortality.

Bosch et al. defined the term "complex pelvic trauma" as any pelvic ring injury with significant concomitant injury to the soft tissues and internal pelvic organs [2]. Open pelvic fractures are a relevant part in the group of complex pelvic trauma, as complication rates were described up to 41.3% for overall complex trauma and 53.2% for open pelvic fractures, respectively, and an overall mortality rate for complex pelvic trauma of 31.1% [3].

The direct communication between the bone and the skin, a rectal, or vaginal wound leads to an increased risk of infectious and septic complications [4, 5].

These injuries predominantly result from high-energy trauma mechanism with a high rate of concomitant injuries and unstable fracture pattern [4–6].

Rothenberger et al. called this fracture type **"a lethal injury"**. Already, in 1978, from a group of 604 patients with pelvic fractures, 3.6% had open fractures, resulting in a mortality rate of 50%, with the open pelvic fracture being the primary cause of death in 73%. In contrast, in patients with closed fracture, only 30% died as a result of the pelvic injury [7].

Perry et al. reported a 4.2% rate of open pelvic fractures with an associated mortality rate of 42%. Hemorrhage, sepsis, and/or renal failure were responsible for mortality [8].

These results lead to a more standardized approach controlling hemorrhage, which resulted in a decreased mortality rate [1]. Prevention of infection was the further main topic of treatment, but associated injuries of the genitourinary tract and pelvic-related nerve injury were responsible for long-term morbidity [9].

Presently, according to less individual experience in treating these injuries, no standardized management algorithm exists.

Open pelvic fractures are rarely observed [10] and present in 1–10% of all admitted pelvic ring fractures, with an average rate of 3% (Table 17.1) [3, 4, 6–8, 11–22].

Table 17.1 Frequency of open pelvic fractures in large samples

Author	Year	No	Open	Freq (%)	Author	Year	No	Open	Freq (%)
Rothenberger [7, 11]	1978	604	22	3.6	Dente [12]	2005	1506	44	2.9
Perry [8]	1980	738	31	4.2	O'Sullivan [13]	2005	174	14	8.0
Hanson [14]	1991	890	43	4.8	Giannoudis [15]	2007	1177	59	5.0
Davidson [16]	1993	957	21	2.2	Hauschild [17]	2008	4291	46	1.1
Gänsslen [3]	1996	2551	77	3.0	Black	2011	3053	52	1.7
Brenneman [4]	1997	1179	44	3.7	Siada [18]	2015	1505	25	1.7
Ferrera [6]	1998	632	17	2.7	Giordano [19]	2016	396	30	7.6
Sriussadaporn [20]	2002	170	16	9.4	Hermans [21]	2018	492	24	4.9

J. Dauwe
Department of Trauma Surgery, University Hospitals Leuven, Leuven, Belgium
e-mail: jan.dauwe@uzleuven.be

A. Gänsslen (✉)
Department of Trauma Surgery, Orthopedics and Hand Surgery, Hospital Wolfsburg, Wolfsburg, Germany

A. Gänsslen et al. (eds.), *Pelvic Ring Fractures*, https://doi.org/10.1007/978-3-030-54730-1_17

17.1 Classification

Several classifications of open pelvic fractures exist, taking several aspects of this injury type into consideration.

Faringer et al. classified open pelvic fractures dependent on the localization of the wounds (Fig. 17.1) [23]:

- Zone I: anterior-lateral from the pubic tubercles, parallel to the inguinal crease to the posterior sacrum (Fig. 17.2)
- Zone II: medial thigh up to the anterior thigh to a line between the SIAS and the medial patella and posterior thigh midline, including the groin creases
- Zone III: posterolateral buttock inferior to the iliac crest

Wounds present in more than one zone were categorized by the zone with the lowest number (Fig. 17.3) [23].

Further definitions include superficial wounds (extending into the subcutaneous fat) or deep wounds (extended to underlying muscle and fascia and degloving injuries).

In 1997, Jones et al. published an open pelvic fractures classification on the basis of pelvic ring stability, perineal and rectal injury [5]:

- Class 1: stable pelvic ring
- Class 2: unstable pelvic ring, no rectal or perineal wound

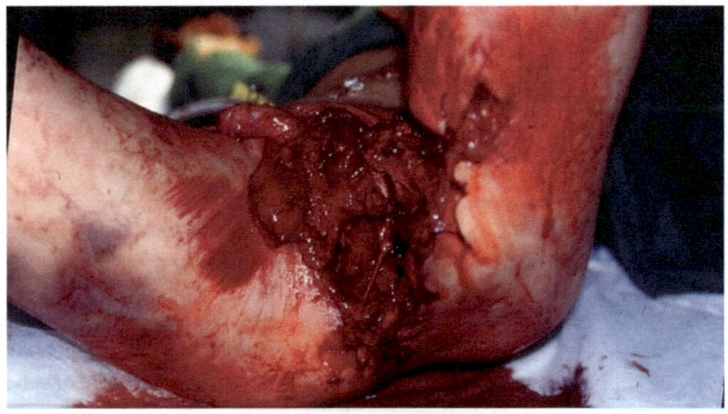

Fig. 17.2 Faringer type I injury

Fig. 17.1 Faringer classification of open pelvic injuries

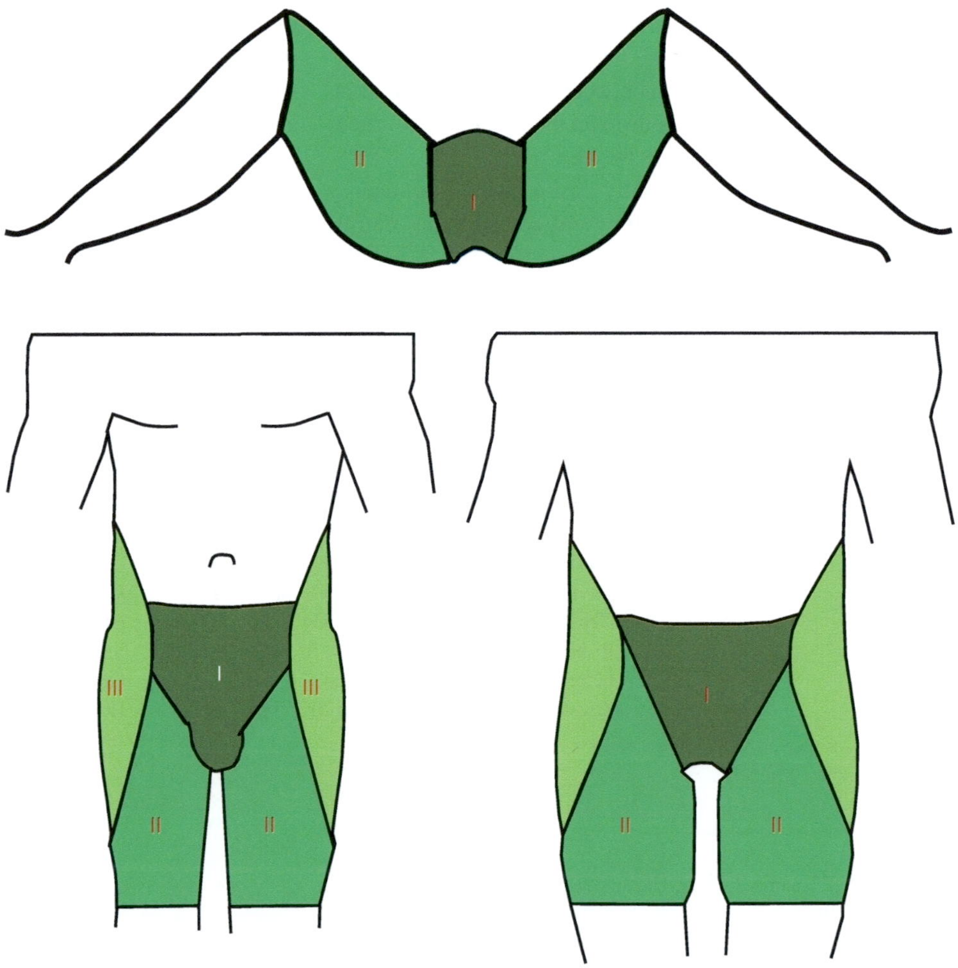

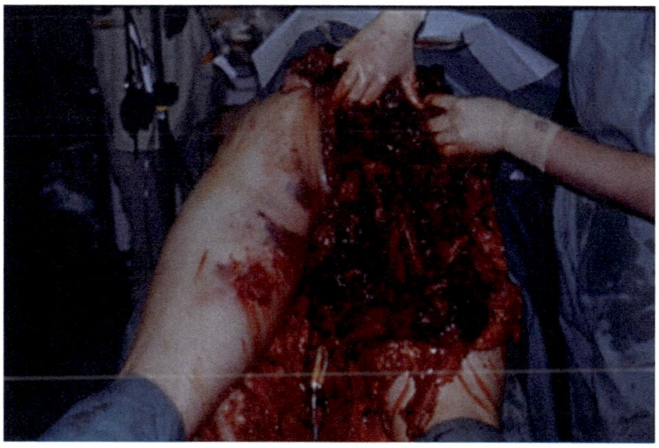

Fig. 17.3 Combined Faringer type I, II, III injury categorized as zone I injury

- Class 3: unstable pelvic ring with rectal or perineal wound

The prognostic value of the Jones-Powell classification was recently confirmed, showing an increased mortality rate from class I to III with 0% to 24% to 38%, respectively [10].

Bircher et al. based their classification on the primary skin lesion, the additional soft-tissue injury and the instability of the pelvic ring according to Tile [24]:

- Type A1: penetrating trauma, type A pelvic ring injury, additional soft-tissue injury, dependent on the missile and its path
- Type A2: "outside in" type A iliac crest fracture, minimal soft-tissue damage
- Type A3: "outside in" type A iliac crest fracture, extensive soft-tissue damage
- Type B1: "inside out" type B2 injury, little external damage, possible genitourinary injury
- Type B2: "inside out" type B2 injury, moderate tissue damage (Morel–Lavallé lesion)
- Type B3: "perineal split" B1 ("open book") fracture
- Type C1: "perineal split" and/or "sacral shear/split" type C injury, moderate/extensive skin loss, complete genitourinary disruption, and rectal lesions with subsequent fecal contamination
- Type C2: "hemipelvic destabilization" type C injury, severe tissue damage, complete urogenital and bowel injury combined with extensive contamination of all tissue layers
- Type C3: "pelvic crush", bilateral complex type C injury, massive damage to soft tissues and intrapelvic organs

Additionally, the grade of the open wound should be classified according to Gustilo and Anderson (Table 17.2) [25]. Some authors proposed to integrate each patient with a wound at the perineal region or rectum involvement into the Gustilo/Anderson III category [1]. The latter injuries were observed in up to 60% [1, 4, 5].

Fu et al. developed a classification for grading of the perineal soft-tissue injury (Table 17.3), integrating the injury characteristics and a resultant treatment protocol [26].

Table 17.2 Gustilo-Anderson classification of open fractures

Grade I	Clean skin opening <1 cm, usually from inside to outside; minimal muscle contusion, simple transverse/short oblique fracture pattern
Grade II	Laceration >1 cm, with extensive soft-tissue damage; minimal to moderate crushing component; simple transverse/short oblique fractures with minimal comminution
Grade III	Extensive soft-tissue damage, incl. muscles, skin and neurovascular structures; often high-energy injury with severe crushing component
Grade IIIA	Extensive soft-tissue laceration, adequate bone coverage; segmental fractures, gunshot injuries, minimal periosteal stripping
Grade IIIB	Extensive soft-tissue injury with periosteal stripping and bone exposure requiring soft-tissue flap closure; usually associated with massive contamination
Grade IIIC	Any type IIIA, B with vascular injury requiring repair

Table 17.3 Classification of perineal soft-tissue injury

Type	Characteristics of injuries	Repair protocols
A. Urogenital zone injuries		
A1	Without urethral injury	Skin graft or flap transplantation without cystostomy
A2	With urethral injury	Skin graft or flap transplantation with cystostomy
B. Anal zone injuries		
B1	Without anorectal injury	Skin graft or flap transplantation without colostomy
B2	With anorectal injury	Skin graft or flap transplantation with colostomy
C. Both urogenital zone and anal zone injuries		
C1	With neither urethral nor anorectal injuries	Skin graft or flap transplantation
C2	With urethral but without anorectal injuries	+ Only cystostomy
C3	With anorectal but without urethral injuries	+ Only colostomy
C4	With both urogenital and anorectal injuries	+ Colostomy *and* cystostomy

17.2 Mortality

Several historical data presented high mortality rates [7, 11, 27, 28]. Grotz et al. reported a 30% rate of mortality from the 1970s to the 1990s [1]. Six reports were analyzed. Four of these showed rates >40%, while two presented rates of 5.7% and 25%, respectively [7–9, 27–29]. Overall, in 148 patients,

Table 17.4 Mortality rates of open pelvic fractures

Author	Year	*N*	Dead	%	Author	Year	*N*	Dead	%
Raffa [28]	1976	16	8	50	Ferrera [6]	1999	17	2	11.8
Maull [27]	1977	12	7	58.3	Mosheiff [30]	1999	15	3	20
Rothenberger [7, 11]	1978	22	11	50	Kudsk [31]	2003	25	8	32
Perry [8]	1980	31	13	41.9	Dente [12]	2005	44	20	45.5
Richardson [9]	1982	35	2	5.7	O'Sullivan [13]	2005	14	4	28.6
Kusminsky [32]	1982	11	3	27.3	Dong [33]	2011	41	10	24.4
Govender [29]	1990	32	8	25	Black [22]	2011	52	10	19.2
Hanson [14]	1991	43	13	30.2	Wei [34]	2012	16	5	31.3
Sinnott [35]	1992	27	4	14.8	Hasankhani [36]	2013	15	2	13.3
Davidson [16]	1993	20	3	15	Cannada [10]	2013	64	15	23.4
Faringer [23]	1994	34	6	17.6	Fu [26]	2015	15	1	6.7
Jones [5]	1997	39	10	25.6	Teixeira [37]	2015	42	15	35.7
Brenneman [4]	1997	44	11	25	Giordano [19]	2016	30	12	40
Woods [38]	1998	60	7	11.7	Song [39]	2017	20	3	15
Pell [40]	1998	18	4	22.2	Siada [18]	2015	25	4	16
Rieger [41]	1999	40	5	12.5	Hermans [21]	2018	24	1	4.2
Michel [42]	1999	11	1	9.1	Moskowitz [43]	2018	14	1	7.1

49 open pelvic fractures were observed, representing a 30.4% mortality rate [1].

Starting in the late 1980s and early 1990s, a more standardized treatment concept on pelvic fractures, including open pelvic fractures was integrated in many trauma centers. This led to a relevant mortality decrease to 18% [1].

Newer data indicated that even today, open pelvic fractures are associated with a relevant mortality rate, which is superior to fractures with a closed soft-tissue envelope [10, 12, 13, 18, 19, 21, 22, 26, 31, 33, 34, 36, 37, 39, 43].

Open fractures are associated with mortality rates between 4 and 60%, with an average rate of 24% (Table 17.4).

17.2.1 Risk Factors of Mortality

The major risk factor during initial treatment of open pelvic fractures is direct hemorrhage, leading to early death [4, 5]. Several further risk factors of mortality were identified [1, 12, 22, 33]:

- *Age*: age >30: 40.9% vs. 5.3% [33], older patients [14].
- *Injury severity* [14]: ISS ≥25: 37% vs. 0% [33]; ISS >35 [19]; >5 associated injuries [22].
- *Revised Trauma Score (RTS)*: low revised trauma score [12]; RTS ≤8: 77.7% vs. 9.4% [33] with the RTS ≤8 as an independent risk factor of mortality
- *Soft-tissue injury*: Jones-Powell classification [19]; size and contamination of the open wound [14]; Faringer zone I or II injuries [12].
- *Gustilo/Anderson grading*: grade III soft-tissue injury [12]; Gustilo III: 57.1% vs. 8% [33].
- *Pelvic ring instability* [5]: vertical shear injuries [12].
- *Abdominal trauma* [12]: intra-abdominal injuries 30% vs. 22.6% [33].
- *Pelvic Organ Injuries*: rectal injury [5] and the necessity of fecal diversion [28]; urogenital injuries 33% vs. 20.7% [33].
- *Traumatic Brain Injury (TBI)*: GCS ≤8: 83.3% vs. 14.2% [33].
- *Hemorrhage control*: necessity of PRBC [7, 8, 41] and angio-embolization [12].

Late death was associated with pelvic sepsis [12] and septic complications (57.1% vs. 17.6%) [33].

17.3 Treatment Open Pelvic Fractures

There is no consensus on how to treat open pelvic fractures [1, 9, 22, 31, 34, 43–45]. Several factors have to be considered to develop a treatment algorithm, including:

- Aggressive resuscitation and (surgical) bleeding control, including local wound packing
- Intravenous antibiotics and tetanus
- Emergency stabilization of the pelvic ring (e.g., external fixation)
- Soft-tissue/wound management: debridement of all devitalized tissues, pulsatile irrigation, no primary wound closure, based on emergency diagnostics (sigmoidoscopy, colostomy, rectal irrigation) and treatment of pelvic organ injuries incl. Fecal or urinary diversion, or both; perineal wound management
- Operative frequent re-debridements with eventual soft-tissue coverage with skin grafts or flaps, or both
- Definitive pelvic fixation strategies
- (Definitive) treatment of associated injuries (urogenital)
- Enteral access and institution of early enteral feeding [31].

17.4 Primary Survey

The patient with an open pelvic fracture is primarily evaluated according to standardized treatment principles, for example, ATLS-protocol [45], as these patients present with a relevant injury severity and concomitant injuries. The mean Injury Severity Score (ISS) in a review of the literature was 29 points [6, 10, 12, 14, 18, 19, 21, 22, 26, 33, 36–38, 43, 46].

Emergency treatment of these injuries already started at the scene. Fixation of the pelvis is routinely performed in all suspected pelvic injuries with pelvic binders (Fig. 17.4) [47].

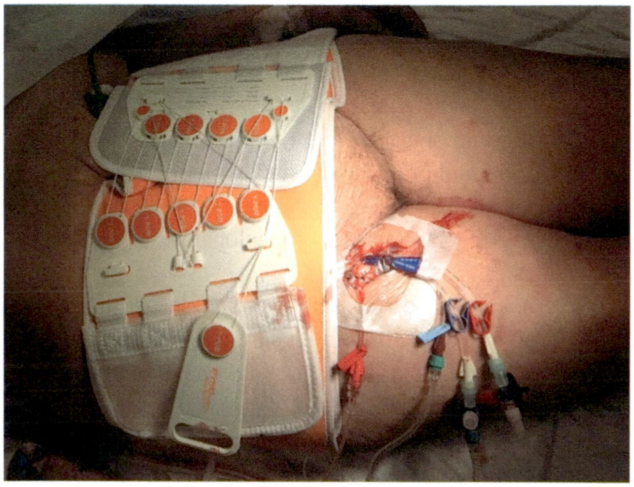

Fig. 17.4 Emergency application of a pelvic binder in a patient with in-hospital diagnosed rectal injury

Not later than in the emergency room (ER), a pelvic binder should be applied [22] and local wound packing is performed to reduce external bleeding (Fig. 17.5) [9]. At that time, all gross contaminants should be removed.

> The most DANGEROUS type of a pelvic fracture is the MISSED one! [48]

Therefore, despite binders being used commonly for pelvic emergency stabilization, inspection of the local skin condition around the pelvis, including the posterior sacral area, integrating the Faringer zones, the perineal area, the vagina and/or rectum and the urethral orifice is mandatory! Additionally, neurovascular assessment should be performed and documented.

All open fractures are by definition contaminated and must be treated as such [49–54]. According to standard guidelines of open fracture treatment, early intravenous administration of antibiotics within 3 h [55] and tetanus immunization should be initiated.

In open fractures, the risk of infection is as high as 10–50% for Gustilo type III fractures [56].

In general, in grade I and II open fractures, the preferred antibiotic agent is Cefazolin 2 g administered for 24 h. In grade III open fractures, without gross contamination, 2 g Ceftriaxone is preferred for 48 h or 24 h after wound closure, while in grade III open fractures, with gross contamination,

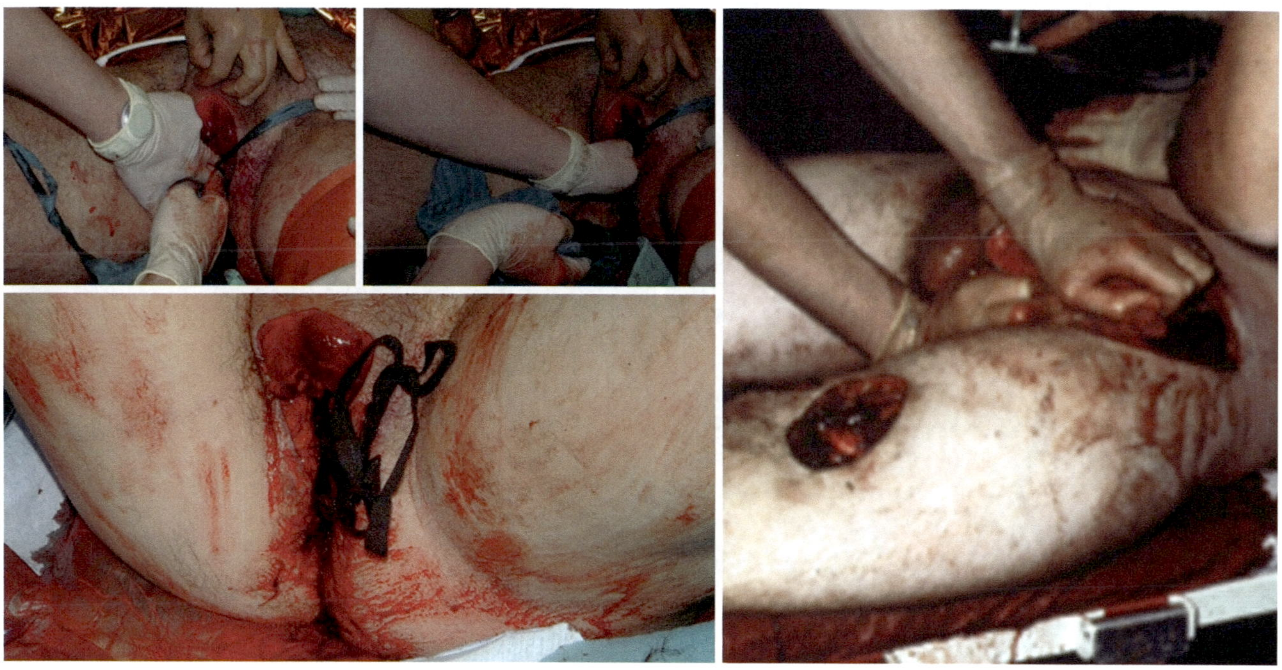

Fig. 17.5 Local manual tamponade or local wound packing to reduce pelvis-related external hemorrhage

2 g Ceftriaxone +500 mg metronidazole is given until 48 h after wound closure [49–52, 54].

A standard pelvic a.p. X-ray is performed in the ER. Depending on the instability type of the pelvic injury, mechanical stabilization is performed [57], depending on the available adjuncts, using standardized treatment options (Fig. 17.6):

- Pelvic binder
- Pelvic sheeting
- Simple external fixators
- Pelvic C-clamp

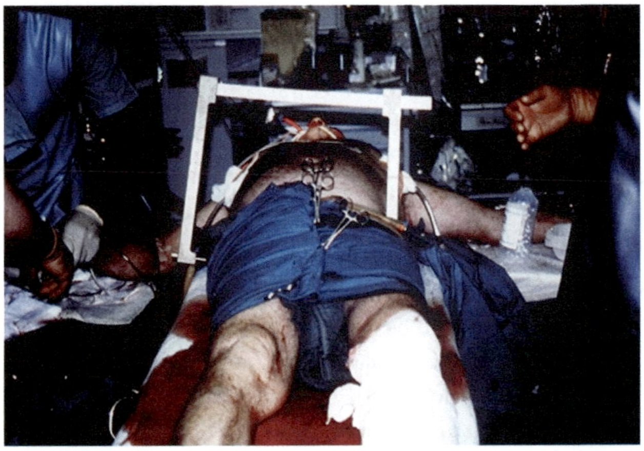

Fig. 17.6 Pelvic C-clamp stabilization of a highly unstable open pelvic injury after primary circumferential sheet application. Source: Pohlemann T, Regel G, Bosch U, Stief Ch, Tscherne H. Kapitel 7: Notfallbehandlung und Komplextrauma, p. 106 (Fig. 7.21c); in: Tscherne H, Pohlemann T (Ed.). Tscherne Unfallchirurgie – Becken und Acetabulum. Springer Verlag Berlin, Heidelberg, New York, 1998

Based on the recent European guidelines on management of major bleeding and coagulopathy following trauma [57], several high-grade recommendations should be integrated into the initial treatment algorithm:

- Initiation of immediate bleeding control procedures in patients presenting with hemorrhagic shock and an identified source of bleeding procedure.
- Early imaging (ultrasonography (eFAST (Fig. 17.7) or contrast-enhanced CT) for the detection of free fluid in patients with suspected torso trauma
- CT assessment for hemodynamically stable patients
- Analysis of special parameters indicating ongoing shock/hemodynamic instability (low initial Hb, serum lactate and/or base deficit measurements)
- Early and repeated monitoring of coagulation ([prothrombin time (PT), activated
- Partial thromboplastin time (APTT) platelet counts and fibrinogen] and/or a viscoelastic method
- Initiation of damage control surgery in the presence of typical triggers (severe coagulopathy, hypothermia, acidosis)
- Mechanical pelvic ring stabilization and additionally in patients with ongoing hemodynamic instability early preperitoneal packing, angiographic embolization and/or surgical bleeding control
- Addition of topical hemostatic agents for venous or moderate arterial bleeding associated with parenchymal injuries

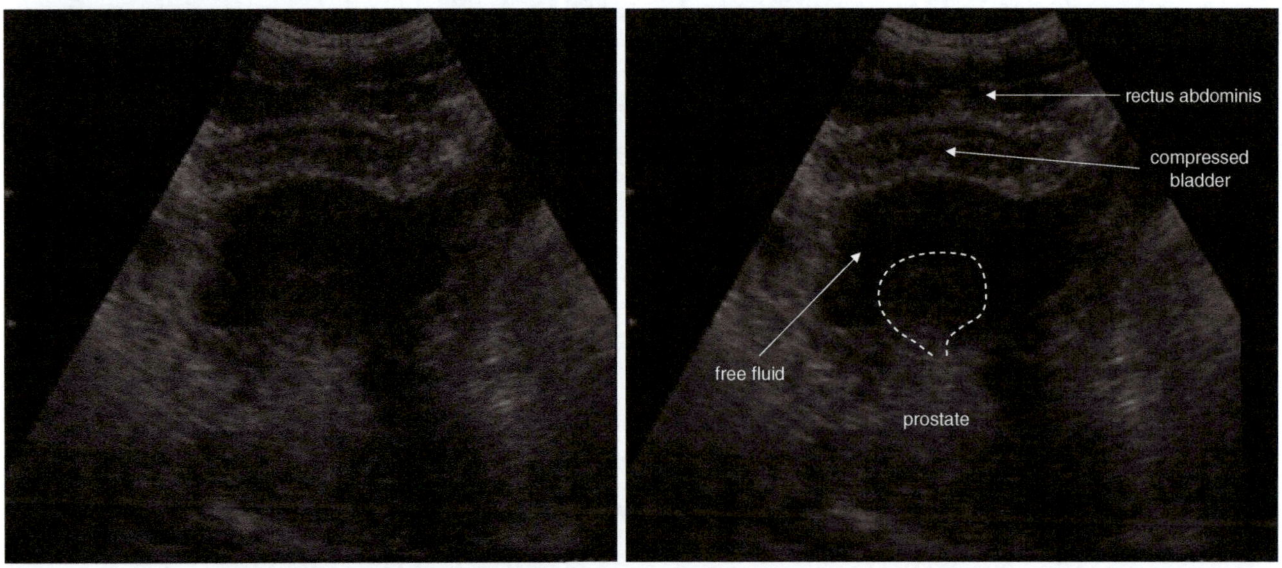

Fig. 17.7 FAST examination reveals relevant retroperitoneal hematoma formation around the prostate

17.5 Hemorrhage Control

Hemorrhage control includes parallel treatment of traumatic induced coagulopathy (TIC) and surgical bleeding control.

17.5.1 TIC Treatment

Monitoring and treatment of TIC should be initiated immediately after admission, using algorithm-based and goal-directed coagulation management [57].

Early administration of plasma (FFP or pathogen-inactivated plasma) in a plasma–RBC ratio of at least 1:2 and fibrinogen concentrate and RBC administration according to hemoglobin level is started, dependent on physiological parameters or according to hospital-directed protocols [57].

Additionally, tranexamic acid should be immediately administered in bleeding patients or patients where significant ongoing bleeding is suspected. Laboratory coagulation parameters and/or viscoelastic tests can support the guidance of TIC-treatment.

Plasma transfusion, fibrinogen concentrate or cryoprecipitate transfusion and platelet transfusion should be considered, dependent on the patient's response and laboratory values. Ionized calcium levels should be monitored during massive transfusion and calcium should be administered until normal levels are present.

In patients under anticoagulants, desmopressin, prothrombin complex concentrate or even off-label use of rFVIIa has to be considered.

Pharmacological thromboprophylaxis within 24 h after bleeding has been controlled is recommended, while, in contrast to historical recommendations, inferior vena cava filters have no role in treating these patients.

In patients with open pelvic fractures, a significant amount of blood products (e.g., Packed Red Blood Cells, PRBC) are administered within the first 24 h of treatment [12, 21, 26, 33, 36, 58]:

- Dente et al. reported, that 73% of all patients with open pelvic fractures required at least 1 PRBC and 37% required ≥10 PRBC, with an average of 11.5 PRBC/24 h [12].
- Dong et al. administered 17.2 PRBCs droning the first 24 h (range: 0–104 PRBCs) [33].
- Hasankhani et al. reported on an average amount of blood transfusion of 8 PRBCs (range: 4–21) [36].
- Fu et al. analyzed 11 patients with perineal soft-tissue injuries and transfused 11.7 units (7–19 units) during the first 24 h [26].
- Hermans et al. transfused 13.2 units (0–30 units) during the first 24 h [21].
- Ramasamy et al. analyzed blast-related open pelvic fractures and had to transfuse an average of 60.31 PRBC's (0–224 PRBC's) [58].

Overall, an average of 13.1 PRBC's was transfused during the first 24 h in recent studies in patients with classical open pelvic fractures, excluding blast-related injuries [12, 21, 26, 33, 36].

17.5.2 Surgical Bleeding Control

Options of surgical bleeding control included mechanical pelvic ring stabilization and hemodynamic stabilization with different options, including packing of external bleeding wounds [9], intrapelvic packing [43, 59–62], angio-embolization and damage control laparotomy [12].

Options for emergency mechanical stabilization of the pelvic ring include application of a pelvic binder, an external fixator or the pelvic C-clamp, but even simple measures, for example, pelvic sheeting or even traction, and internal rotation of both legs can be useful [57]. However, especially, application of a pelvic binder can mask pelvic displacement and instability on the pelvic X-ray or CT [63, 64].

The classical option for bleeding control includes, local tamponade and intrapelvic, extraperitoneal pelvic packing [43, 60–62], angiography and resultant embolization, REBOA or distal aortic or iliac clamping during laparotomy (s. special Chapters).

17.6 Diagnostics

The primary aim in clinically analyzing the pelvic area is to rule out or define concomitant rectal, vaginal, urogenital, or vascular injuries by inspection of all perianal tissues, as this is the most common area of open soft-tissue injury (Fig. 17.8), followed by examination of the vaginal and rectal vault (Fig. 17.9).

The extent of soft-tissue injury is classified according to the Gustilo/Anderson [25] and localization of the open wounds according to Faringer [23].

Anorectal injuries are present in up to 64% [1]. Visible blood at the rectal exit or on rectal examination should lead to suspicion of rectal injury, especially when rectal wall weakness is palpated. Sigmodoiscopy and rigid proctoscopy is then performed (Fig. 17.10) [1]. In stable patients with CT evaluation, indirect signs of bowel injuries include localized extraluminal gas or fluid, hemorrhage, segmental bowel wall thickening, bowel wall discontinuity, and stranding of the mesenteric fat [65–69]. Associated vaginal lacerations can lead to false positive results.

In all suspected injuries of the perineal region, presenting with blood at the perineal orifice (perineal, rectal, or vaginal wounds), a speculum or proctoscopic evaluation should be performed, followed by an adequate debridement and irrigation [44], as septic complications, morbidity, and mortality are associated with these injuries [5].

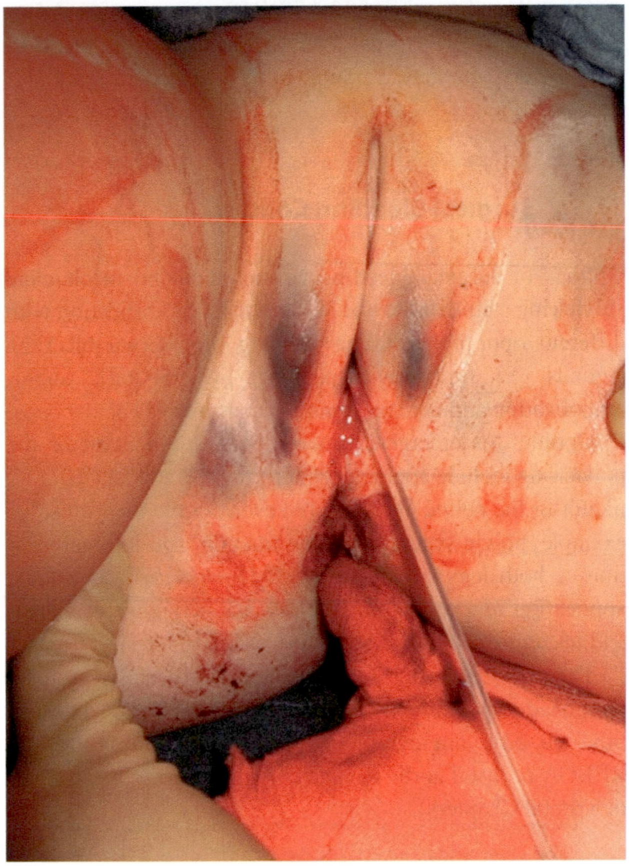

Fig. 17.8 Inspection of the perineal region for (subtle) open injuries

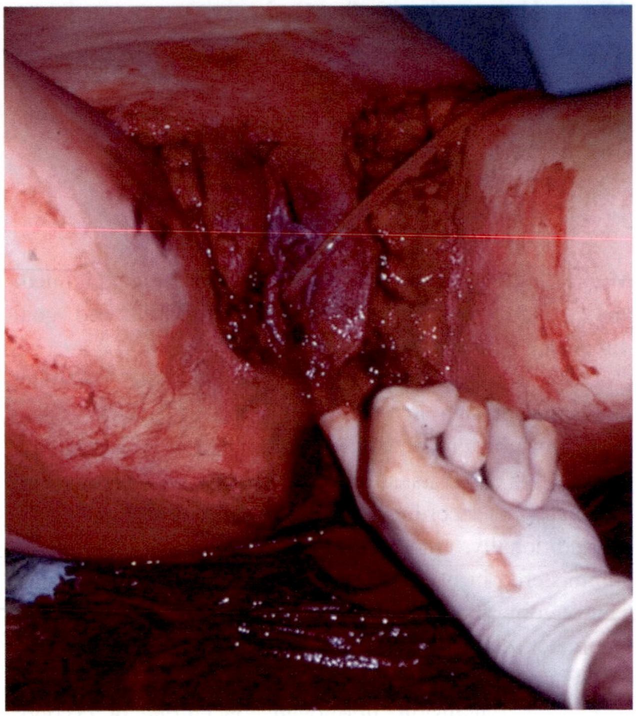

Fig. 17.9 Digital rectal examination: visible blood at the rectal exit or on rectal examination should lead to suspicion of rectal injury, especially when rectal wall weakness is palpated

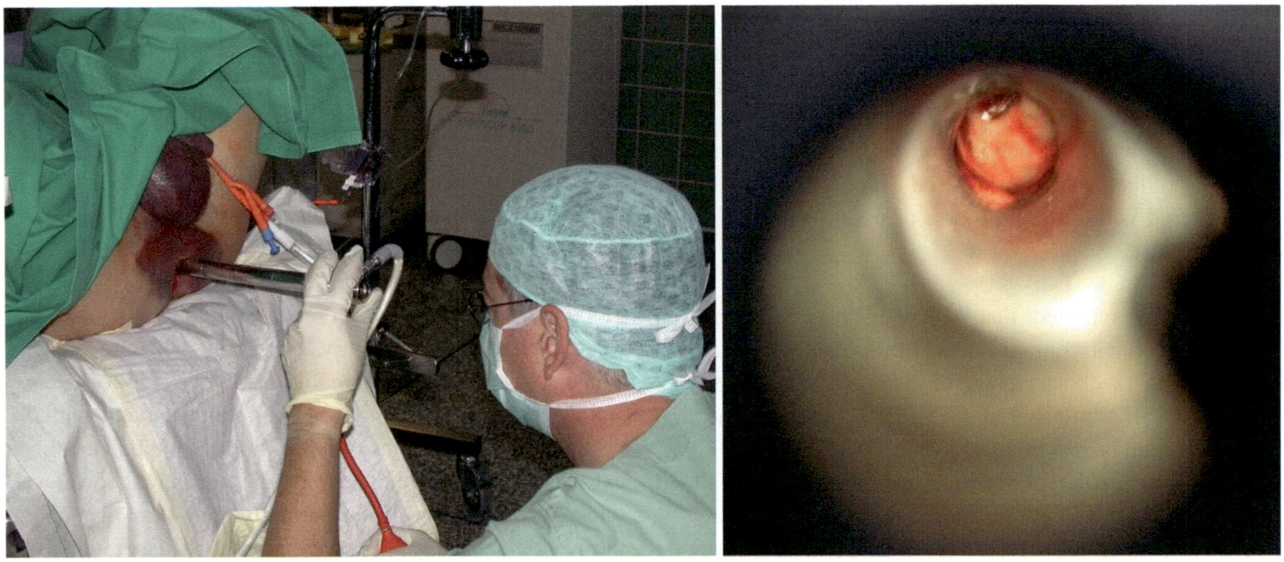

Fig. 17.10 Sigmoidoscopy and rigid proctoscopy to evaluate the rectal injury severity

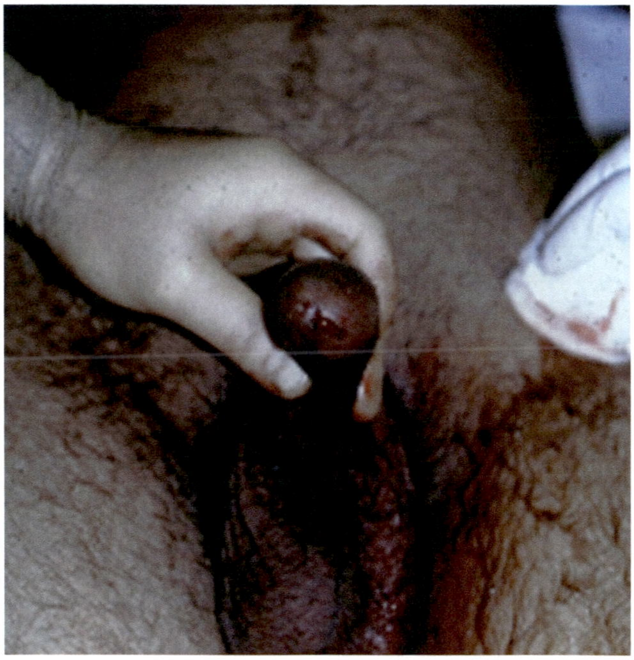

Fig. 17.11 Blood at the urethral meatus in a case with urethra laceration

A retrograde urethrogram is the standard procedure for diagnosis of urethral injury [70–72]. Blood at the urethra meatus is indicative of bladder or urethral injury (Fig. 17.11). Vaginal lacerations are often combined with larger lacerations involving the perineum and rectum. Injuries to the uterus, cervix, or ovaries are often secondary diagnosed, using initial or secondary CT evaluation.

17.7 Associated Injuries

Perry already reported, that concomitant injuries were present in the majority of patients, including head injury, chest injury, abdominal injury, genitourinary injury, major extremity fractures, and neurovascular injuries, with an average of 2.7 additional major injuries per patient [8]. Only two patients presented with isolated open pelvic fractures. Isolated open fractures were observed in 14.1% [10].

Urogenital injuries are expected in approximately 35% (21.2–47.1%) [6, 14, 16, 23, 26, 29, 31, 33, 35, 73].

17.8 Wound Management

Wound management and soft-tissue debridement depends on the grade of open soft-tissue injury. Hanson observed predominantly grade III open wounds according to Gustilo, with a frequency of 74.4%, while a 9.3% rate of Gustilo type I wounds and 16.3% Gustilo type II wounds were seen [14]. Recent studies reported more grade II wounds [18, 21, 33]. Overall, an increase from grade I to grade III has to be expected with [14, 18, 21, 33]:

- 21.1% grade I wounds according to Gustilo/Anderson
- 33.1% grade II wounds according to Gustilo/Anderson
- 45.8% grade III wounds according to Gustilo/Anderson

The localization of these peripelvic wounds, according to Faringer, revealed 39.6% Faringer type I localizations in the perineal area, 21.4% Faringer type II localizations, and 39% Faringer type III localizations [18, 19, 21, 33, 37].

The main principle in wound debridement consists of excision of ALL devitalized tissues except neurovascular bundles to create a wound and a fracture environment close to a closed fracture (Fig. 17.12).

Several steps can be relevant to get an adequate wound cleaning:

- Precleaning (preferably in the anesthetic room) with soap solution and a soft brush
- Regular prepping and draping in the OR
- Application of a tourniquet for optional inflation (not routinely recommended)
- Removal of visible dirt
- Starting a zone-by-zone debridement (layers, compartments, etc.) under periodical irrigation, performing a superficial-to-deep concept
  - Skin debridement until bleeding skin edges are present
  - Subcutaneous fat debridement along fasciotomy lines; often enlargement of the initial wound is necessary; consider a more vulnerable blood supply and the risk of more extensive fat necrosis
  - Muscle debridement with removal of all non-viable muscle fibers (check: color, contractility, consistency, capacity to bleed)
  - Bone debridement: resection of non-viable parts, as less as possible except bone fragments with attached articular cartilage; the latter are thoroughly cleaned, curetted and fixed according to AO-principles with resulting absolute stability as this can lead to revascularization
- Wound lavage/irrigation (Fig. 17.13) is based on the old dogma "The solution to pollution is dilution.", which is still valid; addition of soap, antiseptic agents, or antibiotics are without effect of avoidance of infection; low pressure irrigation is as good as high pressure irrigation and using saline was associated with less re-operation rates compared to soap irrigation [74].

Anglen recommended the following amounts of fluids for irrigation of wounds [75]:

- 3 L for type 1
- 6 L for type 2
- 9 L for type 3

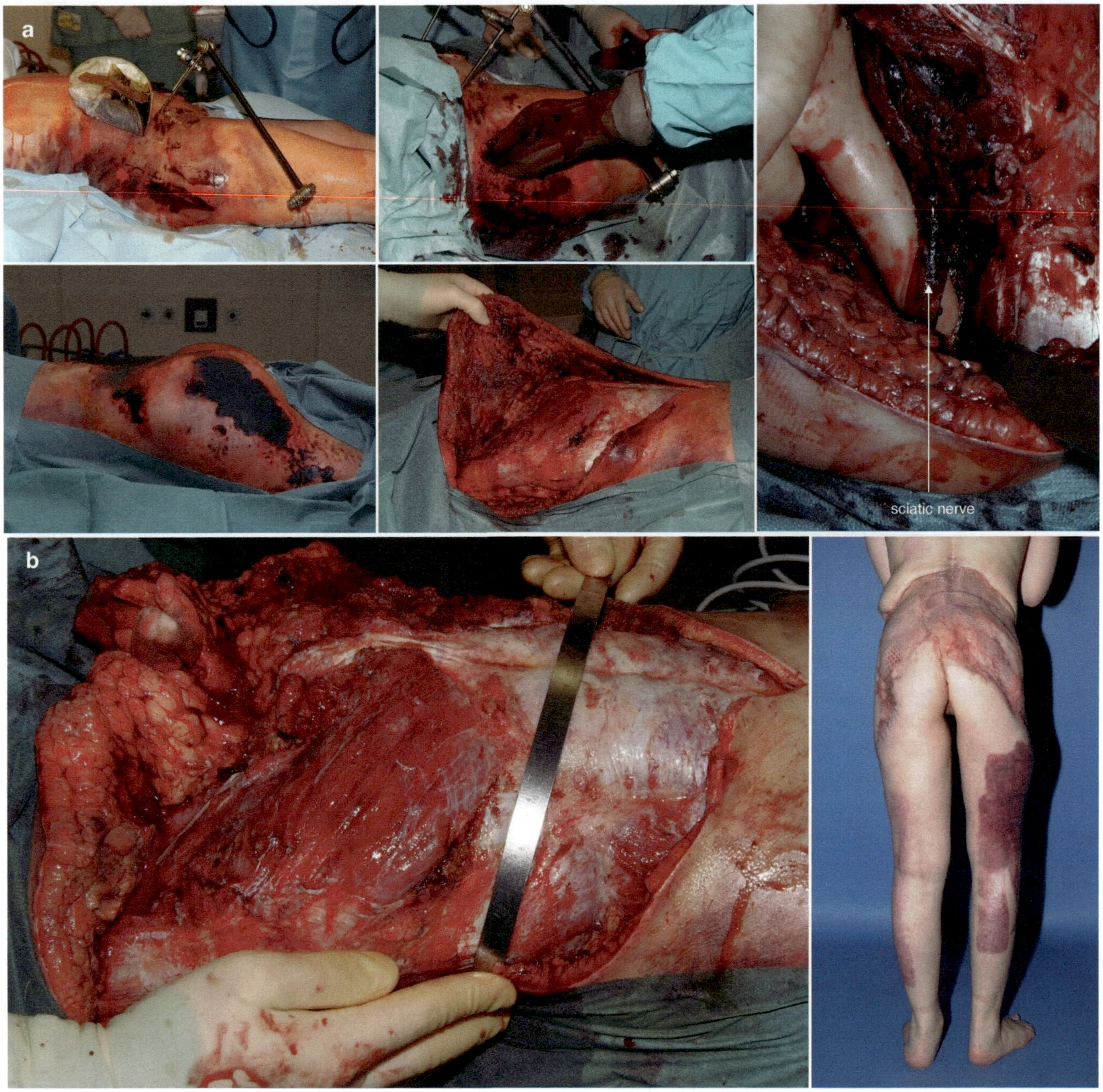

Fig. 17.12 (**a**) Adequate wound debridement and removal of all devitalized soft-tissues is mandatory: neurovascular structures remain intact. (**b**) Secondary skin transplantation is often necessary

Depending on the wound size, especially Faringer type I–III wounds, often higher fluid amounts are necessary.

The decision to close the wound is based on clinical experience, wound size, contamination, et cetera. In the majority of open pelvic fractures, vacuum sealed dressings are preferred, until an adequate wound base is reached [76–80], despite recent data indicate, that the risk of infection was only slightly lower than with standard care [81].

Application of local antibiotic impregnated beads was shown to further reduce the infection rate in severely open fractures [82–85].

A second look is recommended on day 1, with careful irrigation and debridement of secondary soft-tissue necrosis [31]. Grotz et al. highlighted to address early a possible pelvic compartment [1].

Degloving wounds, directly associated with open fractures, are treated by soft-tissue excision and early or secondary skin grafts.

Small skin wounds can be closed after sufficient debridement. Larger wounds can be associated with extensive degloving injuries extending to the Faringer regions. Radical debridement of all necrotic tissues should be performed to

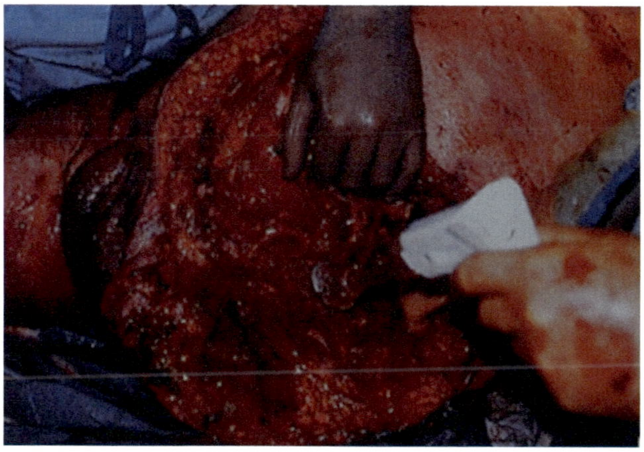

Fig. 17.13 Wound lavage is a basic treatment modality in all open injuries

prevent septic complications until bright-red bleeding can be observed. Daily, at least 48-h re-debridements are recommended to identify early ongoing tissue damage [31].

Kudsk et al. clearly stated, that "skin bridges between degloved areas should be debrided, and under no circumstances should large flaps be closed, because necrotizing infections deep to the flaps are inevitable and difficult to diagnose before the onset of sepsis. Devitalized muscle must be debrided, even if this means that extensive cavities are created in the perineum and perirectal area. Such areas rapidly contract once healing begins" [31].

Exposed bone can be managed with local muscle and skin flaps from the gluteal or thigh region [1, 26].

Fu et al. proposed a two stage concept [26]. After radical debridement of perineal wounds and vacuum sealing drainage for maximum 1 week, to be followed by a repeated debridement and vacuum sealing and deep tissue repair. Definitive wound treatment was then performed with myocutaneous flaps or skin grafting.

17.9 Selective Diverting Colostomy

The concept of fecal diversion was favored to prevent infectious complications. In 1976, Raffa et al. could show a significant decrease in mortality after open pelvic fractures, when early diverting colostomy/ileostomy and a distal rectal washout was performed [28]. This concept was well accepted in the following years [7, 9, 11, 35]. Similarly, Pell et al. demonstrated a reduced mortality and pelvic sepsis rate [40].

Faringer et al., reported a 31% rate of wound sepsis with colostomy and 19% without colostomy and, therefore, concluded that fecal diversion was only indicated in selected patients with open pelvic fractures [23]. It was advocated that all Faringer zone I open pelvic fractures should undergo fecal diversion [4]. This recommendation is supported by other authors [45, 86].

In contrast, already in 1998, Woods et al. stated that fecal diversion was not associated with a lower incidence of abdominopelvic infectious complications and, therefore, fecal diversion was only indicated in a selective group of patients with extensive soft-tissue injury or posterior wounds. The rate of infectious complications was 27% after fecal diversion compared to 17% in patients without diversion, while the mortality rate was identical [38]. The main factor, resulting in pelvic infection, was mechanical instability of the pelvis.

Analysis of fecal diversion in elderly patients with open pelvic fractures revealed, that this patient group was associated with a higher ISS, more abdominal injuries ± intra-abdominal fecal contamination and a higher number of accompanying injuries [87]. It was concluded, despite inconsistent data, that in elderly patients with open pelvic fracture and a severe rectal injury, aggressive fecal diversion is proposed to be the procedure of choice during emergency treatment.

> A diverting colostomy can significantly reduce infective complications and mortality in patients with open pelvic fractures in Faringer zone I/perineal wounds, while Faringer zone II and III injuries do not benefit from colostomy [1, 21].

Delayed colostomy led to a significantly higher rate of pelvic infections [9]. When applying a diverting colostomy or ileostomy, approaches for pelvic ring fixation and suprapubic cystotomy should be considered [4, 23].

17.10 Rectal Injuries

Rectal injuries can be associated with open pelvic injuries. The classical treatment principle comprises diversion, drainage, direct repair, and distal washout [88].

Anorectal injuries are expected in approximately 26% (9.1–64.3%) of patients with open pelvic fractures [10, 12, 14, 16, 21, 23, 26, 29, 31, 33, 35, 73].

These injuries can be associated with pelvic vascular lesions and GU lesions, with resulting high mortality and morbidity [89]. A multidisciplinary management approach is, therefore, required.

Digital rectal examination is unreliable, as up to 77% of these injuries are overlooked. While the specificity of digital rectal examination is 95%, the sensitivity of 24% is minimal [90–92].

Thus, in any suspicious case, rigid proctoscopy or flexible sigmoidoscopy is highly recommended [93].

Several fracture configurations can lead to suspicion of rectal injuries [94]:

- Injury to the pubic symphysis (independent predictor, relative risk [RR] = 3.3)
- Injury to an SI-joint (relative risk [RR] = 2.1)

Fecal diversion by proximal colostomy with or without presacral drainage and primary repair is considered the gold standard in treating traumatic extraperitoneal rectal injuries, while intraperitoneal injuries can be treated like injuries to the colon with primary repair or resection and anastomosis with or without diversion [89, 95, 96].

Distal washout and presacral drainage show reduced evidence, but is still in use [95, 97–99].

In a systematic review of the published literature until the late 1990s, no difference in infection rates were found in patients treated with or without colostomy [100]. All paticnts with a clear diagnosed rectal injury were treated with colostomy and presented with a high infection and mortality rate. Patients with perineal/rectal wounds showed a benefit regarding infectious complications, but it was not distinguished, whether a rectal lesion was present or not.

Colostomy is the keystone of rectal trauma treatment [101].

A loop-type colostomy is favored [98, 101].

Colostomy takedown should be performed early, within 3 months after initiation, as later closure was associated with an increase of complications [98, 102, 103].

In the presence of combined bladder and rectal injuries, one fourth of patients develop rectovesical and rectourethral fistula after penetrating trauma [104]. For these patients, besides rectal debridement, primary repair, and proximal diversion, an omental pedicle flap placed anterior to the rectum can reduce this complication rate [90, 105, 106].

Thus, these concepts can be an option even in blunt trauma cases with combined urogenital and anorectal injuries.

Anal sphincter repair should be initiated, dependent on the hemodynamic status of the patient [98]. In stable patients, primary repair is favored [98, 107]. If sphincteroplasty is considered, delayed reconstruction is recommended. In the presence of massive anorectal lacerations and gross contamination, fecal diversion is favored [107].

Destructed anal sphincter injuries can be treated by delayed abdominal perineal resection [31], while anal tears should be debrided initially and left open. Rectal mucosa tears should be closed after debridement [31].

Song et al. reported on risk factors of infection in 20 patients with rectal injuries [39]. In a univariable analysis, shock, RTS ≤8, GCS ≤8, blood transfusion ≥10 units in the first 24 h, no colostomy, or Gustilo grade III soft-tissue injury were associated with pelvic infection, while in the multivariable analysis, shock and the absence of colostomy were independently associated with pelvic infection.

17.11 Pelvic Ring Treatment

Treatment of the pelvic ring lesions depends on the localization of the accompanying wounds and the instability of the pelvic ring.

Open pelvic fractures with an intact pelvic ring are usually open iliac wing fractures as a result of a direct blow to the ilium. In contrast to unstable pelvic ring disruptions [5, 28], there is an inferior associated bleeding risk and a lower risk for complications and mortality [108]. In this specific injury group, after appropriate resuscitation, treatment can consist of intravenous antibiotics, adequate debridement with wound irrigation, wound packing, and primary or secondary wound closure using an intermediate vacuum system [80, 109].

Most fractures can be treated non-operatively [109], but ORIF can be an option in severely displaced fractures with or without large fragments [80]. To avoid plate fixation, even isolated screw fixation can be an option [110].

In mechanically unstable pelvic ring injuries, ORIF or external fixation is preferred. Classically, after primary temporary external fixation, later definitive fixation is recommended [73, 111, 112].

Dependent on the localization and severity of the accompanying soft-tissue injury, percutaneous limited internal fixation and external fixation was proposed [113].

In many patients, primary pelvic ring stabilization consisted of anterior external fixation ± posterior SI-screw or (percutaneous) plating [10, 36].

17.12 Long-Term Results

Only few results are reported regarding long-term problems after open pelvic fractures (Figs. 17.14 and 17.15):

- Brenneman et al. reported on long-term pain and functional disturbances 4 years after injury in 44 patients [4]; functional complaints included sexual dysfunction, fecal and urinary incontinence, and unhealed fractures; slightly more than half of those who were employed before the injury returned to work.
- Ferrera et al., reported on approximately 50% impaired functions during daily activities; 8/15 patients walked without assistance [6].
- Wei et al. reported results of 11 survivors after a mean of 14 months with no anal incontinence in the patients with an anorectal injury [34].
- Fu et al. analyzed follow-up results in patients after perineal injuries and reported that, after a mean of 16.5 months, no patient revealed complications related to fecal diversion [26].

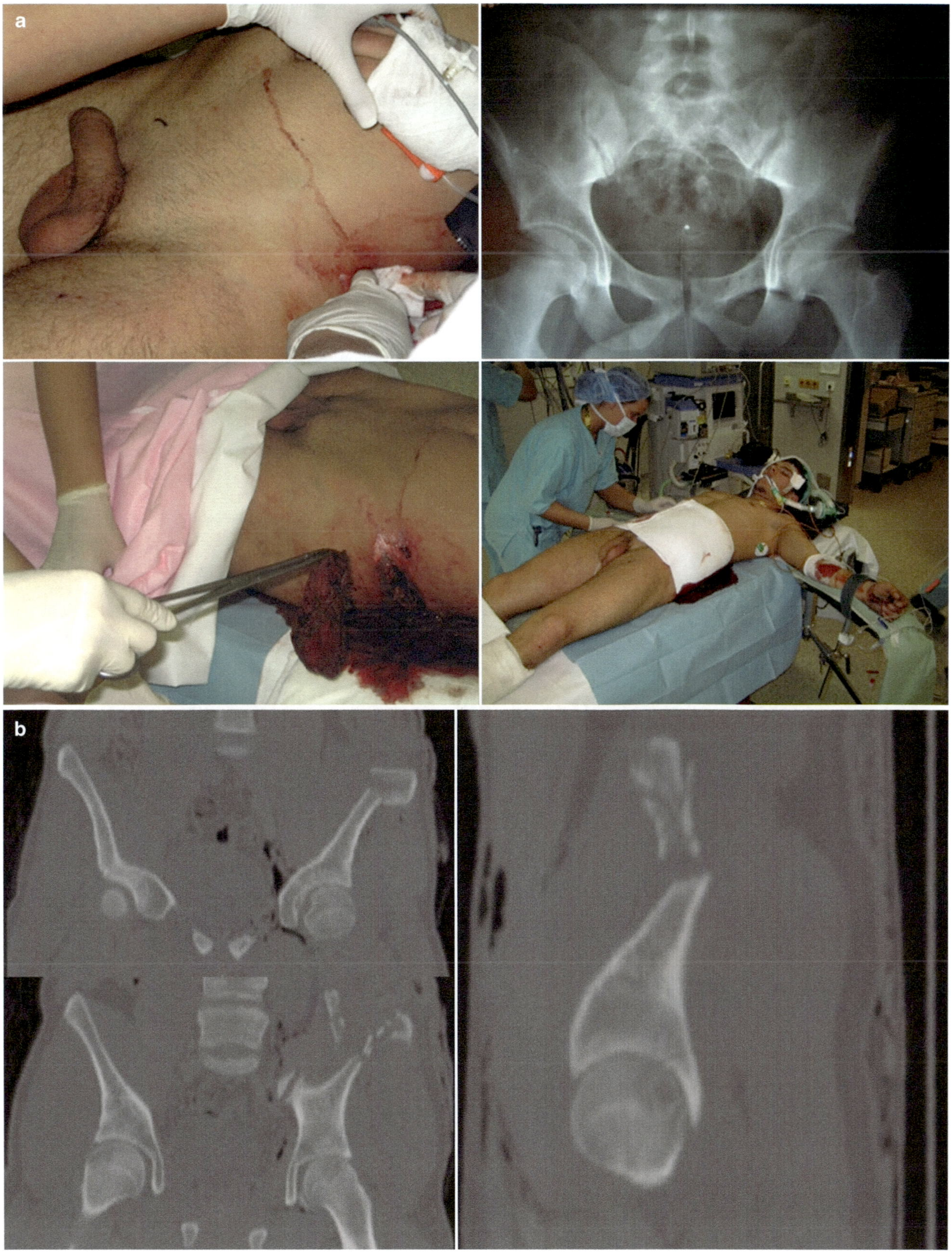

Fig. 17.14 (**a**) Open left ilium fracture with severe dirt in the wound. Initial emergency treatment using a pelvic binder for local compression of the inserted tamponade. (**b**) CT: displaced comminuted iliac wing fracture. (**c**) Primary treatment: local skin excision, extensive debridement of devascularized muscles, and cleaning of the fracture zone. (**d**) Iliac wing screw stabilization and primary wound closure. (**e**) Definitive pelvic a.p. X-ray postoperatively

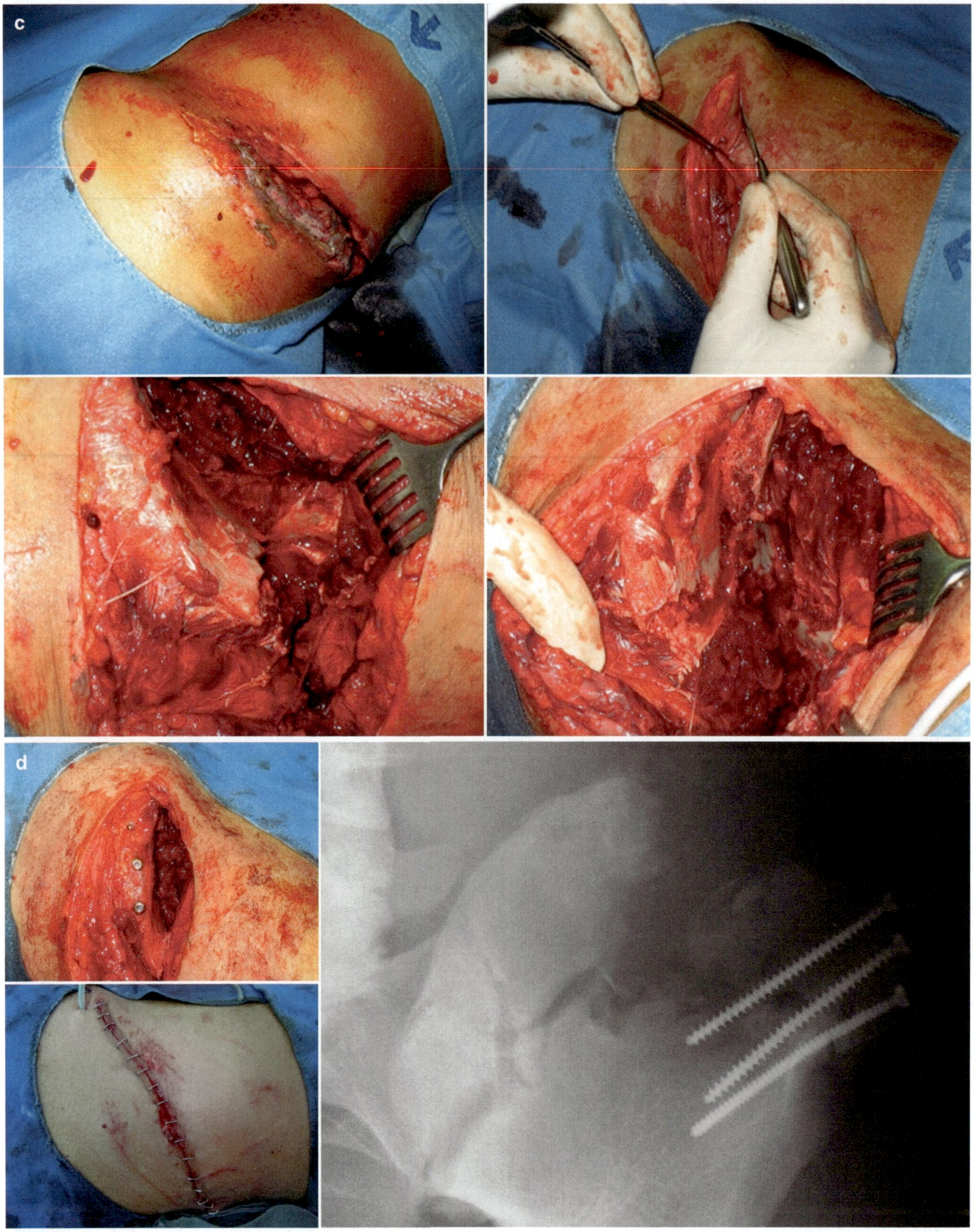

Fig. 17.14 (continued)

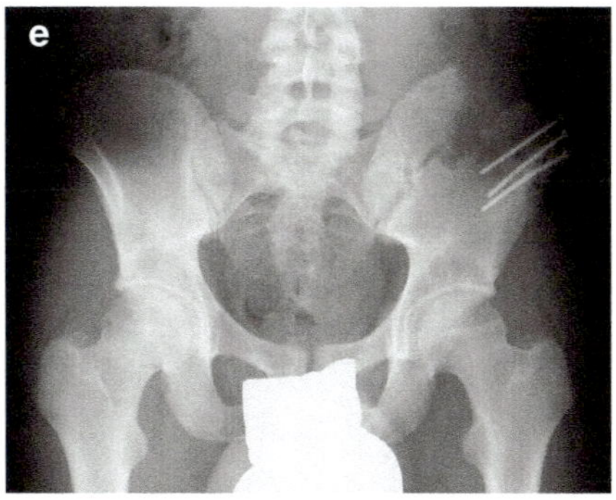

Fig. 17.14 (continued)

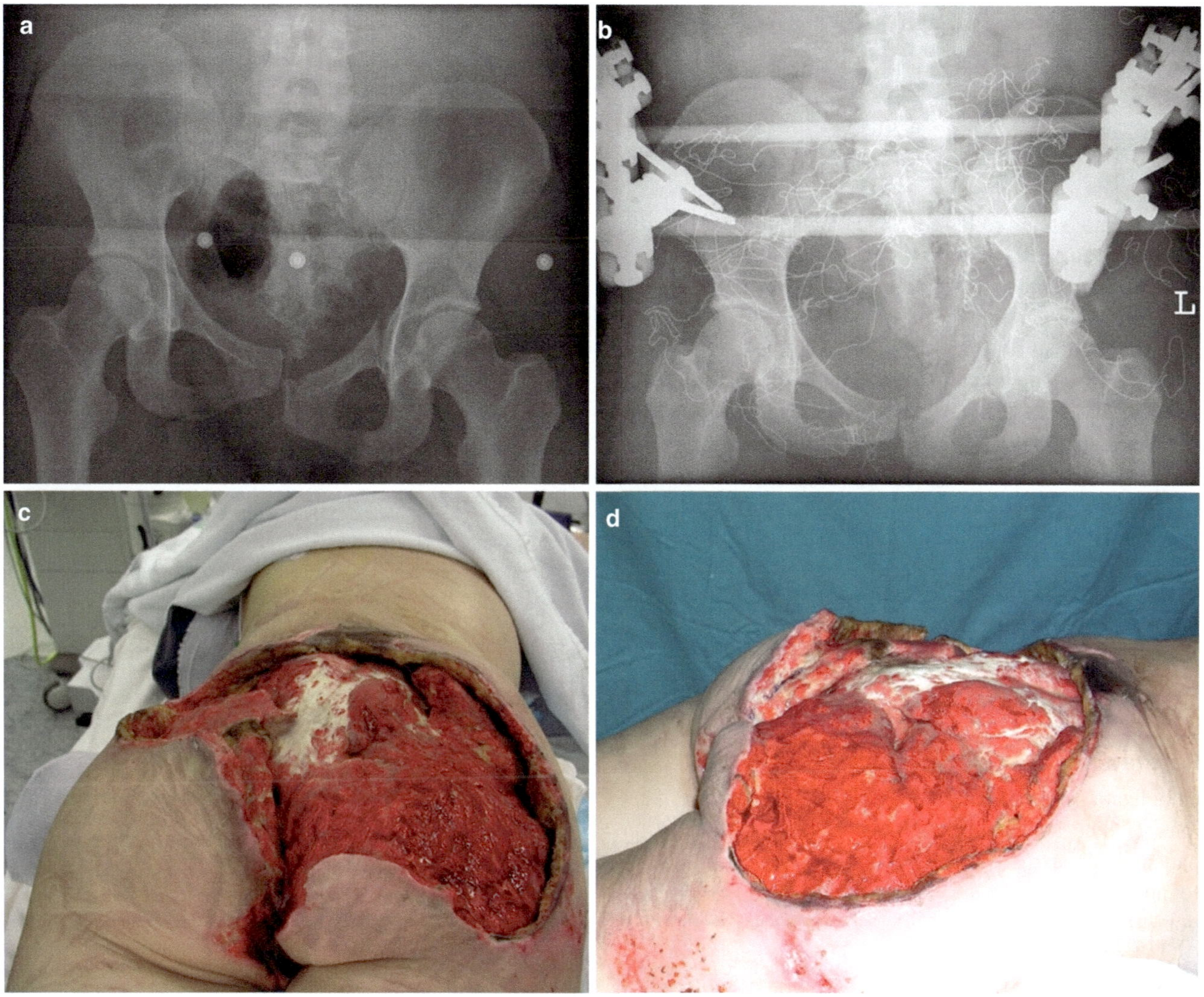

Fig. 17.15 Staged reconstruction of open bilateral transforaminal sacral fractures with symphysis pubis disruption and rami fractures (C3). (**a**) A 26-year-old female cyclist was struck by a bus and sustained an open pelvic fracture. Extended gluteal and perineal soft-tissue injuries developed. An urgent diverting colostomy was performed. (**b**) Closed reduction and external fixation frame were used for emergent skeletal stabilization. Bilateral arterial pelvic bleeding was treated with non-selective angiographic embolization. (**c**, **d**) Skin, subcutaneous fat, and muscle injuries were treated with repeated surgical debridements. (**e**) After three weeks the definitive treatment of pelvic fracture was carried out. The vertical sacral fractures were reduced by mini open control at S1 foramen and fixed with IS-screws, and anterior plating without any infection complications. Skin grafting was used to cover the soft-tissue defect. Later on, plastic surgeons made several local soft-tissue reconstructions. (**f**) Several years later, the patient is satisfied with the situation and is working normally

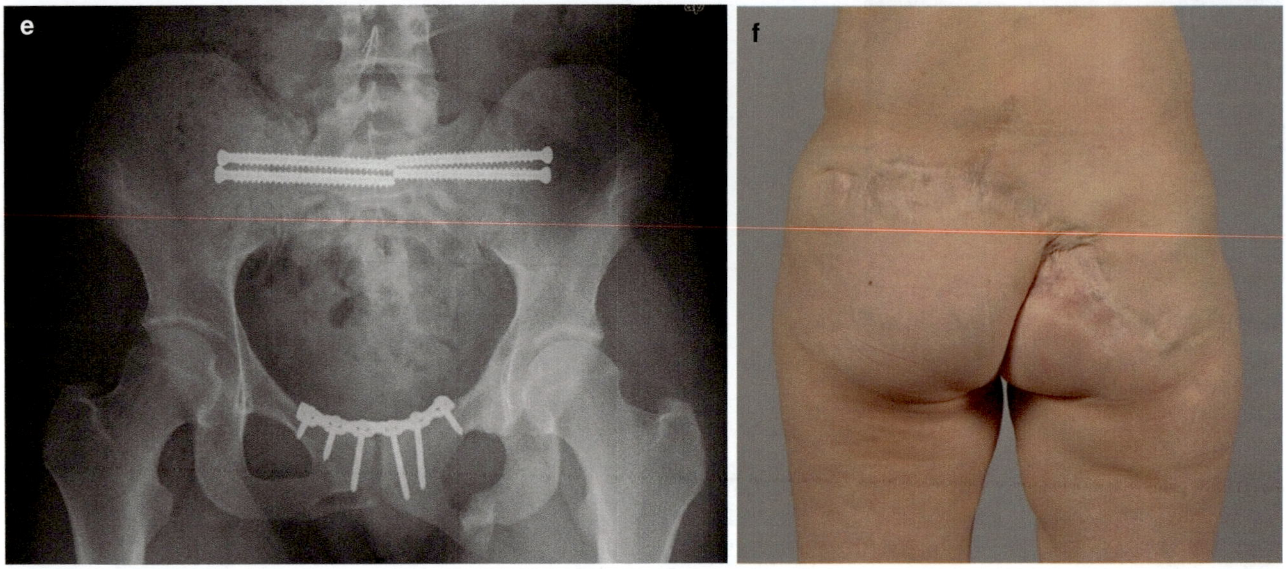

Fig. 17.15 (continued)

- Giordano et al. followed 18 patients after 6 months; 36.6% had satisfactory result and 23.3% an unsatisfactory result according to the EuroQol EQ-5D; the latter patients reported on persistent pain, impotence, active fistula or chronic infection, gait disorders, or decreased sexual intercourse due to coitus pain; signs of post-traumatic stress disorder (PTSD) syndrome and depression were also frequent [19].
- Hermans et al. reported persistent symptoms at 6 months, including impotence, sexual problems, and dyspareunia, while fecal or urinary incontinence was not reported [21].

> Persistent clinical complaints related to pelvic injury are common after open pelvic injuries.

References

1. Grotz M, Allami M, Harwood P, Pape H, Krettek C, Giannoudis P. Open pelvic fractures: epidemiology, current concepts of management and outcome. Injury. 2005;36:1–13.
2. Bosch U, Pohlemann T, Haas N, Tscherne H. Classification and management of complex pelvic trauma. Unfallchirurg. 1992;95:189–96.
3. Gänsslen A, Pohlemann T, Paul C, Lobenhoffer P, Tscherne H. Epidemiology of pelvic ring injuries. Injury. 1996;Suppl. 1(Part 1):13–20.
4. Brenneman F, Katyal D, Boulanger B, Tile M, Redelmeier D. Long-term outcomes in open pelvic fractures. J Trauma. 1997;42(5):773–7.
5. Jones A, Powell J, Kellam J, McCormack R, Dust W, Wimmer P. Open pelvic fractures. A multicentern retrospective analysis. Orthop Clin North Am. 1997;28:345–50.
6. Ferrera PC, Hill DA. Good outcomes of open pelvic fractures. Injury. 1999;30(3):187–90.
7. Rothenberger D, Velasco R, Strate R, Fischer R, Perry J. Open pelvic fractures: a lethal injury. J Trauma. 1978;18(3):184–7.
8. Perry J. Pelvic open fractures. Clin Orthop. 1980;151:41–5.
9. Richardson JD, Harty J, Amin M, Flint LM. Open pelvic fractures. J Trauma. 1982;22(7):533–8.
10. Cannada L, Taylor R, Reddix R, Mullis B, Moghadamian E, Erickson M, Consortium SF. The Jones-Powell classification of open pelvic fractures: a multicenter study evaluating mortality rates. J Trauma Acute Care Surg. 2013;74:901–6.
11. Rothenberger D, Fischer R, Strate R, Velasco R, Perry J. The mortality associated with pelvic fractures. Surgery. 1978;84(3):356–9.
12. Dente C, Feliciano D, Rozycki G, Wyrzykowski A, Nicholas J, Salomone J, Ingram W. The outcome of open pelvic fractures in the modern era. Am J Surg. 2005;190:830–5.
13. O'Sullivan R, White T, Keating J. Major pelvic fractures: identification of patients at high risk. J Bone Joint Surg. 2005;87-B:530–3.
14. Hanson P, Milne J, Chapman M. Open fractures of the pelvis: review of 43 cases. J Bone Joint Surg (Br). 1991;73-B:325–9.
15. Giannoudis P, Grotz M, Tzioupis C, Dinopoulos H, Wells G, Bouamra O, Lecky F. Prevalence of pelvic fractures, associated injuries, and mortality: the United Kingdom perspective. J Trauma. 2007;63:875–83.
16. Davidson B, Simmons G, Williamson P, Buerk C. Pelvic fractures associated with open perineal wounds: a survivable injury. J Trauma. 1993;35(1):36–9.
17. Hauschild O, Strohm P, Culemann U, Pohlemann T, Suedkamp N, Koestler W, Schmal H. Mortality in patients with pelvic fractures: results from the German pelvic injury register. J Trauma. 2008;64:449–55.
18. Siada S, Davis J, Kaups K, Dirks R, Grannis K. Current outcomes of blunt open pelvic fractures: how modern advances in trauma care may decrease mortality. Trauma Surg Acute Care Open. 2017;2:e000136. https://doi.org/10.1136/tsaco-2017-000136. eCollection 2017
19. Giordano V, Koch H, Gasparini S, Serrão de Souza F, Labronici P, do Amaral N. Open pelvic fractures: review of 30 cases. Open Orthop J. 2016;20:772–8.

20. Sriussadaporn S, Sirichindakul B, Pak-Art R, Tharavej C. Pelvic fractures: experience in management of 170 cases at a university hospital in Thailand. J Med Assoc Thail. 2002;85:200–6.
21. Hermans E, Edwards M, Goslings J, Biert J. Open pelvic fracture: the killing fracture? J Orthop Surg Res. 2018;13:83. https://doi.org/10.1186/s13018-018-0793-2.
22. Black E, Lawson C, Scmith S, Daley B. Open pelvic fractures: the University of Tennessee Medical. Center at Knowville Experience over ten years. Iowa Orthop J. 2011;31:193–8.
23. Faringer P, Mullins R, Feliciano P, Duwelius P, Trunkey D. Selective fecal diversion in complex open pelvic fractures from blunt trauma. Arch Surg. 1994;129:958–64.
24. Bircher M, Hargrove R. Is it possible to classify open fractures of the pelvis? Eur J Trauma. 2004;30:74–9.
25. Gustilo R, Anderson J. Prevention of infection in the treatment of one thousand and twenty-five open fractures of long bones. J Bone Joint Surg. 1976;58-A:453–8.
26. Fu G, Wang D, Qin B, Xiang J, Qi J, Li P, Zhu Q, Liu X, Zhu J. Modified 3classification and repair of perineal soft tissue injuries associated with open pelvic fractures. J Reconstr Microsurg. 2015;31:12–9.
27. Maull K, Sachatello C, Ernst C. The deep perineal laceration-an injury frequently associated with open pelvic fractures. J Trauma. 1977;17:685–8.
28. Raffa J, Christensen N. Compound fractures of the pelvis. Am J Surg. 1976;132:282–6.
29. Govender S, Sham A, Singh B. Open pelvic fractures. Injury. 1990;21:373–6.
30. Mosheiff R, Suchar A, Porat S, Shmushkevich A, Segal D, Liebergall M. The crushed open pelvis in children. Injury. 1999;30:14–8.
31. Kudsk K, Hanna M. Management of complex perineal injuries. World J Surg. 2003;27:895–900.
32. Kusmisky R, Shbeeb I, Makos G, Boland J. Blunt pelviperineal injuries. An expanded role for the diverting colostomy. Dis Colon Rectum. 1982;25:787–90.
33. Dong J, Zhou D. Management and outcome of open pelvic fractures: a retrospective study of 41 cases. Injury. 2011;42:1003–7.
34. Wei R, Cao X, Tu D. Clinical treatment of open pelvic fractures associated with perineal injury. [Article in Chinese]. Zhongguo Xiu Fu Chong Jian Wai Ke Za Zhi. 2012;26:550–3.
35. Sinnott R, Rhodes M, Brader A. Open pelvic fractures: an injury for trauma centers. Am J Surg. 1992;163:283–7.
36. Hasankhani E, Omidi-Kashani F. Treatment outcomes of open pelvic fractures associated with extensive perineal injuries. Clin Orthop Surg. 2013;5:263–8.
37. Teixeira F, Netto S, Collet e Silva F, Mori N, Fontes B, Poggetti R, Birolini D, Bernini C, Utiyama E. Complex perineal injuries in blunt trauma patients: the value of a damage control approach. Panam J Trauma Crit Care Emerg Surg. 2015;4:87–95.
38. Woods R, O'Keefe G, Rhee P, Routt M, Maier R. Open pelvic fracture and fecal diversion. Arch Surg. 1998;133(3):281–6.
39. Song W, Zhou D, Xu W, Zhang G, Wang C, Qiu D, Dong J. Factors of pelvic infection and death in patients with open pelvic fractures and rectal injuries. Surg Infect. 2017;18:711–5.
40. Pell M, Flynn W, Seibel R. Is colostomy always necessary in the treatment of open pelvic fractures? J Trauma. 1998;45:371–3.
41. Rieger H, Winde G, Brug E, Senninger N. Open pelvic fracture—an indication for laparotomy? Chirurg. 1998;69:278–83.
42. Michel J, Peter R, Roche B, Vermeulen B, Morel P. Primary surgical care of pelvic fractures with perineal laceration. Swiss Surg. 1999;5:33–7.
43. Moskowitz E, Burlew C, Moore E, Pieracci F, Fox C, Campion E, Lawless R, Cohen M. Preperitoneal pelvic packing is effective for hemorrhage control in open pelvic fractures. Am J Surg. 2018;215:675–7.
44. Collinge C, Tornetta P. Soft tissue injuries associated with pelvic fractures. Orthop Clin North Am. 2004;35:451–6.
45. Govaert G, Siriwardhane M, Hatzifotis M, Malisano L, Schuetz M. Prevention of pelvic sepsis in major open pelviperineal injury. Injury. 2012;43:533–6.
46. Naam N, Brown W, Hurd R, Burdge R, Kaminski D. Major pelvic fractures. Arch Surg. 1983;118:610–7.
47. DGU GTS. Level 3 guideline on the treatment of patients with severe/multiple injuries. Eur J Trauma Emerg Surg. 2018;44:S3–S271.
48. Ward A. AOT Master Course Pelvis. Dubai, UAE: Personal Communication; 2018.
49. Anderson A, Miller A, Bookstaver P. Antimicrobial prophylaxis in open lower extremity fractures. Open Access Emerg Med. 2011;3:7–11.
50. Dunkel N, Pittet D, Tovmirzaeva L, Suvà D, Bernard L, Lew D, Hoffmeyer P, Uçkay I. Short duration of antibiotic prophylaxis in open fractures does not enhance risk of subsequent infection. Bone Joint J. 2013;95-B:831–7.
51. Hauser C, Adams CJ, Eachempati S. Surgical infection society guideline: prophylactic antibiotic use in open fractures: an evidence-based guideline. Surg Infect. 2006;7:379–405.
52. Hoff W, Bonadies J, Cachecho R, Dorlac W. East practice management guidelines work group: update to practice management guidelines for prophylactic antibiotic use in open fractures. J Trauma. 2011;70:751–4.
53. Mundi R, Chaudhry H, Niroopan G, Petrisor B, Bhandari M. Open tibial fractures: updated guidelines for management. JBJS Rev. 2015;3:pii: 01874474-201503020-00003. https://doi.org/10.2106/JBJS.RVW.N.00051.
54. Rodriguez L, Jung H, Goulet J, Cicalo A, Machado-Aranda D, Napolitano L. Evidence-based protocol for prophylactic antibiotics in open fractures: improved antibiotic stewardship with no increase in infection rates. J Trauma Acute Care Surg. 2013;77:400–8.
55. Patzakis M, Wilkins J. Factors influencing infection rate in open fracture wounds. Clin Orthop Relat Res. 1989;243:36–40.
56. Zalavras C, Marcus R, Levin L, Patzakis M. Management of open fractures and subsequent complications. J Bone Joint Surg. 2007;89-A:884–95.
57. Rossaint R, Bouillon B, Cerny V, Coats T, Duranteau J, Fernández-Mondéjar E, Filipescu D, Hunt B, Komadina R, Nardi G, Neugebauer E, Ozier Y, Riddez L, Schultz A, Vincent J, Spahn D. The European guideline on management of major bleeding and coagulopathy following trauma: fourth edition. Crit Care. 2016;20:100.
58. Ramasamy A, Evans S, Kendrew J, Cooper J. The open blast pelvis: the significant burden of management. J Bone Joint Surg. 2012;94-B:829–35.
59. Ertel W, Keel M, Eid K, Platz A, Trentz O. Control of severe hemorrhage using C-clamp and pelvic packing in multiply injured patients with pelvic ring disruption. J Orthop Trauma. 2001;15(7):468–74.
60. Gänsslen A, Giannoudis P, Pape H. Hemorrhage in pelvic fracture: who needs angiography? Curr Opin Crit Care. 2003;9:515–23.
61. Gänsslen A, Hildebrand F, Pohlemann T. Management of hemodynamic unstable patients "in extremis" with pelvic ring fractures. Acta Chir Orthop Traumatol Cechoslov. 2012;79:193–202.
62. Gänsslen A, Krettek C, Pape H, Machtens S. Acute management of pelvic fractures: a european perspective. In: Smith WR, Ziran BH, Morgan SJ, editors. Fractures of the pelvis and acetabulum. New York: Informa Healthcare USA, Inc.; 2007, ISBN-13: 978-0-8247-2846-5.
63. Connolly B, Gerlinger T, Pitcher J. Complete masking of a severe open-book pelvic fracture by a pneumatic antishock garment. J Trauma. 1999;46:340–2.

64. Swartz J, Vaidya R, Hudson I, Oliphant B, Tonnos F. Effect of pelvic binder placement on OTA classification of pelvic ring injuries using computed tomography. Does it mask the injury? J Orthop Trauma. 2016;30:325–30.
65. Bates D, Wasserman M, Malek A, Gorantla V, Anderson S, Soto J, LeBedis C. Multidetector CT of surgically proven blunt bowel and mesenteric injury. Radiographics. 2017;37:613–25.
66. Ebraheim N, Savolaine E, Rusin J, Jackson W, Asensio J. Occult rectal perforation in a major pelvic fracture. J Orthop Trauma. 1988;2:340–3.
67. Shapiro M, Wolverson M. Perforation of the retroperitoneal sigmoid colon secondary to fracture dislocation of the left sacro-iliac joint. J Trauma. 1989;29:694–6.
68. Singh J, Steward M, Booth T, Mukhtar H, Murray D. Evolution of imaging for abdominal perforation. Ann R Coll Surg Engl. 2010;92:182–8.
69. Soto J, Anderson S. Multidetector CT of blunt abdominal trauma. Radiology. 2012;265:678–93.
70. Brandes S. Initial management of anterior and posterior urethral injuries. Urol Clin North Am. 2006;33:87–95.
71. Figler B, Hoffler C, Reisman W, Carney K, Moore T, Feliciano D, Master V. Multi-disciplinary update on pelvic fracture associated bladder and urethral injuries. Injury. 2012;43:1242–9.
72. Rosenstein D, Alsikafi N. Diagnosis and classification of urethral injuries. Urol Clin North Am. 2006;33:73–85.
73. Leenen L, van der Werken C, Schoots F, Goris R. Internal fixation of open unstable pelvic fractures. J Trauma. 1993;35(2):220–5.
74. Bhandari M, Jeray K, Petrisor B, Devereaux P, Heels-Ansdell D, et al. The FLOW Investigators. A trial of wound irrigation in the initial management of open fracture wounds. N Engl J Med. 2015;373:2629–41.
75. Anglen J. Wound irrigation in musculoskeletal injury. JAAOS. 2001;9:219–26.
76. Herscovici JD, Sanders R, Scaduto J, Infante A, Di Pasquale T. Vacuum-assisted wound closure (VAC therapy) for the management of patients with high-energy soft tissue injuries. J Orthop Trauma. 2003;17:683–8.
77. Huang C, Leavitt T, Bayer L, Orgill D. Effect of negative pressure wound therapy on wound healing. Curr Probl Surg. 2014;51:301–31.
78. Liu X, Zhang H, Cen S, Huang C. Negative pressure wound therapy versus conventional wound dressings in treatment of open fractures: a systematic review and meta-analysis. Int J Surg. 2018;53:72–9.
79. Mullner T, Mrkonjic L, Kwasny O, Vecsei V. The use of negative pressure to promote the healing of tissue defects: a clinical trial using the vacuum sealing technique. Br J Plast Surg. 1997;50:194–9.
80. Switzer J, Nork S, Routt M. Comminuted fractures of the iliac wing. J Orthop Trauma. 2000;14:270–6.
81. Costa M, Achten J, Bruce J, Tutton E, Petrou S, Lamb S, Parsons N, Collaboration UW. Pressure wound therapy vs. standard wound management on 12-month disability among adults with severe open fracture of the lower limb: the WOLLF randomized clinical trial. JAMA. 2018;319:2280–8.
82. Henry S, Ostermann P, Seligson D. The prophylactic use of antibiotic impregnated beads in open fractures. J Trauma. 1990;30:11231–8.
83. Henry S, Ostermann P, Seligson D. The antibiotic bead pouch technique. The management of severe compound fractures. Clin Orthop. 1993;295:54–62.
84. Morgenstern M, Vallejo A, McNally M, Moriarty T, Ferguson J, Nijs S, Metsemakers W. The effect of local antibiotic prophylaxis when treating open limb fractures: a systematic review and meta-analysis. Bone Joint Res. 2018;7:447–56.
85. Ostermann P, Seligson D, Henry S. Local antibiotic therapy for severe open fractures. A review of 1085 consecutive cases. J Bone Joint Surg. 1995;77-B:93–7.
86. Van Wessem K, Mackay P, King K, Balogh Z. Selective faecal diversion in open pelvic fractures: reassessment based on recent experience. Injury. 2012;43:522–5.
87. Tsugawa K, Koyanagi N, Hashizume M, Ayukawa K, Wada H, Tomikawa M, Sugimachi K. New therapeutic strategy of open pelvic fracture associated with rectal injury in 43 patients over 60 years of age. Hepato-Gastroenterology. 2002;49:1275–80.
88. Lavenson G, Cohen A. Management of rectal injuries. Am J Surg. 1971;122:226–30.
89. Choi W. Management of colorectal trauma. J Korean Soc Coloproctol. 2011;27:166–73.
90. Crispen P, Kansas B, Pieri P, Fisher C, Gaughan J, Pathak A, et al. Immediate postoperative complications of combined penetrating rectal and bladder injuries. J Trauma. 2007;62:325–9.
91. Herzig D. Care of the patient with anorectal trauma. Clin Colon Rectal Surg. 2012;25:210–3.
92. Shlamovitz G, Mower W, Bergman J, Crisp J, DeVore H, Hardy D, et al. Poor test characteristics for the digital rectal examination in trauma patients. Ann Emerg Med. 2007;50:25–33.
93. Ross G, Dodd O, Lipham J, Campbell J. Rectal perforation in unstable pelvic fractures: the use of flexible sigmoidoscopy. Injury. 2001;32:67–8.
94. Aihara R, Blansfield J, Millham F, LaMorte W, Hirsch E. Fracture locations influence the likelihood of rectal and lower urinary tract injuries in patients sustaining pelvic fractures. J Trauma. 2002;52:205–8.
95. Johnson E, Steele S. Evidence-based management of colorectal trauma. J Gastrointest Surg. 2013;17:12–9.
96. Wu K, Posluszny J, Branch J, Dray E, Blackwell R, Hannick J, Luchette F. Trauma to the pelvis: injuries to the rectum and genitourinary organs. Curr Trauma Rep. 2015;1:8–15.
97. Gonzalez R, Falimirski M, Holevar M. The role of presacral drainage in the management of penetrating rectal injuries. J Trauma. 1998;45:656–61.
98. Petrone P, Velandia W, Dziakova J, Marini C. Treatment of complex perineal trauma. A review of the literature. Cir Esp. 2016;94:313–22.
99. Steele S, Maykel J, Johnson E. Traumatic injury of the colon and rectum: the evidence vs. dogma. Dis Colon Rectum. 2011;54:1184–201.
100. Lunsjo K, Abu-Zidan F. Does colostomy prevent infection in open blunt pelvic fractures? A systematic review. J Trauma. 2006;60:1145–8.
101. Berne J, Velmahos G, Chan L, Asensio J, Demetriades D. The high morbidity of colostomy closure after trauma: further support for the primary repair of colon injuries. Surgery. 1998;123:157–64.
102. Sola J, Bender J, Buchman T. Morbidity and timing of colostomy closure in trauma patients. Injury. 1993;24:438–40.
103. Velmahos G, Degiannis E, Wells M, Souter I, Saadia R. Early closure of colostomies in trauma patients—a prospective randomized trial. Surgery. 1995;118:815–20.
104. Franko E, Ivatury R, Schwalb D. Combined penetrating rectal and genitourinary injuries: a challenge in management. J Trauma. 1993;34:347–53.

105. Kuy S, Codner P, Guralnick M, Dua A, Paul J. Combined rectovesicular injuries from low velocity penetrating trauma in an adult. WMJ. 2013;112:32–334.
106. Pereira B, Reis L, Calderan T, de Campos C, Fraga G. Penetrating bladder trauma: a high risk factor for associated rectal injury. Ther Adv Urol. 2014;2014:386280.
107. Hashish A. Perineal trauma in children: a standardized management approach. Ann Ped Surg. 2011;7:55–60.
108. Bucholz R. The pathological anatomy of malgaigne fracture-dislocations of the pelvis. J Bone Joint Surg. 1981;63-A(3):400–4.
109. Abrassart S, Stern R, Peter R. Morbidity associated with isolated iliac wing fractures. J Trauma. 2009;66:200–3.
110. Cole P, Jamil M, Jacobson A, Hill B. "The skiver screw": a useful fixation technique for iliac wing fractures. J Orthop Trauma. 2015;29:231–4.
111. Browner BD, Cole JD, Graham JM, Bondurant FJ, Nunchuck BS, Colter HB. Delayed posterior internal fixation of unstable pelvic fractures. J Trauma. 1987;27(9):998–1006.
112. Gylling SF, Ward RE, Holcroft JW, Bray TJ, Chapman MW. Immediate external fixation of unstable pelvic fractures. Am J Surg. 1985;150(6):721–4.
113. Chen L, Zhang G, Wu Y, Guo X, Yuan W. Percutaneous limited internal fixation combined with external fixation to treat open pelvic fractures concomitant with perineal lacerations. Orthopedics. 2011;34:827–31.

Morel-Lavallée Lesions

18

Bernd Füchtmeier, Franz Müller, Stephan Grechenig, and Axel Gänsslen

Morel-Lavallée first described a closed degloving injury [1]. Letournel and Judet referred to the classical Morel-Lavallée lesion (MLL), which is a closed internal degloving injury over the greater trochanter [2].

Closed degloving injuries are uncommon and often overlooked, especially in the multiply-injured patient. Correct treatment is essential to avoid relevant morbidity.

18.1 Definition

The MLL is defined as a closed internal degloving injury associated with a pelvic trauma, where the subcutaneous tissue is torn away from the underlying fascia, creating a cavity filled with hematoma and liquefied fat, resulting from the disruption of arteries perforating through the fascia [3, 4].

18.2 Frequency

Letournel reported first data on the frequency of this lesion in acetabular fractures as a result of a direct blow to the greater trochanter [2]. A rate of 8.3% was reported. Steiner observed 2.5% MLL's with pelvic ring injuries and 0.6% with acetabular fractures [5]. In a retrospective analysis on patients with pelvic ring fractures, CT evaluation revealed ML lesions in 182 of 1493 patients (12.2%) [6].

> MLL can be expected in 2–12% after pelvic ring injuries. CT identifies higher rates.

18.3 Localization

MLL can be present at different localizations. The typical expected area after sustaining pelvic or acetabular injuries is the greater trochanteric area (Fig. 18.1). Additionally, the flank and lumbodorsal regions can be involved [3].

Large lesions can additionally involve the thigh, the sacro-gluteal, hypogastric, or inguinal areas or even up to the abdomen [5, 7]. In a CT analysis, the main locations were the lateral thigh and almost all other MLLs were observed posterior at the flank or lumbar region [6].

In a systematic review of 204 ML lesions, independent of additional pelvic fractures, the main locations were the greater trochanteric area in 30.4%, the thigh in 20.1% and the pelvis in 18.6%, while the gluteal and the lumbosacral regions were only reported in 6.4% and 3.4%, respectively [8].

The mean surface area was 30 × 12 cm in MLL's around the pelvis [9].

> The greater trochanteric and thigh areas are predominantly involved in pelvic and acetabular fractures [10].

B. Füchtmeier
Department of Trauma Surgery, Hospital Barmherzige Brüder, Regensburg, Germany
e-mail: Bernd.Fuechtmeier@barmherzige-regensburg.de

F. Müller
Department of Trauma Surgery, Orthopaedics and Sports Medicine, Hospital Barmherzige Brüder Regensburg, Regensburg, Germany

S. Grechenig
Department of Orthopedics and Trauma Surgery, AUVA Trauma Hospital Klagenfurt, Klagenfurt, Austria

Department of Trauma Surgery, University Hospital Regensburg, Regensburg, Germany

A. Gänsslen (✉)
Department of Trauma Surgery, Orthopedics and Hand Surgery, Hospital Wolfsburg, Wolfsburg, Germany

A. Gänsslen et al. (eds.), *Pelvic Ring Fractures*, https://doi.org/10.1007/978-3-030-54730-1_18

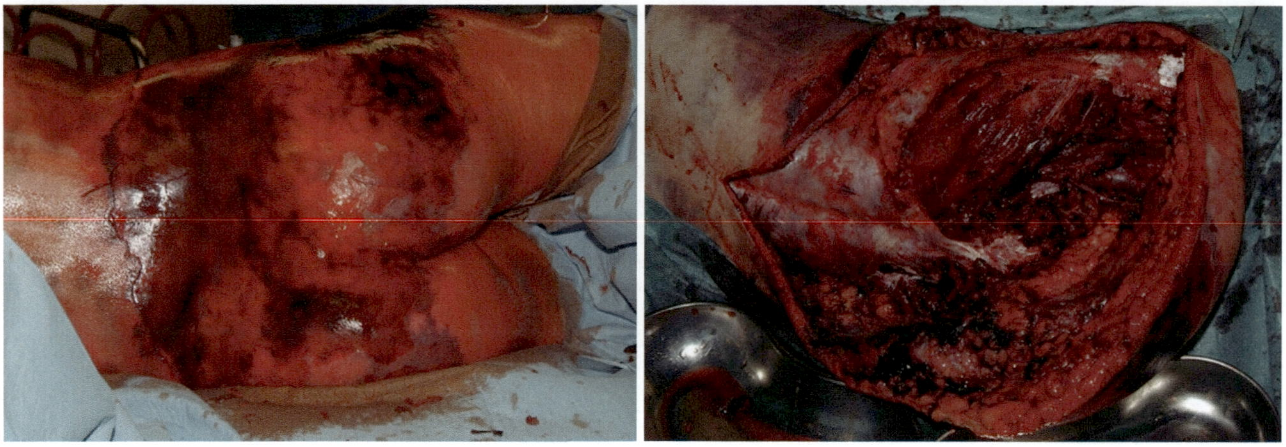

Fig. 18.1 Typical localization of a Morel-Levallée lesion at the greater trochanteric and sacroiliac area in a pelvic ring roll-over injury with severe destruction of the underlying soft-tissues and muscles

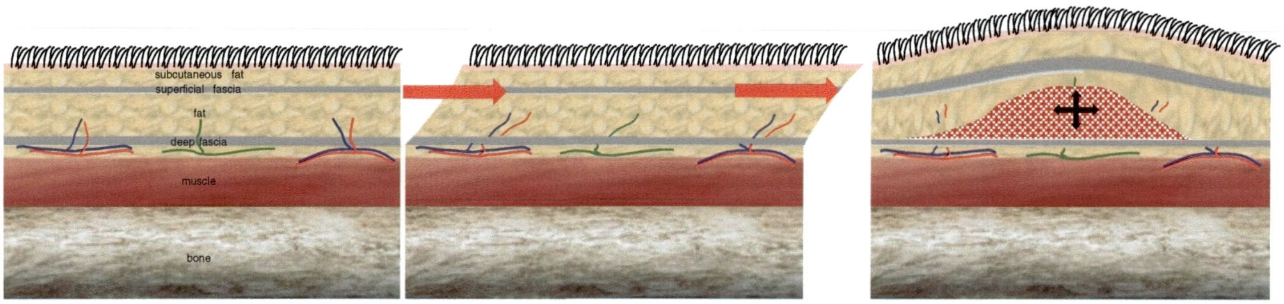

Fig. 18.2 Mechanism of MLL acc. to Bonilla-Yoon et al. Emerg Radiol 2014. Shearing between the subdermal plane and the fascia leads to a distended cavity

18.4 Pathophysiology

An MLL develops after localized abrupt trauma to the peripelvic region, resulting in an additional shearing mechanism between the skin and the fascia.

This leads to a traumatic separation of the skin and/or subcutaneous fat from the underlying fascia, for example, the iliotibial tract, the gluteal or lumbosacral fascia [10].

Disruption of the subdermal capillaries and lymphatics leads to suprafascial hemorrhage, lymphatic fluid, debris, and subdermal fat, resulting in a distended cavity (Fig. 18.2). Necrosis of the fatty and soft tissue necrosis can be present, which increases the risk of infection. Additionally, the involved skin can become necrotic as a result of direct trauma or secondary due to significant MLL cavity swelling, resulting in skin ischemia [4, 11].

> The reduced soft-tissue perfusion can lead to epidermiolysis, necrosis, and infection.

Dependent on additional subdermal arterial injury, accumulation of these contents may develop fast or slow, when only lymphatics are involved.

During the next days, resorption of the hemorrhagic elements takes part, which changes to the presence of serosanguinous fluid and a progressive fibrous encapsulation. The latter impairs fluid resorption and long-term presence of the MLL [12, 13].

Subacute or chronic lesions are associated with a resulting inflammatory reaction, which supports the development of a peripheral fibrous capsule [3, 13–18].

When surgery is performed through an MLL, there is an additional risk of cutaneous flap necrosis [19]. Even external fixation pins should be avoided, whenever possible.

18.5 Clinical Diagnostics

The diagnosis of an MLL is made by physical examination and confirmed during surgery. Typical clinical signs include [4, 5, 10, 12, 13, 20–22]:

- Presence of a soft fluctuant area
- Decreased cutaneous sensation, due to disruption of the subdermal afferent nerves
- Local skin contusion
- Ecchymosis around the pelvic ring
- Tire marks
- Friction burns
- Skin hypermobility
- Contour deformity (late sign)
- Fever and hyperleukocytosis
- Pain

In uncertain clinical situations, preoperative confirmation of such a lesion can be made by needle aspiration of the suspected area [4, 9].

Secondary dermal signs include a dry and cracking skin, discoloration, and secondary necrosis [23].

18.6 Radiographic Diagnostics

The principle detecting tool for MLL's is still clinical suspicion and clinical examination in trauma patients with pelvic fractures.

Several modalities are available for radiographically detecting and confirming MML's (Fig. 18.3). In all modalities, a variable imaging appearance is observed, often as an oval or fusiform cystic structure filled with fluid, and some internal complexity due to intralesional septa [15].

18.6.1 Ultrasound

Ultrasonographic is a non-specific modality and can show the following characteristics of Morel-Lavallée lesions [24]:

- Fluid collection between the deep fat and fascia [24].
- Variable appearance (more homogeneous and flat or fusiform) [24].
- Compressible [24], without flow on color Doppler [10].
- Most often hypoechoic than anechoic [24].
- More heterogeneous than homogeneous [24].
- Echogenic nodules [18, 25].

In the acute phase, within the first month after injury, a more heterogeneous echogenicity is observed, and the MLL presents with irregular margins and a lobular shape. In more chronic lesions, the fluid is more homogeneous and hypoechoic with smooth margins and flat or fusiform shape and a trend to pseudocapsules [10, 16, 24]. Mobile debris with no internal vascular flow can also be seen [10].

18.6.2 Magnetic Resonance Imaging (MRI)

MRI is referred to the diagnostic imaging modality of choice, due to its high contrast resolution, multiplanar acquisition, and presentage of greater anatomic details [15, 16].

Morel-Lavallée lesions present on MRI as hypo- or hyperintense lesions with low signal intensity relative to

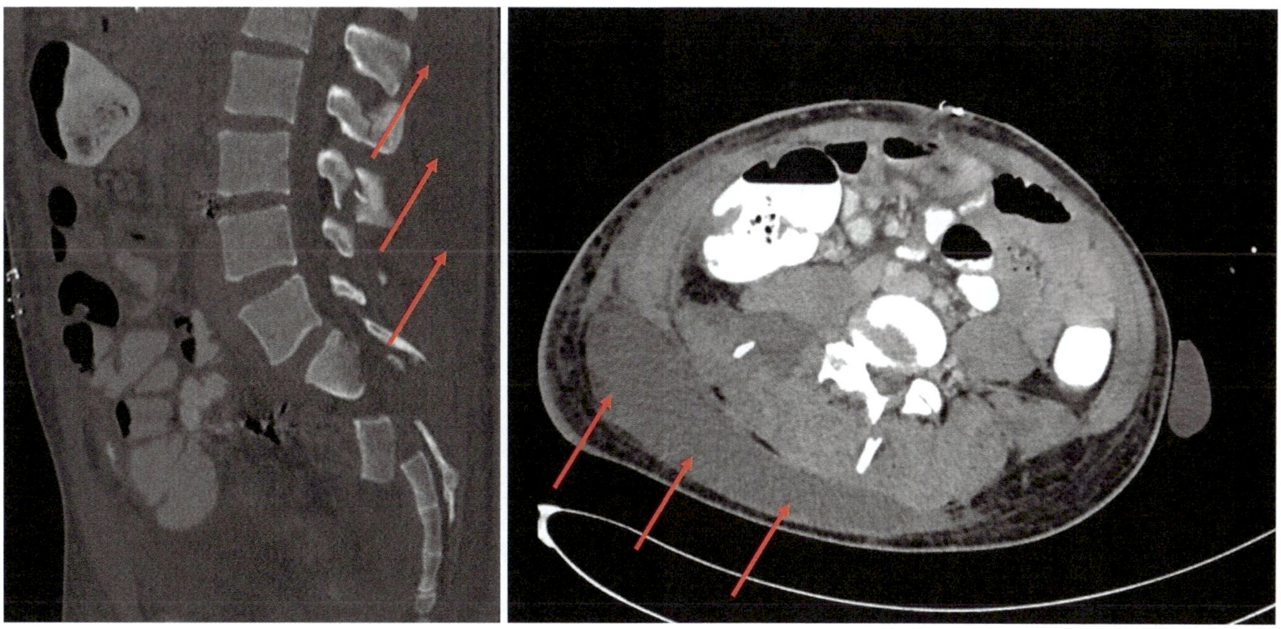

Fig. 18.3 CT diagnosis of an MLL after high-energy fall

muscle on T1-weighted sequences as a result of the presence of methemoglobin (subacute hematoma) and usually hyperintense, high signal intensity on T2-weighted sequences [16].

In the acute setting, blood or lymphatic MR signals are present, presenting with a heterogeneous signal intensity. The surrounding muscles and soft tissues can show edema formation (STIR sequences) [10, 15, 16].

With increasing re-absorption of the primary fluid contents, a more serosanguinous fluid, water-like MRI signal is observed [10].

Chronic lesion present with a hypointense fibrous capsule, sometimes with a pseudonodular appearance along the fascia [10, 15, 26].

18.6.3 Computed Tomography (CT)

Whole body CT with imaging of the pelvic region is usually performed in all patients sustaining significant trauma. An MLL is sometimes apparent on the preoperative CT scan [27]. Therefore, in the emergency setting of acute trauma, CT is the initial modality of choice [28].

McKenzie et al. distinguished acute, subacute, and chronic lesions using CT analysis [28].

- Acute: mostly hyperdense (30 Hounsfield units (HU)), 72% lenticular shape, no capsule, poorly/moderate marginated; 2/3 blood content, 28% blood and fluid; 28% internal fat globule or fat septation.
- Subacute: hypodense attenuation (16 HU); 71% lenticular, 29% oval shaped; 43% at least partial capsule; no capsular enhancement; content: 43% fluid, 29% blood/fluid; 28% add. Fat; 57% internal fat globule or fat septation.
- Chronic: 6HU attenuation; all with complete capsule with pseudocapsular enhancement.

18.7 Classification

Mellado and Bencardino tried to classify MML's (Fig. 18.4) [15]. Under immediate considerations, type I, II lesions are most relevant (Fig. 18.3):

- Type I: = seroma; homogeneous, hypointense on T1 weighted Image (T1WI) and hyperintense on T2 Weighted Images (T2W2), no presence of a capsule
- Type II: = subacute hematoma; homogeneous, hyperintense on both T1WI and T2WI (methemoglobin appearance)
- Type III: = chronic organizing hematoma; hypointense on T1WI and heterogeneous hypointense/isointense on T2WI with capsular formation; already capsular enhancement can be visible (=neovascularization and granulation tissue in organizing hematoma)
- Type IV: hypointense on T1WI and hyperintense on T2W2; no capsule
- Type V: perifascial pseudonodular lesion with variable T1 and T2 signal intensity

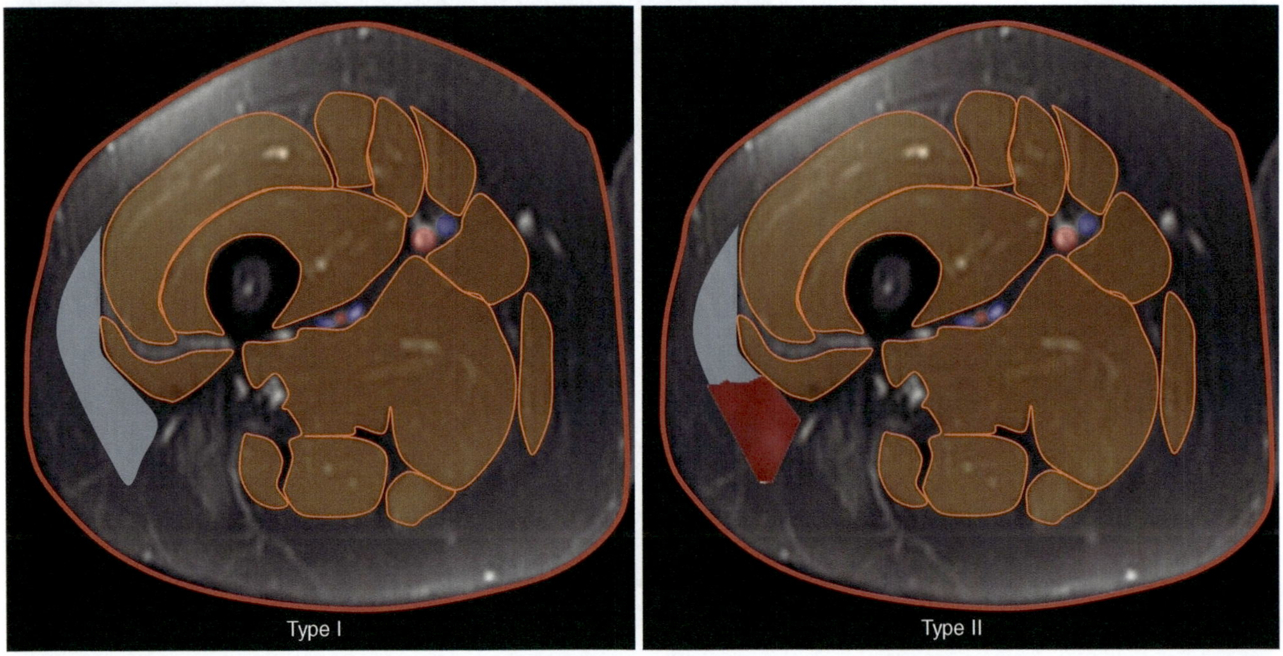

Fig. 18.4 Classification of MLL's according to Mellado and Bencardino

- Type VI: infected lesion; possible sinus tract formation, internal septations, thick enhancing capsule

Distinguishing acute from chronic lesions based on the presence or absence of a capsular formation is more practically.

18.8 Bacteriological Analysis

Hak et al. stated, that intraoperative bacteriological cultures were positive in 46%, independent of the time from injury to debridement, and three patients developed deep infections [3].

Typical bacteria, which will be found, include Staphylococcus aureus, Enterobacter, and Staphylococcus epidermidis [9], Staphylococcus Aureus, Enterobacter cloacae, Acinobacter baumannii, Pseudomonas aeruginosa, Escherichia coli [5].

18.9 Treatment

Letournel and Judet proposed early aspiration or decompression of these lesions [2]. Hudson et al. recommended hematoma evacuation through small incisions, wound irrigation, drainage, and compression banding, while in the presence of severe contour deformity, open wound treatment was favored [4]. A mean of 120 mL blood and necrotic fat was evacuated (15–800 mL).

Helfet and Schmeling supported the evacuation concept using a larger incision with primary closure or closure after 48 h [29]. Several adjuncts were proposed, including aspiration, injection of sclerosing agents (e.g., tetracycline), deep fascial fenestration, compression dressings, and prolonged closed surgical drainage [4, 11, 30, 31].

In general, debridement of all necrotic material is essential in each treatment concept to avoid infection. In delayed diagnosed lesions, >3 days post-injury, open debridement and dead space reduction with serial debridements, as necessary, is recommended [3, 11, 27, 29].

In 2013, Shen et al. analyzed the existing literature (21 articles) of Morel-Lavallée lesions with and without additional pelvic ring fractures in a systematic review [32]. Twelve articles, which include pelvic ring fractures, were part of this analysis [3, 5, 9, 33–41].

Surgical treatment was superior to conservative therapy. In patients with pelvic ring or acetabular fractures, either minimal invasive percutaneous procedures or open debridement with dead space closure technique are both sufficient, while in patients without additional fractures, sclerodesis should be considered. The formation of a fibrosis capsule influences the treatment decision.

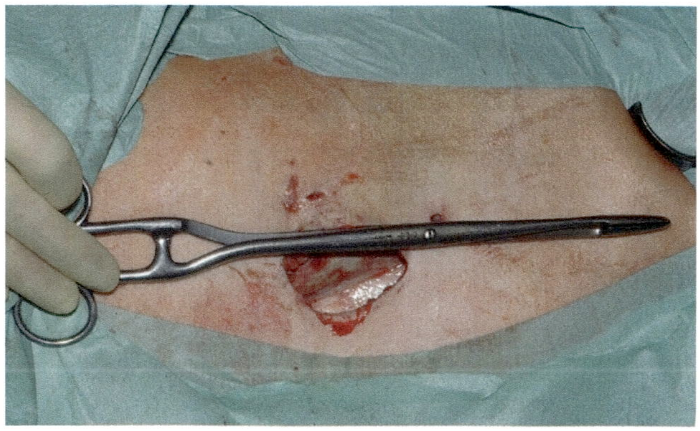

Fig. 18.5 Minimal invasive treatment of an MLL using a percutaneous approach

18.9.1 Minimal Invasive Procedures (Fig. 18.5)

Harma et al. proposed a conservative approach with compressive elastic bandages. Except for one patient with sacral decubitus ulcer due to delayed diagnosis, all lesions healed (loss of fluctuation and elicitation of the normal mobility of the injured skin) after an average of 6 weeks [35].

Tseng et al. reported on 19 patients with MLL's. Percutaneous debridement using 2–3 small 2 cm incisions at the proximal, distal, and posterior area of the lesion included hematoma evacuation, washing out and debridement of necrotic fat using a plastic brush and wound irrigation until the fluid presented clear [9]. Primary wound closure was performed after inserting a suction drainage. The inserted drain was removed, when drainage was <30 mL within 24 h, which was normally observed between 3–8 days. During drain presence, antibiotics were continued.

Zhong et al. used a percutaneous approach with several 2 cm incisions. Suction and irrigations were performed through these incisions. In some cases, a plastic brush supported debridement. All patients received intravenous antibiotics (cefuroxime). Drain removal was performed, when the drainage was <30 mL for a 24-h period [22].

Recently, endoscopic treatment was considered as an option with additional subcutaneous suturing for dead space closure [42].

18.9.2 Open Debridement (Fig. 18.6)

Hak et al. proposed open debridement of the degloved areas with an incision centrally above the degloved area to avoid skin necrosis [3], as the blood supply of the skin is from the dermal and subcutaneous vascular plexus after injury-related dissection of the perforating vessel [43]. Excessive subcutaneous fat debridement should be avoided for skin flap survival [3]. Wounds were not fully closed, even after already

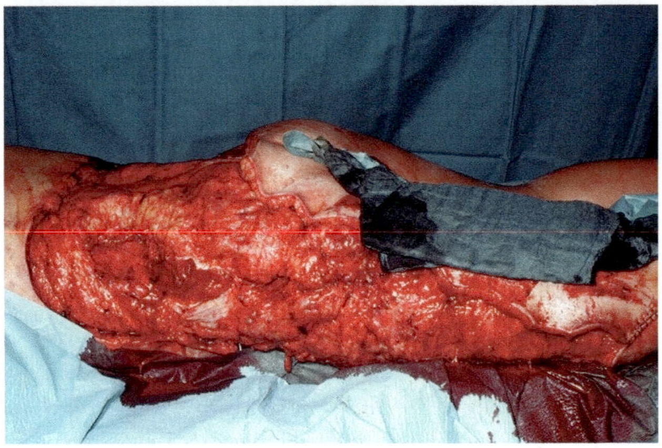

Fig. 18.6 Open debridement of a large MLL with secondary skin grafting

performed osteosynthesis (distal part of the Kocher-Langenbeck approach). Routine prophylactic antibiotics are administered, covering gram-positive organisms. Daily dressing changes are performed until adequate granulation tissue is visible, which is the basis for secondary wound closure.

Carlson et al. performed a longitudinal incision at the mid-portion of the lesion and the classical debridement is performed until healthy, bleeding surfaces were present, followed by approximation of the skin flaps to the fascia for dead space reduction [33]. Two possibilities for dead space reduction were described, depending on the size of the subcutaneous fat layer:

- In patients with a thick subcutaneous fat layer, fascial-fat-tissue absorbable sutures or fascio-dermal sutures were placed.
- In patients with less subcutaneous fat, fascio-cutaneous sutures are placed over dental bolsters.

Additional drains were placed into large spaces, which were typically removed after 2–5 days, when the fluid output was <30 mL/12 h. Prophylactic antibiotics (first generation cephalosporin) are recommended while the drains are in place.

Herscovici et al. introduced the concept of vacuum-assisted wound closure (VAC) in these severe soft-tissue injuries [44]. The historical recommendation to leave the wound open after debridement and hematoma evacuation to reduce the risk of a tissue necrosis was changed with increasing understanding of VAC treatments. VAC-therapy resulted in a high rate of uneventful healing [37].

The VAC-concept was presented in detail by Köhler et al. [36]. A central skin incision of 3–4 cm, directly above the lesion, was performed. After hematoma evacuation, the lesion size was identified using a large clamp and microbiological samples were taken. Definitive treatment was followed with full length incision, debridement, hemostasis, and extensive irrigation and insertion of a complete fitting V.A.C.® GranuFoam™ dressing by avoiding a tamponade effect.

Re-debridement were proposed every 48–72 h until the drainage was reduced to <30 mL/24 h. Definitive wound closure was performed over two large-lumen drains, when the wound was sterile. Optional, wound space narrowing was performed using subcutaneous sutures.

In chronic lesions (>3 weeks old) addition to the standard debridement, fascial debridement is essential [33]. As fluid output can be present for several weeks, the drains are let in place until drainage stops, which can be observed suddenly [33].

When planning ML-incisions, definitive treatment incisions should already be considered. Wei et al. observed no disadvantage, when ML lesions treatment was performed during osteosynthesis of the additional pelvic ring or acetabular injury [45]. Thus, debridements can be performed before or during osteosynthesis of the pelvic ring or acetabular injury [2, 3, 46].

> The majority of surgeons favor a more open approach with extensive debridement of Morel-Lavallée lesions, even during primary osteosynthesis.

18.9.3 Optional Adjuncts

Sclerodesis is especially an option in delayed or chronic lesions. Several promising reports are published.

Demirel et al., proposed surgical drainage, soft tissues reattachment with a synthetic glue, followed by compressive bandage and reported unaffected healing within 5 weeks [34].

Isaacson et al. presented a case with successful alcohol sclerodesis of an ML lesion after percutaneous debridement. 10 mL of dehydrated alcohol was injected and left in place for 10 min before fluid aspiration was performed and a drain was inserted [47].

Penaud et al. successfully treated 5 patients with this concept. The effect of alcohol injection is proposed to result in tissue necrosis due to protein coagulation, hyperosmolar cell destruction, and some antibactericidal effects [48].

Bansal et al. recommended Doxycycline sclerodesis in chronic ML lesions and reported on overall successful results in 16 patients [49].

Nickerson et al. presented their experience from the Mayo clinic on 79 patients with lesion of different locations [50]. Approximately 40% of all lesions with an underlying fracture of the thigh, hip, and/or flank showed recurrence of the lesion. Interestingly, operative and non-operative treatments showed no significant differences, but no detailed analysis was integrated regarding localization of these lesions.

Isolated aspiration was associated with a 59% recurrence rate compared to 19% and 15% after non-operative and operative treatments, respectively. Aspiration >50 mL was an identified risk factor. Thus, operative treatment should then be considered.

18.10 Risk Factors

Some risk factors for MLL's were reported.

MLL's are frequently observed after motorcycle collisions and motor vehicle accidents [6].

Carlson et al. reported on a BMI ≥ 25 as a risk factor [6, 33].

Special fracture types were identified as potential risk factors. Spino-pelvic dissociation injuries [6, 51] and vertical shear injuries were more often associated with MLL's compared to lateral compression and AP compression patterns [6].

> In pelvic and acetabular fractures, early diagnosed lesions (<2 days) can sufficiently be treated using a percutaneous approach with accompanying fracture stabilization. Open debridement is proposed for lesions diagnosed after 2 days [52].

References

1. Morel-Lavallee. Decollements traumatiques de la peau et des couches sous-jacentes. Arch Gen Med. 1863;1:20–38, 172–200, 300–332.
2. Letournel E, Judet R. Fractures of the acetabulum. 2nd ed. Berlin, Germany: Springer-Verlag; 1993.
3. Hak D, Olson S, Matta J. Diagnosis and management of closed internal degloving injuries associated with pelvic and acetabular fractures: the Morel-Lavallee lesion. J Trauma. 1997;42:1046–51.
4. Hudson D, Knottenbelt J, Krige J. Closed degloving injuries: results following conservative surgery. Plast Reconstr Surg. 1992;89:863–55.
5. Steiner C, Trentz O, Labler L. Management of Morel-Lavallee lesion associated with pelvic and/or acetabular fractures. Eur J Trauma Emerg Surg. 2008;34:554–60.
6. Beckmann N, Cai C. CT incidence of Morel-Lavallee lesions in patients with pelvic fractures: a 4-year experience at a level 1 trauma center. Emerg Radiol. 2016;23:615–21.
7. Tresley J, Jose J, Saraf-Lavi E, Sklar E. Sacral Morel-Lavallée Lesion: a not-so-rare diagnosis. Neuroradiol J. 2014;27:755–8.
8. Vanhegan I, Dala-Ali B, Verhelst L, Mallucci P, Haddad F. The Morel-Lavallee lesion as a rare differential diagnosis for recalcitrant bursitis of the knee: case report and literature review. Case Rep Orthop. 2012;593:193.
9. Tseng S, Tornetta P III. Percutaneous management of Morel-Lavallee Lesions. J Bone Joint Surg Am. 2006;88:92–6.
10. McLean K, Popovic S. Morel-Lavallée lesion: AIRP best cases in radiologic-pathologic correlation. Radiographics. 2017;37:190–6.
11. Kottmeier S, Wilson S, Born C, Hanks G, Innacone W, DeLong W. Surgical management of soft tissue lesions associated with pelvic ring injury. Clin Orthop Relat Res. 1996;329:446–53.
12. Bonilla-Yoon I, Masih S, Patel D, White E, Levine B, Chow K, Gottsegen C, Matcuk GJ. The Morel-Lavallée lesion: pathophysiology, clinical presentation, imaging features, and treatment options. Emerg Radiol. 2014;21:35–43.
13. Moriarty J, Borrero C, Kavanagh E. A rare cause of calf swelling: the Morel-Lavallee lesion. Ir J Med Sci. 2011;180:265–8.
14. Kalaci A, Karazincir S, Yanat A. Long-standing Morel-Lavallée lesion of the thigh simulating a neoplasm. Clin Imaging. 2007;31:287–91.
15. Mellado J, Bencardino J. Morel-Lavallee lesion: review with emphasis on MR imaging. Magn Reson Imaging Clin N Am. 2005;13:775–82.
16. Mellado J, Perez del Palomar L, Diaz L, Ramos A, Sauri A. Long-standing Morel-Lavallee lesions of the trochanteric region and proximal thigh: MRI features in five patients. AJR Am J Roentgenol. 2004;182:1289–94.
17. Nair A, Nazar P, Sekhar R, Ramachandran P, Moorthy S. Morel-Lavallée lesion: a closed degloving injury that requires real attention. Indian J Radiol Imaging. 2014;24:288–90.
18. Parra J, Fernandez M, Encinas B, Rico M. Morel-Lavallee effusions in the thigh. Skelet Radiol. 1997;26:239–41.
19. Routt M, Simonian P, Ballmer F. A rational approach to pelvic trauma—resuscitation and early definitive stabilization. Clin Orthop. 1995;318:61–74.
20. Letts R. Degloving injuries in children. J Pediatr Orthop. 1986;6:93–7.
21. Tsur A, Galin A, Kogan L, Loberant N. Morel-Lavallee syndrome after crush injury. Harefuah. 2006;145:111–3.
22. Zhong B, Zhang C, Luo C. Percutaneous drainage of Morel-Lavallée lesions when the diagnosis is delayed. Can J Surg. 2014;57:356–7.
23. Diviti S, Gupta N, Hooda K, Sharma K, Lo L. Morel-Lavallee lesions-review of pathophysiology, clinical findings, imaging findings and management. J Clin Diagn Res. 2017;11:TE01–4.
24. Neal C, Jacobson J, Brandon C, Kalume-Brigido M, Morag Y, Girish G. Sonography of Morel-Lavallée lesions. J Ultrasound Med. 2008;27:1077–81.
25. Mukherjee K, Perrin S, Hughes P. Morel-Lavallee lesion in an adolescent with ultrasound and MRI correlation. Skelet Radiol. 2007;36(Suppl 1):S43–5.
26. Robertson N, Anwar I, Nayagam K, Katz R, Farrant J, Holloway B, Marmnery H. Imaging characteristics of the Morel Lavallee Lesion. Poster No. P-0100. ESSR: EPOS; 2014.
27. Collinge C, Tornetta P III. Soft tissue injuries associated with pelvic fractures. Orthop Clin North Am. 2004;35:451–6.
28. McKenzie G, Niederhauser B, Collins M, Howe B. CT characteristics of Morel-Lavallée lesions: an under-recognized but significant finding in acute trauma imaging. Skelet Radiol. 2016;45:1053–60.
29. Helfet D, Schmeling G. Chapter: complications. In: Tile M, editor. Fractures of the pelvis and acetabulum. 2nd ed. Baltimore, MD: Williams and Wilkins; 1995. p. 451–67.
30. Helfet D, Schmeling G, Kudsk K, Sheldon G, Walton R. Degloving injuries of the extremities and torso. J Trauma. 1981;21:835–9.

31. Matta J. Surgical treatment of acetabular fractures. In: Browner BD, Jupiter JB, Levine AM, Trafton PG, editors. Skeletal trauma. Philadelphia, PA: WB Saunders; 1992. p. 899–922.
32. Shen C, Peng J, Chen X. Efficacy of treatment in peri-pelvic Morel–Lavallee lesion: a systematic review of the literature. Arch Orthop Trauma Surg. 2013;133:635–40.
33. Carlson D, Simmons J, Sando W, Wber T, Clements B. Morel-Lavale'e lesions treated with debridement and meticulous dead space closure: surgical technique. J Orthop Trauma. 2007;21:140–4.
34. Demirel M, Dereboy F, Ozturk A, Turhan E, Yazar T. Morel-Lavallee lesion. Results of surgical drainage with the use of synthetic glue. Saudi Med J. 2007;28:65–7.
35. Harma A, Inan M, Ertem K. The Morel-Lavallée lesion: a conservative approach to closed degloving injuries. Acta Orthop Traumatol Turc. 2004;38:270–3.
36. Köhler D, Pohlemann T. Perative Therapie der peripelvinen Morel-Lavallée-Läsion. Orthop Traumatol. 2011;23:15–20.
37. Labler L, Trentz O. The use of vacuum assisted closure (VAC™) in soft tissue injuries after high energy pelvic trauma. Langenbecks Arch Chir. 2007;392:601–9.
38. Luria S, Applbaum Y, Weil Y, Liebergall M, Peyser A. Talc sclerodhesis of persistent Morel-Lavallee lesions (posttraumatic pseudocysts): case report of 4 patients. J Orthop Trauma. 2006;20:435–8.
39. Phillips T, Jeffcote B, Collopy D. Bilateral Morel-Lavallee lesions after complex pelvic trauma: a case report. J Trauma. 2008;65:708–11.
40. Suzuki T, Hak D, Ziran B, Adams S, Stahel P, Morgan S, Smith W. Outcome and complications of posterior transiliac plating for vertically unstable sacral fractures. Injury. 2009;40:405–9.
41. Tran W, Foran J, Wang M, Schwartz A. Postsurgical bleeding following treatment of a chronic Morel-Lavallee lesion. Orthopedics. 2008;31:814.
42. Kim S. Endoscopic treatment of Morel-Lavallee lesion. Injury. 2016;47:1064–6.
43. Cormack G, Lamberty B. The blood supply of the thigh skin. Plast Reconstr Surg. 1985;75:342–54.
44. Herscovici DJ, Sanders R, Scaduto J, Infante A, DiPasquale T. Vacuum-assisted wound closure (VAC therapy) for the management of patients with high-energy soft tissue injuries. J Orthop Trauma. 2003;17:683–8.
45. Wei D, Wang Y, Yuan J, Tang X, Zhang B, Lu B, Tan B. One-stage operation for pelvis and acetabular fractures combined with Morel-Lavallée injury by internal fixation associated with vacuum sealing drainage. [Article in Chinese]. Zhongguo Xiu Fu Chong Jian Wai Ke Za Zhi. 2014;28:38–42.
46. Helfet D, Schmeling G. Management of complex acetabular fractures through single non-extensile exposures. Clin Orthop Relat Res. 1994;305:58–68.
47. IIsaacson A, Stavas J. Image-guided drainage and sclerodesis of a Morel-Lavallee lesion. J Vasc Interv Radiol. 2013;24:605–6.
48. Penaud A, Quignon R, Danin A, Bahé L, Zakine G. Alcohol sclerodhesis: an innovative treatment for chronic Morel-Lavalle'e lesions. J Plast Reconstr Aesthet Surg. 2011;64:e262–4.
49. Bansal A, Bhatia N, Singh A, Kumar Singh A. Doxycycline sclerodesis as a treatment option for persistent Morel-Lavalle'e lesions. Injury. 2013;44:66–9.
50. Nickerson T, Zielinski M, Jenkins D, Schiller H. The Mayo Clinic experience with Morel-Lavallée lesions: establishment of a practice management guideline. J Trauma Acute Care Surg. 2014;76:493–7.
51. Dodwad S, Niedermeier S, Yu E, Ferguson T, Klineberg E, Khan S. The Morel-Lavallée lesion revisited: management in spinopelvic dissociation. Spine J. 2015;15:e45–51.
52. Becker C, Kammerlander C, Greiner A, Sommer F, Linhart C, Böcker W, Rubenbauer B, Weidert S. Diagnostic and treatment strategies in Morel-Lavallee lesions in the spinal column and pelvis. Z Orthop Unfall. 2018;156(5):541–6.

Pelvic Compartment Syndrome

19

Axel Gänsslen and Stephan Grechenig

The significance of the pelvic compartment syndrome is based on the potential ischemic nerve damage of mainly the sciatic and the femoral nerves (while the obturator nerve is infrequently involved) and ischemic large muscle involvement after pelvic (crush) injuries [1, 2].

The true incidence of fracture-related pelvic compartment syndromes is unknown, as only case reports were published. An injury to the pelvis rarely results in a compartment syndrome, since after high-energy trauma to the pelvis, severe displacement results in rupture of all relevant "compartment boundaries". Significant soft tissue damage, however, can lead to large hematomas and swelling of the entire pelvic region [3].

Traumatic gluteal compartment syndrome accounts for 20% of all pelvic compartment syndromes [4]. Gluteal vessel injury associated with pelvic fracture is one of the reasons [5]. Immediate complications can include infection, acute renal failure, and even death, while only 50% of patients showed full recovery [6].

In a systematic review of traumatic compartment syndromes, based on the definition by Hessmann et al. (ureteral obstruction, intrapelvic pressure increase), non-traumatic cases also were included [7]. Thus the incidence remains still unclear.

A. Gänsslen (✉)
Department of Trauma Surgery, Orthopedics and Hand Surgery, Hospital Wolfsburg, Wolfsburg, Germany

S. Grechenig
Department of Orthopedics and Trauma Surgery, AUVA Trauma Hospital Klagenfurt, Klagenfurt, Austria

Department of Trauma Surgery, University Hospital Regensburg, Regensburg, Germany

19.1 Definition

The pelvic compartment syndrome shows an increased intracompartmental pressure in peripelvic muscles above a critical level in one or more of the pelvic muscular compartments.

Additionally, anuria, with resulting renal organ failure, due to ureteral compression is described as an intrapelvic compartment syndrome [8–11].

19.2 Anatomy

Several compartments are present in the peripelvic area. The main muscular compartments include the

- Iliopsoas compartment
- Gluteus medius and minimus compartments
- Gluteus maximus compartment
- Tensor fasciae latae compartment

Additionally, anuria, with resulting renal organ failure, due to ureteral compression is described as an intrapelvic compartment syndrome of the true pelvis after significant bleeding to the intrapelvic vasculature [9].

19.2.1 Iliopsoas Compartment

The extraperitoneal iliopsoas compartment (Fig. 19.1) is surrounded by the iliopsoas fascia and includes three muscles [12, 13], which function as flexors of the thigh and the trunk:

- Greater psoas muscle: originates from the transverse process of T12 and the lumbar vertebrae, merging with the iliac muscle at the level of L5-S2
- Smaller psoas muscle: anterior to the psoas major muscle: arises from the T12-L1 vertebral bodies, inserting with along and flat tendon at the iliopectineal eminence

A. Gänsslen et al. (eds.), *Pelvic Ring Fractures*, https://doi.org/10.1007/978-3-030-54730-1_19

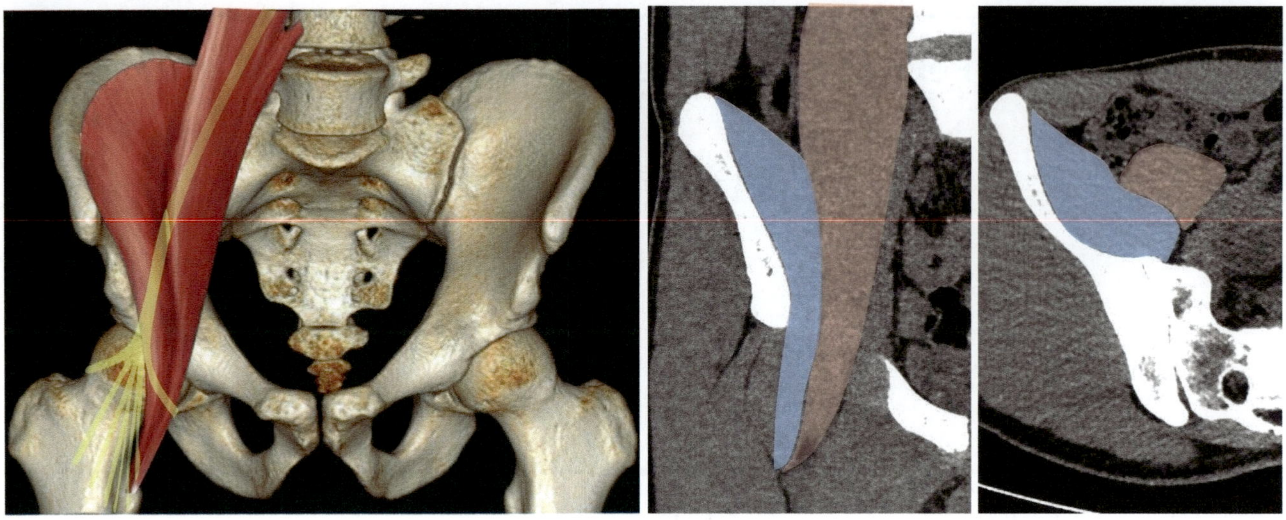

Fig. 19.1 Iliopsoas compartment with the femoral nerve (iliacus muscle (blue), psoas major muscle (red))

- Iliacus muscle: arises from the iliac wing and fossa

The resulting iliopsoas muscle inserts with a thick tendon at the lesser trochanter of the femur [14]. The anterior fascia corresponds to the thickened abdominal transversalis fascia.

The femoral nerve courses obliquely through the greater psoas muscle to its lateral border [15, 16] to further run between the greater psoas and iliac muscles, leaving the pelvis through the lacuna musculorum to the anterior thigh.

The blood supply of the femoral nerve is physiologically impaired between these muscles [17], which can result in ischemic damage with paralysis of the quadriceps femoris muscle and corresponding sensoric deficits at the distal, anterior thigh and the anterior-medial region of the lower leg [15, 16]. Even the saphenus nerve can be affected.

The obturator nerve runs along the medial greater psoas muscle, where it penetrates the fascia to leave the pelvis through the obturator canal.

CT evaluation can show hyperdense muscular enlargement and potential active bleeding [12, 13].

19.2.2 Gluteus Medius and Minimus Compartment

The gluteus medius and minimus compartment presents with its medial border, consisting of the outer ilium and its lateral fascial border to the gluteus maximus fascia (Fig. 19.2). The additional gluteus maximus compartment posteriorly and the tensor fasciae latae compartment anteriorly is present.

Muscle ischemia and compartment pressure elevation can result in sciatic nerve damage and damage to the gluteal nerves.

19.2.3 Gluteus Maximus Compartment (Fig. 19.3)

The gluteus maximus arises from the outer iliac surface and the posterior iliac crest to insert at the posterior-medial proximal femur with a broad tendon. Pressure elevation in this compartment can lead to muscle necrosis and lesions to the posterior cutaneous femoral clunii inferior nerves. Close to both gluteal compartments, the sciatic nerve leaves the pelvis through the greater sciatic notch and through the piriformis muscle to run below the inferior gluteus maximus border between the hamstrings.

19.2.4 Tensor Fasciae Latae Compartment (Fig. 19.4)

The tensor fasciae latae compartment includes only this muscle. A chronic compartment is described in the literature [18], while traumatic compartment syndrome is unusual.

19.2.5 Intrapelvic Compartment

There is no exact osteofascial compartment integrating the true pelvis and thus the retroperitoneal space.

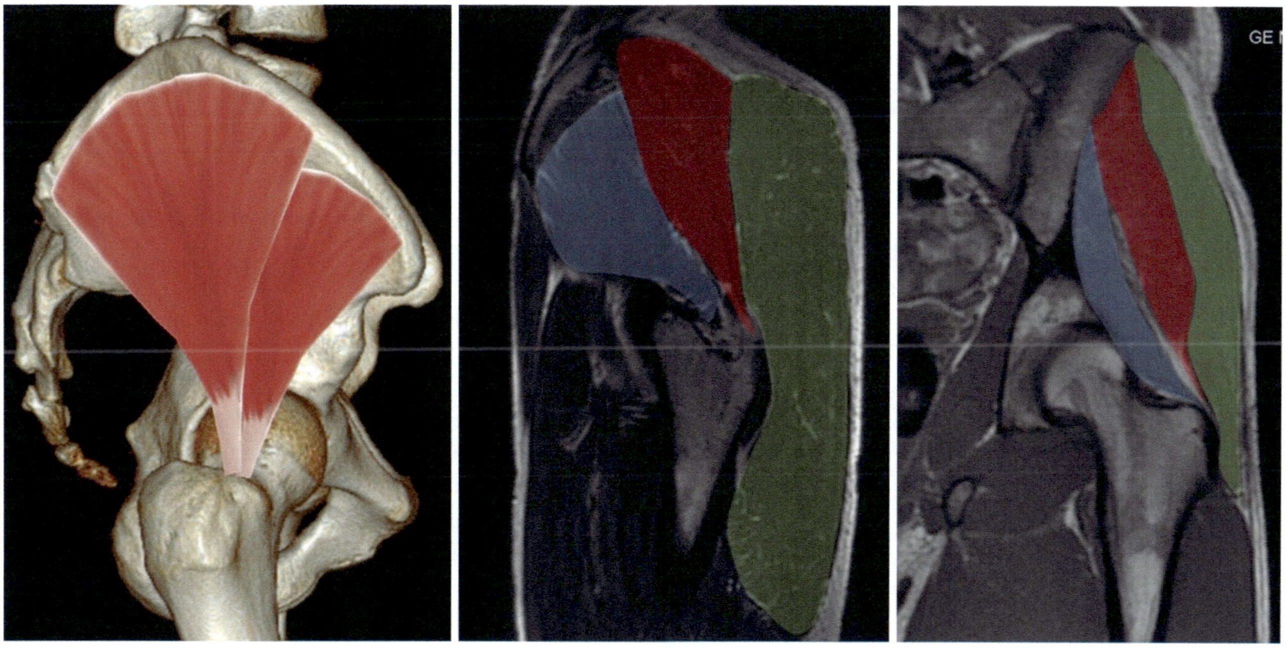

Fig. 19.2 Gluteus medius/minimus compartment: gluteus minimus (blue), gluteus medius (red), and gluteus maximus (green)

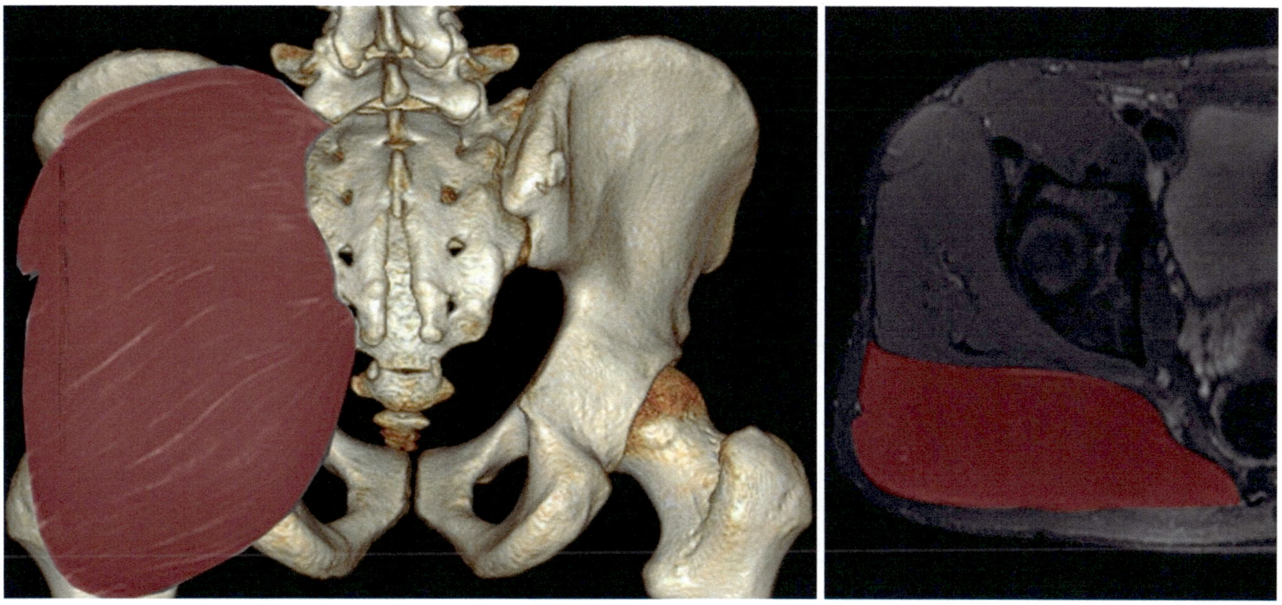

Fig. 19.3 Gluteus maximus compartment

Bleeding within the true pelvis from the extended venous perivisceral plexus can lead to relevant retroperitoneal bleeding (Fig. 19.5). In unstable pelvic fractures, a complete disruption of the retroperitoneal muscle compartments can be present [19], which can lead to uncontrolled hemorrhage creeping cranially above the psoas muscle or along the gluteal muscles, with the risk of exsanguination or pelvic and abdominal compartment syndromes [20]. This phenomenon was therefore called "chimney effect" [21]. Clinically, these injuries can

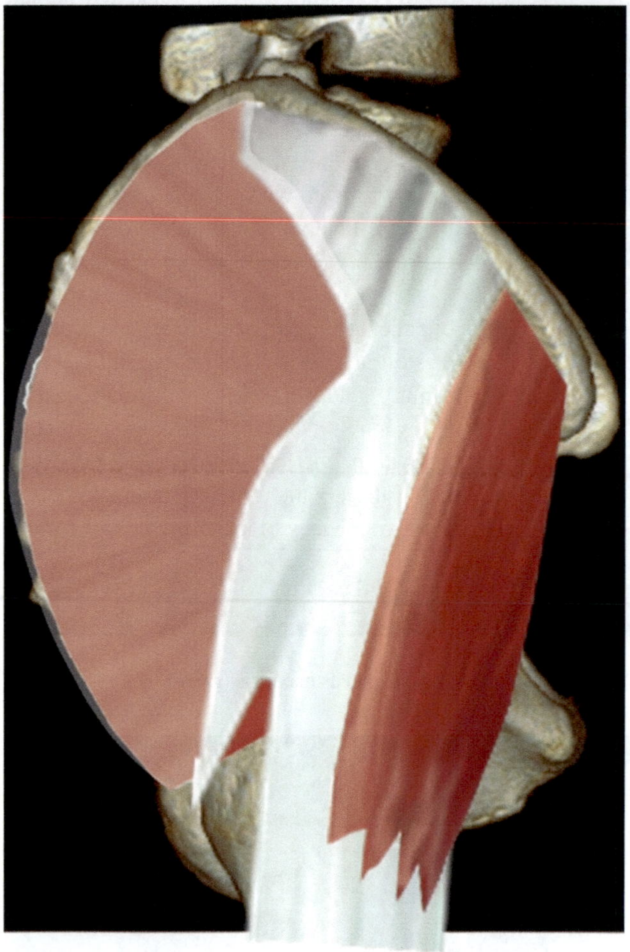

Fig. 19.4 Tensor fasciae latae compartment

mimic abdominal injuries, as the retroperitoneum is not a closed space.

Therefore, a self-limiting, pressure-induced tamponade cannot be expected [19, 22].

19.2.6 Abdominal Compartment Syndrome (ACS)

Retroperitoneal bleeding and the consequences of resulting shock can lead to an additional abdominal compartment syndrome.

An ACS is defined as an intra-abdominal pressure (IAP) increase >20 mmHg (with or without an abdominal perfusion pressure (mean arterial pressure—IAP) <60 mmHg) associated with a new organ dysfunction/failure of the kidney, gut, lung, liver, heart system, or CNS [23]. It can be combined with a significant pressure increase in the thoracic compartment, called polycompartment syndrome [23].

19.3 Diagnostic Signs

In addition to typical subjective clinical symptoms, such as pain out of proportion to the injury, muscle weakness, palpable increased compartment pressure, and hardening of the affected muscles, subfascial tissue pressure measurement is the most important aid for detection of gluteal, tensor fasciae latae and some iliopsoas compartment syndromes.

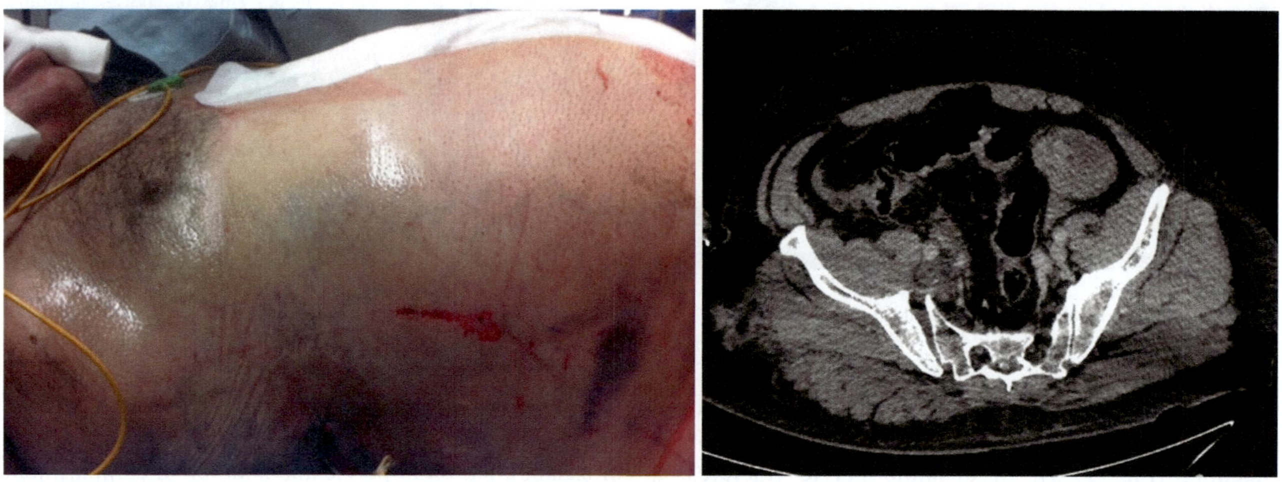

Fig. 19.5 Intrapelvic compartment: significant right intrapelvic hematoma formation

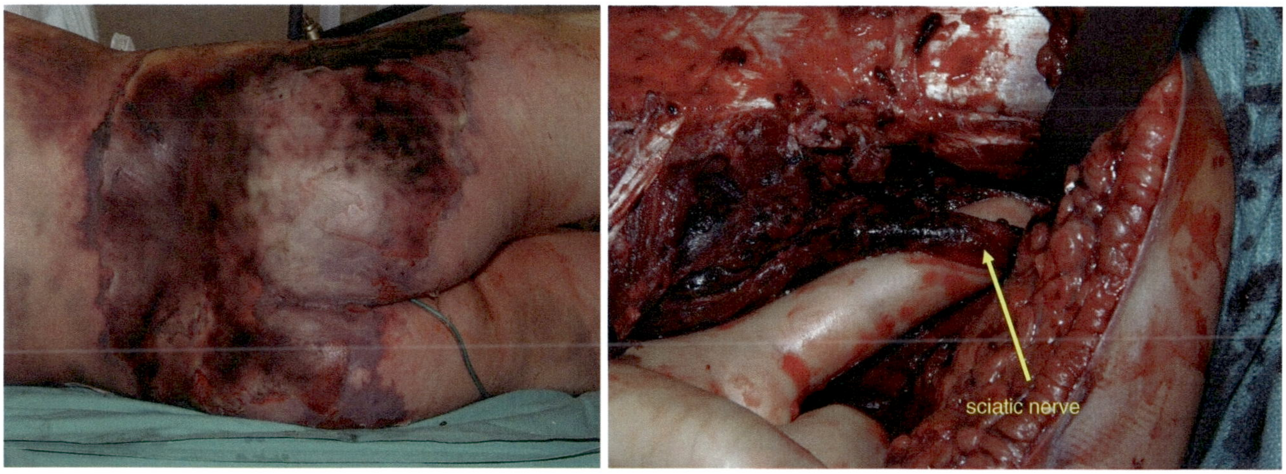

Fig. 19.6 Gluteus maximus compartment after roll-over mechanism with an additional Morel-Lavallée lesion: the sciatic nerve found in the operative field

In a systematic literature review of gluteal compartment syndromes, nearly half were diagnosed measuring compartmental pressures, the others by clinical examination (Fig. 19.6) [4].

The iliopsoas compartment can also be analyzed by ultrasound and better by pelvic CT, which typically shows muscle swelling, hematoma formation, or even contrast media blush.

Admission laboratory should include creatine phosphokinase (CPK) and lactate dehydrogenase (LDH). Increased levels suggest muscle death and tissue damage [24] and are indirect signs of a compartment syndrome.

19.4 Treatment

Early and aggressive dermatofasciotomy is clearly indicated in traumatic pelvic compartment syndrome [15, 16]:

- Gluteal compartment syndrome: depending on the localization of the main injury site, the Kocher-Langenbeck approach is favored; alternatively, the modified Gibson approach can be used; an additional incision parallel to the iliac crest can be considered [15]; it is crucial to also open the gluteus medius and minimus fascia; a systematic review reported 71% fasciotomies and 29% conservative treatment [4]; relevant surgical steps include [3]:
  - Complete evacuation of the gluteal hematoma,
  - Identification and control of the source of bleeding,
  - Complete fasciotomy of all gluteal muscles, usually with epimysiotomy,
  - Careful debridement of already necrotic tissues.
- Iliopsoas compartment: an extraperitoneal approach can be used [25] or, in bilateral compartment syndromes, a transperitoneal approach is recommended [15]; the anterolateral approach to the iliac fossa is favored [26], with an extraperitoneal dissection of the psoas fascia.
- Tensor fasciae latae compartment: this compartment can be approached using part of the Smith-Peterson approach, which, additionally, can release the tension within the iliacus compartment.
- Intrapelvic/retroperitoneal compartment: early surgical evacuation of hematomas, vascular revision, ureteral decompression, and/or temporary nephrostomy [27], while isolated nephrostomy was considered inferior for restoration of renal function [28].

Depending on the extent of wound retraction, vacuum-assisted closure techniques can be used until complete wound closure is possible.

19.5 Pelvic Fracture-Associated Compartment Syndrome

Bosch et al. described two cases with a gluteal pelvic compartment treated conservatively and surgically syndrome [15, 16].

Ureteral obstruction due to massive intra- and retroperitoneal hematoma after pelvic ring or acetabular fractures was reported in several cases [8, 10, 11, 28].

Hessmann et al. reported three cases with bilateral ureteral obstruction, resulting in anuria with renal organ failure [9, 28]. It was stated, that ureteral compression becomes clinically relevant often earliest after 24–48 h and can thus be distinguished from shock-related anuria [27, 28]. In these cases, fracture stabilization and retroperitoneal hematoma evacuation with ureteral decompression is recommended [27–29].

The primary location of the obstruction occurs usually close to the insertion of the ureter into the bladder wall due to hematoma-induced ureteral kinking or intramural [28]. An additional abdominal compartment syndrome has to be considered [7].

Diaz Dilernia et al., reported on a 70-year-old man sustaining an anterior-posterior compression pelvic injury type C1.2 after being run over by a truck, who presented after secondary transfer (emergency treatment consisted of standard external fixation) with local pelvic swelling, scrotal hematoma and senso-motoric deficits consistent with sciatic nerve palsy. A high intra-compartmental pressure of 46 mmHg was measured in the gluteus maximus compartment. Additionally, acute kidney failure with anuria developed. Immediate fasciotomy of all three gluteal muscles was performed with vacuum-assisted wound closure. The sciatic nerve palsy persisted at 1-year follow-up [24].

Songur et al. presented a 21-year-old male patient after a fall from 2 m height with a C-type pelvic ring injury. Within 2 h, he developed gluteal compartment syndrome, which was treated by emergency fasciotomy with evacuation of 800 mL hematoma. Ongoing hemodynamic instability led to further diagnostics, which identified a superior gluteal artery disruption as the cause of bleeding. Unselected angiography was successful for hemodynamic stabilization [5].

An accompanying ACS should be treated immediately by decompression laparotomy in combination with a balanced volume resuscitation using crystalloid, colloid, vasoactive medications, while avoiding excessive fluid resuscitation [23, 30].

Summary

Pelvic compartment syndrome is a rare entity and most commonly involves the gluteal muscular compartment.

Anuria with resulting renal organ failure, due to ureteral compression is considered an intrapelvic compartment syndrome, which has to be distinguished from abdominal compartment syndrome.

Early fasciotomy, hematoma evacuation, vascular revision, retroperitoneal decompression and/or ureteral decompression are indicated.

References

1. Neal W, Schmalzried T, Eckardt J. Diagnosis and treatment of buttock compartment syndromes. In: American Academy of Orthopaedic Surgeons (Hrsg) 56th Annual Meeting of American Academy of Orthopaedic Surgeons, Las Vegas. February 9–14, 1989, p. 130.
2. Szyszkowitz R, Reschauer R. Ätiologie, pathophysiologie und lokalisation des kompartment-syndroms. Unfallheilkunde. 1982;85:126.
3. Pohlemann T, Regel G, Bosch U, Stief C, Tscherne H. Chapter 1.7: Notfallbehandlung und Komplextrauma. In: Tscherne H, Pohlemann T, editors. Tscherne Unfallchirurgie: Becken und Acetabulum. Berlin, Heidelberg, New York: Springer; 1998. p. 89–116.
4. Henson J, Roberts C, Giannoudis P. Gluteal compartment syndrome. Acta Orthop Belg. 2009;75:147–52.
5. Songur M, Şahin E, Zehir S, Oz I, Kalem M. Gluteal compartment syndrome secondary to superior gluteal artery injury following pelvis fracture: a case report and review of literature. Turk J Emerg Med. 2016;16:29–31.
6. MacLean J, Wustrack R, Kandemir U. Compartment syndrome of thigh. Tech Orthop. 2012;27:47–52.
7. Ojike N, Roberts C, Giannoudis P. Pelvic compartment syndrome: a systematic review. Ata Orthop Belg. 2012;78:6–10.
8. Flint P, Allen C. Pelvic fracture complicated by bilateral ureteral obstruction: case report. J Trauma. 1994;36:285–7.
9. Hessmann M, Rommens P. Does the intrapelvic compartment syndrome exist? Acta Chir Belg. 1998;98(1):18–22.
10. Nihal A, Fairbank A, Palmer S, Bircher M. Acute bilateral ureteric obstruction complicating pelvic fractures. Injury. 1994;25(5):328–30.
11. Rothenberger D, Fischer R, Strate R, Velasco R, Perry J. The mortality associated with pelvic fractures. Surgery. 1978;84(3):356–9.
12. Muttarak M, Peh W. CT of unusual iliopsoas compartment lesions. Radiographics. 2000;20:S53–60.
13. Torres G, Cernigliaro J, Abbitt P, Mergo P, Hellein V, Fernandez S, Ros P. Iliopsoas compartment: normal anatomy and pathologic processes. Radiographics. 1995;15:1285–97.
14. Van Dyke J, Hollev H, Anderson S. Review of the iliopsoas anatomy and pathology. Radiographics. 1987;7:53–85.
15. Bosch U. Das Kompartmentsyndrom am Becken. Unfallchirurg. 1991;94:244–8.
16. Bosch U, Tscherne H. The pelvic compartment syndrome. Arch Orthop Trauma Surg. 1992;111(6):314–7.
17. Young M, Norris J. Femoral neuropathy during anticoagulant therapy. Neurology. 1976;26:1173–5.
18. Rydholm U, Brun A, Ekelund L, Rydholm A. Chronic compartmental syndrome in the tensor fasciae latae muscle. Clin Orthop Relat Res. 1983;177:169–71.
19. Grimm M, Vrahas M, Thomas K. Pressure-volume characteristics of the intact and disrupted pelvic retroperitoneum. J Trauma. 1998;44(3):454–9.
20. Gänsslen A, Giannoudis P, Pape H. Hemorrhage in pelvic fracture: who needs angiography? Curr Opin Crit Care. 2003;9:515–23.
21. Trentz O, Bühren V, Friedl H. Beckenverletzungen Chirurg. 1989;60:639–48.
22. Downs A, Dhalla S. Hemorrhage and pelvic fractures. Can J Surg. 1988;31(2):89–90.
23. Kirkpatrick A, Roberts D, De Waele J, Jaeschke R, Malbrain M, De Keulenaer B, Duchesne J, Bjorck M, Leppaniemi A, Ejike J, Sugrue M, Cheatham M, Ivatury R, Ball C, Reintam Blaser A, Regli A, Balogh Z, D'Amours S, Debergh D, Kaplan M, Kimball E, Olvera C, The Pediatric Guidelines Sub-Committee for the World Society of the Abdominal Compartment Syndrome. Intra-abdominal hypertension and the abdominal compartment syndrome: updated consensus definitions and clinical practice guidelines from the World

Society of the Abdominal Compartment Syndrome. Intensive Care Med. 2013;39:1190–206.
24. Diaz Dilernia F, Zaidenberg E, Gamsie S, Taype Zamboni D, Carabelli G, Barla J, Sancineto C. Gluteal compartment syndrome secondary to pelvic trauma case. Rep Orthop. 2016;2016:2780295. https://doi.org/10.1155/2016/2780295.
25. Al-Zamil A, Christenson J. Psoas muscle hematoma—an acute compartment syndrome. Vasa. 1988;17:4.
26. Riska E, Vin Bonsdorff H, Hakkinen S, Jaroma H, Kiviluato O, Paavilainen T. Operative control of massive haemorrhage in comminuted pelvic fractures. Int Orthop. 1979;3:141–4.
27. Michek J, Zelnícek P, Vrastyák J, Kubacák J, Wendsche P, Filipinský J, Sutorý M. Does a pelvic compartment exist? Personal experience. Rozhl Chir. 2000;79:568–70.
28. Hessmann M, Rommens P. Bilateral ureteral obstruction and renal failure caused by massive retroperitoneal hematoma: is there a pelvic compartment syndrome analogous to abdominal compartment syndrome? J Orthop Trauma. 1998;12(8):553–7.
29. Malbrain M, De Laet I. A new concept: the polycompartment syndrome—Part 2. Int J Intens Care. 2009;16:24–31.
30. Roberts D, Ball C, Kirkpatrick A. Increased pressure within the abdominal compartment: intra-abdominal hypertension and the abdominal compartment syndrome. Curr Opin Crit Care. 2016;22:174–85.

20 Traumatic Hemipelvectomy

Bore Bakota, Mario Staresinic, and Axel Gänsslen

With ongoing improvements of the prehospital care, an increasing number of severely injured patients survive their injury and are transferred from the scene into the hospital.

One of the worst injuries in the pelvic area is the Traumatic Hemipelvectomy (TH). The TH is a rare, however, life-threatening injury.

Thus, TH is associated with a high mortality. Theodor Billroth first reported a case of traumatic hemipelvectomy in 1889 (cited in: [1]). The patient survived only 6 h post-injury. The following reports in the literature mostly described single cases of surviving patients (Table 20.1). Only few data are available analyzing consecutive cases.

The management of these severely injured patients places great stress on the resuscitation team. Patient management should be aggressive from the start (Figs. 20.1 and 20.2).

20.1 Definition

Lipkowitz et al. defined the TH as a "unique type of an open pelvic fracture with wide separation of one innominate bone from the pubic symphysis and sacrum, extensive disruption of the soft-tissues in the inguinal area, avulsion of the external iliac vessels, and severe stretch injury or disruption of the femoral and sciatic nerves [2–4]" [5].

Here, it is already mentioned that vascular injury is often more severe than neurological injury.

Rieger et al. defined this injury as "an extreme and near-lethal form of an open pelvic fracture" [6], while Pohlemann et al. defined traumatic hemipelvectomy as an "unstable ligamentous or osseous hemipelvic injury with rupture of the pelvic neurovascular bundle (open or closed integuments)" [7].

Cavadas et al. distinguished between complete or incomplete injuries, with complete injuries being more infrequent than incomplete injuries [8].

Teebken et al. reported a case of a bilateral complete hemipelvic dissociation with a unilateral complete injury to the external iliac artery and an incomplete lumbosacral plexus lesion with closed soft-tissue on this hemipelvic side [9]. Thus, this injury can be present even with closed soft-tissues.

> There is no accepted definition of a traumatic hemipelvectomy.

We recommend the following definition of a traumatic hemipelvectomy:

> A traumatic hemipelvectomy is a unilateral (rarely bilateral) pelvic ring type C-injury with an at least III° pelvic vascular injury (iliac external artery, affecting limb perfusion) in combination with an at least partial lumbosacral plexus injury. An open soft-tissue injury is not mandatorily present [10].

20.2 Epidemiology

There is insufficient knowledge on epidemiological data of TH, as the majority of reports are dealing with survivors of this injury, while no adequate analyses were performed on consecutive case series.

There are only three studies on consecutive cases of TH, analyzed from a whole group of pelvic ring injury patients [7, 11, 12]:

B. Bakota
Department of Orthopaedics and Trauma, Medical University of Graz, Graz, Austria

M. Staresinic
General and Sports Trauma Department, University Hospital Merkur Zagreb, Zagreb, Croatia

A. Gänsslen (✉)
Department of Trauma Surgery, Orthopedics and Hand Surgery, Hospital Wolfsburg, Wolfsburg, Germany

A. Gänsslen et al. (eds.), *Pelvic Ring Fractures*, https://doi.org/10.1007/978-3-030-54730-1_20

Table 20.1 Data on patients after traumatic hemipelvectomy

Author	Year	Age	Sex	Deb.	Vasc.	IF	FK	RT	Col.	St-rec.	p.o. rec	Closure	Rev.	Sec. proc.
McPherson	1960	22	m	+	lig	–	–	–	+	n.r.	n.r.	sec	+	
McLean	1962	23	m	+	n.r.	–	+	+	+	Adapt	+	prim	–	
Wade	1965	20	m	+	n.r.	–	–	–	+	–	+	prim	–	
Wade	1964	14	m	+	lig	–	–	–	+	+	–	prim	–	
Palvolgyi	1969	27	m	+	n.r.	–	–	–	+	Adapt	–	sec	+	
Johansson	1971	17	m	+	lig	–	–	–	–	+	+	prim	–	
Ganapathy	1973	17	m	+	lig	–	+	–	+	+	–	prim	+	
Orcutt	1974	20	f	+	n.r.	–	–	–	–	+	–	sec	+	Skin graft
Meester	1975	26	m	+	lig	–	+	–	–	+	+	prim	+	
Oppenheim	1977	28	m	+	lig	–	+	–	+	+	+	prim	+	
Maull	1977	25	m	+	n.r.	–	–	–	+	+	–	sec	+	
Maull	1977	16	m	+	n.r.	–	+	–	+	+	–	sec	+	
Maull	1977	36	m	+	n.r.	–	+	–	+	+	–	sec	+	HP
Siemens	1977	31	m	+	n.r.	–	+	–	+	+	–	sec	+	
Wyndham	1978	20	m	+	lig	–	–	–	sec	+	+	sec	+	
Rodriguez	1983	20	m	+	lig	–	–	–	+	Adapt	–	sec	+	
Rodriguez	1983	17	m	+	lig	–	+	–	+	–	–	prim	+	
Evans	1984	16	m	+	n.r.	–	+	–	+	+	+	prim	–	
Sattel	1984	21	f	+	lig	–	–	–	+	+	–	prim	+	Skin graft
Sattel	1984	21	m	+	n.r.	–	–	–	–	+	–	prim	+	Skin graft
Lipkowitz	1985	7	m	+	lig	–	+	–	+	+	+	prim	+	
Danisi	1985	32	f	+	n.r.	–	–	–	+	+	–	sec	+	
Cooper	1987	14	m	+	lig	+	+	–	+	+	+	sec	+	HP
Ikpeme	1987	18	m	+	lig	–	–	+	+	+	+	sec	+	
Moore	1987	22	f	+	lig	–	–	–	+	+	–	sec	+	
Nichter	1988	8	m	+	lig	–	+	–	–	+	+	sec	+	
Smejkal	1988	25	m	+	lig	+	–	–	+	+	+	sec	+	HP
Smejkal	1988	22	m	+	emb	–	–	–	sec	+	–	sec	+	HP
Walker	1989	20	f	+	lig	–	+	–	+	+	–	prim	–	
Klasen	1989	24	m	+	lig	–	–	–	+	+	–	prim	–	
Klasen	1989	28	m	+	None	+	+	–	+	+	–	sec	+	HP
Klasen	1989	7	m	+	n.r.	–	+	–	–	+	–	prim	+	Skin graft
Beal	1989	24	m	+	None	+	+	–	+	+	–	sec	+	HP
Beal	1989	28	m	+	lig	–	–	–	+	–	–	sec	+	
Beal	1989	26	m	+	None	+	–	–	+	–	–	sec	+	HP
Wand	1990	19	m	+	n.r.	–	+	–	–	–	–	sec	+	
Klingman	1991	26	f	+	lig	–	+	–	+	+	+	prim	–	
Klingman	1991	29	f	+	lig	–	–	–	+	+	+	prim	+	
Spiers	1991	30	m	+	lig	–	–	–	+	+	–	prim	+	Infection
Smith	1991	26	m	+	n.r.	–	+	–	–	+	–	prim	+	
Dendrinos	1992	26	f	+	n.r.	–	–	–	–	+	–	sec	+	
Raftos	1994	26	m	+	lig	–	–	–	+	+	+	prim	+	
Pohlemann	1996	11	m	+	recon	+	–	–	n.r.	–	+	sec	+	HP
Pohlemann	1996	16	m	+	recon	+	+	–	n.r.	–	+	sec	+	HP
Pohlemann	1996	21	m	+	n.r.	+	–	–	+	–	+	sec	+	HP
Pohlemann	1996	20	m	+	Pack	–	–	–	–	–	–	–		
Pohlemann	1996	36	m	+	n.r.	+	–	+	+	+	+	sec	+	HP
Pohlemann	1996	29	m	+	lig	–	–	–	+	–	+	sec	+	
Pohlemann	1996	50	m	+	n.r.	–	–	–	–	+	–	prim	–	
Pohlemann	1996	3	m	+	n.r.	–	–	–	+	+	–	sec	+	HP
Pohlemann	1996	6	m	+	lig	–	–	–	–	+	–	prim	–	
Pohlemann	1996	7	m	+	lig	–	–	–	–	+	–	prim	–	
Ossewarde	1997	14	m	+	lig	–	+	–	+	–	–	sec	+	Skin graft

Table 20.1 (continued)

Author	Year	Age	Sex	Deb.	Vasc.	IF	FK	RT	Col.	St-rec.	p.o. rec	Closure	Rev.	Sec. proc.
Cho	1999	28	m	+	lig	–	+	–	+	–	+	sec	+	
Hutagalung	2001	25	f	+	n.r.	–	+	–	+	+	–	prim	–	
Losch	2001	21	f	+	n.r.	–	–	–	+	+	–	prim	+	
Losch	2001	21	m	+	n.r.	–	–	–	–	+	–	prim	+	
Schoderbek	2005	20	f	+	emb	+								sec trans
Kauvar	2005	26	f	+	lig	–	–	–	+	–	–	sec	+	
Labler	2005	29	m											
Labler	2005	22	m											HP
Labler	2005	75	m											
Labler	2005	22	m											
Labler	2005	33	m											
Labler	2005	24	m											
Labler	2005	13	m											
Labler	2005	18	m											HP
Labler	2005	33	m											
Osti	2006	21	f	+	recon	+	–	–	–	–	–	sec	+	
Gonzales	2006	21 m	f	+	recon									sec trans
Heineck	2006	16	m	+	recon	+	–	–	–	–	–	sec	+	HP
Yalniz	2007	27	m	+	lig	–	–	+	+	+	–	prim	+	
Cavadas	2008	18	m	+	n.r.	–	–	–	+	+	–	prim	–	
Daub	2008	21	m	+	lig	–	–	–	+	+	–	sec	+	
Williams	2009	21	m	+	recon	–	–	–	sec	–	–	sec	+	HP
Lasurt	2010	22	f	+	lig	–	–	–	+	+	+	prim	–	
Calonge	2010	9	m	+	n.r.	–	+	–	+	+	–	prim	+	
Calonge	2010	18 m	f	+	lig	–	+	+	–	+	+	prim	+	Skin graft
Schuitema	2010	21	m	+	recon	+	–	–	n.r.	–	–	sec	+	HP
Wansbrough	2011	23	m	+	lig	–	+	–	+	+	+	sec	+	HP
Timmers	2012	33	m	+	lig	–	+	–	sec	–	–	sec	+	
Timmers	2012	17	m	+	lig	–	+	–	sec	+	–	prim	+	Infection
Thomas	2012	38	m	+	n.r.	–	+	–	sec	–	–	sec	+	
Faisham	2012	16	m	+	n.r.	–	–	–	+	+	–	prim	+	
Walcher	2013	30	m	+	recon	+	–	+	+	+	–	sec	+	
Kayalar	2014	40	m	+	lig	–	–	–	+	+	–	prim	–	
Salomon	2014	20	m	+	n.r.	–	–	–	+	+	–	prim	+	
Ricci	2014	25	m	+	lig	–	–	–	+	+	+	prim		
Pansard	2014	33	m	+	lig	–	–	–	sec	+	–	prim	+	
Haim	2015	16 m	m	+	recon	–	–	–	–	–	–	sec	+	HP
Rouemliotis	2015	40	f	+	lig	–	–	–	–	+	+	sec	+	
Müller-Höcker	2017	18	f	+	lig	–	–	–	–	+	–	prim	+	
Smith	2017	21	f	+	lig	–	+	–	+	+	+	prim	+	
Ghimire	2018	19	f	+	lig	–	–	–	+	–	+	sec	+	Skin graft
Yildrim	2018	16	m	+	n.r.	–	–	–	+	+	+	prim	–	

m male, *f* female, *deb.* debridement, *vasc.* vascular, *FK* Foley or suprapubic catheter, *RT* rectal tube, *col.* colostomy, *st-rec.* soft-tissue reconstruction, *p.o. rec.* pelvic organ reconstruction, *lig* ligation, *emb* embolization, *prim* primary, *sec* secondary, *n.r.* not recorded, *rev* secondary wound revisions, *sec. proc.* secondary procedures

- Pohlemann et al. analyzed 2002 patients with pelvic ring injuries, treated between 1972 and 1994. In this group, 11 patients suffered traumatic hemipelvectomies (0.5%) [7].
- Labler et al. reported a higher incidence of 2.4% from a group of 373 pelvic ring injuries, of which nine fulfilled the criteria of traumatic hemipelvectomy, treated between 1998 and 2004 [11].
- Wang et al. analyzed 917 patients with pelvic ring fractures, treated between 2000 and 2011, and observed nine cases (1%) with a TH (2× complete, 7× partial) [12].

Combining these data leads to an overall incidence of 0.9% (29/3292 cases).

Overall a TH is a very rare injury.

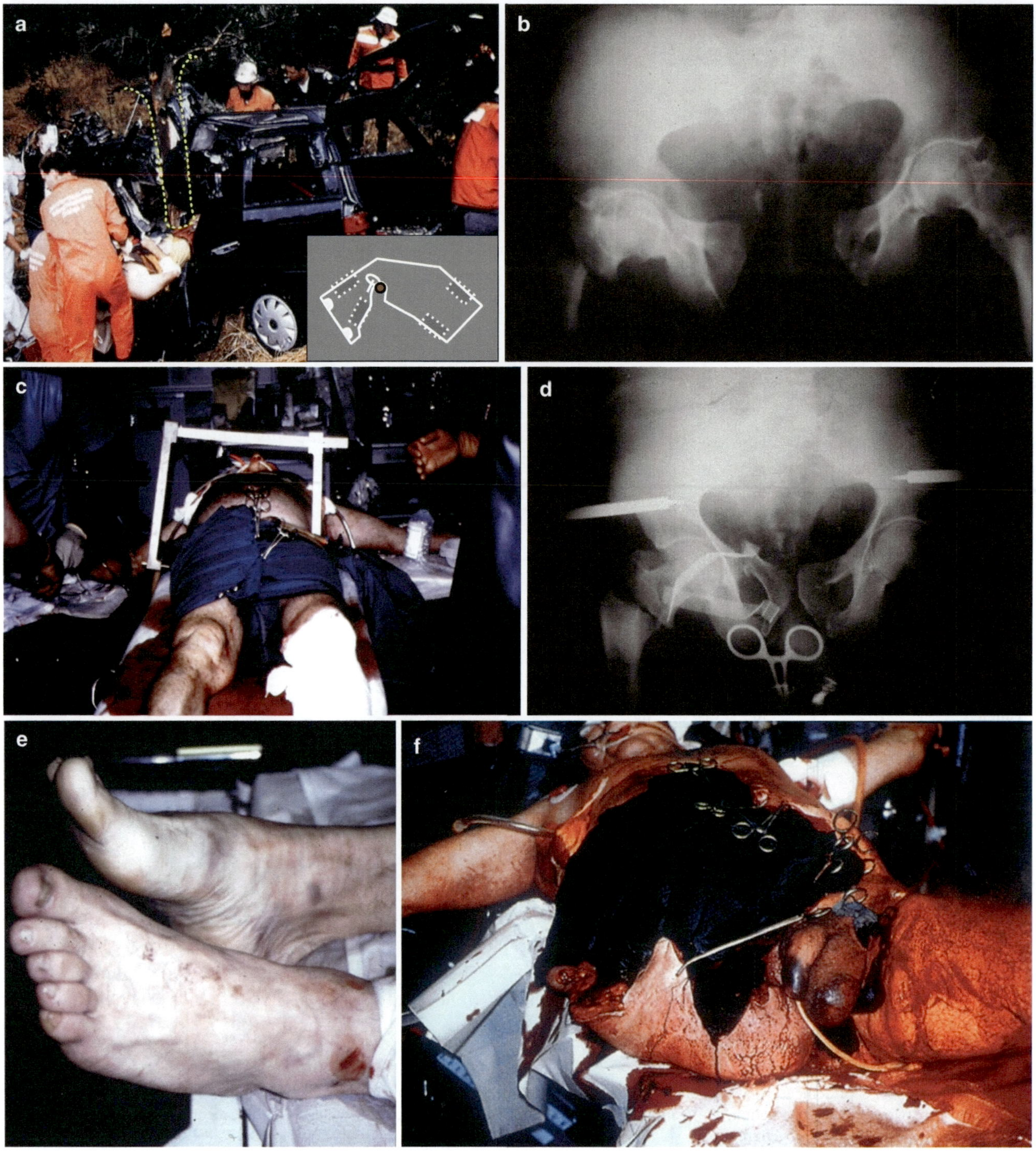

Fig. 20.1 (**a**) MVA with constriction of the driver between a tree and part of the car. (**b**) Primary pelvic a.p. X-ray showing a complete right hemipelvic dislocation (APC III), a left open-book injury (APC II), and bilateral proximal femur fractures. (**c**) Immediate emergency stabilization of the open pelvic injury with a sheet and the pelvic C-clamp. (**d**) Post-reduction pelvic a.p. X-ray showing a near anatomic reduction. (**e**) Clinically, the right foot was pale without peripheral pulses. (**f**) Immediate completion of the hemipelvectomy was performed with open wound treatment. (**g**) Several re-debridements were neccessary, until wound closure was performed using skin grafts. (**h**) Intermediate X-ray showing the hemiplevectomy status and clinical follow-up after 1 year with full mobilization using a hemipelvic prosthesis and crutches. The patient was socially full integrated without psychological sequelae. Source: Pohlemann T, Regel G, Bosch U, Stief Ch, Tscherne H. Kapitel 7: Notfallbehandlung und Komplextrauma, p. 106–107 (Fig. 7.21); in: Tscherne H, Pohlemann T (Eds.). Tscherne Unfallchirurgie – Becken und Acetabulum. Springer Verlag Berlin, Heidelberg, New York, 1998

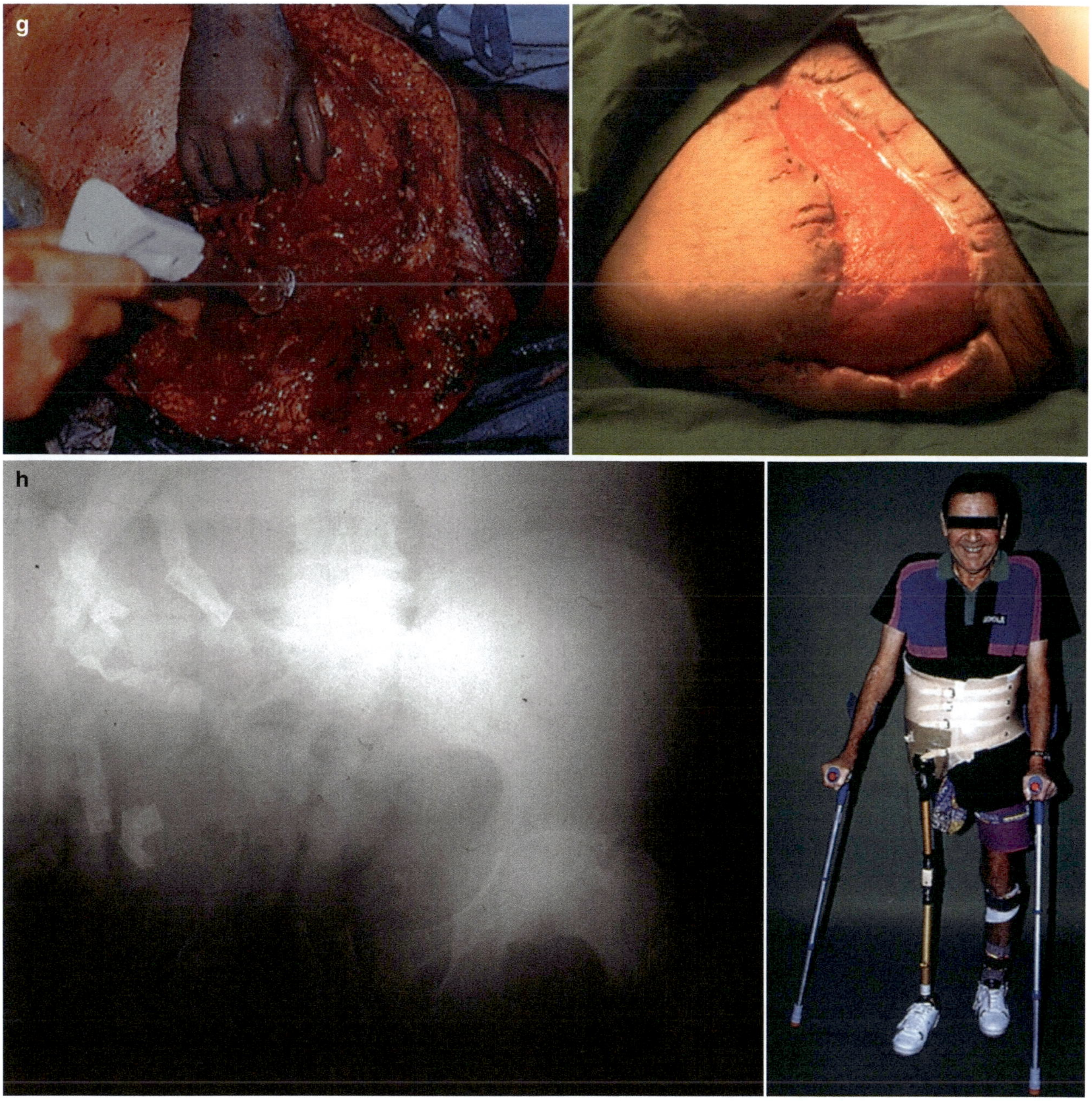

Fig. 20.1 (continued)

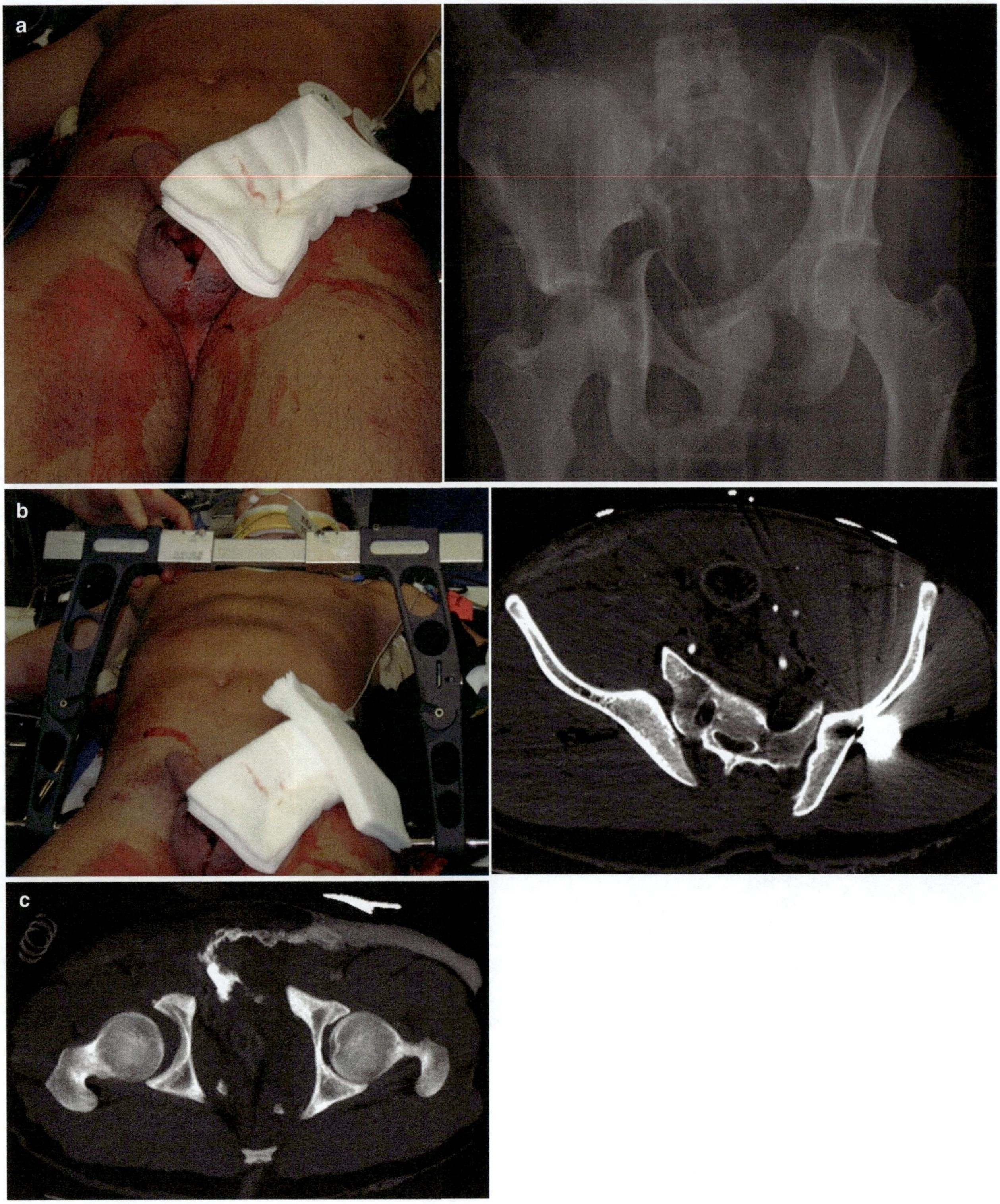

Fig. 20.2 (**a**) 18-year-old man after a motorcycle accident with an open injury of the left groin and an open scrotum injury. The initial pelvic X-ray showed bilateral SI-joint disruption, pubic symphysis disruption, and a right transverse acetabular fracture. (**b**) After C-clamp application and hemodynamic stabilization, the CT-scan revealed insufficient posterior pelvic ring reduction. (**c**) Additionally, an extraperitoneal bladder disruption was found. (**d**) A complete transection of the external iliac artery was diagnosed using angio-CT examination. (**e**) Emergency mechanical pelvic ring stabilization consisted of bilateral SI-joint plating (first window of the ilioinguinal approach) followed by pelvic packing and symphyseal plating as a damage control procedure within 75 min after hospital admission. Additionally, vascular reconstruction was performed using an autologous reversed saphenous vein bypass from the right iliac bifurcation to the proximal common femoral artery and bladder reconstruction. (**f**) Postoperative 3D CT showing the malreduced SI-joints (aim of emergency stabilization was stability and not reduction) and the displaced acetabular fracture. The pelvic X-ray after 14 day shows definitive stabilization of the pelvic ring and the acetabular fracture with anatomic reconstruction of the right hemipelvis and minimal remaining displacement of the left SI-joint

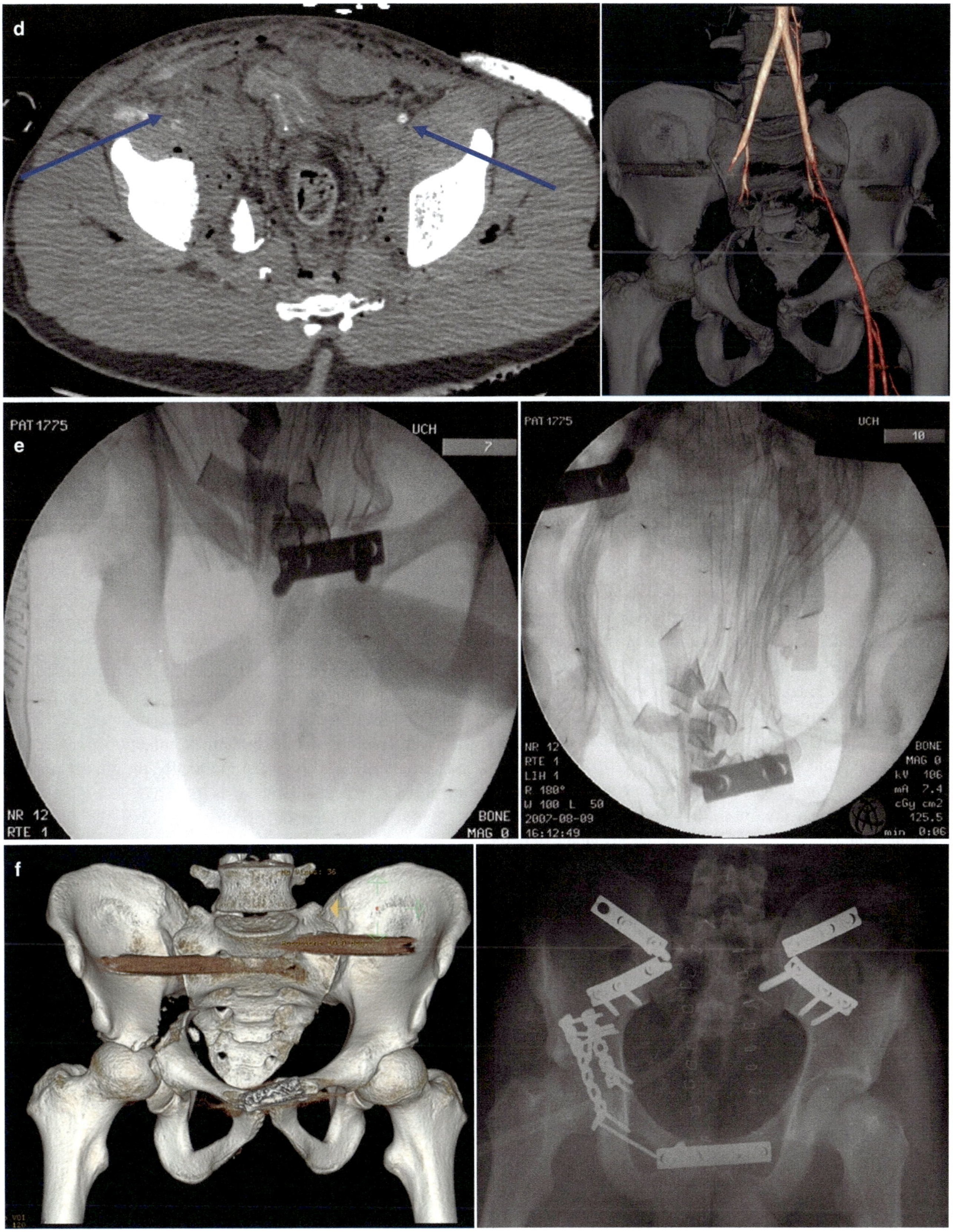

Fig. 20.2 (continued)

Pohlemann et al. observed 11 cases in 23 years (1 case every 2.1 years) [7], Labler et al. reported nine cases in 7 years (1 case every 9.3 months) [11] and Wang et al. reported nine cases in 12 years (1 case every 16 months) [12].

20.3 Mechanism of Injury

Beal et al. summarized the literature and observed three main injury mechanisms [13]:

- Lower extremity forced hyperabduction combined with external rotation (e.g. unrestrained cyclist/motorcyclist)
- Traction-type extremity avulsion from the fixed pelvis during agricultural/machine injuries
- Crush (roll-over) mechanism.

20.4 Treatment Recommendations

Initially, patient resuscitation according to a standardized shock room protocol (e.g. ATLS protocol [14, 15]) is performed.

Specific emergency treatment should focus on hemorrhage control [16, 17], which is usually performed by immediate surgical debridement and wound exploration [18, 19].

Lasurt et al. believed that, in complete TH, higher survival rates can be expected, as "retraction of the vessels, which is possible after complete transection allowing closure by muscular contraction" is more common than after incomplete TH, where this mechanism is not working [20]. Additionally, incomplete TH can be associated with ongoing bleeding, as bleeding is harder to control [21].

Immediate HP completion has here the advantage of hemorrhage control and secondary infection protection [7, 8, 18, 21].

Colorectal injuries are frequently observed in patients with TH. These injuries are present in 2/3 of the patients [8, 13–15, 18, 20, 22–49]. A colostomy is, therefore, an important part of the initial management for protection of sepsis and infection or even secondary wound breakdown. Standards of rectal injury treatment should be considered [24, 26, 30, 50, 51].

> Damage control treatment should, therefore, focus on bleeding and contamination control.

Definitive repairs can be postponed to secondary procedures. As the peritoneum is often lacerated and muscles of the abdominal wall are disrupted, their sealing effect is disturbed, leading to further risk of bleeding complications. Compromised hemodynamics in the unstable pelvic ring injuries are first mechanically stabilized [16, 17, 52]. As already mentioned, in TH patients, completion of the TH allows for bleeding and contamination control.

> Colostomy is effective for adequate fecal diversion [53].

Adequate urine drainage should additionally be performed by simple measures, including use of a conventional bladder catheter, suprapubic drainage, or bilateral nephrostomy [54, 55].

Genital injuries are usually not life-threatening and can, therefore, be treated by local bleeding control (packing, etc.), irrigation, debridement, and VAC therapy [53].

Regarding wound management, after excessive local debridement of all devitalized soft-tissues, it remains unclear, whether a primary or secondary wound closure should be performed [2, 5, 6, 27]. Often a large posterior gluteal flap is created by the injury, which can be used for wound reduction or even primary wound flap closure.

Split-thickness skin grafts are often necessary in the further treatment phase, even after primary closure [8].

In the initial management period, it is often difficult to analyze the vitality of the involved muscles. The iliopsoas is often involved/transected with development of secondary necrosis, resulting in re-debridement, infection, or even sepsis [2, 6, 12, 33, 43, 56–58]. Additionally, the gluteal muscles are at risk for secondary necrosis [6, 7, 57].

Based on experience of survivors from the literature, treatment should include:

1. Damage control treatment of exsanguination/shock/hemorrhage
2. Completion of the hemipelvectomy
3. Damage control treatment for protection of infection (debridement)
4. Damage control treatment for protection of infection (colostomy)
5. Adequate wound care (primary/secondary closure)
6. Low-level planning of re-debridements

20.5 Mortality

Data from consecutive reports are available from four studies:

- Pohlemann et al. reported seven deaths in the group of 11 patients with a TH (63.6%) [7].

- Labler et al. reported seven deaths from their group of nine patients (77.8%) [11].
- Wang et al. reported four survivors from their nine cases (55.5% mortality) [12].
- Wu et al. analyzed four patients with a TH and reported a mortality rate of 50% [59].

The overall mortality rate after TH is still high with an average of 63.6%, based on four case series [7, 11, 12, 59].

20.6 Literature Review of Traumatic Hemipelvectomies

Analysis of the existing literature revealed that predominantly case reports were published on isolated patients or small patient groups sustaining traumatic hemipelvectomies (HP). Only a few series analyzed consecutive case series and HP as a result of blast injuries.

The following review focusses on

- Case reports
- Consecutive case series
- Military-related traumatic HP

The available literature was analyzed for sex, age, injury mechanism, prehospital care, pelvic ring classification, hemipelvectomy classification, the initial hemodynamic status, the extremity status, concomitant pelvic, local muscular, abdominal and neurovascular injuries, associated injuries, initial treatment, transfusion requirements, complications, secondary procedures, definitive wound management, discharge data, and follow-up evaluations.

20.7 Traumatic Hemipelvectomy (Case Reports)

Overall, data on 103 cases were published in the literature.

20.7.1 Demographic Data

Twenty patients were females (19.4%) [20, 23, 31, 34, 35, 38, 40, 41, 45, 58, 60–68], while 83 were males (80.6%) [1, 2, 4, 5, 7, 8, 11, 13, 18, 21, 23, 25, 27, 29, 32, 33, 35, 37, 39, 43–47, 49, 57, 60, 69–89]. The mean age was 22.5 years (1–75 years). No age difference was observed between male and female patients (22.5 years). The rate of pediatric patients (<15 years) was 13.6%.

20.7.2 Mechanism of Injury

Different injury mechanisms were responsible in sustaining traumatic HP:

- Fall from great heights [20, 32].
- Motorcycle injuries (not further specified) [2, 7, 13, 18, 19, 22, 27, 28, 35, 41, 45, 46, 49, 71, 74, 81, 84].
- Motorcycle collision against a car/truck [1, 2, 4, 18, 21, 23, 43, 47, 57, 61, 65, 80, 82].
- Motor vehicle accidents (patient in the motor vehicle) [31, 37, 40, 48, 60, 64, 66, 72, 90].
- Pedestrian struck by a car (including two cases riding a bicycle) [4, 7, 13, 34, 38, 39, 56, 58, 60, 69, 76, 77, 85, 91, 92].
- Roll-over mechanism [5, 7, 25, 29, 63, 68, 70, 73, 74, 83].
- Extremity pull-out mechanisms (winch, trapping) [33, 75, 87–89].
- Crush mechanism [47, 62, 86].
- Blade injuries [8, 34, 78].
- Blunt injuries [44, 79].

Labler et al. additionally reported that, in six of their cases, the cause of the injury was a traffic accident and three sustained accidents at work [11].

Overall, the predominant injury mechanisms were motorcycle injuries and injuries in patients without adequate protection (pedestrians, roll-over mechanisms).

20.7.3 Prehospital Care

Only a few data are available regarding prehospital treatment of these injuries. In the majority of cases, local tamponade, wound packing, or manual compression was performed [4, 5, 18, 20, 27, 38, 39, 44, 49, 60, 62, 64, 65, 76, 77, 80, 82, 85, 87]. Further treatment of bleeding control included pelvic bandage [29], PASG/MAST [34, 47, 78] and direct vessel clamping [18, 84].

20.7.4 Pelvic Ring Injury Classification

In 74 patients, the injury localization was reported [1, 2, 4, 5, 7, 8, 18–21, 23, 25, 27, 29, 31–35, 37–41, 43–49, 57, 60, 62–66, 69–80, 82, 83, 85–88]. The majority of patients (*n* = 43) presented with a left-sided traumatic HP (58.6%). Twenty-nine patients had a right-sided injury (41.4%). Two patients had bilateral HP injuries [68, 70] and two patients sustained a hemicorporectomy [7, 68].

The traumatic HP could be classified into:

- 29× Complete traumatic HP (31.2%) [4, 7, 8, 11, 18, 20, 25, 27, 29, 31–34, 38, 40, 43, 49, 60, 62, 64, 75–77, 79, 80, 87–89].
- 21× Near total traumatic HP (very small remaining soft-tissues) (22.6%) [1, 2, 5, 13, 18, 21, 33–35, 39, 45, 56, 60, 61, 63, 71, 74, 78, 81].
- 43× Incomplete traumatic HP (relevant remaining soft-tissues) (46.2%) [2, 4, 7, 11, 13, 19, 23, 33, 35, 37, 41, 44, 46–48, 57, 58, 65, 66, 69, 72–74, 82–86].

According to the pelvic ring classification (Tile), per definition all patients had type C-injuries.

The typical HP pelvic ring injury is a C1.2 c5 injury with a complete unilateral complete disruption of the SI-joint, in combination with a separation of the pubic symphysis [1, 2, 4, 7, 8, 18, 20, 21, 23, 27, 31–35, 38, 39, 41, 43–45, 47, 49, 57, 60, 63–66, 70, 71, 74, 76–78, 80, 86, 87].

The posterior pelvic ring injury could be classified in 70 cases [1, 2, 4, 5, 7, 8, 18, 20, 21, 23, 27, 29, 31–35, 38, 39, 41, 43–45, 47–49, 56, 57, 60–66, 69–78, 80, 82, 83, 86–88]:

- 1× Type C-injury.
- 1× C1.1 Injury (complete iliac fracture).
- 62× C1.2 Injury (SI-joint dislocation).
- 3× C2 Injuries (ipsilateral type C-injury and contralateral type B injury).
- 3× Bilateral type C-injuries.

Williams et al. reported a case of a both column acetabular fracture resulting in a hemipelvectomy [19].

The anterior pelvic ring injury was predominantly a symphyseal separation in 70.6%. Further types of anterior pelvic ring injuries included:

- 5× Ipsilateral pubic rami fractures.
- 1× Contralateral pubic rami fractures.
- 2× Bilateral pubic rami fractures.
- 3× Ipsilateral pubic rami fractures + symphyseal disruption.
- 9× Contralateral pubic rami fractures + symphyseal disruption.

Overall, the pubic symphysis was significantly displaced in 88.2%.

20.7.5 Hemodynamic Status

Inconsistent data are available regarding the presence of hemorrhagic shock and injury severity. In 65 patients, some initial data (emergency department) were reported in terms of systolic blood pressure (sBP), heart rate (HR), shock index (SI), base deficit (BD), cardio-pulmonary resuscitation (CPR), hemoglobin concentration (Hb), Injury Severity Score (ISS), and the presence of bleeding.

Ninety-eight point three percent of patients were in relevant hemodynamic compromise at admission (59/60 patients). Data on sBP were available in 41 patients [2, 4, 5, 7, 18, 20, 21, 23, 25, 27, 32, 34, 38, 39, 44, 46–49, 57, 68, 71, 73, 76–78, 80, 82, 88]. Except for four patients, all presented with an sBP of ≤90 mmHg (90.2%). The mean sBP at admission was 57 mmHg. Nine patients had an unobtainable blood pressure and, in further ten patients, the sBP was ≤60 mmHg. The mean HR was 107/min.

In 18 patients, both parameters were available (four patients with unobtainable sBP excluded), which led to calculation of the SI [2, 18, 20, 23, 32, 34, 38, 44, 47, 49, 68, 71, 73, 78, 88]. The mean sBP was 76 mmHg, the HR was 122/min, resulting in an average shock index of 1.6.

In six patients, CPR was immediately necessary during admission [29, 39, 47, 63, 74, 77].

In 14 patients, the bleeding status was documented. Active bleeding was observed in half of these patients [2, 4, 5, 25, 27, 32, 40, 46, 68, 73, 77, 87, 88].

In 11 patients, the ISS was documented. The average ISS was 46.5 points [7, 32, 65].

The mean BD in nine patients was −7.8 mmol/L [7, 43, 88] and the mean Hb concentration in 13 patients was 6.15 g/dL [7, 32, 34, 57, 78].

20.7.6 Neurovascular Status of the Extremity

In 78 cases, a combined neurovascular injury was reported [1, 2, 4, 5, 7, 8, 13, 18, 20, 21, 23, 27, 29, 31–35, 38–41, 43, 44, 46, 47, 49, 56–58, 60–64, 66, 68–78, 80–89]. In further 19 cases, a relevant injury to pelvic vessels was recorded without specifying a neurological injury [2, 7, 11, 19, 25, 37, 45, 65, 74, 79].

The vascular injury was further distinguished into injuries to the common iliac vessels (CIAV), the iliac internal vessels (IIAV) and the iliac external vessels (IEAV). In 71 cases, a more detailed description of the vascular lesion was reported:

- 2 Combined CIAV, IIAV, and IEAV injuries [18, 71].
- 3 Combined CIAV and IEAV injuries [18, 35, 47].
- 7 Combined IIAV and IEAV injuries [21, 32, 37, 58, 66, 69, 82].

- 13 Isolated CIAV injuries [7, 23, 29, 35, 41, 44, 45, 64, 72, 78].
- 1 Isolated IIAV injury [73].
- 45 Isolated IEAV injuries [1, 2, 4, 5, 7, 13, 19, 25, 27, 31, 33, 34, 38–40, 45–47, 56, 57, 61, 63, 65, 68, 70, 76, 77, 79–81, 84, 87, 88].

The neurological injury was additionally further specified. Typically, it was distinguished between lumbosacral plexus lesions and transection of the femoral or the sciatic nerve.

- 45 Cases with a lumbosacral plexus lesion [7, 8, 13, 18, 20, 21, 23, 33–35, 38, 46, 56, 57, 61, 64, 68, 70, 71, 73, 77, 78, 80, 83].
- 5 Cases with a combined sciatic and femoral nerve lesion [18, 60, 72, 82, 84].
- 7 Cases with an isolated sciatic nerve transection [1, 4, 5, 58, 87, 88].
- 6 Cases with an isolated femoral nerve transection [7, 43, 82, 85, 86].

Overall, 18 CIAV injuries, 10 IIAV injuries, and 57 IEAV injuries were reported. Additionally, 13 femoral artery or vein transections were reported [7, 20, 47, 48, 66, 70, 75, 76, 82, 83, 85, 88]. These were combined with iliac vessel transection in seven cases.

20.8 Intrapelvic Organ Injuries

Only few case reports described the accompanying muscle injury in detail and, therefore, were excluded from further analysis. All analyzed cases had open wounds in the pelvic region.

Overall, the presence or absence of concomitant injuries to intrapelvic organs or soft-tissues were reported in 90 cases [1, 2, 4, 5, 7, 8, 11, 13, 18–21, 23, 25, 27, 29, 31–35, 37–41, 43–49, 57, 58, 60–66, 68–85, 87–89].

In 14 cases (15.5%), no pelvic organ or soft-tissue injury except the open injury of the traumatic hemipelvectomy with muscle injury was reported [19, 21, 23, 31, 32, 41, 61, 63–66, 81, 82, 84], leaving 76 cases with additional relevant pelvic organ injury (84.5%).

Overall, the following rates of pelvic organ/Soft-tissue injuries were observed:

- 28.9% ($n = 22$) bladder injuries [7, 11, 18, 34, 43, 47, 58, 68, 72, 75, 76, 82, 83, 85, 87].
- 40.8% ($n = 32$) urethra injuries [2, 5, 7, 11, 13, 18, 25, 29, 33, 46, 48, 49, 60, 70, 74, 75, 77, 79, 80, 85, 87, 89].
- 67.1% ($n = 51$) rectum or anal sphincter injuries [2, 4, 5, 7, 8, 11, 13, 18, 20, 25, 33–35, 37, 38, 40, 45, 47, 49, 58, 60, 62, 68–71, 74, 75, 77, 80, 82, 83, 87, 88].
- 5.3% ($n = 4$) ureter injuries [7, 18, 25, 69].

Of these 76 patients, 65 were male and male-specific injury rates were as follows:

- 7.7% ($n = 5$) prostate injuries [7, 18, 25, 27, 87].
- 43.1% ($n = 28$) scrotal injuries [1, 2, 4, 5, 7, 13, 18, 33, 37, 43, 44, 69, 73, 77–80, 87–89].
- 20% ($n = 13$) penis injuries [2, 4, 7, 18, 27, 33, 49, 60, 76, 77, 80, 87, 89].
- 38.5% ($n = 25$) injuries of the testes [2, 5, 7, 8, 13, 18, 25, 27, 29, 33, 39, 43, 57, 69, 76, 77, 80].

Of these 76 patients, 11 were female and female-specific injury rates were as follows:

- 27.3% ($n = 3$) vulva injuries [20, 38, 62].
- 36.4% ($n = 4$) vagina injuries [20, 34, 68, 82].
- 9.1% ($n = 1$) uterus injury [58].
- In 26 cases, an isolated intrapelvic organ injury was seen, while in 50 cases (65.7%), at least two pelvic organs were involved.

20.9 Concomitant Abdominal Injuries

Data on concomitant injuries of the abdomen were reported in 96 cases. In 68 cases, no concomitant intra-abdominal injury was observed [1, 2, 4, 5, 7, 8, 11, 13, 18–21, 23, 25, 27, 31–33, 35, 37, 39, 41, 44–49, 56, 57, 60–66, 69, 71, 73, 74, 77–80, 82–85, 88, 89], despite two patients having a lacerated peritoneum [82, 89].

In 28 cases, an injury was observed [7, 11, 29, 34, 38, 40, 43, 47, 58, 60, 68, 70, 72, 74–76, 81, 87]:

- 13/25 Had an open laceration of the peritoneum [7, 11, 29, 34, 38, 40, 43, 47, 58, 60, 68, 70, 72, 74–76, 81, 87].
- 7/28 Presented with abdominal content evisceration [7, 34, 40, 47, 58, 60].
- 15/28 Presented with an injury of the colon [7, 11, 34, 43, 47, 58, 70, 72, 75].
- 15/28 Presented with an injury of the small bowel [7, 34, 68, 76].
- 2/28 Had an exposure of the kidney without kidney laceration [29, 87].
- 3/28 Had a splenic injury [7, 38].
- 1/28 Had a liver laceration [7].

20.10 Associated Injuries

In 96 cases, data on associated injuries were reported [1, 2, 4, 5, 7, 8, 11, 13, 18–21, 23, 25, 27, 29, 31–35, 37–41, 43–49, 56–58, 60–66, 68–85, 87–89]. Of these, in 51 cases, relevant injuries were recorded [2, 5, 7, 8, 11, 13, 18–21, 23, 25, 27,

31, 33–35, 37, 38, 40, 41, 45, 46, 56, 57, 61, 65, 66, 70, 71, 73–75, 79, 83, 84]:

- 9× Head injury.
- 2× Face trauma.
- 10× Chest trauma.
- 13× Upper extremity injuries (fractures, dislocation, amputations).
- 30× Lower extremity injuries (fractures, dislocation, amputations).
- 1× Spine trauma.

20.11 Shock Management

There are some data on perioperative transfusion requirements [5, 7, 11, 13, 18, 21, 23, 25, 33, 46, 48, 68, 78, 87].

On average, 23.7 PRBC were transfused during the initial perioperative treatment phase [5, 7, 11, 13, 18, 21, 23, 25, 33, 46, 48, 78, 87]. Additionally, a mean of 14.5 FFP were transfused [5, 11, 18, 23, 48, 78].

20.12 Management

Due to the heterogeneity of the patients, no standardized initial and secondary treatment can be derived from the literature (Table 20.1).

All patients had initial wound debridement. Vascular treatment consisted of:

In 12 patients, pelvic osteosynthesis was performed, of which, ten patients received secondary hemipelvectomy. In only two patients, the definition of a traumatic hemipelvectomy was stated and a reconstruction of the pelvis was sufficient [41, 83]. Overall, 16 patients received a secondary hemipelvectomy after initial reconstruction of the pelvis.

Vascular treatment included iliac vessel ligation in the majority of patients, while nine patients had vascular reconstruction, two had embolization of the bleeding vessels, and in one case, only a direct packing was performed.

Primary and secondary definitive wound reconstruction was nearly equally distributed. Interestingly, after primary wound closure/reconstruction, more than half of the patients required secondary soft-tissue procedures.

Not every report dealt with the use of antibiotics or tetanus immunization. Many reports stated that at last antibiotic coverage was performed during initial treatment. Recent reports recommended a combination of a Cephalosporin and Metronidazole [18, 32, 43, 83].

Several data are available regarding ongoing transfusion requirements. These data can be distinguished in transfusions (PRBC and FFP) transfused within 12, 24, 36, and 48 h.

- In the analysis by Pohlemann et al., within 12 h after admission, the average volume replacement was 50.4 PRBC [7].
- Within 24 h after admission, the average volume replacement was 36.4 PRBC, 18.3 FFP and 11 TC [7, 57, 61, 74, 80, 88].
- Within 36 h after admission, the average volume replacement was 56.6 PRBC, 30 FFP and 47 TC [34, 47].
- Within 48 h after admission the average volume replacement was 41.7 PRBC and 10 FFP [2, 7, 27, 32, 38, 40].

20.13 Colostomy

In 94 cases, data on performed colostomy were reported [1, 2, 4, 5, 7, 8, 11, 13, 18–21, 23, 25, 27, 29, 31–35, 37–41, 43–49, 56–58, 60–66, 68–85, 87–89].

A colostomy was performed in 74 of these cases (78.7%) [1, 2, 4, 5, 7, 8, 11, 13, 18–21, 23, 25, 27, 31–35, 37, 38, 40, 43–47, 49, 56, 60, 62–64, 66, 68–72, 74, 75, 77–83, 85, 87–89]:

- 16× Unknown type.
- 8× End colostomy.
- 13× Diverting colostomy.
- 2× Ileostomy.
- 14× Sigmoid colostomy.
- 18× Transverse colostomy.
- 3× Secondary colostomy.

20.14 Further Clinical Course

Patients with traumatic hemipelvectomy had an average hospital length of stay (LOS) of 12.9 weeks (range: 2–55 weeks) [1, 2, 4, 5, 7, 8, 13, 18–21, 23, 32, 33, 35, 39–41, 43, 47–49, 57, 63–66, 69, 72–74, 76, 78, 82–84, 87, 88]. Patients with a secondary wound closure had, on average, a 1 week longer LOS.

20.14.1 Follow-Up

In 34 cases, a prosthetic replacement was recorded, which was often used [1, 4, 5, 7, 8, 13, 19, 21, 27, 29, 32–34, 37, 40, 45–47, 49, 57, 60–62, 69, 72, 73, 77, 78, 82, 85, 87, 88].

In 21 patients, crutches were used [2, 5, 13, 20, 34, 37, 41, 46, 61, 62, 69, 72–74, 83, 88].

Nine patients used both a hemipelvectomy prosthesis and crutches [5, 34, 37, 46, 61, 62, 69, 72, 73].

Three patients developed significant heterotopic bone formation [73, 80, 85]; in one patient, a significant re-ossification of the hemipelvis occurred with large formation of new bone [85].

Two patients developed significant scoliosis with [20, 35], with pelvic tilting deformity.

Five patients died secondary due to several reasons: 1× pulmonary embolism, 1× sepsis, 2× suicide, 1× unknown [7, 35, 68, 74, 87].

In 21 patients, a follow-up of at least 1 year after trauma was reported, after a mean of 3.7 years (range: 1–13 years) [7, 18, 29, 32, 33, 41, 60, 61, 72, 73, 76, 80, 82, 84, 85, 88]. No detailed follow-up evaluation was performed, only descriptive data were available:

- 15 Patients had hemipelvic prosthetic replacement in use, 5 patients used crutches with overall, 18 patients using walking supports.
- 11 Were socially integrated and one was socially isolated.
- 7 Reported on pelvis-related complaints, while six had no pelvis-related problems.
- 2 Had significant psychological problems, while seven were psychologically stable.

There is only one study focusing on long-term results after hemipelvectomy and hip disarticulation due to tumor resection, trauma, infections, neurogenic illness, or peripheral artery disease, using a questionnaire analysis [42]:

- 62.5% Reported on phantom pain.
- 5.4% Had scar related pain.
- 30.4% Reported no pain.
- 38.1% Reported bladder dysfunction after hemipelvectomy.
- 26.8% Reported on low back pain.
- 67.9% Used a hemipelvic prosthesis.
- 58.9% Used a wheelchair.
- 82.1% Used crutches.
- 42.9% Used sitting supports.

20.15 Combat-Related Traumatic Hemipelvectomy

In the military [93] and terror environment [67], high-energy, explosive blast injuries can additionally lead to traumatic hemipelvectomies.

The injury mechanism clearly differs from that of blunt trauma cases, sustained during agricultural, motorcycle, crush, or motor vehicle accidents.

Recent experience with this type of HP was gained by military experience.

Alleyrand et al. reported, in 2012, from their experience of blast-related traumatic hemipelvectomies [94]. Most often, secondary completion of the HP was performed, as the majority of patients arrived at definitive care hospitals between 5 and 10 days after trauma. The mangled extremity was usually already treated with proximal amputation or at the level of the hip joint. Patients can present with existing relevant wound necrosis or even infection, making completion of the hemipelvis a resultant option.

Of interest, these injuries are often accompanied by contralateral mangled lower extremity injuries with subsequent amputation and relevant injury to the non-dominant (non-weapon holding) upper extremity.

> War-related blast traumatic HP often present with bilateral mangled lower extremities and at least one severely injured upper extremity.

The described standard in treating these catastrophic injuries is based on the concept described for blunt trauma hemipelvectomies:

- Administration of broad-spectrum antibiotics and tetanus prophylaxis
- No wound exploration outside the operating room
- Application of direct pressure
- Aggressive resuscitation with blood or component products
- Consideration of proximal, intra-abdominal vascular control
- Direct vascular control:
  - Ligation of avulsed or transected vessels including potential ligation of the contralateral hypogastric artery in complete injuries.
  - Consideration of angio-embolization in incomplete or closed injuries
- Application of a suprapubic catheter
- Consideration of primary urogenital or abdominal injury repair
- Creation of a diverting colostomy and distal colonic washout to reduce fecal contamination
- Early hemipelvectomy completion
- Aggressive wound debridement, especially evaluation of the iliopsoas, quadratus lumborum, and retroperitoneal and paraspinous muscles
- Treatment of the lethal triad of deaths: coagulopathy, acidosis, and hypothermia
- Wound size reduction using a fasciocutaneous or myocutaneous fillet flap, if possible, or consideration of free tissue transfer donated from the distal tissue of the affected (amputated) lower extremity
- Avoidance of primary wound closure.

Postoperative, frequent, and additional debridements are often necessary, as the degree of soft-tissue injury is more severe in blast-related injuries.

Lessons learned from blast-related traumatic hemipelvectomies include [93, 95]:

- Complete injuries often present with minor active bleeding, due to vascular/arterial spasm and vessel retraction with subsequent thrombosis.
- Incomplete injuries and blast injuries present with a higher bleeding risk as vascular spasm is infrequent.
- An additional contralateral amputation of a mangled extremity can lead to relevant pressure sources and ulcers (prolonged phase of immobilization).
- Preservation of as much iliac bone as possible for increase of the weight bearing surface (avoid SI-joint disarticulation) compared to tumor surgery, with secondary screw fixation of the SI-joint [94, 96].
- Depending on the fracture type, a subtotal hemipelvectomy is favored.
- Nerve roots emerging directly at the level of the sacral foramina should be divided with caution to avoid potential contamination of the cerebro-spinal fluid with resultant risk of meningitis [2, 4].
- Avoid primary wound closure.
- Place as much intact skin and subcutaneous tissue over the weight bearing areas.
- Avoid reconstruction using the rectus abdominus muscle (reduced peritoneal support), the latissimus dorsi muscle (impaired use of a wheelchair).

In a recent analysis of consecutive blast-related TH, a mortality rate of 15.4% was reported [94].

20.16 Technique of Hemipelvectomy

The technique of performing a hemipelvectomy is based on experience in tumor surgery [36, 97].

In 1977, Wu et al. reported on their technique of hindquarter amputation (= hemipelvectomy) in 19 cases with bone and soft-tissue tumors [97]. A five-step procedure was described.

With increasing understanding of the pelvic anatomy and experience in large tumor resection around the pelvis, this basic concept was modified by experienced tumor surgeons, resulting in the description of an anterior or posterior flap hemipelvectomy [98, 99].

As in patients with traumatic hemipelvectomy, often a complete leg avulsion or an open pelvic fracture with wounds along the inguinal and perineal crease are observed, a posterior flap hemipelvectomy is often initially performed.

20.17 Posterior Flap Hemipelvectomy

In tumor surgery, a five-step procedure is recommended [36, 99]. The patient is positioned in a semi-floppy position allowing a supine, an abducted-supine, and a slight floppy semi-lateral position.

Malawer recommended a three-step skin incision, consisting of a classical ilioinguinal incision, a perineal incision starting at the pubic symphysis along the inferior pubic ramus up to the ischial tuberosity, and a vertical incision from the iliac crest to the greater trochanter reaching the gluteal fold to connect with the perineal incision from medial. This incision is a modification of the technique described by Wu et al., which consists of four main incisions.

20.18 Skin Incision

The skin incision consists of four parts, including an ilioinguinal incision, a perineal crease incision, a gluteal fold incision, and the straight lateral incision [97].

20.19 Ilioinguinal Approach

The classical ilioinguinal approach is used to explore the intrapelvic retroperitoneal area. In the standard supine position, the abdominal muscles are detached from the iliac crest and the inguinal ligament and the rectus abdominus muscle is detached from the upper pubic rami. Above the inguinal ligament, the external iliac vessels, the femoral nerve, and the psoas muscle are ligated or transected. Mobilization of the peritoneum with the abdominal content proximal and medially allows identification of the common and internal iliac vessels. The ureter remains on the peritoneal reflection. The bladder is mobilized medially and the pubic symphysis is dissected under protection of the bladder and the urethra.

20.20 Perineal Approach

The perineal incision is performed with the surgeon standing between both abducted legs. It starts at the pubic tubercle running along the perineal crease parallel to the inferior pubic ramus up to the ischial tuberosity, where it ends at the beginning of the gluteal fold. Along the inferior ramus the ischiorectal space is exposed.

The pubic symphysis is dissected under protection of the bladder and the distal urethra using a large malleable and, in trauma cases, a subperiosteal detachment of the adjacent muscles from the pubic bone is performed. The sacrotuberous ligament is also released at its insertion.

20.20.1 Anatomy of the Ischiorectal Fossa (Ischiorectal Space) [100, 101]

The ischiorectal fossa is a triangular-shaped space with a lateral border, consisting of the obturator bone segment with the obturator internus muscle and a medial border, consisting of the levator ani and the external sphincter muscles. Posterior, the sacrotuberous ligament and gluteus maximus muscle border this space. Its apex, which is located approximately 5 cm proximal to the ischial tuberosity, is formed by the junction of the levator ani muscle and the obturator fascia.

Besides fatty tissue and lymphatics, the ischiorectal fossa contains the pudendal neurovascular bundle and inferior rectal neurovascular structures.

20.21 Posterior Flap Creation

The posterior gluteal flap is dissected in a semi-lateral position under some flexion and adduction of the extremity.

The perineal incision is extended parallel to the gluteal fold (inferior border of the gluteus maximus muscle) until reaching the greater trochanter and a vertical incision from the greater trochanteric area to the iliac crest at the level of the SI-joint is performed. A posterior fasciocutaneous flap is created along the iliotibial band and the greater trochanter towards the SI-joint.

Posteriorly, the remaining abdominal muscles, the quadratus lumborum and the erector spinae muscles are released from their insertions at the posterior iliac bone. A gluteus maximus muscle flap is created by mobilizing the muscle near its insertion at the linea aspera. The piriformis is released from its sacral origin and the sciatic nerve is dissected near the greater sciatic notch. The SI-joint is then dissected and mobilized and the pelvic floor ligaments are fully dissected.

> Whenever possible, a myocutaneous gluteus maximus flap should be developed to reduce the risk of flap necrosis.

20.22 Completion of Hemipelvectomy

In tumor surgery, the next step consists of dissecting the SI-joint. In traumatic cases, most often a complete hemipelvic dissociation is present with a complete injury (type C) of the SI-joint and, therefore, further dissection of the joint is not necessary. During mobilization of the hemipelvis, the peritoneal content is retracted medially and superiorly to avoid injury, as the peritoneum is often intact. The previously transected iliac vessels and the ureter are protected.

In rare cases of an attached iliac bone to an intact SI-joint, the ilium fracture is debrided and left in place for later prosthetic aftercare. If possible, the inferior gluteal vessels should be preserved.

The obturator neurovascular bundle is then dissected from anterior (ilioinguinal approach).

20.23 Inguinal Canal Reconstruction

In the initial trauma situation, the wound is left open or closed over a vacuum system. In stable hemodynamics, an inguinal canal reconstruction can be performed by suturing the lower medial corner of the gluteus maximus aponeurosis to the rectus abdominis and the medial portion of the abdominal muscles.

References

1. Spiers JP, Croce MA, Fabian TC. Traumatic hemipelvectomy. J Tenn Med Assoc. 1991;84(8):383–4.
2. Rodriguez MG, Phillips T, Conn AK, Cox EF. Traumatic hemipelvectomy: report of two survivors and review. J Trauma. 1983;23(7):615–20.
3. Turnbull H. A case of traumatic hindquarter amputation. Br J Surg. 1978;65:390.
4. Wade F, Macksood W. Traumatic hemipelvectomy: report of two cases with rectal involvement. J Trauma. 1965;5:554–62.
5. Lipkowitz G, Phillips T, Coren C, Spero C, Glassberg K, Tolete VF. Hemipelvectomy, a lifesaving operation in severe open pelvic injury in childhood. J Trauma. 1985;25(9):823–7.
6. Rieger H, Dietl KH. Traumatic hemipelvectomy: an update. J Trauma. 1998;45(2):422–6.
7. Pohlemann T, Paul C, Gänsslen A, Regel G, Tscherne H. Traumatic hemipelvectomy. Experiences with 11 cases. Unfallchirurg. 1996;99:304–12.
8. Cavadas P, Landín L. Traumatic complete hemipelvectomy treated with a free fillet flap. J Trauma. 2008;65:1551.
9. Teebken O, Lotz J, Gänsslen A, Pichlmaier A. Bilateral iliac artery dissection following severe complex unstable pelvic fracture. Interact Cardiovasc Thorac Surg. 2008;7:515–6.
10. Gänsslen A. Traumatic hemipelvectomy presentation. Graz: AO Trauma Course; 2018.

11. Labler L, Trentz O, Keel M. Traumatic Hemipelvectomy. Eur J Trauma. 2005;31:543–50.
12. Wang G, Zhou D, Shen W, Xin M, He J, Li Q, Tan G. Management of partial traumatic hemipelvectomy. Orthopedics. 2013;36:1340–5.
13. Beal SL, Blaisdell FW. Traumatic hemipelvectomy: a catastrophic injury. J Trauma. 1989;29(10):1346–51.
14. ATLS. Advanced Trauma Life Support program for doctors, 8th edn. 9th ed. Chicago: American College of Surgeons; 2012.
15. ATLS. Advanced Trauma Life Support program for doctors, 8th edn. 10th ed. Chicago: American College of Surgeons; 2016.
16. Rossaint R, Bouillon B, Cerny V, Coats T, Duranteau J, Fernández-Mondéjar E, Filipescu D, Hunt B, Komadina R, Nardi G, Neugebauer E, Ozier Y, Riddez L, Schultz A, Vincent J, Spahn D. The European guideline on management of major bleeding and coagulopathy following trauma: fourth edition. Crit Care. 2016;20:100.
17. Spahn D, Bouillon B, Cerny V, Duranteau J, Filipescu D, Hunt B, Komadina R, Maegele M, Nardi G, Riddez L, Samama C, Vincent J, Rossaint R. The European guideline on management of major bleeding and coagulopathy following trauma: fifth edition. Crit Care. 2019;23(1):98. https://doi.org/10.1186/s13054-019-2347-3.
18. Timmers T, Tiren D, Hulstaert P, Schellekens P, Leenen L. Traumatic hemipelvectomy: improvements in the last decennia illustrated by 2 case reports. Int J Surg Case Rep. 2012;3:246–52.
19. Williams D, Masood U, Norton M. A case of traumatic hemipelvectomy. Injury Extra. 2009;40:99–100.
20. Lasurt S, Combalia-Aleu A. Complete traumatic hemipelvectomy: report of a case after 19 years of follow-up. Injury. 2010;41:874–82.
21. Pansard R, Morais E, Alves A, Ramos Neto E, Copetti H, Lazzari B, Ribeiro T. Traumatic Hemipelvectomy: a rare and catastrophic injury: a case report. JBJS Case Connect. 2014;4:e44–e4. https://doi.org/10.2106/JBJS.CC.M.00252.
22. Chappel R, Herregods P, Gevaert M, Mortier G. Traumatic hemipelvectomy, case report. Med Phys. 1986;9:79–83.
23. Daub C, Jörger G, Kumle B, Thielemann F. Hemipelvektomie—eine Lösung bei Beckenzerreißung. Unfallchirurg. 2008;111:545.
24. Demetriades D, Salim A. Colon and rectal trauma and rectal foreign bodies. In: Wolff BG, et al., editors. The ASCRS textbook of colon and rectal surgery. New York: Springer; 2007. p. 322–34. ISBN-13: 978-0387-24846-2.
25. Evans RJ, Foss FE. Traumatic hemipelvectomy in combination with traumatic amputation of an upper extremity. J Trauma. 1984;24(4):342–5.
26. Ibn Majdoub Hassani K, Ait Laalim S, Benjelloun EB, Toughrai I, Mazaz K. Anorectal avulsion: an exceptional rectal trauma. World J Emerg Surg. 2013;8:40. https://doi.org/10.1186/1749-7922-8-40.
27. Ikpeme JO, Craig RP. Traumatic hemipelvectomy: a further case report and comments on management. Injury. 1987;18(3):206–10.
28. Jahn R, Heinrich P. Traumatic hemipelvectomy. Rare survival of accident sequela. Zentralbl Chir. 1990;115:631–4.
29. Johansson H, Olerud S. Traumatic hemipelvectomy in a ten-year-old boy. J Bone Joint Surg Am. 1971;53(1):170–2.
30. Joos A, Herold A, Palma P, Post S. Pfählungsverletzungen des Anus und des Rektums. Chirurg. 2006;77:781–9.
31. Kauvar D, Baskin T, Hayda R, Martin R. Complete traumatic hemipelvectomy resulting from roadside guardrail penetration of a motor vehicle. Injury Extra. 2005;36:454–7.
32. Kayalar M, Gürbüz Y, Süğün T, Kaplan I. Traumatic hemipelvectomy: case presentation. Acta Orthop Traumatol Turc. 2014;48:226.
33. Klasen HJ, Ten DH. Traumatic hemipelvectomy. J Bone Joint Surg (Br). 1989;71(2):291–5.
34. Klingman RR, Smith P, Stromberg B, Valentine J, Goebel M. Traumatic hemipelvectomy. Ann Plast Surg. 1991;27(2):156–63.
35. Losch A, Stankovic P, Stürmer K. Traumatische Hemipelvektomie und die postoperative Lebensqualität. Bericht über 2 Fälle 18 Jahre nach dem Trauma. Unfallchirurgie. 2001;104:91–4.
36. Malawer M, Henshaw R. Posterior flap hemipelvectomy. In: Malawer MM, Sugarbaker PH, editors. Musculoskeletal cancer surgery—treatment of sarcomas and allied disease. Amsterdam: Kluwer Academic Publishers; 2001. p. 319–36.
37. McPherson J. Traumatic hindquarter amputation. J Med Ass GA. 1960;49:494–5.
38. Moore WM, Brown JJ, Haynes JL, Viamontes L. Traumatic hemipelvectomy. J Trauma. 1987;27(5):570–2.
39. Nichter LS, Bolton LL, Rink D. Bony and soft tissue reconstruction and rehabilitation following traumatic hemipelvectomy, exsanguination and cardiac arrest. Ann Plast Surg. 1988;20(4):326–30.
40. Orcutt TW, Emerson CJ, Rhamy RK, Cocke WJ. Reconstruction and rehabilitation following traumatic hemipelvectomy and brachial plexus injury. J Trauma. 1974;14(8):695–704.
41. Osti M, Mittler C, Putzke M, Benedetto K. Traumatic hemipelvectomy: a report of successful reimplantation. Injury. 2006;37:1015–8.
42. Preiser T, Zaghdoud L, Schipper S. Das Leben nach einer Amputation im Bereich des Beckens. Eine Befragung von 56 Betroffenen. Orthopädie Technik. 2017;6:50–5.
43. Ricci S, Salesi M, Ricci P, Stagnitti F, Massoni F. Traumatic hemipelvectomy: surgical and medical-legal aspects. J Forensic Biomech. 2014;5:117. https://doi.org/10.4172/2090-2697.1000117.
44. Salamon T, Kassis S, Lerner A. Hemipelvectomy images of loss caused by war. BMJ Case Rep. 2014;2014:pii: bcr2014204479. https://doi.org/10.1136/bcr-2014-204479.
45. Sattel W, Stankovic P. Traumatische Hemiplevektomie - Bericht über 2 Fälle. Unfallchirurgie. 1984;10(4):213–5.
46. Siemens R, Flint LJ. Traumatic hemipelvectomy: a case report. J Trauma. 1977;17(3):245–7.
47. Smejkal R, Izant T, Born C, Delong W, Schwab W, Ross SE. Pelvic crush injuries with occlusion of the iliac artery. J Trauma. 1988;28(10):1479–82.
48. Smith A, Flinn D, Jang Y, Faulkner A, Dinnan K. Traumatic Hemipelvectomy with a contralateral unstable pelvis and acetabular fracture: a case report and review of the literature. JBJS Case Connect. 2017;7:e52. https://doi.org/10.2106/JBJS.CC.16.00211.
49. Thomas B, Dart B, Maxwell R. Split down the middle: a functional survivor of complete traumatic hemipelvectomy. J Trauma Acute Care Surg. 2012;72:E117. https://doi.org/10.1097/TA.0b013e31824442d4.
50. Ahern D, Kelly M, Courtney D, Rausa E, Winter D. The management of penetrating rectal and anal trauma: a systematic review. Injury. 2017;48:1133–8.
51. Cleary R, Pomerantz R, Lampman R. Colon and rectal injuries. Dis Colon Rectum. 2006;49:1203–22.
52. Gänsslen A, Hildebrand F, Pohlemann T. Management of hemodynamic unstable patients "in extremis" with pelvic ring fractures. Acta Chir Orthop Traumatol Cechoslov. 2012;79:193–202.
53. Petrone P, Velandia W, Dziaková J, Marini C. Treatment of complex perineal trauma. A review of the literature. Cir Esp. 2016;94:313–22.
54. Morey A, Brandes S, Dugi DR, Armstrong J, Breyer B, Broghammer J, Erickson B, Holzbeierlein J, Hudak S, Pruitt J, Reston J, Santucci R, Smith TR, Wessells H, Assocation AU. Urotrauma: AUA guideline. J Urol. 2014;192:327–35.
55. Smith Tr, Coburn M. Damage control maneuvers for urologic trauma. Urol Clin North Am. 2013;40:343–50.
56. Danisi FJ, Stromberg BV. Traumatic hemipelvectomy. Plast Reconstr Surg. 1985;76(6):945–7.
57. Heineck J, Seifert S, Rammelt S, Biewener A, Grass R, Zwipp H. Traumatische Hemipelvektomie Unfallchirurg. 2006;109:411–6.

58. Roumeliotis G, Ignatiuk A, Liew A, Llen M, Boyd K. Hemipelvis reconstruction in trauma: a case report and review. Plast Surg Case Studies. 2015;1:62–4.
59. Wu T, Wu X, Zhang X, Wu C, Zhang Y, Peng A. Management of traumatic hemipelvectomy: an institutional experience on four consecutive cases. Scand J Trauma Resusc Emerg Med. 2013;21:64. https://doi.org/10.1186/1757-7241-21-64.
60. Calonge W, Alova I, Ramos M, Martínez L, Lortat-Jacob S, Ochoa de Castro A, Lottmann H. Traumatic hemipelvectomy in children: report on 2 survivors with urological involvement. J Pediatr Surg. 2010;45:2260.
61. Dendrinos D, Koronias D, Papagiannopoulos G. Traumatic hemipelvectomy. A case report and comments on associated injuries. Acta Orthop Trauma Surg. 1992;111:293–5.
62. Ghimire N, Yan Z, Fang Y, Chirume W, Yang Y. Management of traumatic hemipelvectomy through ERAS pathway: a case report. Medicine (Baltimore). 2018;97:e12251. https://doi.org/10.1097/MD.0000000000012251.
63. González F, Amador E, Andrés Camilo Abril Aguilar A, Villamarín F, Amador Gutiérrez J, Vargas O. Traumatic hemipelvectomia in one year old girl. Report of case. Rev Fac Med Univ Nac Colomb. 2006;54:48–52.
64. Hutagalung E, Qomarrudin Q. Traumatic hemipelvectomy (amputae). Report of one case. Med J Indones. 2001;10:169–73.
65. Müller-Höcker C, Chuck N, Piewtsch U. Surviving major trauma with hemipelvectomy. J Anesth Inten Care Med. 2017;1:JAICM.MS.ID.555567.
66. Schoderbek R, Battaglia T, Dorf E, Kahler D. Traumatic hemipelvectomy: case report and literature review. Arch Orthop Trauma Surg. 2005;125:358–62.
67. Smith S, Devine M, Taddeo J, McAlister V. Injury profile suffered by targets of antipersonnel improvised explosive devices: prospective cohort study. BMJ Open. 2017;7:e014697. https://doi.org/10.1136/bmjopen-2016-014697.
68. Walker SJ, Johnson RH. Traumatic hemisomato-tmesis: a case report and review of the literature. Arch Emerg Med. 1989;6(1):66–9.
69. Cho K, Kang Y, Ahn J, Yoo T. Traumatic hemipelvectomy before body image has developed. Yonsai Med J. 1999;40:80–3.
70. Cooper M, Waterhouse N. Reconstruction of the pelvis using a composite island flap salveged from the remaining leg. Ann Plast Surg. 1987;19(3):276–83.
71. Faisham W, Azman W, Muzaffer T, Muslim D, Azhar A, Yahya M. Traumatic hemipelvectomy with free gluteus Maximus fillet flap covers—a case report. Maly Orthop J. 2012;6:37–9.
72. Ganapathy D. A report of traumatic hindquarter amputation. Injury. 1973;5:51–3.
73. Haim S, Laufer Y, Leonid K, Daniel G, Yechiel S, Zeev Z, Yury G, Asher K, Michal E. Hemipelvectomy after severe pelvic injury in factor VII deficiency toddler. Injury. 2015;46:1178.
74. Maull K, Sachatello C, Ernst C. The deep perineal laceration-an injury frequently associated with open pelvic fractures. J Trauma. 1977;17:685–8.
75. McLean E. Avulsion of the hindquarter. J Bone Joint Surg (Br). 1962;44:384–5.
76. Meester GL, Myerley WH. Traumatic hemipelvectomy: case report and literature review. J Trauma. 1975;15(6):541–5.
77. Oppenheim W, Tricker J, Smith R. Traumatic hemipeivectomy the tenth survivor: a case report and a review of the literature. Injury. 1977;9:307–12.
78. Ossewaarde S. Case study: traumatic Hemipelvectomy. Int J Trauma Nurs. 1997;3:13–7.
79. Palvolgyi M. Traumas hemipelvektia. Orv Hetil. 1969;110:970–13.
80. Raftos J, Ethell A, Bye W, Giles J, Cameron-Strange A. Traumatic hemipelvectomy associated with contralateral hip dislocation: case report. J Trauma. 1994;36(4):583–8.
81. Schuitema O, Mathijssen I, Mureau M. Reconstruction of an extensive traumatic hemipelvectomy defect using a free lower leg fillet flap. J Plast Reconstr Aesthet Surg. 2010;63:116–7.
82. Smith RJ. Hemipelvectomy for trauma: case report. J Natl Med Assoc. 1991;83(3):265–8.
83. Walcher F, Lustenberger T, Schmandra T, Byhahn C, Laurer H, Bingold T, Schweigkofler U, Winckler B, Walter G, Marzi I. First successful complete replantation of a traumatic hemipelvectomy: follow-up after 30 months. Injury. 2013;44:1252–6.
84. Wand JS. Traumatic hemipelvectomy without visceral injury. J Bone Joint Surg. 1990;72-B(2):327–8.
85. Wansbrough G, Boyne N, Pollard C. Re-ossification of the pelvis following hemipelvectomy for trauma. J Bone Joint Surg (Br). 2011;93:269–72.
86. Weiss W, Egan M, Amundson D. Traumatic hemipelvectomy: a survivable injury. Mil Med. 1994;159:164–6.
87. Wyndham N. A case of traumatic hindquarter amputation. The late Harley Turnbull. Br J Surg. 1978;65:390–2.
88. Yalniz E, Ciftdemir M, Durukan T. Traumatic Hemipelvectomy: a case report and a review of the literature. Eur J Trauma Emerg Surg. 2007;33:306–9.
89. Yildrim M, Dadaci M, Baycar Z, Ince B. Reconstruction and Management of Traumatic Hemipelvectomy: a case report. Emerg Med Open Access. 2018;8:381.
90. Torterolo E, Farcic A, Fernandez-Perdomo G, Luksemburg J, Bergalli L, Goller W. Traumatische hemipelvektomie. Akt Chir. 1976;2:309–16.
91. Glorion C, el Helou S, Lortat-Jacob S, Revillon Y, Vincent M, Rigault P. Traumatic amputation of the lower limb and traumatic hemipelvectomy. Report of 2 cases in children and review of the literature. Rev Chir Orthop Reparatrice Appar Mot. 1993;79:670–6.
92. Sham A, Spencer R. Traumatic hemipelvectomy. South African J Surg. 1988;69:79–81.
93. D'Alleyrand J, Fleming M, Gordon W, Andersen R, Potter B. Combat-related hemipelvectomy. J Surg Orthop Adv. 2012;21:38–43.
94. D'Alleyrand J, Lewandowski L, Forsberg J, Gordon W, Fleming M, Mullis B, Andersen R, Potter B. Combat-related hemipelvectomy: 14 cases, a review of the literature and lessons learned. J Orthop Trauma. 2015;29:493–8.
95. Giannou C, Baldan M, Molde Å. War Surgery—Volume 2: Working with limited resources in armed conflict and other situations of violence. Geneva: International Committee of the Red Cross; 2013.
96. Tintle S, Keeling J, Shawen S, Forsberg J, Potter B. Traumatic and trauma-related amputations: part I: general principles and lower-extremity amputations. J Bone Joint Surg Am. 2010;92:1852–2868.
97. Wu K, Guise E, Frost H, Mitchell C. The surgical technique for hindquarter amputation: a report of 19 cases. Acta Orthop Scand. 1977;48:479–86.
98. Malawer M, Wittig J. Chapter 20: Anterior flap hemipelvectomy. In: Malawer MM, Wittig JC, Bickels J, editors. Operative techniques in orthopaedic surgical oncology. Philadelphia, PA: Lippincott Williams & Wilkins; 2012.
99. Malawer M, Wittig J. Chapter 21: Posterior flap hemipelvectomy. In: Malawer MM, Wittig JC, Bickels J, editors. Operative techniques in orthopaedic surgical oncology. Philadelphia, PA: Lippincott Williams & Wilkins; 2012.
100. Arbelo-Cruz N, Lisanti C, Walker K, Schwope R, Bui-Mansfield L, Reiter M. Anatomy and pathology of the Ischiorectal Fossa. CDR. 2016;39:1–8.
101. Llauger J, Palmer J, Pérez C, Monill J, Ribé J, Moreno A. The normal and pathologic ischiorectal fossa at CT and MR imaging. Radiographics. 1998;18:61–82.

Urological Trauma

21

Axel Gänsslen and Stephan Grechenig

Clear recommendations are available to treat pelvic fracture associated urological trauma. In most cases, injury to the bladder and/or urethra is observed and, therefore, these entities are discussed in detail according to recent guidelines [1–3].

21.1 Bladder Trauma

Bladder injuries, in combination with pelvic ring fractures, are common, depending on the amount of forces acting on the pelvis, most often after motor vehicle accidents, falls, pelvic crush injuries, and blows to the lower abdomen [4–7].

In 60–90% of blunt trauma patients bladder injuries present with an additional pelvic fracture or intra-abdominal injuries [8]. In contrast, the overall rate of bladder injuries associated with pelvic fractures is only 3.6% [4, 6].

Bladder injuries present in decreasing rates as extraperitoneal, intraperitoneal, and combined intra- and extraperitoneal ruptures [5, 6, 8]. A combination of bladder and urethral injuries is observed in 4–15% [4, 5].

While almost all extraperitoneal ruptures are associated with pelvic fractures [7], intraperitoneal ruptures, more often, occur due to a sudden rise of the intravesical pressure.

Only 35% of bladder lacerations are located at the fracture area, while 65% are observed opposite of the fracture zone according to the "coup-contrecoup principle" [9].

Extraperitoneal bladder injury is most often the result of a shearing of the anterolateral bladder wall near the bladder base, more rarely due to direct fragment penetration [5]. Pelvic ring injuries with a fracture displacement >1 cm, a symphyseal disruption >1 cm, and pubic rami fractures are often associated with a bladder rupture [4, 10].

Intraperitoneal ruptures are most often caused by a blow to the pelvis or lower abdomen. The bladder dome is the weakest point and, therefore, the predominant injury site, with a full bladder being a risk factor [5]. In contrast to extraperitoneal lacerations, intraperitoneal ruptures are associated with pelvic fractures in 75% and are more frequently observed in polytraumatized patients, resulting in an increased mortality [11].

Approximately 5–10% of the bladder ruptures have a combined intra- and extraperitoneal injury pattern. In 20–50%, an additional urethral injury is present [12].

The most common clinical sign is a macrohematuria [5, 7]. Further signs include inability to void [5, 13], abdominal tenderness [7], suprapubic bruising [5, 13], abdominal distension [5, 13], swelling of scrotum, perineum, abdominal wall and/or thighs [5], uremia and elevated creatinine level [5] and, rarely, lower abdominal, perineal, and buttock wounds in penetrating injuries [13, 14].

The combination of a pelvic ring fracture with visible hematuria [15] should always lead to further imaging [5, 15].

Cystography is the preferred diagnostic modality for traumatic bladder injury (Fig. 21.1) [16, 17], performed by plain or CT cystography, both with a high sensitivity (90–95%) and specificity (100%) [7, 18]. Computed tomography cystography is preferred in the trauma patient to exclude or confirm further injuries [5].

Extraperitoneal bladder ruptures usually present as flame-shaped areas of contrast extravasation in the perivesical soft tissues [5], while intraperitoneal ruptures are observed with free contrast medium in the abdomen, highlighting bowel loops or other organs [5, 19].

Sandler et al. classified urinary bladder injury into five subtypes, based on cystographic evaluation (Figs. 21.2, 21.3, and 21.4) [20]:

A. Gänsslen (✉)
Department of Trauma Surgery, Orthopedics and Hand Surgery, Hospital Wolfsburg, Wolfsburg, Germany

S. Grechenig
Department of Orthopedics and Trauma Surgery, AUVA Trauma Hospital Klagenfurt, Klagenfurt, Austria

Department of Trauma Surgery, University Hospital Regensburg, Regensburg, Germany

A. Gänsslen et al. (eds.), *Pelvic Ring Fractures*, https://doi.org/10.1007/978-3-030-54730-1_21

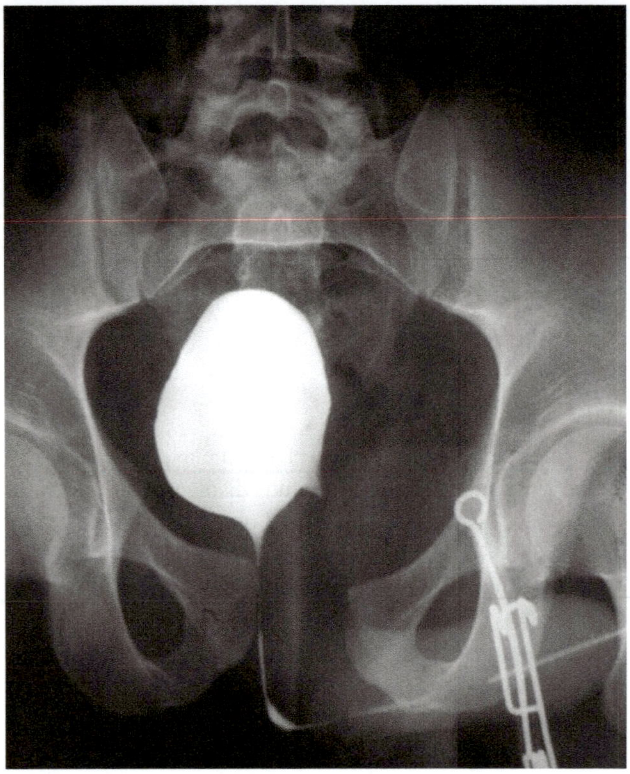

Fig. 21.1 Cystography in suspected traumatic bladder injury

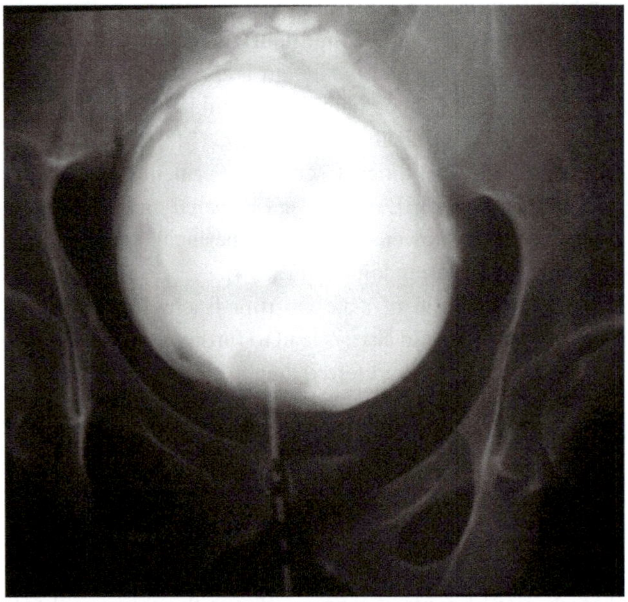

Fig. 21.2 Cystography of a type II intraperitoneal bladder rupture

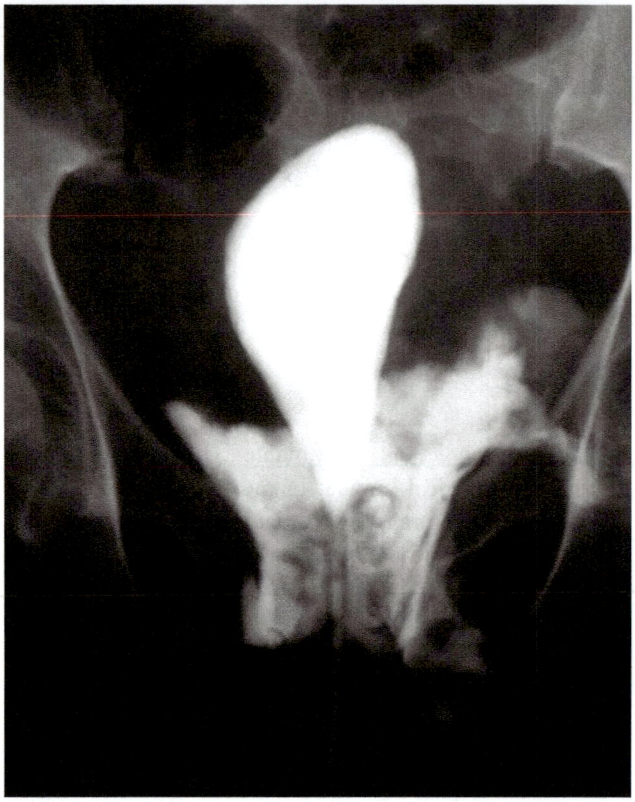

Fig. 21.3 Cystography of a type IVa extraperitoneal bladder rupture

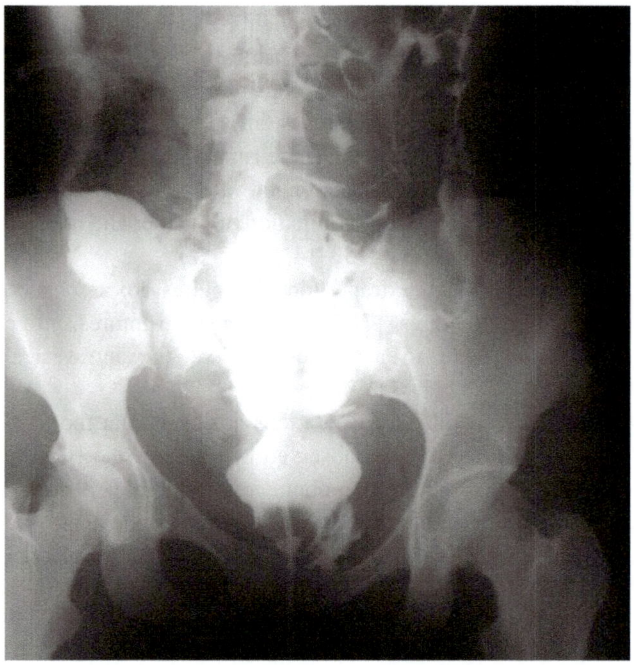

Fig. 21.4 Cystography of a type V combined intraperitoneal and extraperitoneal bladder rupture

- Type I: bladder contusion—incomplete rupture of the mucosa without cystographic abnormalities
- Type II: intraperitoneal rupture—contrast media in paracolic intraperitoneal spaces
- Type III: interstitial bladder injury—extremely rare, contrast media in the urinary bladder wall without extravasation
- Type IVa: simple extraperitoneal rupture—contrast media extravasation limited to the extraperitoneal part of the true pelvis
- Type IVb: complex extraperitoneal rupture—contrast media extravasation additionally within the anterior abdominal wall, the penis, the scrotum or the perineum indicating disruption of fascial structures within the true pelvis
- Type V: combined intraperitoneal and extraperitoneal bladder rupture

The "Organ Injury Scaling Committee" of the "American Association for the Surgery of Trauma" (AAST) presented an anatomical classification [21]:

- Grade I: bladder contusion with intramural hematoma and interstitial laceration of the mucous membrane
- Grade II: extraperitoneal bladder wall injury <2 cm
- Grade III: extraperitoneal bladder wall injury >2 cm or intraperitoneal urinary bladder injury <2 cm
- Grade IV: intraperitoneal bladder wall injury >2 cm
- Grade V: intra- or extraperitoneal bladder wall injury with involvement of the bladder neck or trigonum

Uncomplicated extraperitoneal blunt bladder injuries can sufficiently be treated conservatively by clinical observation, continuous bladder drainage, and antibiotic prophylaxis [5]. Surgical management is indicated with bladder neck involvement, perforation by bone fragments, concomitant rectal injury, or bladder entrapment at fracture sites [5, 13]. When open reduction of anterior pelvic ring injuries is performed, the accompanying bladder rupture should also be treated to prevent infections [5–8], by two-layer vesicorraphy (mucosa-detrusor) with absorbable sutures [5, 9, 22, 23].

Intraperitoneal ruptures should always be treated surgically [5, 13] as urine extravasation can lead to peritonitis, sepsis, and death [8].

In penetrating trauma, emergency exploration, debridement of devitalized bladder soft tissues, and primary bladder repair is recommended [14, 24] under antibiotic prophylaxis [24]. A midline exploratory cystotomy is performed to inspect the bladder wall and the distal ureters [5, 14].

In perineal avulsion injuries, with or without bladder tissue loss, a bladder wall substitute is recommended [25], as, otherwise, primary repair can lead to tension-related bladder wall necrosis.

21.2 Urethral Trauma

Straddle injuries of the pelvis often result in urethral injuries of the urethral bulbus [26], while the penile urethra is less commonly injured. Penetrating injuries are rare [14].

Clinical signs of urethral injuries in male patients include blood at the meatus, inability to void, hematuria, and dysuria. In the case of partial rupture, scrotal, perineal, and/or penile swelling, high-riding or impalpable prostate on rectal examination, and, as an indirect sign, the difficulty/inability to insert a catheter [2].

In female patients, blood at the urethral meatus and/or vaginal introitus, inability to void, labial swelling, vaginal laceration and hematuria in the case of partial rupture can be signs of urethral injuries [2].

The preferred diagnostic modality is the retrograde urethrography [26–28] to distinguish between anterior and posterior injury and between partial and complete injury. Alternatively, urethroscopy should be considered in acute urethral injury [26, 29, 30] or CT-evaluation after contrast media application (Fig. 21.5). In contrast, due to the short urethra in females, urethroscopy and vaginoscopy are favored as primary diagnostic tools [26, 28, 29].

The male anterior urethra is composed of the penile and bulbar urethra up to the urogenital diaphragm. Injuries to this area are more uncommon with additional pelvic fractures, while posterior urethral lesions include injuries between the diaphragm and internal urethral orifice in the trigone of the bladder.

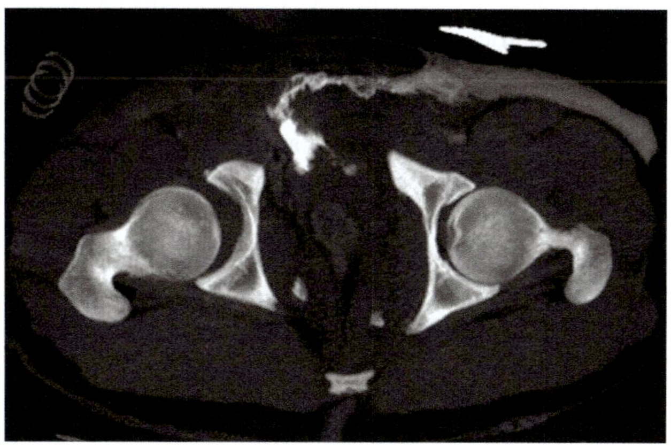

Fig. 21.5 CT-Cystography of a urethral rupture

The AAST classification of urethral injuries includes five degrees of severity [21]:

- Grade I: contusion—blood on the external urethra meatus; normal urethrogram
- Grade II: urethral elongation without extravasation in urethrography
- Grade III: partial rupture—extravasation of contrast media with accumulation of contrast agent in the bladder
- Grade IV: complete rupture—extravasation without contrast enhancement in the urinary bladder; urethral separation <2 cm
- Grade V: complete transection with urethral separation >2 cm or extension to the prostate or vagina

Anterior urethral injuries often are associated with bulbus contusion and, therefore, early reconstructive procedures were associated with worse outcomes [2].

Blunt posterior urethral injuries are more frequent. Regarding treatment, complete and partial ruptures should be distinguished and the time of possible intervention, which include immediate treatment within 48 h, delayed primary treatment between 2 days and 2 weeks, and deferred treatment after >3 months [26, 29].

In all urgent situations, suprapubic catheterization under direct visualization during laparotomy or using ultrasound guidance is favored, until classical urethral catheterization can be achieved [26, 28, 29, 31, 32].

Partial posterior urethral ruptures can sufficiently be treated by suprapubic or urethral catheterization [30–35]. Secondary strictures can be adequately treated by urethrotomy or urethroplasty [34, 35].

Complete posterior urethral ruptures are more difficult to treat. Acute treatment includes acute catheter realignment, exploration and primary repair, and isolated indirect treatment using suprapubic catheterization [2].

Acute catheter realignment avoids urethral distraction and can prevent strictures with a lower stricture rate than with suprapubic catheterization. Secondary restoration of urethral continuity is even simplified after stricture development [2].

In contrast, primary repair is associated with the risk of uncontrolled re-bleeding and high rates of impotence, incontinence, and secondary strictures [26, 36]. Also, endoscopic realignment procedures are not without risk, with reported 14–79% stricture rates and 10–55% impotence rates, while incontinence is uncommon (5%) [27, 34, 37].

Delayed primary realignment consists of primary suprapubic catheterization followed by endoscopic realignment [36, 38].

Deferred treatment nearly always has to deal with some posterior obliteration, which can be treated by urethroplasty or, with more worse results, with endoscopic incision [2].

Female urethral injuries are less common and are treated by early exploration and primary transvaginal repair [2].

References

1. Kitrey N, Djakovic N, Gonsalves M, Kuehhas F, Lumen N, Serafetinidis E, Sharma D, Summerton D. EAU guidelines on urological trauma. Arnhem: European Association of Urology; 2016.
2. Lumen N, Kuehhas F, Djakovic N, Kitrey N, Serafetinidis E, Sharma D, Summerton D. Review of the current management of lower urinary tract injuries by the EAU Trauma Guidelines Panel. Eur Urol. 2015;67:925–9.
3. Morey A, Brandes S, Dugi D III, Armstrong J, Breyer B, Broghammer J, Erickson B, Holzbeierlein J, Hudak S, Pruitt J, Reston J, Santucci R, Smit T III, Wessells H. Urotrauma: AUA guideline. Linthicum Heights: American Urological Association (AUA) Guideline; 2014.
4. Bjurlin M, Fantus R, Mellett M, Goble S. Genitourinary injuries in pelvic fracture morbidity and mortality using the National Trauma Data Bank. J Trauma. 2009;67:1033–9.
5. Gomez R, Ceballos L, Coburn M, Corriere JJ, Dixon C, Lobel B, McAninch J. Consensus statement on bladder injuries. BJU Int. 2004;94:27–32.
6. Pereira B, de Campos C, Calderan T, Reis L, Fraga G. Bladder injuries after external trauma: 20 years experience report in a population-based cross-sectional view. World J Urol. 2013;31:913–7.
7. Wirth G, Peter R, Poletti P, Iselin C. Advances in the management of blunt traumatic bladder rupture: experience with 36 cases. BJU Int. 2010;106:1344–9.
8. Deibert C, Spencer B. The association between operative repair of bladder injury and improved survival: results from the National Trauma Data Bank. J Urol. 2011;186:151–5.
9. Corriere JJ, Sandler C. Mechanisms of injury, patterns of extravasation and management of extraperitoneal bladder rupture due to blunt trauma. J Urol. 1988;139:43–4.
10. Avey G, Blackmore C, Wessells H, Wright J, Talner L. Radiographic and clinical predictors of bladder rupture in blunt trauma patients with pelvic fracture. Acta Radiol. 2006;13:573–9.
11. Peters P. Intraperitoneal rupture of the bladder. Urol Clin North Am. 1989;16:279–82.
12. Siemer S, Russ F, Mutschler W, Zwergel T. Verletzungen des harnableitenden Systems und Management im Rahmen des Polytraumas. Urologe A. 1997;36:513–22.
13. Tonkin J, Tisdale B, Jordan G. Assessment and initial management of urologic trauma. Med Clin North Am. 2011;95:245–51.
14. Cinman N, McAninch J, Porten S, Myers J, Blaschko S, Bagga H, Breyer B. Gunshot wounds to the lower urinary tract: a single-institution experience. J Trauma Acute Care Surg. 2013;74:725–30.
15. Morey A, Iverson A, Swan A, Harmon W, Spore S, Bhayani S, Brandes S. Bladder rupture after blunt trauma: guidelines for diagnostic imaging. J Trauma. 2001;51:683–6.
16. Lehnert B, Sadro C, Monroe E, Moshiri M. Lower male genitourinary trauma: a pictorial review. Emerg Radiol. 2014;21:67–74.
17. Patel B, Gayer G. Imaging of iatrogenic complications of the urinary tract: kidneys, ureters, and bladder. Radiol Clin North Am. 2014;52:1101–016.
18. Quagliano P, Delair S, Malhotra A. Diagnosis of blunt bladder injury: a prospective comparative study of computed tomography cystography and conventional retrograde cystography. J Trauma. 2006;61:410–21.
19. Alperin M, Mantia-Smaldone G, Sagan E. Conservative management of postoperatively diagnosed cystotomy. Urology. 2009;73:e17–9.
20. Sandler C, Hall J, Rodriguez M, Corriere JJ. Bladder injury in blunt pelvic trauma. Radiology. 1986;158:633–8.
21. Moore E, Cogbill T, Jurkovich G, McAninch J, Champion H, Gennarelli T, Malangoni M, Shackford S, Trafton P. Organ injury

scaling. III: chest wall, abdominal vascular, ureter, bladder, and urethra. J Trauma. 1992;33:337–9.
22. Fabozzi S, Schlossberg S, Jordan G. Urological trauma. Curr Opin Urol. 1995;5:127–32.
23. Thomas C, McAnnich J. Bladder trauma. AUA update series. 1989;8:242–7.
24. Al-Azzawi I, Koraitim M. Lower genitourinary trauma in modern warfare: the experience from civil violence in Iraq. Injury. 2014;45:885–8890.
25. Wu C, Lin C, Lin C. One-stage posttraumatic bladder reconstruction and soft-tissue coverage of the lower abdomen or perineum. Ann Plast Surg. 2010;64:65–8.
26. Brandes S. Initial management of anterior and posterior urethral injuries. Urol Clin North Am. 2006;33:87–95.
27. Figler B, Hoffler C, Reisman W, Carney K, Moore T, Feliciano D, Master V. Multi-disciplinary update on pelvic fracture associated bladder and urethral injuries. Injury. 2012;43:1242–9.
28. Rosenstein D, Alsikafi N. Diagnosis and classification of urethral injuries. Urol Clin North Am. 2006;33:73–85.
29. Chapple C, Barbagli G, Jordan G, Mundy A, Rodrigues-Netto N, Pansadoro V, McAninch J. Consensus statement on urethral trauma. BJU Int. 2004;93:1195–202.
30. Kielb S, Voeltz Z, Wolf J. Evaluation and management of traumatic posterior urethral disruption with flexible cystourethroscopy. J Trauma. 2001;50:36–40.
31. Mundy A, Andrich D. Urethral trauma. Part I: introduction, history, anatomy, pathology, assessment and emergency management. BJU Int. 2011;108:310–27.
32. Mundy A, Andrich D. Urethral trauma. Part II: types of injury and their management. BJU Int. 2011;108:630–50.
33. Koraitim M. Effect of early realignment on length and delayed repair of postpelvic fracture urethral injury. Urology. 2012;79:912–5.
34. Leddy L, Vanni A, Wessells H, Voelzke B. Outcomes of endoscopic realignment of pelvic fracture associated urethral injuries at a level 1 trauma center. J Urol. 2012;188:174–8.
35. Mouraviev V, Coburn M, Santucci R. The treatment of posterior urethral disruption associated with pelvic fractures: comparative experience of early realignment versus delayed urethroplasty. J Urol. 2005;173:873–6.
36. Koraitim M. Pelvic fracture urethral injuries: evaluation of various methods of management. J Urol. 1996;156:1288–91.
37. Sofer M, Mabjeesh N, Ben-Chaim J, Aviram G, Bar-Yosef Y, Matzkin H, Kaver I. Long-term results of early endoscopic realignment of complete posterior urethral disruption. J Endourol. 2010;24:1117–21.
38. Moudouni S, Patard J, Manunta A, Guiraud P, Lobel B, Guille F. Early endoscopic realignment of post-traumatic posterior urethral disruption. Urology. 2001;57:628–32.

Part III

Treatment of Pelvic Ring Injuries

Principles of Treatment of Pelvic Ring Injuries

22

Jan Lindahl and Axel Gänsslen

22.1 Treatment Concept

The incidence of pelvic fractures is estimated to be 17–35/100,000 individuals/year [1–6], with a 2–3-fold higher incidence in the elderly population [7, 8].

In Finland, pelvic ring disruptions account for 1% of fractures that require hospitalization among people ≥16 years [9]. Among multiple-trauma patients, up to 25% present with pelvic ring injuries [5, 10–12].

Unstable pelvic ring disruptions are relatively rare injuries, but they constitute a major cause of death and disability in high-energy polytrauma patients [13–17]. High-energy pelvic ring disruptions are frequently associated with multiple concomitant injuries. In those cases, hemorrhage, head injury, pelvic soft tissue trauma (open fractures with or without rectal or vaginal injuries), and primary systemic complications contribute to the high mortality rates [18–22]. However, pelvic fracture-associated urinary tract injuries and closed Morel-Lavallée degloving soft tissue injuries do not influence acute mortality, instead they may contribute to later morbidity [23].

Nevertheless, successful treatment of pelvic fractures remains one of the most challenging clinical problems associated with the management of blunt trauma patients.

The last decades have been a time of rapid progress in the control of pelvic fracture-related mortality and morbidity [13]. A better understanding of the anatomic features of these fractures, and an awareness of potential major, exsanguinating arterial hemorrhage have led to multidisciplinary approaches for controlling bleeding and temporarily stabilizing the pelvic ring [24].

Pelvic fracture management has undergone a remarkable evolution during the last five decades:

- <1970s Non-operative management
- 1970s External fixation became popular [25–27]
- 1980s Methods of ORIF were introduced [28–32]
- 1990s Mini-invasive percutaneous fixation techniques [33–36]
- Today Internal fixation the preferred treatment for posterior and anterior injured elements in type C pelvic ring injuries [14, 37, 38]

After the original description of a fracture-dislocation of the hemipelvis by Malgaigne in the nineteenth century [39, 40], non-operative treatment methods have been described.

These treatments involve combinations of bed rest, skeletal traction, closed reduction, a pelvic sling, and hip spica cast immobilization [17, 41–43]. None of these treatments permit early mobilization of the patient.

In the presence of prolonged bed rest, a high incidence of serious pulmonary, urinary, and psychological problems have been documented [44]. The non-operative modalities of treatment for unstable pelvic injuries have also been associated with serious chronic disabilities, such as a significant leg length discrepancy, severe lower back problems, markedly displaced non-unions, and, in women, obstetric problems [44–46].

Slätis and Huittinen performed late follow-ups for 65 of 163 Malgaigne fracture dislocations. They noted a 46% incidence of late sequelae, including oblique inclination of the pelvis upon sitting, a pelvic limp, disabling sacroiliac pain, signs of persistent damage to the lumbosacral plexus, and lower back pain [17].

Räf followed up 65 patients with double vertical pelvic fractures (type C injury) treated with non-operative methods [47]. They found a more favorable outcome in cases where the posterior pelvic ring injury passed through the posterior ilium. When the posterior injury ran through the SI-joint, a large proportion of patients had persistent back pain. Patients with sacral fractures often had persistent nerve injury in the leg (sacral plexus injury) and genitourinary disturbances.

After non-operative treatment methods, approximately 40–60% of patients with pelvic fractures reported persistent pain, and only half of these patients reached their previous working level [45, 48–51]. Many of these late complications

J. Lindahl
Orthopaedics and Trauma Surgery, Helsinki University Hospital, Helsinki, Finland

A. Gänsslen (✉)
Department of Trauma Surgery, Orthopedics and Hand Surgery, Hospital Wolfsburg, Wolfsburg, Germany

A. Gänsslen et al. (eds.), *Pelvic Ring Fractures*, https://doi.org/10.1007/978-3-030-54730-1_22

were attributable to inadequate reduction of the hemipelvis dislocation [52].

Non-operative management of (unstable) pelvic ring injuries is associated with a relevant complication and morbidity rates.

In the late 1970s, anterior external fixation devices became popular for treating unstable pelvic ring injuries. Patients definitively treated with anterior external fixation frames showed better early results compared to patients that received conservative treatment [25–27, 53, 54]. The use of a trapezoid compression frame markedly diminished the severity of fracture pain, due to stabilization of the fracture fragments [27, 55].

An anterior external fixation frame can restore pelvic bony stability in some, but not all, pelvic fracture types [29]. It has been well established that an anterior external frame is beneficial for treating AP compression pelvic ring instability (type B open book injuries) [56]. However, this approach cannot produce sufficient posterior compression across the sacroiliac joint for adequate stabilization of the posterior pelvis. Moreover, later biomechanical and clinical studies showed that anterior external frames did not restore sufficient stability to an unstable type C disruption of the pelvic ring; treated patients could not ambulate without risking redisplacement of the fracture, even when no weight was carried on the affected side [29, 51, 57, 58].

The advantage of an external fixator is that it is easy to apply. External fixators can be used when internal fixation is hazardous for injuries of the anterior pelvic ring, due to potential contamination from rectal or abdominal injuries. External fixation devices are also easy to remove. A disadvantage is that, because they are external devices, they can interfere with sitting and mobilization. Pin sites require care, and pin site infections are typical. Additionally, it is difficult to obtain and maintain an anatomical reduction of anterior and posterior pelvic ring injuries with an anterior frame.

The various anterior external fixation frames are relatively similar in stability. Ponsen et al. compared the stiffness of several current anterior external fixation systems with that of an aluminium replica of the human pelvis with a type C injury [59]. They found that all the tested external fixators provided low stability.

However, the single bar systems were stiffer and performed better than frame configurations. The difference in performance was attributed to the use of 6-mm pins instead of 5-mm pins; that is, two 6-mm pins provided 15% more stiffness than three 5-mm pins, and to the fact that the single bar systems employed stiffer bars than the more slender rods used in the frames. Other factors were not significant, including the placement of the pins in a cranial (iliac crest) or ventral (AIIS) location.

However, biomechanical and clinical studies showed that these frames had limitations, when used for the most unstable pelvic injuries [29, 51, 57, 58].

External fixation of pelvic fractures increased the rate of acceptable results, but was still associated with reduced overall stability.

Prior to the 1980s, operative treatments for pelvic fractures were the exception to the rule. In 1913, Albin Lambotte (1866–1955), the father of modern osteosynthesis, published a book that described different operative techniques for pelvic stabilization [60]. These techniques included cerclage wiring of the symphysis pubis, sacral bar osteosynthesis, iliosacral screw fixation, and retrograde screw fixation of pubic rami fractures [61]. After recognizing the correlation between late deformities, instabilities, and severe pain, the common opinion gradually changed.

Currently, a century after the work of Lambotte, internal fixation is the preferred treatment for unstable pelvic ring disruptions.

In type C pelvic injuries, the anterior and posterior parts of the pelvic ring are disrupted, which leads to vertical translational and rotational instability. The goals of treatment are realignment, restoration of pelvic ring stability, and decompression of the sacral plexus nerve roots, when indicated. Biomechanical studies have shown that, in type C injuries, the best stability can be achieved by internal fixation of the posterior and anterior pelvic ring injuries [51, 62]. Thus, methods of open reduction and internal fixation (ORIF) were introduced [21, 28, 30–32, 63, 64]. More recently, closed reduction and percutaneous screw fixation techniques have been developed [33–36].

Various methods for pelvic fracture stabilization have been described. Internal fixation has become the preferred treatment for unstable posterior pelvic ring injuries [30, 38, 64, 65]; however, indications for fixation of anterior pelvic ring injuries have been a controversial issue [28, 35, 36, 66]. Many studies have focused on emergency management and initial treatment, but there is a lack of adequate follow-up studies on pelvic ring injuries.

The overall aim of surgical treatment for unstable pelvic ring injuries is to restore the pelvic anatomy, thus allowing normal function with a low rate of complications.

It is difficult to evaluate the efficacy of surgical stabilization of the pelvic ring based on published long-term studies, because different treatment concepts have been used and the majority of studies used non-comparable evaluation parameters. Additionally, no standardized measurement instrument exists to analyze the clinical and radiological data acquired for assessing pelvic ring injuries.

In a systematic review of the English literature over the last 30 years, Papakostidis et al. concluded that "the current literature is insufficient to provide clear evidence for clinical decision-making in regards to the optimal treatment of unstable pelvic ring injuries".

Presently, there is no consensus on the optimal fixation technique of the pelvic ring, neither for posterior injuries [14, 67, 68] nor for anterior ring injuries [28, 30, 69].

Present recommendations from literature analysis allow the following conclusions:

- Fixation of all the injured elements of the pelvic ring in type C injuries yield better anatomical results compared to more non-operative therapeutic strategies [14]
- Type C injuries [37, 38, 67, 70–72]
  - reasons for unsatisfactory functional results include fracture malreduction, loss of reduction, and permanent lumbosacral plexus injury
  - 30–50% of patients suffer from significant persistent pain and have sexual or urogenital disturbances
  - an excellent or good overall functional result can be expected in 70–80%
  - 65–90% healing with residual displacement <5 mm is observed, depending on the type of pelvic ring stabilization
  - studies support the concept of combined anterior and posterior stabilization
- Open-book Type B injuries [70–74]
  - moderate disability and 30–40% relevant persistent pain can be expected, despite a high rate of anatomical healing
  - 70–90% excellent and good functional results when symphyseal plating is performed
  - single external fixation seems to lead to worse results in open-book injuries
- Lateral compression Type B injuries [70, 71, 75]
  - a low rate of permanent pain (5–15%) can be expected, despite anatomical healing of the pelvis in only 70–75%
  - an excellent or good overall functional result is observed in 75–90%

In summary, successful treatment of pelvic fractures remains one of the most challenging clinical problems in the management of patients with blunt trauma.

There is a wide range of completely different types of pelvic ring injury and different treatment concepts are used to treat those injuries. It is still unknown, whether to start fixation first at the anterior or posterior pelvic ring.

A stability-based concept of pelvic ring stabilization seems to be advantageous.

22.2 Aftercare

No uniform postoperative treatment concept for pelvic ring injuries exists.

It is completely unclear how to deal with unilateral or bilateral injuries regarding partial or full weight bearing (when and how) and if a stabilization-dependent mobilization is required.

Based on the AOTrauma Book on Pelvic Ring injuries [76], the following recommendations can be found:

- *Type A injuries*: adequate postoperative antibiotics, deep vein prophylaxis, mobilization with a physiotherapist, appropriate nursing care (posterior wounds (?)), attention to potential pressure effects, but no comments on X-ray re-evaluation were stated.
- *Type B1 open book injuries*: immediate mobilization from bed to chair, weight bearing on the surgeons preference, weight bearing as tolerated (minor B1 injuries), 6–8 weeks partial weight bearing (more unstable pattern), physical therapy to avoid muscle atrophy, no abdominal strengthening for 6 weeks, X-rays at 6, 12, 24 weeks.
- *Type B2 injuries*: protected weight bearing on the side of posterior ring injury, X-rays, when the patient mobilizes to ensure maintained reduction and full weight bearing after 8–12 weeks.

- *Type B3 and C injuries*: air mattress, frequent turning (soft-tissues), DVT prophylaxis, mobilization to chair and on crutches, isometric exercises (abdominal, buttocks, lower extremity muscles); in bilateral injuries 6–8 weeks restricted chair mobilization, followed by 6 weeks assisted ambulation.
- *Sacral fractures*: detailed and daily wound inspection, partial weight bearing after drainage removal; full weight bearing after an expected healing time of 8–12 weeks; X-ray control after 6 and 12 weeks, and after 6 and 12 months.
- *Lumbopelvic stabilization (spinopelvic)*: immediate progressive weight bearing or weight bearing as tolerated; X-ray control at 1, 4, 8 and 12 weeks.
- *Lumbopelvic injury (percutaneous iliosacral screw)*: 2–3 months non-weight bearing in thoraco-lumbar-sacral orthosis; x-ray control at 1, 4, 8, and 12 weeks.

Overall, a fracture type dependent postoperative care concept is presented with the lack, that not every possible part of after-treatment is sufficiently described (e.g. X-ray control, length and type of mobilization, etc.) and no data are available how to perform conservative treatment.

Analysis of published reports on these fracture types resulted in conflicting recommendations!

Type B1 open book injuries: Several authors did NOT report on their after-treatment [72, 74, 77], while Pohlemann et al. recommended partial weight bearing (1/5 BW) for 8–12 weeks and X-rays after start of mobilization, prior to discharge, and at 3 months, respectively [78], and Lindahl et al. recommended mobilization on crutches during the first week postoperatively [71].

In LC lateral compression injuries (type B2), non-weight-bearing for 3 months corresponding to the ipsilateral posterior pelvic injury was recommended, and when weight bearing was initiated, a formal therapy was instituted working on ROM, strengthening, and conditioning. Follow-up X-rays were performed after 2, 6, and 12 weeks, 6 months, 1 year, and 2 years, respectively [79]. Lindahl et al. again recommended early mobilization on crutches during the first week postoperatively [71].

For type C-injuries, depending on the chosen posterior treatment concept, some data on aftercare are available.

Type C-injuries with ilio-iliacal plate stabilization: after initial sit-up and turning, active or passive exercises are initiated once pain was tolerated, and crutch-assisted walking with partial weight bearing was allowed. The start of partial weight bearing differs between authors and was initiated immediately or after 2, 3, 4, or 6 weeks, while full weight bearing was started after 6, 10, or 12 weeks (after radiological healing), respectively. Re-evaluation of fracture healing using X-rays was proposed after 3, 6, 10, and 12 weeks, and after 6 months and 1 year [67, 80–85].

After TIFI stabilization of type C-injuries (transiliacal internal fixator), partial weight bearing was started after 2 or 5 weeks [86, 87], while in geriatric patients, full weight bearing was initiated already on day 1 [88].

Only few proposals are published regarding complete SI-joint dislocations, treated with anterior plate osteosynthesis. Partial weight bearing of the injured side with 15 kg BW for 8–12 weeks was followed by full weight bearing after (8–)12 weeks and X-ray controls were recommended after 1 and 14 days and after 3 and 6 months [89, 90].

Despite its frequent use, only sparse and indifferent data on after-treatment after iliosacral screw fixation of posterior pelvic ring injuries are available.

Partial weight bearing with 15 kg BW was allowed for 6 or 8–12 weeks with corresponding full weight bearing, pain dependent after 6 or 8–12 weeks. X-rays were analyzed for reduction control and fracture healing after 1 day and after 3 and 6 months [91, 92]. In contrast, full weight bearing was allowed once straight leg rise on the affected side was possible [93].

Only for spinopelvic stabilization of unstable sacral fractures, a more or less standardized aftercare concept can be gained from published data, with typically immediate weight bearing or weight bearing as tolerated [94–97]. X-ray control was proposed after 1, 4, 8, and 12 weeks, respectively.

Presently, it is completely unknown if standardized concepts are necessary. No adequate definition of touch bearing, partial and full weight bearing is available and, from the scientific basis, no correlations exist with implant failure rates or type of osteosynthesis.

Thus, the aftercare of patients with pelvic ring injuries is insufficiently described in the available literature.

Interestingly, historical aftercare in patients with uncemented total hip arthroplasty for long time was accepted with 3 months of partial weight bearing to avoid secondary shortening, while today, even in supra-geriatric patients, immediate full weight bearing is initiated. As these patients are normally not able to restrict their weight bearing, even after pelvic ring stabilizations, full weight bearing is performed early [88].

Therefore, the recommendations regarding aftercare after surgical stabilization of the pelvic ring in the following chapters are only author-dependent guidances and are NOT based on scientific evidence.

References

1. Balogh Z, King K, Mackay P, McDougall D, Mackenzie S, Evans J, Lyons T, Deane S. The epidemiology of pelvic ring fractures: a population-based study. J Trauma. 2007;63:1066–73.
2. Court-Brown C, Caesar B. Epidemiology of adult fractures: a review. Injury. 2006;37:691–7.
3. Menon M, Walker J, Court-Brown C. The epidemiology of fractures in adolescents with reference to social deprivation. J Bone Joint Surg Br. 2008;90:1482–6.
4. Muir L, Boot D, Gorman D, Teanby D. The epidemiology of pelvic fractures in the Mersey region. Injury. 1996;27(3):199–204.
5. Ragnarsson B, Jacobsson B. Epidemiology of pelvic fractures in a swedish county. Acta Orthop Scand. 1992;63(3):297–300.
6. Verbeek D, Ponsen K, Fiocco M, Amodio S, Leenen L, Goslings J. Pelvic fractures in the Netherlands: epidemiology, characteristics and risk factors for in-hospital mortality in the older and younger population. Eur J Orthop Surg Traumatol. 2018;28:197–205.
7. Court-Brown C, McQueen M. Global forum: fractures in the elderly. J Bone Joint Surg Am. 2016;98:e36.
8. Kannus P, Parkkari J, Niemi S, Sievänen H. Low-trauma pelvic fractures in elderly finns in 1970-2013. Calcif Tissue Int. 2015;97:577–80.
9. Somersalo A, Paloneva J, Kautiainen H, Lönnroos E, Heinänen M, Kiviranta I. Incidence of fractures requiring inpatient care. Acta Orthop. 2014;85:525–30.
10. Gänsslen A, Pohlemann T, Paul C, Lobenhoffer P, Tscherne H. Epidemiology of pelvic ring injuries. Injury. 1996;27(Suppl 1):13–20.
11. Giannoudis P, Grotz M, Tzioupis C, Dinopoulos H, Wells G, Bouamra O, Lecky F. Prevalence of pelvic fractures, associated injuries, and mortality: the United Kingdom perspective. J Trauma. 2007;63:875–83.
12. Matewski D, Szymkowiak E, Bilinski P. Analysis of management of patients with multiple injuries of the locomotor system. Int Orthop. 2008;32:753–8.
13. Hauschild O, Strohm P, Culemann U, Pohlemann T, Suedkamp N, Koestler W, Schmal H. Mortality in patients with pelvic fractures: results from the German pelvic injury register. J Trauma. 2008;64:449–55.
14. Papakostidis C, Kanakaris N, Kontakis G, Giannoudis P. Pelvic ring disruptions: treatment modalities and analysis of outcomes. Int Orthop. 2009;33:329–38.
15. Rothenberger D, Fischer R, Perry J. Major vascular injuries secondary to pelvic fractures: an unsolved clinical problem. Am J Surg. 1978;136:660–2.
16. Rothenberger D, Fischer R, Strate R, Velasco R, Perry J. The mortality associated with pelvic fractures. Surgery. 1978;84(3):356–9.
17. Slätis P, Huittinen V. Double vertical fractures of the pelvis: a report on 163 patients. Acta Chir Scand. 1972;138:799–807.
18. Burgess A, Eastridge B, Young J, Ellison T, Ellison P, Poka A, Bathon G, Brumback R. Pelvic ring disruption: effective classification systems and treatment protocols. J Trauma. 1990;30(7):848–56.
19. Holstein J, Culemann U, Pohlemann T, Holstein JH, Culemann U, Pohlemann T. Working group mortality in pelvic fracture patients. Clin Orthop. 2012;470:2090–7.
20. Mucha PJ, Welch TJ. Hemorrhage in major pelvic fractures. Surg Clin North Am. 1988;68(4):757–73.
21. Pohlemann T, Bosch U, Gänsslen A, Tscherne H. The Hannover experience in management of pelvic fractures. Clin Orthop. 1994;305:69–80.
22. Tscherne H, Pohlemann T, Gansslen A. Classification, staging, urgency and indications in pelvic injuries. Zentralbl Chir. 2000;125(9):717–24.
23. Lynch T, Martinez-Pineiro L, Plas E, Serafetinides E, Turkeri L, Santucci R, Hohenfellner M. EAU guidelines on urological trauma. Eur Urol. 2005;47:1–15.
24. Flint L, Cryer H. Pelvic fracture: the last 50 years. J Trauma. 2010;69:483–8.
25. Lansinger O, Karlsson J, Berg U, Mare K. Unstable fractures of the pelvis treated with a trapezoid compression frame. Acta Orthop Scand. 1984;55:325–9.
26. Slätis P, Karaharju E. External fixation of the pelvic girdle with a trapezoid compression frame. Injury. 1975;7:53–6.
27. Slätis P, Kraharju E. External fixation of unstable pelvic fractures: experiences in 22 patients treated with a trapezoid compression frame. Clin Orthop. 1980;151:73–9.
28. Hirvensalo E, Lindahl J, Böstman O. A new approach to the internal fixation of unstable pelvic fractures. Clin Orthop. 1993;297:28–32.
29. Kellam J. The role of external fixation in pelvic disruptions. Clin Orthop. 1989;241:66–82.
30. Matta J, Saucedo T. Internal fixation of pelvic ring fractures. Clin Orthop. 1989;242:83–97.
31. Tile M. Pelvic ring fractures: should they be fixed? J Bone Joint Surg. 1988;70-B:1–12.
32. Ward E, Tomasin J, van der Griend R. Open reduction and internal fixation of vertical shear pelvic fractures. J Trauma. 1987;27(3):291–5.
33. Ebraheim NA, Rusin JJ, Coombs RJ, Jackson WT, Holiday B. Percutaneous computed-tomography-stabilization of pelvic fractures: preliminary report. J Orthop Trauma. 1987;1(3):197–204.
34. Routt M. Fixation of pelvic ring disruptions. Orthopaedic knowledge update trauma. Published by AAOS; 1996. p. 241–8.
35. Routt M, Kregor P, Simonian P, Mayo K. Early results of percutaneous iliosacral screws placed with the patient in the supine position. J Orthop Trauma. 1995;9(3):207–14.
36. Routt M, Simonian P. Internal fixation of pelvic ring disruptions. Injury. 1996;27(Suppl 2):20–30.
37. Lindahl J, Hirvensalo E. Outcome of operatively treated type-C injuries of the pelvic ring. Acta Orthop. 2005;76:667–78.
38. Tornetta P, Matta J. Outcome of operatively treated unstable posterior pelvic ring disruptions. Clin Orthop. 1996;329:186–93.
39. Malgaigne J. Traites des fractures et des luxations. Paris: J.B. Balliere; 1847.
40. Malgaigne J. Die Knochenbrüche und Verrenkungen für praktische Aerzte, Wundärzte und Studirende. Erster Band: Knochenbrüche. (deutsche Übersetzung der französischen Ausgabe von 1847). Bearbeitet von Burger C, editor. Stuttgart: Rieger'sche Verlagsbuchhandlung; 1850.
41. Holdsworth F. Dislocation and fracture-dislocation of the pelvis. J Bone Joint Surg. 1948;30-B(3):461–6.
42. Peltier L. Complications associated with fractures of the pelvis. J Bone Joint Surg. 1965;47A:1060–9.
43. Semba R, Yasukawa K, Gustillo R. Critical analysis of results 53 Malgaigne fractures of the pelvis. J Trauma. 1983;23(6):535–7.
44. Trunkey D, Chapman M, Lim R, Dunphy J. Management of pelvic fractures in blunt trauma injury. J Trauma. 1974;14:912–23.
45. Henderson R. The long-term result of nonoperatively treated major pelvic disruption. J Orthop Trauma. 1989;3(1):41–7.
46. Langloh N, Johnson E Jr, Jackson C. Traumatic sacroiliac disruptions. J Trauma. 1972;12:931–5.
47. Räf L. Double vertical fractures of the pelvis. Acta Chir Scand. 1966;131:298–305.
48. Fell M, Meißner A, Rahmanzadeh R. Langzeitergebnisse nach konservativer Behandlung von Beckenringverletzungen und Konsequenzen für das heutige Mangement. Zentr Bl Chir. 1995;120:899–903.
49. Pohlemann T, Gänsslen A, Schellwald O, Culemann U, Tscherne H. Outcome after pelvic ring injuries. Injury. 1996;27(Suppl 2):S-B31–8.

50. Tile M. Pelvic fractures: operative versus nonoperative treatment. Orthop Clin North Am. 1980;11(3):423–64.
51. Tile M. Fractures of the pelvis and acetabulum. 2nd ed. Baltimore: Williams & Wilkins; 1995.
52. Bucholz R. The pathological anatomy of malgaigne fracture-dislocations of the pelvis. J Bone Joint Surg. 1981;63-A(3):400–4.
53. Carabalona P, Rabichong P, Bonnel F, Peruchon E, Peguret F. Apports du fixateur externe dans le disjonctions du pubis and de l'articulation sacro-iliaque. Montpell Chir. 1973;19:61–70.
54. Gunterberg B, Goldie I, Slätis P. Fixation of pelvic fractures and dislocations. Acta Orthop Scand. 1978;49:278–86.
55. Karaharju E, Slätis P. External fixation of double vertical pelvic fractures with a trapezoid compression frame. Injury. 1978;10:142–5.
56. Gilliland M, Ward R, Barton R, Miller P, Duke J. Factors affecting mortality in pelvic fractures. J Trauma. 1982;22(8):691–3.
57. Mears D, Fu F. External fixation in pelvic fractures. Orthop Clin North Am. 1980;11:465–79.
58. Wild J, Hanson G, Tullos H. Unstable fractures of the pelvis treated by external fixation. J Bone Joint Surg. 1982;64-A(7):1010–9.
59. Ponsen K, van Dijke G, Joosse P, Snijders C. External fixators for pelvic fractures. Comparison of the stiffness of current systems. Acta Orthop Scand. 2003;74:165–71.
60. Lambotte A. Chirurgie opératoire des fractures. répité. Bruxelles. 1948;1913:126–44. Société Franco-Belge D'Editions Scientifiques.
61. Rommens P, Tile M. A short history of pelvic trauma surgery. Part 1; The pelvic ring: from Malgaigne to the present. AO Dialoque. 2003;16(28–30).
62. Leighton R, Waddell J, Bray T, Chapman M, Simpson L, Martin R, Sharkey N. Biomechanical testing of new and old fixation devices for vertical shear fractures of the pelvis. J Orthop Trauma. 1991;5(3):313–7.
63. Goldstein A, Phillips T, Sclafani S, Scalea T, Duncan A, Goldstein J, Panetta T, Shaftan G. Early open reduction and internal fixation of the disrupted pelvic ring. J Trauma. 1986;26(4):325–33.
64. Kellam JF, McMurtry RY, Paley D, Tile M. The unstable pelvic fracture—operative treatment. Orthop Clin North Am. 1987;18(1):25–41.
65. Pohlemann T, Tscherne H. Die operative Therapie von Sakrumfrakturen. Oper Orthop Traumatol. 1996;8(1):55–72.
66. Matta J, Tornetta P. Internal fixation of unstable pelvic ring injuries. Clin Orthop. 1996;329:129–40.
67. Suzuki T, Hak D, Ziran B, Adams S, Stahel P, Morgan S, Smith W. Outcome and complications of posterior transiliac plating for vertically unstable sacral fractures. Injury. 2009;40:405–9.
68. van Zwienen C, van den Bosch E, van Dijke G, Snijders C, van Vugt A. Cyclic loading of sacroiliac screws in Tile C pelvic fractures. J Trauma. 2005;58:1029–34.
69. Simonian P, Schwappach J, Routt M, Agnew S, Harrington R, Tencer A. Evaluation of new plate designs for symphysis pubis internal fixation. J Trauma. 1996;41(3):498–502.
70. Gänsslen A, Lindahl J. Evaluation tools and outcomes after osteosynthesis of unstable type B and C pelvic ring injuries. Acta Chir Orthop Traumatol Cechoslov. 2013;80:305–20.
71. Lindahl J, Hirvensalo E, Bostman O, Santavirta S. Failure of reduction with an external fixator in the management of injuries of the pelvic ring. Long-term evaluation of 110 patients. J Bone Joint Surg Br. 1999;81(6):955–62.
72. Rommens PM, Hessmann MH. Staged reconstruction of pelvic ring disruption: differences in morbidity, mortality, radiologic results, and functional outcomes between B1, B2/B3, and C-type lesions. J Orthop Trauma. 2002;16(2):92–8.
73. Gruen G, Leit M, Gruen R, Garrison H, Auble T, Peitzman A. Functional outcome of patients with unstable pelvic ring fractures stabilized with open reduction and internal fixation. J Trauma. 1995;39(5):838–44.
74. van Loon P, Kuhn S, Hofmann A, Hessmann M, Rommens P. Radiological analysis, operative management and functional outcome of open book pelvic lesions: a 13-year cohort study. Injury. 2011;42:1012–9.
75. Laflamme G, Delisle J, Rouleau D, Uzel A, Leduc S. Lateral compression fractures of the superior pubic ramus with intra-articular extension. J Bone Joint Surg. 2009;91-B:1208–12.
76. Tile M, Helfe DL, Kellam JF, Vrahas M, editors. AO trauma, fractures of the pelvis and acetabulum (AO): principles and methods of management. 4th ed. AO Education AO Foundation; 2015.
77. Rommens P, Gercek E, Hansen M, Hessmann M. [Mortality, morbidity and functional outcome after open book and lateral compression lesions of the pelvic ring. A retrospective analysis of 100 type B pelvic ring lesions according to Tile's classification]. Unfallchirurg. 2003;106:542–9.
78. Pohlemann T, Gänsslen A. Die Operation der Symphysensprengung. Oper Orthop Traumatol. 1999;11:149–59.
79. Hoffmann M, Jones C, Sietsema D. Persistent impairment after surgically treated lateral compression pelvic injury. Clin Orthop Relat Res. 2012;470:2161–72.
80. Ayoub M, Gad H, Seleem O. Standalone percutaneous transiliac plating of vertically unstable sacral fractures: outcomes, complications, and recommendations. Eur Spine J. 2016;25:1153–62.
81. Chen W, Hou Z, Su Y, Smith W, Liporace F, Zhang Y. Treatment of posterior pelvic ring disruptions using a minimally invasive adjustable plate. Injury. 2013;44:975–80.
82. Dolati B, Larndorfer R, Krappinger D, Rosenberger R. Stabilization of the posterior pelvic ring with a slide-insertion plate. Oper Orthop Traumatol. 2007;19:16–31.
83. Hao T, Changwei Y, Qiulin Z. Treatment of posterior pelvic ring injuries with minimally invasive percutaneous plate osteosynthesis. Int Orthop. 2009;33:1435–9.
84. Kobbe P, Hockertz I, Sellei R, Reilmann H, Hockertz T. Minimally invasive stabilisation of posterior pelvic-ring instabilities with a transiliac locked compression plate. Int Orthop. 2012;36:159–64.
85. Krappinger D, Larndorfer R, Struve P, Rosenberger R, Arora R, Blauth M. Minimally invasive transiliac plate osteosynthesis for type C injuries of the pelvic ring: a clinical and radiological follow-up. J Orthop Trauma. 2007;21:595–602.
86. Dienstknecht T, Berner A, Lenich A, Nerlich M, Fuechtmeier B. A minimally invasive stabilizing system for dorsal pelvic ring injuries. Clin Orthop. 2011;469:3209–17.
87. Salášek M, Pavelka T. [Minimally invasive fixation of the pelvic ring with a transiliacal internal fixator]. Acta Chir Orthop Traumatol Cechoslov. 2012;79:335–40.
88. Schmitz P, Baumann F, Grechenig S, Gaensslen A, Nerlich M, Müller M. The cement-augmented transiliacal internal fixator (caT-IFI): an innovative surgical technique for stabilization of fragility fractures of the pelvis. Injury. 2015;46(Suppl 4):S114–20.
89. Gänsslen A, Pohlemann T, Krettek C. [Internal fixation of sacroiliac joint disruption]. Oper Orthop Traumatol. 2005;17:281–95.
90. Ragnarsson B, Olerud C, Olerud S. Anterior square-plate fixation of sacroiliac disruption. Acta Orthop Scand. 1993;64(2):138–42.
91. Gänsslen A, Hüfner T, Krettek C. Percutaneous iliosacral screw fixation of unstable pelvic injuries by conventional fluoroscopy. Oper Orthop Traumatol. 2006;18:225–44.
92. Rysavý M, Pavelka T, Khayarin M, Dzupa V. Iliosacral screw fixation of the unstable pelvic ring injuries. Acta Chir Orthop Traumatol Cechoslov. 2010;77:209–14.

93. Khaled S, Soliman O, Wahed M. Functional outcome of unstable pelvic ring injuries after iliosacral screw fixation: single versus two screw fixation. Eur J Trauma Emerg Surg. 2015;41:387–9.
94. Bellabarba C, Schildhauer T, Vaccaro A, Chapman J. Complications associated with surgical stabilization of high-grade sacral fracture dislocations with spino-pelvic instability. Spine. 2006;31:S80–8.
95. Schildhauer T, Bellabarba C, Nork S, Barei D, Routt JM, Chapman J. Decompression and lumbopelvic fixation for sacral fracture-dislocations with spino-pelvic dissociation. J Orthop Trauma. 2006;20:447–57.
96. Schroeder G, Savage J, Patel A, Stover M. Spinopelvic fixation in complex sacral fractures. J Bone Joint Surg Rev. 2015;3(3):e4. https://doi.org/10.2106/JBJS.RVW.N.00007.
97. Williams S, Quinnan S. Percutaneous lumbopelvic fixation for reduction and stabilization of sacral fractures with spinopelvic dissociation patterns. J Orthop Trauma. 2016;30:e318–24.

Symphyseal Disruption

23

Axel Gänsslen, Jan Lindahl, and Wolfgang Grechenig

A symphyseal disruption is part of a pelvic ring injury and, therefore, treatment should always additionally consider the posterior pelvic ring injury. Trafton stated that a symphyseal diastasis can sufficiently be fixed by open reduction and internal fixation when an associated posterior injury is properly fixed [1].

The historical standard in treating symphyseal disruption was a nonoperative treatment using the sling method ("Beckenschwebe") (Fig. 23.1) [2, 3]. Although patients were mobilized only after 12 weeks, good clinical outcomes were achieved [2].

Symphyseal ruptures were probably the first surgical interventions performed on the pelvic ring. Already in 1911, Finsterer treated an older symphysis rupture by using an aluminum-bronze wire [4], and Lambotte described a dynamic technique using a wire cerclage or a screw osteosynthesis (Fig. 23.2) [5].

In 1973, Sharp was the first to report a series of five cases with plate osteosynthesis for treating traumatic symphysis disruption. Interestingly, the initial treatment in this series had been conducted 10 years prior, and an "anatomic" plate design (angled four-hole plate) had been used [6].

Historically, different stabilization techniques were proposed including cerclage stabilization around screws [7], resorbable wire fixation techniques [8–10], or steel cables [11, 12]. Rubel et al. reported a case of endoscopic fixation of the pubic symphysis [13].

The present gold standard is symphyseal plating [14–21] due to excellent biomechanical results [22–24] despite new developments also show encouraging results, including endoscopic-assisted stabilization methods [25].

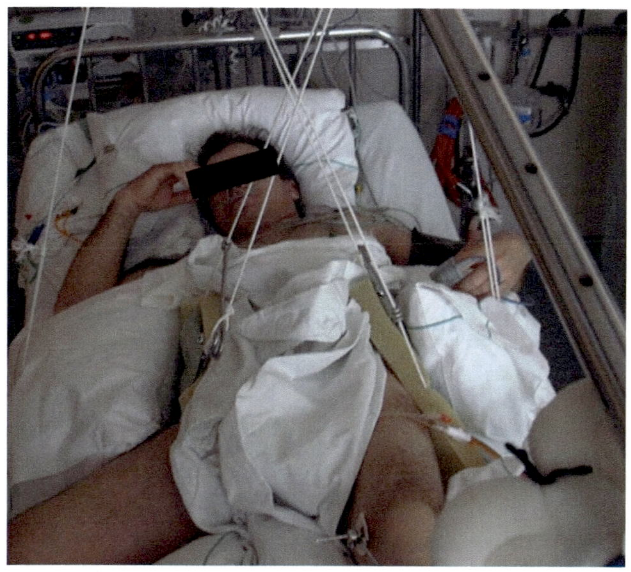

Fig. 23.1 Conservative treatment of pelvic ring injuries using a pelvic sling

23.1 Biomechanical Data

The biomechanical relevance of the pubic symphysis regarding the overall pelvic ring stability was analyzed in detail by Marvin Tile and coworkers (Fig. 23.3).

Dissection of the symphysis leads to an approximate reduction of overall ring stiffness of 40% [24]. Correspondingly, in type C injuries, overall pelvic stability is significantly increased with anterior internal fixation [26]. Disruption forces were reported to be between 1000 and 3000 N [27].

Early biomechanical data indicate that symphyseal plating showed higher pelvic ring stiffness compared to external fixation [28] and significantly reduces displacement in type

A. Gänsslen (✉)
Department of Trauma Surgery, Orthopedics and Hand Surgery, Hospital Wolfsburg, Wolfsburg, Germany

J. Lindahl
Orthopaedics and Trauma Surgery, Helsinki University Hospital, Helsinki, Finland

W. Grechenig
Department of Orthopaedics and Trauma, Medical University of Graz, Graz, Austria
e-mail: wolfgang.grechenig@medunigraz.at

A. Gänsslen et al. (eds.), *Pelvic Ring Fractures*, https://doi.org/10.1007/978-3-030-54730-1_23

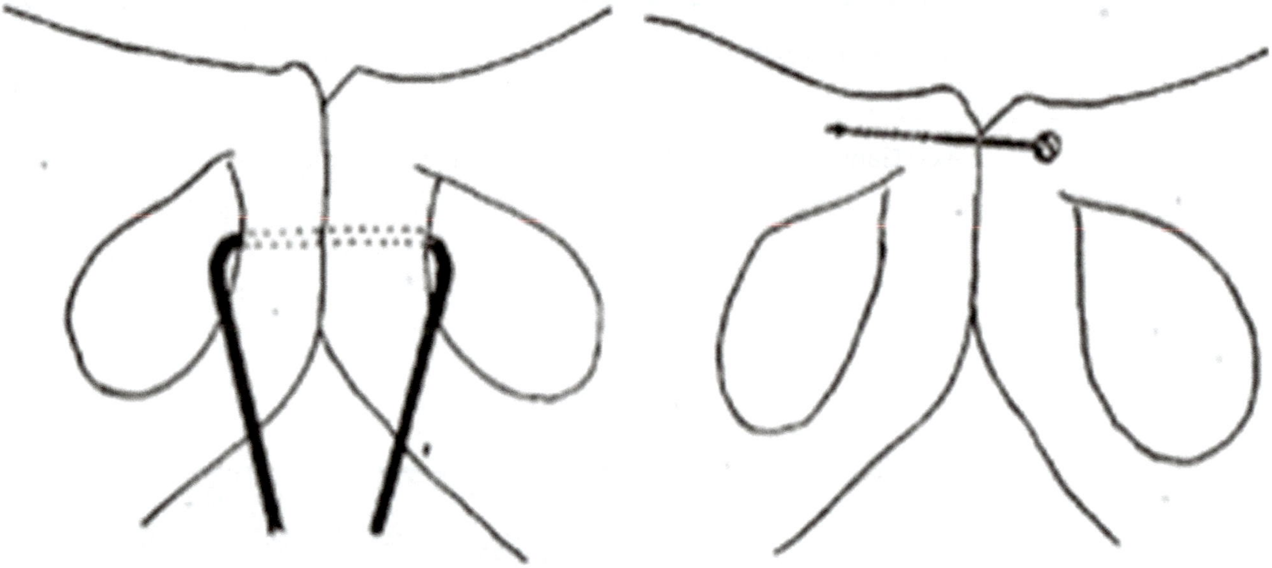

Fig. 23.2 Lambotte's recommendation of surgical treatment of the disrupted pubic symphysis

Fig. 23.3 According to Marvin Tile, dissection of the pubic symphysis results in approximately 40% less stiffness of the pelvic ring

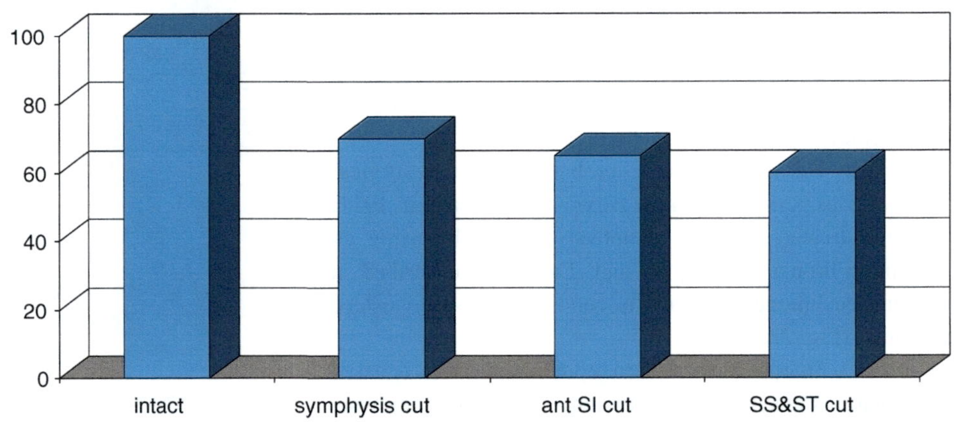

C injuries [29]. Using two symphyseal plates further increased the construct stiffness [30] (Fig. 23.4a–c).

Ecke et al. in 1984 investigated four different surgical symphyseal stabilization methods in a type C1.2 injury in 25 fresh human cadaver pelves. Interestingly, the anterior reconstruction plates first failed, despite posterior screw osteosynthesis. Best results were achieved when using a symphyseal DC plate combined with posterior tension band wiring of the SI joint [8].

Varga et al. compared double symphyseal plating with 4.5-mm reconstruction plates with wire stabilization around two 6.5-mm fully threaded cancellous screws and absorbable sutures in eight type C cadaveric pelves [31]. The tests resulted in significantly lesser symphyseal motion when using wires compared to the other two fixations methods. However, these measurements were not evaluated in a simulated gait condition.

In a cadaveric analysis of seven fresh cadavers using a double-leg stance model, Simonian et al. compared different plate configurations to test the stability of these constructs in a B1 injury model [32]. All tested plate systems, even a box-type plate, showed comparable stability with only minimal symphyseal motion [32].

In a dynamic experimental investigation, DC plates (4.5 mm four-hole DC) were compared with reconstruction plates (4.5 mm five holes), cerclage wires, and PDS bandings under gait simulation conditions [33]. Neither wire cerclages nor PDS banding achieved sufficient stabilization of sym-

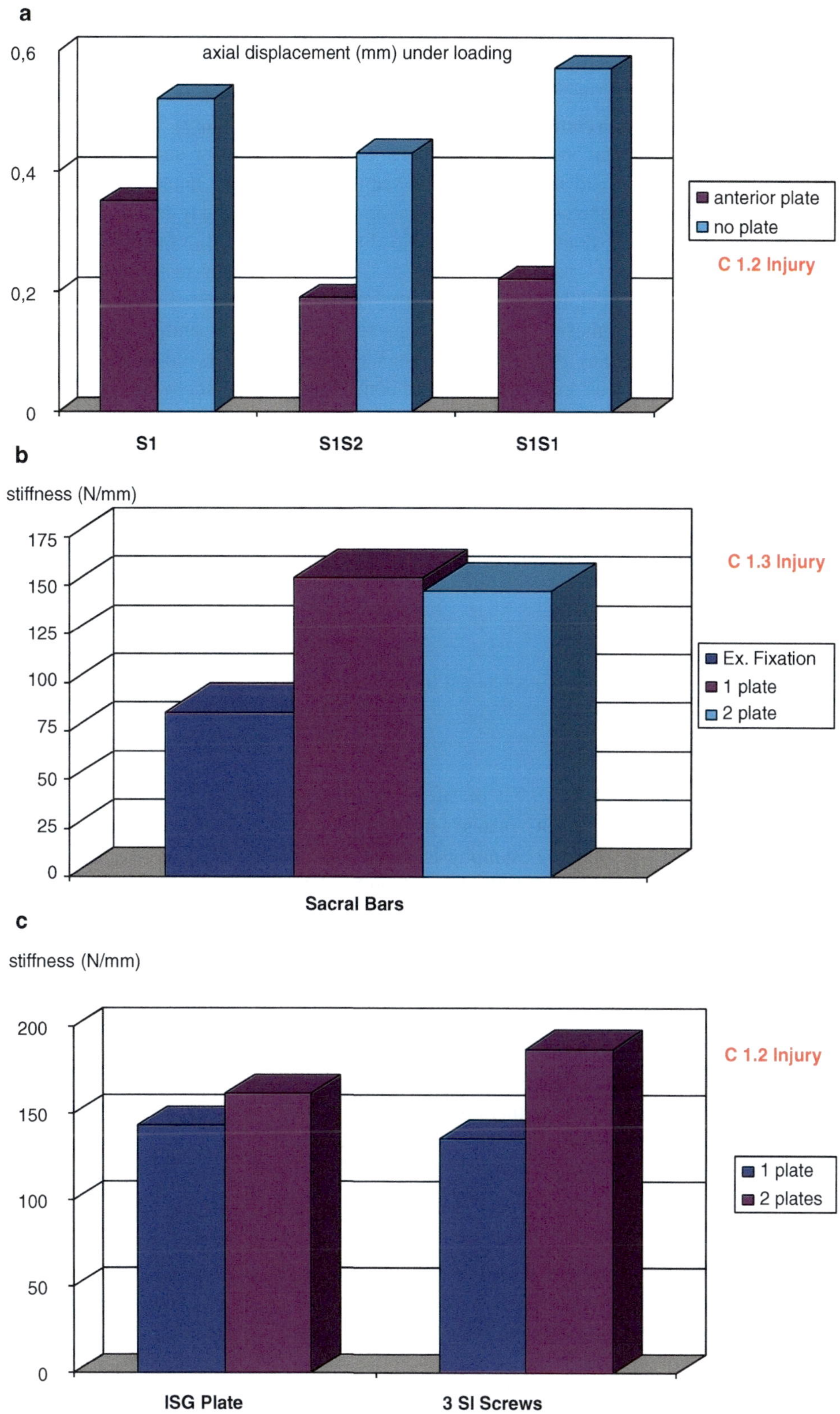

Fig. 23.4 (**a**) Symphyseal plating significantly increases pelvic ring stability in a C1.2 injury model. (**b**) Symphyseal plating resulted in significant higher stiffness compared to external fixation in a type C sacral fracture model. (**c**) Two symphyseal plates were associated with the highest stiffness in a C1.2 injury model

physeal ruptures. In contrast, a sufficient primary stabilization could be achieved when using DC or reconstruction plates, although progressive loosening was observed in osteoporotic bone.

Daily et al. performed a comparative biomechanical study on locking (four-hole unicortical locking plate, four-hole bicortical locking plate) and nonlocking plate stabilization (four-hole bicortical compression plate) of an open-book type B injury simulating double-leg stance. No difference could be observed [34].

Recently, Cano-Luis et al. biomechanically analyzed percutaneous screw osteosynthesis with two crossing screws in open-book type B1 injuries in a double–leg stance model [35]. Percutaneous screw osteosynthesis showed comparable displacements as to the intact pelvis.

Prasarn et al. performed another biomechanical study using a single-leg stance simulation, comparing locked and unlocked 4-hole plating in a type B injury [36]. Locking plates showed no advantage over unlocked plates.

No advantage of locking plates could also be confirmed in osteopenic bones [37, 38].

Locking plates show no biomechanical advantage to standard plating techniques.

Pizanis et al. analyzed the effect of lateral prebending comparing standard 4.5 mm DC plates with the 3.5 mm "combi-hole" and interlocking symphysis plate in an unmounted plastic pelvic model [39]. Lateral prebending resulted in biomechanical optimization regarding contact area, especially when 3.5 mm prebended plates were used and fixed with a medial DC effect and lateral locking stabilization.

Plate osteosynthesis is sufficient to restore symphyseal stability. Lateral prebending further optimizes the contact area of the plate to the bone. Locking plates show no relevant biomechanical advantage.

Finite element studies confirmed these results [40].

Yao et al. developed a three-dimensional finite element model of a Tile type B1 injury and simulated symphyseal osteosynthesis with a single superior plate, a double plate, single cannulated screw, and crossed dual- and parallel dual-cannulated screws [41]. Double-leg stance, single-leg stance, and rotation forces were simulated. The highest stiffnesses were observed with parallel and crossed screws, while a single implant and parallel screws showed failure tendency under single-leg stance conditions. Parallel screws were optimal in dual-leg simulations. Crossing screws resulted in decreased shearing forces under single-leg stance conditions.

In a further finite element study, Yag et al. compared five fixation methods to stabilize a pubic symphysis diastasis (Tile B1 injury). The authors used a single superior plate, a combined superior and anterior plate, a single cannulated screw, cross dual-cannulated screws, and parallel dual-cannulated screws. The study demonstrated that a single implant and parallel screws tended to fail. The best anterior and posterior pelvic stabilizations were achieved by a dual implant fixation [42].

Yu et al. analyzed a finite element model of a Tile type B1 injury and simulated symphyseal stabilization comparing percutaneous cannulated screw fixation and reconstruction plate screw fixation [40]. Both fixation methods adequately stabilized the symphysis with comparable biomechanical properties.

Finite element analyses indicate adequate symphyseal stabilization even with percutaneous screw stabilization methods.

23.2 Indication

Classical indications for plate stabilization of the pubic symphysis include several type B and type Cinjuries of the pelvic ring:

- Symphyseal diastasis as part of a Tile type B injury of the pelvic ring (>2.5 cm diastasis corresponds to a clinical "instability") [43]
- Symphyseal diastasis as part of a Tile type C injury of the pelvic ring in addition to posterior pelvic ring stabilization [43]

In contrast, external fixation is limited to cases that need emergency stabilization without an indication for laparotomy [1] as, in general, long healing times are expected [43]. The results after definitive treatment of symphyseal disruption with an external fixator alone led to unacceptable results [44].

The potential of additional bleeding should be considered. Baqué et al. performed a cadaveric analysis and found that symphyseal widening of 5 cm was associated with a 20.8% increase of pelvic volume in a bilateral open-book injury model with venous laceration of the ilio-lumbar vein in 60% [45].

Matta and others recommended anterior fixation prior to posterior fixation if no obturator foramen or acetabular fractures were present [46, 47].

23.3 Contraindications

Contraindications include stable pelvic fractures (type A, few type B injuries) and a reduced general patient condition [43].

23.4 Patient Positioning

The patient is positioned on a radiolucent OR table in the standard supine position allowing standard intraoperative x-ray examination including AP view of the pelvis, inlet- and outlet views. A transurethral bladder catheter is inserted to reduce the risk of accidental bladder injuries.

Moreover, the patient's genital area must be covered appropriately using a simple fourfold cover, and the patient's legs must not be disinfected separately or positioned in a specific manner.

23.5 Incision

There are two possible skin incisions to get access to the pubic symphysis (Fig. 23.5) [1]:

- Vertical midline incisions (if laparotomy is required)
- Transverse Pfannenstiel incisions [48–50], placed 2 cm above the symphysis [46]

The Pfannenstiel incision is favored as it is more esthetic [43]. The incision is marked approximately 1–2 cm proximal to the usually well palpable pubic tubercles, often not exceeding lateral to the tubercles. An incisional length of 7–10 cm is sufficient (Fig. 23.5). Dissection of the spermatic cord/round ligament is usually not necessary. In obese patients, the vertical incision is often easier and offers comparable results [51].

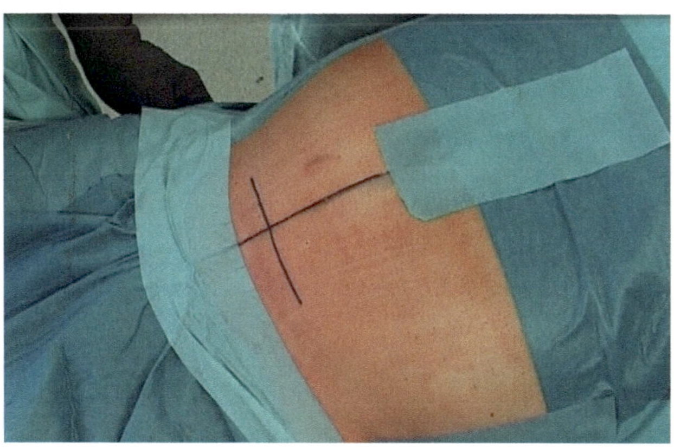

Fig. 23.5 Two possible incisions for symphyseal plating: the transverse (standard) Pfannestiel incision and the longitudinal incision

23.6 Superficial Dissection

The subcutaneous tissue is dissected parallel to the skin incision until the abdominal midline (linea alba/white line) is identified (Fig. 23.6). Splitting the anterior layer of the linea alba is performed with the scalpel in the midline, and after identification, both rectus abdominis muscle bellies are identified and mobilized laterally (Fig. 23.6).

The posterior layer of the linea alba is identified and perforated bluntly near the symphysis using the finger to open the space of Rezzi. The bladder is protected using a protecting spatula (Fig. 23.7). The insertions of the rectus abdominis muscles could be incompletely detached from the pubis on their inner aspects [1], whereas their lateral and outer parts of attachments are left intact.

23.7 Deep Dissection

After inserting a bladder-protecting spatula, a good view of the broadly separated pubic symphysis can be easily identified with visualization of the unilaterally torn pubic disk after hematoma evacuation. Subsequently, temporary tamponade against the bladder is established by using abdominal swabs (and/or similar items) (Fig. 23.8). There is a potential risk of bladder injury during incorrect dissection. If a bladder injury occurs, a two-layer bladder wall reconstruction is usually performed.

Hohmann retractors are inserted close to the pubic tubercles without complete release of the rectus sheath, respecting the spermatic cords/round ligament, the obturator neurovascular bundle, and the external iliac vessels [1]. Injuries to the spermatic cord due to brisk hook insertion are potentially possible as there is close relationship to these structures [52]. A close relationship of the spermatic cord directly lateral to the pubic tubercle was identified during cadaveric dissection with an average distance of 0.8 mm (Fig. 23.9).

Regarding the fibrocartilaginous disk, it was a standard recommendation to only perform minimal debridement [1]. Recently, Lybrand et al. compared 96 patients with APC II and III injuries, stabilized with anterior symphyseal plating (six-hole plate). Fifty patients had symphyseal cartilage removal. The postoperative symphyseal gap was lower compared to disk retention. The implant failure rate was lower after cartilage excision in the APC II group (7% vs. 19% implant breakage, 13% vs. 42% screw loosening/breakage, 20% vs. 61% combined problems), whereas after type APC III injuries no significant implant failure rate was observed in both groups. Overall, comparing disk excision and disk retaining treatment, after disk excision implant failure rates were lower (16% vs. 35% screw loosening, 4% vs. 17% plate breakage, 20% vs. 52% combined failures) [53].

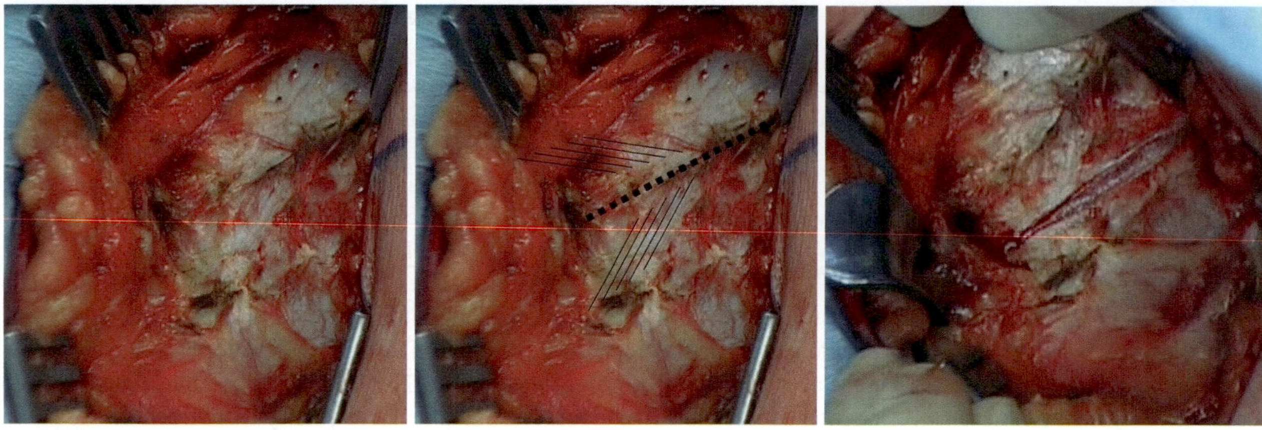

Fig. 23.6 Identification of the midline and fascial incision

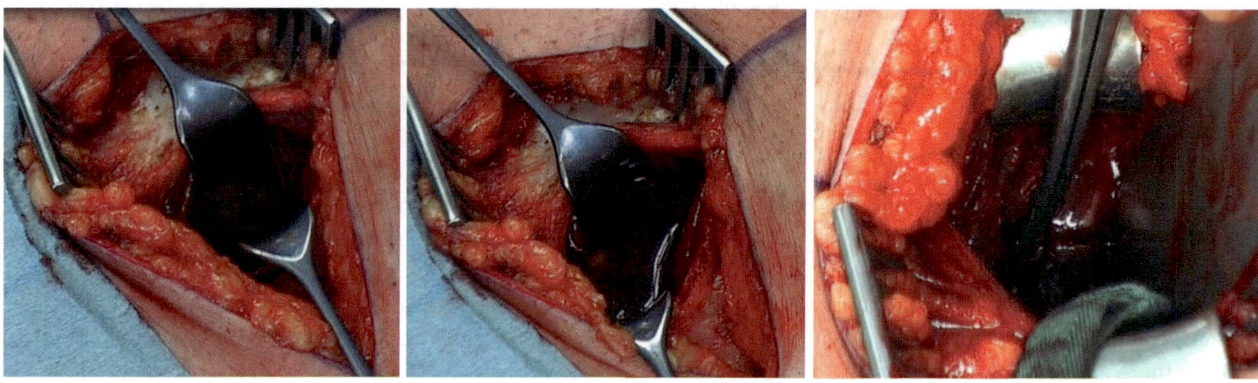

Fig. 23.7 Mobilization of both rectus abdominis muscles and opening of the retrosymphyseal space

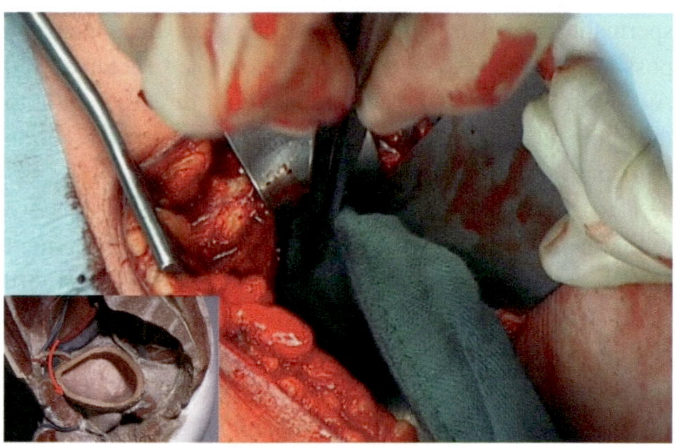

Fig. 23.8 Bladder protection using a spatula and a retrosymphyseal tamponade

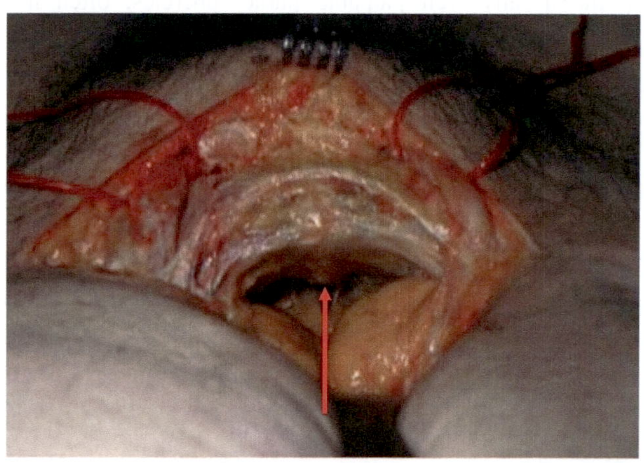

Fig. 23.9 Relation of the spermatic cord in males relative to the symphyseal dissection. Symphyseal midline (retrosymphyseal buldge, arrow)

23.8 Reduction

The typical displacement of an open-book injury consists of external rotation of the affected hemipelvis with resulting distalization of the superior ramus (Fig. 23.10) [54].

Thus, reduction maneuvers should aim on internal rotation, anterior-posterior, and vertical reduction.

Internal rotation of the leg is performed, which can be supported by Schanz screw insertion into the iliac bone at the level of the AIIS, ASIS, or iliac crest in a joy stick technique or by applying a distractor (Fig. 23.11). In type C injuries, length can be regained with distal traction [1].

A pointed reduction forceps can be placed either into the obturator foramen or superior near the pubic tubercles for compression of the symphysis (Fig. 23.12a, c) [43, 55]. Compensation of a "vertical offset" can be achieved by "tilting" the reduction forceps (Fig. 23.12b) [43]. Vertical reduction can be also achieved using a ball spike pusher at the superior pubic ramus.

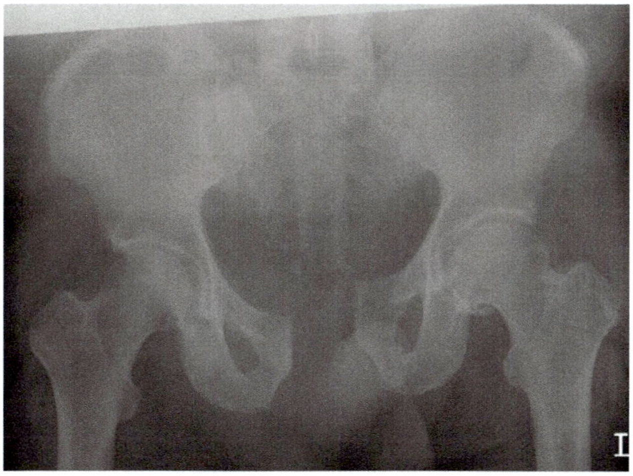

Fig. 23.10 Radiological triad in a right open-book injury: presence of a distalized upper pubic ramus, a widened iliac wing widening, and a smaller obturator foramen

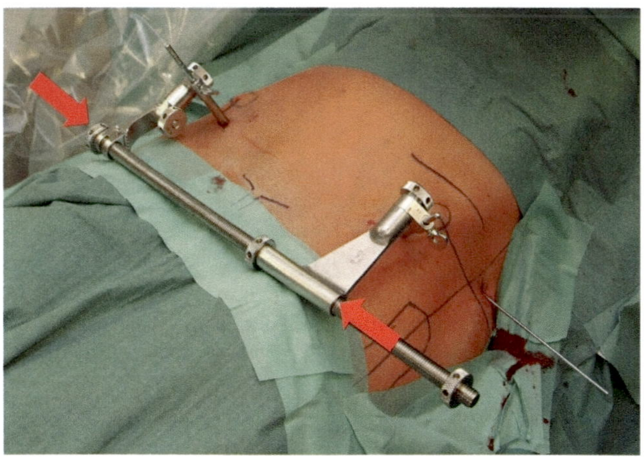

Fig. 23.11 Compression reduction using a distractor

Alternatively, compression is achieved using a Farabeuf or Jungbluth clamp connected to two 3.5 mm screws, which are inserted from anterior to posterior at each superior pubic ramus medial to the pubic tubercles (Fig. 23.13a, b). The reduced screw hold has to be considered.

When the "vertical offset" cannot be compensated using these maneuvers or is only incompletely achieved, an indirect reduction with the plate can be helpful. The plate is fixed on the unaffected side, and vertical displacement can be corrected by tightening the plate screws on the affected side (Fig. 23.14).

Reduction is then radiographically confirmed in the standard three x-ray planes.

23.9 Plate Osteosynthesis

A single plate is reliable for fixation of the symphysis pubis [46]. Historically, two-hole dynamic compression plates were proposed, acting as a tension band construct to allow a small amount of normal motion [56].

> Multiple hole plate fixation is the gold standard for treatment of symphyseal disruptions [57].

Sagi et al. stated that two-hole fixation was inadequate compared to multiple hole plate fixation with higher implant failure rates (33% vs. 12%) and malunions (57% vs. 15%) [58]. Using the Young-Burgess classification, no clear data were available regarding instability-dependent posterior fixation of specific fractures types.

Locked plates were associated with fixation failure. Moed et al. presented six cases with several failure types: implant loosening, complete construct pullout, screw breakage, screw loosening, and outbacking of screws [59].

In a clinical series of 11 patients with different injury types according to Young-Burgess, five showed loosening at the screw–bone interface with resultant minor loss of reduction and implant breakage, all without clinical impairments at follow-up of 2.5 months [60].

> As the symphysis shows physiological movements, potentially locking constructs are possibly too stiff for symphyseal fixation.

The plate is positioned posterior to the pubic tubercle and posterior to the insertion of the rectus abdominis muscle on top of the superior ramus (Fig. 23.15).

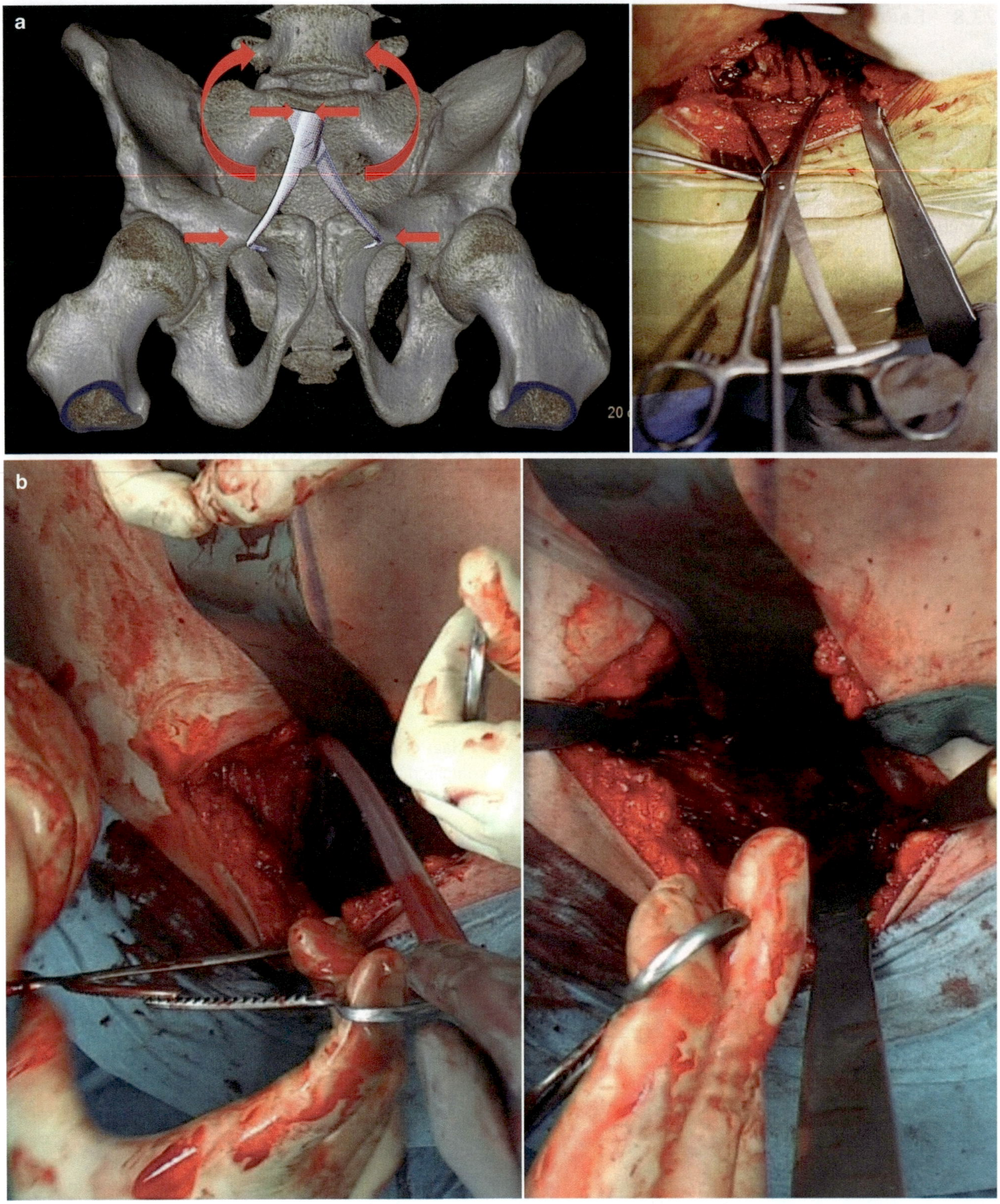

Fig. 23.12 (**a**) Reduction of a displaced pubic symphysis using the pointed reduction forceps from anterior. (**b**) Clinical example of symphyseal reduction using the pointed reduction forceps. Note: tilting of the clamp arms to reduce vertical/posterior displacement. (**c**) Clinical example of symphyseal reduction by compressing the pointed reduction forceps

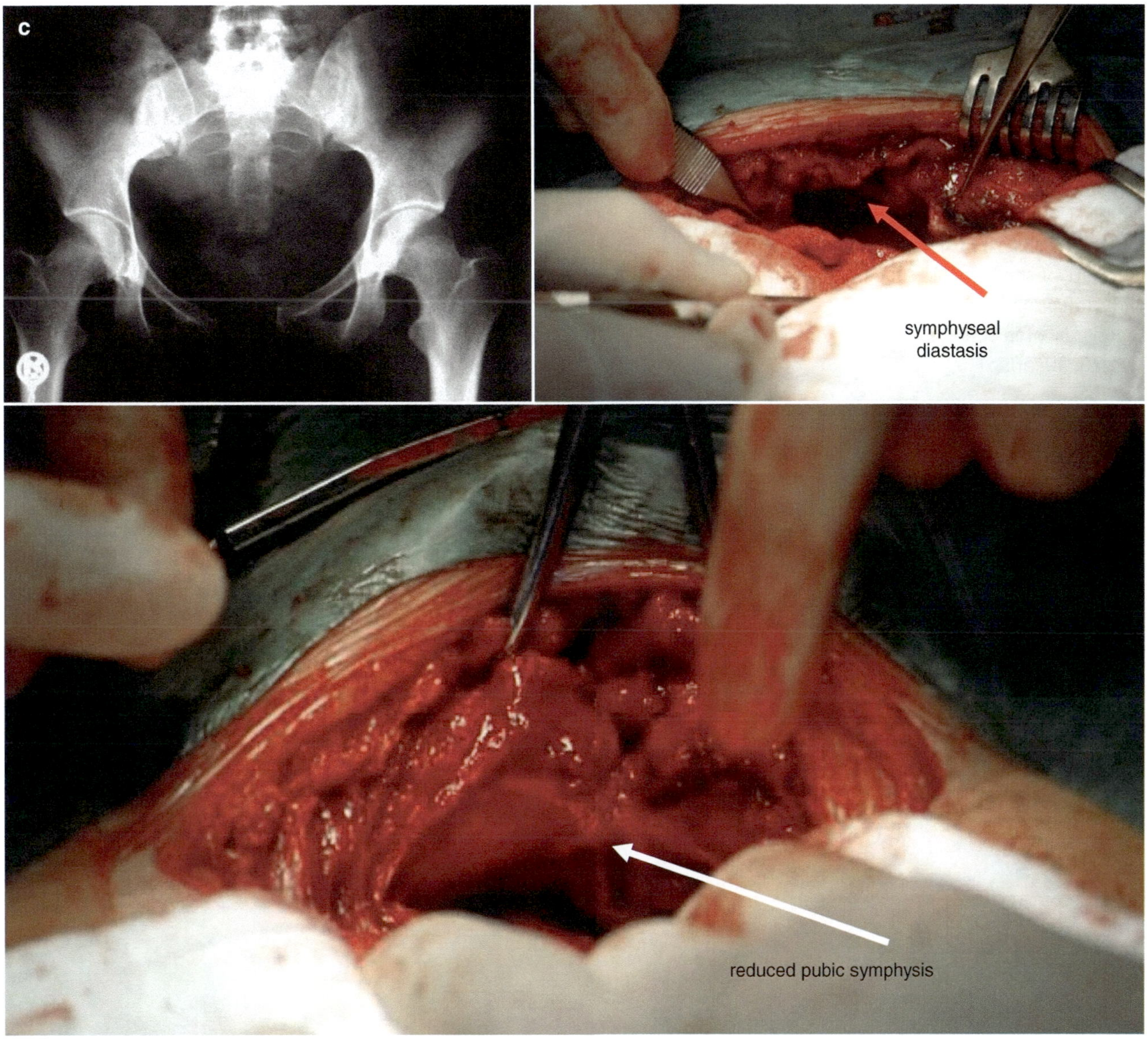

Fig. 23.12 (continued)

The exact localization of the pubic disk can be recognized by palpating the posterior symphyseal surface. Here, a bulge is palpable in nearly all patients, even in young patients.

Pohlemann et al. proposed the small 4.5 mm four-hole DC plate. The lateral plate ends have often to be bent down about 10–15° for optimal screw direction. The medial screws are inserted parallel to the symphysis using the compression technique of the plate (Fig. 23.16). Oscillating drilling is performed under digital guidance using the index or long finger to protect periosseous structures (Fig. 23.17). If insufficient holding power is achieved, cancellous fully threaded screws can be used.

The lateral screws are orientated obliquely toward the inserted tip of each medial screw (Fig. 23.18). Screws lengths between 50 and 70 mm are often possible. Also, cancellous screws can be used [43].

There is a potential risk of vaginal impingement in women if these screws are too long (Fig. 23.19).

Matta proposed a treatment algorithm for combined symphyseal and pubic rami fractures using curved pelvic plates with 3.5 mm screws [46], Extension of the Pfannenstiel approach is necessary. Often a classical intrapelvic approach is used (Fig. 23.20):

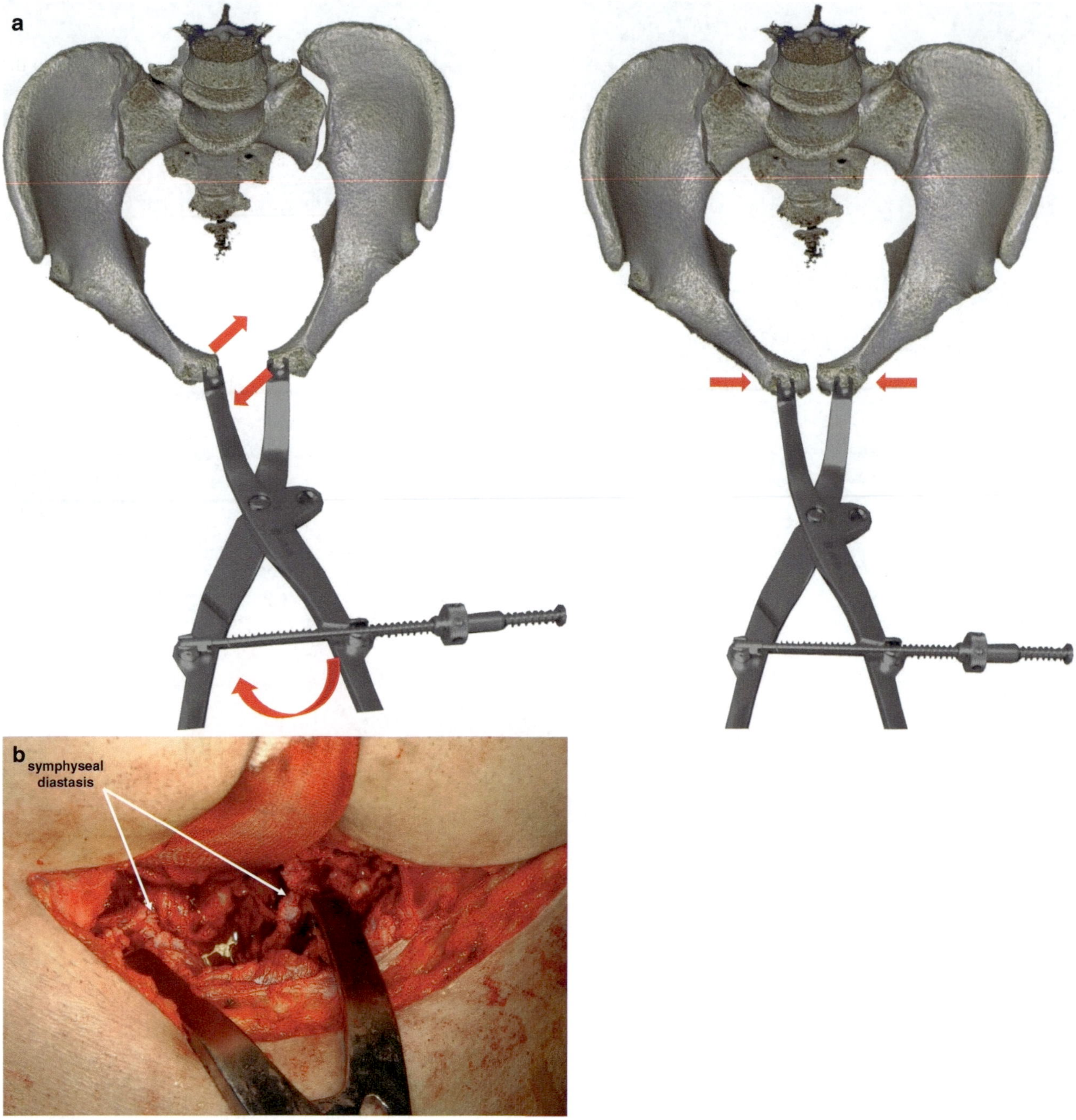

Fig. 23.13 (**a**) Redcution of the pubic symphysis using the Jungbluth clamp from anterior. Note: This clamp also allows distraction and tilting. (**b**:) Clinical application of the Jungbluth clamp from anterior

- Symphysis dislocation combined with minor displaced unilateral or bilateral ramus fractures → isolated symphyseal fixation
- Displaced associated ramus fractures (>20 mm) and symphyseal disruption → 6-hole plate
- Medial/lateral ramus fractures in association with a symphysis dislocation → >6-hole plate (Fig. 23.21)

Today, anatomically preshaped plates are in use. For optimizing stability, different screw orientations are recommended.

During the screw drilling process, the index finger is positioned at the inner cortex of the pubic bone and the pubic disk to control the drill direction (Fig. 23.17).

Intraoperative x-rays (AP, inlet, outlet) confirm the quality of reduction, the screw length, and the plate position.

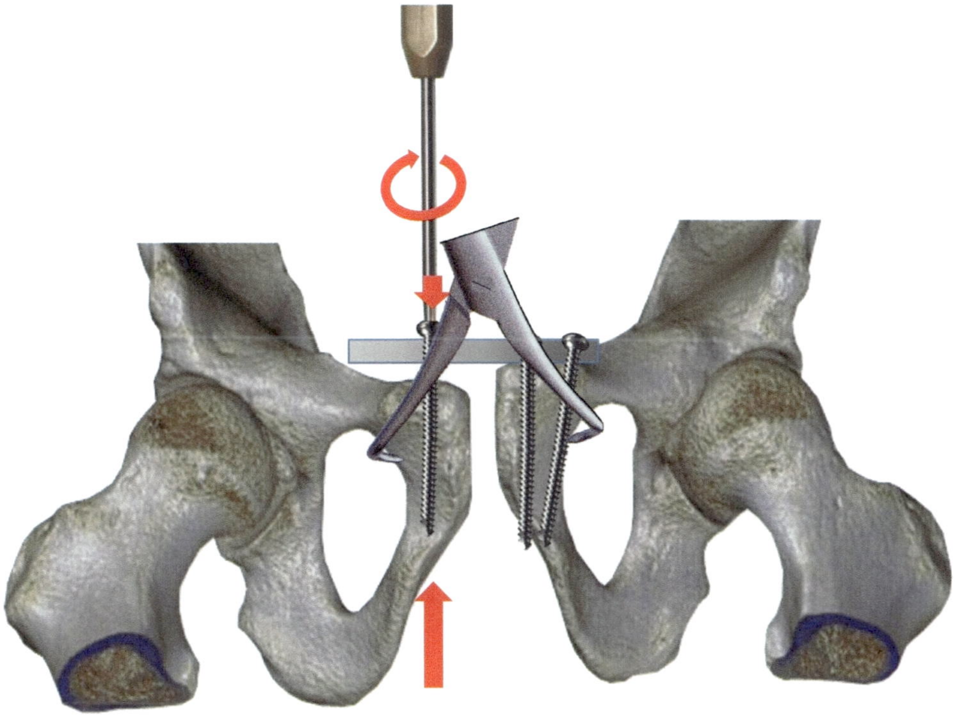

Fig. 23.14 Reduction of the pubic symphysis using the plate

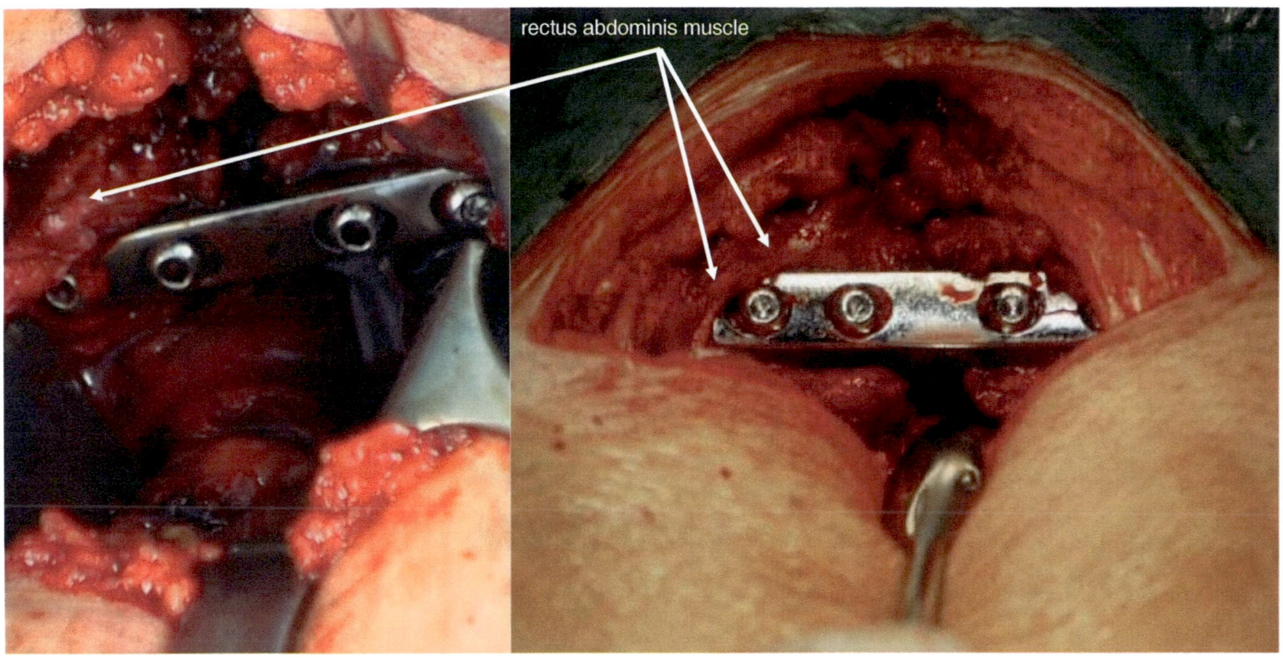

Fig. 23.15 Plate position posterior to the rectus abdominis insertion

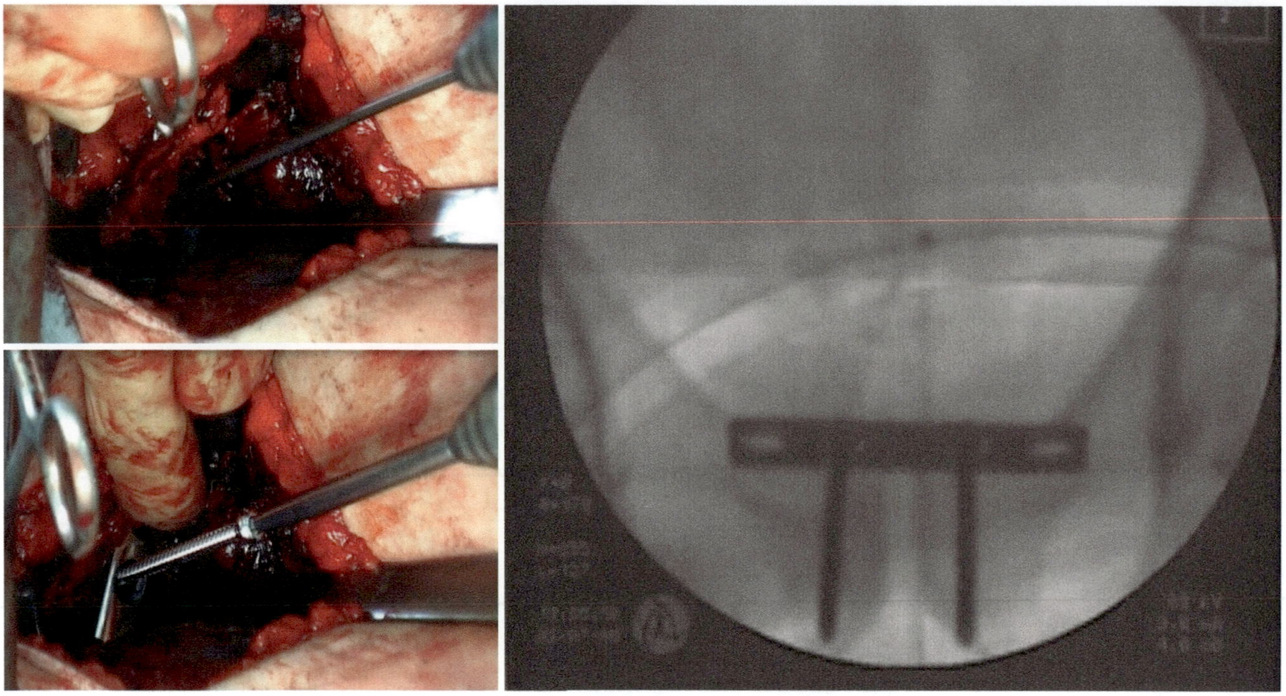

Fig. 23.16 Parallel screw orientation near the symphyseal space

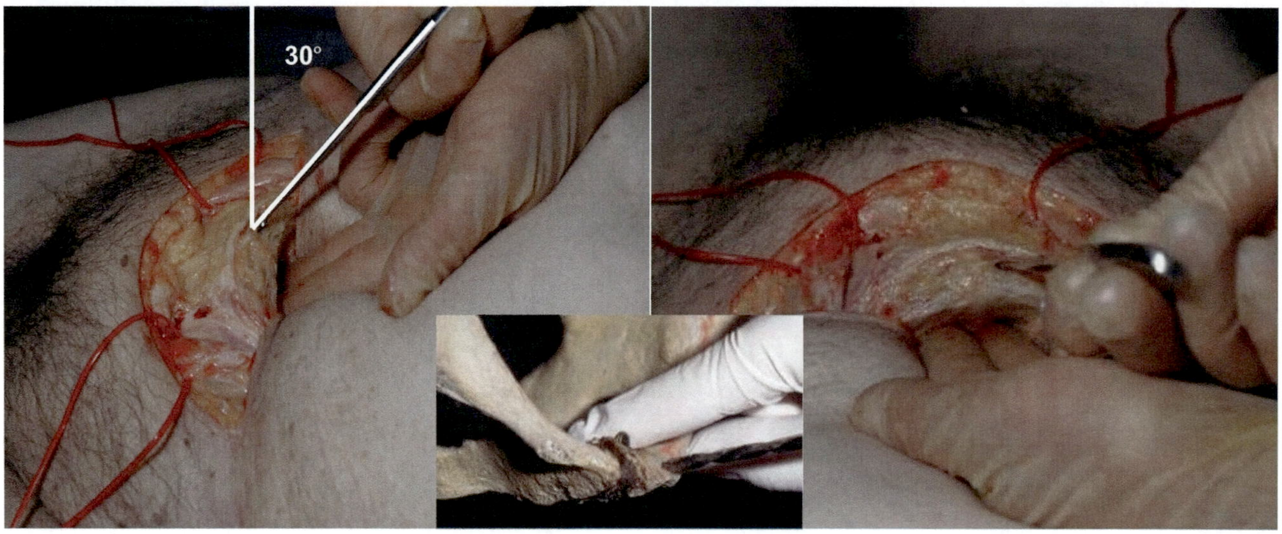

Fig. 23.17 Digital guidance of the drilling procedure to avoid intrapelvic screw positioning

An additional anterior plate ("box plate," Figs. 23.22 and 23.23) can be used to increase the overall stability, either from extra- or intrapelvic.

23.10 Wound Closure

After wound irrigation, closure starts with refixation of the eventually torn rectus abdominis muscle. In case of extensive ruptures, additional transosseous sutures can be necessary. A 12Ch drain is inserted into the space of Rezzi, and fascial closure is performed using standard sutures (Fig. 23.24). A subcutaneous suction drain is not required. Subcutaneous stitches and classical Donati skin sutures are inserted.

23.11 Postoperative Care

The wound drain is removed typically after day 1 postoperatively. The transurethral bladder catheter is removed as soon as possible, typically on day 1 or 2 postoperatively.

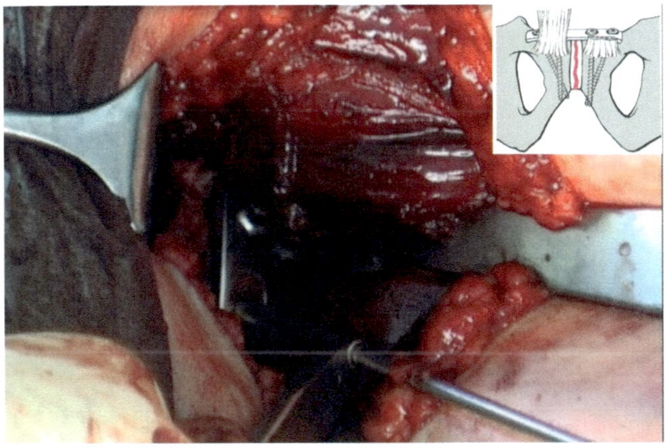

Fig. 23.18 Oblique screw orientation lateral to the midline

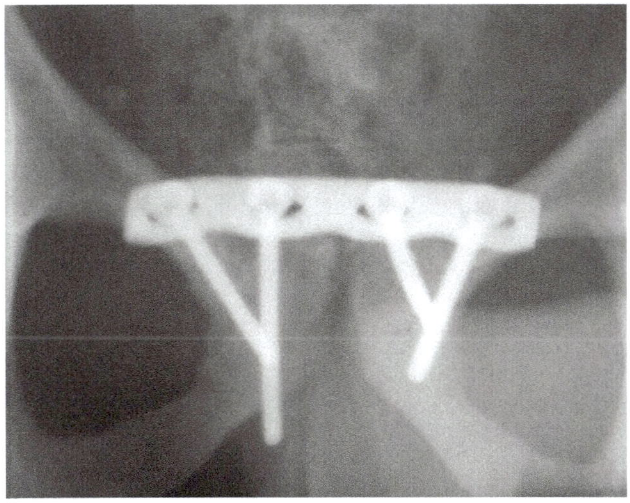

Fig. 23.19 Subsymphyseal soft tissue impingement due to a too-long screw

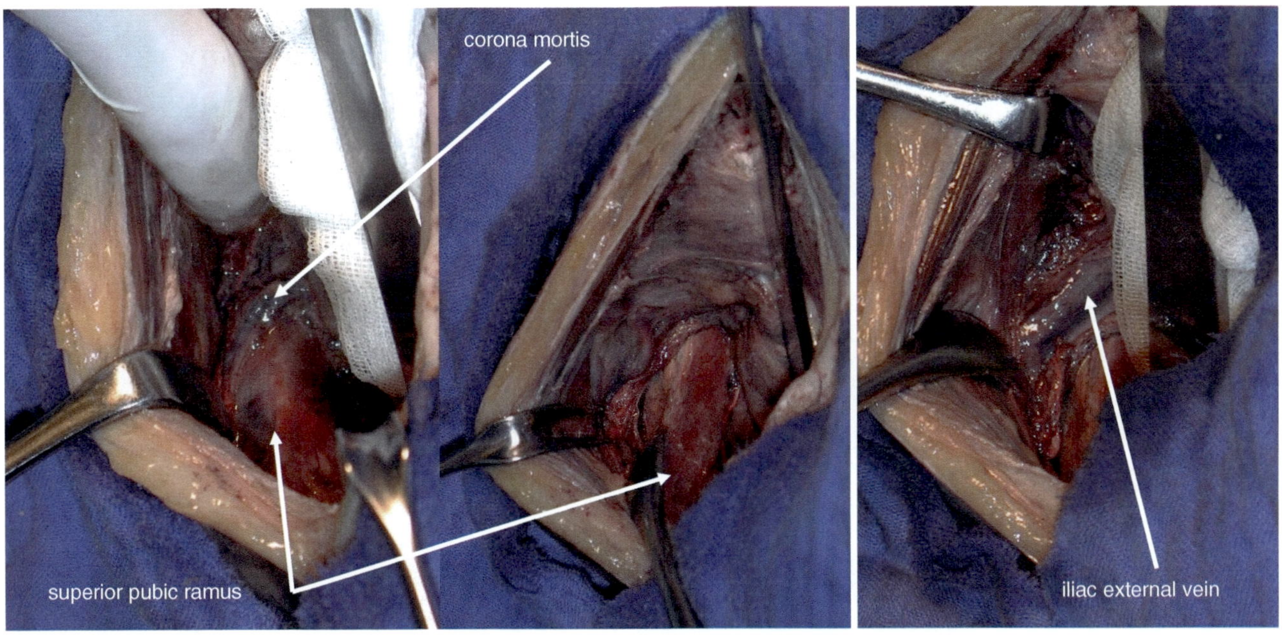

Fig. 23.20 Extension of the Pfannestiel approach to an intrapelvic approach with identification of the corona mortis and the eternal iliac vessels

A postoperative AP x-ray of the pelvis is performed and follow-up x-rays are recommended at 6 and 12 weeks.

In unilateral lesions, partial weight bearing on the injured side (injured sacroiliac joint) with 15 kg body weight for 6 weeks is recommended. DVT prophylaxis according to implemented guidelines is performed.

If both posterior pelvic sides are involved, mobilization should be restricted to short walking trips with crutches within pain limits during the first 6–8 weeks.

23.12 New Stabilization Techniques

Mu et al. reported on the option of percutaneous screw fixation of symphyseal injury supported by Iso-C 3D computer navigation with one horizontal or two crossing 7.3 mm cannulated screws in eight patients with type B and type C injuries [61].

Chen et al. compared percutaneous screw fixation with 7.3 mm cannulated compression screws in 45 patients with

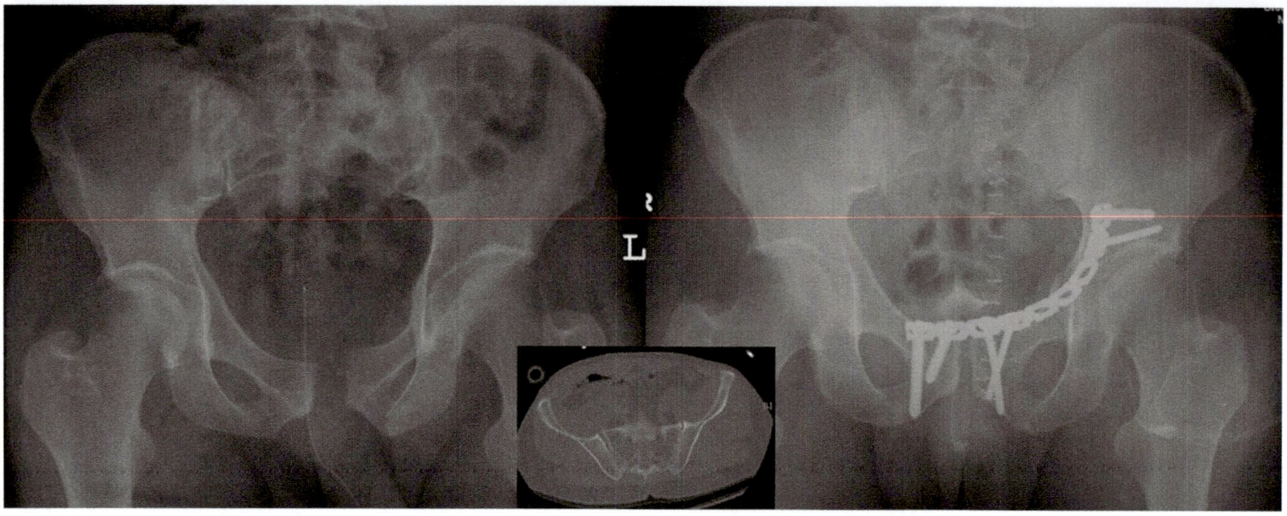

Fig. 23.21 Lateral extension of the plate in a combined symphyseal disruption and upper pubic rami fracture

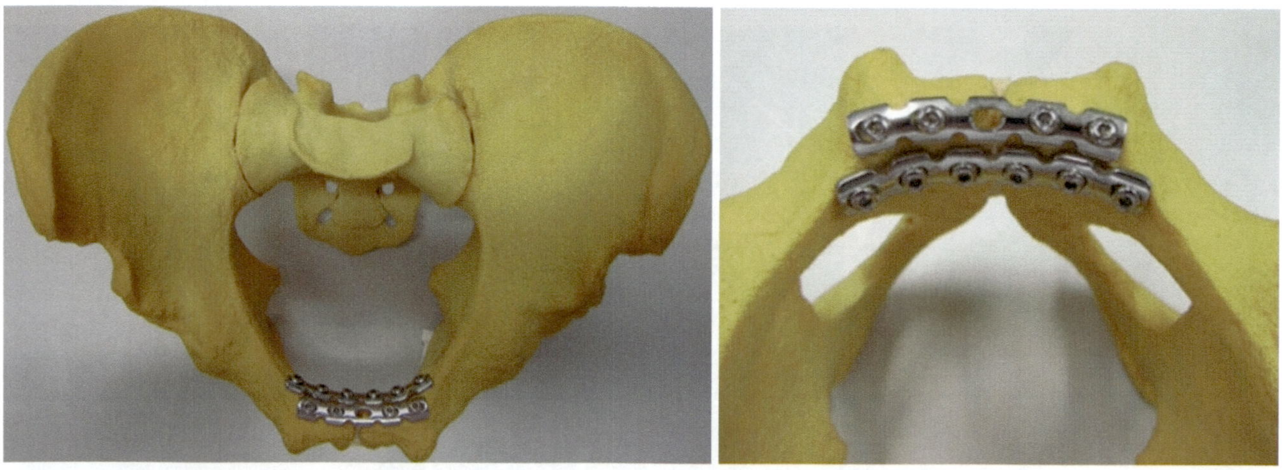

Fig. 23.22 Intrapelvic "box plate" principle

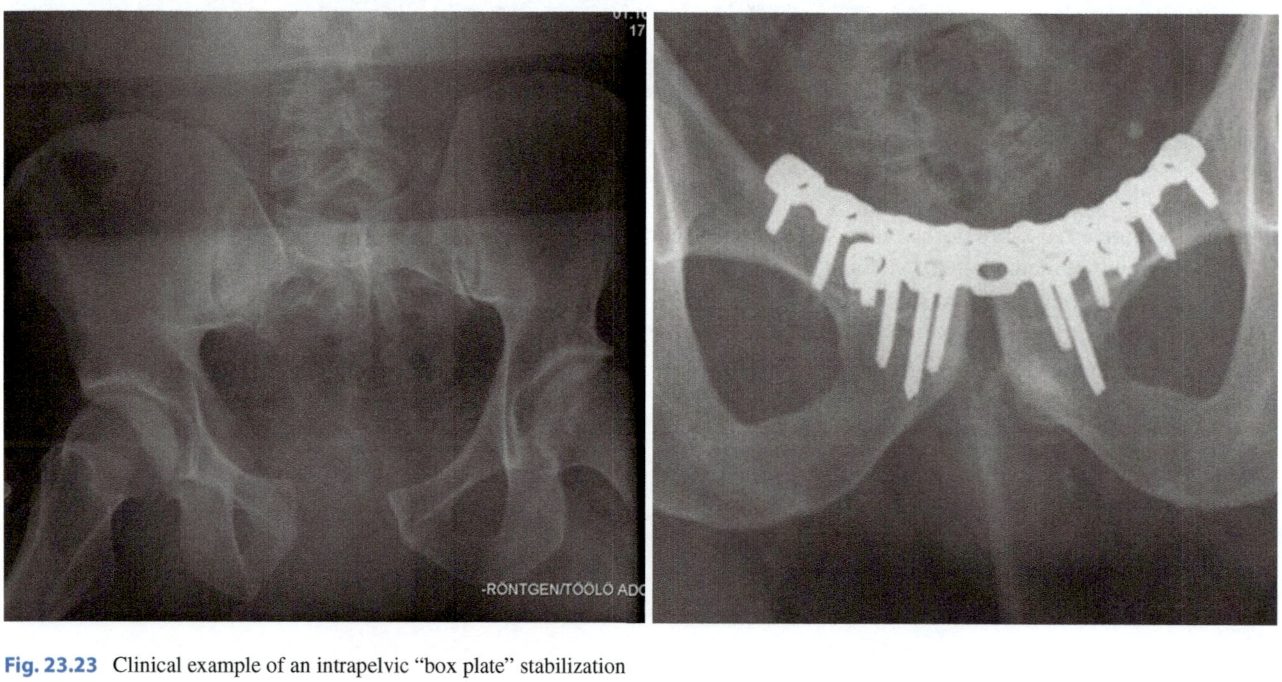

Fig. 23.23 Clinical example of an intrapelvic "box plate" stabilization

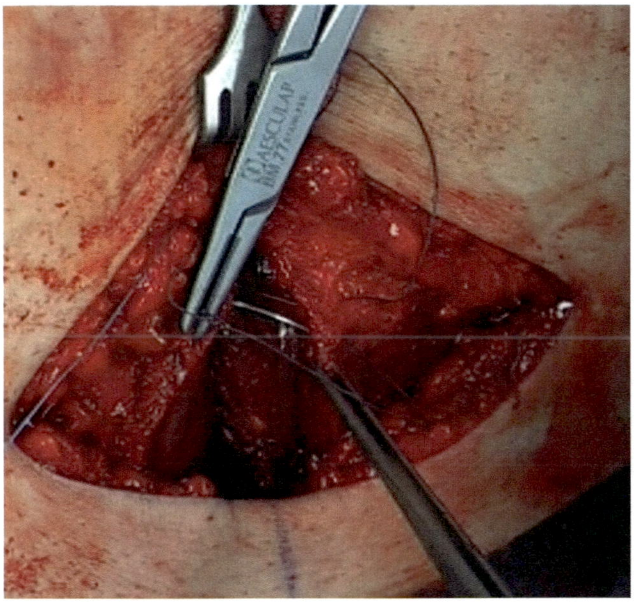

Fig. 23.24 Fascial closure

standard plate osteosynthesis (one reconstruction plate) and reported on lower iatrogenic injury rates and better functional outcome with comparable strength of fixation [62]. Blood loss (18.3 mL vs. 157 mL), incision length (1.7 cm vs. 7.9 cm), implant failure rate (12.2% vs. 19%), malunion rate (19.5% vs. 33.3%), and the percentage of impotence in male patients (3.4% vs. 15%) were lesser than in patients with plate osteosynthesis, while residual displacement/quality of reduction was comparable. At follow-up of 21 months, 56.1% and 29.3% showed excellent and good functional results according to the Majeed Score, respectively.

Percutaneous screw fixation techniques were also biomechanically effective [35].

23.13 Technique of Percutaneous Screw Fixation [61]

Percutaneous Schanz pin insertion into both iliac crests was performed to preliminarily reduce the external rotation displacement.

Under C-arm control in the AP, inlet, and outlet views, a horizontal K-wire placed parallel to the superior pubic border was percutaneously inserted through the symphysis. The entry and exit points are defined at the junction between the pubic tubercle and superior ramus of pubis. After overdrilling, a short-threaded 7.3 mm screw was inserted with or without a washer.

Ten patients with TightRope® fixation complemented by an external fixator were analyzed. Time of surgery was 48.5 min. No change of postoperative symphyseal width was observed at an average of 15 months. One infection and one fixation failure were observed. The functional outcome according to the Majeed Score was graded good to excellent in all cases with an average satisfaction score of 8.1 points [63].

Further 16 patients were stabilized with percutaneous screw fixation. Time of surgery was 27.3 min. No change of postoperative symphyseal width was observed at an average of 15 months. No infection but three fixation failures were observed, one requiring revision. The functional outcome according to the Majeed Score was graded good to excellent in all but one case with an average satisfaction score of 8.3 points [63].

Stabilization of the pubic symphysis using an internal fixator (INFIX) in 24 patients resulted in symphyseal space reduction to 10.7 mm compared to 7 mm using classical plate stabilization. The median Majeed Score was 84 points [64].

23.14 Results (Figs. 23.25 and 23.26)

Weber et al. analyzed 22 patients with isolated B1 injuries (open-book, no posterior vertical instability) using a combined reconstruction plate osteosynthesis and tension band wiring [65]. Follow-up was performed after at least 1 year (average 4 years, range 1–9 years) using the German Pelvic Outcome Score with a clinical and radiological analysis. Of these, 40.9% reported pain. The absence of pain was associated with an excellent outcome.

Pohlemann et al. reported on 21 patients with type B1 injuries without additional relevant peripelvic soft tissue injury [43]. Surgery was performed, on an average, after 4 days with a mean blood loss of 45 mL (20–160 mL) and an average surgery time of 47 min (20–75 min). In all patients, an anatomic reduction could be achieved. No intraoperative complications occurred, while one deep infection was treated surgically. Four patients complained of urological disturbances: one micturition complaint and two of erectile dysfunction which were completely resolved, while one patient developed a urethral stricture.

Spagnolo et al. reported on 16 patients with symphyseal injury without clear data on the posterior lesions, treated with double plating (box-type plating) [66]. Ninety percent showed anatomical pelvic reconstruction. One patient developed a pulmonary embolism, while no infections or implant failure was observed. Three patients reported on symphyseal pain. Overall, excellent results were observed in 90% and good results in 10%.

Aggarwal et al. analyzed 19 patients with different open-book AP compression injuries (1x APC I, 13x APC II, 5x APC III) according to Young-Burgess [67]. In 17 patients, follow-up analysis was possible after a mean of 2.9 years. After APC II injuries (type B acc. to Tile), the clinical out-

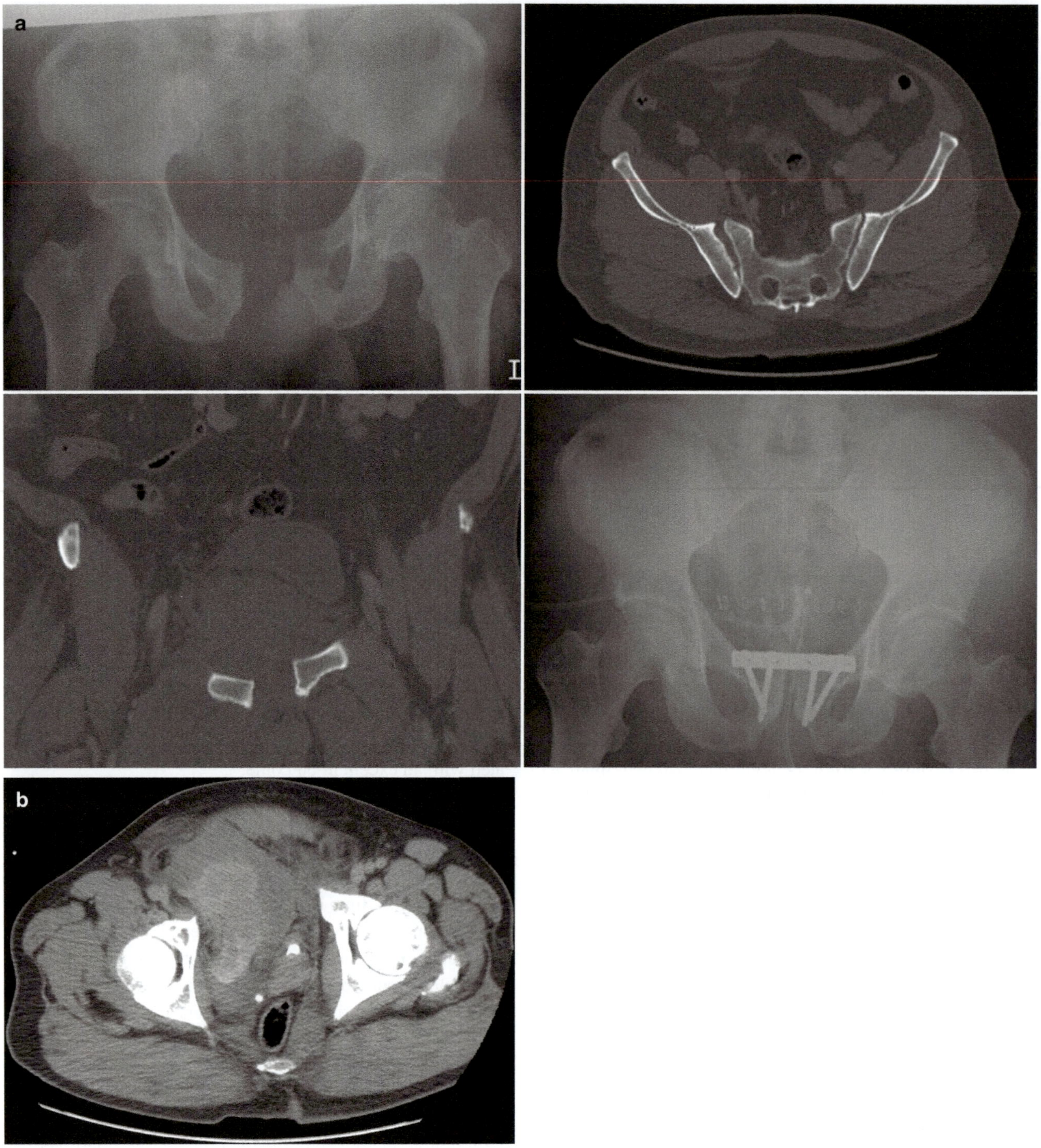

Fig. 23.25 (a) Classical right open-book injury with unstable hemodynamics, immediately stabilized with a 4.5 mm four-hole DC plate. (b) Note: the large intrapelvic hematoma formation due to injury of the prevescical venous plexus

come according to the Majeed Score was only excellent or good in 53.8% (1× excellent, 6× good, 4× fair, 2× poor). The radiographic result was excellent (<5 mm) in two patients (15.4%) and good (6–10 mm) in eight patients (61.5%). There was a tendency to better clinical results after single symphyseal plating, while double plating resulted in better radiological results.

Putnis et al. analyzed 49 patients with internal fixation of the symphysis using different plate constructs including single and double plating of different lengths [68]. No infectious complications were recorded. Of these, 30.6% showed some implant failure (screw loosening or breakage), which developed up to 1 year postoperatively. Double plating was not associated with implant movement. Overall, loss of

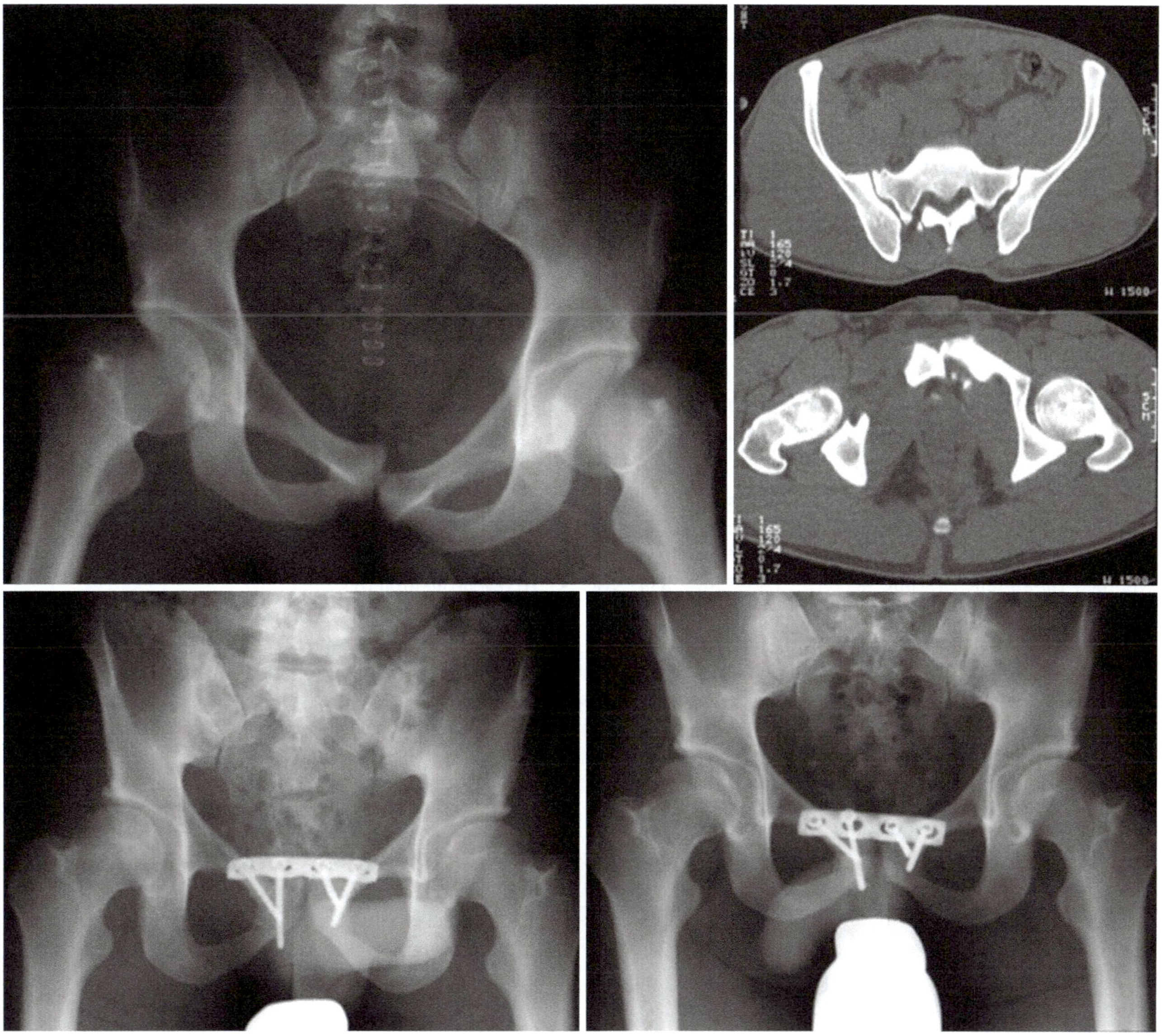

Fig. 23.26 Lateral compression injury with a locked pubic symphysis, treated with a small 4.5 mm, four-hole DC plate. Follow-up shows screw loosening after 1 year.

reduction was observed in 12.2%. Using the SF-12 scoring, after plate osteosynthesis of different fracture entities, physical health was impaired. After 1 year, 15 patients (37%) reported no pain, 29% had mild or very mild pain, 27% moderate pain, and 3 patients reported (7%) severe pain. The mean subjective physical function score was 69%. Daily activities were relevantly affected in 20%. Walking disturbances were reported in 51%.

Van Loon et al. presented midterm results of 38 open-book lesions. All but one patient was treated with open reduction and internal fixation of the symphysis pubis [69]. The functional outcome was excellent after a median of 84 months with a mean Majeed Score of 96. However, compared with the SF-36 score of the normal German population, the mean value of the "role-physical" and the "physical function" categories were significantly lower for patients treated with an open-book lesion.

Chen et al. analyzed 45 patients with standard plate osteosynthesis (one reconstruction plate) [62]. Blood loss was 157 mL, incision length 7.9 cm, implant failure rate 19%, malunion rate 33.3%, and the percentage of impotence in the male patients 15%. At follow-up of 21 months, 24.4% and 57.1% showed excellent and good functional results according to the Majeed Score, respectively.

Comparable results were reported using an open Endobutton technique [70].

Adams et al. analyzed 25 patients with 18 APC II, 2 APC III, 5 LC-, and 1 VS injury, stabilized with 8–10-hole reconstruction plates [51]. The average blood loss was 244 mL. One patient developed postoperative infection (4%).

Yu et al. compared 24 patients with percutaneous screw osteosynthesis of a Tile type B1 injury and 27 patients with reconstruction plate stabilization [40]. As expected, intraoperative blood loss, operative time, and the incision length were significantly less than after ORIF, while the quality of reduction was comparable. In each group two cases of implant failure were observed, and one wound infection occurred in the ORIF group.

After a mean follow-up of 29 months, patients with percutaneous stabilization presented with 95.8% good and excellent results (Majeed Score) compared to 92.6% in the ORIF group.

Jain et al. performed an outcome study on 15 patients with 9 APC II and 6 APC III injuries. APC II injuries were fixed anteriorly with DC- and reconstruction plates, while APC III injuries had additional posterior sacroiliac screw fixation [71]. Anterior fixation was performed first. APC II injuries showed good and excellent functional results (Majeed Score) after at least 1 year in 89% and good to excellent radiological results in 77%, while after APC III injuries 83% good and excellent clinical and radiological results were observed. No implant failure was seen.

Lybrand et al. evaluated 54 patients with 35 APC II and 19 type III injuries at an average follow-up of 7 years (minimum 2 years) using the EuroQol five dimensions (EQ5D), EuroQol health index, Visual Analog Score (VAS) pain, Majeed Pelvic Score, and change in work status [72]. A tendency for slightly better outcome was observed regarding APC II injuries. Implant loosening was observed in 19 patients, with two requiring revision.

Plate stabilization of the pubic symphysis in 28 patients resulted in symphyseal space reduction to 7 mm compared to 10.7 mm using the INFIX concept. The median Majeed Score was 77.7 points [64].

23.15 Symphyseal Widening

There is usually some secondary widening of the symphyseal space after osteosynthesis of a symphyseal disruption. Lybrand et al. Observed a 1–2 mm increase until union occurred, also after disk removal or disk retaining procedures [53].

23.16 Complications

Weber et al. reported on 1 septic implant removal and 1 DVT in 22 patients after combined reconstruction-plate osteosynthesis and tension band wiring [65].

Pohlemann et al. reported five complications after plate osteosynthesis in 21 patients [43]. One deep infection was treated by debridement and screw change. Micturition disturbances and erectile dysfunction were observed in four patients of which one erectile dysfunction persisted. Follow-up analysis of 20 patients found that 11 patients reported no pain and three reported on slight pelvic pain. One patient presented with a rectus abdominis hernia, not requiring further treatment. All pelves anatomically healed, while in nine patients some heterotopic bone formation was observed near the symphysis. Overall, 66.7% were graded excellent and 26.7% good using the German Pelvic Outcome Score (POS) [73].

Raman et al. performed a literature review of 482 patients with symphyseal internal stabilization and reported an overall complication rate of 7.5% [74]. Analyzing only larger series (>10 patients) and trauma cases including the above-cited reports and a further analysis, the following rates were found [43, 65, 74, 75]:

- 3.6% infections
- 3.7% implant failure (Fig. 23.20)
- 9.7% residual pain
- 10.0% urogenital dysfunction

Recent analyses of the literature indicate an infection rate after symphyseal plating of 4.3% [40, 51, 60, 62, 64, 66–68, 75, 76].

23.17 Rectus Hernia

A rectus hernia is a rare consequence of surgical stabilization of the pubic symphysis.

Restoration of the abdominal wall and anatomical refixation of torn abdominal wall muscles are the primary treatment aims [77].

Often when a rectus abdominis muscle injury is observed on the injured side, at least a partial rectus insertional injury is present. Rarely, bony avulsion injuries can be present. If dissected muscles are not adequately fixed to the upper pubic rami periosteum, retraction and atrophy can develop, which lead to retraction to the flanks [78]. Lack of anterior abdominal wall muscle function can lead to increased lumbar lordosis with concomitant back pain [78].

Open-book external rotation injuries can additionally result in bladder herniation due to injury of the puboprostatic and pubovesical ligaments and the pelvic fascia [79].

Surgical reconstruction is performed predominantly using plastic meshes [80, 81]. The risk of wound infections, mesh migration, or enteric fistulas should be considered [82].

Only a few case reports are found in the literature:

- Pohlemann et al. reported on one rectus herniation after four-hole plate stabilization [43].
- Another case was reported by Del Frari et al. who performed an osseous refixation of the rectus abdominis muscles with Mersilene bands [83].
- Cantu et al. reported a case with reconstruction using a prolene mesh without reattaching the muscles [84].
- Seckiner et al. treated a bladder herniation with a cortico-cancellous bone allograft for occlusion of the persistent symphyseal diastasis and a prolene mesh anterior fascial rectus muscle reconstruction [85].
- Bartlett et al. reported on a case of anchor refixation of the torn rectus abdominis muscles after bladder herniation [86].

> Anterior abdominal wall herniations, including bladder herniation, are rare complications associated with internal osteosynthesis of symphyseal disruption. Several reconstructive options exist.

23.18 Implant Removal

Historically, implant removal was frequently performed after plate osteosynthesis of the disrupted pubic symphysis.

Weber et al. analyzed 22 patients with pubic symphysis disruption treated with combined reconstructionplate osteosynthesis and tension band wiring. In 45.5% implant removal was performed after an average of 15.7 months (3–42 months) [65]. Metal removal had no influence on the clinical and radiological long-term results.

Pohlemann et al. recommended implant removal after 6–12 months in all cases due to physiological movements of the symphysis [43].

Raman et al. performed a literature review on 482 patients with symphyseal internal stabilization on implant removal and stated that no consensus could be derived for routine implant removal [74]. A 7.5% complication rate was observed with implant removal with infection the most common complication.

Giannoudis et al. analyzed 74 patients after symphyseal plating. Implant removal was performed in only four patients (5.4%) in an observational period of 41 months [75]. It was stated, that routine removal of the plate is not essential while in women of childbearing age, no clear data were available.

Collinge et al. retrospectively reviewed 126 patients with type B and type C injuries treated with anterior plate fixation using a four- or six-hole 3.5 mm plate without locking screws [76]. All type C injuries additionally had posterior stabilization, while type B injuries were fixed posteriorly in 30%. In 75%, radiographic hardware failure was detected at an average follow-up of 12.2 months, including screw loosening/breakage (71% screw loosening, 5% screw breakage, 7% plate breakage, and 17% combined screw loosening/breakage). Even in type B injuries, 74% implant failure rate was observed. After type C injuries this rate was 77%. During follow-up of these patients, symphyseal gap increased from 4.9 to 8.5 mm.

Morris et al. retrospectively reviewed 148 patients with symphyseal disruption, fixed with plates, treated using three different plating systems. In three cases, double plating was performed [87]. After a minimum follow-up of 12 months, implant breakage was observed in 43%. Of these patients, 96.8% were asymptomatic. In only 3% of patients, revision surgery was indicated.

There is often some secondary widening of the symphyseal space after osteosynthesis of a symphyseal disruption. Lybrand et al. observed 1–2 mm increase until union occurred, also after disk removal or disk retaining procedures [53].

> Late fixation failure, e.g., symphyseal widening ± fixation failure, is considered a benign condition as few patients need revision surgery [76, 87].

In a series of 37 patients with symphyseal plating (3× type A, 24× type B, 10× type C injuries, 76% posterior fixation), 29.7% rate of symphyseal implant failure was detected [88]. The quality of the reduction was excellent in 38% (≤5 mm), good in 27% (6–10 mm), and insufficient in 36% (>10 mm) according to Lindahl [44]. The SF-36 score was not significantly affected by implant failure, while the Majeed Score showed a tendency of better results after implant failure (83 vs. 72 points).

23.19 Failure Rates

Lybrand et al. compared 96 patients with APC II and III injuries, stabilized with anterior symphyseal plating (six-hole plate). Fifty patients had symphyseal cartilage removal. The postoperative symphyseal gap was lower compared to disk retention. The implant failure rate was lower after cartilage excision in the APC II group (7% vs. 19% implant breakage, 13% vs. 42% screw loosening/breakage, 20% vs. 61% combined problems), whereas after type APC III injuries no significant implant failure rate was observed in both groups. Overall, comparing disk excision and disk retaining treatment, after disk excision implant failure rates were lower (16% vs. 35% screw loosening, 4% vs. 17% plate breakage, 20% vs. 52% combined failures) [53].

Eastman et al. analyzed 126 patients treated with symphyseal plate stabilization and additional iliosacral screw fixation. Of these, 11.1% presented with early fixation failure after an average of 29 days. Overall, 30.9% sustained implant failure at an average of 92.4 days. Revision was performed in only 5.1% [89].

In an analysis of 134 patients with APC II injuries, 92 (69%) had combined anterior and posterior fixation (3.5 mm six-hole symphyseal plate, 7.0 or 7.3 mm iliosacral screw) and 42 (31%) had isolated anterior plate osteosynthesis. Fixation failure and malunion occurred more frequently after isolated anterior fixation (40% vs. 5%, 36% vs. 1%), respectively [90].

23.20 Locked Pubic Symphysis

Lateral compression forces can rarely result in symphyseal overlapping ("locked pubic symphysis") (Fig. 23.21). Only few papers have dealt with this condition.

Recently, Bontanioglu et al. performed a literature overview with a case and presented an open reduction technique [91]. After bilateral iliac compression, resulting in injury mobility, reduction is performed using a curved elevator placed in the obturator foramen to act as a lever arm. Of 13 cases, 53.8% were associated with a urethral injury. Treatment consisted of pure closed reduction in three cases and primary open reduction in four cases. In the remaining patients, closed reduction failed and open reduction was necessary. Thus, in 77% open reduction has to be performed.

Internal fixation is favored using plates, especially if the symphysis is unstable following reduction [91, 92]. External fixation is considered optional for distraction in lateral compression type injuries [93].

23.21 Comparison Analyses

Several reports compared different stabilization methods. The following results were obtained:

- Combined tension band wiring and symphyseal plate fixation were superior to isolated plate fixation in terms of radiological outcome, hardware loosening, and revision surgery [47].
- Plate stabilization was superior to INFIX in terms of reduction quality [64].
- Percutaneous screw fixation is as strong as plate fixation but offers the advantage of less iatrogenic injuries and a better functional outcome [62].
- TightRope® + external fixator showed similar outcomes to percutaneous cannulated screw fixation [63].

23.22 Summary

Traumatic symphyseal disruption should be treated surgically, irrespective of existing posterior pelvic ring damage. Plate osteosynthesis is still the gold standard with at least two screws on each side. The plate type does not interfere with long-term results. A high rate of implant failures should be expected, but most often without surgical and clinical consequences. Thus, routine implant removal is not necessary.

References

1. Trafton P. Fixation of the pubic symphysis. Oper Tech Orthop. 1993;3:13–8.
2. Holdsworth F. Dislocation and fracture-dislocation of the pelvis. J Bone Joint Surg. 1948;30-B(3):461–6.
3. Theiss E. Traumatic symphyseal dislocation and their reposition. Chirurg. 1964;35:41–2.
4. Finsterer H. Über Beckenluxationen. Dtsch Z Chir. 1911;110:191–210.
5. Lambotte A. Chirurgie opératoire des fractures. répité, vol. 1913. Bruxelles: Société Franco-Belge D'Editions Scientifiques; 1948. p. 126–44.
6. Sparp I. Plate fixation of disrupted symphysis pubis. Preliminary report. J Bone Joint Surg. 1973;55B:618–20.
7. Dolati B. Die operative Versorgung der Symphysenruptur. Unfallchirurgie. 1985;11:223–7.
8. Ecke H, Burger H, Hofmann D, Nazari P, Maier K. Stabilitätsprüfung verschiedener Osteosyntheseverfahren nach Symphysenruptur und Sprengung der Ileosacralfuge. Langenbecks Arch Chir. 1984;84:195–9.
9. Ecke H, Patzak H, Hofmann D. Überbrückungszuggurtungen zur Wiederherstellung rupturierter Amphiarthrosen am Beckenring. Unfallchirurgie. 1991;17:335–42.
10. Hofmann D, Ecke H, Burger H, Nazari P, Maier K, Pabst W. Festigkeitsuntersuchung verschiedener Osteosyntheseverfahren bei Symphysenruptur und Sprengung der Iliosacralfuge. Hefte zur Unfallheilkunde, 1985. Heft 174. p. 75–8.
11. Labitzke R. Drahtseile und intraossäre Druckverteilungshülsen in der Chirurgie. Chirurg. 1982;53:741–3.
12. Labitzke R, Witzel U. Biomechanische Grundlagen und Technik der elastischen Hülsen-Seil-Verspannung der Beckenruptur. Hefte zur Unfallheilkunde. Heft 181. 1986. p. 622–4.
13. Rubel I, Roberts C, Hemling B, Seligson D. Endoscopic fixation of the symphysis pubis. Osteosynthese Int. 1999;7:204–8.
14. Berner W, Oestern H, Tscherne H. Die hintere Beckenringluxation—eine Indikation zur Operation. Hefte zur Unfallheilkunde, 1984. Heft 164. p. 286–91.
15. Fink D, Möseneder H. Offene Symphysensprengung mit primärer Verplattung. Hefte zur Unfallheilkunde, 1974. Heft 124. p. 292–3.
16. Hierholzer G, Gras U. Verletzungen des Beckens und seiner Bandverbindungen. Hefte zur Unfallheilkunde, 1984. Heft 164. p. 181–7.
17. Kellam JF, McMurtry RY, Paley D, Tile M. The unstable pelvic fracture—operative treatment. Orthop Clin North Am. 1987;18(1):25–41.
18. Kinzl L, Burri C, Wörsdörfer O. Operative Therapie bei Beckenfugenzerreißungen. Hefte zur Unfallheilkunde. Heft 164. 1984. p. 222–3.

19. Lange R, Hansen S. Pelvic ring disruptions with symphysis pubis diastasis—indications, technique and limitations of anterior internal fixation. Clin Orthop. 1985;201:130–7.
20. Olerud S, Walheim G. Symphysiodesis with a new compression plate. Acta Orthop Scand. 1984;55:315–8.
21. Tile M, Burry C, Poigenfürst J. Pelvis. In: Müller M, et al., editors. Manual of internal fixation. Berlin, Heidelberg, New York: Springer; 1991. p. 485–500.
22. Meißner A. Biomechanik und Stabilisierung der Symphyse. Berlin: Freie Universität; 1989.
23. Meißner A, Breyer H, Ramanzadeh R. Experimentelle Untersuchungen zur Beweglichkeit in der Symphyse. Hefte Unfallheilk. 1986;181:79–82.
24. Tile M. Fractures of the pelvis and acetabulum. 2nd ed. Baltimore: Williams & Wilkins; 1995.
25. Trulson A, Küper M, Trulson I, Minarski C, Grünwald L, Hirt B, Stöckle U, Stuby F. Endoscopic approach to the quadrilateral plate (EAQUAL): a new endoscopic approach for plate osteosynthesis of the pelvic ring and acetabulum—a cadaver study. Z Orthop Unfall. 2018;157(1):22–8. https://doi.org/10.1055/a-0621-9570. (German).
26. McBroom R, Tile M. Disruption of the pelvic ring. Orthop Trans. 1982;6:493.
27. Lehmann U. Belastungsmessung an der Symphysis pubis, normale Belastung und Plattenosteosynthese. Inaugural Dissertation. Hannover. 1990.
28. Stocks G, Gablel D, Noble P, Hanson G, Tullos H. Anterior and posterior internal fixation of vertical shear fractures of the pelvis. J Orthop Res. 1991;9:237–45.
29. Sagi H, Ordway N, DiPasquale T. Biomechanical analysis of fixation for vertically unstable sacroiliac dislocations with Iliosacral screws and symphyseal plating. J Orthop Trauma. 2004;18:138–43.
30. Leighton R, Waddell J, Bray T, Chapman M, Simpson L, Martin R, Sharkey N. Biomechanical testing of new and old fixation devices for vertical shear fractures of the pelvis. J Orthop Trauma. 1991;5(3):313–7.
31. Varga E. Comparison of different methods of internal symphyseal fixations in unstable pelvic ring injuries: a biomechanical study. Surgery of the Pelvis and Acetabulum: The second International Consensus Pittsburgh. October 21–27, 1994.
32. Simonian P, Schwappach J, Routt M, Agnew S, Harrington R, Tencer A. Evaluation of new plate designs for symphysis pubis internal fixation. J Trauma. 1996;41(3):498–502.
33. Meißner A, Fell M, Wilk R, Boenick U, Rahmanzadeh R. Vergleich interner Stabilisierungsverfahren für die Symphyse im multidirektionalen dynamischen Gangbedingungssimulator. Unfallchirurg. 1998;101(1):18–25.
34. Daily B, Chong A, Buhr B, Greesion C, Cooke F. Locking and nonlocking plate fixation pubic symphysis diastasis management. Am J Orthop. 2012;41:540–5.
35. Cano-Luis P, Giráldez-Sanchez M, Martínez-Reina J, Serrano-Escalante F, Galleguillos-Rioboo C, Lázaro-Gonzálvez A, García-Rodríguez J, Navarro A. Biomechanical analysis of a new minimally invasive system for osteosynthesis of pubis symphysis disruption. Injury. 2012;43:20–7.
36. Prasarn M, Zych G, Gaski G, Baria D, Kaimrajh D, Milne T, Laytta L. Biomechanical study of 4-hole pubic symphyseal plating: locked versus unlocked constructs. Orthopedics. 2012;35:e1028–32.
37. Grimshaw C, Bledsoe J, Moed B. Locked versus standard unlocked plating of the pubic symphysis: a cadaver biomechanical study. J Orthop Trauma. 2012;26:402–6.
38. Moed B, O'Boynick C, Bledsoe J. Locked versus standard unlocked plating of the symphysis pubis in a Typ-C plevic injury: a cadaver biomechanical study. Injury. 2014;45:748–51.
39. Pizanis A, Garcia P, Santelmann M, Culemann U, Pohlemann T. Reduction and fixation capabilities of different plate designs for pubic symphysis disruption: a biomechanical comparison. Injury. 2013;44:183–8.
40. Yu K, Hong J, Guo X, Zhou D. Comparison of reconstruction plate screw fixation and percutaneous cannulated screw fixation in treatment of Tile B1 type pubic symphysis diastasis: a finite element analysis and 10-year clinical experience. J Orthop Surg Res. 2015;10:151.
41. Yao F, He Y, Qian H, Zhou D, Li Q. Comparison of biomechanical characteristics and pelvic ring stability using different fixation methods to treat pubic symphysis diastasis. A finite element study. Medicine. 2015;94:e2207.
42. Yag F, He Y, Qian H, Zhou D, Li Q. Comparison of biomechanical characteristics and pelvic ring stability using different fixation methods to treat pubic symphysis diastasis: a finite element study. Medicine. 2015;94:e2207.
43. Pohlemann T, Gänsslen A. Die Operation der Symphysensprengung. Oper Orthop Traumatol. 1999;11:149–59.
44. Lindahl J, Hirvensalo E, Bostman O, Santavirta S. Failure of reduction with an external fixator in the management of injuries of the pelvic ring. Long-term evaluation of 110 patients. J Bone Joint Surg Br. 1999;81(6):955–62.
45. Baqué P, Trojani C, Delotte J, Seéjor E, Senni-Buratti M, Baqué F, Bourgeon A. Anatomical consequences of "open-book" pelvic ring disruption. A cadaver experimental study. Surg Radiol Anat. 2005;27:487–90.
46. Matta J. Indications for anterior fixation of pelvic fractures. Clin Orthop. 1996;329:88–96.
47. Park M, Yoon S, Choi S, Lee K. Is there a clinical benefit of additional tension band wiring in plate fixation of the symphysis? BMC Musculoskelet Disord. 2017;18:40. https://doi.org/10.1186/s12891-017-1418-3.
48. Kisielinski K, Conze J, Murken A, Lenzen N, Klinge U, Schumpelick V. The Pfannenstiel or so called "bikini cut": still effective more than 100 years after first description. Hernia. 2004;8:177–81.
49. Pfannenstiel H. Ueber die Vortheile des suprasymphysären Fascienquerschnitts für die gynäkologischen Köliotomien, zugleich ein Beitrage zu der Indikationstellung der Operationswege. Samm Klin Vorträge (Leipzig). 1900;268:1735.
50. Thiery M, Hermann J. Pfannenstiel (1862–1909) and the Pfannenstiel incision. Gynecol Surg. 2010;7:93–5.
51. Adams M, Scolaro J, Routt M. The pubic midline exposure for symphyseal open reduction and plate fixation. J Orthop Traumatol. 2014;15:195. https://doi.org/10.1007/s10195-014-0296-9.
52. Collinge C, Beltran M. Anatomic relationship between the spermatic cord and the pubic tubercle: are our clamps injuring the cord during symphyseal repair? J Orthop Trauma. 2015;29:290–4.
53. Lybrand K, Kurylo J, Gross J, Templeman D, Tornetta PR. Does removal of the symphyseal cartilage in symphyseal dislocations have any effect on final alignment and implant failure? J Orthop Trauma. 2015;29:470–4.
54. Hefzy MS, Ebraheim N, Mekhail A, Caruntu D, Lin H, Yeasting R. Kinematics of the human pelvis following open book injury. Med Eng Phys. 2003;25(4):259–74.
55. Vrahas M. Fixation of pubic symphysis diastasis and pubic rami fractures. Tech Orthop. 1995;9(4):283–9.
56. Webb L, Gristina A, Wilson J, Rhyne A, Meredith J, Hansen S. Two-hole plate fixation for traumatic symphysis pubis diastasis. J Trauma. 1988;28(6):813–7.
57. Pierce T, Issa K, Callaghan J, Wright C. Traumatic diastasis of the pubic symphysis—a review of fixation method outcomes. Surg Technol Int. 2016;29:165–269.
58. Sagi H, Papp S. Comparative radiographic and clinical outcome of two-hole and multi-hole symphyseal plating. J Orthop Trauma. 2008;22:373–8.

59. Moed B, Grimshaw C, Segina D. Failure of locked design-specific plate fixation of the pubic symphysis: a report of six cases. J Orthop Trauma. 2012;26:e71–5.
60. Hamada A, Pavlou G, Dwyer J, Lim J. Management of pubic symphysis diastasis with locking plates: a report of 11 cases. Injury. 2013;44:947–51.
61. Mu W, Wang H, Zhou D, Yu L, Jia T, Li L. Computer navigated percutaneous screw fixation for traumatic pubic symphysis diastasis of unstable pelvic ring injuries. Chin Med J. 2009;122:1699–703.
62. Chen L, Zhang G, Song D, Guo X, Yuan W. A comparison of percutaneous reduction and screw fixation versus open reduction and plate fixation of traumatic symphysis pubis diastasis. Arch Orthop Trauma Surg. 2012;132:265–70.
63. Feng Y, Hong J, Guo X, Lin C, Ling W, Zhang L, Wang G. Percutaneous fixation of traumatic pubic symphysis diastasis using a TightRope and external fixator versus using a cannulated screw. J Orthop Surg Res. 2016;11:62.
64. Vaidya R, Martin A, Roth M, Nasr K, Gheraibeh P, Tonnos F. INFIX versus plating for pelvic fractures with disruption of the symphysis pubis. Int Orthop. 2017;41:1671–8.
65. Weber K, Vock B, Müller W, Wentzensen A. Rupture of the pubic symphysis: diagnosis, treatment and clinical outcome. Ann Saudi Med. 1999;19:544–6.
66. Spagnolo R, Pace F, Bonalumi M, Capitani D. Anterior pelvic ring fractures: a proposal of a variant of osteosynthesis of the pubic symphysis. Eur J Orthop Surg Traumatol. 2010;21:33. https://doi.org/10.1007/s00590-010-0651-3.
67. Aggarwal S, Bali K, Krishnan V, Kumar V, Meena D, Sen R. Management outcomes in pubic diastasis: our experience with 19 patients. J Orthop Surg. 2011;6:21.
68. Putnis S, Pearce R, Wali U, Bircher M, Rickman M. Open reduction and internal fixation of a traumatic diastasis of the pubic symphysis. J Bone Joint Surg Br. 2011;93:78–84.
69. Van Loon P, Kuhn S, Hofmann A, Hessmann M, Rommens P. Radiological analysis, operative management and functional outcome of open book pelvic lesions: a 13-year cohort study. Injury. 2011;42:1012–9.
70. Chen L, Ouyang Y, Huang G, Lu X, Ye X, Hong J. Endobutton technique for dynamic fixation of traumatic symphysis pubis disruption. Acta Orthop Belg. 2013;79:54–9.
71. Jain M, Runu R, Kumar S, Kumar M. Outcome of plate osteosynthesis in pubic diastasis: an experience of tertiary care centre. Indian J Orthop Surg. 2016;2:326–30.
72. Lybrand K, Bell A, Rodericks D, Templeman D, Tornetta PR. APC Injuries with symphyseal fixation: what affects outcome? J Orthop Trauma. 2017;31:27–30.
73. Pohlemann T, Gänsslen A, Schellwald O, Culemann U, Tscherne H. Ergebnisbeurteilung nach instabilen Verletzungen des Beckenrings. Unfallchirurg. 1996;99(4):249–59.
74. Raman R, Roberts C, Pape H, Giannoudis P. Implant retention and removal after internal fixation of the symphysis pubis. Injury. 2005;36:827–31.
75. Giannoudis P, Chalidis B, Roberts C. Internal fixation of traumatic diastasis of pubic symphysis: is plate removal essential? Arch Orthop Trauma Surg. 2008;128:325–31.
76. Collinge C, Archdeacon M, Dulaney-Cripe E, Moed B. Radiographic changes of implant failure after plating for pubic symphysis diastasis: an underappreciated reality? Clin Orthop. 2012;470:2148–53.
77. DiBello J, Moore J, DiBello JN Jr, Moore JH Jr. Sliding myofascial flap of the rectus abdominis muscles for the closure of recurrent ventral hernias. Plast Reconstr Surg. 1996;98:464–9.
78. Flament J, Rices J. Major incisional hernia. In: Chevrel JP, editor. Hernias and surgery of the abdominal wall. 2nd ed. Berlin, Heidelberg, New York: Springer; 1998. p. 128–58.
79. Fallon B, Wendt J, Hawtrey C. Urological injury and assessment in patients with fractured pelvis. J Urol. 1984;131:712–3.
80. Jaques L, Gloviczki P, Patterson D, Sarr M. Successful repair of an unusual hernia associated with traumatic pubic diastasis. Mayo Clin Proc. 1988;63(5):492–5.
81. Sharma A, Jain P, Shaw C, Sedman P. Successful laparoscopic repair of a traumatic pubic symphysis hernia. Surg Endosc. 2004;18:345–9.
82. Schumpelick V, Conze J, Klinge U. Preperitoneal mesh-plasty in incisional hernia repair. A comparative retrospective study of 272 operated incisional hernias. Chirurg. 1996;67:1028–35.
83. Del Frari B, Larndorfer R, Piz-Katzer H. Abriss der geraden Bauchmuskeln der Symphyse nach Symphysenruptur—Möglichkeit der Wiederherstellung. Unfallchirurg. 2008;111:845. https://doi.org/10.1007/s00113-008-1412-1.
84. Cantu R, Poka A. Traumatic abdominal hernia and lateral compression type 1 pelvic fracture: a case report. J Orthop Trauma. 2006;20:289–91.
85. Seckiner I, Keser S, Bayar A, Yesilli C, Mungan A. Successful repair of a bladder herniation after old traumatic pubic symphysis diastasis using bone graft and hernia mesh. Arch Orthop Trauma Surg. 2007;127:655–7.
86. Bartlett C, Ali A, Helfet D. Bladder incarceration in a traumatic symphysis pubis diastasis treated with external fixation: a case report and review of the literature. J Orthop Trauma. 1998;12:64–7.
87. Morris S, Loveridge J, Smart D, Ward A, Chesser T. Is fixation failure after plate fixation of the symphysis pubis clinically important? Clin Orthop. 2012;470:2154–60.
88. Frietman B, Verbeek J, Biert J, Frölke J. The effect of implant failure after symphyseal plating on functional outcome and general health. J Orthop Trauma. 2016;30:336–9.
89. Eastman J, Krieg J, Routt MJ. Early failure of symphysis pubis plating. Injury. 2016;47:1707–12.
90. Avilucea F, Whiting P, Mir H. Posterior fixation of APC-2 pelvic ring injuries decreases rates of anterior plate failure and malunion. J Bone Joint Surg Am. 2016;98:944–51.
91. Botanlioglu H, Bisel N, Kaynak G, Ünlü M. Open reduction technique for overlapping and locked pubic symphysis. Acta Orthop Traumatol Turc. 2012;46:77–81.
92. Sreesobh K, Sageer A, Raffic M. Locked overlapping dislocation of the pubic symphysis into the obturator foramen: a case report. J Orthop Surg (Hong Kong). 2006;14:200–3.
93. Bellabarba C, Ricci WM, Bolhofner BR. Distraction external fixation in lateral compression pelvic fractures. J Orthop Trauma. 2000;14(7):475–82.

Retrograde Pubic Rami Screw

24

Franz Müller, Bernd Füchtmeier, Axel Gänsslen, and Jan Lindahl

Fractures of the pubic rami are the most commonly observed injuries in pelvic ring fractures [1]. Direct surgical stabilization of these fractures is rarely performed. The surrounding muscles, e.g., the internal and external obturator and adductor muscles, and the thick periosteal layer allow rapid bone healing with early adequate callus formation within 3–4 weeks [2].

Historically, most commonly, external fixation is performed for emergency stabilization or definitive treatment of the anterior pelvic ring [1, 3–7], when ramus fractures are present, while symphyseal disruption is best treated by plating.

Alternatively, transpubic screw fixation [8–10] or open reduction and plate fixation was recommended [11–15].

More than 100 years ago, Albin Lambotte already illustrated and proposed intramedullary splinting of the public ramus but did not actually perform the procedure [16]. Routt et al. described the percutaneous technique of screw application in 1995 and reported first results in 26 patients [9]. Today, percutaneous and open procedures of transpubic screw fixation are implemented [8–10], or with continual intraoperative visualization techniques cannulated screws can also be inserted [17, 18].

F. Müller
Department of Trauma Surgery, Orthopaedics and Sports Medicine, Hospital Barmherzige Brüder Regensburg, Regensburg, Germany

B. Füchtmeier
Krankenhaus Barmherzige Brüder, Klinik für Unfallchirurgie, Regensburg, Germany
e-mail: Bernd.Fuechtmeier@barmherzige-regensburg.de

A. Gänsslen (✉)
Department of Trauma Surgery, Orthopedics and Hand Surgery, Hospital Wolfsburg, Wolfsburg, Germany

J. Lindahl
Orthopaedics and Trauma Surgery, Helsinki University Hospital, Helsinki, Finland

24.1 Indications

Indication for retrograde superior pubic rami screw fixation include [19]:

- Displaced and/or unstable upper pubic rami fractures as part of type B and type C pelvic injuries
- Posteriorly displaced upper pubic ramus fractures, when there is a risk of fracture-related, secondary complications (tilt fractures or pubic spike) [20, 21]
- Stabilization of the anterior column of the acetabulum in isolated fractures of the anterior column
- Additional internal fixation as part of the management of acetabular fractures with transverse components combined with stabilization of the posterior column
- Symptomatic nonunions of the superior ramus [22, 23]

24.2 Surgical Anatomy of the Superior Pubic Ramus

Knowledge of the anatomy of the superior pubic ramus is essential for adequate screw application. The size and width of the superior ramus differ interindividually and the optimal entry point have to be clearly defined [24].

Several anatomic and radiographic analyses were performed for optimal intraoperative understanding.

The anatomical osseous corridor for the superior ramus screw is typically the distal part of the full anterior column screw corridor (Fig. 24.1).

The superior border is extremely variable due to several bony landmarks. It starts at the pubic symphysis. The first few centimeters extend laterally to the pubic tubercle, the insertion of the inguinal ligament. Medially, a ridge on top of the superior ramus becomes visible (pecten ossis pubis) and is the origin of the strong superior periosteum. The pecten ossis pubis, together with the arcuate line medially, forms the iliopectineal line, which is the medial border of the anterior column. Lateral to the pecten ossis pubis, a grove is visible, where the iliac external vessels course to the outer side of the

A. Gänsslen et al. (eds.), *Pelvic Ring Fractures*, https://doi.org/10.1007/978-3-030-54730-1_24

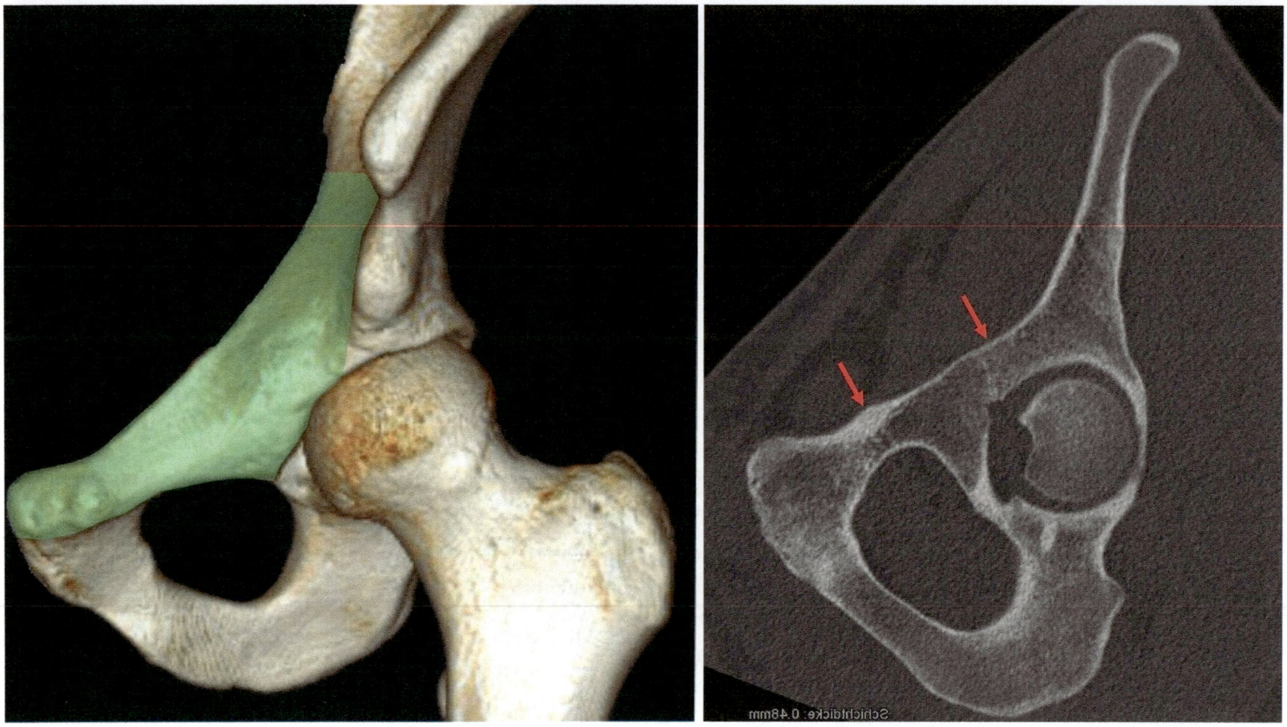

Fig. 24.1 Anatomical osseous corridor for a retrograde superior ramus screw

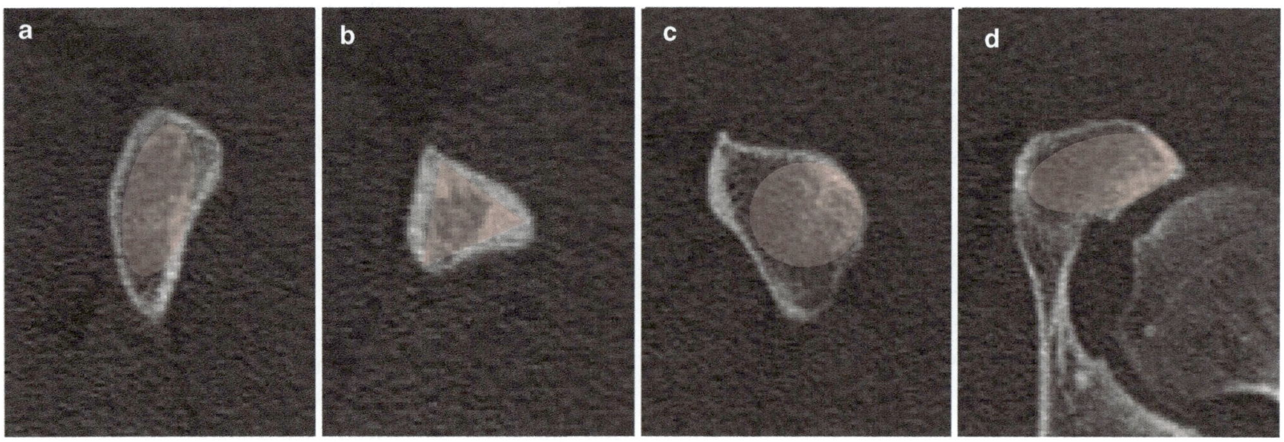

Fig. 24.2 Change of the transverse shape of the upper pubic ramus: parasymphyseal (**a**), mid-ramus (**b**), area of the iliopectineal eminence (**c**), and iliopsoas gutter (**d**)

pelvic area. Medial to the anterior acetabular rim, the iliopectineal eminence becomes prominent, the insertion of the iliopectineal fascia, which divides the muscular from the vascular lacuna. The iliopectineal eminence is a thickened bone part opposite to the anterior horn of the acetabulum. Posterior to the iliopectineal eminence, the iliopsoas groove (iliopsoas gutter) is present, which ends at the level of the AIIS.

Relevant surrounding anatomical structures include the corona mortis, the obturator canal with the obturator neurovascular bundle, and the iliac external vessels.

The transverse shape of the upper pubic ramus differs from anterior to posterior [24, 25] (Fig. 24.2):

- Parasymphyseal: elliptical
- Mid-ramus: triangular
- Iliopectineal eminence: circular
- Iliopsoas gutter: ovoid

Quan et al. analyzed CT data from 40 adult hips. Based on their analysis and clinical experience, 6.5–7.3 mm screws with a length of 60–70 mm were recommended for male patients and 4.5–6.5 mm screws with a length of 70–80 mm for female patients [26].

24.3 Biomechanics

Combined anterior and posterior pelvic ring stabilization allows for optimal stability of the disrupted pelvic ring [27]. Several reports analyzed biomechanical stability of superior ramus fixation.

In a finite element pelvic model, operative fixation of pubic rami fractures with retrograde pubic screw fixation or suprapectineal plate stabilization resulted in decreased fracture movements at the anterior and posterior pelvis [28].

Simonian et al. performed superior/inferior pubic rami osteotomies and unilateral anterior SI-joint injuries with pelvic floor ligament dissection (APC II fracture model) in six fresh-frozen cadaveric pelvic specimens [10].

Isolated stabilization of the anterior pelvic ring was performed, including stabilization with a ten-hole 3.5 mm reconstruction plate fixed with four or six screws and with 80 mm and 130 mm long 4.5 mm retrograde medullary superior pubic ramus cortical screws. No relevant difference between the stabilization methods was detected; especially, longer implants resulted not in increased stiffness.

In a simulated OTA 61-B2.1, LCI injury on plastic pelvic models, after posterior stabilization with two fully threaded, 7.3 mm cannulated iliosacral S1 and S2 screws, supraacetabular external fixation was compared with 7.3 mm partially threaded retrograde superior pubic ramus screw fixation. Screw fixation was 160–180% superior to external fixation [29].

Acklin et al. compared superior pubic ramus fixation with either a 7.3 mm cannulated retrograde screw or a ten-hole 3.5 mm reconstruction plate in 12 human cadaveric pelvis with low bone mineral density [30]. The overall stiffness was lower with screw fixation. Implant failure consisted of screw cutting-out vs. plate bending. In osteoporotic bone, plate stabilization should therefore be considered.

Acklin et al. also compared 7.3 mm cannulated screw fixation with one screw with stabilization of the pubic ramus with two 3.5 mm pelvic cortex screws [31]. Only a tendency of less displacement was observed using 7.3 mm screws. Thus, pubic both stabilization techniques showed comparable results in osteoporotic bone, while the two-screw technique was less demanding.

> Superior pubic ramus screw fixation as an adjunct to posterior stabilization allows for adequate biomechanical stability.

24.4 Classification of Upper Pubic Rami Fractures

The well-accepted classification scheme is the Nakatani system (Fig. 24.3) [32]:

• Zone I	Medial to the obturator foramen
• Zone II	Between Zones I and III
• Zone III	Lateral to the obturator foramen

24.5 Cannulated Upper Pubic Rami Screw Fixation

Mosheiff et al. described the percutaneous approach for cannulated upper pubic rami screw fixation in detail [17].

24.5.1 Positioning and Draping

In the standard supine position on a radiolucent table, a lumbosacral support is advocated to allow easier manipulation. Draping includes the whole pelvic area with low perineal access.

Three radiographic standard views are necessary to adequately identify the anterior and superior ramus [17, 32]: pelvic inlet view, inlet-iliac oblique view, and obturator-outlet view. The C-arm is positioned ipsilateral, while the surgeon is standing contralateral to the fracture site.

24.5.2 Incision

A stab incision is made near the contralateral pubic tubercle followed by subcutaneous dissection until the pubic tubercle can be indirectly palpated using the drill sleeve of the drill bit [17]. Routt et al. recommend the parasymphyseal bone medial to the pectineal tuberosity at its anteromedial corner [24].

24.5.3 Entry Point

A detailed analysis of the existing literature for retrograde screw application was analyzed by Gänsslen et al. for anterior column screw fixation [33]. In summary, the following results were obtained:

- The distance to the center of the pubic symphysis was between 18 and 28 mm [34]
- The distance between this entry point and the pubic tubercle was 14–17 mm [34, 35].
- An overall maximum bone corridor length of 110–130 mm can be expected, influenced by the localization of the fracture [35–40].

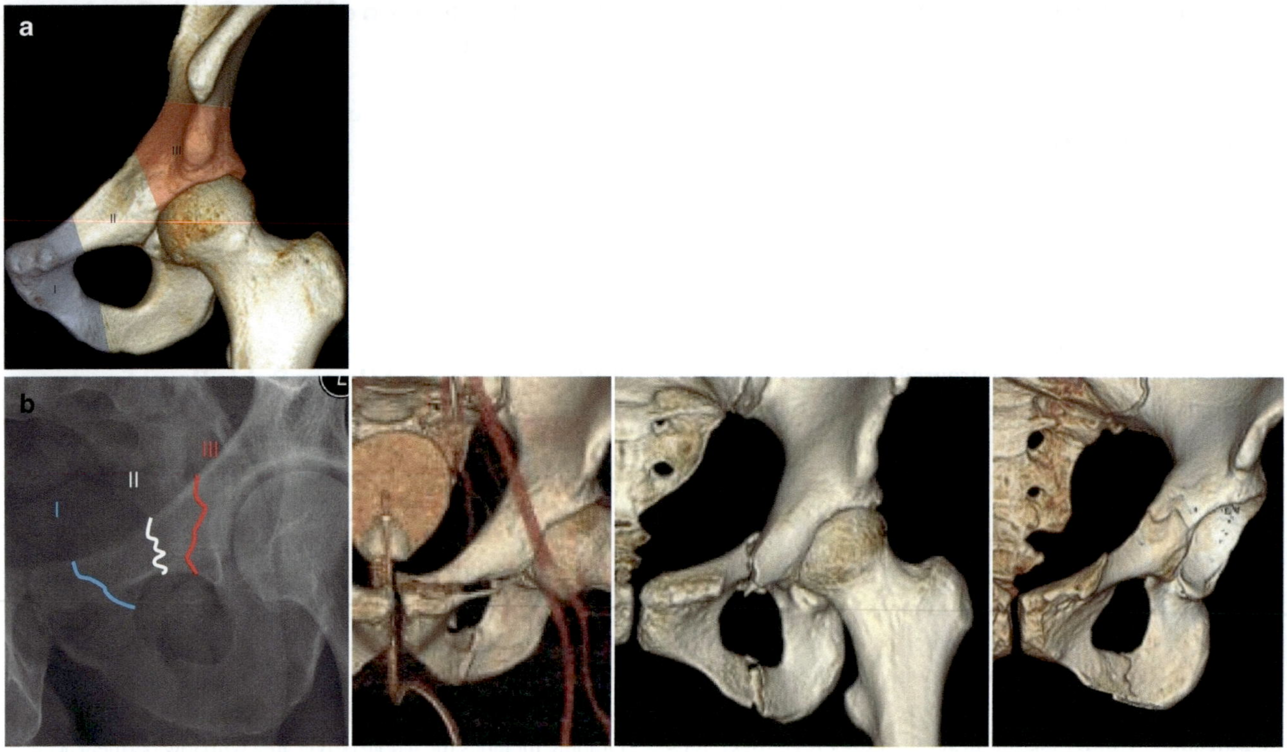

Fig. 24.3 (**a**) Nakatani classification of upper pubic rami fractures. (**b**) Radiographic examples of the Nakatani classification of upper pubic rami fractures

- The most narrowest isthmus of the superior ramus is located between the iliopsoas gutter and obturator neurovascular canal [39, 41] and, depending on the type of measurement, is sized between 10 and 14 mm [25, 35–38, 40–43].
- The laterally directed angle to the sagittal plane was approximately 50° [26, 40], the vertically directed angle to the horizontal plane was approximately 66° [40], and an 8° orientation to the coronal plane were considered optimal [26].
- The distal, anterior slope of the pubic tubercle is the optimal location; the insertion site should be placed as far laterally as the fracture line allows in order to get a more favorable angle in direction to the acetabulum; the screw is inserted parallel to the pectineal line continuing into the linea terminalis [19].

24.5.4 Intraoperative Radiography

The superior ramus anatomy is highly variable due to the different obliquity and curvature of the ramus in the anteroposterior and the coronal planes [24].

Standard radiographic projections include [24, 33] (Fig. 24.4):

- Standard pelvic-inlet view (PI)
- Combined obturator oblique outlet view (COOO)
- Combined iliac oblique inlet view (CIOI)
- Axial anterior column screw view [43]
- Gun barrel view [44]

Due to the variability of the medullary pathway, no standardized C-arm position can be recommended.

Eastman et al. favored a step-by-step procedure of intraoperative imaging for retrograde screw application [24]:

- True anteroposterior (AP) pelvic view, with a centered symphysis on the coccyx
- PI view to identify the entry point (tangential beam to the posterior surface of the superior pubic ramus, which is typically located posterior to the inferior ramus; tilt: approximately 15–35°)
- COOO view (C-arm tilted approximately 30–40° to the pelvic outlet and 20–30° to the obturator oblique) confirms the proximal and periacetabular position of the bone corridor (cranial, caudal, and lateral ramus); the view is optimal, when the beam is orientated tangential to the lateral supraacetabular iliac cortical bone

24.5.5 Pelvic Inlet View

The pelvic inlet view (PIV) can exclude medial cortex penetration [32]. Overlapping of the superior and inferior pubic rami was supposed to be either helpful [18, 45] or should be

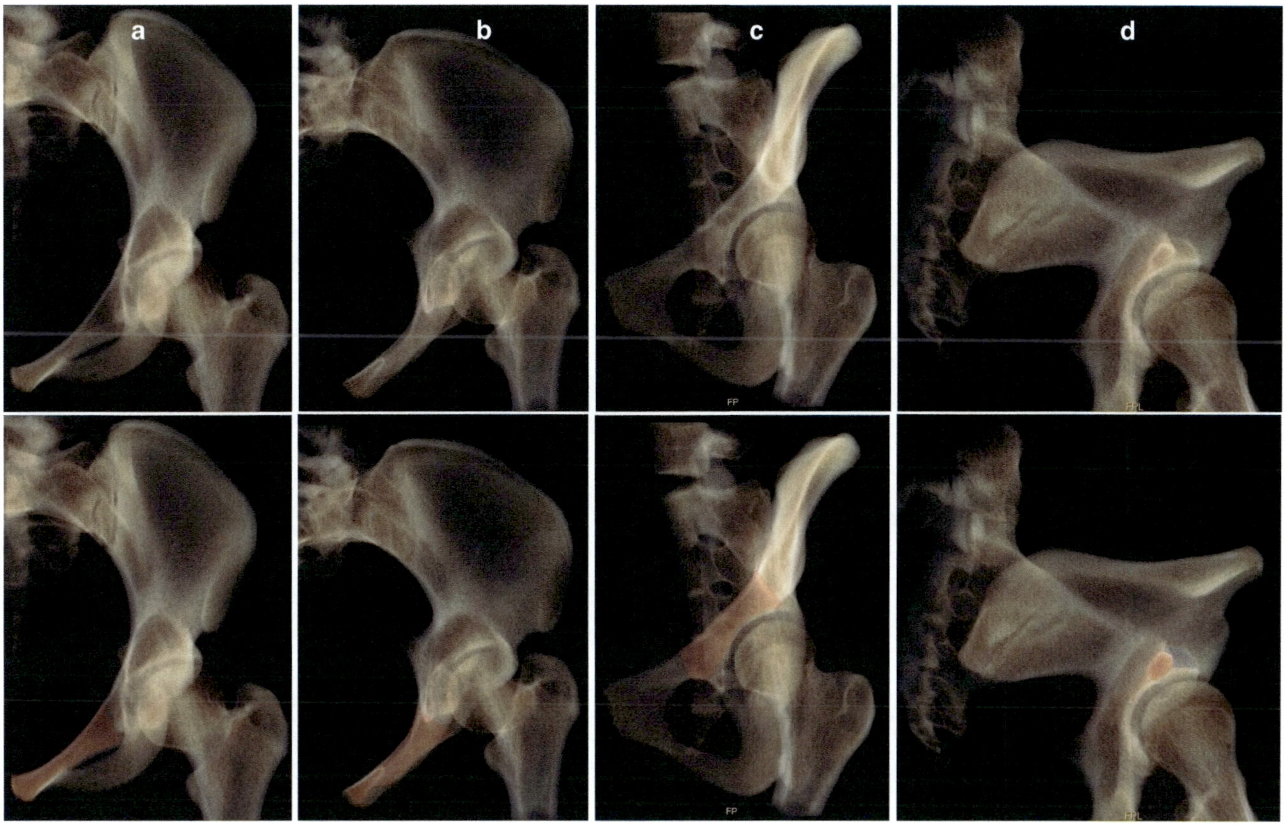

Fig. 24.4 Standard radiographic projections to control the intraoperative screw course: pelvic a.p. view (**a**), pelvic Inlet (**b**), combined obturator oblique Outlet (**c**), and axial anterior column screw view (**d**)

avoided [24, 46]. The entry point for a retrograde superior ramus screw is typically at the pubic tubercle on the PIV. Variations are possible, depending on fracture localization and necessary screw length (Fig. 24.4).

24.5.6 The Combined Obturator Oblique Outlet View (COOO)

The COOO is performed to exclude hip joint penetration and of a superior extraosseous pathway. Starting with the outlet configuration, the maximum width of the bone corridor between the joint and the iliopectineal eminence should be obtained (Fig. 24.4).

24.5.7 Axial Anterior Column Screw View

Recently, a new intraoperative image view was described for analysis of sufficient screw position in anterior column screws.

The C-arm is tilted approximately 35° toward the contralateral hip joint to result in an iliac oblique view and is then rotated toward the feet for an extended outlet image. Superior to the joint area ("sourcil"), an oval track image gradually appears [43] (Fig. 24.4).

To confirm the intraosseous pathway, careful radiopaque contrast medium application into the screw corridor can be performed [45].

24.5.8 Implants

Primarily, 3.5 or 4.5 mm cortical bone screws are used. Larger diameter screws (6.5 mm, 7.0 mm or even 7.3 mm) should be inserted only in exceptional cases depending on a detailed CT analysis.

24.5.9 Guide Wire and Screw Insertion

Mosheiff et al. described several steps for optimal screw insertion [17] (Fig. 24.5):

- Central insertion of a 2.4 mm guidewire into the first 1–2 cm of the upper pubic ramus
- Guidewire orientation is approximated 45° from medial to lateral, and at an angle of 40° to the horizontal plane

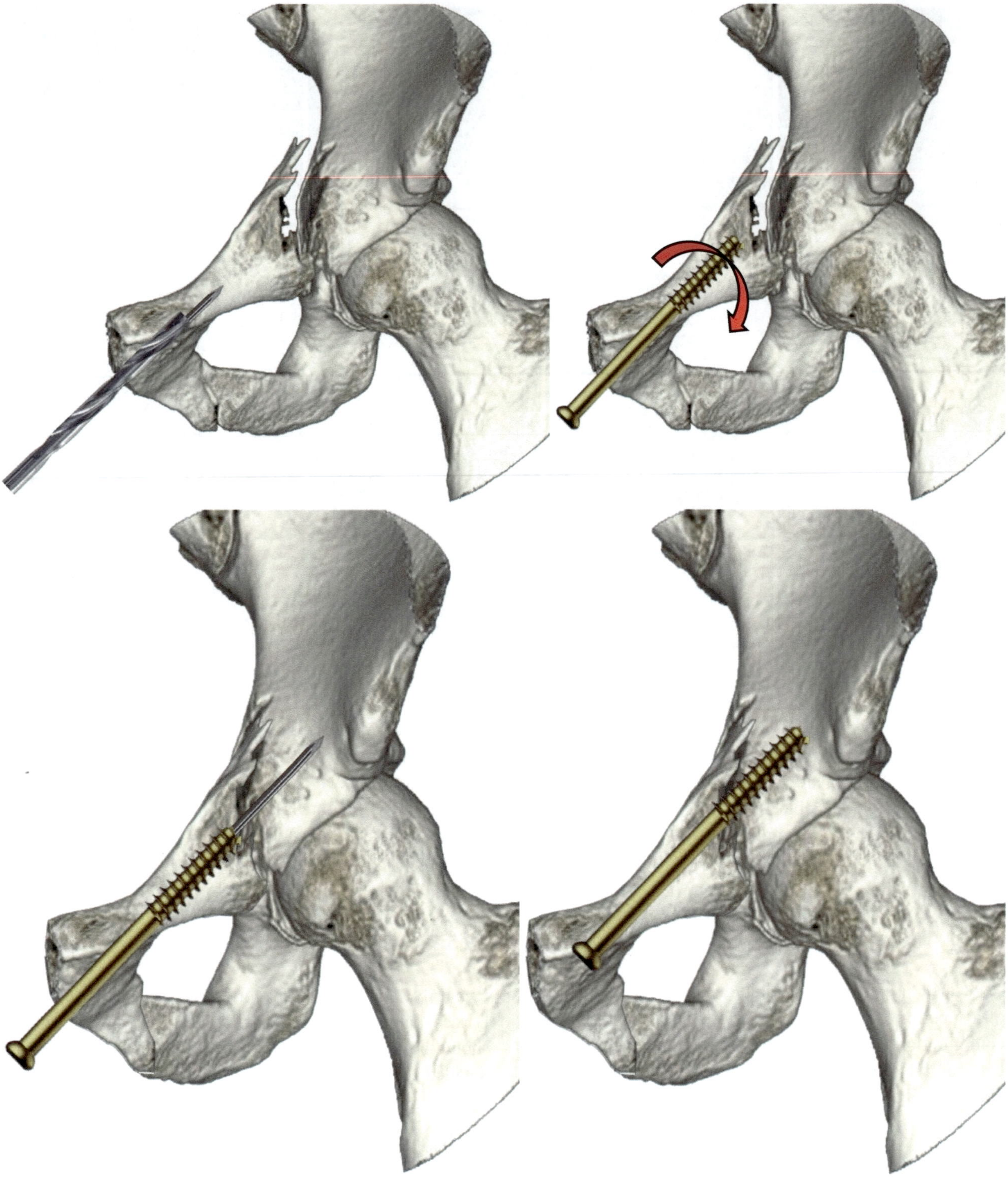

Fig. 24.5 Possible technique of reduction and screw application (details: see text)

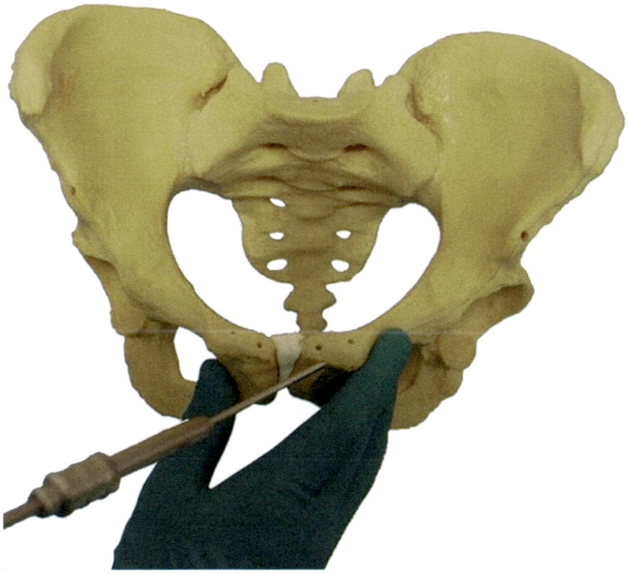

Fig. 24.6 Starting point and guide wire orientation with digital control

downward (Fig. 24.6) [47] or the guide is aimed just posterior and inferior to the anterior-inferior iliac spine [32]
- Opening of the cortex is performed using a 4.7 mm cannulated drill
- A temporary 6.5 mm cannulated screw is advanced to the fracture site
- The screw is used for reduction of the fracture
- The guidewire is directed over the fracture zone into the proximal-lateral fragment area
- Removal of the temporary screw
- Length/depth measurement
- Over-drilling with penetration of the outer cortex of the ilium (drilling should be performed in an oscillating or "pushing" technique [9, 19])
- Insertion of a new cannulated screw

During the procedure, alternating between the PI and COOO views is recommended [24].

Eastman et al. proposed a 3.5 mm drilling until reaching the fracture area, followed by a 2.5 mm drill bit to cross the fracture zone [24].

As a modification, the retrograde-antegrade-retrograde technique is used, if retrograde intramedullary guidewire insertion over the fracture zone is not possible [24, 48]. After starting retrograde, the classical antegrade approach is used to guide the wire to and over the fracture zone until penetrating the anterior ramus cortex using the pelvic inlet and COOO views. Definitive fixation is performed using a retrograde screw.

24.5.10 Risks

Starting lateral to the pubic tubercle takes the spermatic cord and genital branch of the genitofemoral nerve at risk [49, 50].

24.5.11 Tips and Tricks

A bent tip guidewire technique can be used to optimize the intraosseous pathway for retrograde screw insertion using a 2.0 mm Kirschner wire [51].

24.6 Results (Table 24.1)

Routt et al. analyzed 26 patients treated with open or percutaneous applied superior ramus screws. In two cases, retrograde placement of a screw was not possible. One screw was displaced superior to the pubic ramus. One patient experienced symptomatic screw malposition requiring revision. All fractures healed and no infections developed [9].

Mouhsine et al. stabilized 21 consecutive geriatric patients with minimal or undisplaced (<2 mm) acetabular fractures treated with combined percutaneous retrograde anterior and posterior column screws [47]. At 3.5 years, no secondary displacement, hip joint degeneration, or screw failure was observed, and 89% had good to excellent clinical results (Merle d'Aubigné Score).

Table 24.1 Results due to retrograde rami pubic screws

Year	Author	No.	Infection	Revisions	Outcome
1995	Routt	26	0%	4%	Ramus screw is advocated with caution
2006	Gänsslen	16	6%	6%	All but one fracture healed
2008	Starr	82	0%	0%	Loss of reduction: 15%
2012	Winkelhagen	6	0	0	Pain improvement

Starr et al. analyzed 145 upper pubic rami fractures stabilized using percutaneous antegrade and retrograde techniques [32]. Loss of reduction was present in 15 fractures and was associated with higher patient's age, female gender, and retrograde screw insertion. However, no patient sustained neurologic, vascular, or urologic injuries.

Winkelhagen et al. reported on six geriatric patients with isolated pubic ramus fractures after failed nonoperative mobilization [18]. All patients clinically improved, but long-term results were not stated.

24.7 Open Upper Pubic Rami Screw Fixation

Gänsslen et al. described the technique of open reduction and direct screw fixation of upper pubic rami fractures [19].

Patient positioning, draping, and x-ray procedures are comparable to the percutaneous technique.

24.7.1 Surgical Technique

A (small) Pfannenstiel incision is performed, orientated toward the injured side approximately 1 cm proximal to the easily palpable pubic tubercles. The classical dissection is performed to enter the space of Rezzii, and the medial upper pubic ramus is palpated just posterior to the fracture zone. After exposure, the fracture may be directly manipulated with bone-holding forceps or a pointed reduction forceps. The reaming procedure is "guided" by palpation along the medial pubic ramus. Drilling is performed under fluoroscopy control using the index finger for optimal orientation. The screw primarily acts as a positioning screw.

In cases of displaced posterior ring injuries, initial reduction of the posterior ring may help to indirectly reduce the ramus fractures.

24.7.2 Results

Gänsslen et al. analyzed 16 patients with two type A injuries, 6 patients with type B injuries, and 8 patients with type C injuries of the pelvic ring [19]. No intraoperative complications occurred. One patient developed chronic infection and recurrent fistula at the pubic ramus requiring surgical revisions and implant removal. All other fractures healed within 3 months.

24.8 Postoperative Management

Typically, partial weight bearing of the injured side with 15 kg BW for 3–6 weeks is recommended, starting on the second postoperative day.

24.9 Errors, Hazards, and Potential Complications

Injury to the bladder can occur due to insufficient bladder mobilization or incorrect dissection. The external iliac vessels are at risk in cases of superior cortical penetration and a risk of articular joint perforation exists in cases of inferior cortical penetration. Loss of reduction/instability is possible when using too short screws [19]. Loss of reduction is possible also in comminuted superior pubic rami fractures.

24.10 Conclusions

Intramedullary fixation of the upper pubic ramus (Figs. 24.7 and 24.8) can be technically demanding and sometimes impossible to perform due to anatomic abnormalities.

Therefore, preoperative planning using CT is mandatory. Biomechanically, the type and length of the screw are without advantage, while additional anterior pelvic ring fixation improves overall pelvic ring stability.

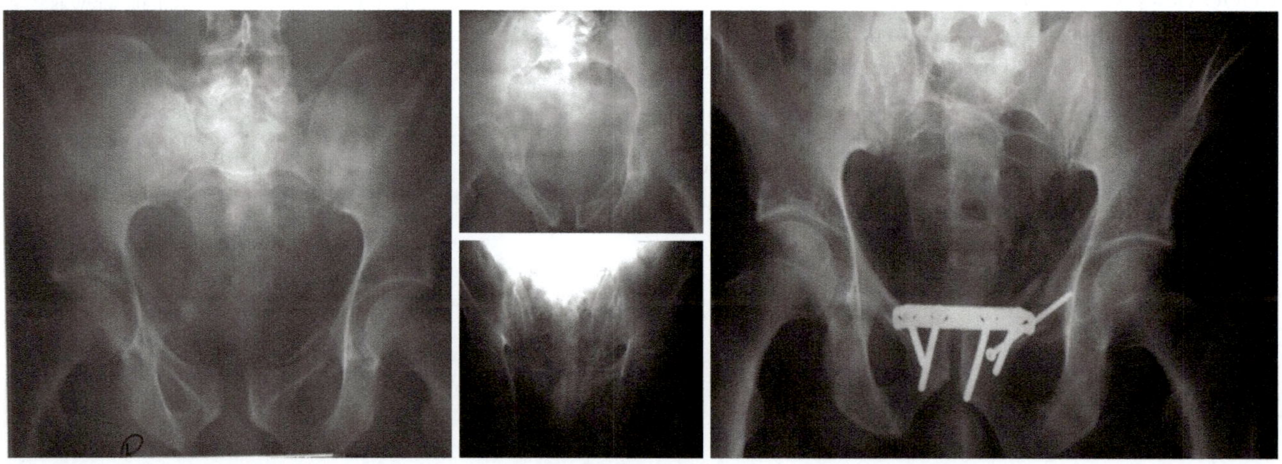

Fig. 24.7 Case of a short retrograde inserted upper pubic ramus screw

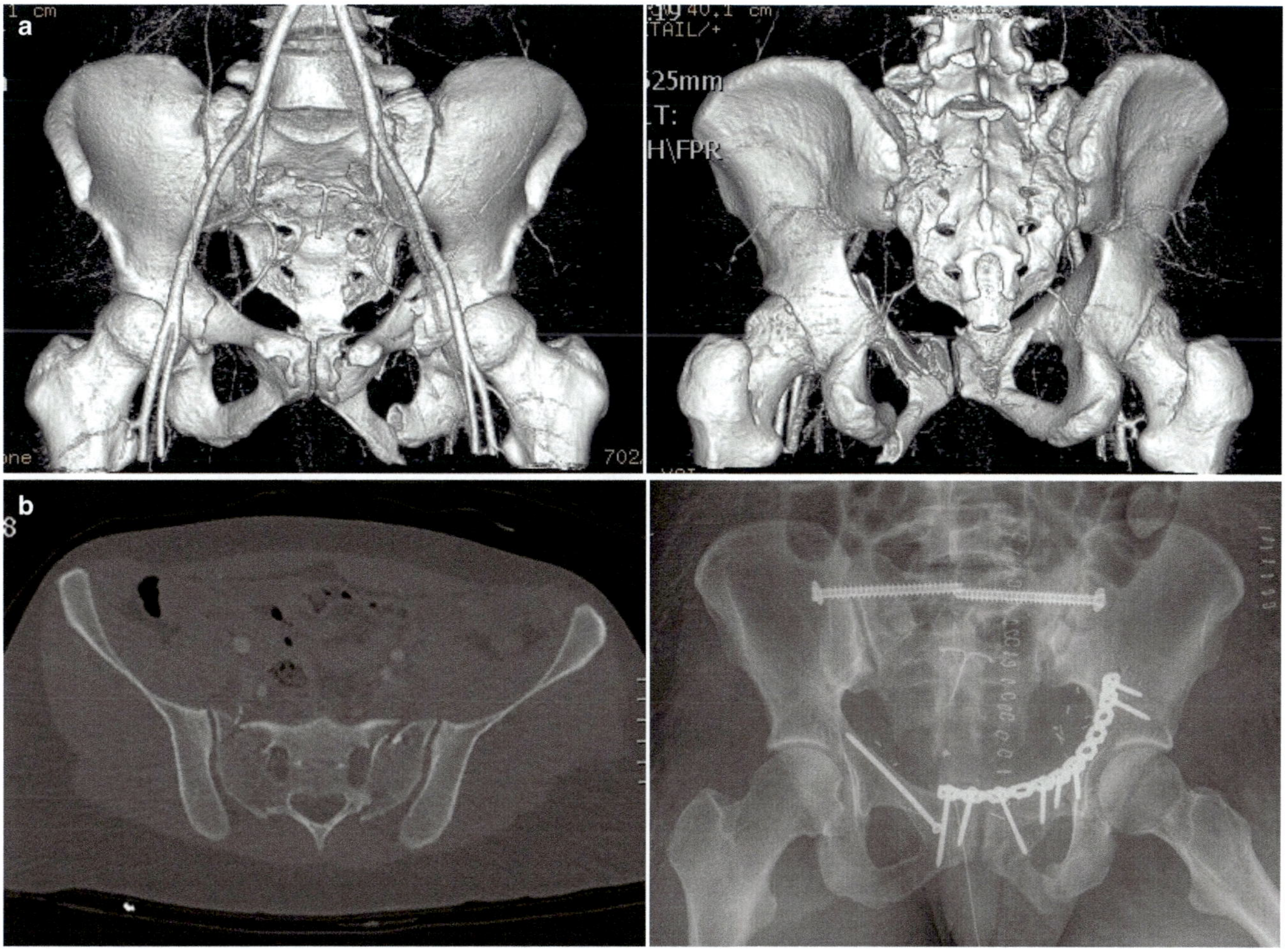

Fig. 24.8 (**a**) Retrograde pubic rami screw fixation on one side and plating on the other side in C3 pelvic ring fracture. A33-year-old female sustained bilateral pubic rami fractures and bilateral sacral fractures in a car-pedestrian accident. (**b**) First stage consisted of retrograde superior pubic rami screw fixation, and simultaneous open reduction and plate fixation of contralateral duplex pubic rami fractures through a low midline approach. The second stage was percutaneous iliosacral screw fixation of the minimally displaced vertical sacral fractures

References

1. Pohlemann T, Gänsslen A, Hartung S, für die Arbeitsgruppe Becken, H.T., H., Beckenverletzungen/Pelvic Injuries. Hefte zu "Der Unfallchirurg". Heft 266. 1998.
2. Tscherne H, Pohlemann T. Tscherne Unfallchirurgie: Becken und Acetabulum. Berlin, Heidelberg, New York: Springer; 1998.
3. Bellabarba C, Ricci WM, Bolhofner BR. Distraction external fixation in lateral compression pelvic fractures. J Orthop Trauma. 2000;14(7):475–82.
4. Gylling SF, Ward RE, Holcroft JW, Bray TJ, Chapman MW. Immediate external fixation of unstable pelvic fractures. Am J Surg. 1985;150(6):721–4.
5. Hofmann G, Bredow J. Spätergebnisse der Beckenringverletzungen-Behandlung mit dem Fixateur externe. Hefte Unfallheilk. 1986;181:612–8.
6. Kellam J. The role of external fixation in pelvic disruptions. Clin Orthop. 1989;241:66–82.
7. Lindahl J, Hirvensalo E, Bostman O, Santavirta S. Failure of reduction with an external fixator in the management of injuries of the pelvic ring. Long-term evaluation of 110 patients. J Bone Joint Surg Br. 1999;81(6):955–62.
8. Pohlemann T, Bosch U, Gänsslen A, Tscherne H. The Hannover experience in management of pelvic fractures. Clin Orthop. 1994;305:69–80.
9. Routt M, Simonian P, Grujic L. The retrograde medullary superior pubic ramus screw for the treatment of anterior pelvic ring disruptions: a new technique. J Orthop Trauma. 1995;9(1):35–40.
10. Simonian P, Routt M, Harrington R, Tencer A. Internal fixation of the unstable anterior pelvic ring: a biomechanical comparison of standard plating techniques and the retrograde medullary superior pubic ramus screw. J Orthop Trauma. 1994;8(6):476–82.
11. Ertel W, von Lüdinghausen M, Trentz O. Becken. In: Platzer W, Trentz O, editors. Posttraumatische Defekt- und Weichteilsanierung. Schädel, Wirbelsäule, Becken. Stuttgart, New York: Thieme; 1997. p. 414–557.
12. Felenda M, Dittel K. Instabile Beckenringverletzungen: Klassifikation—Behandlungsstrategie. Akt Traumatol. 1993;23:263–71.
13. Hirvensalo E, Lindahl J, Böstman O. A new approach to the internal fixation of unstable pelvic fractures. Clin Orthop. 1993;297:28–32.
14. Mears D, Rubash H. External and internal fixation of the pelvic ring. AAOS Instr Course Lect. 1984;33:144–58.
15. Trentz O, Bühren V, Friedl H. Beckenverletzungen. Chirurg. 1989;60:639–48.

16. Lambotte A. Chirurgie opératoire des fractures. répité, vol. 1913. Bruxelles: Société Franco-Belge D'Editions Scientifiques; 1948. p. 126–44.
17. Mosheiff R, Liebergall M. Maneuvering the retrograde medullary screw in pubic ramus fractures. J Orthop Trauma. 2002;16:594–6.
18. Winkelhagen J, van den Bekerom M, Bolhuis H, Hogervorst M. Preliminary results of cannulated screw fixation for isolated pubic ramus fractures. Strategies Trauma Limb Reconstr. 2012;7:87–91.
19. Gänsslen A, Krettek C. Retrograde transpubic screw fixation of transpubic instabilities. Oper Orthop Traumatol. 2006;18:330–40.
20. Kiefer S, Kleinfeld F. Die ungewöhnliche Komplikation nach Schambeinastfraktur: traumatische Dünndarmperforation. Akt Traumatol. 1994;24(3):81–2.
21. Tile M. Pelvic ring fractures: should they be fixed? J Bone Joint Surg. 1988;70-B:1–12.
22. Akagi M, Ikeda N, Fukiage K, Nakamura T. A modification of the retrograde medullary screw for the treatment of bilateral pubic ramus nonunions: a case report. J Orthop Trauma. 2002;16:431–3.
23. Altman G, Altman D, Routt MJ. Symptomatic hypertrophic pubic ramus nonunion treated with a retrograde medullary screw. J Orthop Trauma. 2000;14:582–5.
24. Eastman J, Chip Routt MJ. Intramedullary fixation techniques for the anterior pelvic ring. J Orthop Trauma. 2018;32:4–13.
25. Ji X, Bi C, Wang F, Jiang Y, Wang D, Wang Q. Digital anatomical measurements of safe screw placement at superior border of the arcuate line for acetabular fractures. BMC Musculoskelet Disord. 2015;16:55.
26. Quan Q, Hong L, Chang B, Liu R, Zhang Y, Zhao Q, Lu S. A radiographic simulation study of fixed superior pubis ramus fractures with retrograde screw insertion. J Orthop. 2016;13:364–8.
27. Tile M. Fractures of the pelvis and acetabulum. Baltimore: Williams & Wilkins; 1984.
28. Bodzay T, Sztrinkai G, Pajor S, Gál T, Jónás Z, Erdös P, Váradi K. Does surgically fixation of pubic fracture increase the stability of the operated posterior pelvis? Eklem Hastalık Cerrahisi. 2014;25:91–5.
29. Krajca J, Kim H, Nascone J, Manson T, Boulton C, Hsieh A, O'Toole R. Biomechanical analysis of mechanically unstable pelvic fractures: retrograde superior pubic ramus screw versus anterior external fixation. OTA, Scientific Poster #83; Tampa, FL; Date: October 15–18, 2014.
30. Acklin Y, Zderic I, Buschbaum J, Varga P, Inzana J, Grechenig S, Richards R, Gueorguiev B, Schmitz P. Biomechanical comparison of plate and screw fixation in anterior pelvic ring fractures with low bone mineral density. Injury. 2016;47:1456–60.
31. Acklin Y, Zderic I, Grechenig S, Richards R, Schmitz P, Gueorguiev B. Are two retrograde 3.5 mm screws superior to one 7.3 mm screw for anterior pelvic ring fixation in bones with low bone mineral densitiy? Bone Joint Res. 2017;6:8–13.
32. Starr A, Nakatani T, Reinert C, Cederberg K. Superior pubic ramus fractures fixed with percutaneous screws: what predicts fixation failure? J Orthop Trauma. 2008;22:81–7.
33. Gänsslen A, Hildebrand F, Klebingat M, Nerlich M, Lindahl J. Chapter 22: Special screws and views. In: Gänsslen A, Müller M, Nerlich M, Lindahl J, Hrsg. Acetabular fractures: diagnosis, indications, treatment strategies. New York: Thieme; 2017. ISBN-13: 978-3132415607.
34. Dienstknecht T, Müller M, Sellei R, Nerlich M, Pfeifer C, Krutsch W, Fuechtmeier B, Berner A. Percutaneous screw placement in acetabular posterior column surgery: gender differences in implant positioning. Injury. 2014;45:715–20.
35. Chen K, Wang G, Cao L, Zhang M. Differences of percutaneous retrograde screw fixation of anterior column acetabular fractures between male and female: a study of 164 virtual three-dimensional models. Injury. 2009;40:10676–1072.
36. Chacko A, Mostert P, Snyckers C, Ismail F. Measurement of acetabular column sizes for guiding percutaneous fixation of acetabular fractures in the South African population. EPOS, Eur Soc Radiol. Poster No.: C-0758. 2013.
37. Pichler W, Puchwein P, Clement H, Grechenig C, Grechenig W. Percutaneous fixation of acetabular fractures: computer assisted determination of safe zones, angles and lengths for screw insertion. Suomen Ortop Traumatol. 2013;36:94–100.
38. Puchwein P, Enninghorst N, Sisak K, Ortner T, Schildhauer T, Balogh Z, Pichler W. Percutaneous fixation of acetabular fractures: computer-assisted determination of safe zones, angles and lengths for screw insertion. Arch Orthop Trauma Surg. 2012;132:805–11.
39. Shahulhameed A, Roberts C, Pomeroy C, Acland R, Giannoudis P. Mapping the columns of the acetabulum—implications for percutaneous fixation. Injury. 2010;41:339–42.
40. Suzuki T, Soma K, Shindo M, Minehara H, Itoman M. Anatomic study for pubic medullary screw insertion. J Orthop Surg (Hong Kong). 2008;16:321–5.
41. Attias N, Lindsey R, Starr A, Borer D, Bridges K, Hipp J. The use of a virtual three-dimensional model to evaluate the intraosseous space available for percutaneous screw fixation of acetabular fractures. J Bone Joint Surg. 2005;87-Br:1520–3.
42. Bi C, Ji X, Wang F, Wang D, Wang Q. Digital anatomical measurements and crucial bending areas of the fixation route along the inferior border of the arcuate line for pelvic and acetabular fractures. BMC Musculoskelet Disord. 2016;17:125.
43. Zheng Z, Wu W, Yu X, Pan J, Latif M, Hou Z, Zhang Y. Axial view of acetabular anterior column: a new X-ray projection of percutaneous screw placement. Arch Orthop Trauma Surg. 2015;135:187–92.
44. Quercetti NR, Horne B, DiPaolo Z, Prayson M. Gun barrel view of the anterior pelvic ring for percutaneous anterior column or superior pubic ramus screw placement. Eur J Orthop Surg Traumatol. 2017;27:695–704.
45. Vioreanu M, Mulhall K. Intra-operative imaging technique to aid safe placement of screws in percutaneous fixation of pelvic and acetabular fractures. Acta Orthop Belg. 2011;77:398–401.
46. Bishop J, Routt M. Osseous fixation pathways in pelvic and acetabular fracture surgery: osteology, radiology, and clinical applications. J Trauma Acute Care Surg. 2012;72:1502–9.
47. Mouhsine E, Garofalo R, Borens O, Wettstein M, Blanc C, Fischer J, Moretti B, Leyvraz P. Percutaneous retrograde screwing for stabilisation of acetabular fractures. Injury. 2005;36:1330–6.
48. Weatherby D, Chip Routt MJ, Eastman J. The retrograde-antegrade-retrograde technique for successful placement of a retrograde superior ramus screw. J Orthop Trauma. 2017;31:224–9.
49. Collinge C, Beltran M. Anatomic relationship between the spermatic cord and the pubic tubercle: are our clamps injuring the cord during symphyseal repair? J Orthop Trauma. 2015;29:290–4.
50. Firoozabadi R, Stafford P, Routt M. Risk of spermatic cord injury during anterior pelvic ring and acetabular surgery: an anatomical study. Arch Bone Jt Surg. 2015;3:269–73.
51. Scolaro J, Routt M. Intraosseous correction of misdirected cannulated screws and fracture malalignment using a bent tip 2.0 mm guidewire: technique and indications. Arch Orthop Trauma Surg. 2013;133:883–7.

External Fixation

25

Franz Müller, Axel Gänsslen, and Jan Lindahl

In the late 1970s and early 1980s, unstable pelvic ring injuries were predominantly fixed using external skeletal fixation [1–8]. Various devices were used to stabilize even complex fracture situations, including open fractures, infected nonunions, and even accompanying acetabular fractures [2, 9, 10].

Mears and Fu extended the external fixator application even to complex combined pelvic ring and acetabular fractures (Fig. 25.1) and introduced a transpelvic application, connecting the posterior pelvis with the anterior pelvis [4]. The fixator bars were inserted completely transosseous through the ilium and a connected posterior to the buttock and classically anterior (Fig. 25.1).

To address the weight-bearing posterior pelvic ring, several constructs were developed to gain some compression even to the posterior pelvis (e.g., the Slätis construction (Fig. 25.2) [8] and the Egbers construction [11]).

The biomechanical efficiency of these constructs could be confirmed in several analyses [3, 12], but more complex fixator constructs failed to significantly increase overall pelvic ring stability [13].

Until recently, external fixation is the most commonly recommended treatment concept for surgical stabilization of the pelvic ring in emergency situations [14–22]. Its main advantage is easy handling and common availability.

Despite biomechanical data indicating insufficient stability while weight bearing for some configurations of external fixation, in emergency situations mechanical stability is the primary treatment aim [15, 17, 22]. Interestingly, simple anterior bar fixators showed better biomechanical stability than complex frames [23].

> The basic concept of external fixation included an anterior metallic compression frame anchored to the pelvic ring with half pins inserted into the anterior iliac crests [3, 4].

Thus, a simple and quickly applicable external fixator is favored in contrast to complex fixator configurations to effectively control pelvic hemorrhage [24].

Jeanneret and Ruflin introduced the concept of a simple one bar percutaneous anterior fixator [25]. This concept of simple supraacetabular fixation is favored [24, 25] as biomechanical and experimental data indicate superior holding power of Schanz screws in the supraacetabular region compared to iliac crest application [26–28]. Additionally, superior soft-tissue coverage is present.

25.1 External Fixation Options

Several external fixation strategies are reported, including iliac crest fixation, subcristal fixation, supraacetabular fixation, and combined fixation strategies.

25.1.1 Iliac Crest Fixation

Historically, the iliac crest route with insertion of 2–3 pins into the iliac crest was favored for decades. The optimal entry point is located at the border between the anterior and middle third of the iliac crest. Here, a bony thickening is always present, which forms the iliac tuberosity (Fig. 25.3) and which is located approximately 4–8 cm posterior to the ASIS.

F. Müller
Department of Trauma Surgery, Orthopaedics and Sports Medicine, Hospital Barmherzige Brüder Regensburg, Regensburg, Germany

A. Gänsslen (✉)
Department of Trauma Surgery, Orthopedics and Hand Surgery, Hospital Wolfsburg, Wolfsburg, Germany

J. Lindahl
Orthopaedics and Trauma Surgery, Helsinki University Hospital, Helsinki, Finland

A. Gänsslen et al. (eds.), *Pelvic Ring Fractures*, https://doi.org/10.1007/978-3-030-54730-1_25

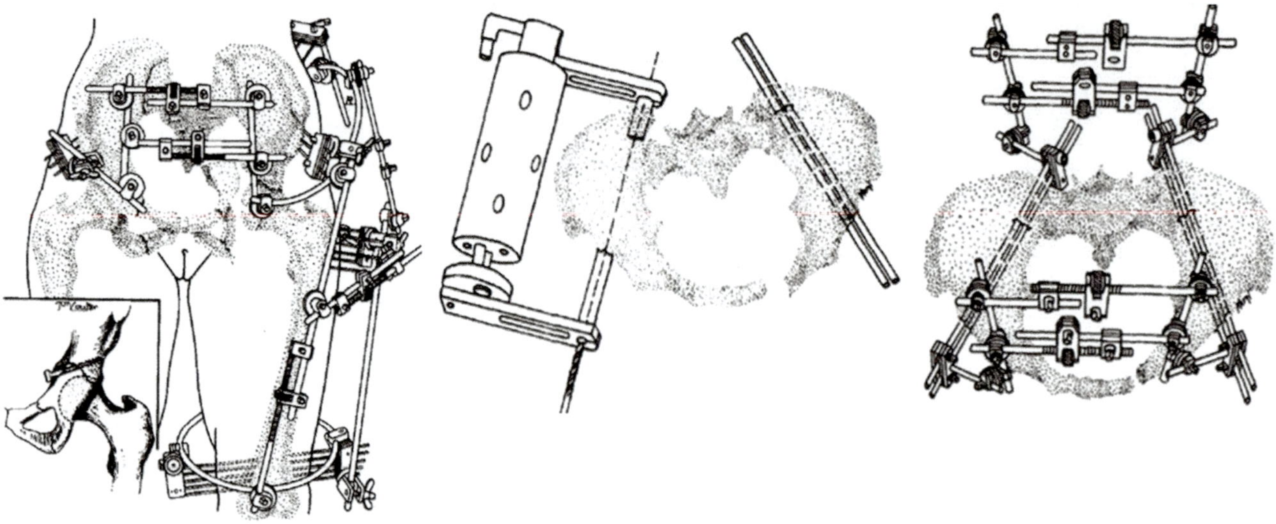

Fig. 25.1 Combined pelvic ring and acetabular fixation, transfixing the hip joint with a pelvic-femoral fixator (left) and the transpelvic fixator, with posterior and anterior horizontal connections [39]

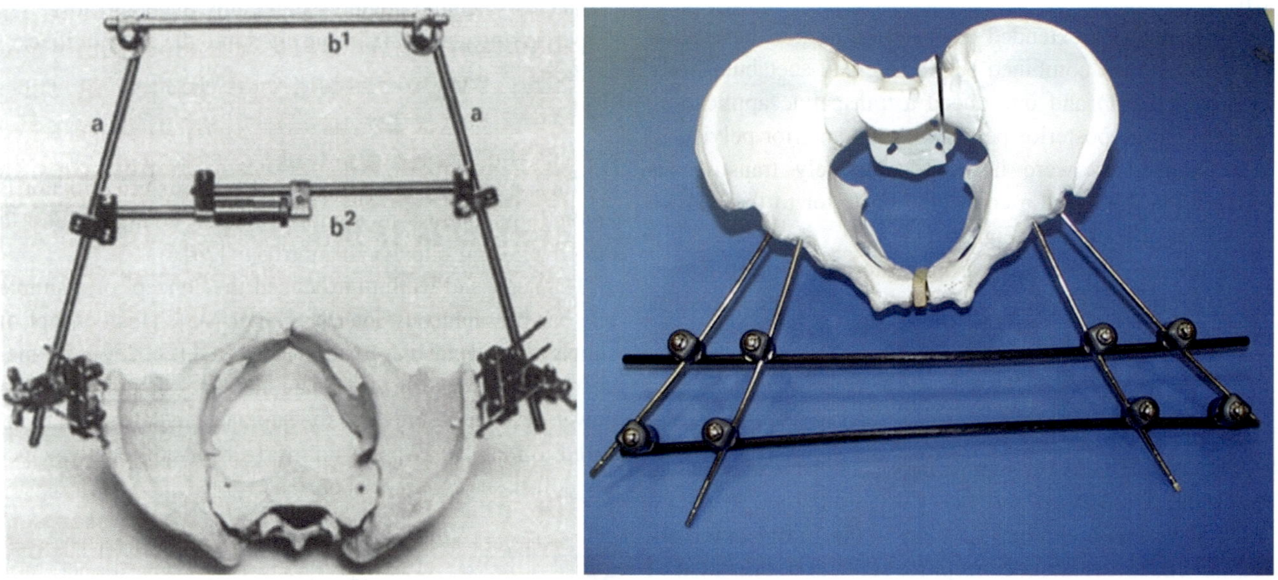

Fig. 25.2 Slätis trapezoidal fixator (left) and the modified Egbers fixator (right) allowing posterior pelvic ring compression

This area is relatively thick and includes a slightly angulated bone corridor running from the iliac crest to the supraacetabular region. This landmark is of surgical relevance during pelvic ring external fixation techniques. Here, the strong bone structure allows sufficient holding forces for pin application in an iliac external fixator [24].

In acute cases, a percutaneous pin insertion technique is preferred, and two pins are inserted at each side (Fig. 25.4). Alternatively, a small 1–2 cm incision is chosen. Whenever possible, three 5 mm pins are recommended to ensure better stability.

For optimal screw insertion, the iliac bone is palpated with an instrument [29], a Kirschner wire [30], or digitally (Fig. 25.5). By drilling, only the cortex is perforated and the Schanz screws are then introduced into the drill hole and further advanced between the two layers of the iliac bone without further predrilling.

Advantages of the iliac crest route include fast application during damage control surgery and no necessity of image intensification. Potential disadvantages are the small anatomical bone corridor, a high incidence of screw misplace-

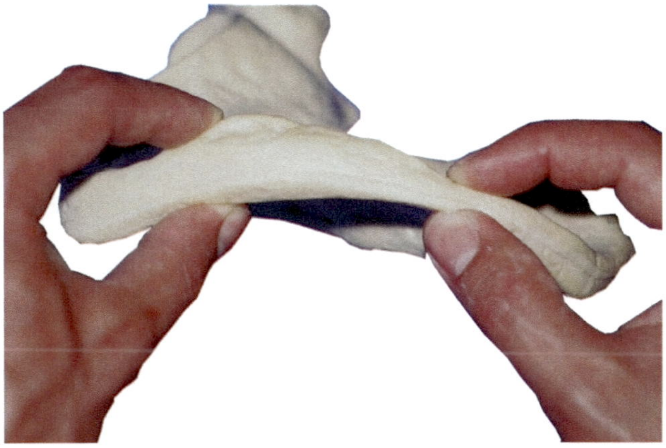

Fig. 25.3 Iliac crest thickening (iliac tuberosity) for iliac crest Schanz pin insertion

ment (Fig. 25.5), necessity of multiple pins (Fig. 25.6) to ensure adequate stability, and a higher failure rate [31].

25.1.2 Subcristal Fixation

A further option for adequate Schanz screws insertion was recently proposed: the subcristal screw insertion (Fig. 25.7).

Solomon et al. performed a cadaver and CT analysis of the subcristal bone corridor [32]. The mean length from the ASIS to the iliac tuberosity on top of the iliac crest was 62 mm; the mean width was 11 mm.

The first clinical experience was reported on 20 patients [33]. The fixators were removed on average after 10.7 weeks. Except 20% ($n = 4$) superficial pin track infections, suffi-

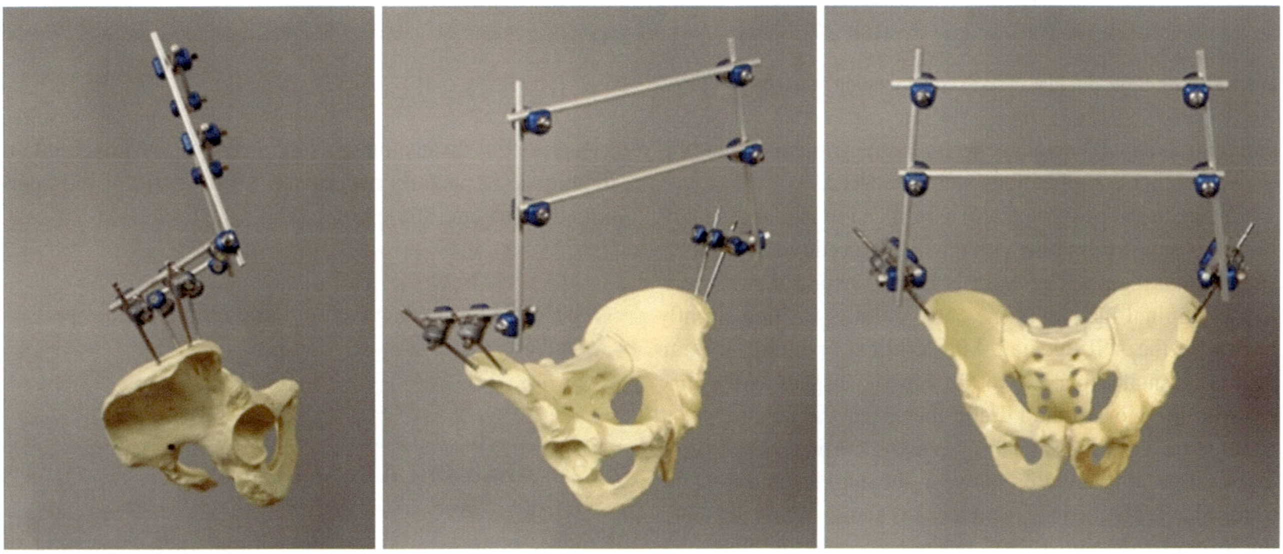

Fig. 25.4 Iliac crest external fixator

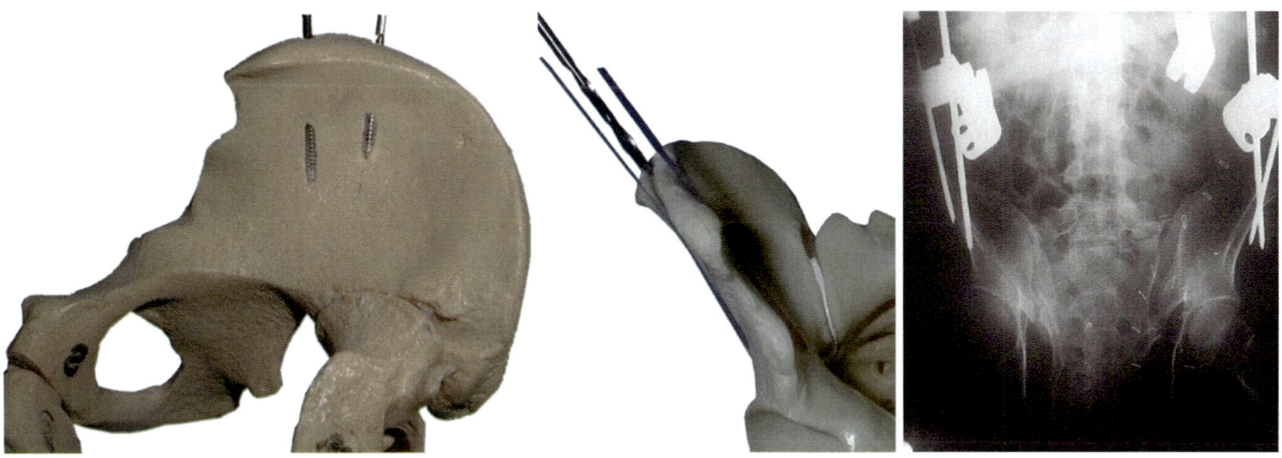

Fig. 25.5 Due to the thin bone structure, malplacement of Schanz pins is possible with internal or external bone perforation, which can be avoided by "palpation" of the outer and inner iliac surface

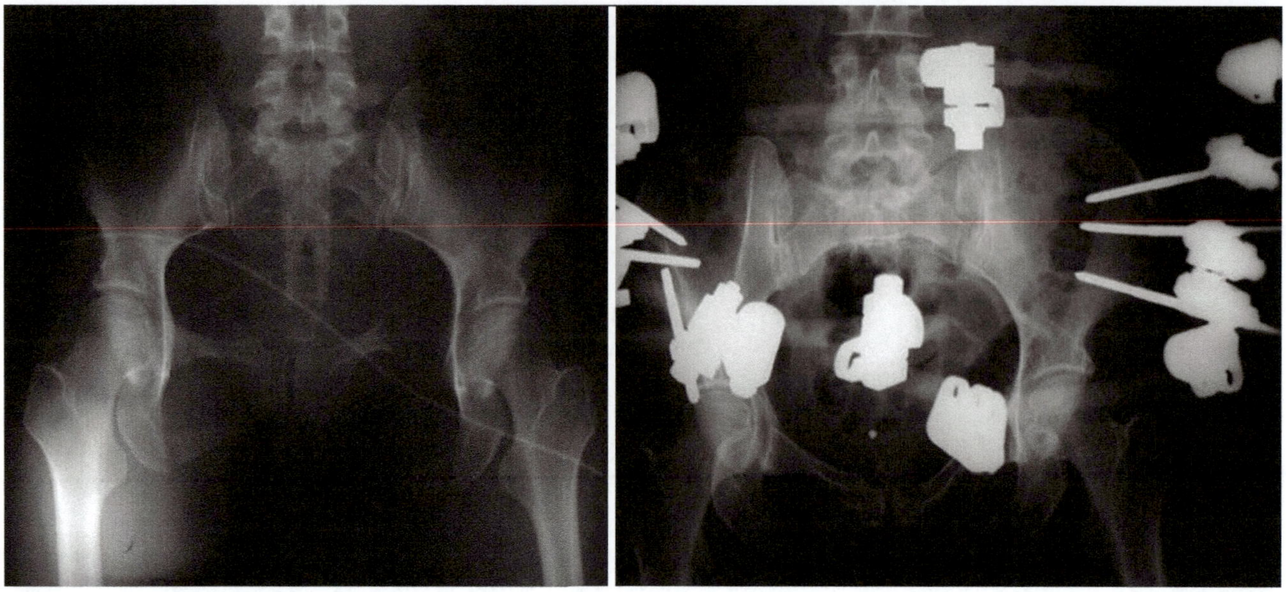

Fig. 25.6 Multiple pin iliac crest external fixation in a type B-injury

ciently treated with standard wound management and antibiotics, no other complications were observed.

In the supine position, 2 cm skin incision is marked starting from the ASIS in line with the iliac crest down toward the subinguinal region. The ASIS is bluntly exposed superficial to the inguinal ligament. The entry point is verified slightly medial to the ASIS center. After cortical opening, 4.0 mm drill is orientated parallel to the superior aspect of the iliac crest in direction to the IT, and thereafter the Schanz pin is inserted by slow speed drilling to avoid cortical penetration. The change of orientation between the anterior and the posterior iliac crest corridor, which is angulated highly variable, but is approximately 20–40°, has to be considered.

25.1.3 Supraacetabular Fixation

The supraacetabular bone corridor gives sufficient and even better holding power than the iliac route [11, 26]. Sufficient soft-tissue coverage leads to a reduced pin site infection rate [24]. This route is considered safe, simple, and effective [34] as it is easier to close a book from the front than the top [29].

The proposed main advantages include [31, 34]:

- Firmer pin anchorage to the bone (tighter spongiosis)
- Single pin sufficiency
- Greater insertion depth
- Possibility of large diameter (up to 6 mm) pin usage
- Greater stability in the posterior pelvic ring
- Lower risk of bone perforation
- Lower risk of infection
- More freedom in concomitant abdominal operations
- Optimized patient comfort, especially while sitting

A potential disadvantage is the necessity of image intensification [31]. In daily experience, x-ray control is only performed at the end of the procedure.

> The supraacetabular fixation route represents the gold standard.

25.2 Anatomical Considerations

The iliac bone is a "ring-shaped" construct, consisting of three rings: the iliac ring, the acetabular ring, and the obturator ring [35].

The stabilizing bone structures for external fixation are located at the rim of the "iliac ring" [36]. Centrally, at the iliac fossa, the bone thickness is only few millimeters thick or may even be completely absent. This bony anatomical background is the basis for safe placement of Schanz screws for external fixation.

Iliac pin placement can be associated with pin malplacement, presenting with pin penetration outside the ilium to gluteal or iliac fossa [37, 38].

The supracetabular bone corridor was clinically and radiographically identified to be a strong and sufficiently thick bone structure for the simple insertion of Schanz screws and lumbo-pelvic screws [24, 25, 39, 40].

Four relevant landmarks are the bases for the iliac ring segment [24]:

- The superior part of the iliac ring, representing the iliac crest, extends from the anterior superior iliac spine (ASIS) to the posterior superior iliac spine (PSIS).

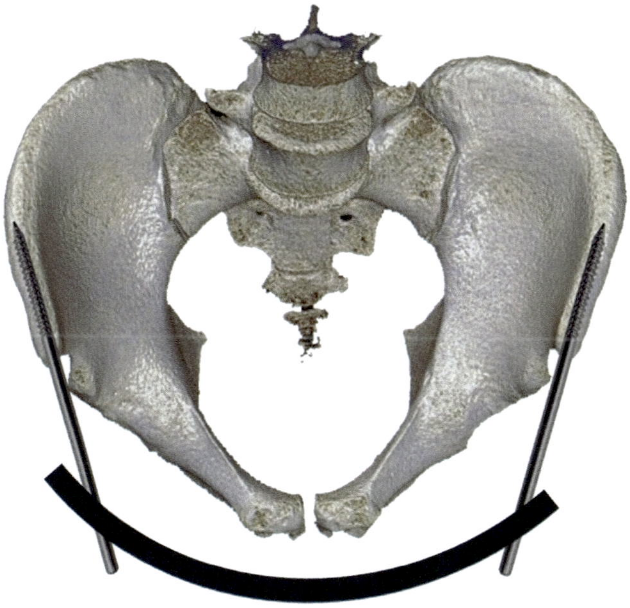

Fig. 25.7 Subcristal external fixation concept

- The anterior border is the thick and strong bone segment from the ASIS to the pelvic brim, superior to the joint just inferior to the anterior inferior iliac spine (AIIS); good bone quality is present in 2–3 cm corridor.
- The inferior part of the supraacetabular corridor is located superior to the greater sciatic notch starting at the AIIS and ending at the posterior inferior iliac spine (PIIS) or the PSIS; this AIIS-PIIS bone corridor has a length of approximately 85–100 mm, and the AIIS-PSIS bone corridor has a length of approximately 128–141 mm [39, 40].
- The posterior part consists of the strong bone between the PIIS and the PSIS; this bone segment is approximately 2–3 cm thick and has an anterior enlargement of up to 2 cm up to the posterior gluteal line [35].

Overall, parallel to the iliopectineal line in the horizontal plane, this bone corridor shows a length of approximately 3 × 15 cm, which can easily be confirmed on CT scans (Fig. 25.8). To obtain the maximal screw length and, therefore, an optimal screw purchase, a drill orientation from lateral to medial of approximately 20° must be selected for the Schanz screw (Fig. 25.9) [41].

In the frontal plane, the cancellous triangular-shaped area above the iliopectineal line is orientated slightly caudal. Drilling direction is therefore inclined approximately 10–20° caudally (Fig. 25.9) [41].

The capsule of the hip originates on average 16 mm (11–20 mm) superior to the anterior rim of the acetabulum [42]. On an AP x-ray, this rim is represented by the acetabular "sourcil" [43]. To avoid intraarticular screw placement, a distance of approximately 1.5–2 cm cranial to the anterior rim of the acetabulum should therefore be selected. Clinically, this optimal starting point corresponds to a position just cranial to the tip of the AIIS (Fig. 25.10).

The position of the lateral femoral cutaneous nerve should be known (Fig. 25.11). Its trunk normally exits the pelvis below the inguinal ligament approximately 15–20 mm medial to the anterior superior iliac spine and then divides into several branches approximately 5 cm caudal to the anterior superior iliac spine [44–46].

4–13% of the nerves show relevant variations with courses up to 5 cm lateral to the ASIS. Consequently, the LCFN is at risk during too superior incisions [47–51].

25.3 Indications

Classical indications for supraacetabular external fixation include:

- Emergency stabilization of unstable type B and type C pelvic ring fractures [15, 17, 22, 24, 52]
- Temporary stabilization of unstable pelvic ring fractures, particularly in patients in poor general condition or with local soft-tissue damage, the latter being a relatively contraindication
- Definitive treatment of type B injuries with pubic rami fractures [24, 52]; symphyseal dislocations are more effectively treated with internal osteosynthesis [52–55]
- Distraction of the pelvic inlet in lateral compression fractures [53]
- Definitive treatment of the anterior pelvic ring in type C injuries with pubic fracture instability after or before posterior internal stabilization [55, 56]
- Adjunct stabilization of internal fixation [55, 56]
- Stabilization of pelvic ring fractures in children [57, 58]
- Stabilization of pelvic ring fractures after infection of internal osteosynthesis [59]
- Immobilization of (unstable) pubic fractures for pain control [60]

Stabilizations of type C injuries (complete posterior pelvic instability) are associated with a risk of secondary displacements with an exclusive anterior external fixation [52, 55, 61].

25.4 Contraindications

Contraindications for supraacetabular pin placement include [24]:

- Poor general condition
- Local soft-tissue damage
- Local infection

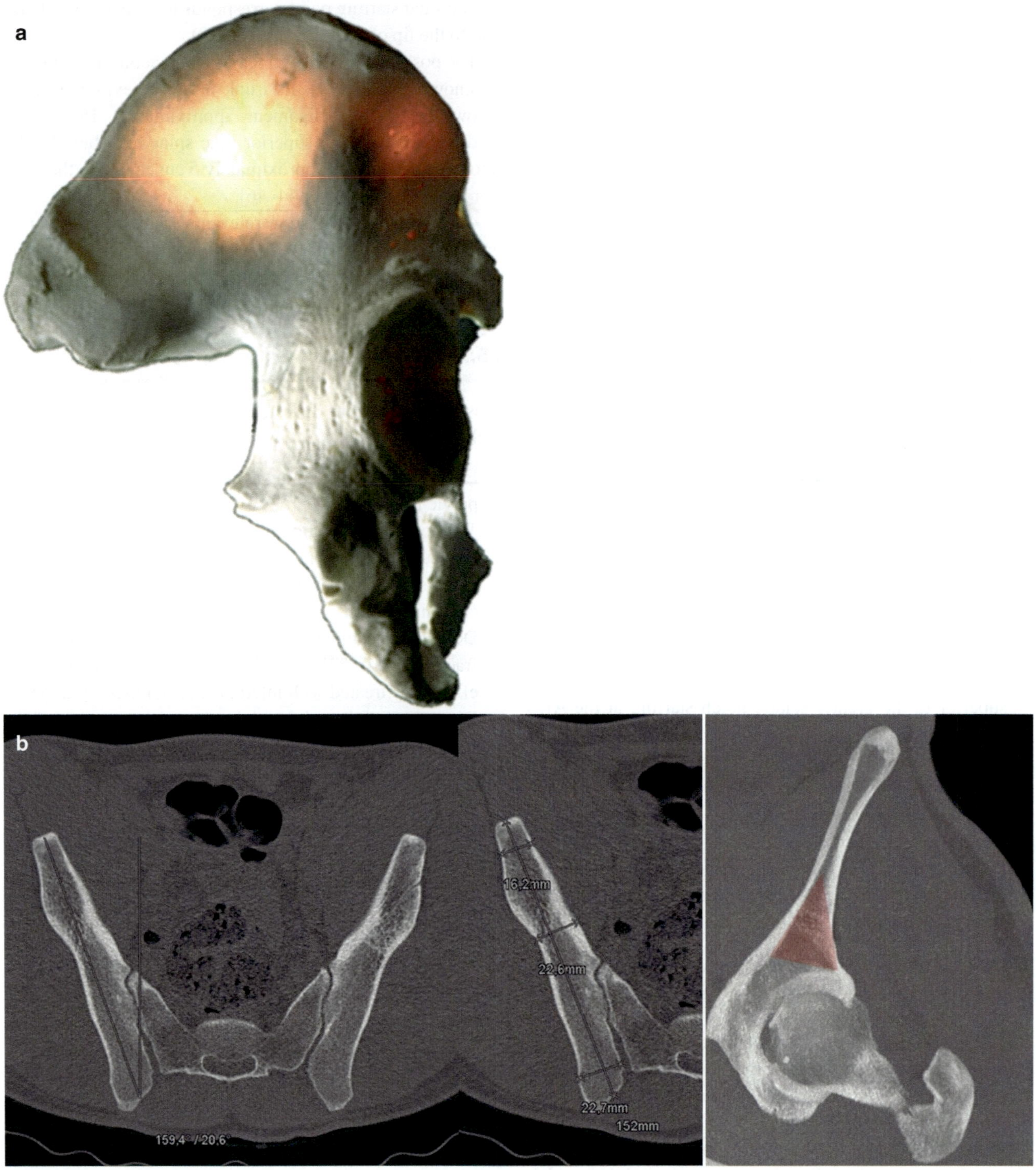

Fig. 25.8 (a) Bone model, identifying the supraacetabular bone corridor. (b) CT-anatomy of the supraacetabular bone corridor for supraacetabular pin insertion

25.5 Preoperative Considerations

Standard pelvic radiographs, e.g., AP pelvic x-ray, and if necessary oblique views (inlet and outlet views) or computed tomography are recommended.

Prophylactic antibiotics are generally not necessary as a percutaneous approach or minimally invasive approach is chosen.

The patient has to be informed about usual surgical risks, the risk of thromboembolic complications, potential wound

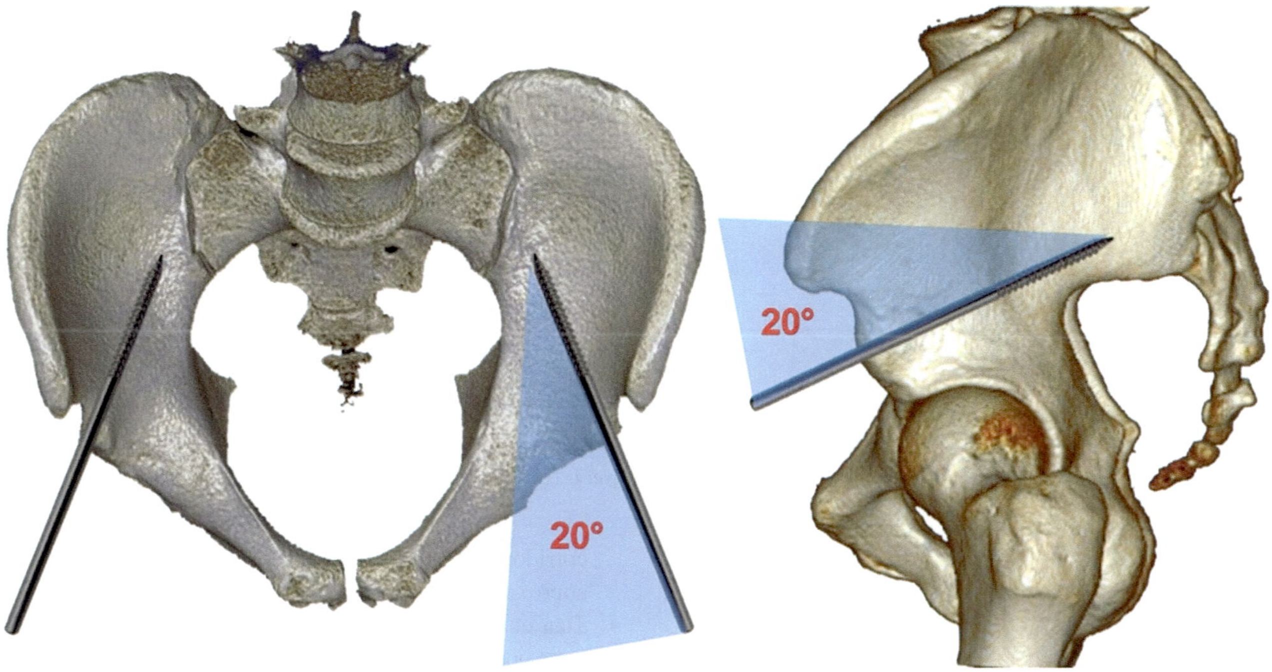

Fig. 25.9 Orientation of the Schanz screws: in the horizontal plane a 20° external position and in the sagittal plane a 20° inferior rotation is recommended

infection and possible (most often temporary) injury to the lateral femoral cutaneous nerve, screw misplacements, particularly intraarticular implant positioning of the hip joint, and perforation of the iliac bone.

25.6 Patient Positioning

Surgery is performed under general anesthesia in the standard supine position on a radiolucent operation table allowing the standard pelvic and acetabular (Judet) views.

Free draping of the lower limb on the side of the injured pelvis is optional for allowing easier reduction maneuvers, depending on the displacement.

Draping is performed so that the anterior superior iliac spine and symphysis can be clearly palpated. The potential course of the femoral vessels is marked with a colored pen.

25.7 Incision

After palpation of the ASIS and marking the ASIS, the suspected 2 cm long incision is drawn obliquely approximately 2 cm distal and 2 cm medial from the ASIS (Fig. 25.12).

Typically, the AIIS can easily palpated at this level, even in obese patients. A slightly lateral incision is recommended to consider the proposed pin direction. Malposition can lead to soft tissue tension after reduction.

If pelvic compression is planned in external rotation injuries, the approach should preferably be rather more medial [24]. After skin incision with scalpel, spreading of the soft tissues is performed bluntly using a clamp or a scissors, while at the same time palpating the anterior inferior iliac spine.

25.8 Deep Dissection

To avoid injury to the LCFN, only further blunt dissection is recommended (Fig. 25.12). Complete, visible exposure of the anterior inferior iliac spine is usually not necessary and should only be performed when the anatomy of the hemipelvis remains unclear. An incisional extend to 5 cm can then be performed. Even through the 2 cm standard incision, the AIIS can easily palpated.

25.9 Cortical Opening and Screw Direction

The basis of cortical opening is to establish the correct entry point and consider the direction of the drilling. Prior to cortical opening, it can be helpful to palpate the medial iliac fossa and the outer lateral gluteal side of the ilium starting at the level of the AIIS.

Knowledge of the anatomy of the bone corridor is crucial:

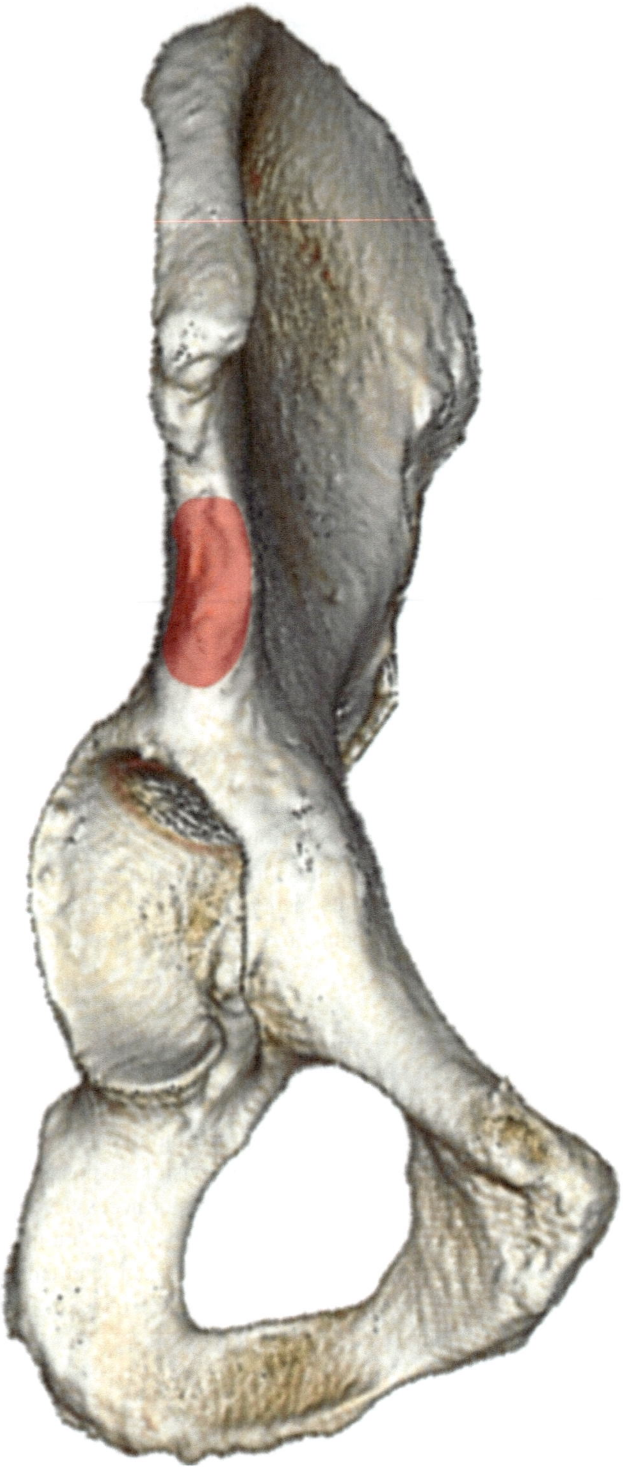

Fig. 25.10 Localization of the optimal Schanz pin entry point, respecting the capsular insertion of the hip joint

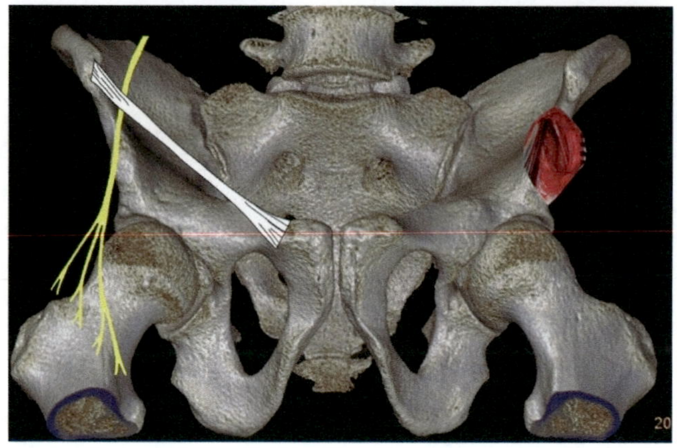

Fig. 25.11 Anatomical course of the Lateral Cutaneous Femoral Nerve (LCFN)

- Wang et al. analyzed the bony anatomy of supraacetabular external fixation on 120 normal pelvic CT scans [62]. In the sagittal plane, an angle of 22–23° was measured, while in the horizontal plane an angle of 20–23° was measured. The maximum and minimum width of the bone corridor in the plane between the AIIS and PSIS were approximately 27 mm and 16 mm, respectively.
- Tian et al. analyzed 18 cadaver pelves and measured the bone corridor length from the PSIS to AIIS and from the PIIS to the AIIS together with the sagittal angle of the bone corridor at three levels [63]. Male pelves had a slightly longer canal length (135 vs. 125 mm) while the angulation was comparable (26° vs. 25°).
- Solomon et al. performed a CT analysis of the horizontal supraacetabular angulation and stated an average value of 23.85° [32].

> In the supine position, the direction of cortical opening is inclined approximately 20° caudally and 20° laterally (Fig. 25.13).

The correct position can be additionally analyzed using fluoroscopy (obturator view or combined obturator oblique–outlet view (Fig. 25.14) [35, 40]) to ensure safe extraarticular positioning of the Schanz screw. Respecting the mentioned angles, from clinical practice no fluoroscopy is mandatory at this stage.

> The entry point is on top of the AIIS [24] or slightly proximal [64].

It is sufficient to only open the cortex or to perform a drilling with a depth of 1–2 cm as the Schanz screw will "find" its path between the iliac laminae. For longer drill corridors, oscillating drilling using the "hammer" technique is recommended.

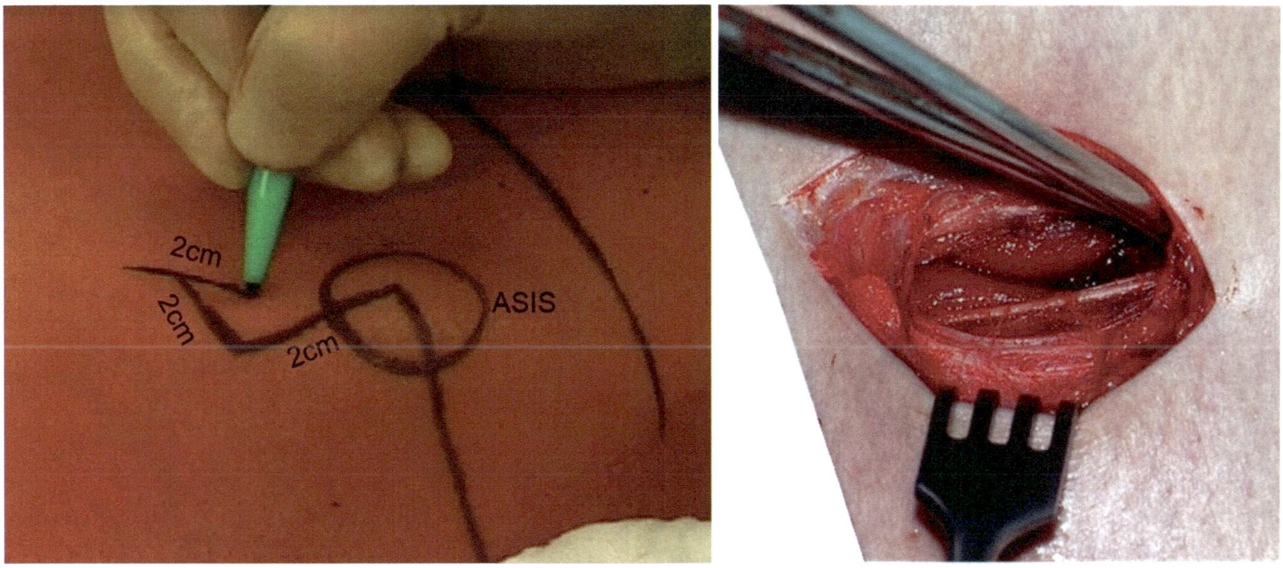

Fig. 25.12 A 2 cm skin incision is made 2 cm distal and 2 cm medial to the Anterior Superior Iliac Spine (ASIS). By blunt dissection, injury to the LCFN can be avoided

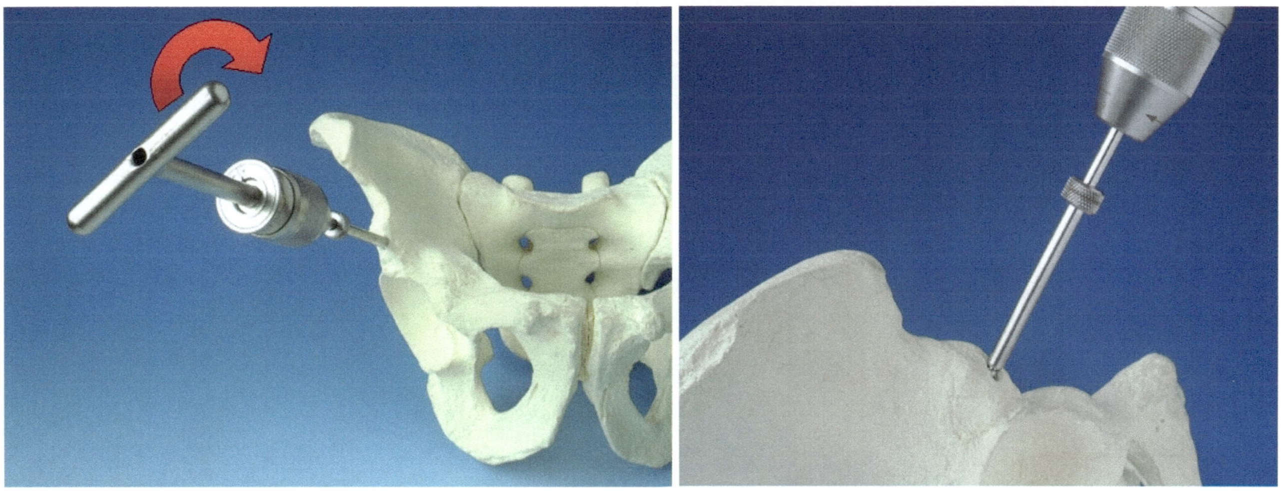

Fig. 25.13 Pin orientation on a pelvic model

The Schanz screw is then inserted through the outer drill sleeve to avoid potential injury to the LCFN. The Schanz screw is advanced as far as possible until a firm purchase is noticed.

After bilateral Schanz screw insertion, closed reduction maneuvers are performed, if necessary, using leg traction and medial rotation of the leg or with assistance of the Schanz screws in a “joystick” technique.

In severe internal rotation deformities, a standard distractor can be applied to the Schanz pins to correct the deformity (Fig. 25.15).

The reduction is then maintained by the connecting rod. A curved carbon rod is preferred (Fig. 25.16) as it avoids interference during radiologic examinations and discomfort to the patient. The carbon rod should be placed as close to the body as possible, respecting the individual anterior abdominal wall anatomy, not to disturb during sitting (Fig. 25.17). A tube-to-tube construct can avoid soft-tissue complications (Fig. 25.18).

Finally, the tension-free passage of the Schanz screws through the skin has to be checked (change in position due to the reduction). Consequently, the incision should be enlarged, if necessary. Partial skin closure is only necessary after large incisions.

In rare situations, a two-pin fixation is possible as the bone corridor in the frontal plane is usually sufficient in height (Fig. 25.19). The second Schanz screw is directed more horizontal close to the first screw, usually between the

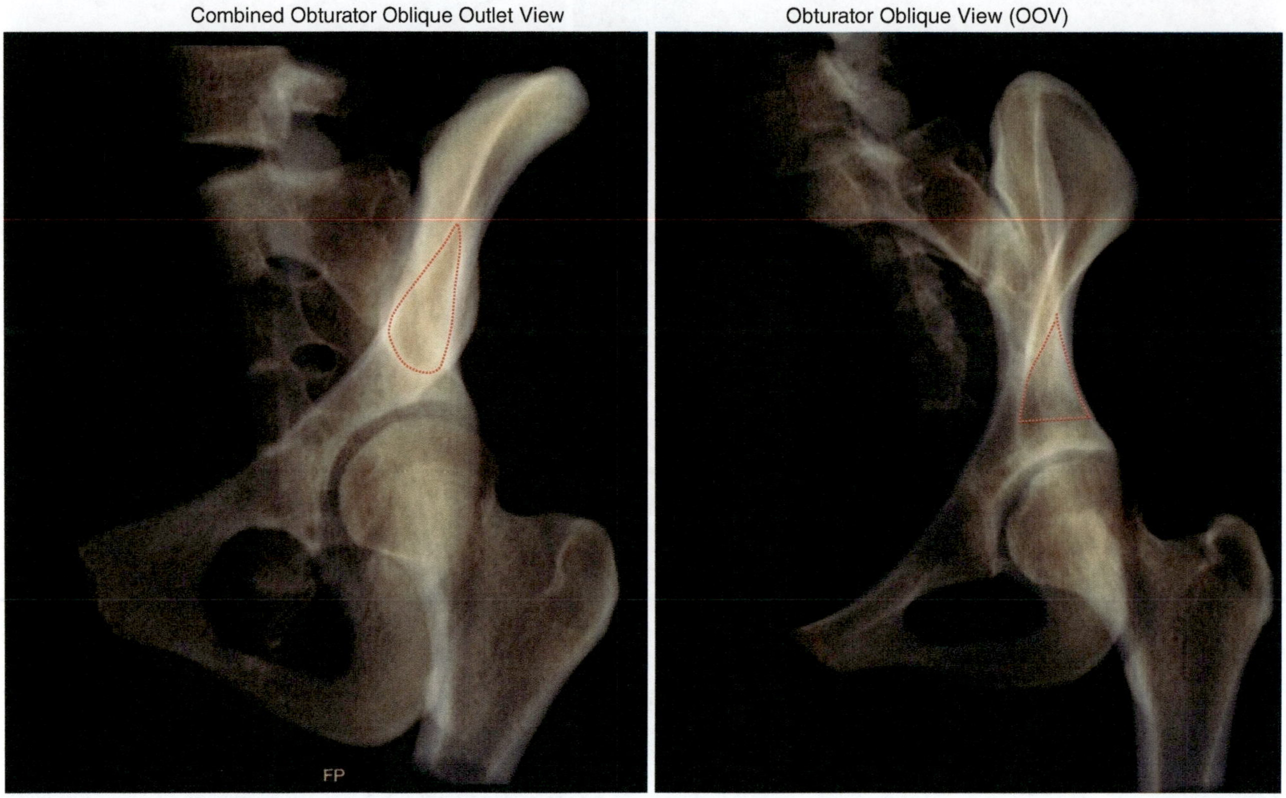

Fig. 25.14 Intraoperative x-rays to confirm optimal pin placement

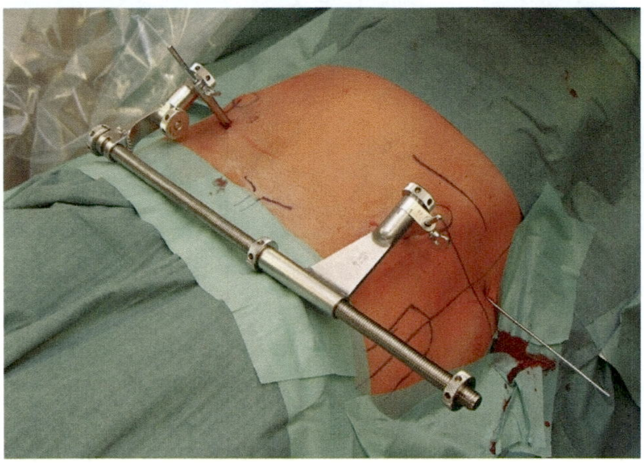

Fig. 25.15 A distractor can be used in severe internal rotation deformities to correct the pelvic anatomy

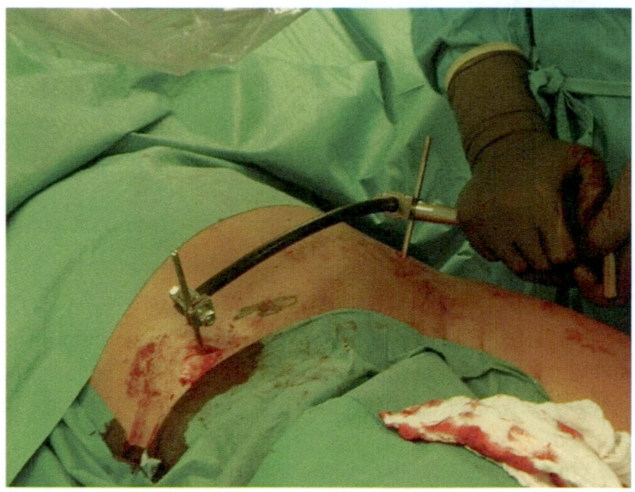

Fig. 25.16 Final application of a curved carbon connecting rod

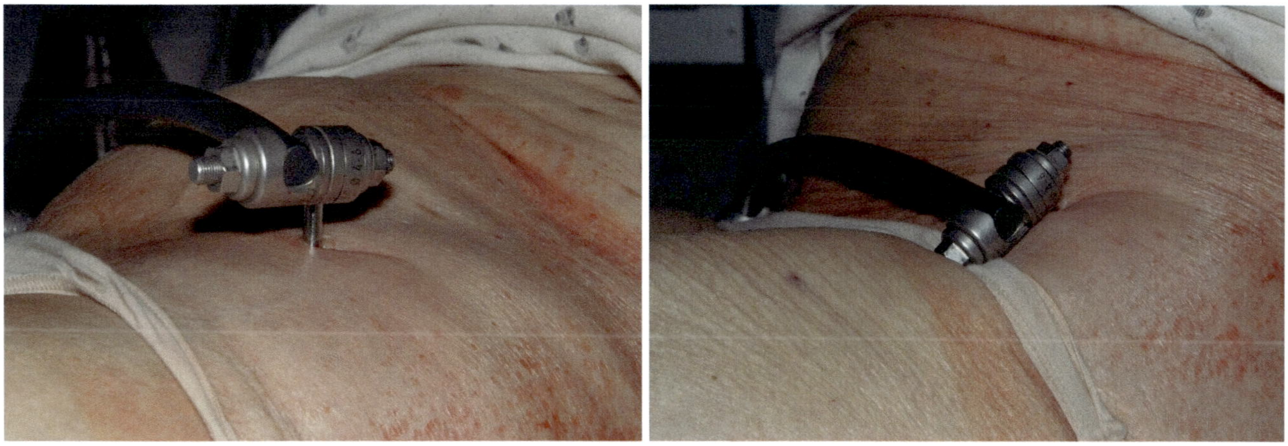

Fig. 25.17 A too close application to the skin (left) of the curved rod can result in soft-tissue impingement during sitting (right)

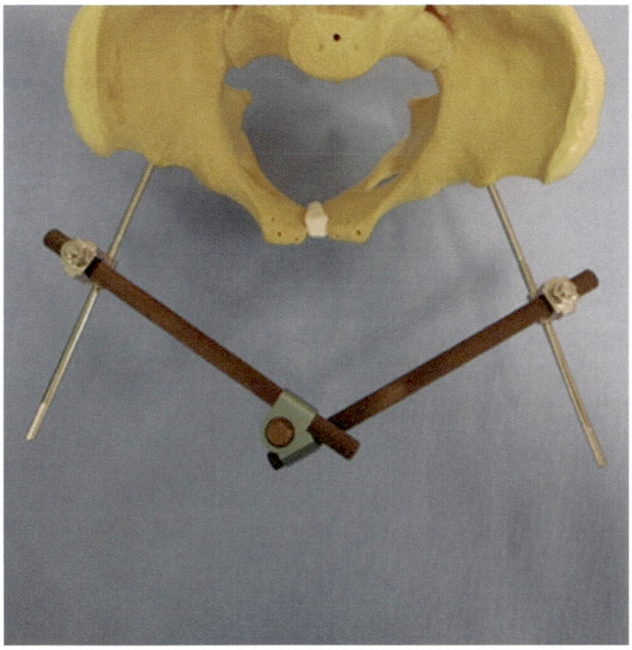

Fig. 25.18 A tube-to-tube construct can avoid soft-tissue complications

ASIS and AIIS. For better verification of the screw position, imaging should be done using the ALA view. The supraacetabular position should be given preference for biomechanical reasons [26].

Alternatively, the iliac Schanz screw insertion can be performed. Here, 1–2 cm skin incision is made approximately 3 cm posterior to the ASIS to avoid injury to the LCFN, which infrequently can run lateral to the ASIS. For optimal screw insertion, the iliac bone is palpated with an instrument [29], a Kirschner wire [30], or digitally. Again, only the cortex is perforated by the drill bit, and the Schanz screw is then introduced into the drill hole and further advanced between the two laminae of the iliac bone without predrilling.

25.10 Radiographic Check-Up

To check the position of the implant and the quality of reduction, a pelvic AP radiograph and bilateral combined obturator oblique outlet views are taken while still in the operating room (Fig. 25.20).

25.11 Wound Closure

Adaptive suturing is performed only, if the skin wound gaps. Wound drainage is not necessary. For wound dressing, a compress is placed around the Schanz screw.

25.12 Postoperative Management

A postoperative AP x-ray is performed for documentation. Further views are not necessary. A radiologic control (pelvic AP view) is additionally performed after 3 months to state definitive healing.

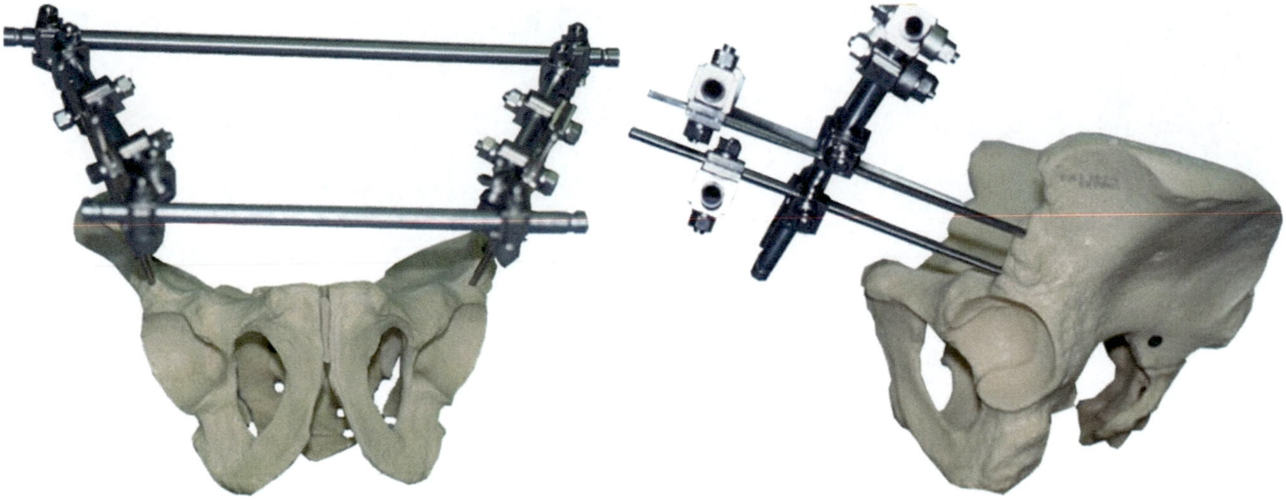

Fig. 25.19 Two-pin supraacetabular fixation

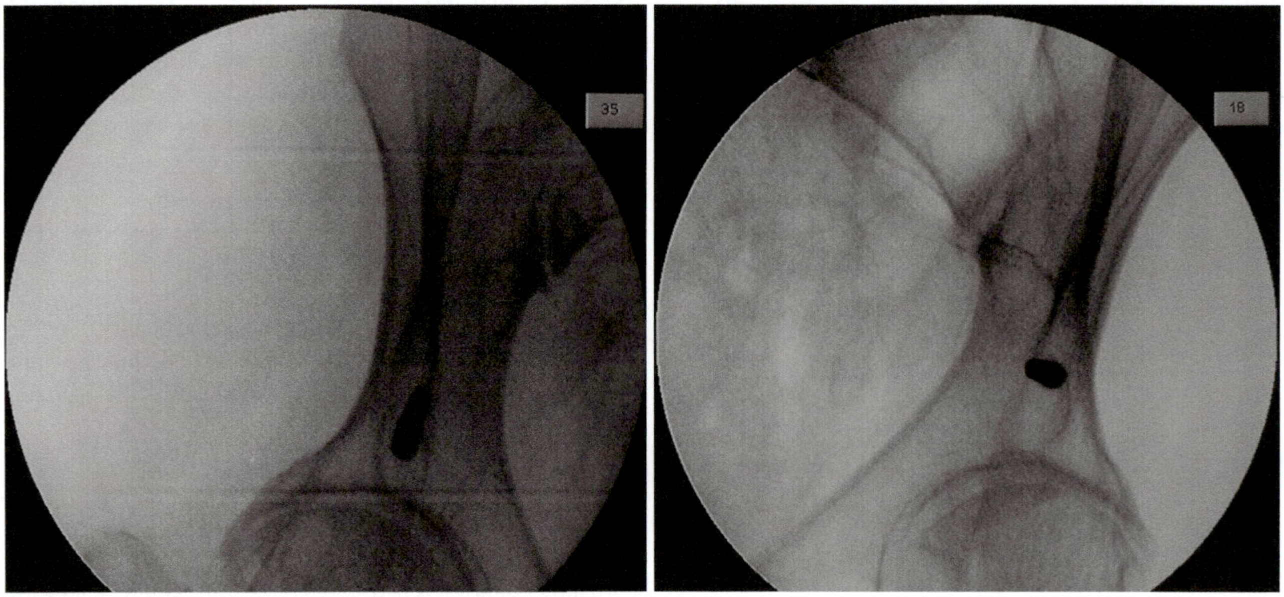

Fig. 25.20 Intraoperative x-rays show optimal pin position between the iliac cortices

In type B injuries, partial weight bearing (15 kg) on the posteriorly injured side for 3–4 weeks using forearm crutches starts at the second postoperative day.

in type C injuries, partial weight bearing (15 kg) on the posteriorly injured side for 4–6 weeks using forearm crutches starts at the second postoperative day.

Standard prophylactic antithrombotic treatment is recommended until partial weight bearing is performed according to standard regimens, e.g., enoxaparin twice daily according to body weight until full mobilization.

Daily local wound cleansing of the pin sites and change of sterile dressing is performed after education the patient. Possible sutures are removed after 10–14 days.

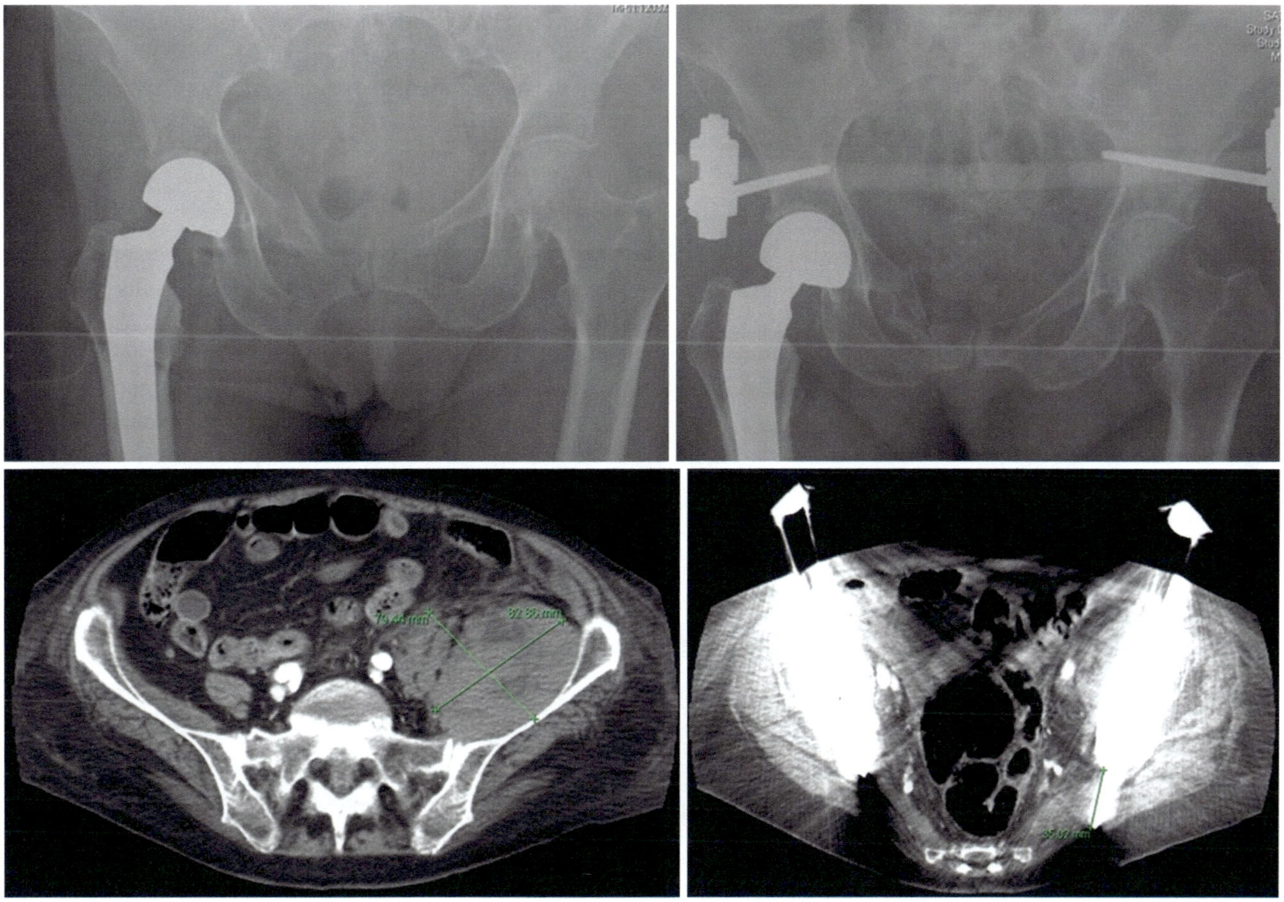

Fig. 25.21 Case with intrapelvic pin perforation, resulting in significant iliacus hematoma, requiring revision surgery

25.13 Implant Removal

Due to the excellent muscle coverage in the area of the pubic ramus (internal and external obturator muscle, adductors) and the usual thick periosteal layer including periosteal thickening ("Cooper's ligament"), a rapid bone healing can be expected. Thus, already after 3 or a maximum of 4 weeks, clinical healing can be expected to allow full weight.

The connecting rod of the external fixator is therefore loosened after 3 weeks, and the injury is tested for stability by manipulation at the Schanz screws. If the patient complains of pain at the fracture sites during this maneuver, the fixator is left in place for a further week; otherwise it is removed.

Only in rare cases, when a symphyseal disruption was definitively treated with a fixator, the external fixator is left in place for a total of 3 months, as the symphysis requires longer healing times.

The Schanz screws are removed in the outpatient clinic. Routine anesthesia is not necessary [65].

25.14 Complications

Perforation of the iliac bone can be avoided by adequately respecting the anatomy and clear palpation of the AIIS (Fig. 25.21). If the pin is inserted to close to the acetabular "sourcil", a potential risk of joint perforation exists.

The main risk factor of external fixation is occurrence of pin site infection (Fig. 25.22), which is usually treated by local wound care and antibiotics.

Respect to the individual soft-tissue envelope is important to avoid skin complications, especially in obese patients (Fig. 25.23).

Lesions of the LCFN are usually temporary lesions, which resolve after pin removal or during further course.

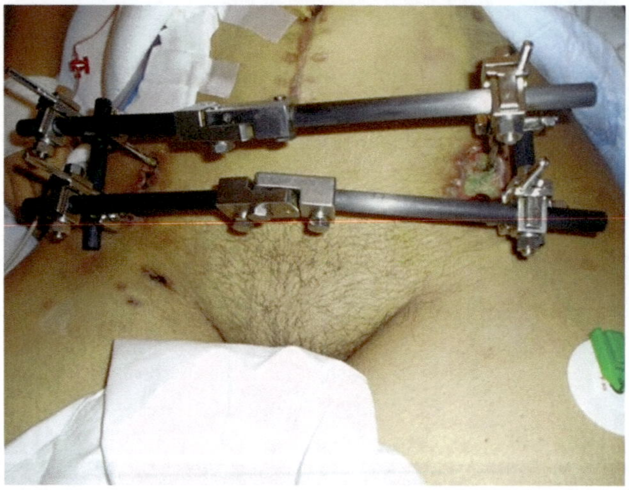

Fig. 25.22 Relevant pin tract infection

A wrong entry point in supraacetabular fixation, too close to the hip joint, can result in intraarticular pin placement, with the potential risk of joint infection and destruction (Fig. 25.24).

25.15 Results

Several reports are dealing with long-term results of external fixation. Only recent reports were analyzed (Fig. 25.25, Tables 25.1 and 25.2).

Lindahl et al. analyzed 70 type B injuries and 40 type C injuries, historically treated with an isolated anterior Slätis external fixator. A high rate of complications were observed (Table 25.1), especially after treatment of open-book type B injuries and nearly all type C injuries [52]. Mason et al. could

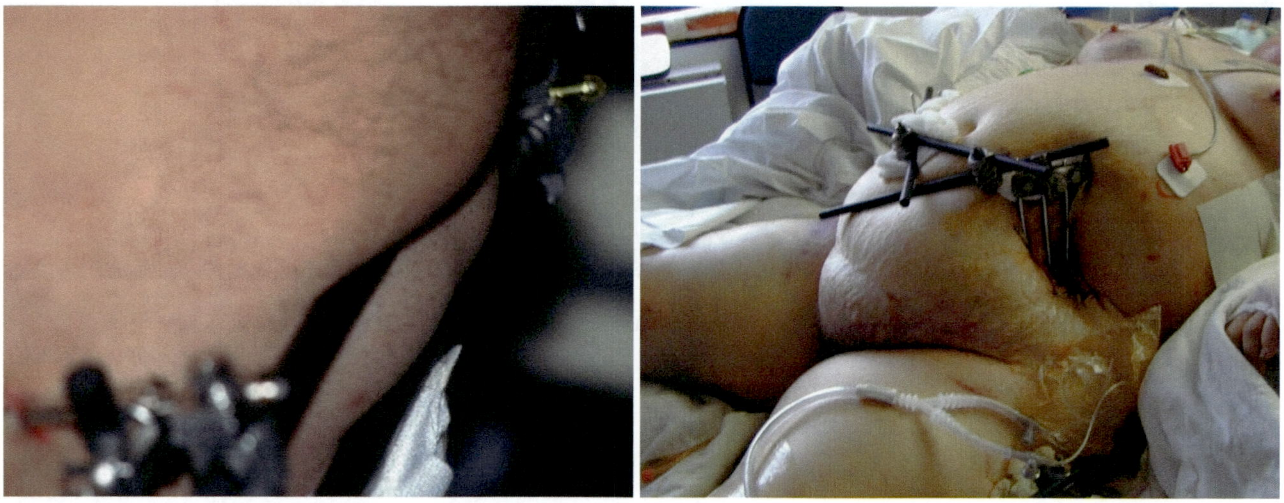

Fig. 25.23 Soft-tissue pressure complication in obese patients

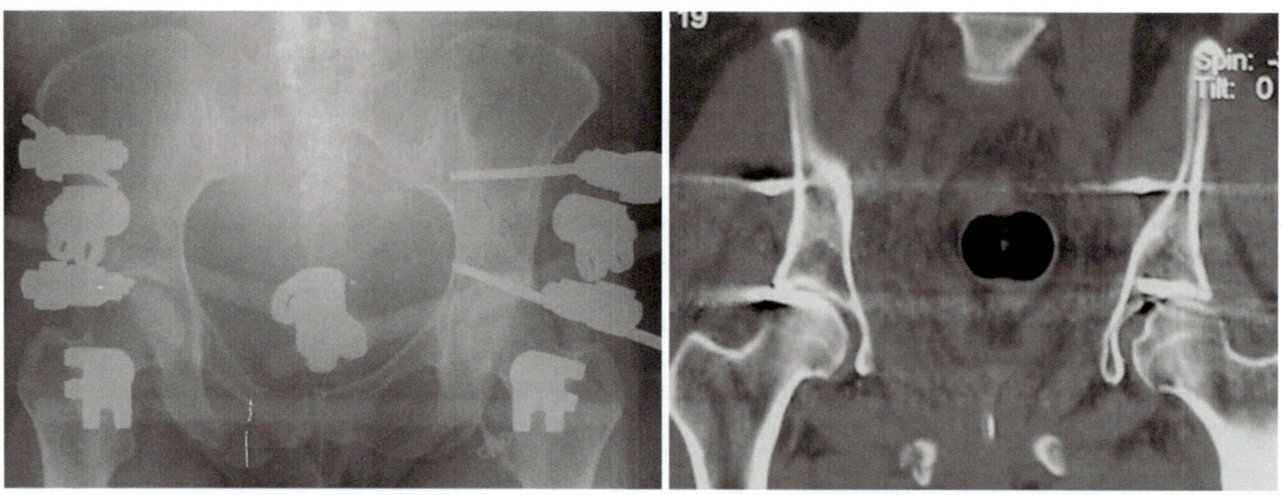

Fig. 25.24 Intraarticular pin placement

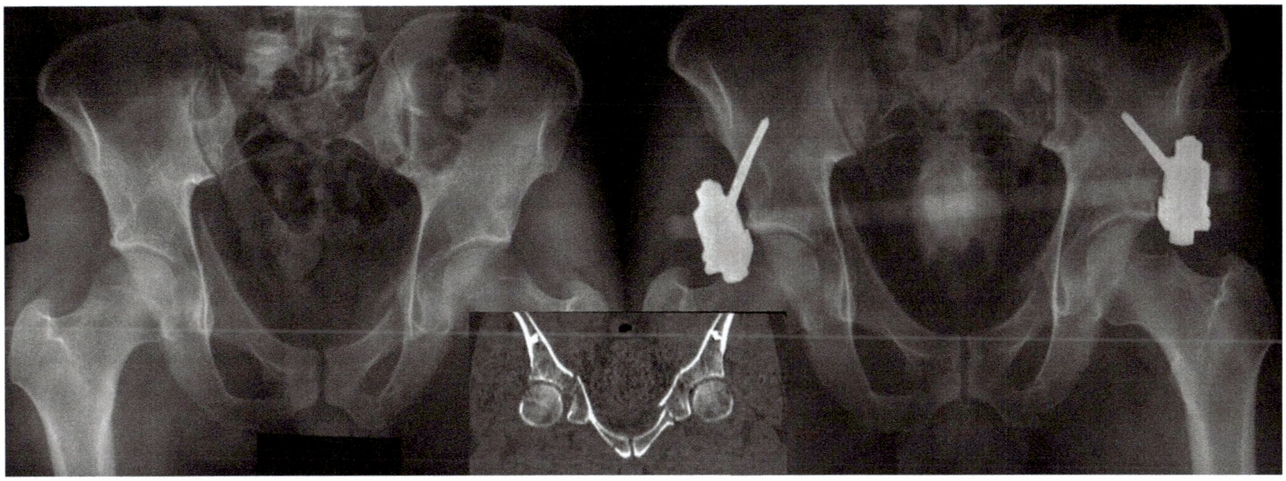

Fig. 25.25 Optimal supraacetabular pin placement in a type B-injury

Table 25.1 Results after iliac crest external fixation

Author	Year	No.	B	C	pO	PSI	LOR	aL	LCFN	Revision	Malunion	Nonunion
Lindahl	1999	110	70	40	0	26	63	2	2	0	64	6
Tucker	2000	40	15	26	32	1	3	3		3		0
Arazi	2000	41	24	17	0	8	2			0	2	
Mason	2005	52	24	28	0	26	4	6		9		
Scaglione	2010	41	35	6	4	13		7	0	3		0
Vecsei	2010	28	10	18	4	2/20			2/20		1/20	
Mitchell	2013	129	?	?	0	20						

loc location, *IC* iliac crest, *pO* posterior osteosynthesis, *PSI* pin site infection, *LOR* loss of reduction, *aL* aseptic loosening

Table 25.2 Results after supraacetabular external fixation

Author	Year	No.	B	C	pO	PSI	LOR	aL	LCFN	Revision	Malunion	Nonunion
Bellabarba	2001	14			0	4	0	0	1	0		0
Gänsslen	2005	20	20	0	0	0	0	0	2	0		
Gänsslen	2005	25	0	25	21	0	0	0	1	0	0	1
Gänsslen	2013	25	25	0	0	2	0	1	0	0	0	0
McDonald	2017	52				10			3			

show that temporary fixation was associated with less complications than definitive treatment (21% vs. 62%) of pelvic ring injuries [66].

Recently, Wardle et al. performed a systematic review and analyzed the difference between anterior internal and anterior external definitive fixations [67].

Internal fixation was associated with less residual displacement and lower rates of loss of reduction, delayed union, and malunion. Additionally, superficial infections were less common while the rate of deep infections was similar. It was stated that pin tract infections were not included in the infection analysis. No data were reported regarding fracture classification and additional posterior pelvic ring stabilization.

25.16 Summary

Iliac crest application is associated with higher complications rates compared to the supraacetabular fixation route.

Overall, several conclusions can be stated from the literature [24, 52, 66]:

- External fixation is useful in the acute phase of resuscitation
- Temporary use of external fixation is safe and effective
- External fixation is of limited value in the definitive treatment of an unstable type C injury
- External fixation is of limited value in the definitive treatment of type B open-book injuries
- External fixation is usually unnecessary in minimally displaced lateral compression injuries
- Definitive treatment is associated with a high rate of infection and aseptic pin loosening

Appendix

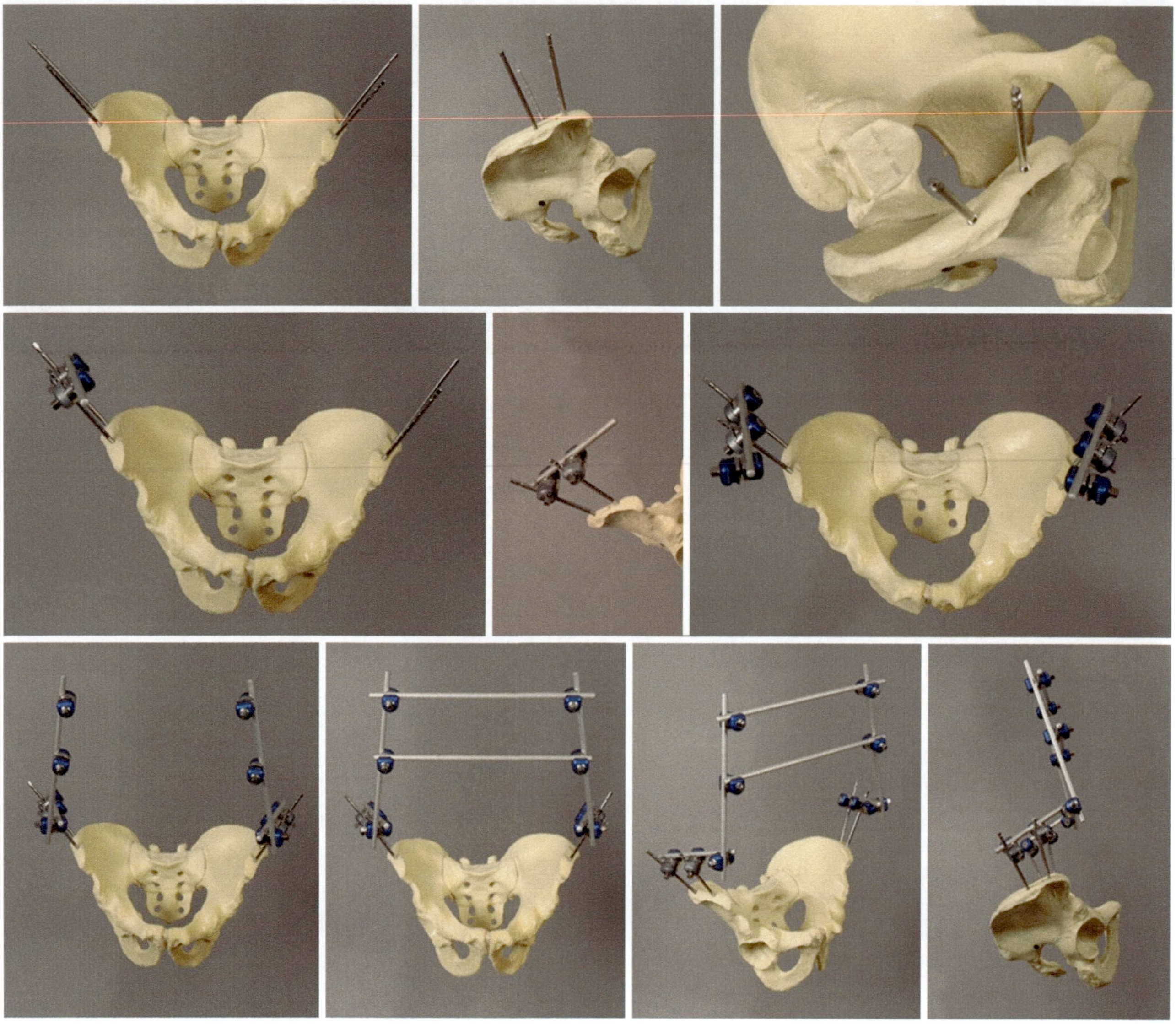

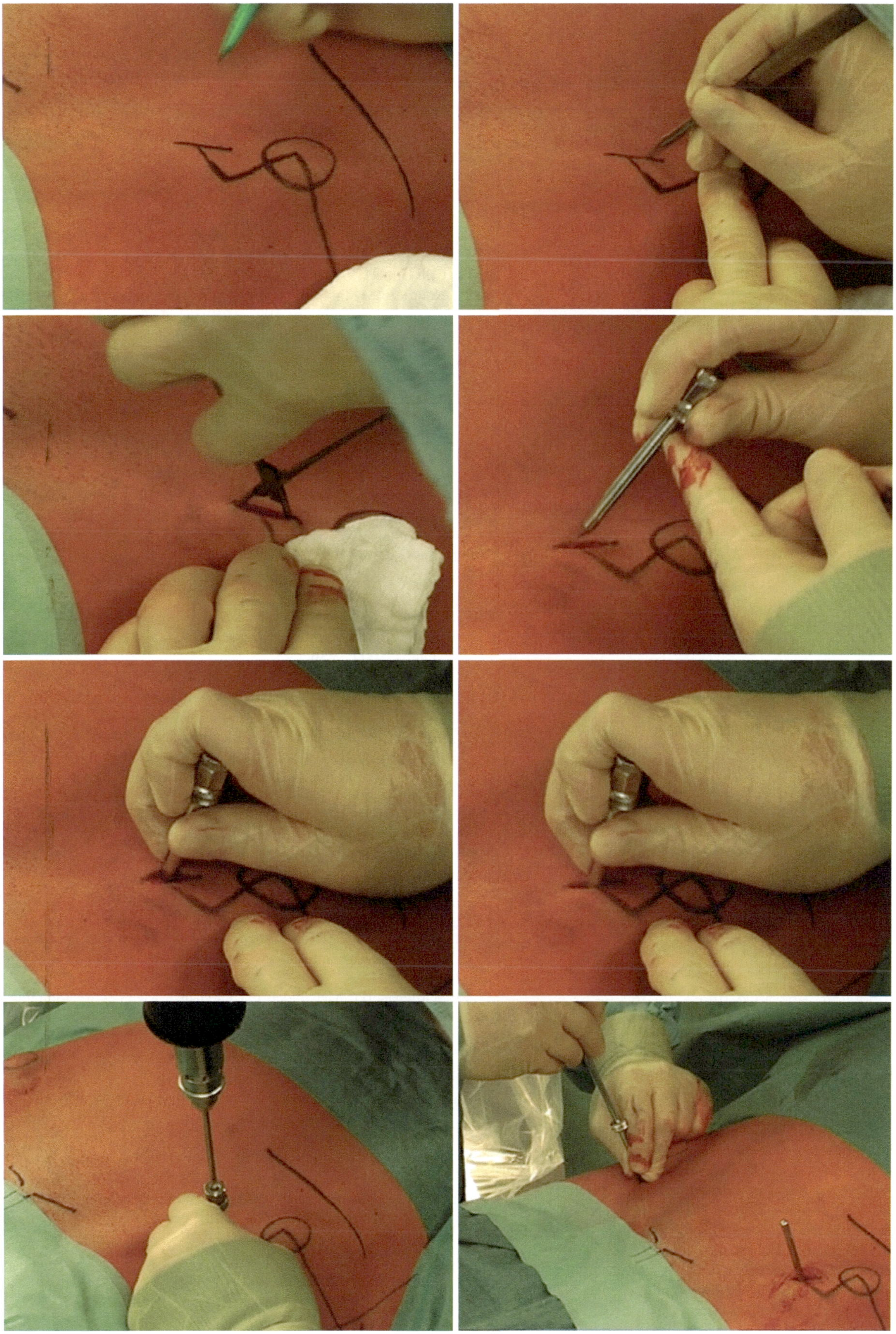

References

1. Carabalona P, Rabichong P, Bonnel F, Peruchon E, Peguret F. Apports du fixateur externe dans le disjonctions du pubis and de l'articulation sacro-iliaque. Montpell Chir. 1973;19:61–70.
2. Karaharju E, Slätis P. External fixation of double vertical pelvic fractures with a trapezoid compression frame. Injury. 1978;10:142–5.
3. Mears D, Fu F. External fixation in pelvic fractures. Orthop Clin North Am. 1980;11:465–79.
4. Mears D, Fu F. Modern concepts of external skeletal fixation of the pelvis. Clin Orthop. 1980;151:65–72.
5. Müller K, Müller-Färber J. Die Osteosynthese mit dem Fixateur externe am Becken. Arch Orthop Traumatol Surg. 1978;92:273–83.
6. Müller K, Müller-Färber J. Die Indikation externer und interner Stabilisationsverfahren bei der operativen Versorgung der Beckenringfrakturen. Hefte zur Unfallheilkunde. Heft 164. 1984. p. 216–21.
7. Slätis P, Karaharju E. External fixation of the pelvic girdle with a trapezoid compression frame. Injury. 1975;7:53–6.
8. Slätis P, Kraharju E. External fixation of unstable pelvic fractures: experiences in 22 patients treated with a trapezoid compression frame. Clin Orthop. 1980;151:73–9.
9. Holm C. Treatment of pelvic fractures and dislocations. Clin Orthop. 1973;97:97–107.
10. Kane W. Fractures of the pelvis. In: Rockwood C, Green D, editors. Fractures in adults. Philadelphia: Lippincott; 1975.
11. Egbers H, Draijer F, Havemann D, Zenker W. Stabilisierung des Beckenrings mit Fixatuer externe: biomechanische Untersuchungen und klinische Erfahrungen. Orthopade. 1992;21:363–72.
12. Rubash H, Brown T, Nelson D, Mears D. Comparative mechanical performance of some new devices for fixation of unstable pelvic ring fractures. Med Biol Eng Comput. 1983;21:657–63.
13. Brown T, Stone J, Schuster J, Mears D. External fixation of unstable pelvic ring fractures: comparative rigidity of some current frame configurations. Med Biol Eng Comput. 1982;20:727–33.
14. Burgess A, Eastridge B, Young J, Ellison T, Ellison P, Poka A, Bathon G, Brumback R. Pelvic ring disruption: effective classification systems and treatment protocols. J Trauma. 1990;30(7):848–56.
15. Coccolini F, Stahel P, Montori G, Biffl W, Horer T, Catena F, Kluger Y, Moore E, Peitzman A, Ivatury R, Coimbra R, Fraga G, Pereira B, Rizoli S, Kirkpatrick A, Leppaniemi A, Manfredi R, Magnone S, Chiara O, Solaini L, Ceresoli M, Allievi N, Arvieux C, Velmahos G, Balogh Z, Naidoo N, Weber D, Abu-Zidan F, Sartelli M, Ansaloni L. Pelvic trauma: WSES classification and guidelines. World J Emerg Surg. 2017;12:5. https://doi.org/10.1186/s13017-017-0117-6.
16. Cook R, Keating J, Gillespie I. The role of angiography in the management of haemorrhage from major fractures of the pelvis. J Bone Joint Surg Br. 2002;84(2):178–82.
17. Polytrauma Guideline Update Group. Level 3 guideline on the treatment of patients with severe/multiple injuries. Eur J Trauma Emerg Surg. 2018;44:S3–S271.
18. Gylling SF, Ward RE, Holcroft JW, Bray TJ, Chapman MW. Immediate external fixation of unstable pelvic fractures. Am J Surg. 1985;150(6):721–4.
19. Kellam J. The role of external fixation in pelvic disruptions. Clin Orthop. 1989;241:66–82.
20. Krettek C, Simon R, Tscherne H. Management priorities in patients with polytrauma. Langenbecks Arch Surg. 1998;383(3–4):220–7.
21. Miller P, Moore P, Mansell E, Meredith J, Chang M. External fixation or arteriogram in bleeding pelvic fracture: initial therapy guided by markers of arterial hemorrhage. J Trauma. 2003;54(3):437–43.
22. Rossaint R, Bouillon B, Cerny V, Coats T, Duranteau J, Fernández-Mondéjar E, Filipescu D, Hunt B, Komadina R, Nardi G, Neugebauer E, Ozier Y, Riddez L, Schultz A, Vincent J, Spahn D. The European guideline on management of major bleeding and coagulopathy following trauma: fourth edition. Crit Care. 2016;20:100.
23. Ponsen K, Hoek van Dijke G, Joosse P, Snijders C. External fixators for pelvic fractures: comparison of the stiffness of current systems. Acta Orthop Scand. 2003;74:165–71.
24. Gänsslen A, Pohlemann T, Krettek C. Supraacetabular external fixation for pelvic ring fractures. Oper Orthop Traumatol. 2005;17:296–312.
25. Jeanneret B, Ruflin G. Eine technische Variante des geschlossenen Fixateur externe am Becken. Z Unfallchir Vers med Berufskr. 1988;81(Heft 2):120–5.
26. Kim W, Hearn T, Seleem O, Mahalingam E, Stephen D, Tile M. Effect of pin location on stability of pelvic external fixation. Clin Orthop. 1999;361:237–44.
27. Noordeen M, Taylor B, Briggs T, Lavy C. Pin placement in pelvic external fixation. Injury. 1993;24(9):581–4.
28. Rupp R, Ebraheim N, Jackson W. Anatomic and radiographic considerations in the placement of anterior pelvic external fixator pins. Clin Orthop. 1994;302:213–8.
29. Waikakul S, Kojaranon N, Vanadurongwan V, Harnroongroj T. An aiming device for pin fixation at the iliac crest for external fixation in unstable pelvic fracture. Injury. 1998;29(10):757–62.
30. Tucker M, Nork S, Simonian P, Routt MJ. Simple anterior pelvic external fixation. J Trauma. 2000;49(6):989–94.
31. Stahel P, Mauffrey C, Smith W, McKean J, Hao J, Burlew C, Moore E. External fixation for acute pelvic ring injuries: decision making and technical options. J Trauma Acute Care Surg. 2013;75:882–7.
32. Solomon L, Pohl A, Chehade M, Malcolm A, Howie D, Henneberg M. Surgical anatomy for pelvic external fixation. Clin Anat. 2008;21:674–82.
33. Solomon L, Pohl A, Sukthankar A, Chehade M. The subcristal pelvic external fixator: technique, results, and rationale. J Orthop Trauma. 2009;23:362–9.
34. Apostolov P, Burnev M, Milkov P. Methods and techniques ofd percutaneous external fixation in pelvic fractures. J IMAB. 2011;17:166–71.
35. Gänsslen A, Hildebrand F, Klebingat M, Nerlich M, Lindahl J. Chapter 22: Special screws and views. In: Gänsslen A, et al., editors. Acetabular fractures: diagnosis, indications, treatment strategies. New York: Thieme; 2017. ISBN-13: 978-3132415607.
36. Mollier S. Plastische Anatomie. 2. Auflage, unveränderter Neudruck 1967 ed. München: J.F. Bergmann; 1938.
37. Rubel I, Kloen P, Borens O, Helfet D. External fixation for pelvic ring injuries. Tech Orthop. 2002;17:221–7.
38. Tang P, Meredick R, Prayson M, Gruen G. External fixation of the pelvis. Tech Orthop. 2002;17:228–38.
39. Berry J, Stahurski T, Asher M. Morphometry of the supra sciatic notch intrailiac implant anchor passage. Spine (Phila Pa 1976). 2001;26:143–8.
40. Schildhauer T, McCulloch P, Chapman J, Mann F. Anatomic and radiographic considerations for placement of transiliac screws in lumbopelvic fixations. J Spinal Disord Tech. 2002;15:199–205.
41. Tscherne H, Pohlemann T. Tscherne Unfallchirurgie: Becken und Acetabulum. Berlin, Heidelberg, New York: Springer; 1998.
42. Haidukewych G, Kumar S, Prpa B. Placement of half-pins for supra-acetabular external fixation: an anatomic study. Clin Orthop. 2003;411:269–73.
43. Pauwels F. Atlas zur Biomechanik der gesunden und kranken Hüfte. Berlin, Heidelberg, New York: Springer; 1973.
44. de Ridder V, de Lange S, Popta J. Anatomical variations of the lateral femoral cutaneous nerve and the consequences for surgery. J Orthop Trauma. 1999;13(3):207–11.
45. Hospodar P, Ashman E, Traub J. Anatomic study of the lateral femoral cutaneous nerve with respect to the ilioinguinal surgical dissection. J Orthop Trauma. 1999;13:17–9.

46. Surucu H, Tanyeli E, Sargon M, Karahan S. An anatomic study of the lateral femoral cutaneous nerve. Surg Radiol Anat. 1997;19:307–10.
47. Aszmann OC, Dellon ES, Dellon AL. Anatomical course of the lateral femoral cutaneous nerve and its susceptibility to compression and injury. Plast Reconstr Surg. 1997;100(3):600–4.
48. Kosiyatrakul A, Nuansalee N, Luenam S, Koonchornboon T, Prachaporn S. The anatomical variation of the lateral femoral cutaneous nerve in relation to the anterior superior iliac spine and the iliac crest. Musculoskelet Surg. 2010;94:17–20.
49. Majkrzak A, Johnston J, Kacey D, Zeller J. Variability of the lateral femoral cutaneous nerve: an anatomic basis for planning safe surgical approaches. Clin Anat. 2010;23:304–11.
50. Ropars M, Morandi X, Huten D, Thomazeau H, Berton E, Darnault P. Anatomical study of the lateral femoral cutaneous nerve with special reference to minimally invasive anterior approach for total hip replacement. Surg Radiol Anat. 2009;31:199–204.
51. Üzel M, Akkin S, Tanyeli E, Koebke J. Relationships of the lateral femoral cutaneous nerve to bony landmarks. Clin Orthop. 2011;469:2605–11.
52. Lindahl J, Hirvensalo E, Bostman O, Santavirta S. Failure of reduction with an external fixator in the management of injuries of the pelvic ring. Long-term evaluation of 110 patients. J Bone Joint Surg Br. 1999;81(6):955–62.
53. Bellabarba C, Ricci W, Bolhofner B. Distraction external fixation in lateral compression pelvic fractures. J Orthop Trauma. 2000;14(7):475–82.
54. Pohlemann T, Gänsslen A. Die Operation der Symphysensprengung. Oper Orthop Traumatol. 1999;11:149–59.
55. Pohlemann T, Gänsslen A, Hartung S, für die Arbeitsgruppe Becken, H.T., H, Beckenverletzungen/Pelvic Injuries. Hefte zu "Der Unfallchirurg". Heft 266. 1998.
56. Pohlemann T, Krettek C, Hoffmann R, Culemann U, Gänsslen A. Biomechanischer Vergleich verschiedener Notfallstabilisierungsmaßnahmen am Beckenring. Unfallchirurg. 1994;97(10):503–10.
57. Gänsslen A, Heidari N, Weinberg A. Fractures of the pelvis in children: a review of the literature. Eur J Orthop Surg Traumatol. 2013;23:847–61.
58. Gänsslen A, Hildebrand F, Heidari N, Weinberg A. Pelvic ring injuries in children. Part II: treatment and results. A review of the literature. Acta Chir Orthop Traumatol Cechoslov. 2013;80:241–9.
59. Weber O, Gravius S, Henkel S, Berdel P, Burger C, Wirtz D. Pelvic osseous infections: clinical outcome and surgical treatment. Z Orthop Unfall. 2008;146:510–9.
60. Gänsslen A, Hildebrand F, Krettek C. Supraacetabular external fixation for pain control in geriatric type B pelvic injuries. Acta Chir Orthop Traumatol Cechoslov. 2013;80:101–5.
61. Hofmann G, Bredow J. Spätergebnisse der Beckenringverletzungen-Behandlung mit dem Fixateur externe. Hefte Unfallheilk. 1986;181:612–8.
62. Wang F, Song H, Zhao F, Yang Q, Tang H, Ji X, Wang Q, Wang Z, Wang Q. Supra-acetabular external fixation for pelvic fractures: a digital anatomical study. Clin Anat. 2012;25:503–8.
63. Tian X, Li J, Sheng W, Qu D, Ouyang J, Xu D, Chen S, Ding Z. Morphometry of iliac anchorage for transiliac screws: a cadaver and CT study of the Eastern population. Surg Radiol Anat. 2010;32:455–62.
64. Calafi L, Routt M. Anterior pelvic external fixation: is there an optimal placement for the supra-acetabular pin? Am J Orthop. 2013;42:125–7.
65. Ryder S, Gorczyca J. Routine removal of external fixators without anesthesia. J Orthop Trauma. 2007;21:571–3.
66. Mason W, Khan S, James C, Chesser T, Ward A. Complications of temporary and definitive external fixation of pelvic ring injuries. Injury. 2005;36:599–604.
67. Wardle B, Eslick G, Sunner P. Internal versus external fixation of the anterior component in unstable fractures of the pelvic ring: pooled results from a systematic review. Eur J Trauma Emerg Surg. 2016;42:635–43.

Subcutaneous Anterior Pelvic Fixation

26

Bernd Füchtmeier, Franz Müller, and Axel Gänsslen

During the last 10 years, two new innovative concepts of anterior pelvic ring fixation were introduced based on a minimal invasive percutaneous basis to avoid external hardware placement:

- Subcutaneous anterior pelvic internal fixator fixation (SAPIF)
- Subcutaneous anterior pelvic internal plate fixation (SAPIP)

The optimal indication includes displaced anterior rami fractures as part of a pelvic ring injury while isolated symphyseal separations are considered better for open reduction and internal fixation [1, 2].

Contraindications include severe soft tissue injury at the anterior pelvis, traumatic urologic or general surgery wounds, and cases requiring emergency anterior stabilization of the pelvic ring, especially in hemodynamically unstable patients [1]. The posterior pelvic ring injury is usually stabilized first [1–3].

26.1 Subcutaneous Anterior Pelvic Internal Fixator Fixation (SAPIF)

In 2009, Kuttner et al. introduced the concept of a subcutaneous fixator (pelvic subcutaneous cross-over internal fixator, SVFI) based on the classical concept of a supraacetabular external fixator [2]. Indications included the typical indications for anterior pelvic ring injuries, except that symphyseal plating was favored [2].

26.1.1 Surgical Technique

In the supine position, a 3–4 cm incision is made over the iliac crest just two fingers posterior to the ASIS followed by sharp/blunt dissection of the anterior abdominal wall muscles medially to reach the medial supraacetabular bone. The course of the lateral cutaneous femoral nerve (LCFN) has to be respected. On each side, a polyaxial pedicle screw is inserted into the medial (intrapelvic) bone just 1–2 cm medial to the AIIS. Screw lengths of 45–60 mm are considered sufficient.

Dissection of the horizontal subcutaneous layer is performed bluntly using a curved forceps. A plastic tube is inserted into the resulting tunnel, acting as a space holder, followed by insertion of the definitive prebended titanium rod. Classical anterior pelvic ring reduction maneuvers are used until definitive fixation of the construct is performed. Polyaxial 3D heads are then connected to the pedicle screws, and their pods and the fixator rod is finally fixed to both pedicle screws.

26.1.2 Results

This concept was used in 22 patients (21 type C injuries, 1 type B injury) after additional posterior lumbopelvic distraction osteosynthesis. The mean OR time was 41 min. Nineteen patients were followed up for an average of 2.5 years. All anterior injuries healed uneventful. Of these, 52.6% presented with anatomical healing and 42.1% had healing in <10 mm malhealing. No nonunions were observed. The functional results were rated good and excellent in 52.6%. Subjective anterior impairments were reported in 21.1%.

B. Füchtmeier
Department of Trauma Surgery, Orthopaedics and Sports Medicine, Hospital Barmherzige Brüder, Regensburg, Germany
e-mail: Bernd.Fuechtmeier@barmherzige-regensburg.de

F. Müller
Department of Trauma Surgery, Orthopaedics and Sports Medicine, Hospital Barmherzige Brüder Regensburg, Regensburg, Germany

A. Gänsslen (✉)
Department of Trauma Surgery, Orthopedics and Hand Surgery, Hospital Wolfsburg, Wolfsburg, Germany

A. Gänsslen et al. (eds.), *Pelvic Ring Fractures*, https://doi.org/10.1007/978-3-030-54730-1_26

Relevant complications occurred in two patients: 1× implant loosening and 1× subcutaneous wound infection. In seven cases, a transient LCFN lesion was present with complete recovery within 6 months [2].

In the meantime, several other groups used such a concept [1, 3–15]. The authors used different acronyms, e.g., anterior pelvic internal fixation (APIF) and internal fixator (INFIX).

Gardner et al. and Vaidya et al. proposed a similar concept. The pedicle screws are percutaneously inserted into the classical external fixator bone corridor [16] starting at the AIIS [3, 10]. A contoured rod is inserted subcutaneously, tunneled anterior to the fascia, and then connected to the pedicle screws.

The results of these comparable procedures are summarized in Table 26.1 [2, 3, 6, 8, 10, 11, 13, 15, 17, 18].

Potentially, the femoral nerve can be at risk when inadequately inserting the fixator [18, 19].

Biomechanical tests showed that the use of monoaxial screws was superior regrading stiffness compared to polyaxial screws [20].

The main conclusions from the literature using the SAPIF are [2–4, 6–15, 17–27]:

- The majority of anterior pelvic ring injuries heal uneventful.
- Good reductions can be achieved in the majority of patients.
- Implant removal is recommended at 3–6 months postoperatively.
- Heterotopic ossification is a common phenomenon at the pedicle screw entry; in a few cases even higher grades were observed.
- Irritation of the LCFN is common and resolves latest after implant removal.
- A few patients show persistent LCFN problems.
- The femoral nerve is in danger; lesions can lead to relevant morbidity.
- Some patients develop anterior ring nonunion.

26.2 Subcutaneous Anterior Pelvic Internal Plate Fixation (SAPIP)

In 2012, additionally, a percutaneous plate application was introduced to stabilize either anterior ramus fractures or symphyseal disruptions ("pelvic bridge fixation") [1]. Two possible fixations options were reported:

- Long reconstruction plates
- Occipitocervical fusion plate-rod hybrid implant with pedicle screw fixation

26.2.1 Anatomical Background

Moazzam et al. performed an anatomical study to analyze the potential risk during dissection to surrounding structures [28].

Dissection of five fresh frozen cadavers was performed, and the relationship between the plates and the lateral femoral cutaneous nerve (LFCN), ilioinguinal nerve (IIN), iliohypogastric nerve (IHN), femoral nerve, femoral artery, femoral vein, genitofemoral nerve, and the spermatic cord/round ligament was analyzed. The mean distance to these structures was all above 1.5 cm. Only the distance between the spermatic cord and the plate was 4 mm in average but was directly visualized during potential surgery.

Table 26.1 Results after internal subcutaneous fixation

Author	Year	No.	OTA	Postfix	OR time	f/u	No.	INF	LCFN	LOR	HO	IR
Kuttner [2]	2009	22	21×C	21	41 min	29 m	19	1[a]	7	1	0	17
Gardner [3]	2012	24	24×C	24	unknown	12 m	13	1[a]	2	0	6	12
Vaidya [10]	2012	24	16×C	16	unknown	19 m	22	0	2	0	unknown	16
Vaidya [11]	2012	96	[b]	unknown	unknown	15 m	91	3	27	3	32	[c]
Müller [8]	2013	36	36	36	30-60 min	18 m	31	2	6	unknown	9	30
Hoskins [6]	2016	21	unknown	19	51 min	12 m	19	3	12		9	19
Wang [15]	2016	26	26×B	0	57.9 min	8.2 m	26	0	2	unknown	unknown	26
Dahill [17]	2017	47	unknown	unknown	unknown	38 m	47	2	34	2	0	45
Fang [18]	2017	43	unknown	unknown	unknown	7.2 m	43	14	1	2	0	21
Vaidya [13]	2017	24	9×C	unknown	unknown			1	1	2	11	

INF infection, *LCFN* lateral cutaneous femoral nerve lesion, *LOR* loss of reduction, *HO* heterotopic ossification, *IR* implant removal
[a]Superficial infection
[b]Unclear
[c]Majority of patients

26.2.2 Surgical Technique

In the supine position on a radiolucent table, long 3.5 mm locking reconstruction plates (14–18 holes) were used [1].

Preoperative planning included precontouring using standardized Sawbone models to fix the plate with at least two screws on each side at the anterior iliac crest and with four holes bridging the pubic symphysis, depending on fracture morphology. In unilateral injuries, even unilateral application can be considered.

After 3 cm incision at the ASIS, as with the SAPIF, subcutaneous tunneling is performed anterior to the external oblique fascia and the rectus sheath and superior to the inguinal ligament, and a precontoured reconstruction plate is inserted.

Depending on the fracture type, two options for plate stabilization are possible:

- Unilateral plate application
  - *Incision*: 3 cm posteriorly orientated incision starting at the ASIS and an additional 6–8 cm Pfannenstiel incision
  - *Dissection*: Blunt development of a unilateral subcutaneous tunnel anterior to the external oblique fascia and the rectus sheath and superior to the inguinal ligament using a finger; identification of the spermatic cord and superior plate positioning to it
  - *Plate insertion*: Insertion of a 14–18-hole precontoured plate, spanned from the anterior iliac crest to the contralateral pubic tubercle
  - *Fixation*: one standard and one locking screw, each at the iliac crest and parallel to the symphysis
- Bilateral plate application
  - *Incision*: Two 3 cm incisions posteriorly orientated starting at both ASIS and an additional 6–8 cm Pfannenstiel incision
  - *Dissection*: Blunt development of a combined bilateral subcutaneous tunnel anterior to the external oblique fascia and the rectus sheath and superior to the inguinal ligament using a finger; identification of the spermatic cord and superior plate positioning to it
  - *First plate insertion*: Insertion of one 14–18-hole precontoured plate, spanned from the anterior iliac crest to the contralateral pubic tubercle
  - *First fixation*: Loose fixation at the iliac crest and plate positioning parallel to the symphysis
  - *Second plate insertion*: Insertion of another 14–18-hole precontoured plate, spanned from the anterior iliac crest to the contralateral pubic tubercle, overlapping the first plate at the symphyseal region
  - *Second fixation*: Loose fixation at the iliac crest, cortical screw fixation of the overlapping plate through the first plate followed by locking screw fixation through both plates parasymphyseally

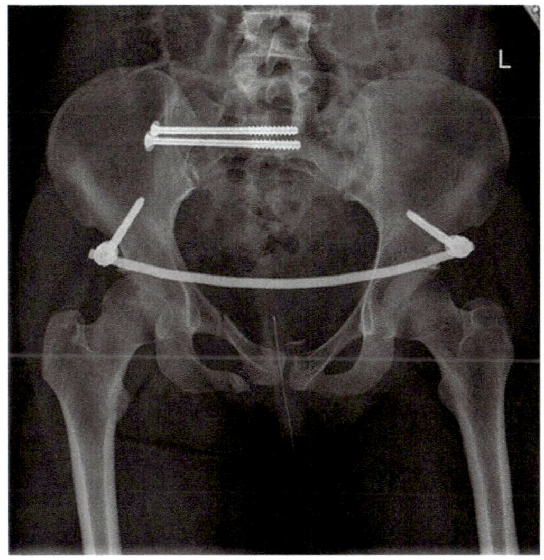

Fig. 26.1 Example of an x-ray of a subcutaneous internal anterior fixator

Alternatively, an occipitocervical spinal polyaxial implant can be used, either uni- or bilaterally.

26.2.3 Results

First clinical results were reported on 24 consecutive patients and compared to 24 patients with standard anterior external fixation [5]. Overall, less wound complications (pin site infections) and less surgical site pain were seen. Additionally, less loss of reduction and less implant loosening were observed. Slightly better postoperative reductions were possible using the internal plates. Implant removal was routinely performed.

> Subcutaneous internal anterior fixator offers a clinical alternative for fixation of displaced anterior pelvic ring injuries (Fig. 26.1).

References

1. Hiesterman T, Hill B, Cole P. Surgical technique: a percutaneous method of subcutaneous fixation for the anterior pelvic ring: the pelvic bridge. Clin Orthop Relat Res. 2012;470(8):2116–23.
2. Kuttner M, Klaiber A, Lorenz T, Fuchtmeier B, Neugebauer R. [The pelvic subcutaneous cross-over internal fixator]. Unfallchirurg. 2009;112(7):661–9.
3. Gardner M, Mehta S, Mirza A, Ricci W. Anterior pelvic reduction and fixation using a subcutaneous internal fixator. J Orthop Trauma. 2012;26(5):314–21.

4. Apivatthakakul T, Rujiwattanapong N. "Anterior subcutaneous pelvic internal fixator (INFIX), is it safe?" A cadaveric study. Injury. 2016;47(10):2077–80.
5. Cole P, Gauger E, Anavian J, Ly T, Morgan R, Heddings A. Anterior pelvic external fixator versus subcutaneous internal fixator in the treatment of anterior ring pelvic fractures. J Orthop Trauma. 2012;26(5):269–77.
6. Hoskins W, Bucknill A, Wong J, Britton E, Judson R, Gumm K, Santos R, Sheehy R, Griffin X. A prospective case series for a minimally invasive internal fixation device for anterior pelvic ring fractures. J Orthop Surg Res. 2016;11(1):135.
7. McDonald E, Theologis A, Horst P, Kandemir U, Pekmezci M. When do anterior external or internal fixators provide additional stability in an unstable (Tile C) pelvic fracture? A biomechanical study. Eur J Trauma Emerg Surg. 2015;41(6):665–71.
8. Muller F, Stosiek W, Zellner M, Neugebauer R, Fuchtmeier B. The anterior subcutaneous internal fixator (ASIF) for unstable pelvic ring fractures: clinical and radiological mid-term results. Int Orthop. 2013;37(11):2239–45.
9. Scheyerer M, Zimmermann S, Osterhoff G, Tiziani S, Simmen H, Wanner G, Werner C. Anterior subcutaneous internal fixation for treatment of unstable pelvic fractures. BMC Res Notes. 2014;7:133.
10. Vaidya R, Colen R, Vigdorchik J, Tonnos F, Sethi A. Treatment of unstable pelvic ring injuries with an internal anterior fixator and posterior fixation: initial clinical series. J Orthop Trauma. 2012;26(1):1–8.
11. Vaidya R, Kubiak E, Bergin P, Dombroski D, Critchlow R, Sethi A, Starr A. Complications of anterior subcutaneous internal fixation for unstable pelvis fractures: a multicenter study. Clin Orthop Relat Res. 2012;470(8):2124–31.
12. Vaidya R, Martin A, Roth M, Nasr K, Gheraibeh P, Tonnos F. INFIX versus plating for pelvic fractures with disruption of the symphysis pubis. Int Orthop. 2017;41(8):1671–8.
13. Vaidya R, Martin A, Roth M, Tonnos F, Oliphant B, Carlson J. Midterm radiographic and functional outcomes of the anterior subcutaneous internal pelvic fixator (INFIX) for pelvic ring injuries. J Orthop Trauma. 2017;31(5):252–9.
14. Vaidya R, Tonnos F, Nasr K, Kanneganti P, Curtis G. The anterior subcutaneous pelvic fixator (INFIX) in an anterior posterior compression type 3 pelvic fracture. J Orthop Trauma. 2016;30(Suppl 2):S21–2.
15. Wang Q, Wang Q, Wang J. Treatment of type B pelvic fracture using anterior subcutaneous internal fixator with triple pedicle screws: a new surgical technique. Arch Orthop Trauma Surg. 2017;137(7):887–93.
16. Gänsslen A, Pohlemann T, Krettek C. [A simple supraacetabular external fixation for pelvic ring fractures]. Oper Orthop Traumatol. 2005;17:296–312.
17. Dahill M, McArthur J, Roberts G, Acharya M, Ward A, Chesser T. The use of an anterior pelvic internal fixator to treat disruptions of the anterior pelvic ring: a report of technique, indications and complications. Bone Joint J. 2017;99-B:1232–6.
18. Fang C, Alabdulrahman H, Pape H. Complications after percutaneous internal fixator for anterior pelvic ring injuries. Int Orthop. 2017;41:1785–90.
19. Hesse D, Kandmir U, Solberg B, Stroh A, Osgood G, Sems S, Collinge C. Femoral nerve palsy after pelvic fracture treated with INFIX: a case series. J Orthop Trauma. 2015;29(3):138–43.
20. Eagan M, Kim H, Manson T, Gary J, Russell J, Hsieh A, O'Toole R, Boulton C. Internal anterior fixators for pelvic ring injuries: do monaxial pedicle screws provide more stiffness than polyaxial pedicle screws? Injury. 2015;46(6):996–1000.
21. Merriman D, Ricci W, McAndrew C, Gardner M. Is application of an internal anterior pelvic fixator anatomically feasible? Clin Orthop Relat Res. 2012;470(8):2111–5.
22. Osterhoff G, Aichner E, Scherer J, Simmen H, Werner C, Feigl G. Anterior subcutaneous internal fixation of the pelvis—what rod-to-bone distance is anatomically optimal? Injury. 2017;48(10):2162–8.
23. Osterhoff G, Tiziani S, Ferguson S, Spreiter G, Scheyerer M, Spinas G, Wanner G, Simmen H, Werner C. Mechanical testing of a device for subcutaneous internal anterior pelvic ring fixation versus external pelvic ring fixation. BMC Musculoskelet Disord. 2014;15:111.
24. Owen M, Tinkler B, Stewart R. Failure and salvage of "INFIX" instrumentation for pelvic ring disruption in a morbidly obese patient. J Orthop Trauma. 2013;27(10):e243–6.
25. Smith A, Malek I, Lewis J, Mohanty K, et al. J Orthop Surg (Hong Kong). 2017;25(1):2309499016684994.
26. Vaidya R, Oliphant B, Jain R, Nasr K, Siwiec R, Onwudiwe N, Sethi A. The bikini area and bikini line as a location for anterior subcutaneous pelvic fixation: an anatomic and clinical investigation. Clin Anat. 2013;26(3):392–9.
27. Vigdorchik J, Esquivel A, Jin X, Yang K, Onwudiwe N, Vaidya R. Biomechanical stability of a supra-acetabular pedicle screw internal fixation device (INFIX) vs external fixation and plates for vertically unstable pelvic fractures. J Orthop Surg Res. 2012;7:31.
28. Moazzam C, Heddings A, Moodie P, Cole P. Anterior pelvic subcutaneous internal fixator application: an anatomic study. J Orthop Trauma. 2012;26(5):263–8.

Ilium Fractures

27

Axel Gänsslen and Jan Dauwe

Fractures of the ilium are rarely observed. These fractures can be part of unstable or stable pelvic ring injuries. The latter is present when the pelvic brim is not involved, e.g., avulsion fractures of the ASIS (see Chap. 37) or iliac crest/iliac fossa fractures. Additionally, iliac fracture dislocations of the SI joint involve the iliac bone (see Chap. 30). In fractures involving the pure ilium, two fracture types can be distinguished (Fig. 27.1):

- Iliac wing fractures
- Longitudinal ilium fractures, starting at the iliac crest, running along the iliac fossa to reach the pelvic brim as the posterior part of an unstable type C injury

27.1 Iliac Wing Fractures

Fractures of the iliac wing are most often the result of a direct blow against the lateral ilium during a fall (Fig. 27.2) or can be present as an insufficiency fracture after bone graft harvesting (Fig. 27.3) or in the geriatric population (Fig. 27.4) or even as stress fractures in runners [1].

A traumatic iliac wing fracture was recognized already in the seventeenth century and was called "Duverney fracture." This fracture was described as a transverse fracture of the ilium [2]. The patient described by Duverney died on day 4 due to septic multiple organ failure.

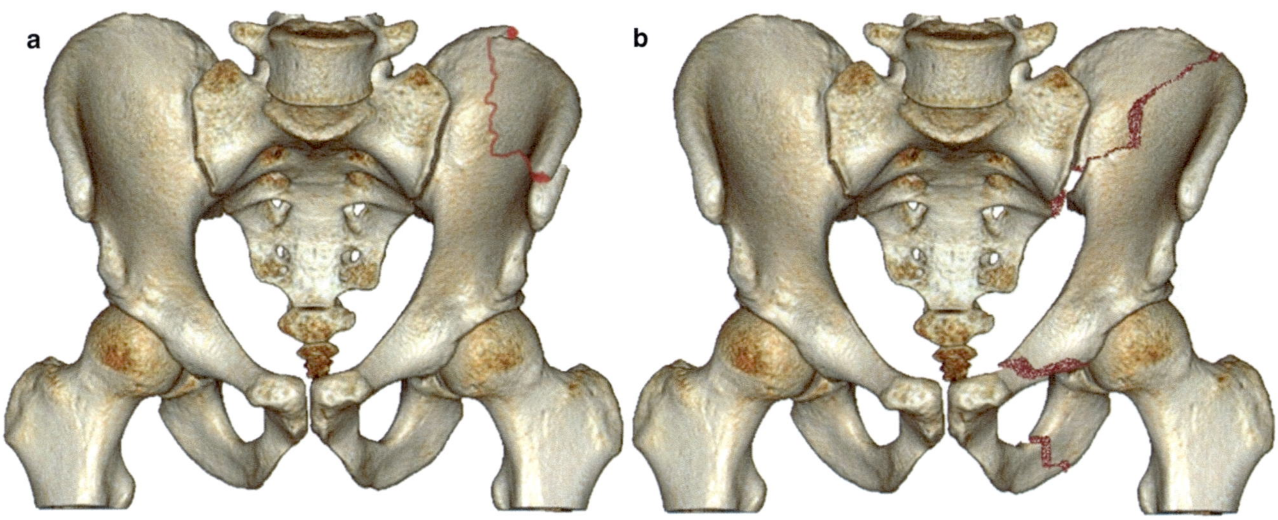

Fig. 27.1 Two types of ilium fractures: iliac wing fracture (**a**) and complete ilium fracture (**b**)

A. Gänsslen (✉)
Department of Trauma Surgery, Orthopedics and Hand Surgery, Hospital Wolfsburg, Wolfsburg, Germany

J. Dauwe
Department of Trauma Surgery, University Hospitals Leuven, Leuven, Belgium
e-mail: jan.dauwe@uzleuven.be

A. Gänsslen et al. (eds.), *Pelvic Ring Fractures*, https://doi.org/10.1007/978-3-030-54730-1_27

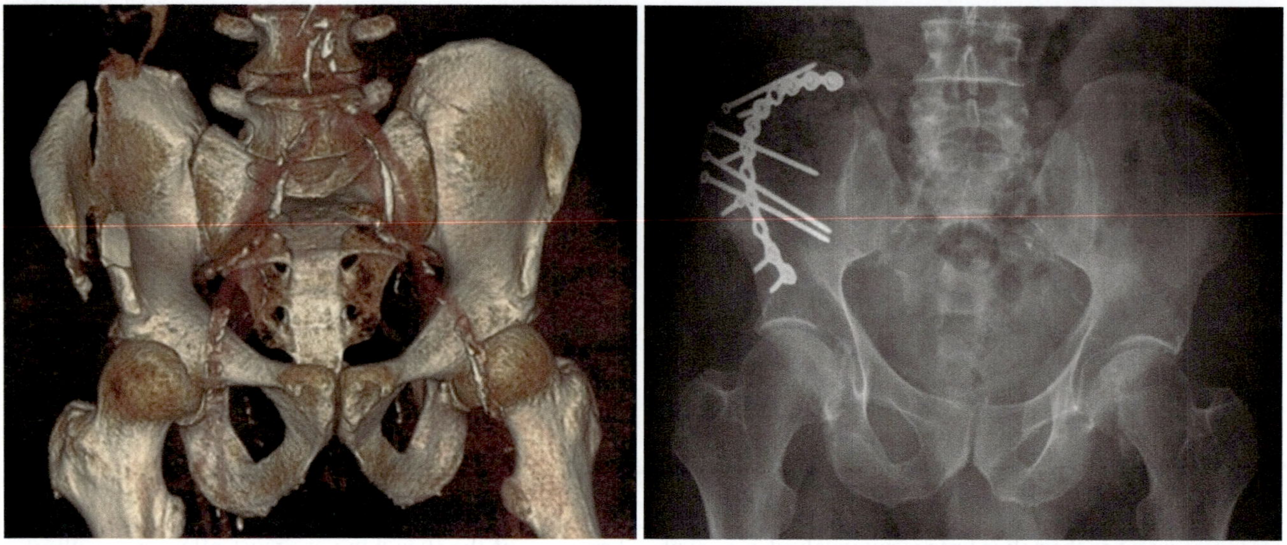

Fig. 27.2 Iliac wing fracture (Duverney's fracture) after a fall onto the right side. Screw osteosynthesis at the iliac crest in combination with iliac fossa plate stabilization resulted in anatomical reconstruction of the iliac wing

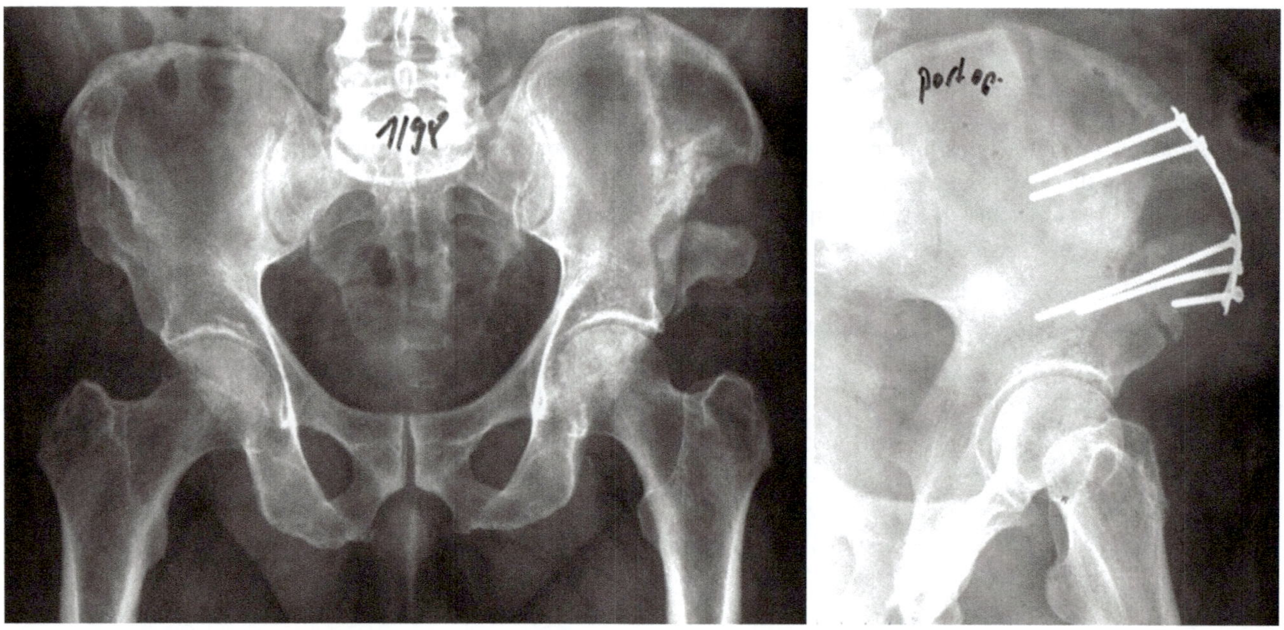

Fig. 27.3 Insufficiency fracture at the left iliac wing after bone graft harvesting. Contour plate stabilization with a 1/3 tubular plate for abdominal muscle refixation was performed

This fracture type is typically stable and, therefore, is a benign injury from the reconstructive standpoint. Thus, conservative treatment is recommended in the majority of cases. Due to the extended forces acting on the pelvis sustaining these injuries, concomitant abdominal, vascular, and/or neurological injuries should be analyzed.

In severely displaced injuries, with large hematoma formation, relevant pain during mobilization or cosmetic disturbance due to the internal rotation deformity, open reduction, and internal fixation should be recommended (Fig. 27.5).

Only two small series analyzed this fracture type.

Switzer et al. reported on 13 patients from a group of 695 survived patients with pelvic ring disruptions (1.9%), which presented with comminuted/displaced ilium fractures after high-energy lateral impacts [3]. All patients sustained additional injuries; the mean ISS was 23 points. Five of these

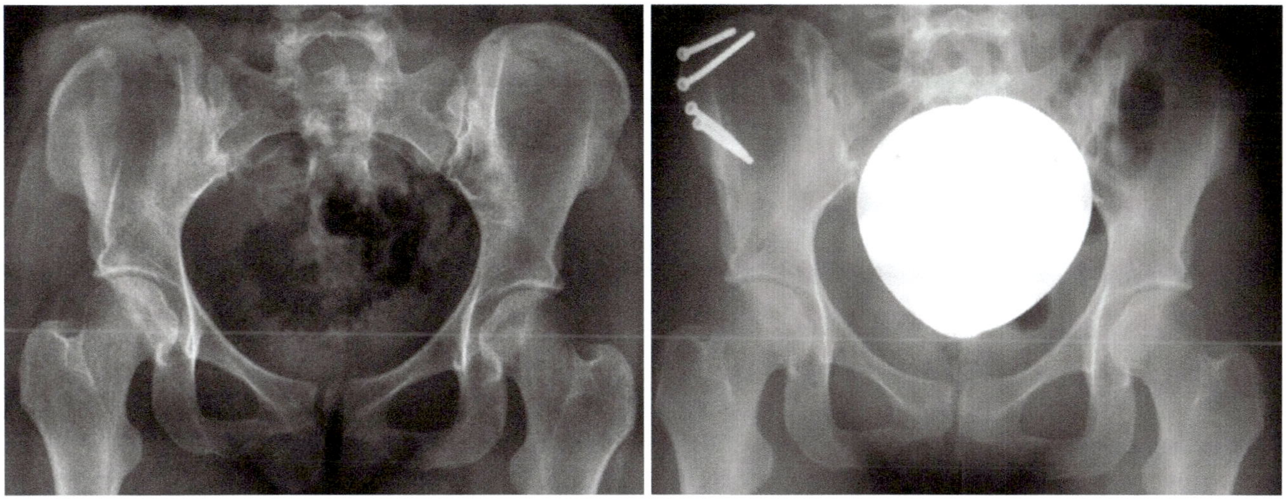

Fig. 27.4 Right iliac wing fracture, stabilized with isolated screws

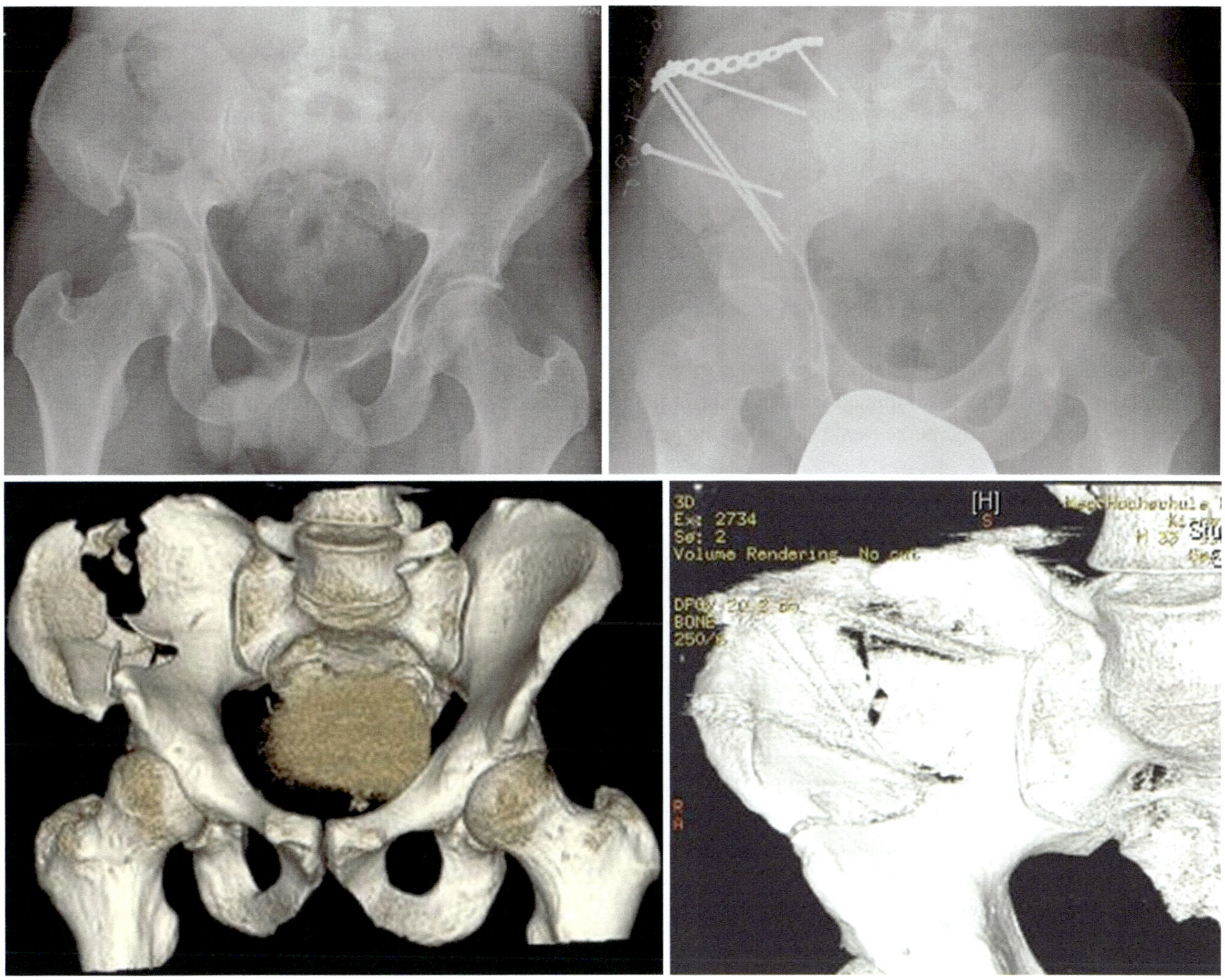

Fig. 27.5 Severely displaced iliac wing fracture, stabilized with a contour plate and screws

patients (0.7%) had isolated iliac wing injuries not involving the pelvic brim/greater sciatic notch. Of these:

- All had degloving injuries (Morel Levallée)
- 3/5 had open fractures
- 1/5 had arterial injury
- All were treated with ORIF (leg screw ± plate)
- 3/5 presented with postoperative complications

Abrassart et al. analyzed 10 iliac wing fractures from a group of 450 polytraumatized patients after high-energy trauma [4]. One isolated injury was observed while the majority sustained additional head, chest, spine, abdomen, urologic, and/or orthopedic injuries. In two patients, ORIF was performed due to bowel compression. Two patients had open fractures.

One case report presented a case with a combined lateral compression injury, resulting in a lumbosacral plexus lesion [5].

> Iliac wing fractures in the younger patient are often associated with relevant soft-tissue injuries, e.g., open fracture, Morel-Levallée lesions and concomitant multiple injuries.

27.2 Longitudinal Ilium Fractures

A longitudinal fracture of the ilium was already described by Malgaigne [6, 7], which was combined with an anterior pelvic ring fracture through the pubic rami or through the pubic symphysis.

Fracture morphology shows a fracture starting variable at the iliac crest and exiting through the greater sciatic notch, with a potential risk of injuring the superior gluteal neurovascular bundle [8].

The excellent muscular coverage around the iliac bone, e.g., the gluteus muscles on the outer ilium and the iliopsoas on the inner surface, leads to some dynamic stabilization. As a consequence, complete iliac fractures are often minor displaced.

These fractures are rare. Switzer et al. reported on eight patients from a group of 695 patients with pelvic ring disruptions after high-energy lateral impacts with combined anterior and posterior injuries (1.1%) [3]. Five of these patients (0.7%) had a fracture extension into the greater sciatic notch. Of these:

- All had local arterial injuries, identified on pelvic angiography.
- Degloving injuries (Morel Levallée) and open fractures were common.
- All were treated with ORIF (leg screw ± plate).

In the geriatric patient group, this fracture type is increasingly observed.

Rommens classified these fractures as IIIa (unilateral) and IVa (bilateral) in their "Comprehensive Classification of Fragility Fractures of the Pelvic Ring." Unilateral fractures were observed in 8.2% while bilateral fractures were uncommon 0.8% Ring [9].

27.3 Indications of Treatment

The decision to stabilize such a fracture depends on the stability of the fracture, independent if there is traumatic or geriatric fracture and the fracture displacement.

27.3.1 Iliac Wing Fractures

As these fractures are often associated with a significant soft-tissue injury (open fracture, Morel-Levallée lesions) due to high-energy trauma, open reduction and internal fixation are usually recommended [3, 4]. In contrast, geriatric fractures after a simple fall may be minor displaced and, therefore, nonoperative treatment is possible.

Displaced fractures extend to the ASIS and, therefore, involve the inguinal ligament, and the sartorius muscle tends to displace further. For these fractures, a relative surgical indication is proposed, especially in the geriatric population [10].

27.3.2 Incomplete Iliac Fractures

Some rare cases present with incomplete ilium fracture. A partial stability of the posterior ring can be expected, and, therefore, nonoperative management should be discussed. It should be considered that nonoperative management is only suitable, if partial weight bearing is possible [10]. Thus, in the geriatric patient group a relative indication of surgical treatment is also recommended [10].

27.3.3 Complete Iliac Fractures

In complete iliac fractures, the integrity of the posterior pelvic ring is impaired, and, therefore, the load transfer from the spine to the lower extremities is significantly disrupted.

These vertical fractures are classified as type C fractures [11], resulting in a posterior discontinuity of the pelvis.

Even in minor displaced fractures, in general, a surgical indication to stabilize these fractures is recommended [8, 10].

27.4 ORIF of Iliac Fractures

Open reduction and internal fixation are most often indicated in displaced ilium fractures. The surgical approach is standardized and described in the literature [10, 12–14].

27.5 Surgical Prerequisites

Surgery is performed after intravenous administration of single-shot antibiotics (second-generation cephalosporin) and, usually, a urinary catheter is inserted. Tranexamic acid may be considered. Usually, significant bleeding is uncommon.

27.6 Patient Positioning

The patient is placed in the standard supine position on a radiolucent table (Fig. 27.6), allowing intraoperative standard x-rays, e.g., pelvis AP views, inlet- and outlet views and obturator oblique and iliac oblique views, respectively. A lumbar or gluteal support can be helpful to elevate the affected hemipelvis.

The image intensifier is positioned on the opposite side of the patient.

27.7 Draping

Draping includes the whole anterior and ipsilateral pelvic region (Fig. 27.6). Additionally, the ipsilateral leg can be completely draped free to allow manipulation to easier support reduction maneuvers.

Additional below-knee support resulting in slight knee and hip flexion can be helpful to release the tension of the iliopsoas muscle, which allows easier reduction and fracture manipulation.

27.8 Landmarks and Surgical Approach

The standard surgical approach is the anterolateral approach to the SI joint (Fig. 27.7), e.g., the Olerud approach or first window of the ilioinguinal approach [13].

First, all relevant landmarks are marked with a pen on the skin: the anterior superior iliac spine (ASIS), the course of the iliac crest, and the iliac tubercle.

A curved incision is made along the iliac crest. The ideal starting point is at the level of the iliac tubercle approximately 5 cm posterior to the ASIS at the iliac tubercle area and runs approximately 1–2 cm lateral to the iliac crest and over its apex in a posterior direction along the iliac crest. Depending on the localization of the fracture, the incision is extended either anterior or posterior as necessary.

The course of the lateral cutaneous femoral nerve has to be considered.

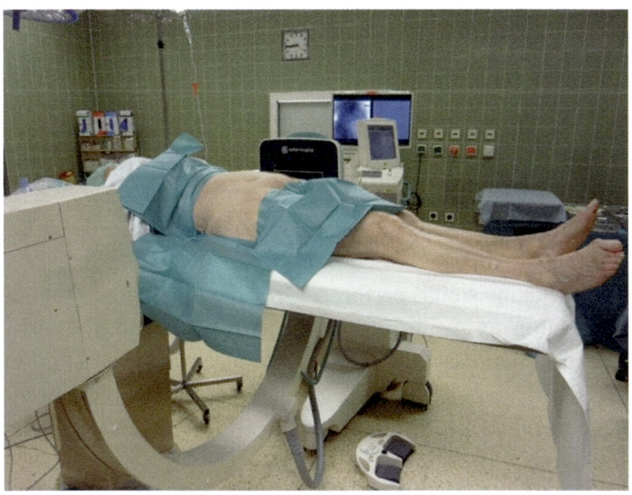

Fig. 27.6 Standard supine positioning on a radiolucent table

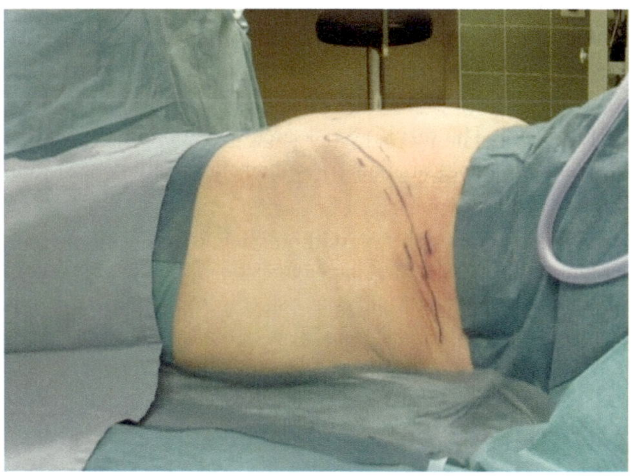

Fig. 27.7 Standard approach: first window of the ilioinguinal approach. Landmarks: ASIS, iliac crest

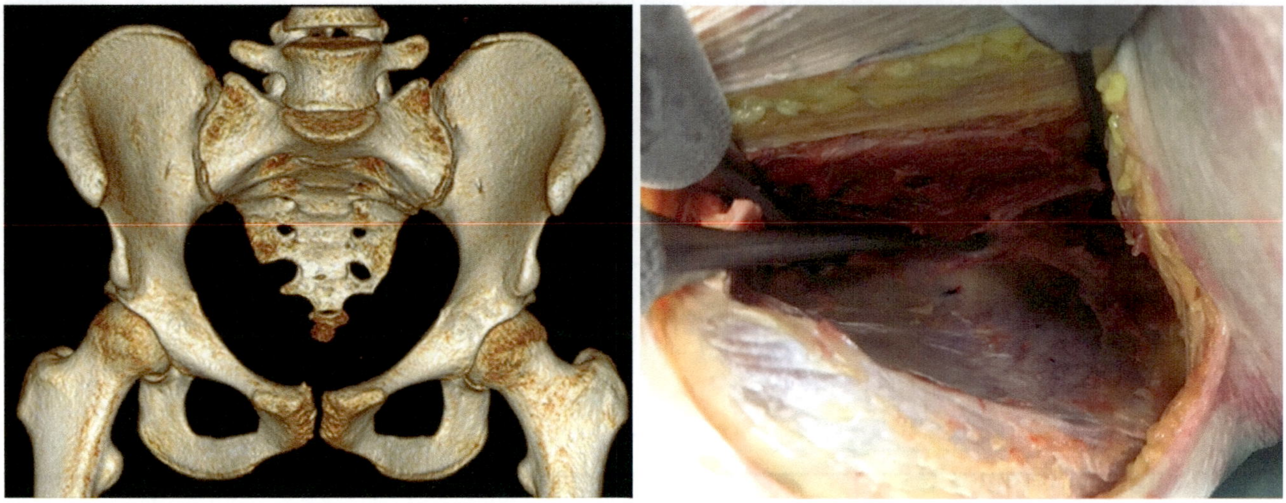

Fig. 27.8 Nutrient foramen at the iliac fossa, which can be responsible for relevant bleeding during subperiosteal dissection in the trauma situation

27.9 Surgical Anatomy

The course of the lateral femoral cutaneous femoral nerve must be considered as its trunk usually leaves the inner pelvis just below the inguinal ligament approximately 15–20 mm medial to the ASIS and then splits into several branches [15–17].

However, a highly variable course is reported with an exit to the outer pelvis up to 5 cm lateral to the ASIS in 4–13%. A too anterior incision (starting close to the ASIS) of the approach may take the nerve risk [18–20].

During dissection through the iliac fossa, the nutrient artery, a branch from the iliolumbar artery, is at risk to be injured, leading to potential relevant bleeding in addition to fracture site bleeding (Fig. 27.8, Appendix) [21].

In a cadaver analysis, Ebraheim et al. located the nutrient foramen 23.5 mm posterior to the starting curve of the iliac cortical density (straight pelvic brim line) and 12.5 mm lateral to the SI joint. The foraminal size was 1.8 mm [21]. Recently, Alla et al. found the foramen 20.1 mm from the nearest point on the pelvic brim and 18 mm from the anterior SI joint [22]. The resulting risk area was found between the typical plate position of anterior plate stabilization of SI joint dislocations.

Further dissection to the SI joint and, if necessary, in particular, during the exposure of the lateral side of the sacral promontory, the lumbosacral trunk is at risk (Fig. 27.9, Appendix). Its distance to the anterior SI joint is only 10 mm [23].

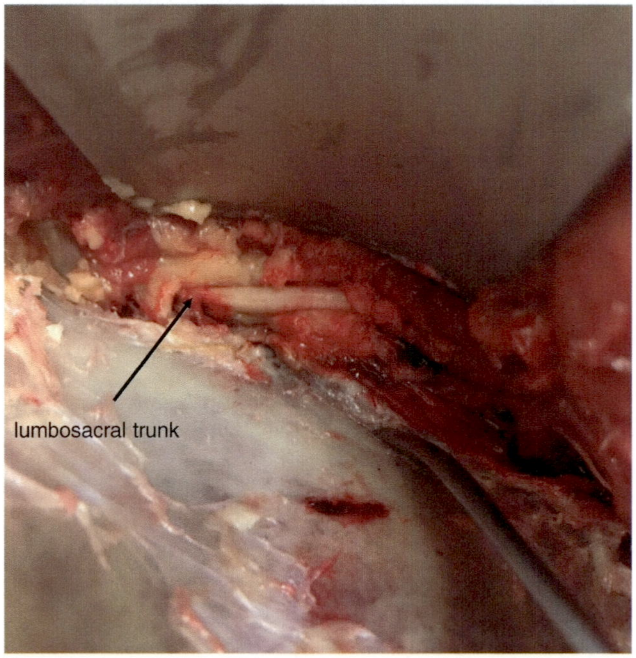

Fig. 27.9 Lumbosacral trunk medial to the SI joint (marked with raspatory)

27.10 Dissection

After dissection of the subcutaneous tissue in line with the skin incision, the connection between the external oblique muscle and the gluteus muscle is identified. The external oblique muscle belly usually extends slightly lateral to the iliac crest (Appendix).

Fascial incision is performed from lateral to medial at this connection to avoid transmuscular dissection, followed by direct subperiostal elevation of this muscle "over-the-top" of the iliac crest to enter the iliac fossa. The entire muscle attachment should be left attached to the periosteum for later refixation.

The iliac fossa is dissected subperiostally, with elevation of the iliacus muscle using a periosteal elevator until reaching the pelvic brim and/or SI joint. Subperiostal dissection

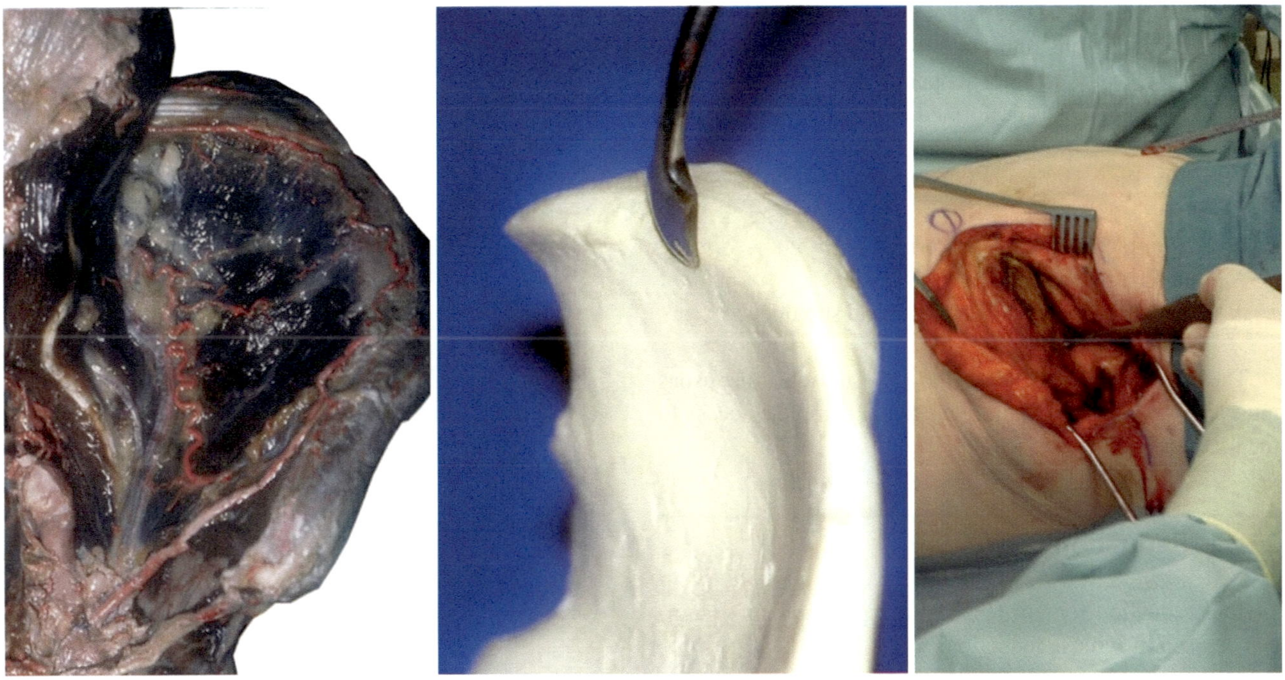

Fig. 27.10 Subperiosteal dissection: protection of the vascular supply near the iliac crest and opening of the iliac fossa using a raspatory

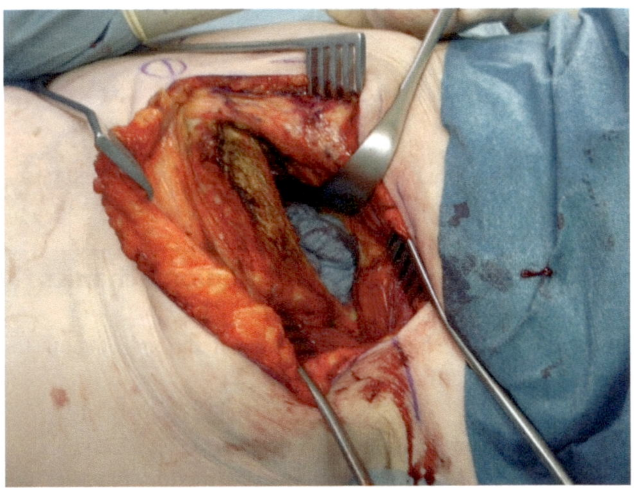

Fig. 27.11 Local tamponade of the iliac fossa

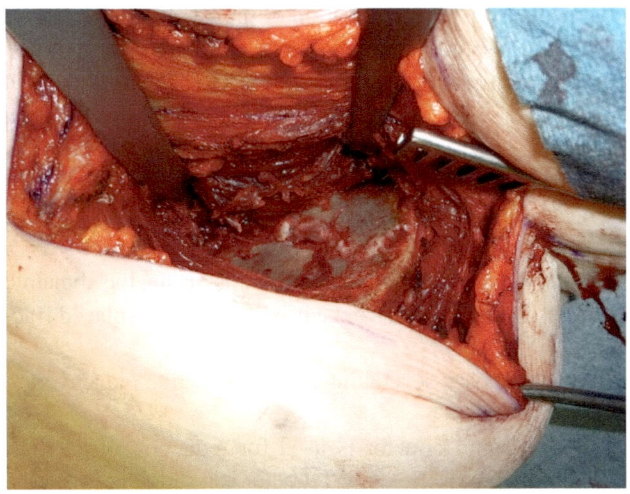

Fig. 27.12 Dissection up to the SI joint. The left retractor is positioned anterior to the SI joint, the right retractor is placed on the lateral sacral shoulder

protects the relevant vascular supply near the iliac crest (Fig. 27.10). As the obturator nerve runs between the iliacus and the psoas muscle, this dissection does not harm the nerve.

Hematoma evacuation is performed which leads to identification of the complete fracture course. Local tamponade reduces blood loss (Fig. 27.11).

Posterior extension usually allows sufficient visualization of the longitudinal fracture. Additional anterior extension of the approach is necessary in some iliac wing fractures to reach the ASIS for optimal placement of screws and plates.

Release of the sartorius muscle and inguinal ligament origin can extend anterior dissection [10].

Near the pelvic brim the nutrient foramen of the nutrient artery is identified (Figs. 27.8, 27.9, and 27.12). Often, relevant bleeding is observed, which can be controlled by closing the foramen with bone wax, temporary local packing, and/or coagulation of the nutrient artery.

The SI joint is easily identified as most often a bony ridge is palpable (Fig. 27.12).

Dissection on the lateral part of the sacrum is only necessary if the fracture line runs close to the SI joint. Then, using a periosteal elevator, a direct subperiosteal dissection on top of the sacral shoulder is performed to lift up and protect the lumbosacral trunk.

Typically, three Hohmann retractors are inserted:

- A blunt retractor at the pelvic brim
- A blunt retractor anterior to the SI joint
- A sharp retractor onto the lateral sacral shoulder

These retractors medialize the iliac muscle, the psoas muscle, and the abdominal organs to get complete access to the iliac fossa.

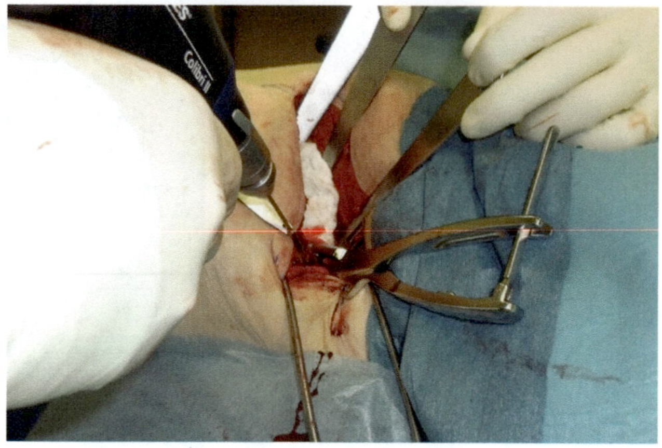

Fig. 27.13 Faraboeuf clamp for reduction near the iliac crest

27.11 Reduction

Various reduction forceps (Weber forceps, Farabeuf clamp) can be used to achieve reduction.

At the iliac crest, different pointed reduction forceps are used for fracture compression. Alternatively, the small Farabeuf forceps can help to manipulate the main fracture fragments (Fig. 27.13). Fixation of the Farabeuf clamp with two 3.5 mm screws at the iliac crest allows reduction of distraction and rotation deformities. It has to be considered that this can lead to interference with the definitive fixation strategy.

Temporary insertion of a Schanz screw at the iliac crest or at the AIIS can allow manipulation of the anterior fragment.

Near the pelvic brim, plate fixation using the dynamic compression technique can be used to reduce displaced fractures (Fig. 27.14).

Mast proposed several interesting reduction maneuvers:

- A Hohmann retractor is used for reduction of ad latus deformities: the tip of the retractor is inserted between the two cortices of the anterior and posterior iliac fragment. After a 180° turn, the curved tip provides a lever for regaining reduction [24].
- Reduction of translation of at a flat bone, e.g. the ilium, can be controlled by manipulation using the "Jungbluth" or Farabeuf pelvic reduction forceps; the Jungbluth clamp is advantageous, as it additionally allows, besides compression, rotation and angulation, distraction of the fracture site [24].

Additionally, Jeffrey Mast used a small (2–3 hole) one-third tubular plate for reducing ad latus deformities. Fixing the plate at the laterally displaced fragment with a screw results in a lateralization of this fragment against the free plate part [25].

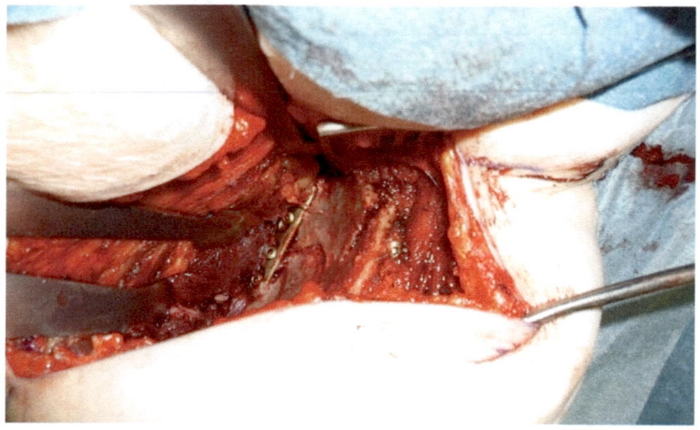

Fig. 27.14 Plate fixation near the pelvic brim parallel to the SI joint

27.12 Fixation Strategies and Biomechanics

Simonian et al. proposed several stabilization concepts for longitudinal iliac fractures [8]:

- Isolated screw fixation at the iliac crest (Fig. 27.4)
- Isolated four-hole 3.5 mm reconstruction plate at the inner iliac surface at the iliac crest
- Two screw fixation strategy: first screw (3.5 mm) at the iliac crest and a second screw (4.5 mm) through the supraacetabular corridor (AIIS to PSIS) (Fig. 27.15)
- Combined screw + plate fixation: one screw fixation (3.5 mm) at the iliac crest and four-hole 3.5 mm reconstruction plate at the pelvic brim (Fig. 27.16)
- Combined screw + plate fixation: four-hole 3.5 mm reconstruction plate at the inner iliac surface at the iliac crest and additional screw fixation (4.5 mm) through the supraacetabular corridor (AIIS to PSIS)
- Two-plate fixation strategy (two four-hole 3.5 mm reconstruction plates): first plate at the inner iliac surface at the iliac crest and a second plate at the pelvic brim (Figs. 27.17, 27.18, and 27.19)

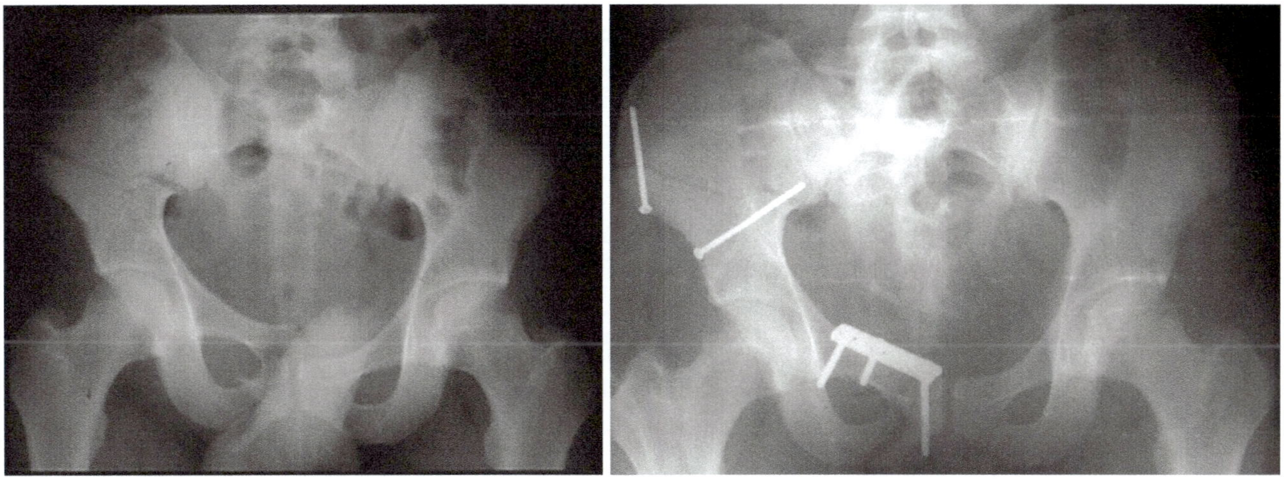

Fig. 27.15 Complete ilium fracture: isolated screw stabilization

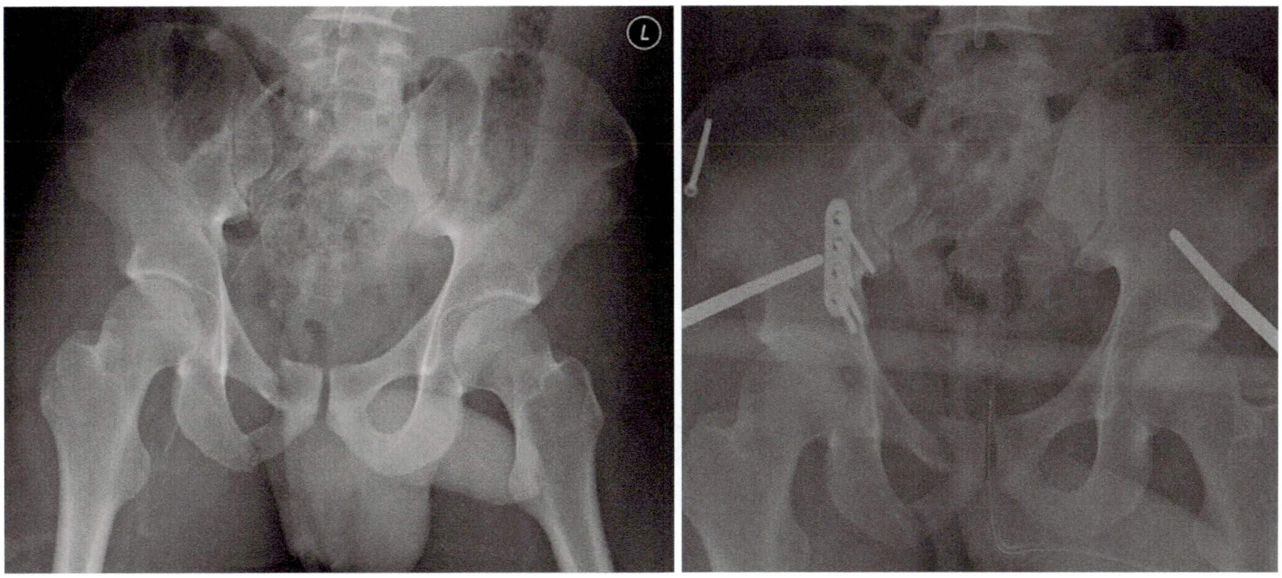

Fig. 27.16 Combined iliac crest screw and pelvic brim plate stabilization of a complete ilium fracture

In the resulting biomechanical analysis, the combined iliac crest screw and pelvic brim plate fixation or the combined iliac crest screw and 4.5 mm pelvic brim lag screw fixation were favored.

The anatomy of the ilium is of major importance to understand options of possible implant positions.

Adequate bone quality is peripherally present at the iliac crest in a curved orientation and vertically at the iliac tubercle. Additionally, the classical supraacetabular bone corridor allows for safe and secure fixation [26].

At the iliac crest, 3.5 mm screw of sufficient length can be inserted in an anterior-to-posterior direction or vice versa starting at the ASIS or at the iliac tubercle. Screw lengths of 60–100 mm are typically possible.

At the pelvic brim, a plate can be fixed parallel to the pelvic brim. Here extreme good bone quality is present, which corresponds to the iliac cortical density near the SI joint. Typically, a small 4–6-hole plate (reconstruction plate or LCP) is used.

In special, simple longitudinal fractures, an anterior-to-posterior directed 4.5 mm or even 7.3 mm (cannulated) screw can fix the fracture just above the pelvic brim, which starts at the AIIS and is directed to the PSIS. Screw lengths of up to 140 mm are possible.

In iliac wing fractures, beside peripheral iliac crest screws, the transverse fracture component can be adressed by screws, which can be inserted at the ASIS in direction to the acetabulum and at the iliac tubercle, running through this local bone corridor [27].

The healing potential of these longitudinal fractures is excellent as the iliac fossa is surrounded by extensive muscles: the iliopsoas on the inner side and the gluteal muscles on the outer side (Fig. 27.20).

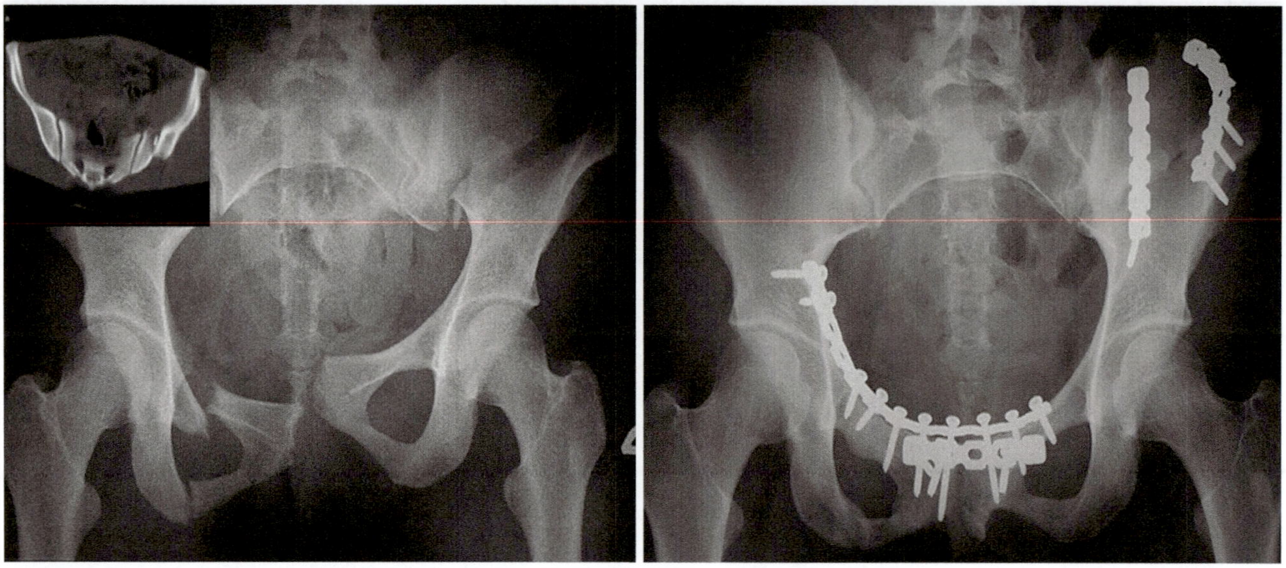

Fig. 27.17 Plate stabilization of a complete ilium fracture

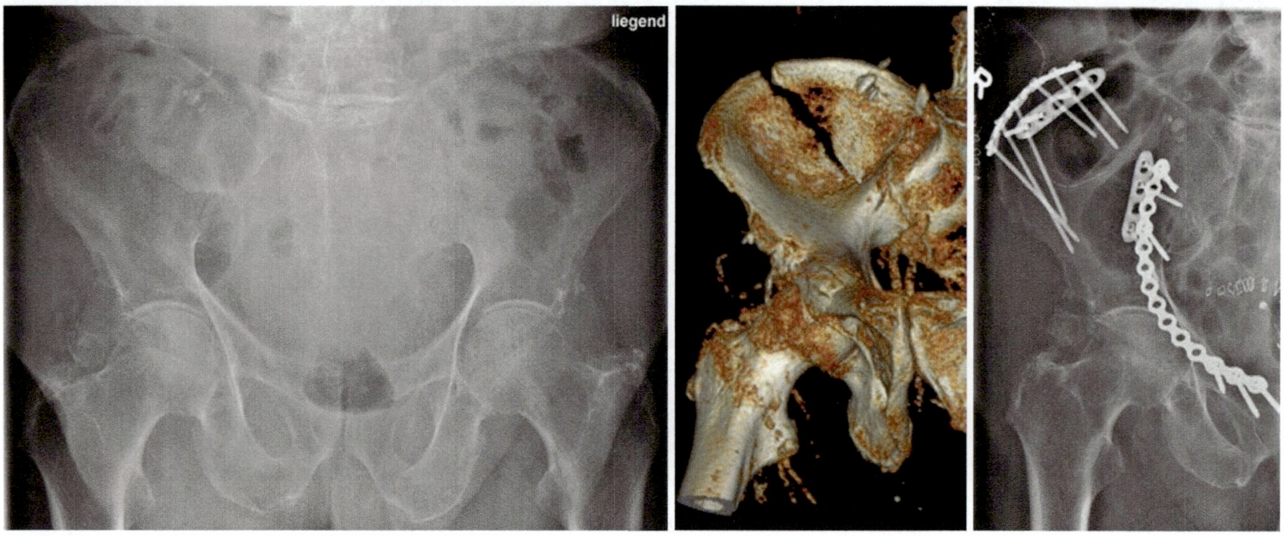

Fig. 27.18 Geriatric patient (87 years) with a complete ilium fracture. Due to his severe osteoporosis, several plates were used to adequately stabilize the ilium

27.13 Wound Closure

Closing the wound is easy as the soft tissues/muscles spontaneously get originally repositioned. Always, a deep suction drain is placed at the iliac fossa. The detached abdominal wall muscles are carefully reattached by direct suturing. Alternatively, transosseous refixation or fixation through plate holes at the iliac crest can support fascial reconstruction. After subcutaneous suturing the skin is closed in a standardized manner.

27.14 Aftercare

Partial weight bearing of the injured side with one-fifth of the body weight is recommended for 6 weeks.

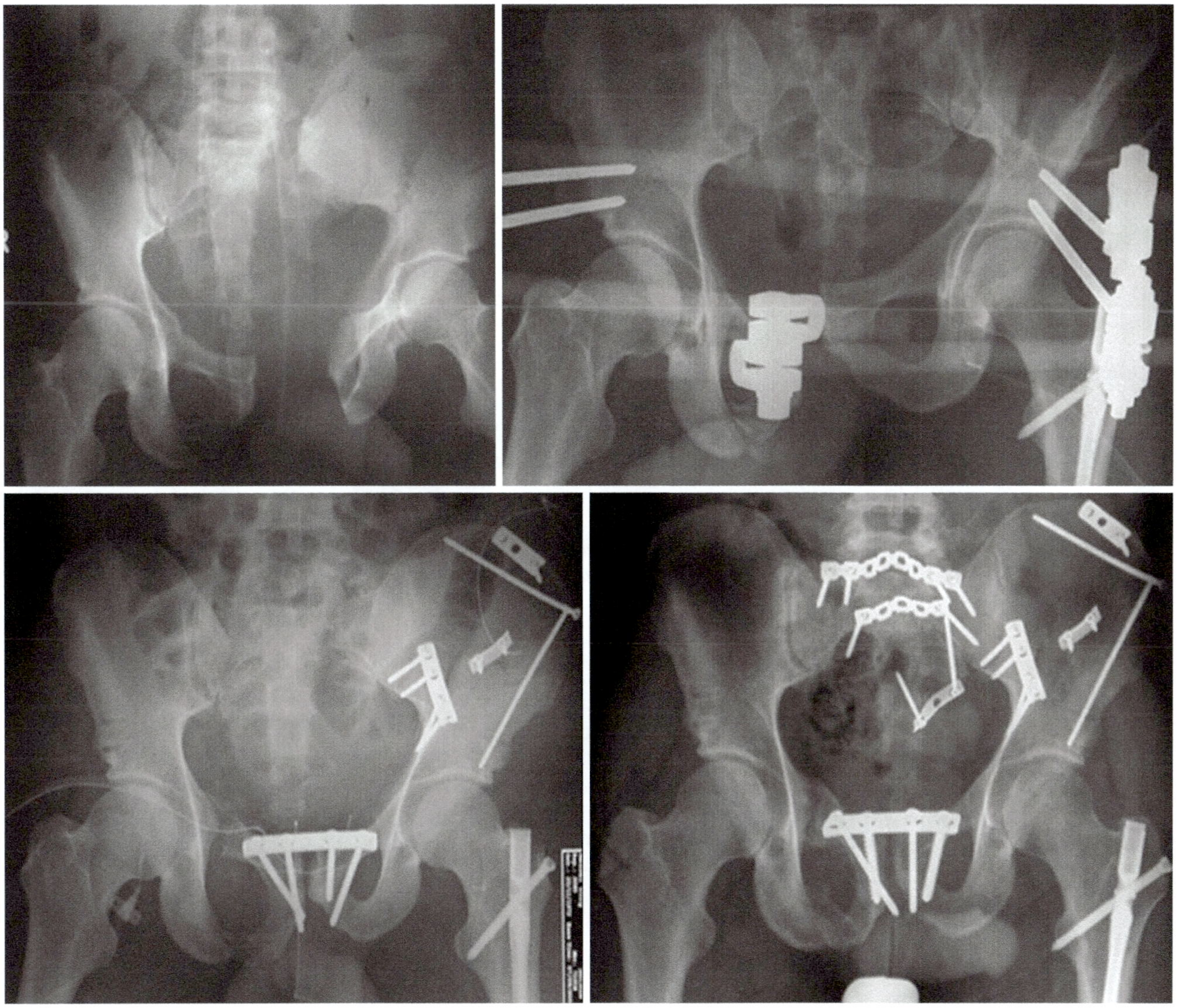

Fig. 27.19 Complete left sacrum and ilium fracture. After emergency stabilization with an external fixator, first reconstruction of the ilium was performed using plates and iliac crest screws with fixation of the pubic symphysis, followed by posterior ORIF of the sacrum using three sacral plates

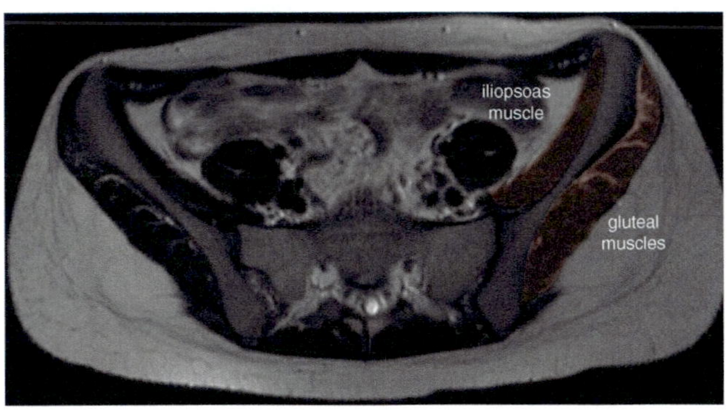

Fig. 27.20 Iliopsoas and gluteal muscles surrounding the iliac fossa

Routine implant removal is not indicated. Disturbing subcutaneous screw heads can lead to partial implant removal.

27.15 Summary

Longitudinal ilium fracture presents with a high rate of accompanying vascular and soft-tissue lesions.

Vertically, type C injuries are usually stabilized using standardized stabilization concepts.

Iliac wing fractures are fixed depending on the amount of displacement and concomitant injuries.

Appendix

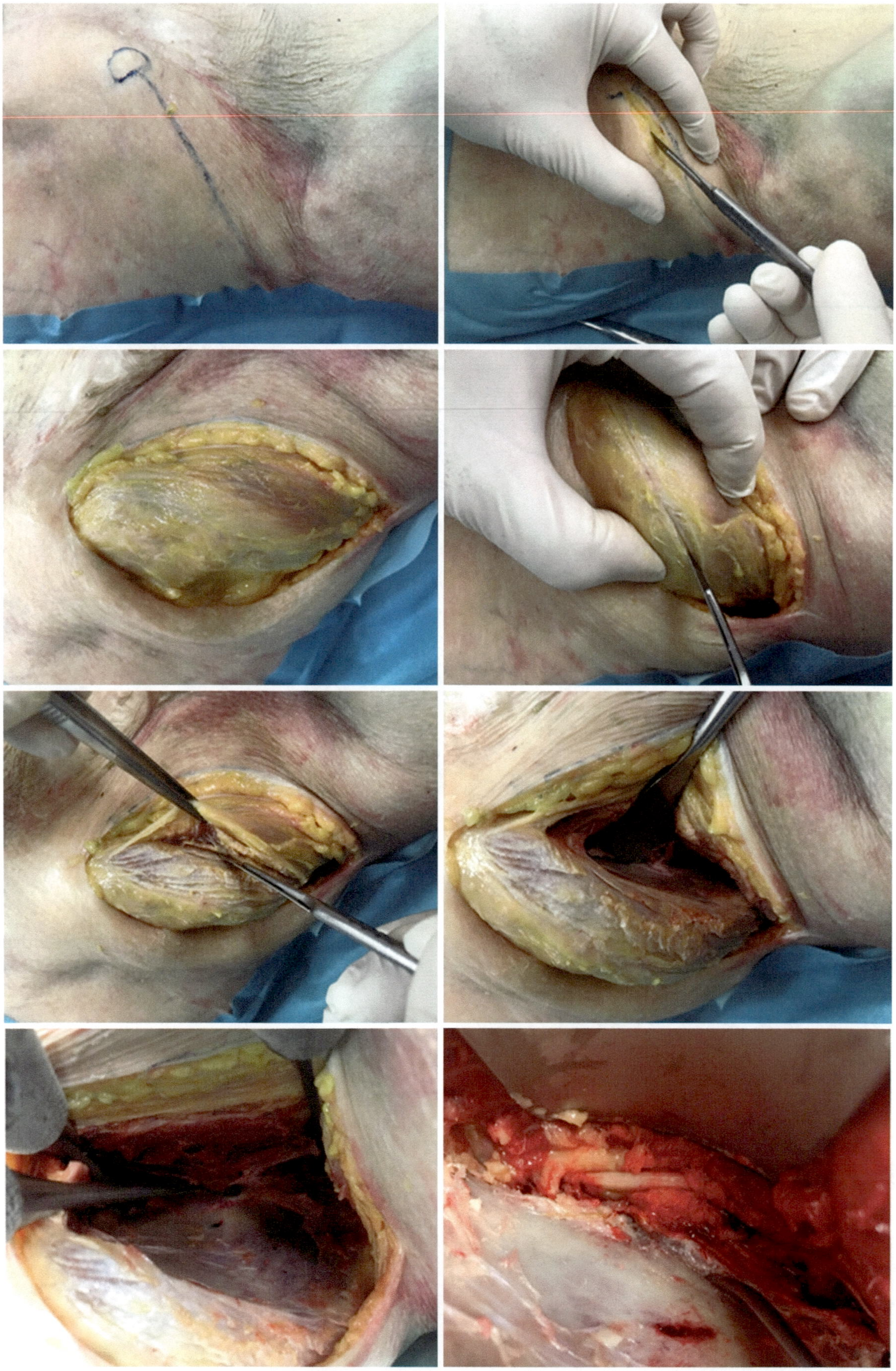

References

1. Amorosa L, Serota A, Berman N, Lorich D, Helfet D. An isolated iliac wing stress fracture in a marathon runner. Am J Orthop (Belle Mead NJ). 2014;43:74–7.
2. Duverney J. Traite de maladies des os, vol. 1. Paris: Bure l'Aiine; 1751. p. 284–5.
3. Switzer JA, Nork SE, Routt ML Jr. Comminuted fractures of the iliac wing. J Orthop Trauma. 2000;14(4):270–6.
4. Abrassart S, Stern R, Peter R. Morbidity associated with isolated iliac wing fractures. J Trauma. 2009;66:200–3.
5. Amr S, Abdel-Meguid K, Kholeif A. Neurologic injury caused by fracture of the iliac wing (Duverney's fracture): case report. J Trauma. 2002;52:370–6.
6. Malgaigne J. Traites des fractures et des luxations. Paris: J.B. Balliere; 1847.
7. Malgaigne J. Die Knochenbrüche und Verrenkungen für praktische Aerzte, Wundärzte und Studirende. Erster Band: Knochenbrüche. (deutsche Übersetzung der französischen Ausgabe von 1847), ed. Bearbeitet von Burger, C. Stuttgart: Rieger'sche Verlagsbuchhandlung; 1850.
8. Simonian P, Routt M, Harrington R, Tencer A. The unstable iliac fracture: a biomechanical evaluation of internal fixation. Injury. 1997;28(7):469–75.
9. Rommens P, Hofmann A. Comprehensive classification of fragility fractures of the pelvic ring: recommendations for surgical treatment. Injury. 2013;44:1733–44.
10. Hessmann M. Plate and screw fixation of the ilium. In: Rommens PM, Hofmann A, editors. Fragility fractures of the pelvis. Berlin: Springer; 2017. https://doi.org/10.1007/978-3-319-66572-6.
11. Tile M. Pelvic ring fractures: should they be fixed? J Bone Joint Surg. 1988;70-B:1–12.
12. Gänsslen A, Pohlemann T, Krettek C. [Internal fixation of sacroiliac joint disruption]. Oper Orthop Traumatol. 2005;17:281–195.
13. Letournel E. Fractures of the pelvis and acetabulum. In: Ninth AFOR Course and Workshop. Paris, France. 1993.
14. Ragnarsson B, Olerud C, Olerud S. Anterior square-plate fixation of sacroiliac disruption. Acta Orthop Scand. 1993;64(2):138–42.
15. de Ridder VA, de Lange S, Popta JV. Anatomical variations of the lateral femoral cutaneous nerve and the consequences for surgery. J Orthop Trauma. 1999;13(3):207–11.
16. Hospodar P, Ashman E, Traub J. Anatomic study of the lateral femoral cutaneous nerve with respect to the ilioinguinal surgical dissection. J Orthop Trauma. 1999;13:17–9.
17. Sürücü H, Tanyeli E, Sargon M, Karahan S. An anatomic study of the lateral femoral cutaneous nerve. Surg Radiol Anat. 1997;19:307–10.
18. Aszmann OC, Dellon ES, Dellon AL. Anatomical course of the lateral femoral cutaneous nerve and its susceptibility to compression and injury. Plast Reconstr Surg. 1997;100(3):600–4.
19. Murata Y, Takahashi K, Yamagata M, Shimada Y, Moriya H. The anatomy of the lateral femoral cutaneous nerve, with special reference to the harvesting of iliac bone graft. J Bone Joint Surg Am. 2000;82(5):746–7.
20. Rosenberger RJ, Loeweneck H, Meyer G. The cutaneous nerves encountered during laparoscopic repair of inguinal hernia: new anatomical findings for the surgeon. Surg Endosc. 2000;14(8):731–5.
21. Ebraheim N, Lu J, Biyani A, Yang H. Anatomic considerations of the principal nutrient foramen and artery on internal surface of the ilium. Surg Radiol Anat. 1997;19:237–9.
22. Alla S, Roberts C, Ojike N. Vascular risk reduction during anterior surgical approach sacroiliac joint plating. Injury. 2013;44:175–7.
23. Ebraheim N, Padanilam T, Waldrop J, Yeasting R. Anatomic consideration in the anterior approach to the sacro-iliac joint. Spine. 1994;19(6):721–5.
24. Mast J, Jakob R, Ganz R. Planning and reduction technique in fractuzre surgery. Berlin, Heidelberg, New York: Springer; 1989. p. 234, 236. ISBN 0-387-16283-6.
25. Mast J. Personal communication. 1996.
26. Gänsslen A, Pohlemann T, Krettek C. [A simple supraacetabular external fixation for pelvic ring fractures]. Oper Orthop Traumatol. 2005;17:296–312.
27. Kim W, Lee S, Kim K, Kwon S, Choi Y. Minimally invasive surgical treatment using 'iliac pillar' screw for isolated iliac wing fractures in geriatric patients: a new challenge. Eur J Trauma Emerg Surg. 2018;45:213–9. https://doi.org/10.1007/s00068-018-1046-0.

28 Anterior Plating of the SI Joint

Jan Lindahl, Axel Gänsslen, and Peter Grechenig

Lambotte in 1913 described a case with symphyseal separation and iliosacral joint injury resulting in a posterior hemipelvic dislocation after a railway accident. This case was treated exclusively by symphyseal wire stabilization through a Pfannenstiel-like approach. No stabilization of the SI joint was performed [1]. However, the option of the iliosacral screw fixation for the injured SI joint was already specified by Lambotte.

Historically, closed reduction techniques and castings or traction treatment were favored for hemipelvic dislocations [2–4].

In a cadaver dissection study on patients that died of trauma injuries, type C injuries with complete disruption of the SI joint (C1.2) were associated with a triplane displacement of the hemipelvis [5]. The displacement was typically cranial, posterior, and externally rotated. They found that a closed reduction with traction and external pelvis manipulation was not possible because the osseous and ligamentous tissues interposed into the joint. Stability of the SI joint is based on accurate reduction and also on sacroiliac geometries that may limit manipulations, such as the concave-convex shape of the opposing joint surfaces in every plane and the small anterior shelf of bone on the ilium [6, 7].

28.1 Historical Experience

The potential first case of an anterior plate stabilization of the SI joint was published in 1985 in a patient with posttraumatic joint disorder [8].

Anterior plate stabilization of a traumatic disrupted SI joint was potentially first described by Olerud et al. and Simpson et al. in 1987.

Simpson et al. first performed anterior staple fixation of a disrupted SI joint and also reported on anterior plate fixation using an anterior retrofascial approach [9]. With their experience, a specially designed four-hole plate was developed. In the same year, Olerud used a comparable plate for fixing SI joints [10].

This treatment principle is indicated for complete uni- or bilateral dislocations of the SI joint with or without iliac fracture. In case of chronic instability or degenerative changes with corresponding symptoms, arthrodesis of the joint may be indicated.

28.2 Principle of Surgery

The principle of anterior plating of the SI joint is based on Olerud's recommendation and consists of a bridging plate osteosynthesis of the SI joint.

28.3 Biomechanics

Marvin Tile's group analyzed type C injuries with combined symphyseal and unilateral SI joint dislocations (OTA 61-C1.2 c5) [11–15]. Anterior plating of the SI joint in combination with anterior ring fixation led to a pelvic ring stiffness of 270 N/mm.

Leighton et al. analyzed unembalmed pelves with a 61-C1.2 c5 injury in a single leg stance simulation [16]. The pubic symphysis was fixed with two plates and the SI joint with a specially designed anterior plate. This concept was

J. Lindahl
Orthopaedics and Trauma Surgery, Helsinki University Hospital, Helsinki, Finland

A. Gänsslen (✉)
Department of Trauma Surgery, Orthopedics and Hand Surgery, Hospital Wolfsburg, Wolfsburg, Germany

P. Grechenig
Division of Macroscopic and Clinical Anatomy, Medical University of Graz, Graz, Austria
e-mail: peter.grechenig@stud.medunigraz.at

A. Gänsslen et al. (eds.), *Pelvic Ring Fractures*, https://doi.org/10.1007/978-3-030-54730-1_28

compared to posterior iliosacral screw fixation. No difference was observed with both posterior stabilization concepts, but stiffness doesn't reach the intact pelvis (35% of the intact pelvis).

Rieger examined this injury type and stabilized the SI joint with three-hole DC plates, iliosacral screws, and sacral bars. Anterior plate fixation resulted in 85% of the stiffness of iliosacral screws [17].

Comstock et al. investigated embalmed cadaver pelves simulating a OTA C-1.2 c1 injury [18]. The anterior ring was not fixed, while the SI joint was fixed using two sacral bars, two anterior SI joint plates, two iliosacral screws, or two iliosacral screws in combination with two sacral bars, respectively. Anterior plating reached 84% of the stiffness of iliosacral screws. Comparable data were found by Yinger et al. [19].

Recently Chen et al. analyzed different posterior stabilization concepts of SI joint fixation in a type C simulation in a single leg stance model. Best results were observed with two three-hole plates at an angle of 60°. The overall stability was comparable to iliosacral screw fixation [20].

The position of the plates is of lesser significance. In both, the parallel and the angled position the load limit was around 100% of body weight [21].

> Anterior SI joint plating seems to be biomechanically equal to iliosacral screw fixation, but biomechanical data are somehow conflicting. However, closed anatomical reduction is achieved in about 50% of cases [22–24] and with increasing displacement a decrease of overall stability is expected [7, 25, 26].

28.4 Surgical Prerequisites

Surgery is performed after intravenous administration of single-shot antibiotics (second-generation cephalosporin) and usually a urinary catheter is inserted. Tranexamic acid (1 g IV) can be considered.

28.5 Patient Positioning

The patient is placed in the standard supine position on a radiolucent table (Fig. 28.1), allowing intraoperative standard x-rays, e.g., pelvis AP views, inlet- and outlet views, and obturator oblique and iliac oblique views, respectively. A lumbar or gluteal support can be helpful to elevate the opposite hemipelvis. The image intensifier is positioned on the opposite side of the patient.

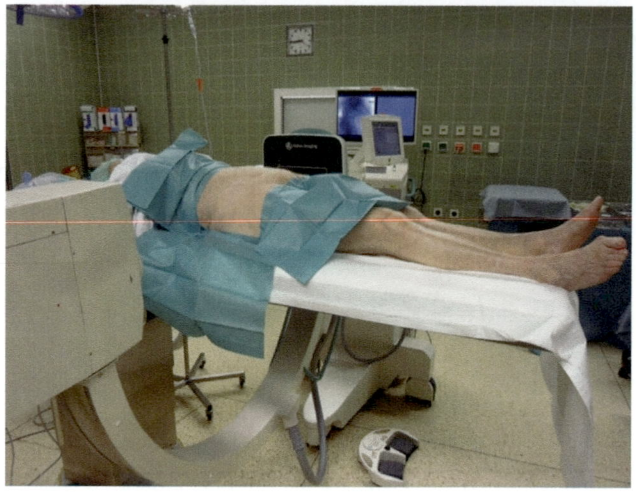

Fig. 28.1 Standard supine positioning on a radiolucent table with draping of the pelvic region

28.6 Draping

Draping includes the whole anterior and ipsilateral pelvic region (Fig. 28.1). Additionally, the ipsilateral leg is usually completely draped free to allow leg manipulation and to support reduction maneuvers.

Additional below knee support, resulting in slight knee and hip flexion, can be helpful to release the tension of the iliopsoas muscle, which allows easier reduction and manipulation.

28.7 Landmarks and Surgical Approach

The standard surgical approach to the SI joint is the anterolateral approach, e.g., the Olerud approach [10] or first window of the ilioinguinal approach [27]. However, this approach was described already in 1941 for debridement of pyogenic infection of the SI joint [28].

First, all relevant landmarks are marked with a pen on the skin: the anterior superior iliac spine (ASIS), the course of the iliac crest, and the iliac tubercle (Fig. 28.2).

A curved incision is made along the iliac crest. The ideal starting point is near the ASIS and runs approximately 1–2 cm lateral to the iliac crest and over its apex in a posterior direction along the iliac crest. Anterior or posterior extension of the approach is possible up to the PSIS or with an osteotomy of the ASIS [29].

The course of the lateral cutaneous femoral nerve (LCFN) has to be considered.

28.8 Surgical Anatomy

The course of the lateral femoral cutaneous femoral nerve must be considered as its trunk usually leaves the inner pelvis just below the inguinal ligament approximately 15–20 mm medial to the ASIS and then splits into several branches [30–32].

However, a highly variable course is reported with an exit to the outer pelvis up to 5 cm lateral to the ASIS in 4–13%.

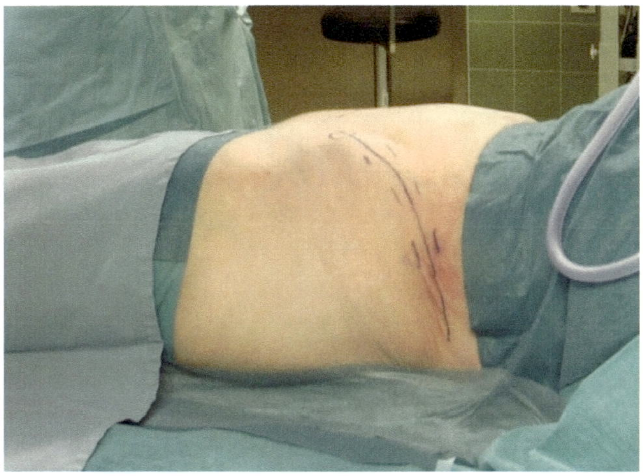

Fig. 28.2 Standard approach: first window of the ilioinguinal approach. Landmarks: ASIS, iliac crest

Thus, a too far anterior extension of the approach may take the nerve at risk [33–35].

During dissection through the iliac fossa, the nutrient artery, a branch from the iliolumbar artery, is at risk to be injured (Fig. 28.3), leading to potential relevant bleeding in addition to fracture site bleeding [36].

In a cadaver analysis, Ebraheim et al. located the nutrient foramen 23.5 mm posterior to the starting curve of the iliac cortical density (straight pelvic brim line) and 12.5 mm lateral to the SI joint. The foraminal size was 1.8 mm. Recently, Alla et al. found the foramen 20.1 mm from the nearest point on the pelvic brim and 18 mm from the anterior SI joint [37]. The resulting risk area was found between the typical plate position of anterior plate stabilization of SI joint dislocations.

Further dissection to the SI joint and, if necessary, in particular, during the exposure of the lateral side of the sacral promontory, the lumbosacral trunk is at risk (Fig. 28.4). Its distance to the anterior SI joint is only 10 mm [38].

The area of the iliac crest is supplied by a vessel coming from the external iliac artery and running along the medial iliac crest just some centimeters below the tip of the iliac crest and a branch of the deep circumflex iliac artery which runs parallel to the iliac crest (Fig. 28.5) [39].

28.9 Dissection

After dissection of the subcutaneous tissue in line with the skin incision, the connection between the external oblique muscle and the gluteus muscle is identified (Fig. 28.6). The

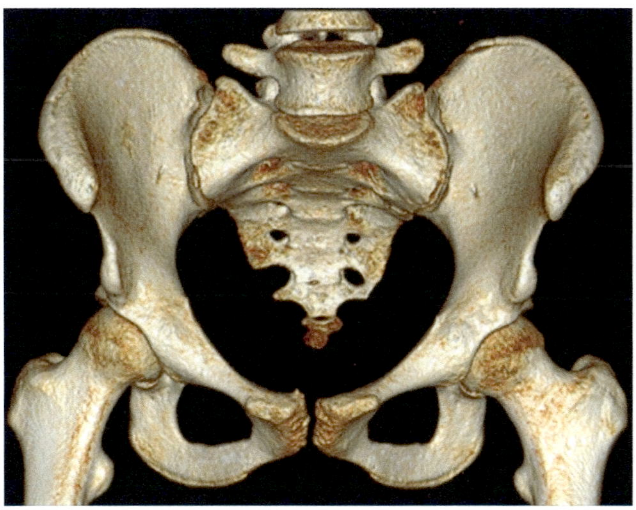

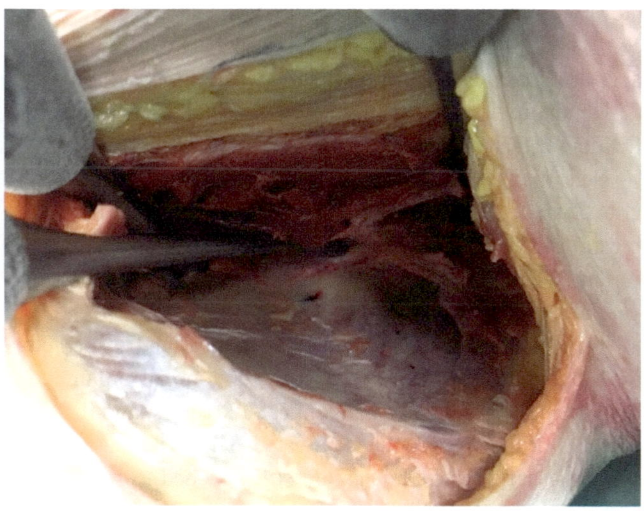

Fig. 28.3 Nutrient foramen at the iliac fossa, which can be responsible for relevant bleeding during subperiosteal dissection in the trauma situation

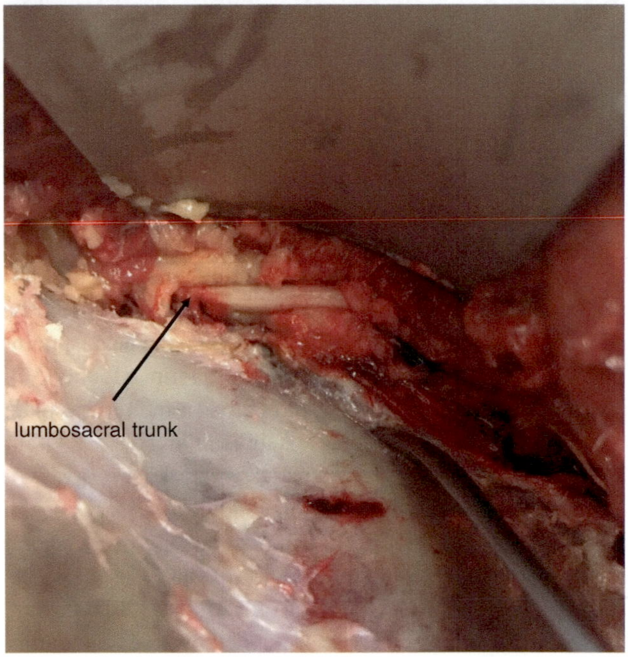

Fig. 28.4 Lumbosacral trunk medial to the SI joint (marked with a raspatory)

external oblique muscle belly usually extends slightly lateral to the iliac crest.

Fascial incision is performed from lateral to medial at this connection to avoid transmuscular dissection, followed by direct subperiosteal elevation of this muscle "over-the-top" of the iliac crest to enter the iliac fossa (see Appendix).

The entire muscle attachment should be left attached to the periosteum for later refixation.

The iliac fossa is dissected along the inner surface of the ilium, with elevation of the iliacus muscle using a periosteal elevator until reaching the pelvic brim and the SI joint (Fig. 28.7). As the obturator nerve runs between the iliacus and the psoas muscle, this dissection will not harm the nerve.

Hematoma evacuation is performed which leads to identification of the complete joint line.

Near the pelvic brim the nutrient foramen of the nutrient artery is identified (Figs. 28.3 and 28.4). Often, relevant bleeding is observed, which can be controlled by closing the foramen with bone wax, temporary local packing, and/or coagulation of the nutrient artery.

The disrupted SI joint is easily identified and inspected. The iliac and psoas muscles and the abdominal organs are held medially using long Langenbeck retractors, and the lateral part of the sacral bone is palpated. The torn anterior and superior sacroiliac ligaments are still attached to the sacral and iliac bone (Fig. 28.8).

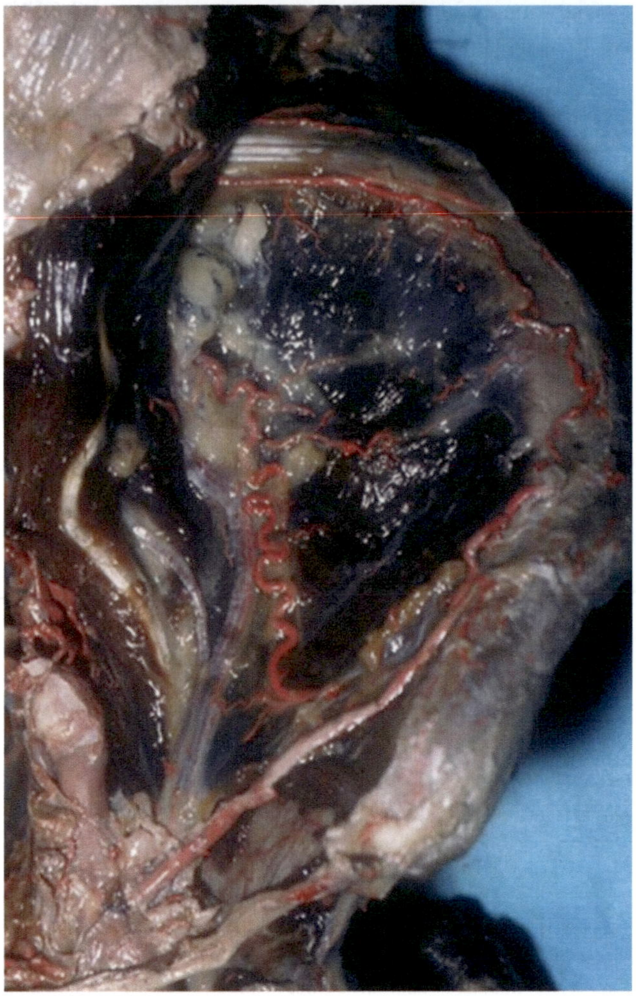

Fig. 28.5 The vascular supply near the iliac crest is visualized

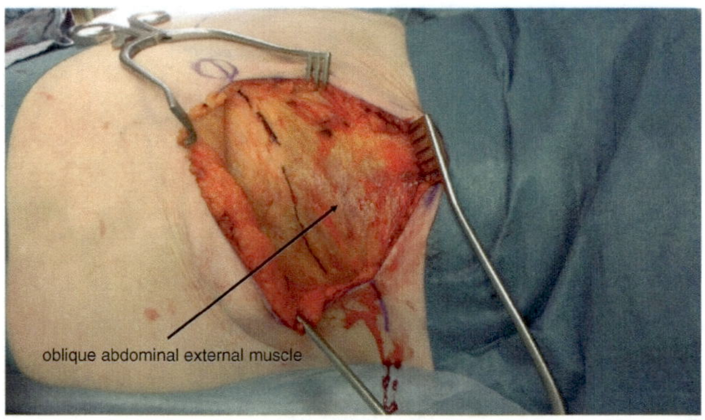

Fig. 28.6 Identification of the oblique external muscle

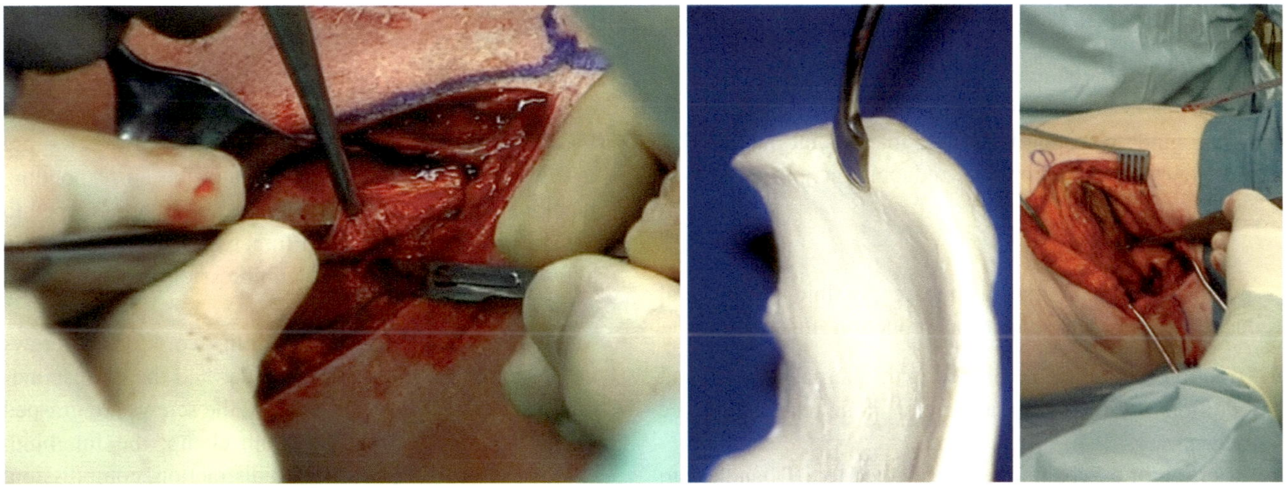

Fig. 28.7 Subperiosteal dissection: protection of the vascular supply near the iliac crest and opening of the iliac fossa using a raspatory

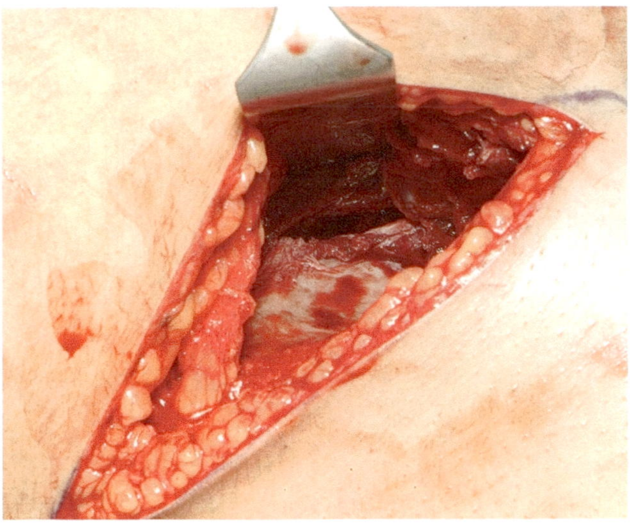

Fig. 28.8 Inspection of the disrupted SI joint. Note the torn ligamentous fibers

Under direct visualization, the sacral periosteum is carefully lifted from the lateral sacral shoulder (sacral ala) using a periosteal elevator. A far medial slippage has to be avoided to protect the lumbosacral trunk (L5 nerve root).

Typically, four Hohmann retractors are inserted (Fig. 28.9):

- A blunt retractor at the posterior sacrum
- A blunt retractor anterior to the SI joint placed at an angle of approximately 60–80° to the plane of the SI joint
- Two sharp retractors are hammered into the sacral ala <15 mm from the joint below the periosteum

These retractors medialize the iliac muscle, the psoas muscle, and the abdominal organs to get complete access to the iliac fossa and the SI joint, especially medial and anterior. Alternatively, 2.5 or 3.0 mm Kirschner wires can be introduced into the lateral sacrum.

28.10 Joint Debridement

Following dissection, the SI joint is widened using an arthrodesis spreader (Fig. 28.10). The joint surface is inspected and debrided under direct vision. Cartilage or osseous fragments are removed. In instances of extensive cartilage damage, preparation for primary joint arthrodesis should be considered.

28.11 Reduction

Reduction can now be performed.

> **Tip**
> Before starting any reduction maneuver, sacral drilling of the screw holes is recommended as this allows direct visualization of the potential screw course and the individual sacral anatomy. Especially, this can be helpful for posterior drilling as the sacral anatomy often presents with a "balcony"-shaped sacrum. After cortical starting, the drill enters the posterior interosseous ligament complex before re-entering the cancellous bone of the posterior-lateral part of the sacrum.

If visualization is poor, a long Kirschner wire is inserted into the SI joint to facilitate anatomical joint orientation.

Tip

Before starting the reduction maneuver, a 2.5–3.0 mm K-wire is inserted from the outer side (e.g., iliosacral screw guide wire) until reaching the SI joint plane for later temporary fixation after reducing the joint.

Various reduction maneuvers are possible and several reduction forceps can support the reduction (Fig. 28.11):

- Traction on the leg, combined with internal rotation and additional direct manual lateral compression of the pelvis.
- Insertion of a Schanz screw connected to a T-handle into the iliac crest at the iliac tubercle or into the anterior supraacetabular corridor for hemipelvic manipulation (joystick technique for reduction).
- Manipulation of the hemipelvis with a Farabeuf forceps or a pointed reduction forceps at the iliac crest.
- Farabeuf forceps reduction: two 4.5 mm screws are inserted into the sacral shoulder and the corresponding iliac bone close to the SI joint; the screws are grasped to the sidearms of the Farabeuf forceps; the Farabeuf clamp allows for controlling of compression, rotation, and cranial-caudal manipulation.
- Small Jungbluth forceps reduction: two 4.5 mm screws are inserted into the sacral shoulder and the corresponding iliac bone close to the SI joint; the screws are grasped to the sidearms of the Jungbluth clamp; the Jungbluth clamp allows for controlling of distraction, compression, rotation, and cranial-caudal manipulation.

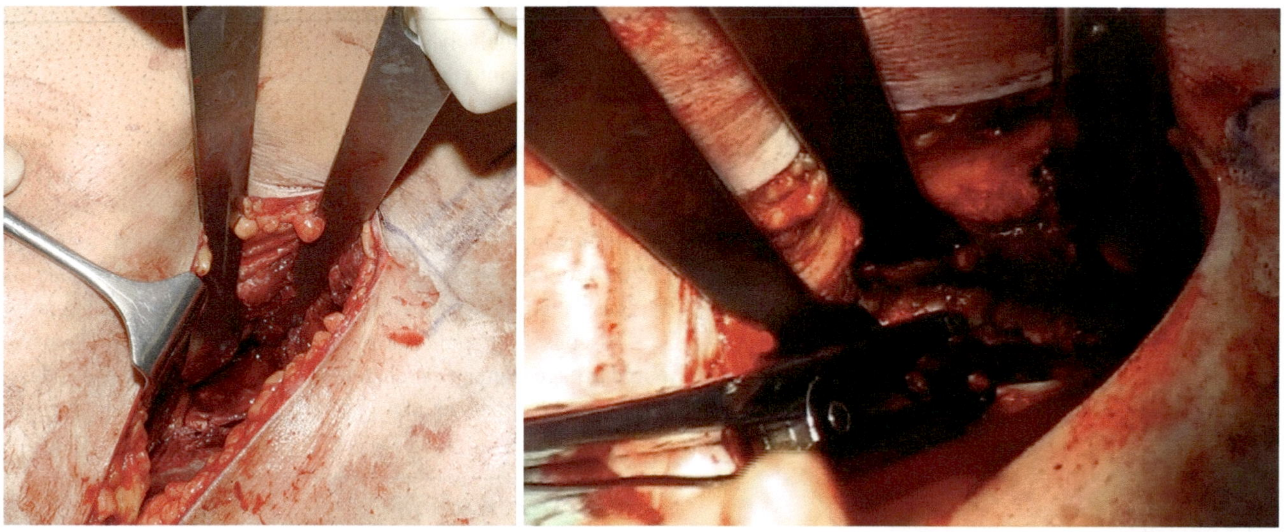

Fig. 28.9 Retractor placement to visualize the SI joint

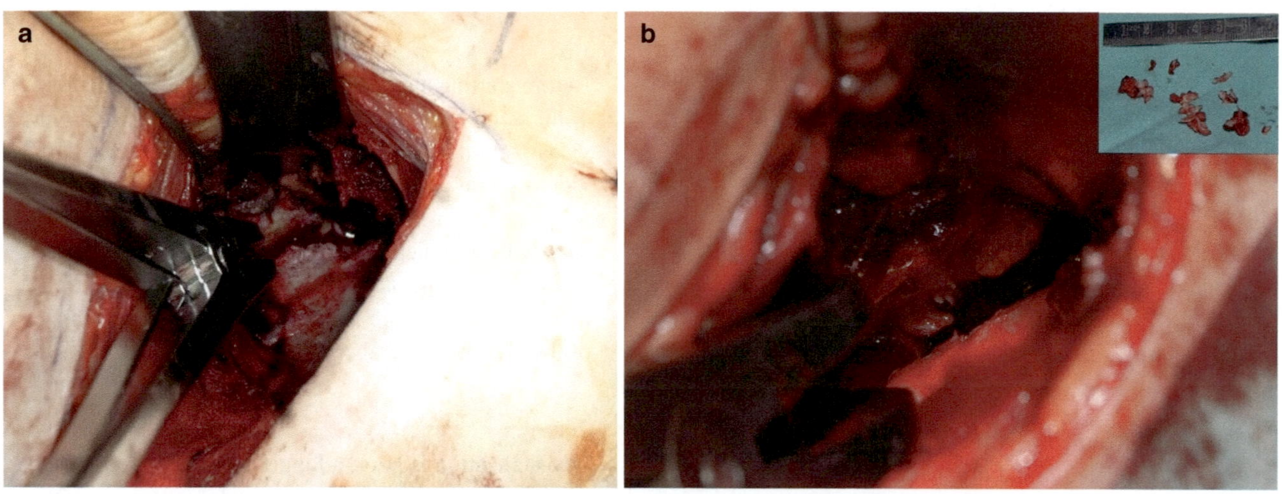

Fig. 28.10 (**a**) Joint opening with a laminar spreader. (**b**) Joint debridement after opening with a laminar spreader

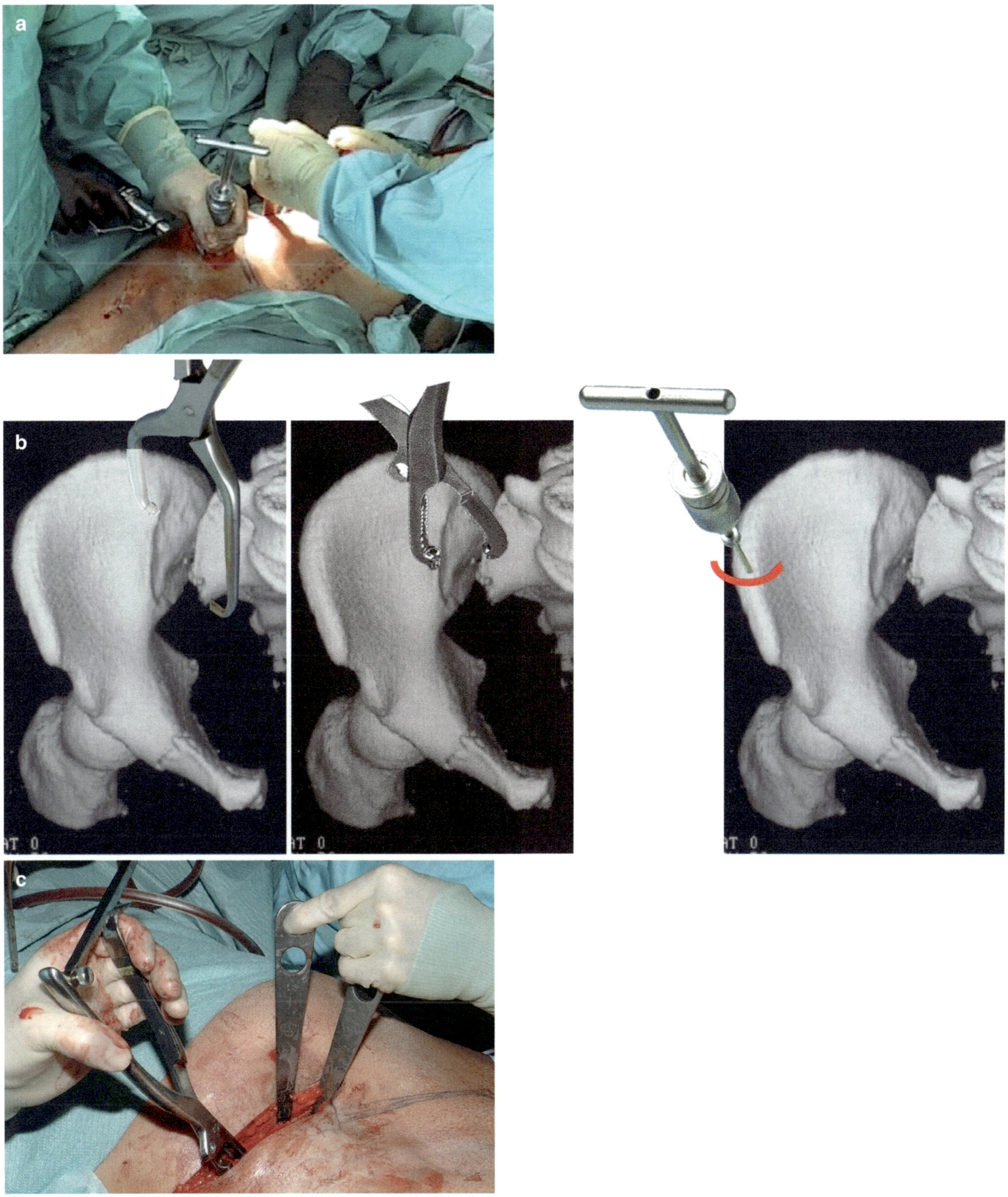

Fig. 28.11 (**a**) Possible reduction aids: percutaneous K-wire fixation of the reduced SI joint after hemipelvic manipulation with a Schanz screw attached to a T-handle. (**b**) Possible reduction aids: asymmetric clamp, Faraboef clamp, and T-Handel with Schanz screw. (**c**) Intraoperative view: manipulation of the hemipelvis using a Faraboef clamp placed at the iliac crest

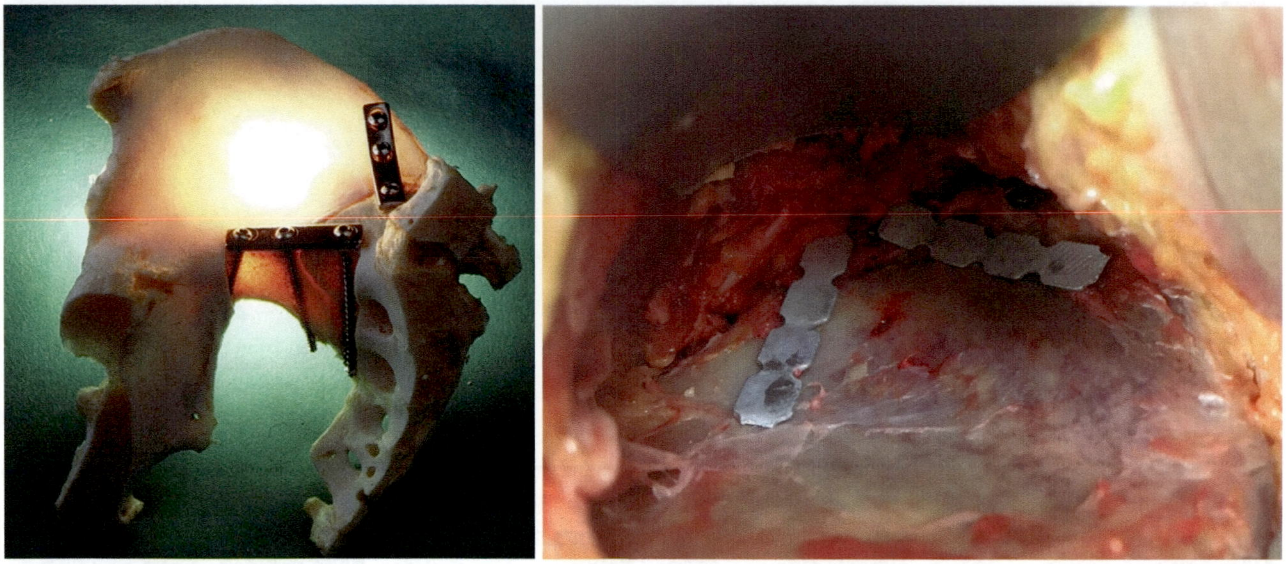

Fig. 28.12 Proposed plate position in an angle of 70–90°

- Indirect reduction using the definitive or a temporary plate: a 4.5 mm plate is fixed into the lateral sacrum; inserting an iliac screw can support reduction of a caudally displaced hemipelvis or vice versa.
- Use of the large asymmetric pointed reduction forceps: the long sidearm is placed to the anterior sacrum, while the shorter sidearm is placed on the outer iliac side.

During all reduction maneuvers close to the joint plane, the position of the definitive plates should already be considered.

28.12 Choice of Implant

Different implants can be used for anterior plate osteosynthesis: parallel 3.5 mm DC plates [13], large (4.5 mm) or small (3.5 mm) reconstruction plates [40–43], or the modified square plate (SI joint plate) [44, 45]. The authors experience is that 3.5 mm reconstruction plates are weak and lead to screw breakage too often.

Narrow three-hole DC plates offer the advantage of a higher level of rigidity in comparison to other types of plates and allow anchorage in the soft sacral bone with 6.5 mm cancellous bone screws [46].

28.13 Fixation Strategies

The orientation of the plates is of minor importance as biomechanical data indicate that the parallel and the angled position do not influence the stability [21].

From the anatomical standpoint, a plate angulation of 60–90° is proposed as this leads to sufficient screw lengths in the iliac bone (Figs. 28.12 and 28.13, Appendix).

Usually, the sacral drilling is already performed prior to reduction. The screws or screw holes used for reduction can be used for final plate fixation. Usually, the plates have to be prebended according to the local anatomy (Fig. 28.14). The first plate is fixed at the sacral side and is orientated closed along the pelvic brim. Thereafter, both iliac screws are drilled and inserted. Anterior screw lengths of up to 50 mm can be achieved in firm bone.

The posterior plate is directed toward the posterior iliac crest. Therefore, for the posterior iliac screws, drilling is directed in a dorsomedial direction. Possible screw lengths of up to 50 mm are achieved.

In some rare cases, supplemental internal fixation can be achieved with a sacroiliac screw placed percutaneously on the same supine position.

28.14 Wound Closure

Closing the wound is easy as the soft tissues/muscles spontaneously get originally repositioned. A deep suction drain placed at the iliac fossa can be considered. The detached abdominal wall muscles are carefully reattached by direct suturing. Alternatively, transosseous refixation or fixation through plate holes at the iliac crest can support fascial reconstruction. After subcutaneous suturing the ski is closed in a standardized manner.

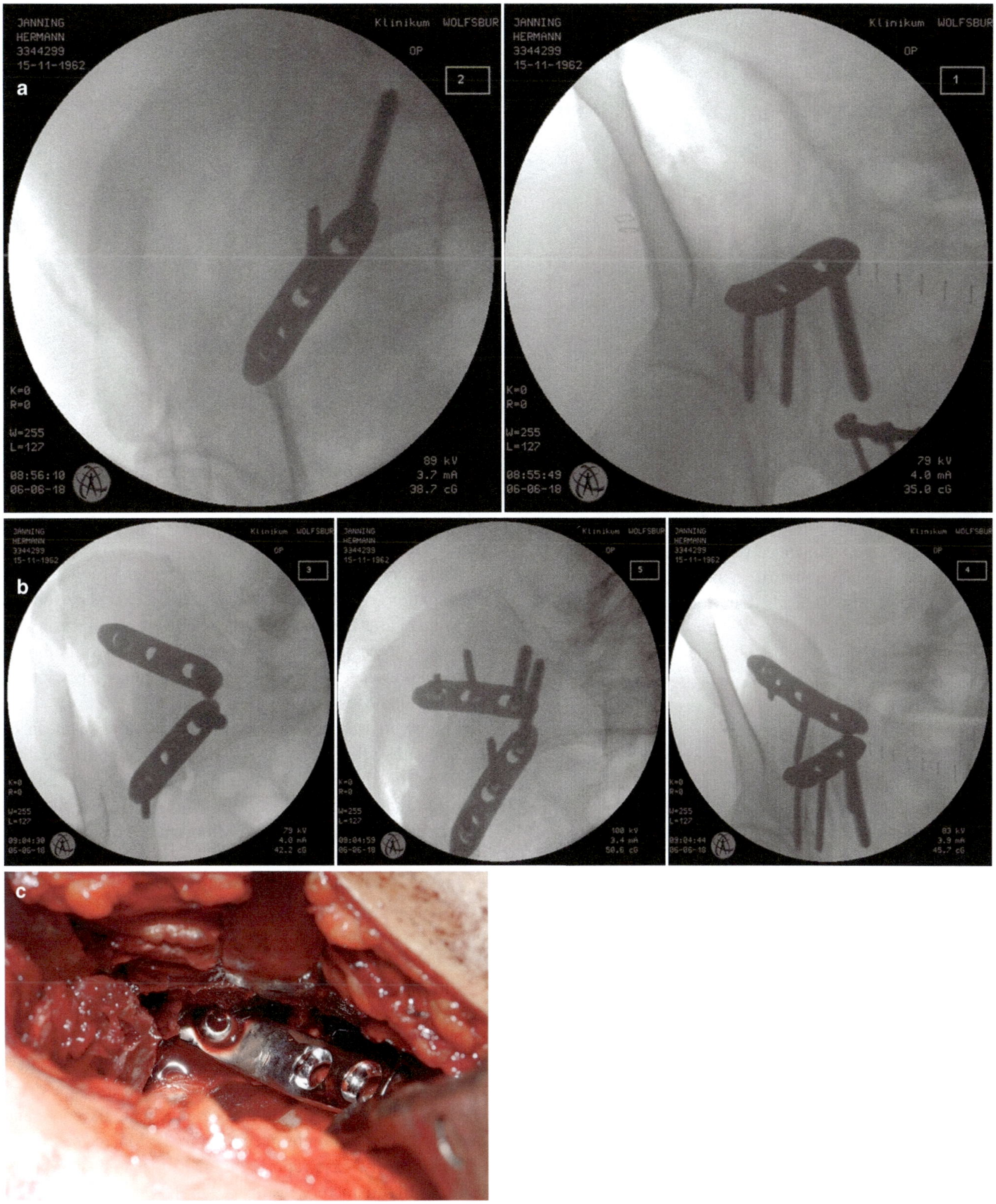

Fig. 28.13 (**a**) Intraoperative views of the plate position after reduction: anterior plate. (**b**) Intraoperative views of the plate position after reduction: both plates. (**c**) Intraoperative view of anterior plate application

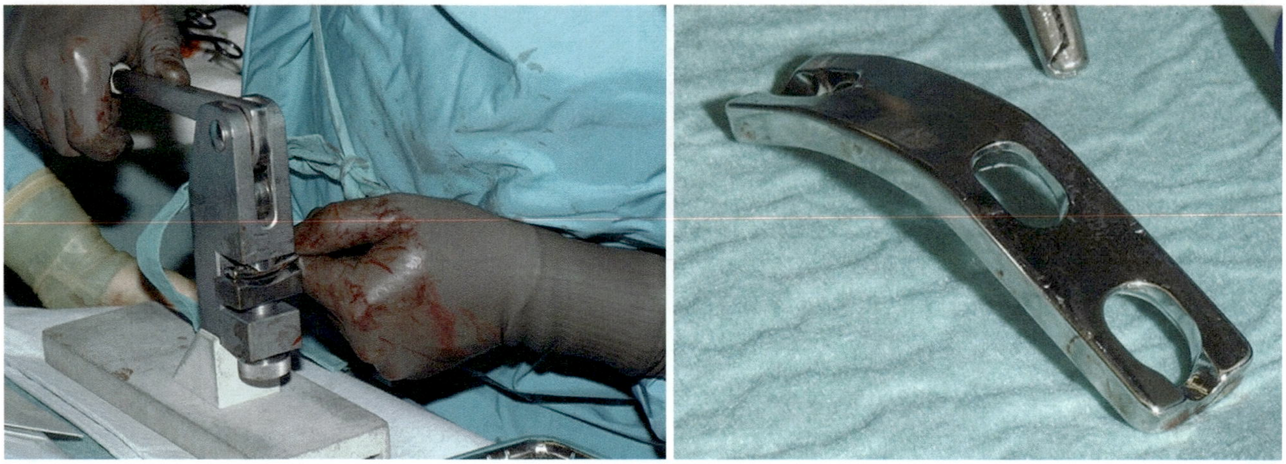

Fig. 28.14 Prebending of the plates

28.15 Aftercare

Partial weight bearing of the injured side with one-fifth of the body weight is recommended for 6 weeks.

Routine implant removal is not indicated. Disturbing subcutaneous screw heads can lead to partial implant removal.

28.16 Results

Clinical data of anterior SI joint plating are sparse (Figs. 28.15, 28.16, and 28.17).

Leighton et al. reported on their multicenter experience with 42 patients and anterior square plate fixation of completely disrupted SI joints [47]. Of these, 100% healing and anatomic reduction in 80% were recorded. No implant failure was observed.

Ragnarsson et al. reported on 23 patients after anterior square plate fixation of the SI joint [45]. Anatomical joint reconstruction was achieved in 82.6%. Surgery-related complications occurred in six patients: 1× seroma, 1× deep infection, 1× lumbosacral plexus injury, 1× LCFN injury, 1× nonunion, and 1× unsatisfactory reduction.

At clinical follow-up after a median of 70 months, two patients had relevant pain (with additional lumbosacral plexus lesion), 17 presented with normal gait, 4 had slight sitting discomfort, and 1 patient had an erectile dysfunction disturbance. No neurological recovery was observed in 10 patients with either a pre- or postoperative neurological deficit. The radiological result revealed no secondary dislocation was observed, and 22 of 23 patients had identical implant position.

Gänsslen et al. reported on 27 patients with disruption of the SI joint [46]. Except for one patient, a high-energy trauma resulted in this injury type. The average ISS (Injury Severity Score) was 23 points (9–50 points). Five patients presented with primary lumbosacral plexus lesion (18.5%). Three patients died (mean ISS 39 points).

The average displacement of the affected SI joint on CT examination was 16 mm (8–30 mm). Surgery was performed on average after 5 days (1–18 days). One deep infection was observed, three patients developed deep vein thrombosis, and two presented with iatrogenic nerve damage (2× lateral femoral cutaneous nerve).

Follow-up was possible in 16 patients after a mean of 63.2 months after injury (1–14 years). Anatomical healing was seen in 81.3%. The remaining patients showed persistent maximum displacement of 2–4 mm on CT examination. No secondary implant failure (loosening, secondary displacement) was observed.

In 9 of 10 patients with follow-up CT examination, degenerative changes of the SI joint were seen: 8× anterior osteophytes, 4× SI joint arthrosis, and 1× joint ankyloses while the contralateral SI joint was "normal" in seven patients.

Elmanawy et al. reported on 10 patients, all after high-energy trauma, who received anterior SI joint plating [48]. Surgery was performed on average after 9 days. All joints healed. Posterior pain was present in three patients at latest follow-up. One patient developed a temporary foot drop. Overall, three patients were graded excellent, six good, and one poor after 12 months according to the Majeed scoring.

Additionally, case reports on anterior plating were published with satisfactory results [49–51].

Recently, several reports compared anterior SI joint plating with iliosacral screw fixation of the disrupted SI joint. These data are not unequivocal.

Li compared 32 patients with iliosacral screw stabilization and 32 patients with anterior plating of Tile type C injuries [52].

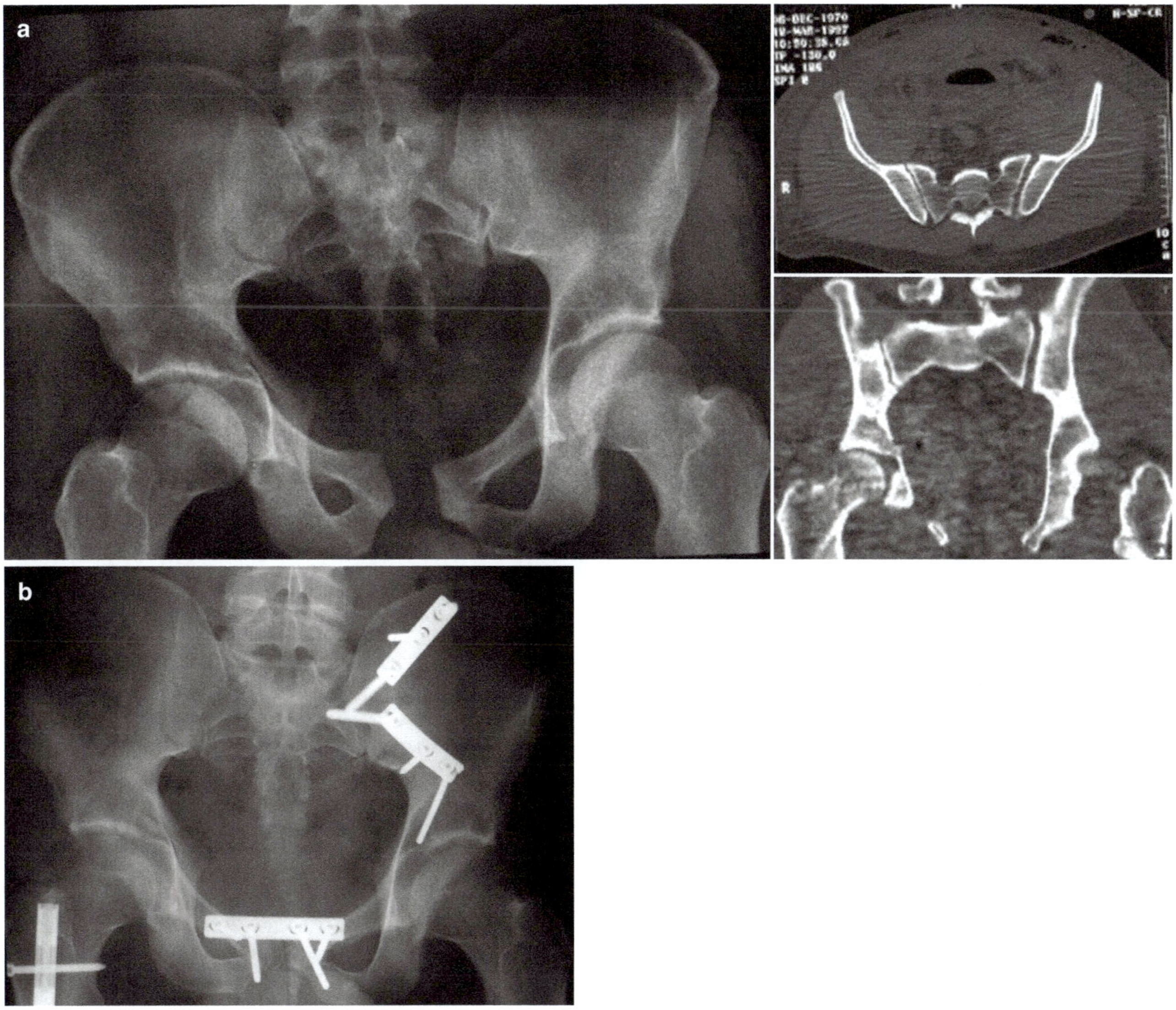

Fig. 28.15 (**a**) Left complete SI joint disruption (indicated on the CT by parallel joint widening) with symphyseal disruption and undisplaced right acetabular fracture. (**b**) Anterior plate stabilization of the SI joint and symphyseal plating. The acetabular fractures were treated conservatively

As expected, operative time, blood loss, wound length, and hospitalization time were significantly minor in the iliosacral screw group. In detail:

- The complication rate was lower after iliosacral screw fixation (3.1% vs. 21.9%).
- The quality of reduction (≤4 mm) was better after iliosacral screw fixation (75% vs. 56.3%).
- Majeed score ≥ 84 points was more common after iliosacral screw fixation (93.8% vs. 75%).

Gu et al. analyzed overall 78 patients with 68 Tile type B and only 10 type C injuries [53]. Of these, 26 patients were treated with iliosacral screw fixation, while 26 were treated with a reconstruction plate or a T plate, and 26 patients were treated with a specially designed anterior SI joint plate. With less data on type C injuries, no relevant statistical evaluation is possible.

Tan et al. compared each 25 patients with type C injuries with either anterior plate fixation or computerized navigated iliosacral screw fixation [54]. After iliosacral screw fixation, fewer complications were observed, while the quality of reduction and functional and clinical scores were comparable.

Zhang et al. compared the results of 38 patients with iliosacral screw stabilization and 32 patients with anterior plating [47]. All injuries healed and no nonunions were observed. The main results include:

- The average blood loss was minor in the iliosacral screw group (287 mL vs. 426 mL).

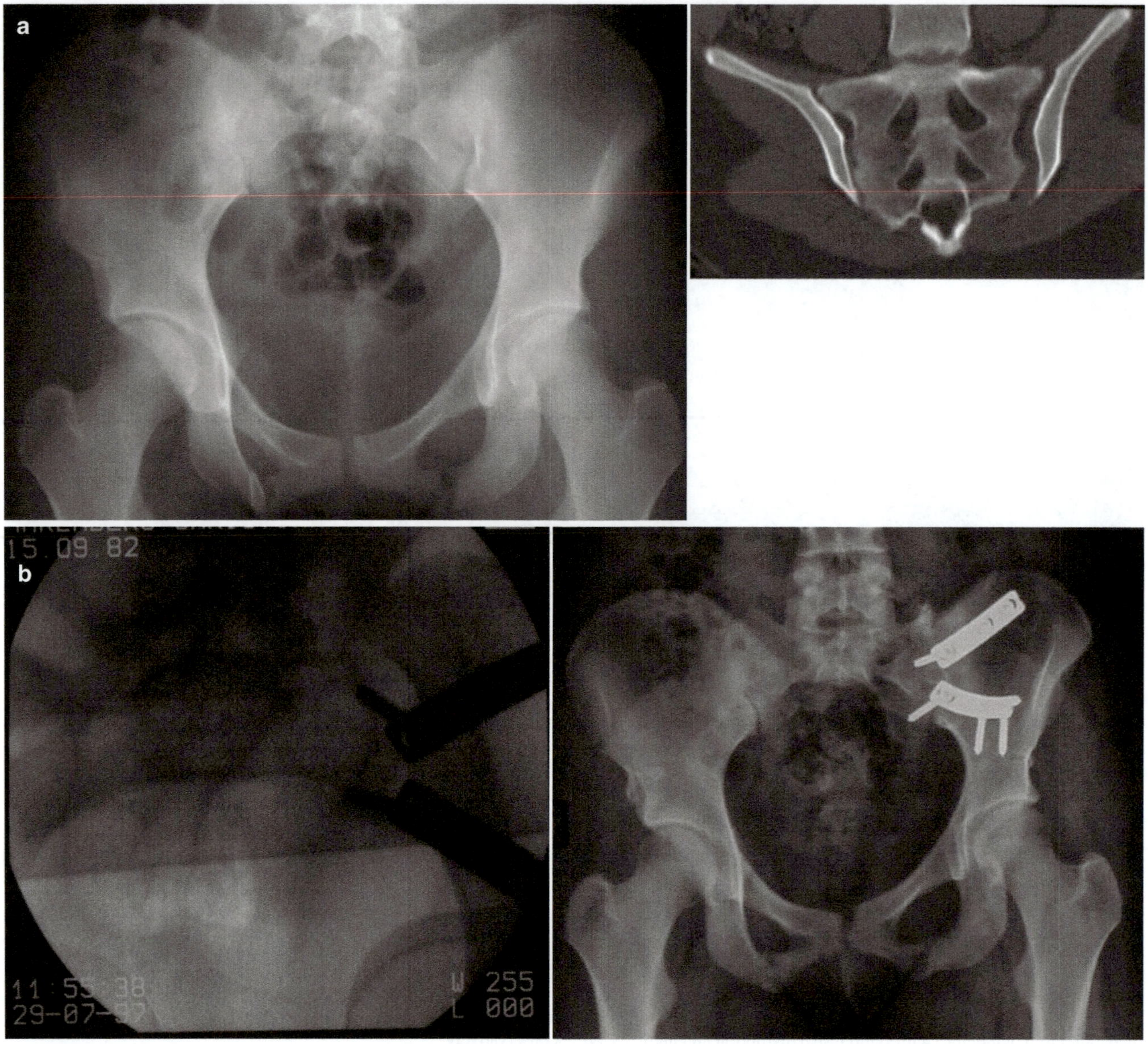

Fig. 28.16 (**a**) Left complete SI joint disruption (confirmed on the CT) bilateral pubic rami fractures. (**b**) Intraoperative view after plating and one-year follow-up x-ray

- The mean fluoroscopy frequency was increased in the iliosacral screw group (15.8 s vs. 3.94 s).
- Satisfactory reductions (<4 mm) were observed in 86.4% (iliosacral) vs. 78.1%.
- Satisfactory outcomes (Majeed ≥84 points) were present in 84.2% vs. 87.5%.
- The complication rate was lower after anterior plating (15.8% vs. 9.4%).

After iliosacral screw fixation, three patients developed iatrogenic lumbosacral plexus injury; one patient had screw loosening without secondary joint dislocation and two soft-tissue infections.

After anterior plate fixation, one patient had screw loosening without secondary joint dislocation, one patient had local hematoma treated by puncture, and one patient suffered from temporary LCFN injury.

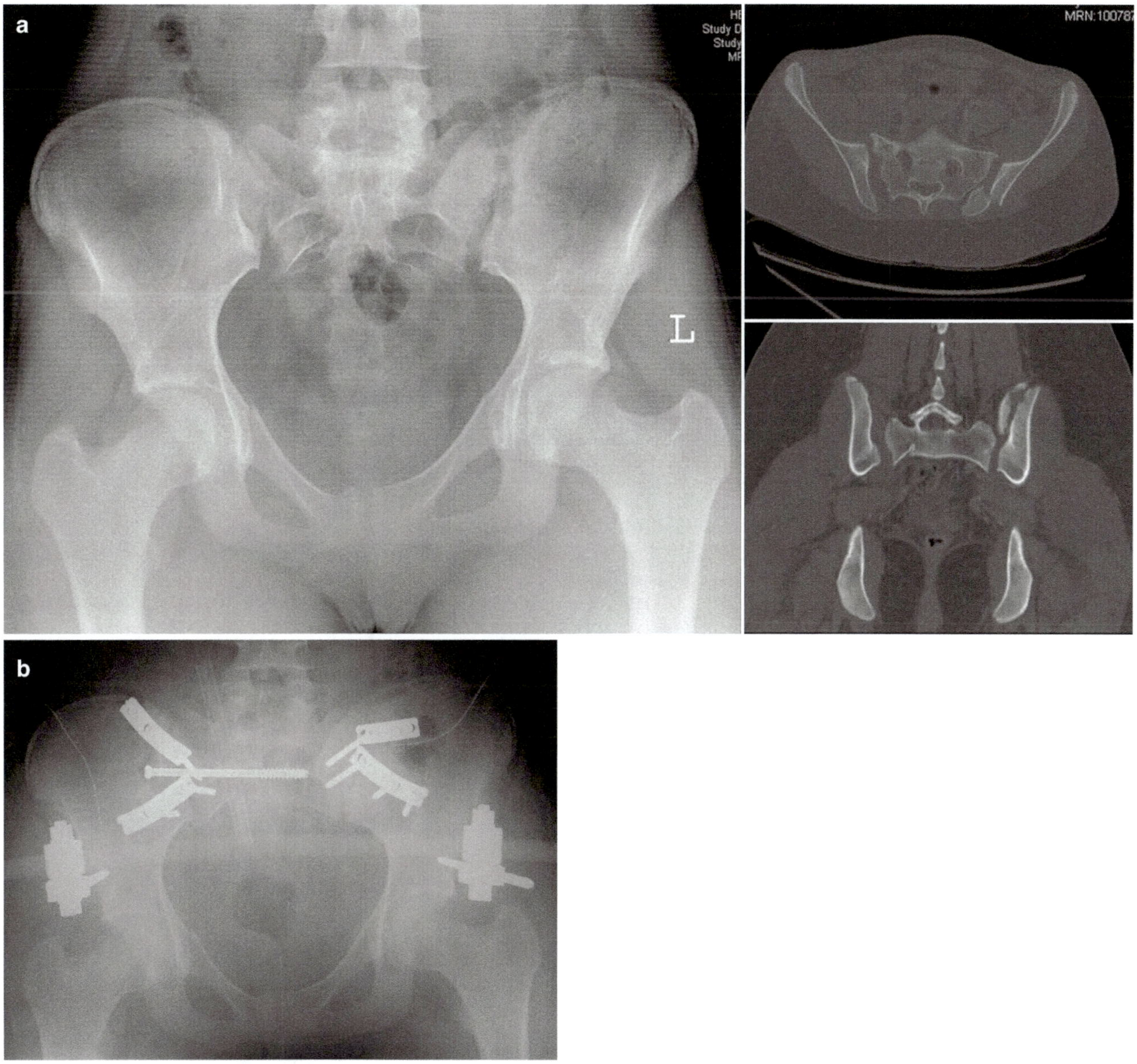

Fig. 28.17 (a) Bilateral SI joint Injury: left crescent fracture and right SI joint dislocation with bilateral anterior rami fractures. (b) Bilateral anterior plating of both SI joints with additional iliosacral screw fixation and anterior external fixation

Anterior plating of the completely disrupted SI joint leads to adequate long-term results with an acceptable complication rate. Anatomical reduction is achieved in approximately 80%. Anatomical reduction is the key for stable fixation because the opposing joint surfaces of the SI joint are concave-convex shaped in every plane.

28.17 Summary

Anterior plate fixation allows for a high rate of anatomical reconstructions under direct visualization of the disrupted joint. It is still a valuable option in stabilizing the posterior pelvis. Anterior approach and anterior plating of the SI joint allow simultaneous reduction and fixation of the symphysis pubis and pubic rami fractures with the patient in the supine position.

Appendix

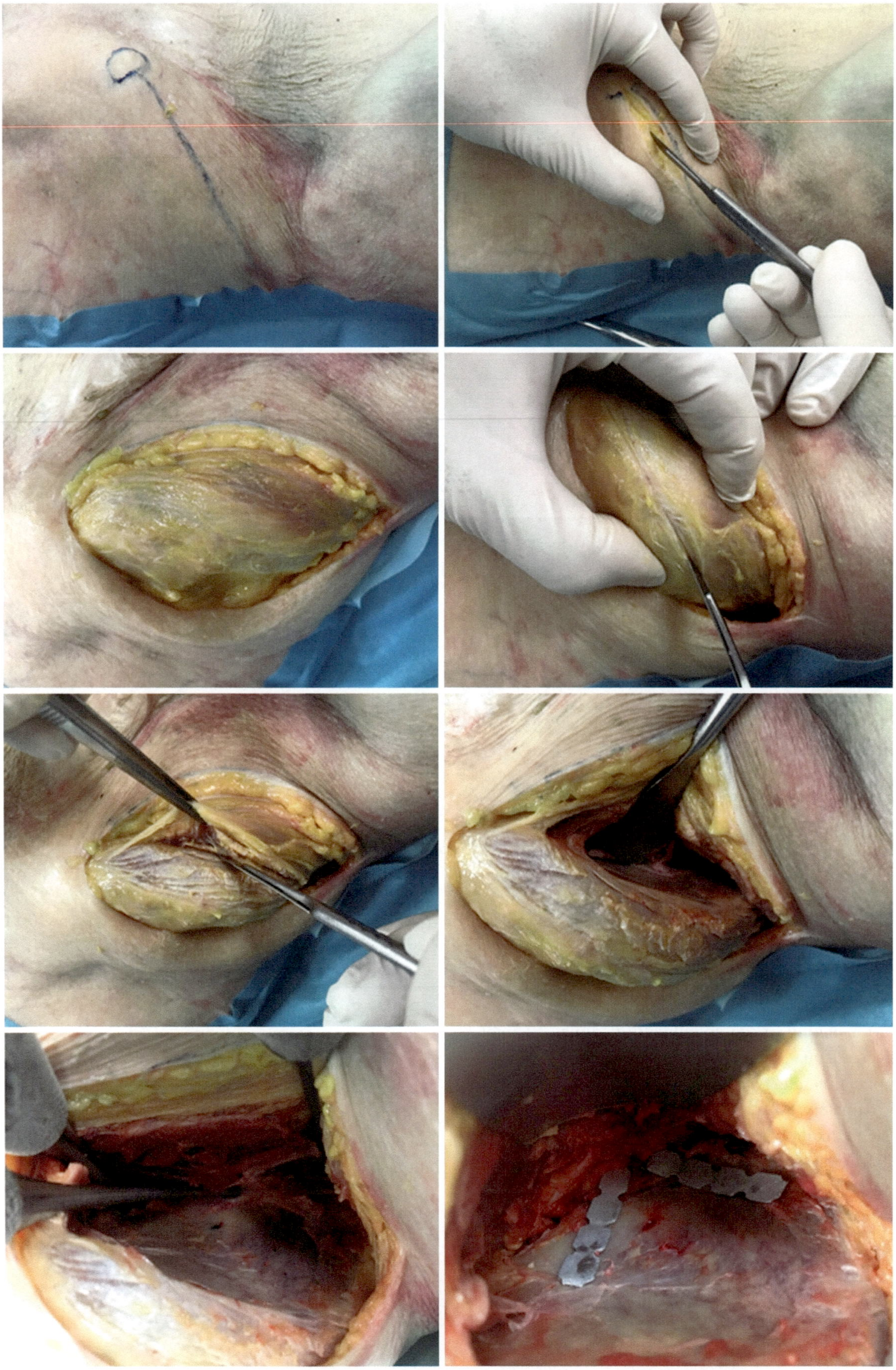

References

1. Lambotte A. Chirurgie opératoire des fractures. répité, vol. 1913. Bruxelles: Société Franco-Belge D'Editions Scientifiques; 1948. p. 126–44.
2. Noland L, Conwell H. Fractures of the pelvis. Surg Gynecol Obstet. 1933;56:522–5.
3. Watson-Jones R. Dislocations and fracture-dislocations of the pelvis. Br J Surg. 1938;25:773–81.
4. Westerborn A. Beiträge zur Kenntnis der der Beckenbrüche und Beckenluxationen. Acta Chir Scand Suppl. 1928;8:80–156.
5. Bucholz R. The pathological anatomy of Malgaigne fracture-dislocations of the pelvis. J Bone Joint Surg. 1981;63-A(3):400–4.
6. Domisse G. Diametric fractures of the pelvis. JBJS. 1960;42(B):432–4443.
7. Shaw J, Eng M, Mino D, Werner F, Eng M, Murray D. Posterior stabilisation of pelvic fractures by use of threated compression rods. Clin Orthop. 1985;192:240–54.
8. Rand J. Anterior sacro-iliac arthrodesis for post-traumatic sacro-iliac arthritis. A case report. J Bone Joint Surg. 1985;67-Am:157–9.
9. Simpson LA, Waddell JP, Leighton RK, Kellam JF, Tile M. Anterior approach and stabilization of the disrupted sacroiliac joint. J Trauma. 1987;27(12):1332–9.
10. Olerud S, Hamberg M. The anterior approach to the dislocated sacroiliac joint. Reduction and fixation with a square plate. In: Noble J, Galasko CSB, editors. Recent development in orthopaedic surgery. Manchester: Manchester University Press; 1987. p. 175–81.
11. Hearn T, Schopfer A, D'Angelo D, Tile M. The effects of ligament sectioning and internal fixation on bending stiffness of the pelvic ring. In: Proceedings of the 13th International Conference on Biomechanics, Perth, Australia. 1991.
12. McBroom R, Tile M. Disruption of the pelvic ring. Orthop Trans. 1982;6:493.
13. Tile M. Fractures of the pelvis and acetabulum. Baltimore: Williams & Wilkins; 1984.
14. Tile M. Fractures of the pelvis and acetabulum. 2nd ed. Baltimore: Williams & Wilkins; 1995.
15. Tile M, Helfet D, Kellam J. Fractures of the pelvis and acetabulum. 3rd ed. Lippincott: Williams and Williams; 2003.
16. Leighton R, Waddell J, Bray T, Chapman M, Simpson L, Martin R, Sharkey N. Biomechanical testing of new and old fixation devices for vertical shear fractures of the pelvis. J Orthop Trauma. 1991;5(3):313–7.
17. Rieger H. Das instabile Becken, Diagnostik, Therapie und Prognose der Beckenringfraktur. München, Bern, Wien, New York: W. Zuckschwerdt Verlag; 1996.
18. Comstock C, van der Meulen M, Marjolein C, Goodman S. Biomechanical comparison of posterior internal fixation techniques for unstable pelvic fractures. J Orthop Trauma. 1996;10:517–22.
19. Yinger K, Scalise J, Olson S, Bay B, Finkemeier C. Biomechanical comparison of posterior pelvic ring fixation. J Orthop Trauma. 2003;17:481–7.
20. Chen W, Pan Z, Chen J. Biomechanical research on anterior double-plate fixation for vertically unstable sacroiliac dislocations. Orthop Surg. 2009;1:127–31.
21. Gänsslen A, Pohlemann T, Culemann U, Krettek C, von Samson F, Tscherne H. Vergleichende dreidimensionale Stabilitätsprüfung verschiedener Osteosynthesen zur SI-Gelenks-Stabilisierung. Swiss Surg. 1996;(Suppl 2):43.
22. Jacob A, Messmer P, Stock K, Suhm N, Baumann B, Regazzoni P, Steinbrich W. Posterior pelvic ring fractures: closed reduction and percutaneous CT-guided sacroiliac screw fixation. Cardiovasc Intervent Radiol. 1997;20:285–94.
23. Lansinger O, Karlsson J, Berg U, Mare K. Unstable fractures of the pelvis treated with a trapezoid compression frame. Acta Orthop Scand. 1984;55:325–9.
24. Sahlstrand T. Disruption of the pelvic ring treated by the external skeletal fixation. J Bone Joint Surg. 1979;61-Am:433–4.
25. Brown T, Stone J, Schuster J, Mears D. External fixation of unstable pelvic ring fractures: comparative rigidity of some current frame configurations. Med Biol Eng Comput. 1982;20:727–33.
26. Rubash H, Brown T, Nelson D, Mears D. Comparative mechanical performance of some new devices for fixation of unstable pelvic ring fractures. Med Biol Eng Comput. 1983;21:657–63.
27. Letournel E. Fractures of the pelvis and acetabulum. In: Ninth AFOR Course and Workshop. Paris, France. 1993.
28. Avila LJ. Primary pyogenic infection of the sacroiliac articulation. A new approach to the joint. J Bone Joint Surg. 1941;23-Am:922–8.
29. Trentz O, Bühren V, Friedl H. Beckenverletzungen. Chirurg. 1989;60:639–48.
30. de Ridder VA, de Lange S, Popta JV. Anatomical variations of the lateral femoral cutaneous nerve and the consequences for surgery. J Orthop Trauma. 1999;13(3):207–11.
31. Hospodar P, Ashman E, Traub J. Anatomic study of the lateral femoral cutaneous nerve with respect to the ilioinguinal surgical dissection. J Orthop Trauma. 1999;13:17–9.
32. Sürücü H, Tanyeli E, Sargon M, Karahan S. An anatomic study of the lateral femoral cutaneous nerve. Surg Radiol Anat. 1997;19:307–10.
33. Aszmann OC, Dellon ES, Dellon AL. Anatomical course of the lateral femoral cutaneous nerve and its susceptibility to compression and injury. Plast Reconstr Surg. 1997;100(3):600–4.
34. Murata Y, Takahashi K, Yamagata M, Shimada Y, Moriya H. The anatomy of the lateral femoral cutaneous nerve, with special reference to the harvesting of iliac bone graft. J Bone Joint Surg Am. 2000;82(5):746–7.
35. Rosenberger RJ, Loeweneck H, Meyer G. The cutaneous nerves encountered during laparoscopic repair of inguinal hernia: new anatomical findings for the surgeon. Surg Endosc. 2000;14(8):731–5.
36. Ebraheim N, Lu J, Biyani A, Yang H. Anatomic considerations of the principal nutrient foramen and artery on internal surface of the ilium. Surg Radiol Anat. 1997;19:237–9.
37. Alla S, Roberts C, Ojike N. Vascular risk reduction during anterior surgical approach sacroiliac joint plating. Injury. 2013;44:175–7.
38. Ebraheim N, Padanilam T, Waldrop J, Yeasting R. Anatomic consideration in the anterior approach to the sacro-iliac joint. Spine. 1994;19(6):721–5.
39. Thein T, Kreidler J, Stocker E, Herrmann M. Morphology and blood supply of the iliac crest applied to jaw reconstruction. Surg Radiol Anat. 1997;19:217–25.
40. Ertel W, von Lüdinghausen M, Trentz O. Becken. In: Platzer W, Trentz O, editors. Posttraumatische Defekt- und Weichteilsanierung. Schädel, Wirbelsäule, Becken. Stuttgart, New York: Thieme; 1997. p. 414–557.
41. Kellam JF, McMurtry RY, Paley D, Tile M. The unstable pelvic fracture—operative treatment. Orthop Clin North Am. 1987;18(1):25–41.
42. Müller-Färber J. Beckenverletzungen. In: Kinzl L, editor. Breitner Chirurgische Operationslehre. München, Wien, Baltimore: Urban & Schwarzenberg; 1993. p. 37–63.
43. Schmit-Neuerburg K, Hartwig T. Osteosyntheseverfahren am dorsalen Beckenring-Plattentechnik. Hefte Unfallheilkunde. 1986;181:566–79.
44. Martin R, Leighton R. Fixation of the sacroiliac joint through the anterior approach. Tech Orthop. 1995;9(4):290–4.
45. Ragnarsson B, Olerud C, Olerud S. Anterior square-plate fixation of sacroiliac disruption. Acta Orthop Scand. 1993;64(2):138–42.
46. Gänsslen A, Pohlemann T, Krettek C. [Internal fixation of sacroiliac joint disruption]. Oper Orthop Traumatol. 2005;17:281–195.
47. Leighton R, Waddell J. Techniques for reduction and posterior fixation through the anterior approach. Clin Orthop. 1996;329:115–20.

48. Elmanawy M, Elshoura S, Youssef S, Salama F. Treatment of sacroiliac joint disruption with anterior stabilization. Egypt Orthop J. 2015;50:45–50.
49. Faisham W, Nawaz A, Joehaimey J, Sallehuddin A, Wan Z. Anterior stabilisation of sacroilliac joint for complex pelvic injuries. Malays J Med Sci. 2009;16:47–51.
50. Teebken O, Lotz J, Gänsslen A, Pichlmaier A. Bilateral iliac artery dissection following severe complex unstable pelvic fracture. Interact Cardiovasc Thorac Surg. 2008;7:515–6.
51. Wright V, Zelle B, Prayson M. Bilateral sacroiliac joint dislocation without associated fracture or anterior pelvic ring injuries. J Orthop Trauma. 2004;18:634–7.
52. Li C. Clinical comparative analysis on unstable pelvic fractures in the treatment with percutaneous sacroiliac screws and sacroiliac joint anterior plate fixation. Eur Rev Med Pharmacol Sci. 2014;18:2704–8.
53. Gu R, Huang W, Yang L, Liu H, Xie K, Huang Z. Comparisons of front plate, percutaneous sacroiliac screws, and sacroiliac anterior papilionaceous plate in fixation of unstable pelvic fractures. Medicine (Baltimore). 2017;96(36):e7775. https://doi.org/10.1097/MD.0000000000007775.
54. Tan Z, Fang Y, Zhang H, Liu L, Xiang Z, Zhong G, Huang F, Wang G. [Efficacy of sacroiliac joint anterior approach with double reconstruction plate and computer assisted navigation percutaneous sacroiliac screw for treating tile C1 pelvic fractures]. Sichuan Da Xue Xue Bao Yi Xue Ban. 2017;48:668–72.

SI Joint: Posterior Reduction and Stabilization

29

Jan Lindahl and Axel Gänsslen

29.1 Posterolateral Approach to the SI Joint

The posterolateral approach, which is based on the original description by Joel Matta [1], described for the treatment of crescent fractures of the posterior pelvic ring can be used also in SI joint (fracture) dislocations [2, 3].

29.1.1 Positioning

Surgery is performed under general anesthesia in the standard prone position. A complete radiolucent table is preferred. Support of the left and right anterior chest and abdomen is recommended. The pelvis is left free, so even after anterior stabilization, e.g., with an external fixator prior to posterior stabilization, positioning is easy.

29.1.2 Draping

The whole or ipsilateral posterior pelvic region, including the buttock, and iliac wing are draped. Depending on the displacement and the side, the lower extremity is additionally draped free [2, 3]. This allows also somatosensory-evoked potential monitoring.

29.1.3 Incision

A curvilinear or longitudinal incision starts 1–2 cm lateral to the top of the iliac crest and runs parallel 1–2 cm lateral to the posterior superior iliac spine (PSIS) and posterior inferior iliac spine (PIIS) (Fig. 29.1) [2–6].

Caudal extension is important when exposure of the greater sciatic notch and the inferior portion of the sacroiliac joint is planned [4].

Incision length must be adequate depending on the fracture morphology to allow medial exposure. Matta recommended an incision starting 5 cm proximal to the iliac crest and ending 5 cm distal to the superior border of the greater sciatic notch [1].

29.1.4 Superficial Dissection

The superficial dissection should be performed in line with the skin incision [4] until the gluteus maximus fascia is identified. Fowler et al. recommended not to create a subcutaneous flap to avoid any dead space, while Matta proposed some subcutaneous mobilization [1]. The gluteus maximus origin is identified at the posterior iliac crest and the sacrum (Fig. 29.2).

29.1.5 Deep Dissection

Sharp incision of the iliac crest periosteum is performed for direct subperiosteal dissection to reflect the gluteus maximus and part of the gluteus medius from the iliac crest, PSIS, PIIS, and the outer surface of the iliac wing (Fig. 29.3). Often some detachment of the gluteus maximus from the posterior and lateral sacral from the underlying multifidus fascia surface is necessary [1].

The localization of the nervi clunii should be considered, as the main medial branch is located approximately 8 cm lateral to the midline and 6.5 cm lateral to the PSIS at the superior iliac crest. The nerve runs through a fascial tunnel and is, therefore, at risk for compression injuries [7].

J. Lindahl
Orthopaedics and Trauma Surgery, Helsinki University Hospital, Helsinki, Finland

A. Gänsslen (✉)
Department of Trauma Surgery, Orthopedics and Hand Surgery, Hospital Wolfsburg, Wolfsburg, Germany

A. Gänsslen et al. (eds.), *Pelvic Ring Fractures*, https://doi.org/10.1007/978-3-030-54730-1_29

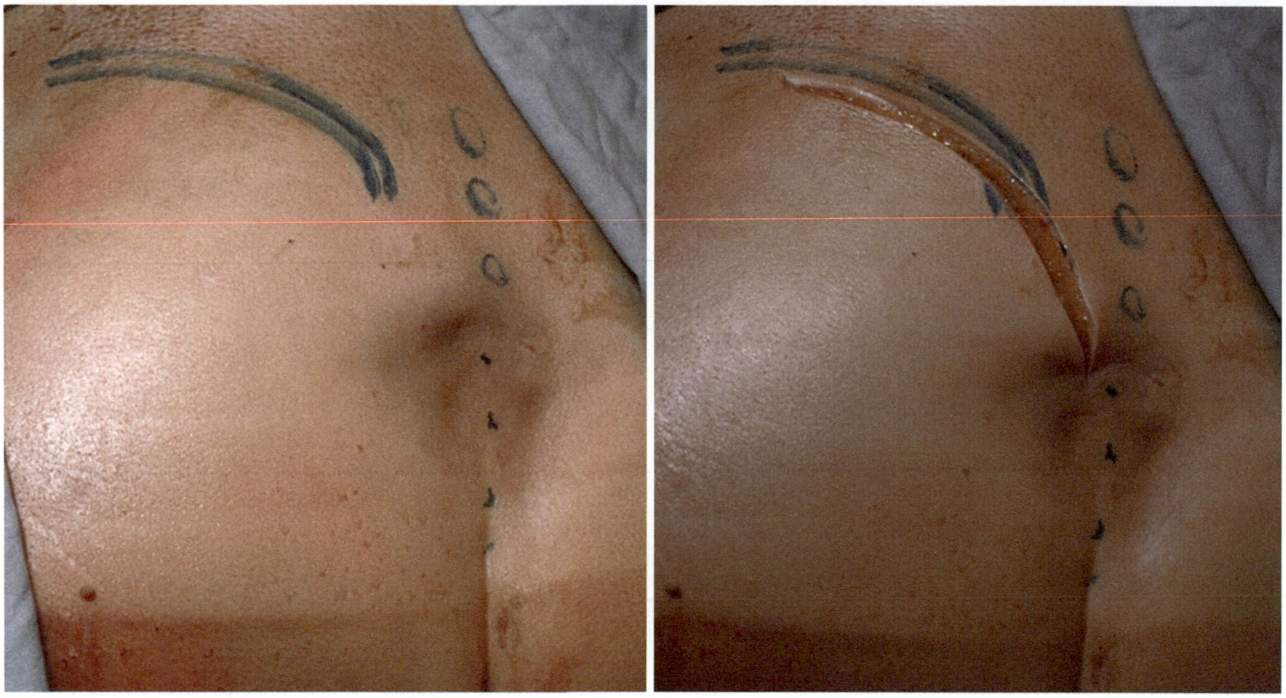

Fig. 29.1 A curvilinear incision is performed in line with the posterior iliac crest

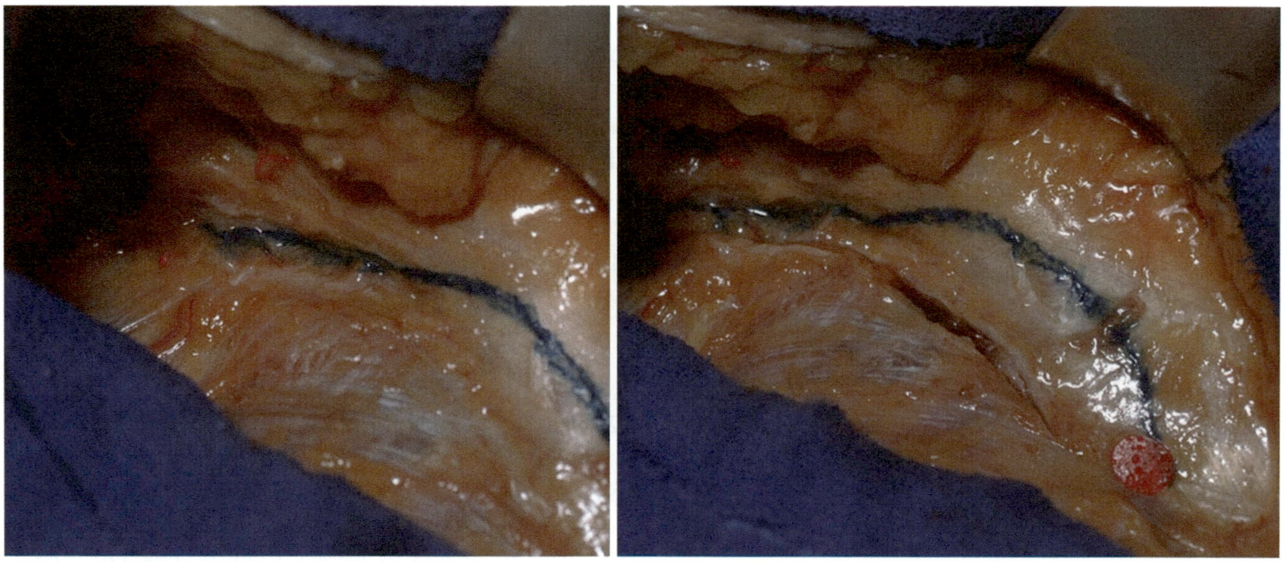

Fig. 29.2 Identification of the posterior iliac crest and fascial incision parallel to the iliac crest to release the gluteus maximus origin

Inferiorly, detachment of the muscle from the sacrotuberous ligament can be necessary (Fig. 29.3). A tendinous strip can be dissected for easier later reconstruction [5].

The fracture morphology determines the lateral and anterior extension of dissection of the abductor complex [4].

Developing a full gluteal flap, based on the superior gluteal neurovascular bundle, is not always necessary in crescent-type fractures. The course of the superior gluteal neurovascular bundle has to be respected.

Exposure of the greater sciatic notch leads to optimal anatomic reduction of the SI joint. Insertion of a curved perios-

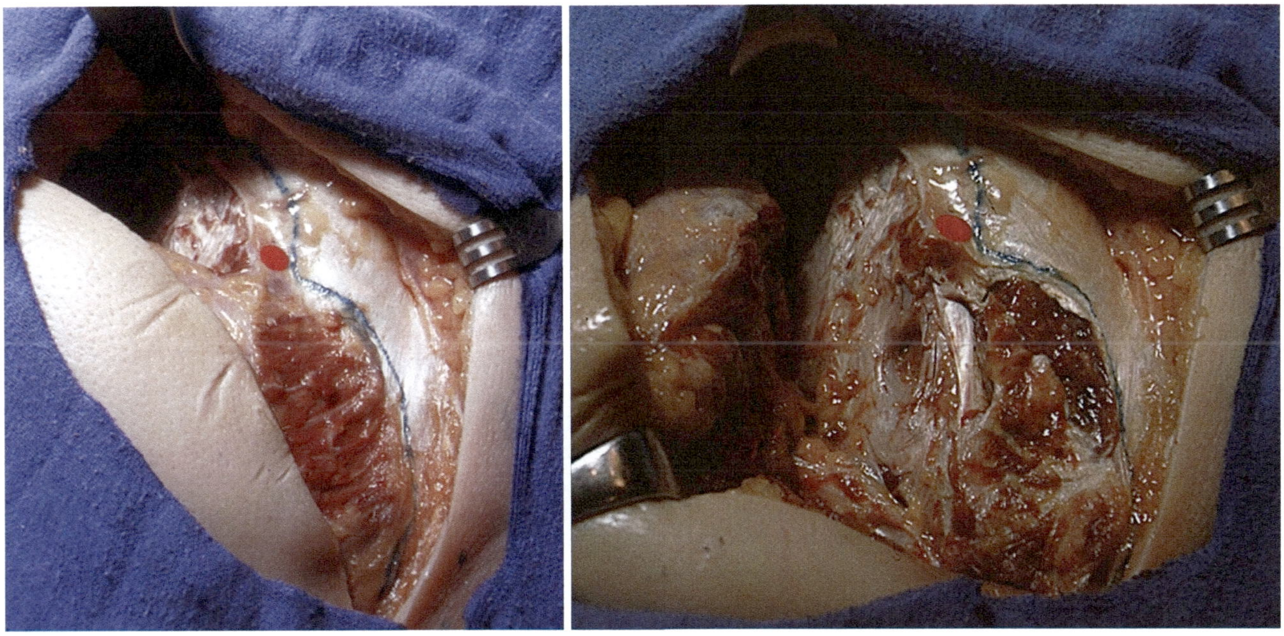

Fig. 29.3 Detachment of the gluteus maximus from the posterior and lateral sacral surface. Inferiorly, detachment of the muscle from the sacrotuberous ligament can be necessary. PSIS (red dot)

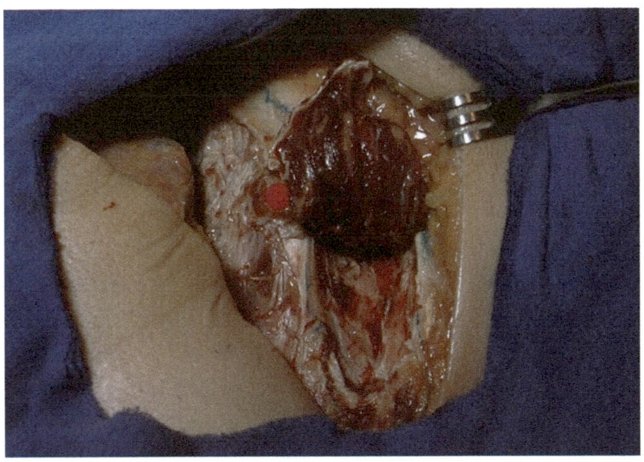

Fig. 29.4 Detailed view of the posterior sacral surface, with complete elevation of the erector trunci muscle. PSIS (red dot)

teal elevator at the anterior aspect of the sacrum after dissecting the piriformis origin can protect the neurovascular bundle. The inferior SI joint becomes visible and the anterior part of the SI joint with the anterior lateral sacral ala can be palpated. Extending the dissection more medially to the PSIS by elevation of the erector spinae from the dorsal sacrum (Fig. 29.4), the posterior sacral foramina can be visualized, which can be helpful to reduce the SI joint part of the injury [5].

29.1.6 Fracture Cleaning

By inserting a laminar spreader into the iliac wing fracture (Fig. 29.5), the disrupted part of the SI joint is visualized, and the joint is debrided.

Inferior dissection to visualize the upper greater sciatic notch can be helpful to control the reduction under digital control.

29.1.7 Reduction

The iliac wing fracture is first reduced under direct visualization. A large Weber reduction forceps can be used, with positioning of one sidearm at the PSIS and the other at the iliac wing (Fig. 29.6). Temporary fixation is possible with one or two 2.0 mm K-wires, inserted from the PSIS across the fracture.

Reduction of the SI joint can be digitally controlled by inserting a finger into the greater sciatic notch. Inserting a reduction forceps (angled ball spike forceps according to Matta) through the greater sciatic notch to the anterior sacrum can reduce the SI joint part of the fracture (Fig. 29.7). The superior gluteal neurovascular bundle and, anterior to the sacrum, the L5 nerve root have to be protected.

Alternatively, medial mobilization of the erector spinae and the multifidi muscles allows SI joint visualization by

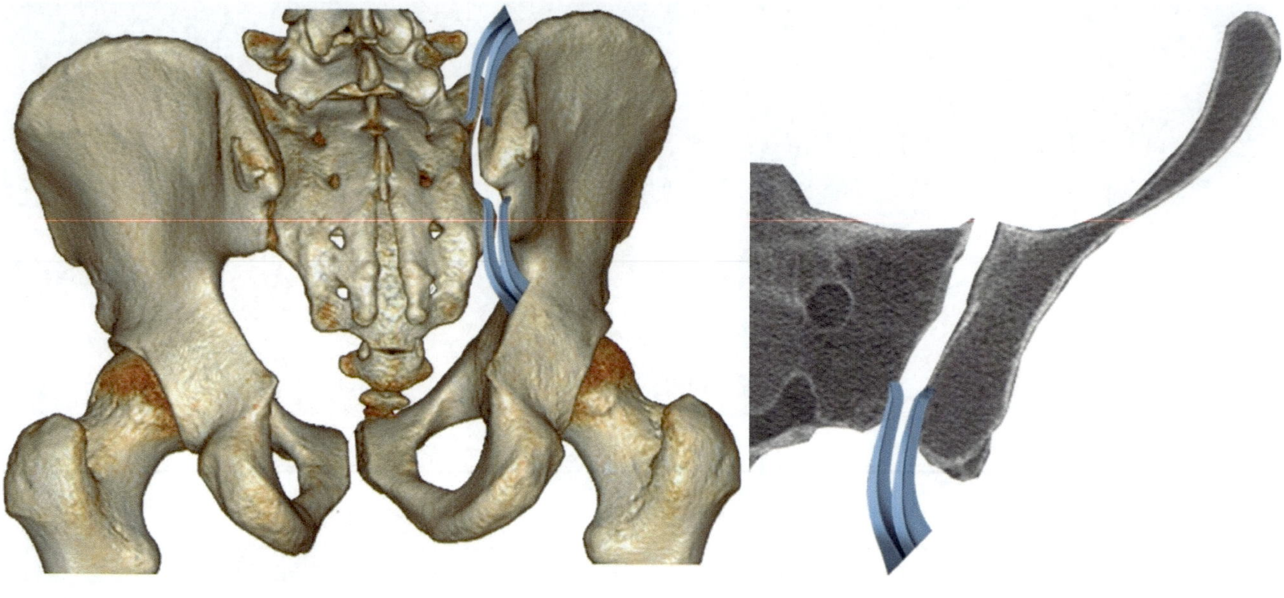

Fig. 29.5 Fracture/joint cleaning by inserting a laminar spreader

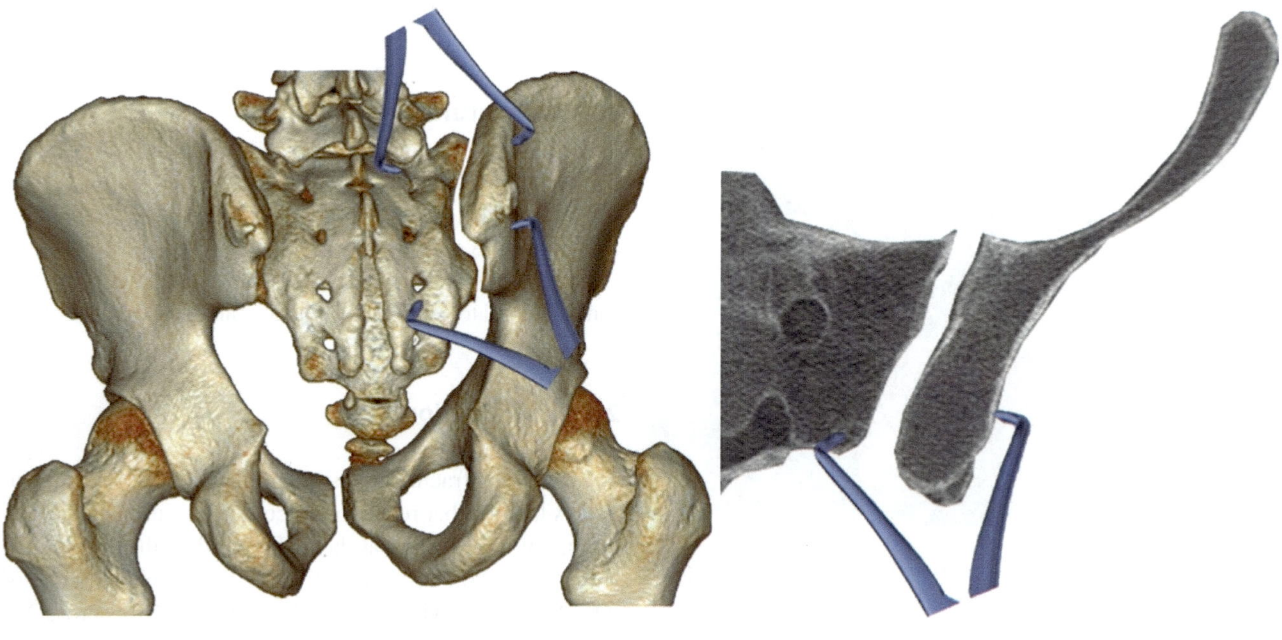

Fig. 29.6 Fracture/joint reduction using a pointed reduction forceps

insertion of laminar spreaders between the sacrum and the PSIS for SI joint debridement.

In additional ilium fractures, reduction at the iliac crest with a pointed reduction forceps can be helpful (Fig. 29.8).

29.1.8 Definitive Fixation

Parallel to the applied K-wires 3.5 or 4.5 mm lag screws are inserted perpendicular to the fracture line. Depending on the bone quality, washers can be useful. Borrelli et al. recommended additional application of two 3.5 mm antiglide plates on the outer iliac surface lateral below the iliac crest and inferior crossing the fracture line (Fig. 29.9).

In type III injuries according to Day, iliosacral screw fixation can be optionally performed.

The entry points on the outer iliac surface can be identified on a connecting line between the iliac crest and the greater sciatic notch, approximately 15 mm anterior to the posterior gluteal line.

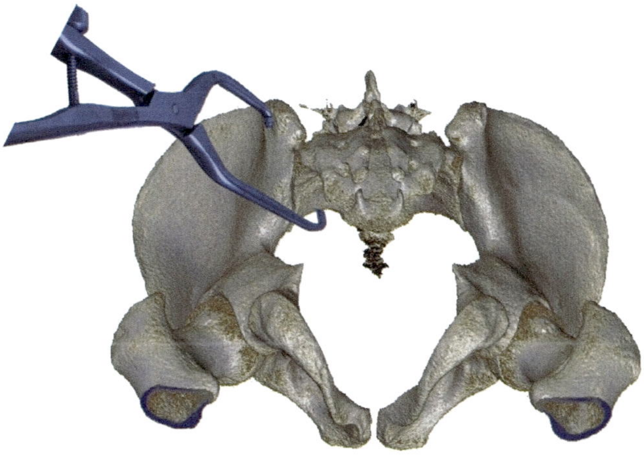

Fig. 29.7 Reduction of the SI joint through the greater sciatic notch with an asymmetric reduction forceps

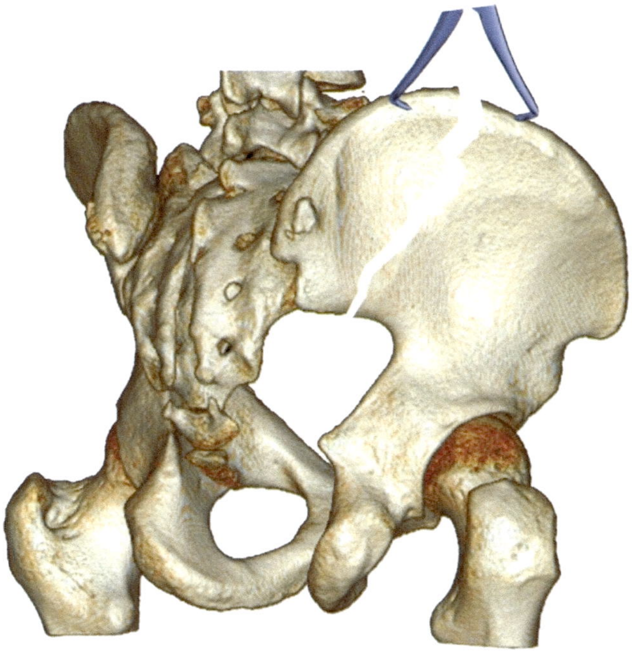

Fig. 29.8 Reduction of an ilium fracture with a pointed reduction forceps at the iliac crest

29.1.9 Wound Closure

After irrigation with a pulsatile irrigation system, drainage is recommended and the fascia of the gluteus maximus muscle is reattached.

29.1.10 Postoperative Course

Standard x-ray imaging is performed and a CT scan can be useful to analyze the quality of reduction in detail.

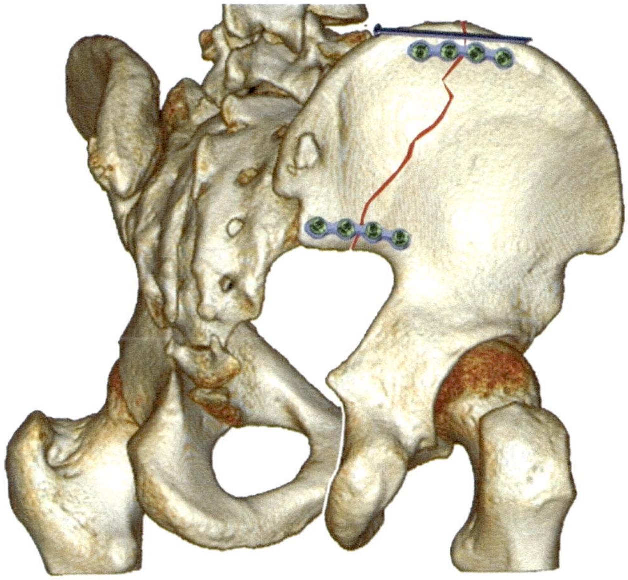

Fig. 29.9 Definitive stabilization at the outer iliac surface with two antiglide plates crossing the fracture line

29.2 Results of Treatment

Borrelli et al. first described their results using this approach in patients with fracture dislocations of the SI joint [2, 3].

Twenty-two patients were treated and run to uneventful healing within 3 months. After an average of 19 months, no loss of reduction, delayed union, nonunion, malunion, nor acute wound problems or neurologic complications developed. One patient presented with osteomyelitis of the iliac wing after 6 months, requiring implant removal, antibiotics, and debridement of the ilium.

French et al. described the technique of this approach but only gave an overview of results of treatment in unstable pelvic ring injuries without relating these results to the chosen approach [5].

29.3 Complications

After the original description of this approach in 1996, it took one decade until relevant scientific data were available. Stöver et al. retrospectively reported on 236 patients from a multicenter study with 268 performed posterior approaches in patients with type C injuries [6].

Approach-related complications included eight deep wound infections (3.4%), requiring debridement and further eight patients had signs of superficial infection. Overall, the rate of deep surgical site infection was between 2.3 and 5.5%.

A further retrospective analysis of 31 patients with 34 acute approaches reported a wound complication rate of 2.94%, while only one deep surgical site infections was reported (3.2%) [4].

The reported infection rates using this approach were comparable to other posterior pelvic procedures reported in the literature.

29.4 Summary

The posterior approach to the SI joint is a valuable approach but not routinely used.

References

1. Matta J. Surgical approaches to fractures of the acetabulum and pelvis. 1989. www.mizuhosi.com.
2. Borrelli J, Koval K, Helfet D. The crescent fracture: a posterior fracture dislocation of the sacroiliac joint. J Orthop Trauma. 1996;10:165–70.
3. Borrelli J, Koval K, Helfet D. Operative stabilization of fracture dislocations of the sacroiliac joint. Clin Orthop Relat Res. 1996;329:141–6.
4. Fowler T, Bishop J, Bellino M. The posterior approach to pelvic ring injuries: a technique for minimizing soft tissue complications. Injury. 2013;44:1780–6.
5. French B, Tornetta P. Transiliosakrale Osteosynthese bei instabilen Verletzugen des hinteren Bekenringes. Oper Orthop Traumatol. 2002;14:29–49.
6. Stöver M, Sims S, Matta J. What is the infection rate of the posterior approach to type C pelvic injuries? Clin Orthop Relat Res. 2012;470:2142–7.
7. Lu J, Ebraheim N, Huntoon M, Heck B, Yeasting R. Anatomic considerations of superior cluneal nerve at posterior iliac crest region. Clin Orthop Relat Res. 1998;347:224–8.

Fracture Dislocations of the SI Joint

30

Axel Gänsslen and Jan Lindahl

There are two possible types of SI joint fracture dislocations:

- Transiliac SI joint fracture dislocation (crescent fracture)
- Transsacral SI joint fracture dislocation

30.1 Crescent Fractures

The crescent fracture was described in the pelvic ring fracture classification by Burgess et al. [1, 2]. The treatment and prognosis of this fracture type were described in detail, and this fracture was defined as a transiliac fracture dislocation of the SI joint (Fig. 30.1), which combines a ligamentous disruption of the inferior part of the SI joint with a vertical fracture line of the posterior ilium, extending from the SI joint and reaching the iliac crest at different levels [3, 4].

A crescent fracture was considered rotationally unstable but vertically stable as the pelvic floor ligaments were suspected to be intact. Operative stabilization was performed using a posterolateral approach in the prone position with lag screws and two antiglide plates on the outer side of the ilium [3, 4].

The follow-up results after a mean of 19 months of 22 patients with unilateral posterior fracture dislocations were described. All fractures healed within 3 months; no loss of reduction, nonunion, malunion, acute wound complications, and neurologic complications were reported, while one patient developed osteomyelitis.

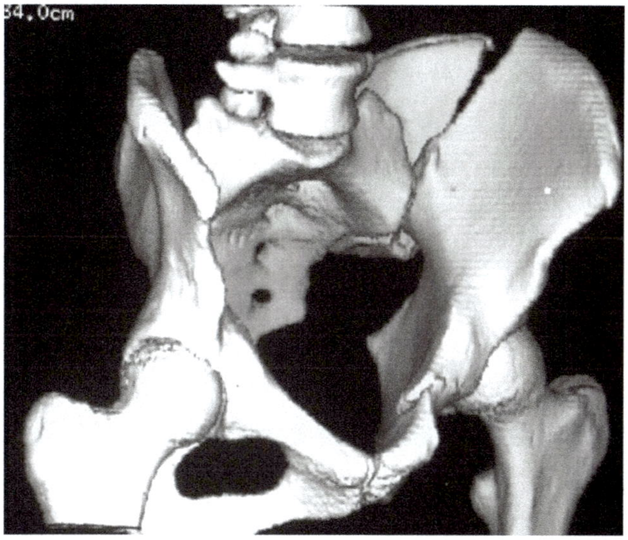

Fig. 30.1 Crescent fracture = transiliac fracture dislocation of the SI joint

30.1.1 Definition

A Crescent Fracture is defined as a combination of a ligamentous disruption of the inferior portion of the sacroiliac joint and a vertical fracture of the posterior ilium that extends from the middle of the sacroiliac joint and exits the iliac crest superiorly. The posterior superior iliac spine remains firmly attached to the sacrum via the superior portion of the posterior ligamentous complex [4].

30.1.2 Classification

Several different fracture types can be distinguished influencing the type of treatment. Day et al. proposed the presently accepted classification with three different fracture types (Fig. 30.2) and resulting treatment recommendation (Table 30.1, Fig. 30.2) [5]:

A. Gänsslen (✉)
Department of Trauma Surgery, Orthopedics and Hand Surgery, Hospital Wolfsburg, Wolfsburg, Germany

J. Lindahl
Orthopaedics and Trauma Surgery, Helsinki University Hospital, Helsinki, Finland

A. Gänsslen et al. (eds.), *Pelvic Ring Fractures*, https://doi.org/10.1007/978-3-030-54730-1_30

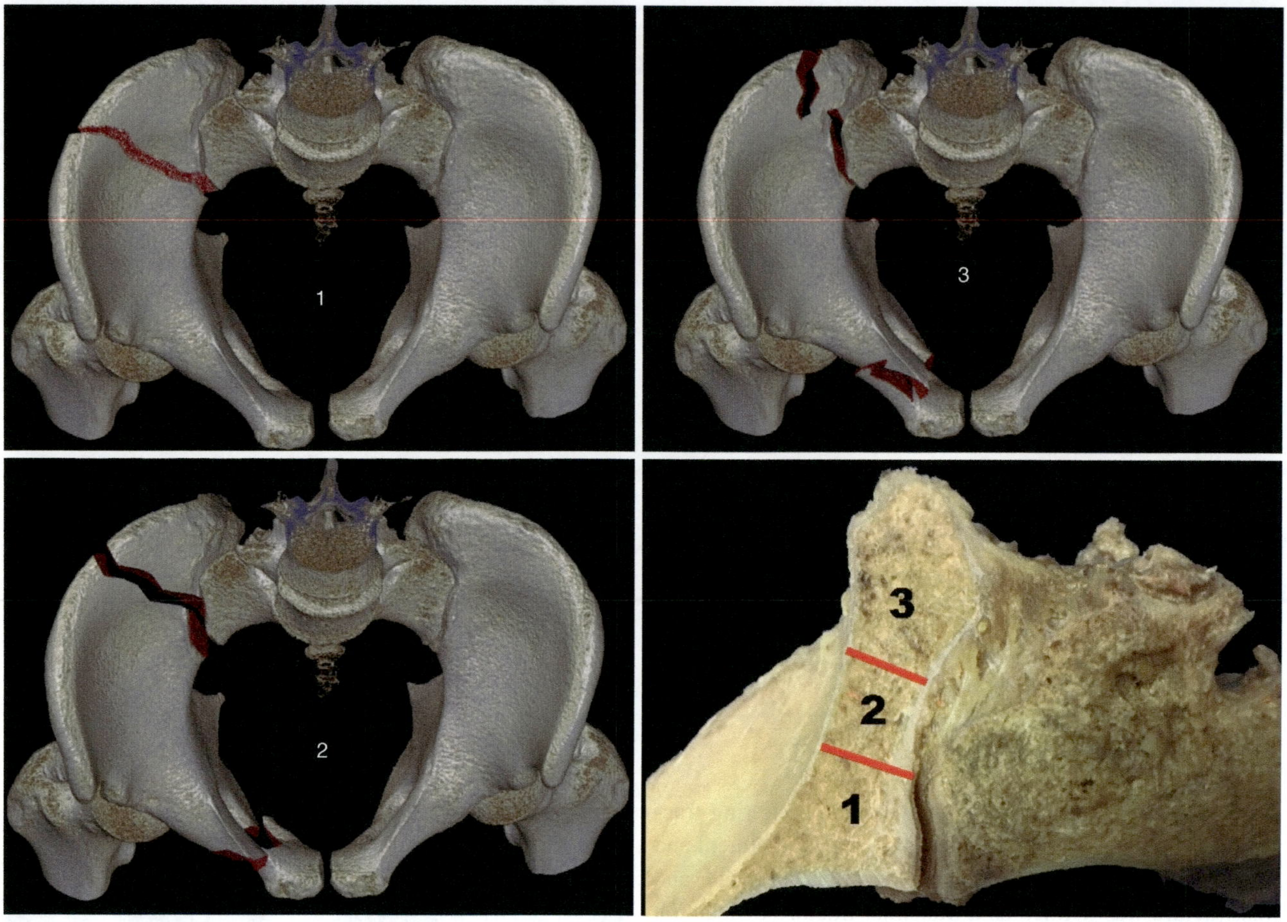

Fig. 30.2 Classification of Crescent fractures (details: see text)

Table 30.1 Day classification of crescent fractures

Type	Definition	Treatment recommendation
I	<1/3 SI joint involvement	Anterolateral approach (first window of ilioinguinal approximately), anterior SI joint plating
II	1/3–2/3 SI joint involvement	Posterior approach (Borrelli), lag screw + antigliding plates
III	>2/3 SI joint involvement	Plan A: closed/percutaneous reduction and iliosacral screw fixation Plan B: anterior SI joint plating techniques

- Type I fracture (Fig. 30.3): <1/3 SI joint involvement; fracture line enters the SI joint at its inferior parts at the level of S2 (Outlet view); large crescent fragment; anterior plate osteosynthesis of the SI joint and the fracture via the anterior-lateral approach (= first window of the ilioinguinal approach) is proposed (Fig. 30.4); reduction is advised to be performed by traction in lower extremity flexion and additional rotation control, using a percutaneously applied Schanz pin inserted at the anterior inferior iliac spine
- Type II fractures: 1/3–2/3 SI joint involvement (Fig. 30.5); fracture line enters the SI joint between the S1 and S2

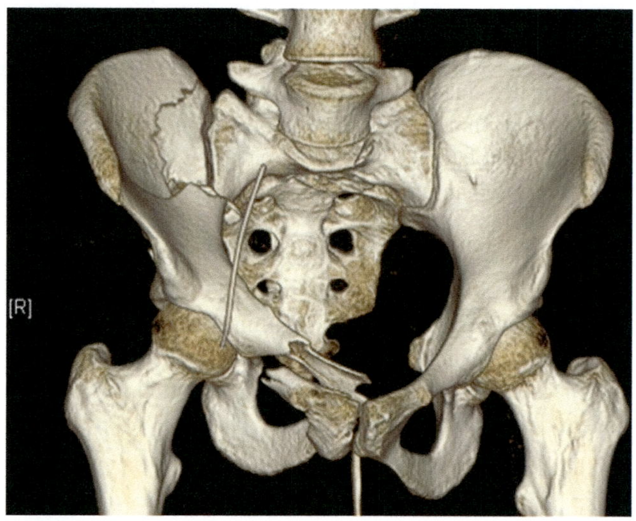

Fig. 30.3 Type I Crescent fractures involving the anterior third of the SI joint

foramina; moderate sized crescent fragment; fixation is recommended using the technique, described by Borrelli et al. [3, 4], by a posterior approach with lag screw fixa-

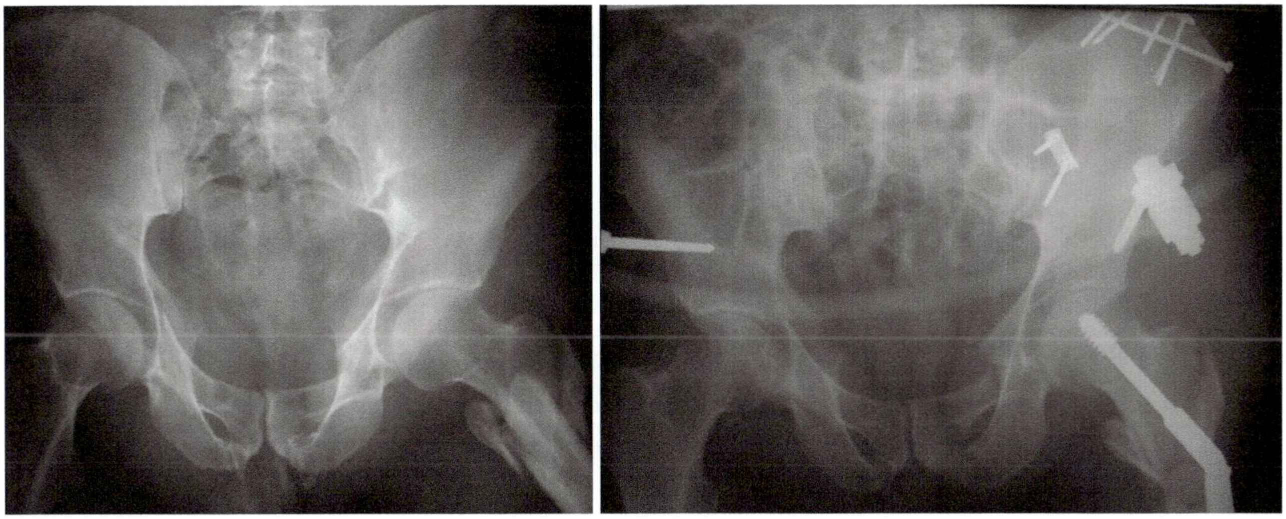

Fig. 30.4 Type I Crescent fracture: ORIF is performed without bridging the SI joint

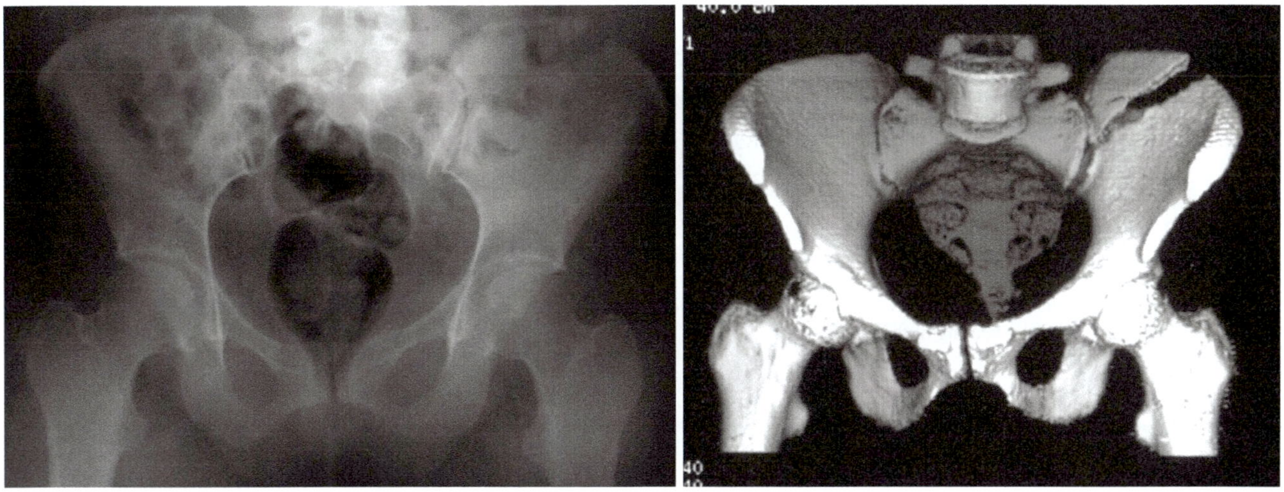

Fig. 30.5 Type II Crescent fractures involving the middle third of the SI joint

tion followed by anti-glide plating with two plates at the iliac crest and inferior at the greater sciatic notch (Fig. 30.6)

- Type III fractures: >2/3 SI joint involvement (Fig. 30.7); fracture line enters the SI joint at the S1 level; small sized, superior crescent fragment; if closed anatomic reduction is possible, percutaneous iliosacral screw fixation s recommended (Fig. 30.8); reduction is supported by skeletal traction using a traction pin placed in the proximal tibia in lower extremity flexion; control of rotational deformity is performed, using a percutaneously applied Schanz pin inserted at the anterior inferior iliac spine or at the iliac crest level; alternatively, stable anterior plate fixation of the disrupted part of the SI joint is possible (Fig. 30.9)

This classification was integrated into the classification of iliosacral injuries described by Tan et al. [6].

According to the Young-Burgess classification, crescent fractures are part of the lateral compression type II injuries and thus considered horizontally unstable but vertically stable [1, 7]. Their frequency was reported to be approximately 13% [8].

In contrast, recent reports indicated that some crescent fractures can be vertically unstable.

Zong et al. reported on four translationally unstable crescent fractures in group of 31 patients (12.9%) [9]. In contrast to the results of Borrelli et al., all patients were stable; these four patients were hemodynamically unstable at admission and were associated with complications from concomitant injuries and presented with higher injury severity.

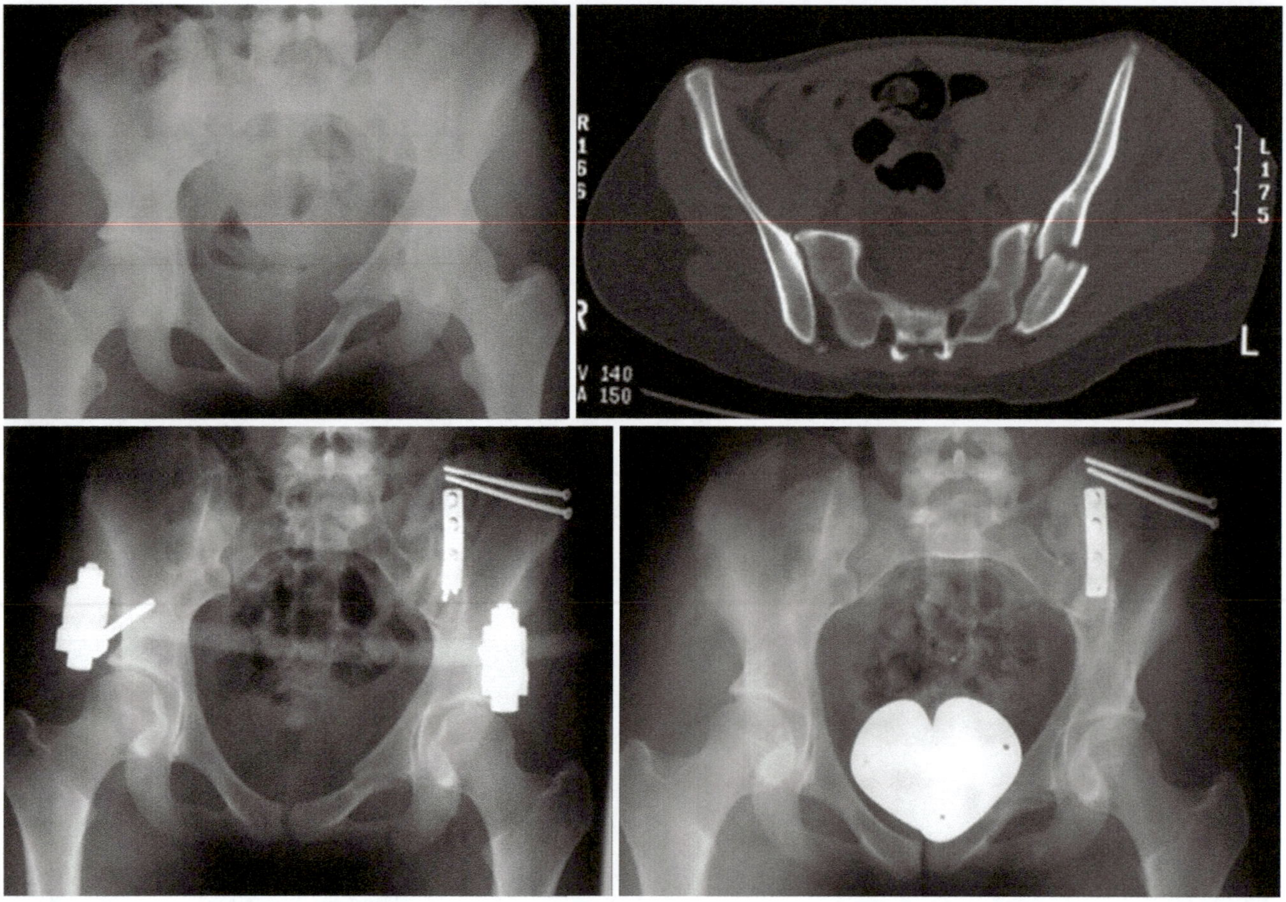

Fig. 30.6 Type II Crescent fracture: ORIF is performed without bridging the SI joint using iliac crest screws and a pelvic brim plate. Follow-up at 4 years shows near anatomic healing of the pelvic ring

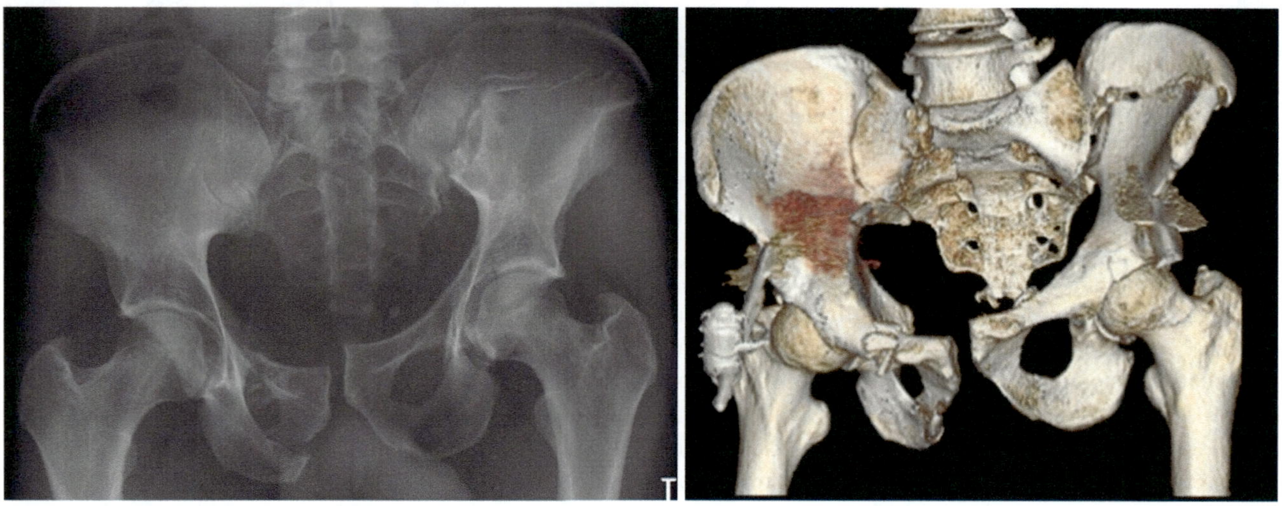

Fig. 30.7 Type III Crescent fractures involving the posterior third of the SI joint

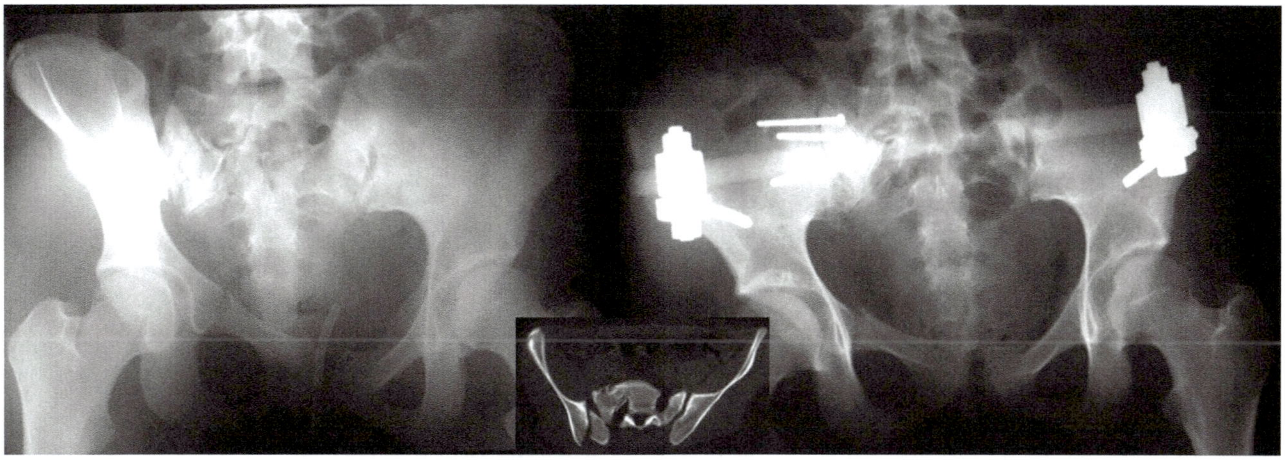

Fig. 30.8 Type III Crescent fractures: posterior screw osteosynthesis of the iliac fragment, resulting in a change from a type C into a type B injury, which was stabilized anteriorly by an external fixator

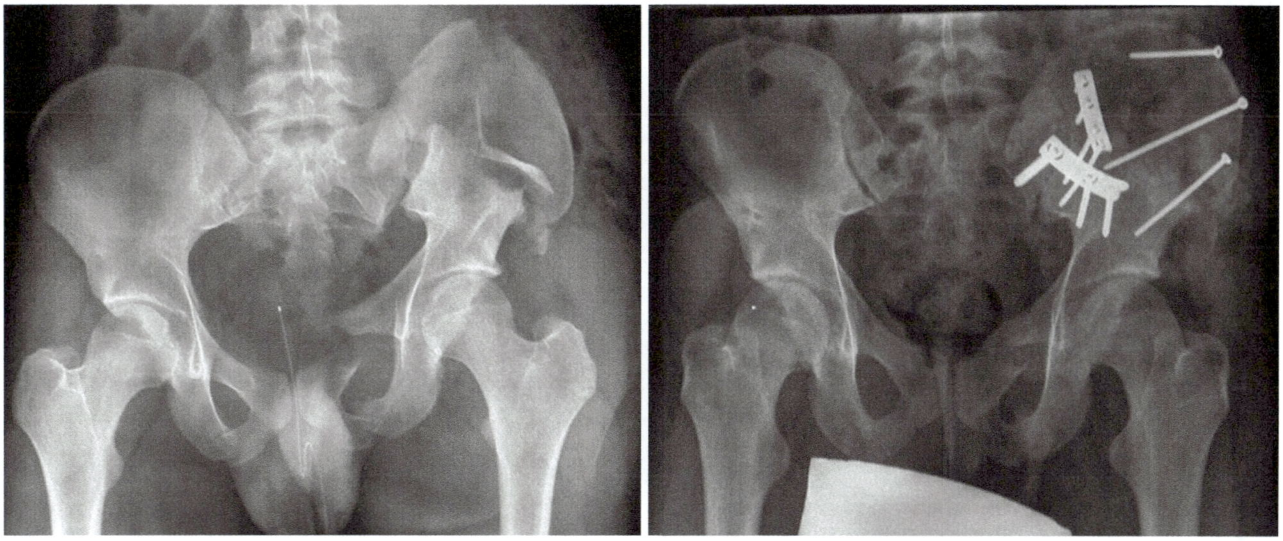

Fig. 30.9 Type III Crescent fractures: combined iliac crest screw osteosynthesis and pelvic brim plate osteosynthesis with one plate bridging the SI joint was performed

Additionally, Park et al. presented a case with vertical instability after a fall from great height [10].

Approximately 30–40% of all crescent fractures are classified as type C-injuries according to Tile [11, 12].

Between 12 and 30% of crescent-type fractures do not fit into the Day classification scheme [13].

30.1.3 Associated Injuries

According to the transferred energy resulting in these pelvic injuries, several concomitant injuries can be present:

- 23–77% head injuries [1, 3, 4]
- 9–33% chest trauma [1, 3, 4]
- 14% abdominal injuries [3]
- 9–33% intrapelvic injuries [1, 3, 4]
- 23% neurological injuries [3]
- 2% neurovascular injuries [13]
- 10% urological injuries [13]

30.1.4 Results

Several reports are dealing with treatment of classical crescent fractures (Figs. 30.10 and 30.11).

Borrelli et al. first reported on 22 patients with unilateral crescent fractures without presenting data of operative details, additional anterior ring stabilization, and functional

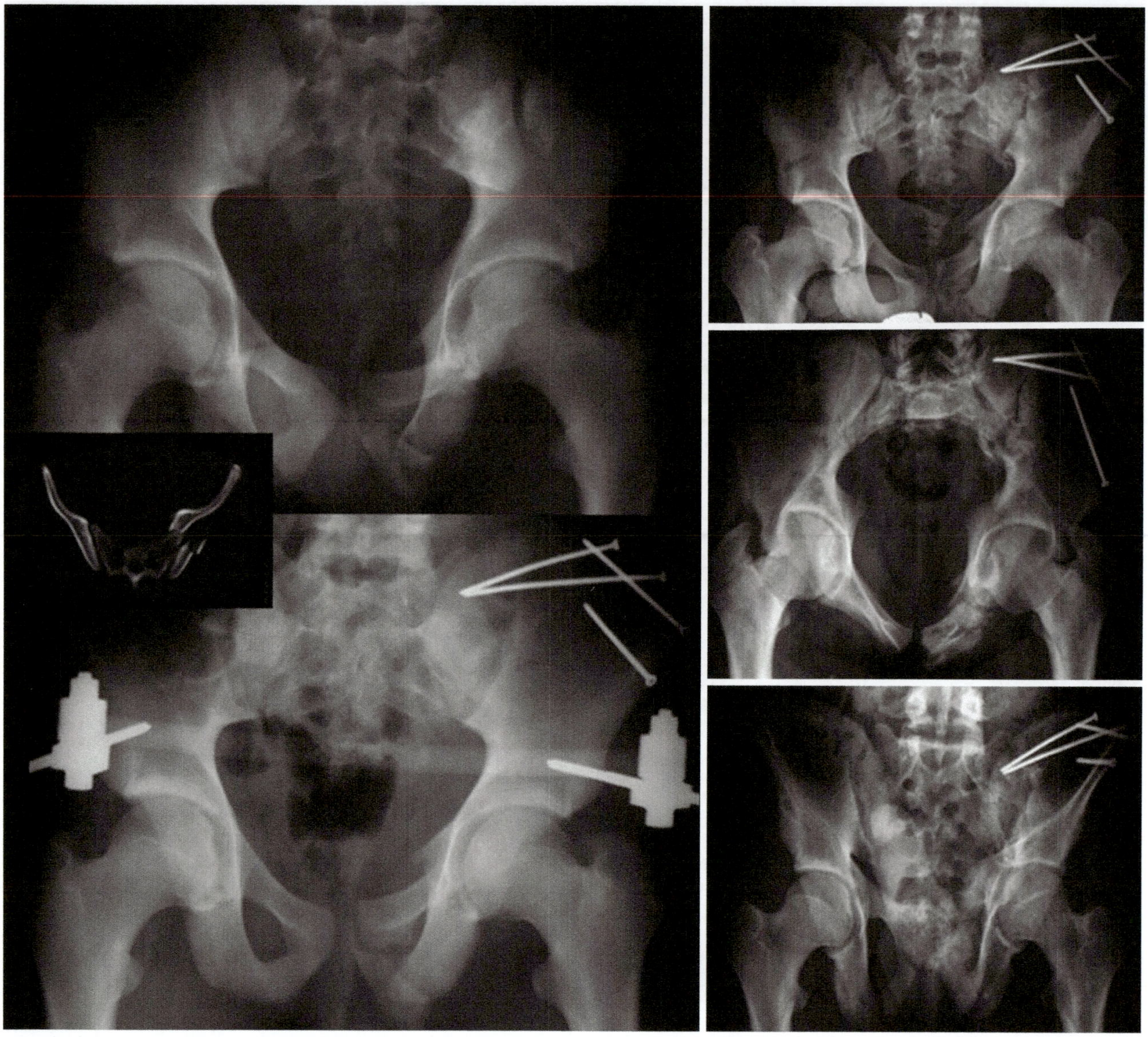

Fig. 30.10 Anterior Crescent fracture with dislocation of the iliac fragment anterior to the sacrum: screw osteosynthesis for near anatomic reduction. Three-year follow-up

results [3, 4]. All fractures healed within 3 months with 95.5% anatomical healing. The complication rate was low (4.5%). One patient developed iliac osteomyelitis, which resolved after debridement, hardware removal, and intravenous antibiotics.

Kim et al. reported on 19 patients (mean age, 47.4 years) with crescent fracture dislocations (7× type I, 9× type II, 3× type III) [14]. Except two patients with nonunion after ORIF, 17 patients healed between 3 and 4 months. Additional anterior pelvic ring fixation was highly recommended for achieving better results. Anatomic posterior reconstruction was achieved in seven cases. The functional result was graded excellent in 9 and 76.5% being satisfactory. Complications related to the posterior osteosynthesis were observed in 3/19 patients.

Menon et al. stated that not every fracture fit into the Day classification scheme [11].

Thus, several case reports are dealing with special crescent fracture configurations.

Stevens et al. presented a case of bilateral posterior sacroiliac fracture dislocations after axial trauma, resulting in anterior sacrum displacement. No anterior pelvic ring was present. This fracture type more corresponds to a spinopelvic dissociation injury than a typical SI joint injury [15].

O'Neill et al. reported on a case of bilateral crescent fractures with bilateral anterior pelvic ring injury [16]. After plate osteosynthesis of the anterior pelvic ring, percutaneous stabilization of the crescent fractures was performed with iliosacral screws and anterior supraacetabular screws. At the

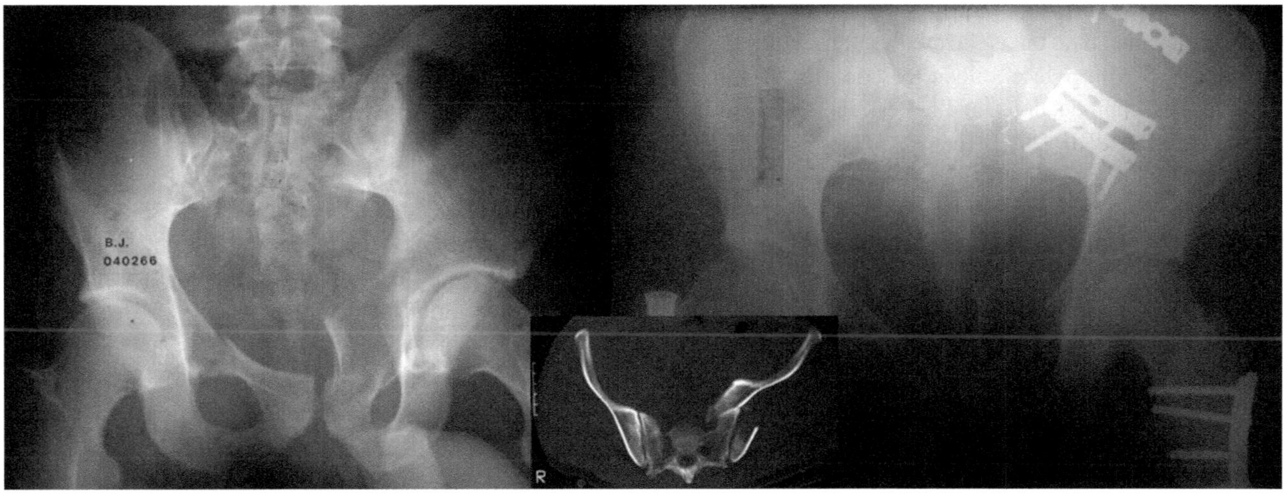

Fig. 30.11 Anterior Crescent fracture with dislocation of the iliac fragment anterior to the sacrum: plate osteosynthesis for near anatomic reduction

16 months follow-up, all fractures were healed and an excellent functional result was reported.

Sobhan et al. reported on five patients (mean age 33 years, four male patients) after high-energy trauma [17]. Two patients developed local infection and one patient had persistent displacement of 2 cm after primary displacement of 55 mm. In this patient surgical delay of 45 days after trauma was reported. After a mean of 40 months, the mean Majeed Score was 87 points.

Larger series were reported during the last years.

Calafi et al. analyzed 100 patients with crescent-type fractures and a follow-up of at least 3 months. There were 57 males and 43 females, the average age was 42 years, and the mean ISS was 25.5. According to Day, 16 type I, 47 type II, and 37 type III crescent fractures were diagnosed. Twelve percent of these injuries did not fit into the Day scheme. Percutaneous iliosacral screw fixation was possible in 60%, which was predominantly performed in type II and III injuries, while type I injuries had ORIF in the majority of cases. At 3 months, no patient suffered from pain or nonunion. Five patients developed malunion [13].

Shui et al. analyzed the treatment in 117 patients [12]. Seventy-three patients with closed reduction and stabilization (group I) were compared with 44 patients treated by ORIF (group II). In group I, anterior pelvic ring stabilization was performed prior to posterior stabilization. The posterior injury was treated depending on the fracture type according to the Day classification. Type I injuries got parallel screw fixation either from anterior or posterior, type II injuries were treated with crossing screws, and type III injuries with iliosacral screws. ORIF was performed using the described techniques using the ilioinguinal or posterior approach.

As expected, group I patients showed less blood loss, less extensive exposure, less duration of surgery, less duration of hospital stay, and a reduced infection rate. The reduction quality showed a postoperative mean displacement of 4.2 mm in group I and 3.6 mm in group II. At latest follow-up (mean 14 months, minimal 6 months), the mean displacement was 6.5 mm in group I and 8.3 mm in group II, indicating some secondary displacement.

The functional outcome according to the Majeed score was superior in group I: 86 points vs. 81 points in group II.

Khaled et al. assessed the clinical results in 43 patients (34 male, 9 female patients) with an average age of 37.3 years after high-energy trauma [18]. These patients were classified according to Young-Burges (21× CM, 22× LC) and Tile (27× type C, 16× type B). According to Day, there were 31.8% type I, 40.9% type II, and 27.3% type III injuries. In 45.5% isolated percutaneous screws were used for stabilization, isolated plate osteosynthesis in 50%, and a combination of both in 4.5%. In 60.4% additional anterior pelvic ring fixation was performed. No information was given regarding "anterior first" or "posterior first." No wound complications, surgery-related neurological complications, or residual rotational deformity were observed. All fractures healed.

At a mean follow-up of 53 months, the mean Majeed Score was 86.2 points, indicating an excellent result. Only two patients showed a poor clinical result. A tendency for better Majeed scores was observed with percutaneous stabilizations.

Recently, Menon et al. reported on ten functional long-term results after a mean of 17 months using the Majeed Score [11]. The average modified Majeed Score was 77.5/96, which are graded as good and excellent, respectively.

> Percutaneous fixation is favored as this concept is associated with reduced blood loss, shorter operative time, less complications, and better functional results compared to ORIF [12, 18].

30.1.5 Anterior Fracture Dislocation (Fig. 30.11)

Magu et al. presented a case with an anterior fracture dislocation with dislocation of the posterior ilium anterior to the sacral ala, associated with a relevant lumbar plexus injury, making nerve root decompression necessary with partial recovery after 14 months [19]. Stabilization was performed with anterior plate stabilization and iliac crest screw osteosynthesis.

Trikha et al. presented four further cases with anterior fracture dislocation of the SI joint [20].

- 26 year old male, MVA, hemodynamically stable (SI = 1); symphyseal disruption; L5 nerve root injury (foot drop); Pfannenstiel incision and first window of ilioinguinal approach; decompression L5 nerve root; anterior SI joint plate osteosynthesis; 2-year follow-up: all pretrauma activities, full nerve recovery
- 28 year old male, pedestrian hit by truck, hemodynamically stable; bilateral posterior injury: right classical posterior fracture dislocation of the SI joint, left anterior crescent fracture; ipsilateral rami fractures; first reduction and fixation of left SI joint via first window; second posterior approach and closed reduction + percutaneous screw fixation right crescent fracture; 18-month follow-up: excellent functional result
- 36 year old male, fall from height, bilateral posterior injury: right anterior crescent fracture type Day III, left classical posterior fracture dislocation of the SI joint; bilateral pubic rami fractures; bilateral anterior plate osteosynthesis; 14-month follow-up: all pretrauma activities
- 29 year old male, fall from height; hemodynamically unstable; multiple injuries; anterior SI joint plating + percutaneous screw fixation of the ilium; 12-month follow-up: unaided walking, no pain

Park et al. reported an excellent clinical result 2.5 years after a fall from great height with vertically unstable crescent fractures treated with anterior SI joint plating and iliac crest screw osteosynthesis [10].

30.1.6 Posterolateral Approach to the SI Joint

The posterolateral approach to the SI joint was described by Borrelli et al. for the treatment of crescent fractures of the posterior pelvic ring [3, 4], which is based on the original description by Joel Matta [21]. However, French et al. clearly recommend anterior pelvic ring stabilization prior to addressing the crescent fracture [22].

30.1.6.1 Positioning

Surgery is performed under general anesthesia in the standard prone position. A complete radiolucent table is preferred. Support of the left and right anterior chest and abdomen is recommended. The pelvis is left free, so even after anterior stabilization, e.g., with an external fixator prior to posterior stabilization, positioning is easy.

30.1.6.2 Draping

The whole or ipsilateral posterior pelvic region, including the buttock, and iliac wing is draped. Depending on the displacement and the side, the lower extremity is additionally draped free [3, 4]. This also allows somatosensory-evoked potential monitoring.

30.1.6.3 Incision

A curvilinear or longitudinal incision starts 1–2 cm lateral to the top of the iliac crest and runs parallel 1–2 cm lateral to the posterior superior iliac spine (PSIS) and posterior inferior iliac spine (PIIS) (Fig. 30.12) [3, 4, 22–24].

Caudal extension is important when exposure of the greater sciatic notch and the inferior portion of the sacroiliac joint is planned [23].

Incision length must be adequate depending on the fracture morphology (Fig. 30.13) to allow medial exposure. Matta recommended an incision starting 5 cm proximal to the iliac crest and ending 5 cm distal to the superior border of the greater sciatic notch [21].

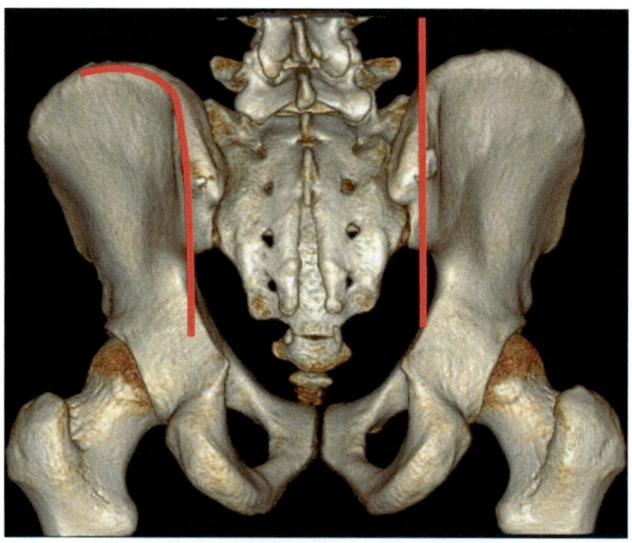

Fig. 30.12 Two possible skin incisions for the posterior approach to the iliac wing and SI joint

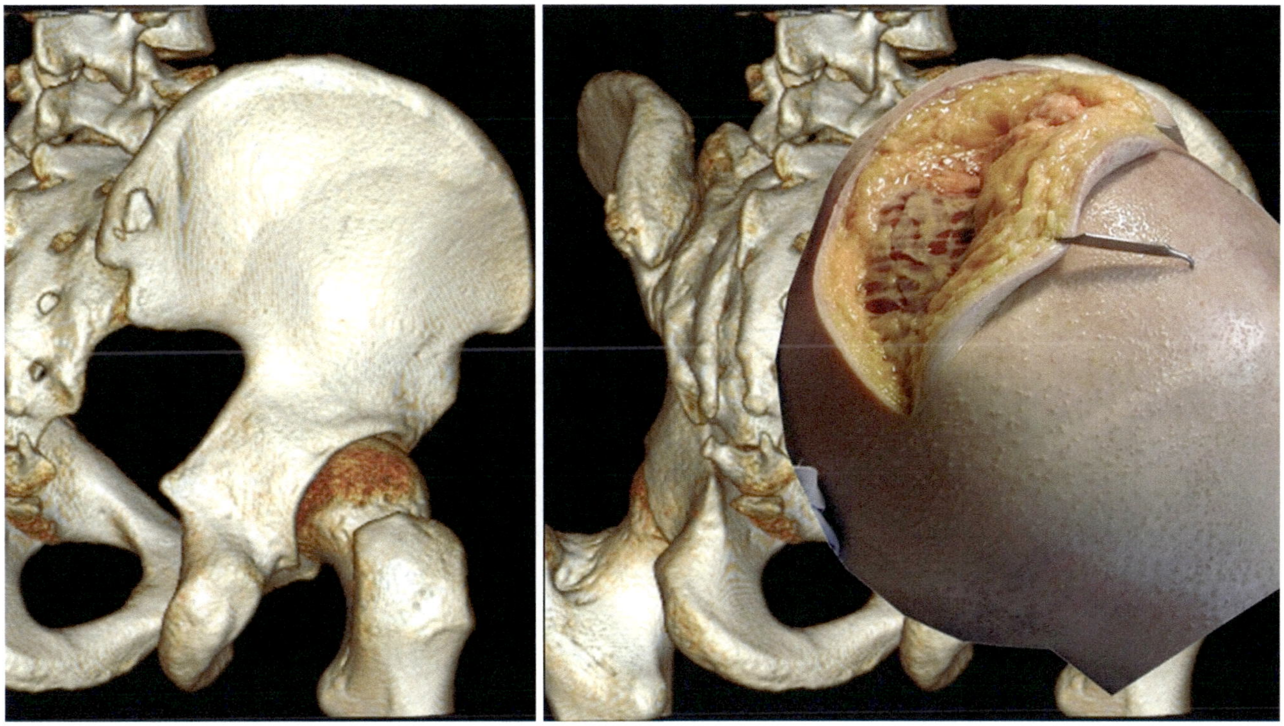

Fig. 30.13 Skin incision, starting at the mid iliac crest and running to the ischial spine

30.1.6.4 Superficial Dissection

The superficial dissection should be performed in line with the skin incision [23] until the gluteus maximus fascia is identified. Fowler et al. recommended not to create a subcutaneous flap to avoid any dead space, while Matta proposed some subcutaneous mobilization [21]. The gluteus maximus origin is identified at the posterior iliac crest and the sacrum (Fig. 30.14).

30.1.6.5 Deep Dissection

Sharp incision of the iliac crest periosteum is performed for direct subperiosteal dissection to reflect the gluteus maximus and part of the gluteus medius from the iliac crest, PSIS, PIIS, and the outer surface of the iliac wing (Fig. 30.14). Often some detachment of the gluteus maximus from the posterior and lateral sacral from the underlying multifidus fascia surface is necessary [21].

The localization of the nervi clunii should be considered as the main medial branch is located approximately 8 cm lateral to the midline and 6.5 cm lateral to the PSIS at the superior iliac crest. The nerve runs through a fascial tunnel and is, therefore, at risk for compression injuries [25].

Inferiorly, detachment of the muscle from the sacrotuberous ligament can be necessary (Fig. 30.15). A tendinous strip can be dissected for easier later reconstruction [22].

The fracture morphology determines the lateral and anterior extension of dissection of the abductor complex [23].

Developing a full gluteal flap, based on the superior gluteal neurovascular bundle, is not always necessary in crescent-type fractures. The course of the superior gluteal neurovascular bundle has to be respected (Fig. 30.15).

Exposure of the greater sciatic notch leads to optimal anatomic reduction of the SI joint. Insertion of a curved periosteal elevator at the anterior aspect of the sacrum after dissecting the piriformis origin can protect the neurovascular bundle. The inferior SI joint becomes visible, and the anterior part of the SI joint with the anterior lateral sacral ala can be palpated (Fig. 30.15).

Extending the dissection more medially to the PSIS by elevation of the erector spinae from the dorsal sacrum (Fig. 30.16), the posterior sacral foramina can be visualized, which can be helpful to reduce the SI joint part of the injury [22].

30.1.6.6 Fracture Cleaning

By inserting a laminar spreader into the iliac wing fracture, the disrupted part of the SI joint is visualized and the joint is debrided.

Inferior dissection to visualize the upper greater sciatic notch can be helpful to control the reduction under digital control.

30.1.6.7 Reduction

The iliac wing fracture is first reduced under direct visualization. A large Weber reduction forceps can be used, with

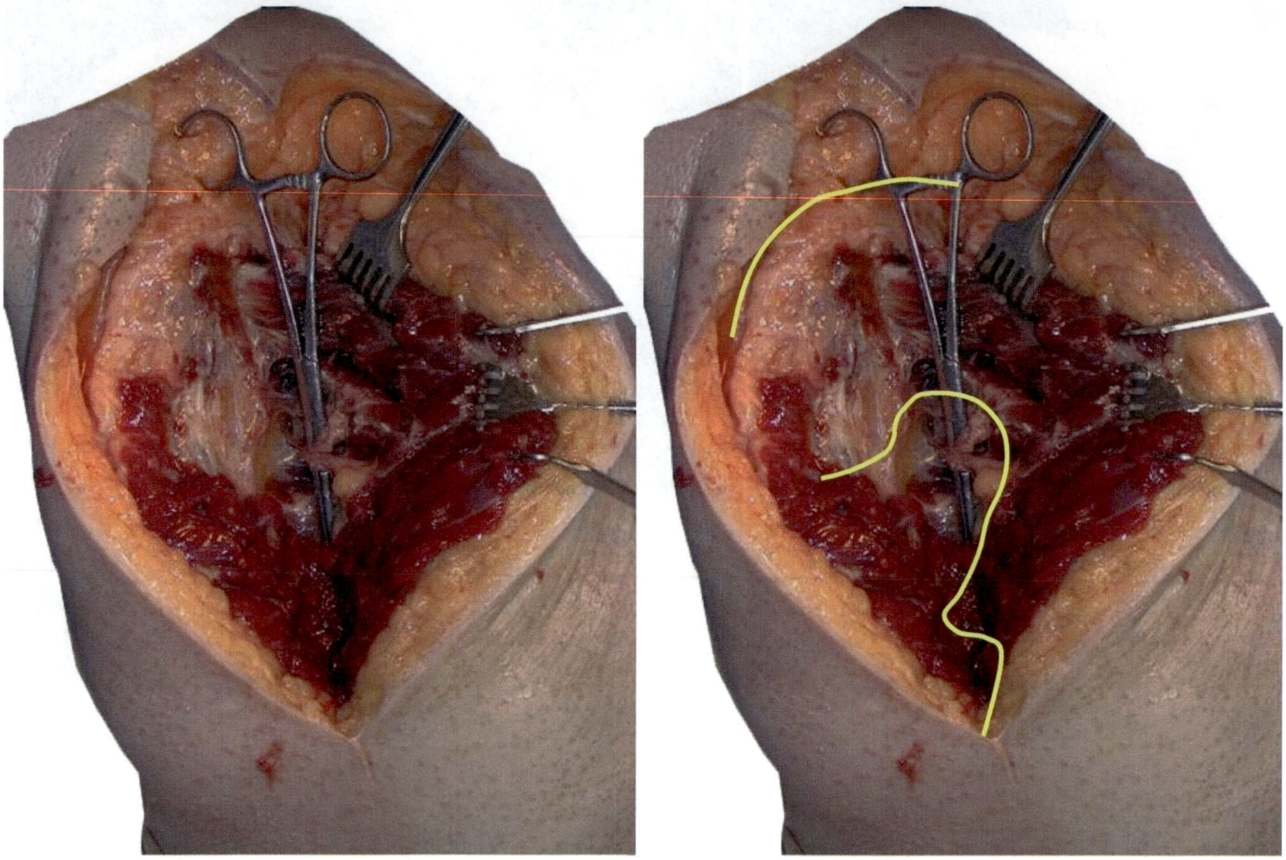

Fig. 30.14 Mobilization/dissection of the gluteus maximus muscle from the iliac crest, the sacrum, and the sacrotuberous ligament. Identification of the greater sciatic notch with the gluteal superior neurovascular bundle undermined

positioning of one sidearm at the PSIS or the iliac crest, depending on the fracture localization, and the other at the iliac wing (Fig. 30.17). Temporary fixation is possible with one or two 2.0 mm K-wires, inserted from the PSIS across the fracture.

Reduction of the SI joint can be digitally controlled by inserting a finger into the greater sciatic notch (Fig. 30.18). Inserting a reduction forceps (angled ball spike forceps according to Matta) through the greater sciatic notch to the anterior sacrum can reduce the SI joint part of the fracture (Fig. 30.19). The superior gluteal neurovascular bundle and, anterior to the sacrum, the L5 nerve root have to be protected.

Alternatively, medial mobilization of the erector spinae and the multifidi muscles allows SI joint visualization by insertion of laminar spreaders between the sacrum and the PSIS for SI joint debridement (Fig. 30.20).

30.1.6.8 Definitive Fixation

Parallel to the applied K-wires 3.5 or 4.5 mm lag screws are inserted perpendicular to the fracture line. Depending on the bone quality, washers can be useful. Borrelli et al. recommended additional application of two 3.5 mm antiglide plates on the outer iliac surface lateral below the iliac crest and inferior crossing the fracture line (Fig. 30.21).

In type III injuries according to Day, iliosacral screw fixation can be optional performed.

The entry points on the outer iliac surface can be identified on a connecting line between the iliac crest and the greater sciatic notch, approximately 15 mm anterior to the posterior gluteal line.

The anatomical basis of this approach is shown in Fig. 30.22.

30.1.6.9 Wound Closure

After irrigation with a pulsatile irrigation system, drainage is recommended and the fascia of the gluteus maximus muscle is reattached.

30.1.6.10 Postoperative Course

Standard x-ray imaging is performed and a CT scan can be useful to analyze the quality of reduction in detail.

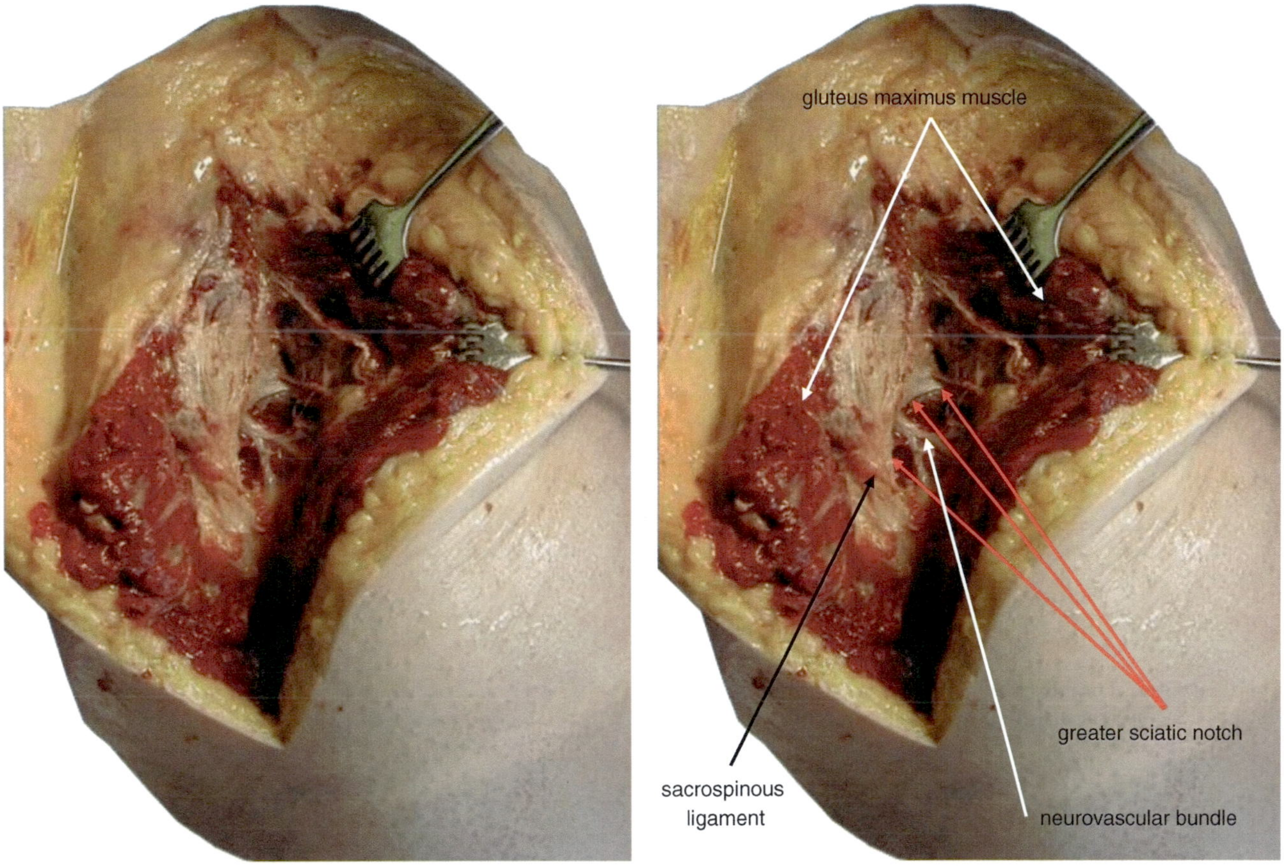

Fig. 30.15 Complete dissection of the gluteus maximus muscle with full exposure of the greater sciatic notch

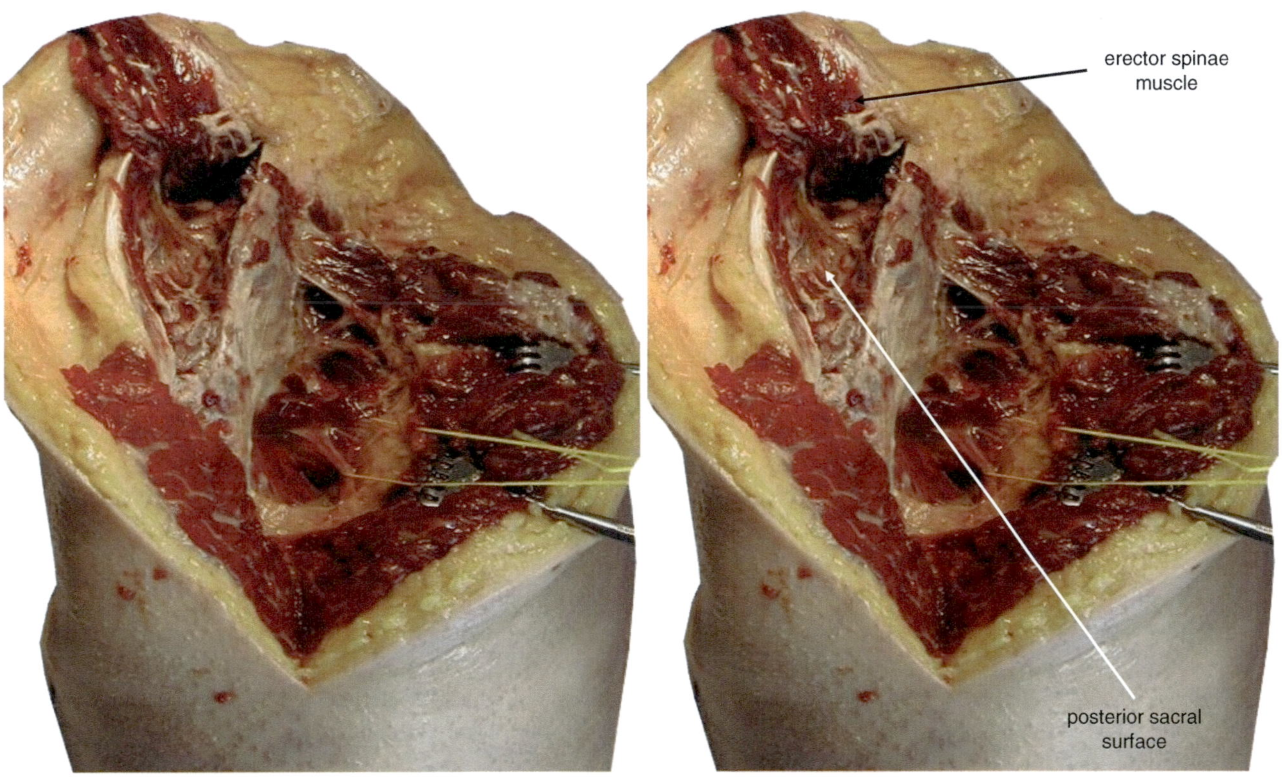

Fig. 30.16 Additional dissection of the erector spinae muscle of the posterior sacral surface for full exposure

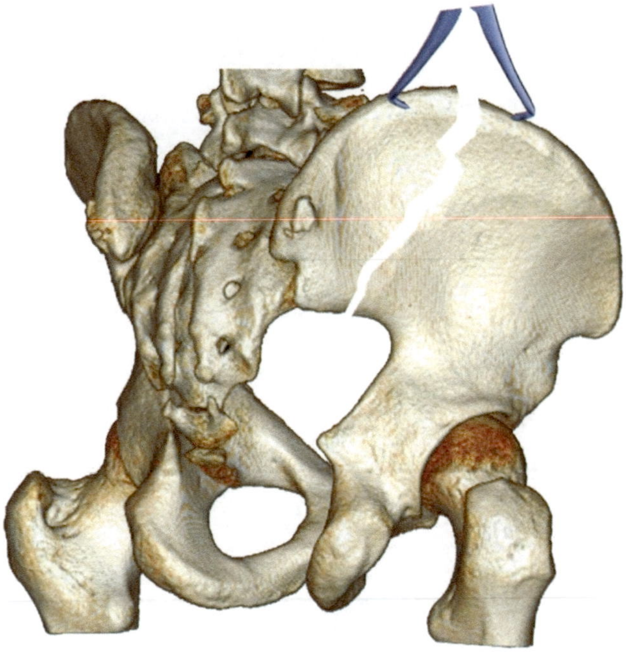

Fig. 30.17 Reduction using a large Weber reduction forceps with positioning of one sidearm at the PSIS and the other at the iliac wing

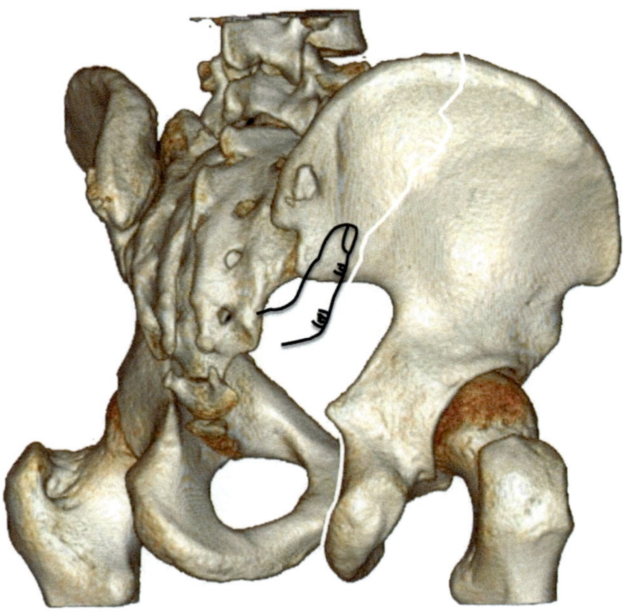

Fig. 30.18 Visualization of the inferior and part of the anterior SI joint and palpation of the anterior lateral sacral surface

30.1.7 Summary

In crescent fractures (Day type I, II, and III):

- Percutaneous iliosacral screw fixation is recommended, if closed anatomic reduction is possible
- Anterior plate fixation of the disrupted part of the SI joint, when open reduction and internal fixation is needed

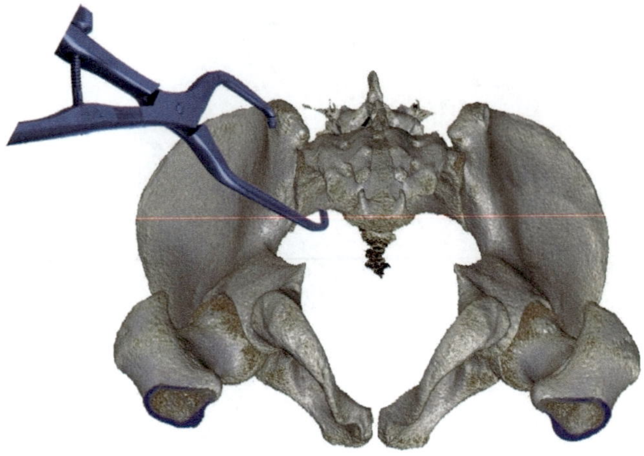

Fig. 30.19 Reduction with an angled ball spike forceps acc. to Matta through the greater sciatic notch to the anterior sacrum

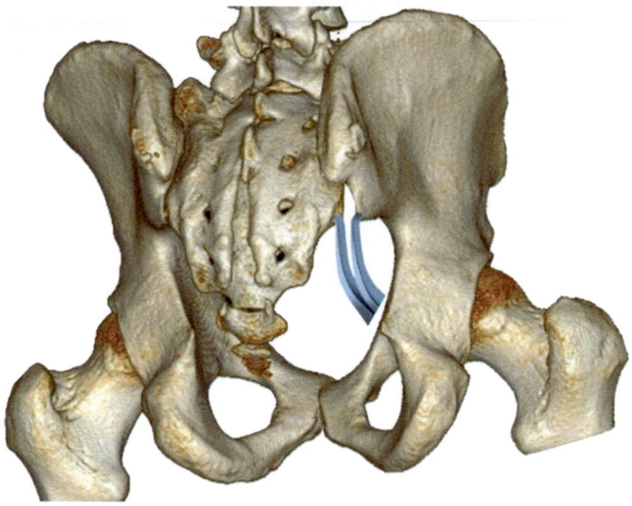

Fig. 30.20 Alternatively, medial mobilization of the erector spinae and the multifidi muscles allows SI joint debridement directly from posterior using a laminar spreader

- Posterior approach with lag screw and plate fixation is associated with more soft-tissue complications

30.2 Transsacral Fracture Dislocation

In contrast to transiliac fracture dislocations, better known as crescent fractures, transsacral fracture dislocations are extremely rare entities in pelvic ring fractures. Accordingly, a clear stabilization concept is missing.

In the literature, no articles are dealing with this specific fracture type. As the posterior ilium is much weaker than the corresponding lateral sacrum (sacral ala), this is the potential reason for this rare frequency.

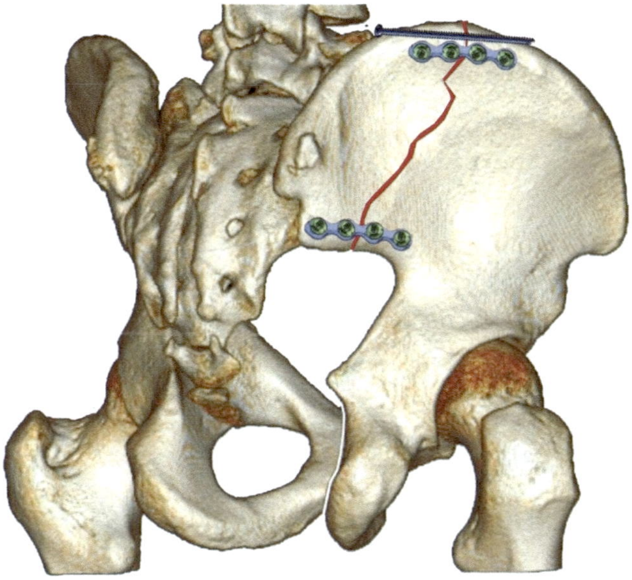

Fig. 30.21 Options for fixation of the ilium fracture from the outer side

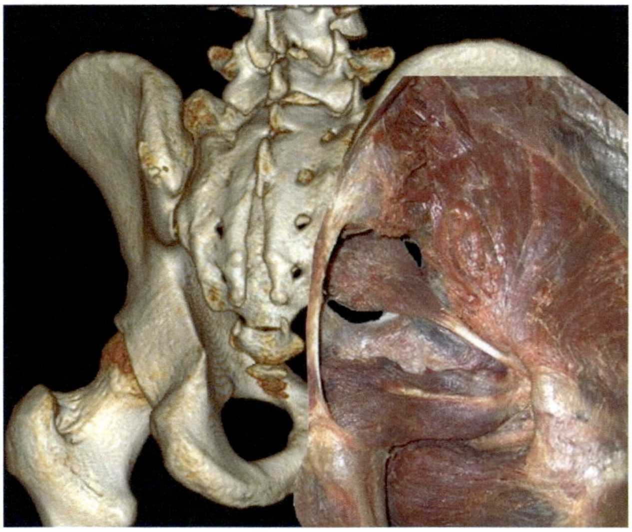

Fig. 30.22 Anatomical basis of the posterior approach

Pohlemann et al. developed a sacral fracture classification scheme, which integrated this fracture type [26, 27]. Type I injuries consists of fractures of the sacral ala. Pohlemann described a subtype with a superior/cranial sacral fragment (type Ia) (Fig. 30.23).

The fracture localization is limited to the cranial part of the sacrum and therefore usually an expression of a transsacral fracture dislocation of the SI joint. This fracture type was observed in 28 patients. Three patients showed injury to the L5/S1 nerve roots without accompanying cauda symptoms. Ten patients presented without neurological deficits and in 15 patients no data on neurological deficits were stated in their patient reports.

Overall, the frequency of this fracture type was 0.9%, with 10.1% presenting with neurological impairments [26].

In the German Multicenter Study Pelvis revealed, this fracture type was observed in 23 patients [28]. In nine cases this injury was classified as a lateral compression injury, representing 7% of all LC-injuries. In 16 cases this injury was classified as a type C injury, representing 13.1% of all type C-injuries. In the group of all pelvic ring injuries ($n = 1356$), this fracture type represents 1.8% of injuries [28].

The following treatment recommendations were stated:

- small sacrum fragments are not reduced as stabilization of the SI joint is performed using anterior plate osteosynthesis (Fig. 30.24) (as for pure SI joint dislocations)
- fracture dislocations with a large sacral fragment are treated by open posterior stabilization of the SI joint as described by French et al. [29], or rarely, open posterior sacral stabilization techniques may be useful

Recently, Murphy et al., showed x-rays of such a case treated by anterior plate osteosynthesis of the SI joint [30].

Due to a lack of experience with this type of injury in the literature, no clear treatment concept can be proposed from the literature.

Own experience guide to three treatment recommendations:

- small anterior or posterior sacrum fragments can be stabilized by anterior SI joint plating (Fig. 30.24)
- in larger fragments screw osteosynthesis is favored (Fig. 30.25)
- in comminuted sacral fractures distraction plate osteosynthesis (ilio-iliacal plating) or lumbopelvic fixation techniques are considered

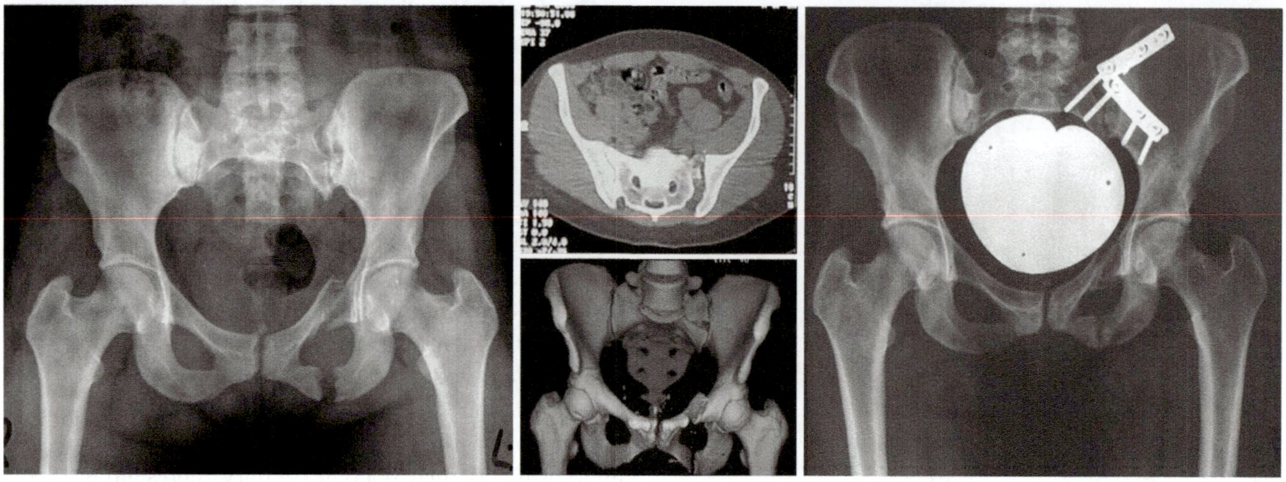

Fig. 30.23 Type Ia sacral injury according to Pohlemann

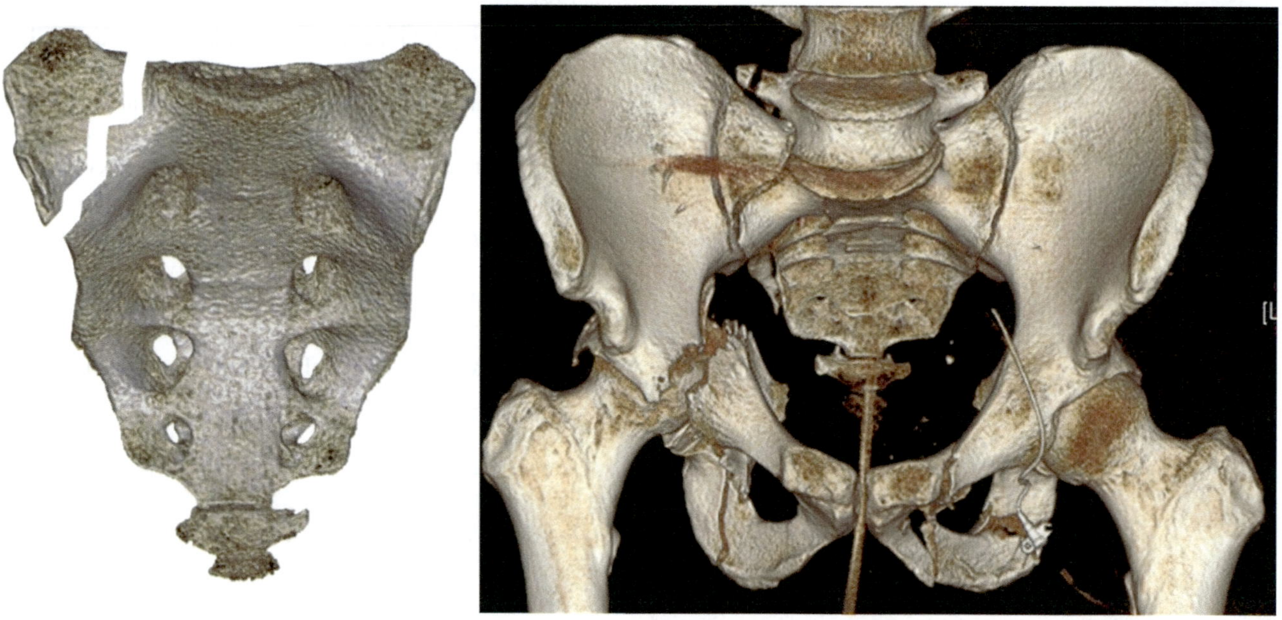

Fig. 30.24 Case of a combined transsacral fracture dislocation and an acetabular fracture, posteriorly treated with anterior SI joint plating

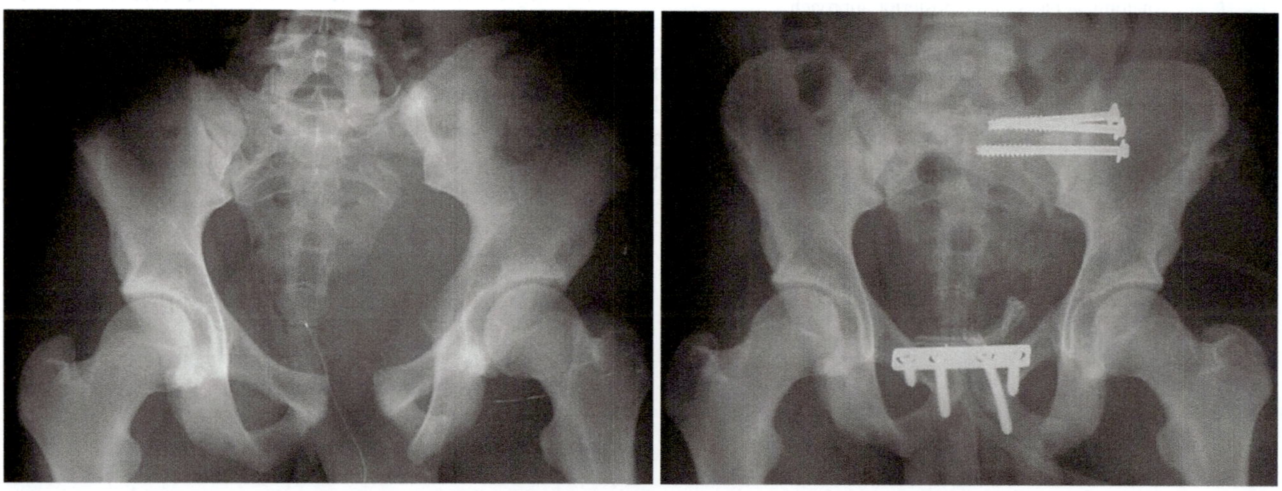

Fig. 30.25 Case of a left sacral fracture dislocation treated with SI-screws

References

1. Burgess A, Eastridge B, Young J, Ellison T, Ellison P, Poka A, Bathon G, Brumback R. Pelvic ring disruption: effective classification systems and treatment protocols. J Trauma. 1990;30(7):848–56.
2. Lange R, Webb L, Mayo K. Efficacy of the anterior approach for fixation of sacroiliac dislocations and fracture-dislocations [Abstract]. J Orthop Trauma. 1990;4:220–1.
3. Borrelli J, Koval K, Helfet D. The crescent fracture: a posterior fracture dislocation of the sacroiliac joint. J Orthop Trauma. 1996;10:165–70.
4. Borrelli J, Koval K, Helfet D. Operative stabilization of fracture dislocations of the sacroiliac joint. Clin Orthop Relat Res. 1996;329:141–6.
5. Day A, Kinmont C, Bircher M, Kumar S. Crescent fracture-dislocation of the sacroiliac joint. A functional classification. J Bone Joint Surg. 2007;89-B:651–8.
6. Tan Z, Huang Z, Li L, Meng W, Liu L, Zhang H, Wang G, Huang F. [Classification and treatment of sacroiliac joint dislocation]. [Article in Chinese]. Sichuan Da Xue Xue Bao Yi Xue Ban. 2017;48:661–7.
7. Young JW, Burgess AR, Brumback RJ, Poka A. Pelvic fractures: value of plain radiography in early assessment and management. Radiology. 1986;160(2):445–51.
8. Weaver M, Bruinsma W, Toney E, Dafford E, Vrahas M. What are the patterns of injury and displacement seen in lateral compression pelvic fractures? Clin Orthop Relat Res. 2012;470:2104–10.
9. Zong Z, Chen S, Jia M, Shen Y, Hua X, Liu D. Posterior iliac crescent fracture-dislocation: is it only rotationally unstable? Orthopedics. 2014;37:435–40.
10. Park S, Lee S, Kim W, Park Y. Atypical pelvic crescent fracture caused by vertical shear force. Hip Pelvis. 2014;26:194–7.
11. Menon K, Suresh S, Kalyanasundaram S, Varughese J. Crescent fractures of the pelvis treated by open reduction and internal fixation: a critique of Day's guidelines. Eur J Orthop Surg Traumatol. 2017;27:1089–95.
12. Shui X, Ying X, Mao C, Feng Y, Chen L, Kong J, Guo X, Wang G. Percutaneous screw fixation of crescent fracture-dislocation of the sacroiliac joint. Orthopedics. 2015;38:976–82.
13. Calafi L, Routt M. Posterior iliac crescent fracture-dislocation: what morphological variations are amenable to iliosacral screw fixation? Injury. 2013;44:194–8.
14. Kim H, Oh C, Kim P, Byun Y, Kim J, Park B, Min W, Lee H. Crescent fracture-dislocation of sacroiliac joint: affecting factors of operative results. J Korean Fracture Soc. 2009;22:71–8.
15. Stevens K, Preston B, Hahn D. Bilateral fracture dislocation of the sacroiliac joint. Skelet Radiol. 1997;26:556–8.
16. O'Neill F, Leonard M, Morris S. A bilateral crescent and anterior ring pelvic fracture sustained by inadvertently performing the 'splits'. J Surg Case Rep. 2012;9:11.
17. Sobhan M, Abrisham S, Vakili M, Saeed Shirdel S. Fixation of sacroiliac joint fractures and fracture-dislocations: a clinical 8 years follow-up study. Arch Bone Jt Surg. 2016;4:381–6.
18. Khaled S, Abdel Karim M, Abdel-Azeem A. Management of crescent fracture–dislocation of the sacroiliac joint: iliosacral screws versus plate fixation. Egypt Orthop J. 2016;51:231–7.
19. Magu N, Singla R, Gogna P, Amanpreetz, Jain N, Aggarwal S. Lumbar plexus injury in an anterior fracture dislocation of sacroiliac joint: a case report and review of literature. Strategies Trauma Limb Reconstr. 2013;8:181–5.
20. Trikha V, Singh V, Kumar V. Anterior fracture dislocation of sacroiliac joint: a rare type of crescent fracture. Indian J Orthop. 2015;49:255–9.
21. Matta J. Surgical approaches to fractures of the acetabulum and pelvis. 1989. www.mizuhosi.com.
22. French B, Tornetta P. Transiliosakrale Osteosynthese bei instabilen Verletzugen des hinteren Bekenringes. Oper Orthop Traumatol. 2002;14:29–49.
23. Fowler T, Bishop J, Bellino M. The posterior approach to pelvic ring injuries: a technique for minimizing soft tissue complications. Injury. 2013;44:1780–6.
24. Stover M, Sims S, Matta J. What is the infection rate of the posterior approach to type C pelvic injuries? Clin Orthop Relat Res. 2012;470:2142–7.
25. Lu J, Ebraheim N, Huntoon M, Heck B, Yeasting R. Anatomic considerations of superior cluneal nerve at posterior iliac crest region. Clin Orthop Relat Res. 1998;347:224–8.
26. Pohlemann T, Gänsslen A, Tscherne H. Die Problematik der Sakrumfraktur, klinische Analyse von 377 Fällen. Orthopade. 1992;21:400–12.
27. Pohlemann T, Gänsslen A, Tscherne H. Die Sakrumfraktur. Unfallchirurg. 2000;103:769–86.
28. Pohlemann T, Gänsslen A, Hartung S, für die Arbeitsgruppe Becken, H.T., H., Beckenverletzungen/Pelvic Injuries. Hefte zu "Der Unfallchirurg". Heft 266. 1998.
29. French B, Tornetta P. Transiliosacral osteosynthesis in unstable injuries of the posterior pelvic ring. Oper Orthop Traumatol. 2002;10:27–46.
30. Murphy C, Gill J, Carrothers A, Hull P. Treatment of displaced sacroiliac fracture using the lateral window for short plate buttress reduction and percutaneous sacroiliac screw fixation. Arch Bone Jt Surg. 2016;4:173–6.

Iliosacral Screw Fixation

31

Axel Gänsslen, Jan Lindahl, and Philipp Kobbe

Historically, iliosacral screw fixation was performed in unstable sacral fractures and SI joint dislocations using CT-guided screw fixation techniques. Nearly one decade later, fluoroscopy-based insertion was favored until today. During the last years, navigation-assisted iliosacral screw placement was used with the aim to optimize safe screw placement, reduction of intraoperative x-ray time, and to reduce overall surgical time.

31.1 Sacral Anatomy for Iliosacral Screw Insertion

The internal sacral architecture with its irregular bone mineral density zones is relevant for understanding the stability of iliosacral screw fixation.

Ebraheim et al. reported the weakest bone zones to be in the lateral sacral alar of S1 and at the level of the junction of S2 and S3, while the strongest bone zone was observed between the S1 and S2 foramina [1].

A CT analysis of the normal sacrum revealed a reduced bone density in typical sacral regions, with lowest bone density paraforaminal lateral and between S1 and S2 [2, 3].

The mean bone mineral density (BMD) of the S1 body was found to be 31.9% higher than that of the sacral alar, and the highest bone mineral density is typically observed near the lateral posterior and lateral anterior part of the S1 body [4].

A DEXA scan analysis found highest cancellous BMD in the anterior two thirds of the S1 body, while the highest cortical BMD was observed anteriorly [5].

Clinical Relevance

The internal bone density can explain specific fracture patterns in traumatic and fragility fractures of the sacrum [6] (Fig. 31.1), and, therefore, specific screw pathways can be recommended.

A typical internal trabecular pattern of the upper sacrum was found by Pal et al., which shows strong trabeculae running from the superior surface of the S1 body to the articular

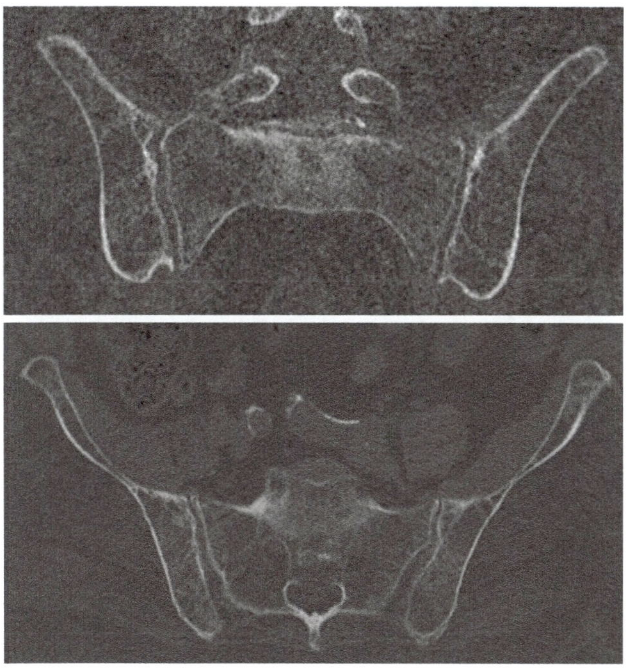

Fig. 31.1 Bone mineral density in the upper sacrum at the S1 level

A. Gänsslen (✉)
Department of Trauma Surgery, Orthopedics and Hand Surgery, Hospital Wolfsburg, Wolfsburg, Germany

J. Lindahl
Orthopaedics and Trauma Surgery, Helsinki University Hospital, Helsinki, Finland

P. Kobbe
Clinic for Accident and Reconstructive Surgery, University Hospital Aachen, Aachen, Germany
e-mail: pkobbe@ukaachen.de

A. Gänsslen et al. (eds.), *Pelvic Ring Fractures*, https://doi.org/10.1007/978-3-030-54730-1_31

surface of the SI joint, from the articular process and the S1 pedicle to the SI joint, from the posterolateral angle of the ala (attachment site of the lumbosacral ligament) to the S1 body, and from the lateral portion of the laminae to the auricular surface [7].

31.1.1 The First Sacral Vestibule

Carlson et al. described the so-called vestibule concept (Fig. 31.2) of the S1 and S2 pedicle anatomy. It was defined as "the smallest area through which an iliosacral screw would pass and was therefore considered the pivotal anatomic landmark for safe iliosacral screw placement" [8].

The sacral alar slope with the attached L5 nerve root represents the superior border of the vestibule while the superior border of the S1 sacral foramen with the S1 nerve root represents the inferior border (Fig. 31.2). Laterally and medially, two bone cones expand from this narrow zone to either the lateral sacral ala and ilium and the S1 vertebral body, respectively [8, 9].

This ovoid-shaped narrow area defines the safe insertion of an iliosacral screw, either perpendicular to the SI joint or to a typically longitudinal sacral fracture. The latter results in a smaller area.

From a clinical perspective, it was shown that sacral fracture malreduction leads to a significant reduction of this safe area/bone corridor [10]. Reilly et al. could show that the cross-sectional fracture contact area decreases by 30%, 56%, 81%, and 90% at 5, 10, 15, and 20 mm of displacement, respectively.

The size of the S1 vestibule was analyzed by Carlson and a mean area of 534mm^2 in males and 450mm^2 in females was reported. At the level of S2 this area was 253mm^2 in males and 213 mm^2 in females, respectively [8].

Gardner et al. reported a 36% smaller vestibule area in dysmorphic sacra: 222mm^2 versus 346mm^2, indicating a more oblique screw orientation [11].

Noojin et al. defined the average diameter of the narrowest part of the vestibule [12]. A mean width of 28.05 mm and a mean height of 27.76 mm were measured in 13 CT scans of the pelvis.

> The first sacral vestibule represents the narrowest zone for iliosacral screw placement and is influenced by fracture displacement and presence of sacral dysmorphism.

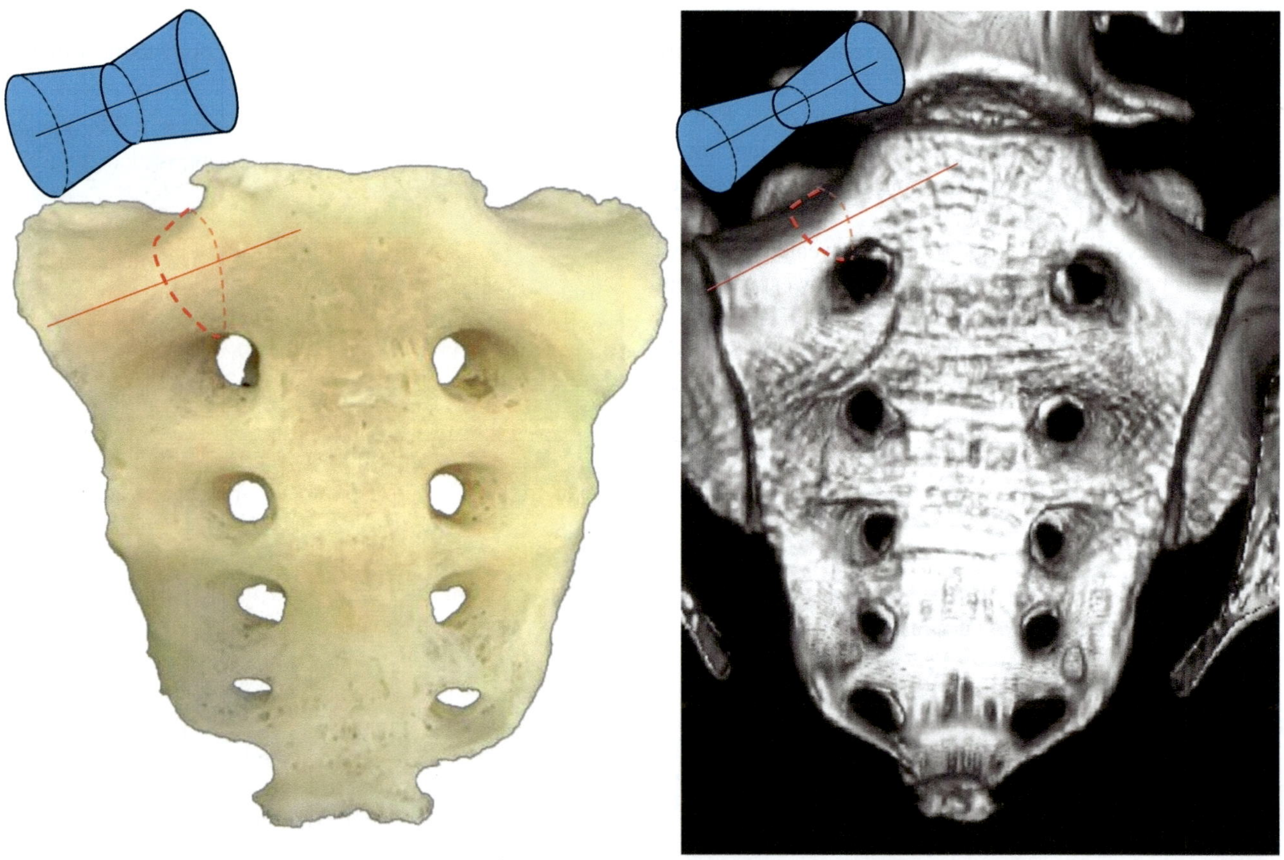

Fig. 31.2 Vestibule concept of the upper sacrum at the level of S1 in a normal (left) and a dysmorphic sacrum (right)

31.1.2 Sacral Dysmorphism

An atypical anatomy of the upper sacrum can be due to lumbosacral transitional vertebrae (Fig. 31.3) and due to sacral dysmorphism (Fig. 31.4).

Sacral dysmorphism can be expected in 14–52% [13–16].

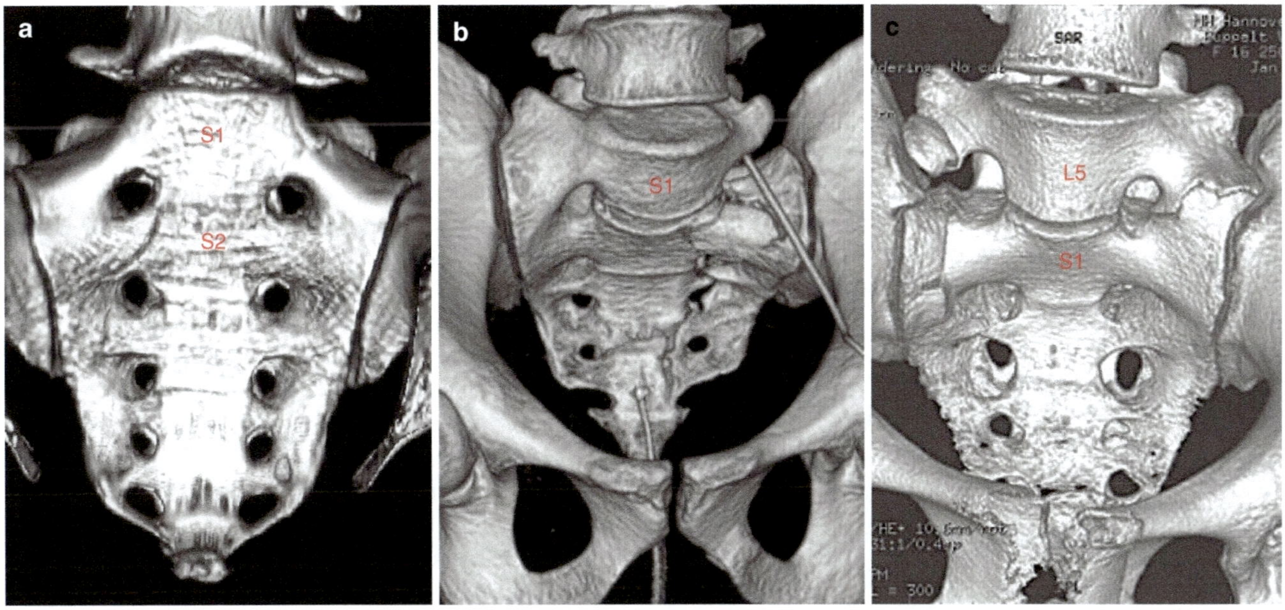

Fig. 31.3 Atypical sacral morphology: sacral dysmorphism (**a**), right hemisacralization (**b**) of the S1-vertebra, and left incomplete sacralization with a dysmorphic fifth lumbar spine (**c**)

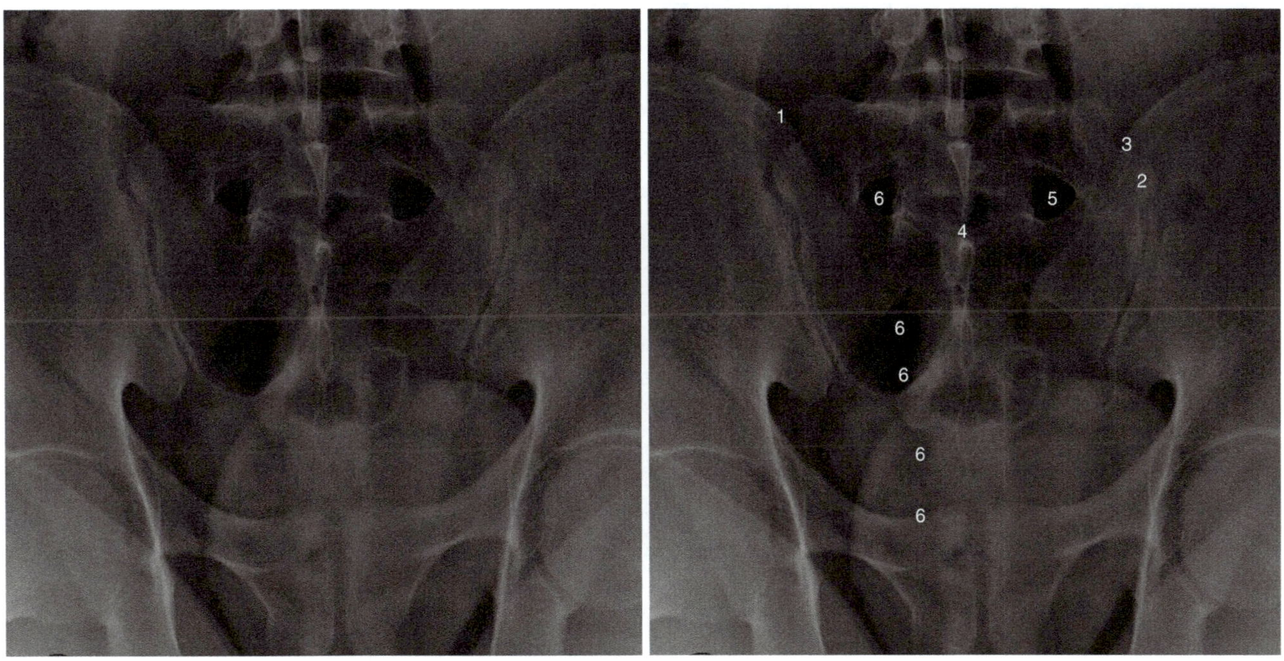

Fig. 31.4 Radiological-anatomical signs of sacral dysmorphism: upper sacral segment not recessed in the pelvis (1), existence of mammillary processes (2), acute alar slope (3), residual disc between the first and second sacral segments (4), noncircular upper sacral neural foramina (5), and five sacral foramina (6)

Routt et al. first described five radiographic-anatomical parameters of sacral dysmorphism (Fig. 31.4) assessed on outlet projections [17, 18]:

- An upper sacral segment superior to the iliosacral connection, thus not recessed within the pelvis
- Presence of mammillary processes
- Acute alar slope
- Residual disc between the first and second sacral segment
- Noncircular upper sacral neural foramina

Additionally, the axial CT scan was analyzed for an iliosacral "tongue-in-groove" sacral type (Fig. 31.5). This anatomical type is characterized by a protrusion of the iliac bone into a corresponding concave shape of the sacrum [17, 18].

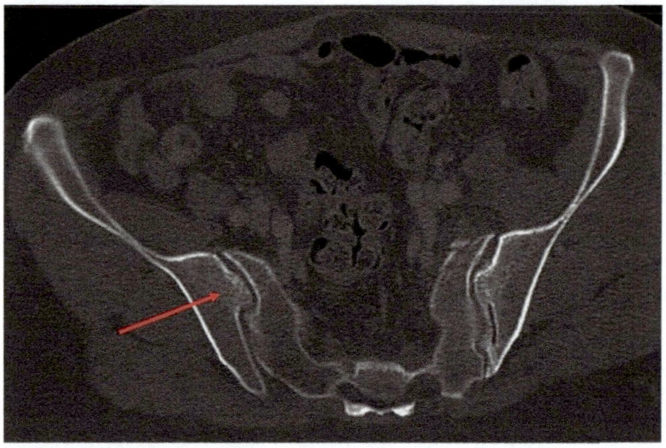

Fig. 31.5 "Tongue-in-groove" sacral type, characterized by a protrusion of the iliac bone into a corresponding concave shape of the sacrum

Recently, additional parameters of sacral dysmorphism were described based on extended radiographic analyses:

- A transsacral corridor <7.5 mm in the axial CT at the S1 level [19]
- Lateral sacral triangle ratio by ≤1.5 [20]
- Sacral dysmorphism score >70 [15]

31.1.3 The Lateral Sacral Triangle

Mendel et al. defined the "lateral sacral triangle" (LST) measurement to allow safe placement of 7.3 mm iliosacral screws into a horizontal bone corridor at the level of S1 (Fig. 31.6) [20].

On a true lateral pelvic view, a triangle is measured with the anterior S1 body height (SBH = distance between the iliac cortical density (ICD) and the most superior anterior promontory), superior anterior to posterior promontory width (PW) and the base consisting of the length of the ICD.

The ratio of SBH and PW of ≤1.5 revealed the possibility of a safe insertion of at least one 7.3 mm screw into the S1 pedicular transverse bone corridor [20, 21].

Additionally, the distance between the superior endplate of S1 (promontory) to the most upper level of the both SI joints (= endplate–joint distance) was analyzed on the outlet view. A small distance was associated with a proposed safe screw insertion.

The sacral dysmorphism score was calculated, which consists of the sum of the S1 coronal angle plus two times the S1 axial angle (Fig. 31.7). It was found that a higher score indicated relevant sacral dysmorphism and a high risk

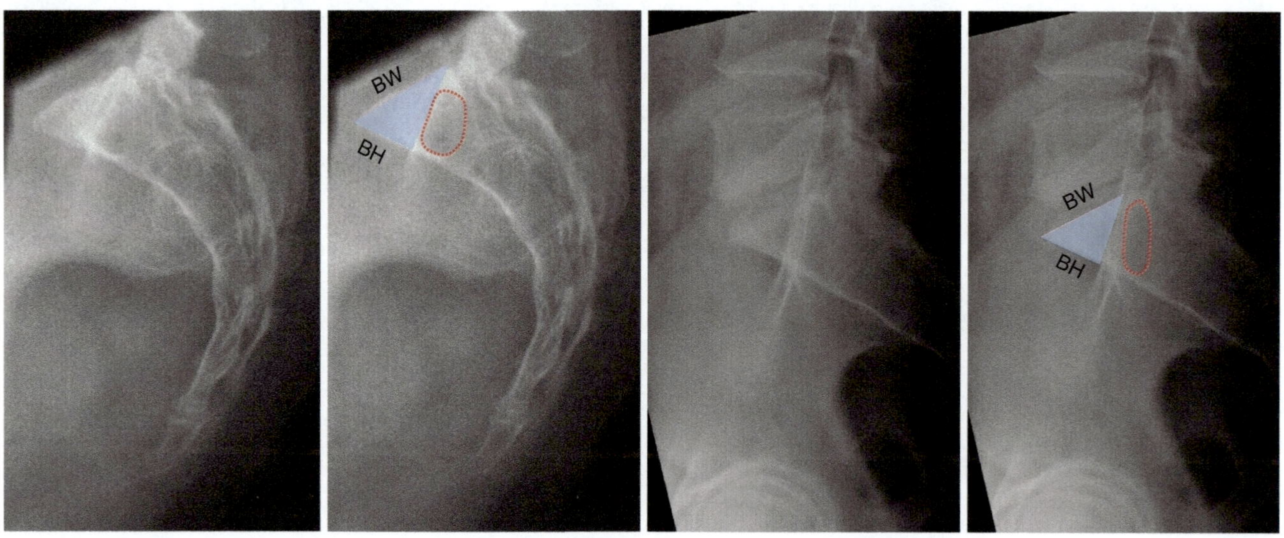

Fig. 31.6 Lateral sacral triangle. Measurement of anterior height (BH) and superior width (BW) of S1. A ratio of BH and BW ≥1.5 (left example) reveals potential safe insertion of at least one 7.3 mm screw into the S1 pedicular transverse bone corridor

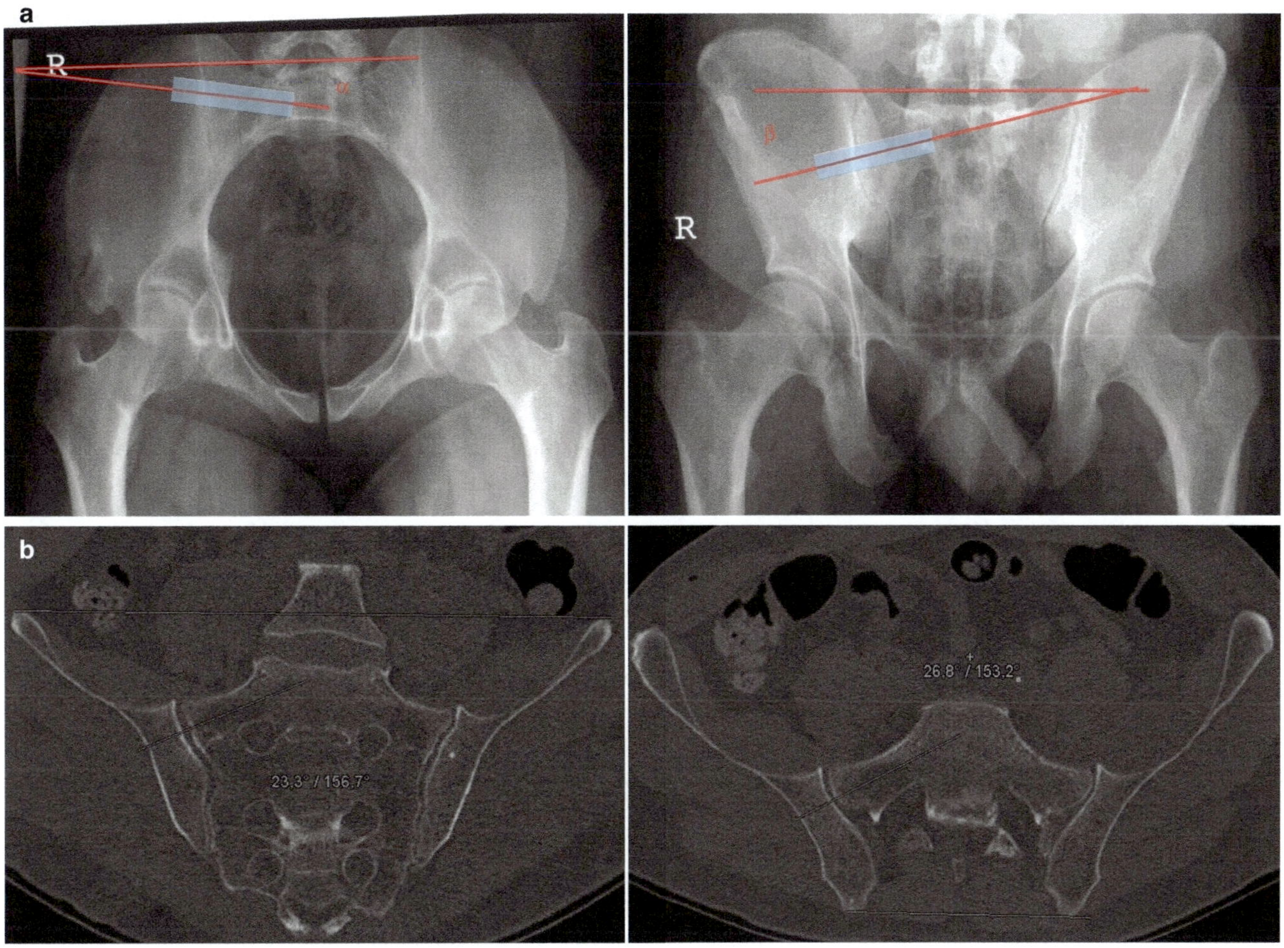

Fig. 31.7 (**a**) S1 Inlet angle (α) and S1 Outlet angle (β). (**b**) Sacral Dysmorphism Score = sum of the S1 coronal angle (left) plus two-times the S1 axial angle (right). A score >70 indicates a high risk of non-intraosseous screw placement via the horizontal route (in this example the score is 76.9°)

of non-intraosseous screw placement in subjects with a dysmorphic score >70 [15].

Goetzen et al. analyzed the upper sacral morphology using 1000 CT data sets with standardized reconstructions of the inlet, outlet, and lateral projections of the sacrum [22]. Three different major morphological types could be identified (Fig. 31.8):

- Ascending type
- Horizontal type
- Descending type

An anterior bilateral notching of the anterior sacral cortex was additionally present in the majority of cases.

Wendt et al. recently analyzed 55 multislice CT scans with sacral dysmorphism [19]. According to established dysmorphism criteria, the frequency of different criteria was as follows:

- 97% acute alar slope (true lateral)
- 79% visible mammillary processes (outlet)
- 76% oval-shaped neuroforamen (outlet)
- 50% sacrum not recessed within the pelvis (outlet)
- 47% residual disc spaces between the upper two sacral segments (outlet)
- 29% “tongue-in-groove” morphology
- 57% with a triangle ratio <1.5 (dysmorphic type)
- 47.4 points dysmorphic score

Several radiographic parameters are available to sufficiently detect and analyze sacral dysmorphism.

31.1.4 Vascular Risks

There is a potential risk of damaging the deep superior branches of superior gluteal artery while inserting iliosacral screws.

Collinge et al. performed a cadaver analysis after SI joint iliosacral screw placement and reported a neurovascu-

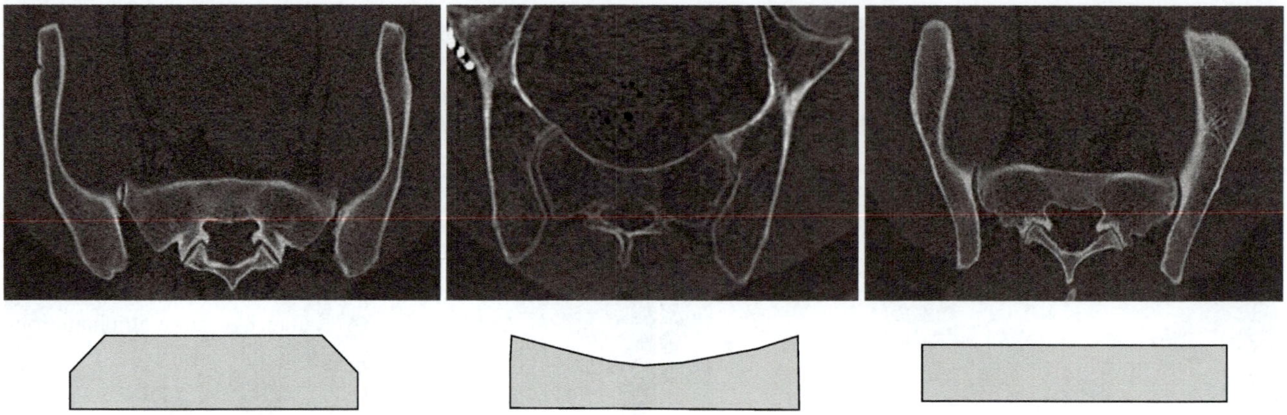

Fig. 31.8 Morphology of the upper sacrum identifying an ascending type, a horizontal, and a descending type. Anterior bilateral notching of the anterior sacral cortex was associated with dysmorphism

lar injury in 17.2% [23]. A close relationship between the screw head and the deep superior branches of the superior gluteal nerve and vessels of 9.1 mm was observed. Zhao et al. reported a 45.1% risk of vascular damage in a CT analysis [24].

In a further CT angiographic analysis of 20 uninjured pelvic data sets, the distance from the superior gluteal artery to the proposed iliosacral screw insertion point on the outer iliac bone was analyzed for oblique SI joint screws and transverse S1 and S2 screws [25]. An average distance of 2.53 cm was found for an iliosacral SI joint screw trajectory. The distance to a transversely orientated screw into the S1 and S2 corridor was 12.4 mm and 23.5 mm, respectively. The S1 transverse screw trajectory can cause superior gluteal nerve injury.

> There is a potential risk of damaging the superior gluteal neurovascular bundle during iliosacral screw insertion, especially at the level of S1.

31.2 SI Joint Screw Corridor Level S1

Routt et al. described the anatomical basis for iliosacral screw fixation of the disrupted SI joint in detail already in 1995. The detailed radiographic analysis of the sacrum including the sacral alar slope and the applied clinical anatomy of the neurovascular structures and of transitional vertebra were described [26].

The orientation of an iliosacral screw at the level of S1 is typically slightly oblique to guide the screw perpendicular to the SI joint plane (Fig. 31.9). The bone corridor for iliosacral screw fixation is bounded anteriorly by the alar cortex and posteriorly by the sacral neural foramen [18].

In a CT analysis, this oblique corridor had a minimum width of 21.7 ± 3.4 mm between the S1 foramen and the anterior cortex of the sacrum [27].

A comparable analysis was performed by Ebraheim et al. in cadavers [28]. Here, the minimum mean corridor depth was 27.8 ± 2.7 mm (range 24-32 mm), while at the level of the SI joint, the depth was 45.8 ± 1.9 mm (range 43-48 mm). A potential screw length of 105.2 ± 5.1 mm (range 92-112 mm) was defined.

Day et al. analyzed the oblique SI joint S1 bone corridor and reported a minimal craniocaudal diameter of the vestibule of 18.9 mm and an anterior-posterior minimal diameter of 10.9 mm for sufficient screw insertion [29].

Okutan et al. measured the anterior-posterior width of the S1 pedicle in cadavers and reported a width of 22.5 ± 2.6 mm in males and 22.2 ± 2.8 mm in females [30].

From a clinical point of view, the screw should be placed perpendicular to the joint plane and tilted slightly upward in the frontal plane of the sacral bone, whereas in the horizontal plane a slightly posterior-anterior screw angulation (Fig. 31.10) is proposed, with a corresponding skin incision entry point, that lies more toward the posterior aspect [31], compared to the sacral fracture screw insertion [28].

Gardner et al. analyzed the oblique screw trajectory in normal and dysplastic sacra at the level of 1 [11]. In dysmorphic sacra, a minimal screw length along the vestibule of at least 75 mm was possible. The CT reconstruction of an Outlet view showed a mean caudal to cranial screw axis orientation of 20.5° in normal and 30.3° in dysmorphic sacra, while the reconstructed Inlet view showed posterior to anterior angulations of 4.2° and 12.9°, respectively.

Wendt et al. recently analyzed 55 multislice CT scans with sacral dysmorphism. In dysmorphic sacra, the CT reconstruction of an outlet view showed a mean caudal to cranial screw axis orientation of 32°, while the reconstructed

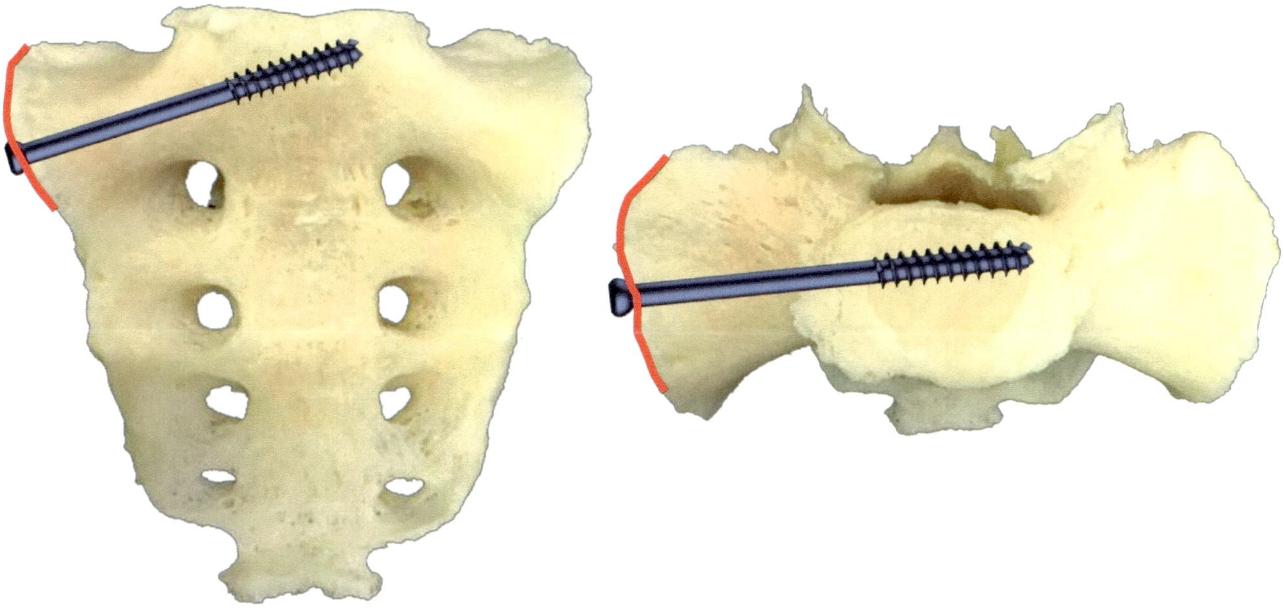

Fig. 31.9 Screw orientation for iliosacral screw fixation in SI joint dislocations, perpendicular to the joint plane

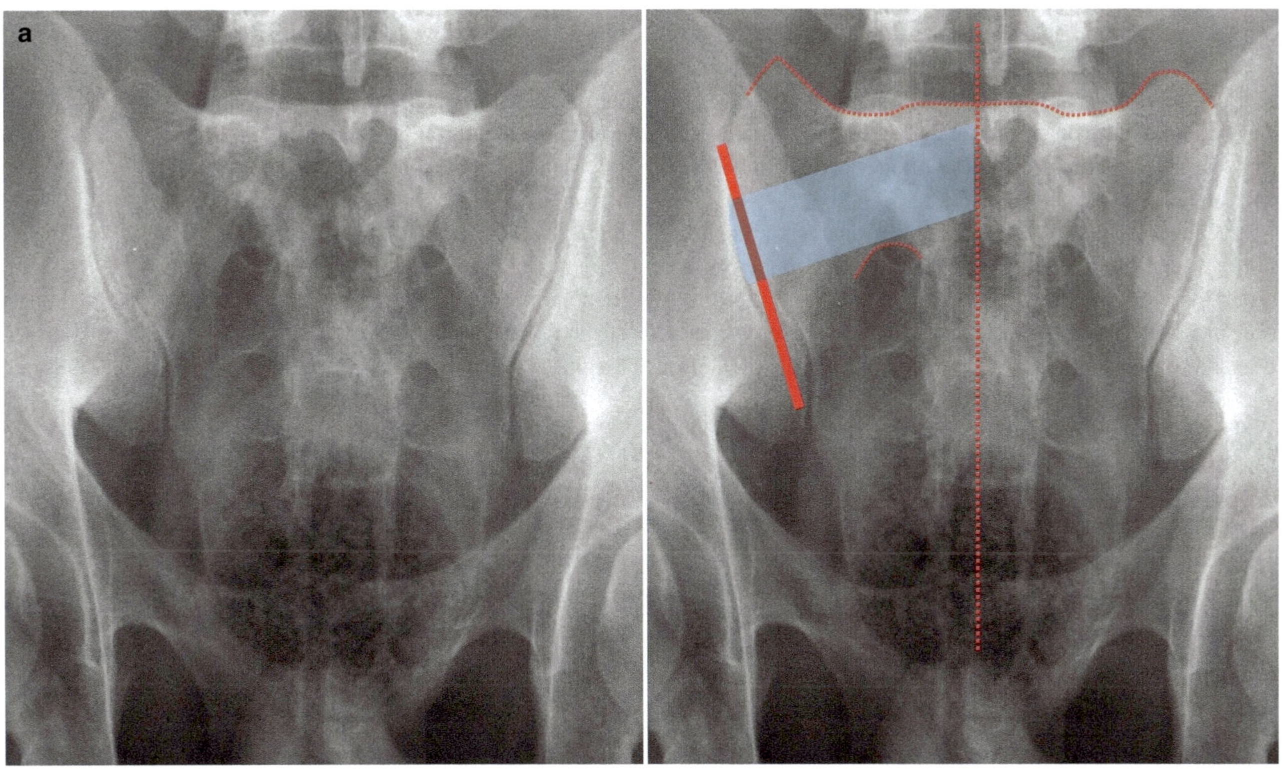

Fig. 31.10 (**a**) Oblique bone corridor for iliosacral screw application in SI joint injuries, perpendicular to the joint line: Outlet view. (**b**) Oblique posterior bone corridor for iliosacral screw application in SI joint injuries, perpendicular to the joint line: Inlet view

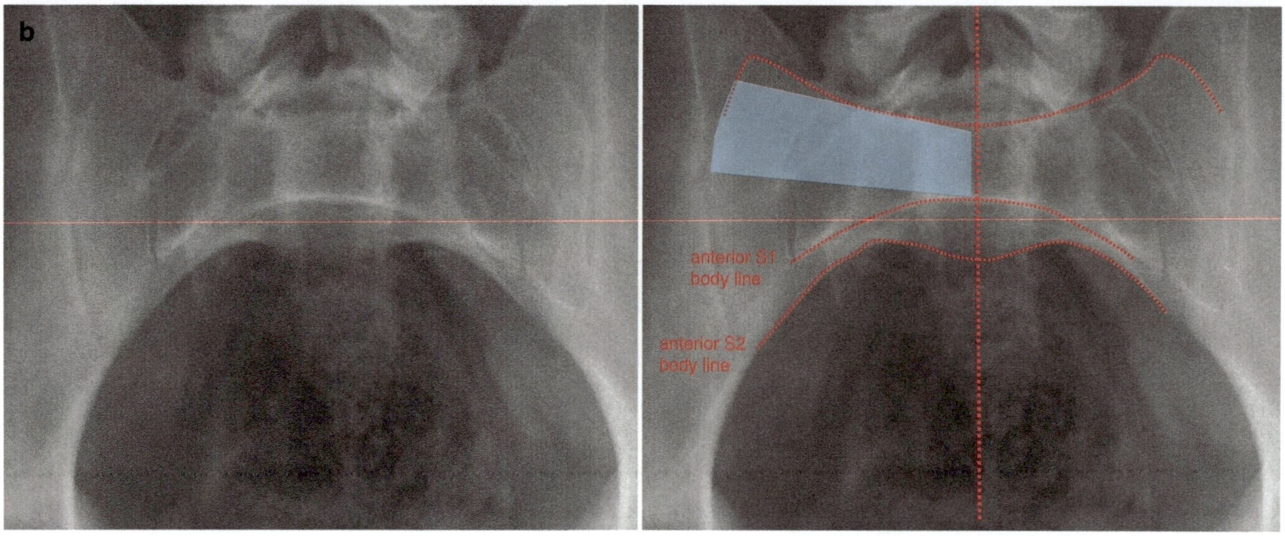

Fig. 31.10 (continued)

inlet view showed posterior to anterior 8° [19]. An in-out-in corridor at the posterior iliosacral recessus, representing a screw path starting at the iliac bone, running through the interosseous sacroiliacal ligaments to enter the sacral body was proposed, which leads to an increased corridor diameter at S1 between 15% and 26% (males vs. females).

A CT analysis from normal and dysmorphic sacra reported an average length of the oblique S1 bone corridor of 98.8 mm and 101.2 mm, respectively [32].

Collinge et al. performed a cadaver analysis after insertion of an iliosacral screw via this SI joint trajectory and reported neurovascular injuries in 17.2% [23]. A close relationship between the screw head and the deep superior branches of the superior gluteal nerve and vessels of 9.1 mm was observed.

The optimal entry point for an oblique S1 screw was identified recently at the level of first sacral foramen, directed toward the opposite upper corner of the first sacral body [32].

31.3 Transverse S1 Bone Corridor

In contrast to the SI joint screw, the orientation of a sacral screw at the level of S1 should be orientated perpendicular to the fracture planes, which is typically a vertical/longitudinal fracture course, and, therefore, the screw has a more horizontal orientation (Fig. 31.11). This technique is also used in unilateral or even bilateral U- or H-shaped sacral fractures [33].

The bone corridor is bounded anteriorly by the alar cortex and posteriorly by the sacral neural foramen [18]. The cranial-caudal narrow area is defined from the superior border of the S1 foramen to the upper margin of the sacral shoulder (Fig. 31.12).

From the clinical perspective, in sacral fractures, the fracture is oriented toward the sagittal plane. The tube-shaped channel for the screw is smallest in diameter at the level of the sacral foramina but then develops into a skittle shape laterally and medially [8, 29].

31.3.1 Morphological Analyses

In a morphological surface analysis of 100 sacral bones, Arman defined the anterior and posterior sacral surface heights of the narrowest area to be 14.81 mm and 20.98 mm, respectively. The sacral pedicle depth was 24.65 mm [34].

A comparable analysis reported anterior and posterior sacral surface heights of 20.74 mm and 20.18 mm, respectively, while the S1 pedicle depth was 23.48 mm [35].

> The narrow morphological surface height of the S1 bone corridor is approximately 2 cm with an S1 pedicle depth of 2.4 cm.

31.3.2 Radiographic Analyses

In a cadaver analysis by Ebraheim et al., the narrowest zone was defined by the anterior and posterior pedicle height on the cadaver and the outlet view [28]. Anatomical measurements showed a larger diameter with an anterior pedicular height of 30.2 ± 3.4 mm (range 24–38 mm) and a

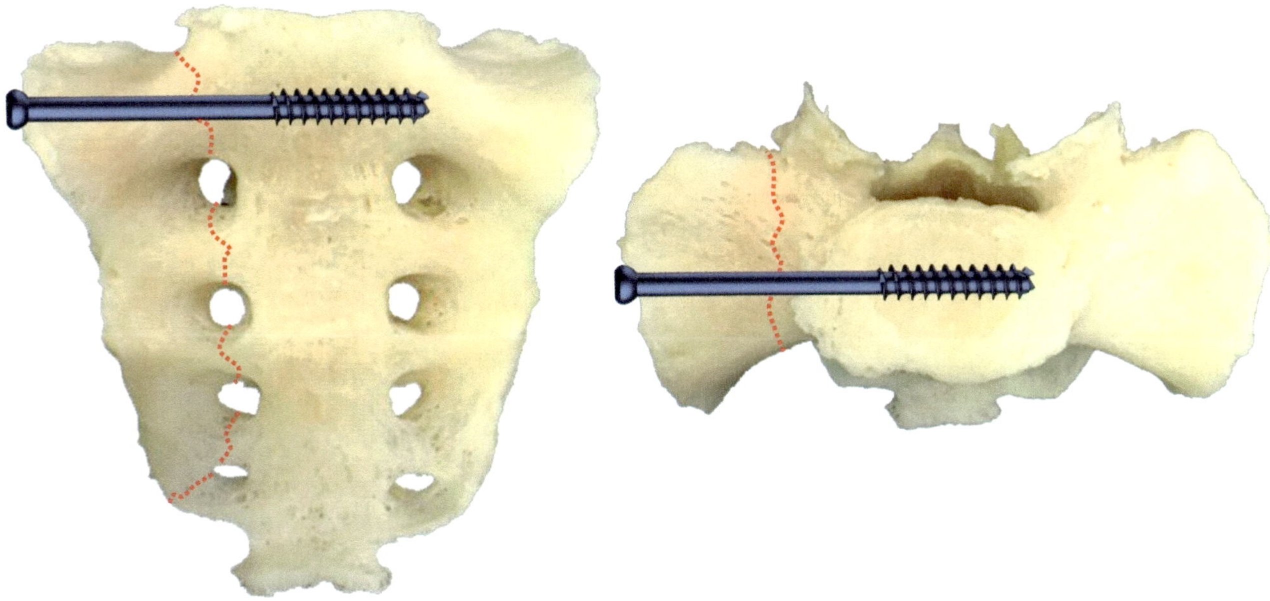

Fig. 31.11 Screw orientation for iliosacral screw fixation in sacral fractures (typical vertical fracture course), perpendicular to the fracture plane

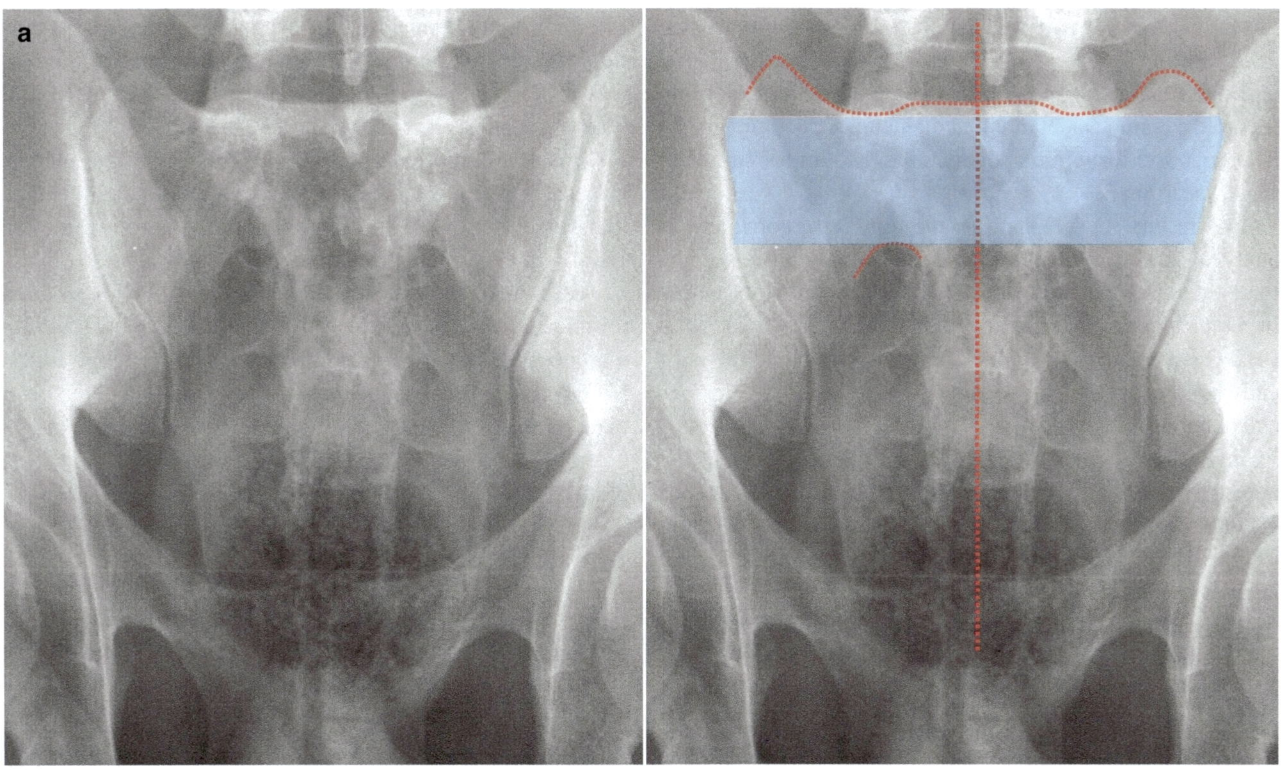

Fig. 31.12 (**a**) Transverse S1 bone corridor for iliosacral screw application in sacral fractures, perpendicular to the most commonly seen vertical fracture orientation: Outlet View. (**b**) Transverse S1 bone corridor for iliosacral screw application in sacral fractures, perpendicular to the most commonly seen vertical fracture orientation: Inlet View

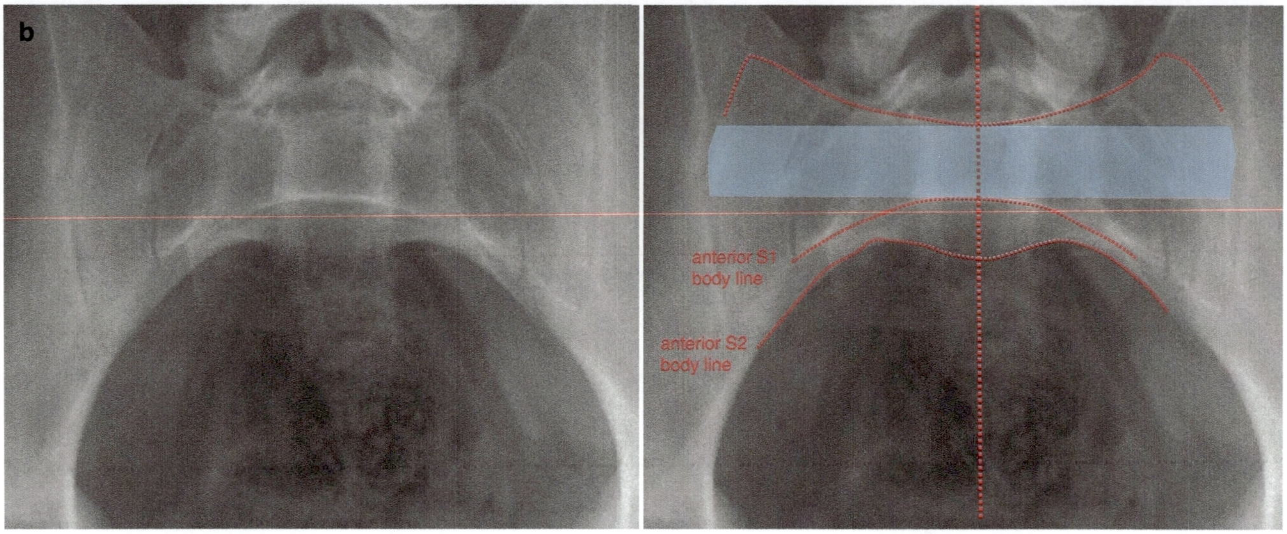

Fig. 31.12 (continued)

posterior pedicular height of 26.1 ± 3.4 mm (range 21–35 mm), while radiographic measurements on the outlet view revealed a narrow zone of 20 ± 2.mm (range 18–25 mm).

Day et al. analyzed the transverse S1 bone corridor and reported a craniocaudal minimal diameter of 26.2 mm and an anterior-posterior minimal diameter of 18 mm for sufficient screw insertion [29].

In a recent 3D CT analysis, the transverse corridor was analyzed, and screw application was primarily influenced by the bilateral sacral isthmus, where the mean corridor height was typically smaller than the width: 13.0 mm vs. 26.7 mm [21]. On average, 3.7 parallel 7.3 mm screws could theoretically be inserted into this corridor. The optimal diameter was calculated to 14.2 mm.

In an analysis of 36 CT data from Chinese people, the anterior-posterior vestibular width (VW) was 25.15 ± 2.91 mm and the superior-inferior vestibular height (VH) was 20.94 ± 3.03 mm, which both were significantly smaller in females [36].

The average vertical diameter of the S1 bone corridor was 13.4 mm; the anterior-posterior (horizontal) diameter was 22.5 mm with a safe zone area of 239.5mm^2. Sacral dysmorphism led to a safe zone area decrease (48.9 mm^2 vs. 278.7mm^2) [37].

31.3.3 Corridor Length

The S1 transverse bone corridor has an average length of 16.3 cm [38]. Females present with smaller S1 corridors. This corridor was large enough to insert an average of four 7.3 mm screws in males and 3.1 screws in females.

In a further CT analysis, the average length of the S1 corridor was determined with 162 mm in males and 155 mm in females [39]. This corridor was present in 63% of males and 66% of females.

Gras et al. reported a corridor length of 164 mm [40]. A CT analysis of normal cadaveric sacral reported an average transverse length of the transverse S1 bone corridor was 151.4 mm [32].

A CT analysis of 280 patients without pelvic fractures revealed a sufficient S1 transverse bone corridor in 89% with a proposed safe screw insertion rate (7.3 mm screw) of 68% [41]. Female specimens had smaller-corridor diameters than male pelves.

- An average 16 cm length of the transverse S1 bone corridor can be expected.
- A “physiological transverse pelvic asymmetry” exists, indicated by bilateral different diameter values of the horizontal S1 bone corridor [21].
- Females present with smaller transverse bone corridors than males.

The optimal entry point for a horizontal S1 screw was identified recently just inferior to the iliac cortical density in the true lateral x-ray [32].

31.4 Transverse S2 Bone Corridor

S2 bone corridors are present in nearly all specimens (Fig. 31.13) while the presence of a transverse S1 corridor depends on the rate of sacral dysmorphism.

Barrick et al. reported a height of the S2 pedicle in the anterior-posterior plane of 17 mm [42]. In a morphological surface analysis of 100 sacral bones, Arman defined the anterior and posterior height of the narrowest area to be 10.54 mm and 15.92 mm, respectively [34]. A comparable analysis reported anterior and posterior sacral surface heights of 11.33 mm and 14.18 mm, respectively [35].

The average vertical diameter of the S2 bone corridor was 15.5 mm; the anterior-posterior (horizontal) diameter was 18.3 mm with a safe zone area of 221.1mm^2. Sacral dysmorphism led to a safe zone area increase (209.6 mm^2 vs. 276.9 mm^2) and a larger vertical diameter [32].

Typically, this transverse bone corridor has an average length of 14.1 cm [38]. Females presented with smaller S2 corridors. This corridor was large enough to insert an average of 2.1 7.3 mm screws in males and 1.8 screws in females.

Gras et al. reported a length of 142 ± 10.2 mm [40]. In a further CT analysis, the average length of the S2 corridor was determined with 137 mm in males and 135 mm in females [39]. This corridor was present in all males and in 87% of females. The interforaminal distance was smaller in females with 12 mm vs. 14 mm.

A CT analysis from normal and dysmorphic sacra reported an average transverse length of the S2 bone corridor of 134.2 mm and 144.6 mm, respectively [32].

A CT analysis of 280 patients without pelvic fractures revealed a sufficient S2 transverse bone corridor in nearly 100% with a proposed safe screw insertion rate (7.3 mm screw) of 88% [41]. Female specimens had smaller-corridor diameters than male pelves.

In a clinical analysis of dysmorphic S1 sacra, the mean length of the S2 pathway was 151.9 mm with the majority of screw inserted centrally into the corridor while 16.6% were rated juxtaforaminal, with contact to the S2 foramen [43].

Gardner et al. analyzed the screw trajectory in normal and dysplastic sacra at the level of S2 and found larger S2 bone corridors in dysmorphic sacra [11]. This association was recently confirmed as a decrease of the S1 corridor size, present in sacral dysmorphism, was correlated with a larger S2 corridor diameter [40, 41].

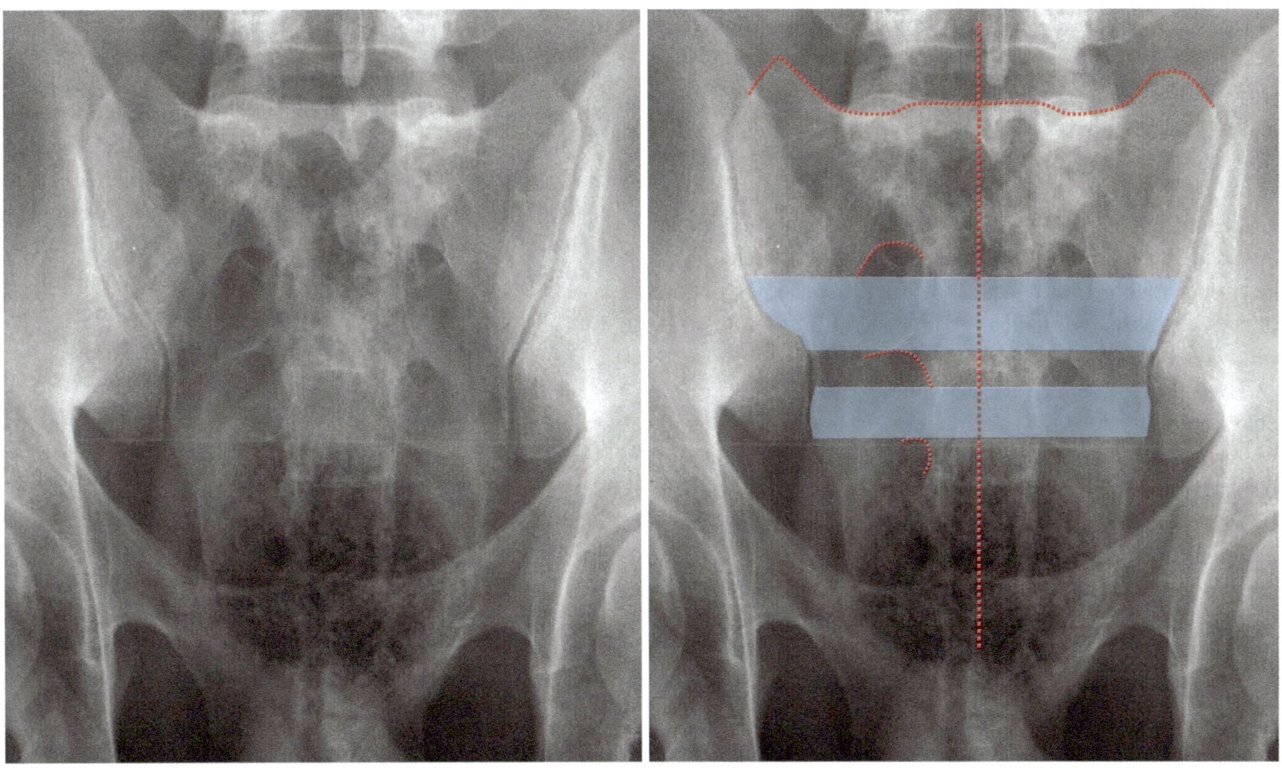

Fig. 31.13 Transverse S2 and S3 bone corridor for iliosacral screw application in sacral fractures, perpendicular to the most commonly seen vertical fracture orientation

The modification of the screw path by Wendt et al. led to an increase of the sufficient S2 bone corridor of 50% [19].

- An average 14 cm length of the transverse S2-bone corridor can be expected.
- Females present with smaller transverse bone corridors than males.
- The corridor is larger in S1 sacral dysmorphism.

The optimal entry point for a horizontal S2 screw was identified recently inferior or slightly anterior to the S1 entry point, which is just inferior to the iliac cortical density [32].

31.5 Transverse S3 Bone Corridor

Dilogo et al. reported a technique of S3 screw application [44]. An oblique direction from superior-cranial to inferior-caudal on the AP view and an oblique direction from anterior to posterior on the lateral projection were proposed.

The transverse S3 bone corridor has an average gender-independent length of 11.6 cm [45]. In only ¼ of analyzed pelves, a 7.3 mm screw could theoretically be safely inserted (Fig. 31.13).

Wagner identified a surgically usable S3 corridor in only 23% when the distal part of the SI joint reached the inferior border of the S3 sacral transverse bone corridor [46].

Eastman et al. analyzed the CT of 250 patients and found an adequate S3 transverse bone corridor, sufficient for a 7.0 mm screw in 15.2% [13]. In nearly 90% sacral dysmorphism was observed, indicating that sacral dysmorphism is often associated with a S3 bone corridor.

Hwang et al. defined the S3 bone corridor size in a CT analysis of 59 adults [47]. A 2 mm larger bone corridor was observed in dysmorphic sacra (9.5 mm craniocaudal diameter, 9.14 mm anterior-posterior diameter) compared to non-dysmorphic sacra (7.71 mm craniocaudal diameter, 7.12 mm anterior-posterior diameter), and the corresponding cross-sectional area was 55.8mm^2 vs. 77.9 mm^{2,} respectively.

- In the presence of S1 sacral dysmorphism, a larger S3 bone corridor can be expected
- A sufficient S3 bone corridor for iliosacral screw application can be expected in 15–25% of cases

31.6 Biomechanics of Iliosacral Screw Fixation

Several biomechanical data are available, testing different posterior pelvic ring instabilities using iliosacral screws.

- Gorczyca et al. analyzed 10 fresh frozen cadaver pelves in a C1.3 injury model (transalar sacrum fracture), simulating a bilateral stance [48]. Stabilization consisted of symphyseal box-plate stabilization and posterior two 6.5 mm iliosacral screws or two sacral bars. The mean strength of the screws was comparable to sacral bars: 819 N vs. 1066 N.
- Culemann et al. performed a displacement analysis in a C1.3 transforaminal fracture model in a single leg stance simulation [49]. After iliosacral screw fixation, rotational displacement around the screw axis was observed.
- Sagi et al. compared different posterior stabilization constructs in a C1.2 c5 injury model simulating a single leg stance; posterior fixation consisted of one and two S1 iliosacral screws and one screw into S1 and S2, respectively, while the pubic symphysis was stabilized with or without a 2-hole plate; all three posterior stabilization methods resulted in a comparable reduction of displacements [50].
- van Swienen et al. analyzed a C3.3 c5 fracture model (bilateral sacral fractures) in 12 specimens, posteriorly fixed with one iliosacral screw in S1, two screws into S1, or one screw in S1 and another screw in S2; no anterior stabilization was performed; two iliosacral screws increased rotation stiffness and resulted in a higher load to failure [51].
- Tabaie et al. analyzed a C1.3.2 c1 injury model; two 7.0 mm iliosacral screws into the S1 body led to higher loads of failure and deformation than one 7.0 mm iliosacral screw and one 7.0 mm transsacral screw [52].
- Dilogo et al. recently analyzed a Synbone C1.3 c5 sacral fracture model in a double-leg stance simulation [53]; the sacral fracture was fixed either by an iliosacral screw into S1 and S2, iliosacral tension band plating, and iliosacral screws into S1, S2, and S3 with different anterior ring stabilization techniques; three iliosacral screws together with the pubic symphysis plate was the most stiff construct.
- van den Bosch et al. analyzed a B1 open book injury and compared the intact pelvis with either anterior stabilization of the pubic symphysis (plate) and additional iliosacral screw fixation. Additional iliosacral screw fixation did not result in less displacement or stiffness increase [54].

Biomechanical data on iliosacral stabilization of the posterior pelvic ring show sufficient stability.

31.7 Oblique Iliosacral Screw Fixation of the Disrupted SI Joint

Stabilization of the disrupted SI joint was probably first described by Lehmann in 1934, who presented a case with a screw stabilization [55].

After closed reduction maneuvers, open reduction in the prone position was performed using a posterior curved approach along the posterior iliac crest with mobilization of the gluteus maximus muscle. Under direct visualization, the screw was inserted respecting the upper neuroforamina, resulting in a screw orientation, which was rated nonoptimal regarding biomechanical principles.

Original text: "Technik: Extensionstisch, Bauchlage. Direkter Zug mit Extensionszange an den Femurcondylen der verletzten Seite und — da an der zerrissenen Symphyse ein Gegenlager nicht angebracht werden konnte — direkter Gegenzug mit Kirschnerdraht am entgegengesetzten Beckenkamm. Nach Anziehen der Extensionsspindel Röntgenkontrolle . Dann Freilegen der Synchondrosis mit einem flachen Bogenschnitt unter teilweisem Ablösen des Glut. max. Nun konnte man bei direkter Sicht die gelungene Reposition kontrollieren. Bei der Verschraubung wurde Rücksicht auf die Zwischenwirbellöcher mit ihren Nerven genommen. Die Richtung der Schraube wurde dadurch im mechanischen Sinne nicht einwandfrei. Trotzdem erfüllte die Schraube ihren Zweck, das gute Repositionsergebnis zu erhalten" [55].

Meyer-Burgdorf reported two further cases with open ("bloody") reduction, without describing the technique in detail [56]. Forty years later, open technology was reintroduced by Emile Letournel in 1978 [57].

The basis of the recent minimally invasive iliosacral screw osteosynthesis was introduced in 1987 by Ebraheim et al. using CT guidance [58]. By improving intraoperative visualization techniques, fluoroscopic and computer-assisted screw insertions were proposed until recently.

The technique of oblique iliosacral screw fixation was described in detail by Chip Routt et al. [59, 60], followed by several modifications reported in the literature.

31.7.1 Indications

The classical indications for oblique iliosacral screw fixation of the disrupted SI joint include pure SI joint dislocations and some sacral fractures [8, 42, 61–64]. Currently, some sacral H- and U-type fractures can successfully be stabilized using iliosacral screws [32, 65].

31.7.2 Patient Positioning

Prone, (semi-)lateral, and supine positioning can be performed (Fig. 31.14) [62, 66–70].

For pure SI joint dislocations, Routt et al. proposed placing the patient on a radiolucent OR table in the supine position (Fig. 31.14) [26]. A lumbopelvic support is advised to enable sufficient posterior access (Fig. 31.15) [31].

Positioning must allow pelvic inlet and outlet views and the true lateral sacral x-ray. Historically, the angulation of pelvic inlet and outlet views in relation to the anterior-posterior plane of the pelvis was described as being 40° in each plane [71].

Recent CT analyses revealed an optimal inlet angulation for the S1 body of approximately 25° and a corresponding

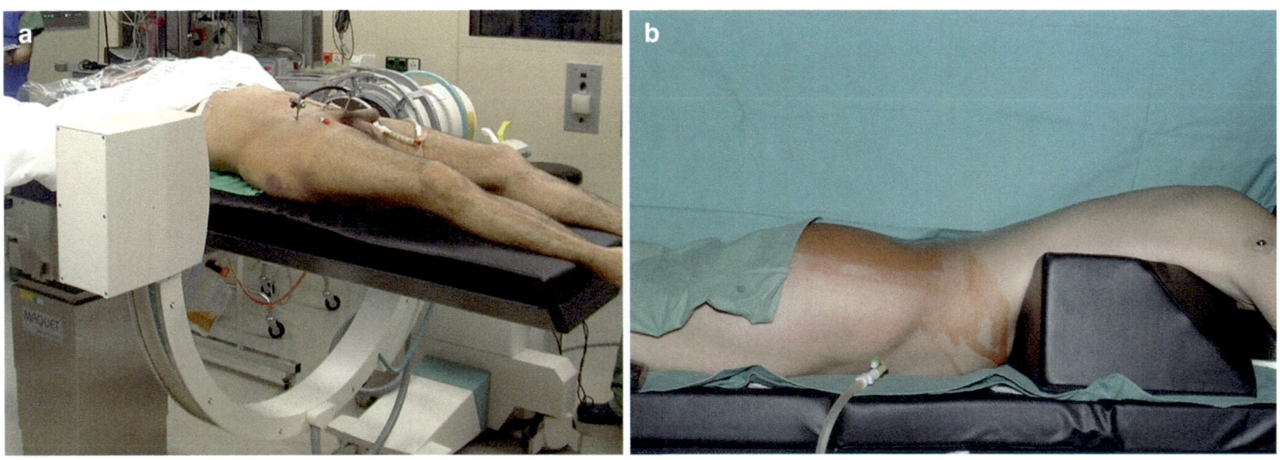

Fig. 31.14 (**a**) Standard supine positioning for iliosacral screw fixation on a radiolucent table. (**b**) Prone positioning as an alternative for iliosacral screw fixation on a radiolucent table

outlet angle of approximately 50° [72–75]. Sacral dysmorphism lead to an increase of the outlet angle of 5° (Fig. 31.16) [73].

From a clinical perspective, the optimum pelvic inlet view is achieved when the first and second sacral bodies directly overlap, while an optimal pelvic outlet view is achieved when the upper border of the pubic symphysis/pubic rami is projected on the second sacral vertebra (Fig. 31.16).

31.7.3 Anesthesiology

General anesthesia is routinely recommended [26]. But even local anesthesia or epidural anesthesia is possible [58, 62, 66, 68, 70].

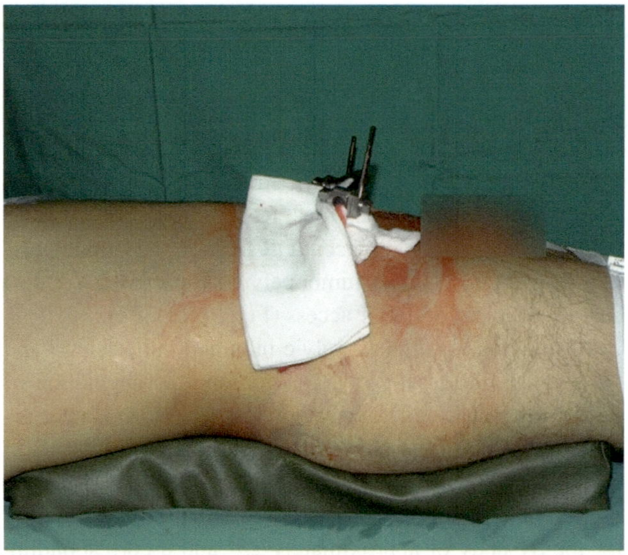

Fig. 31.15 Lumbosacral support to lift-up the pelvic area for easier access to the proposed entry point

In the 1980s and early 1990s, additional somatosensory-evoked potential monitoring was recommended [26, 76, 77].

31.7.4 Draping

The lower abdomen and the affected half of the pelvis are draped (Fig. 31.17). Depending on the amount of displacement and the necessity of reduction, the leg is mobile draped.

31.7.5 Closed Reduction

Routt et al. proposed closed reduction maneuvers of the disrupted SI joint. It was stated that the best intraoperative view is the obturator oblique view (Fig. 31.18) to analyze the reduction of the SI joint [26]. The true inlet view is of additional value to analyze the anterior reduction (Fig. 31.18).

Rotational deformity is difficult to correct [67]. Percutaneous application of Schanz pins at different locations, including the ASIS, AIIS, and the pubic tubercle, (Fig. 31.19) or even the proximal femur, can support closed reduction maneuvers [26].

Cranial and posterior displacements of the posterior hemipelvis can be corrected using longitudinal traction [26, 58, 66, 68]. Ebraheim et al. proposed padding underneath the pelvis or used manual manipulation to support reduction of posterior displacement [58].

Reduction of rotational and flexion deformities can be performed by using an oblique distractor (Fig. 31.20), fixed at the uninjured hemipelvis and connected to the injured hemipelvic iliac crest, allowing distraction and compression.

Routt et al. already stated that closed reduction of complete SI joint dislocations can be hard to achieve, especially when this maneuver is performed later than 24–48 h after

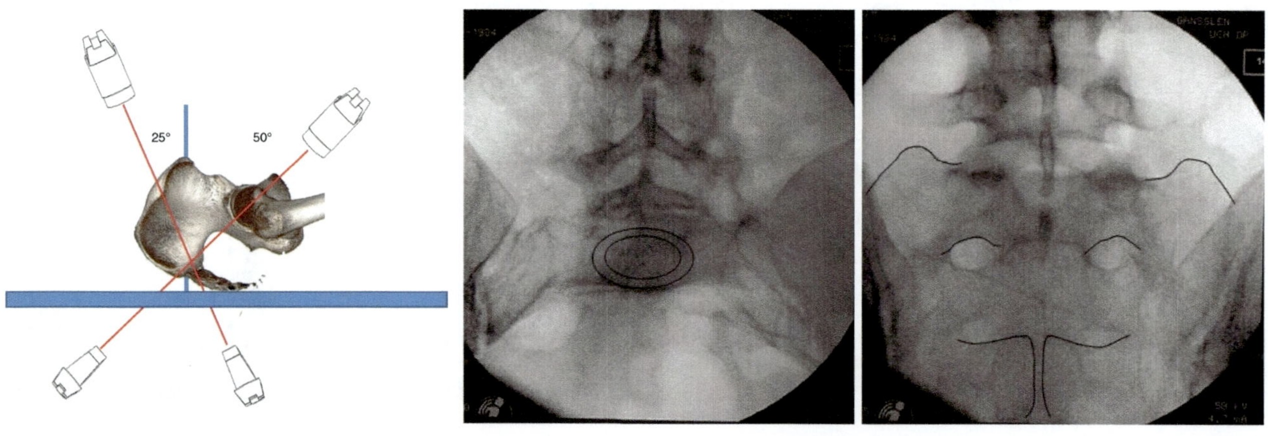

Fig. 31.16 Inlet and Outlet projections with the image intensifier. Ideal Inlet and Outlet projection: the Inlet view shows superimposition of the anterior S1 and S2 cortical lines and oval shape of the vertebral bodies of both vertebrae; an optimal Outlet view is seen, when the superior border of the symphysis is near the second sacral foramen

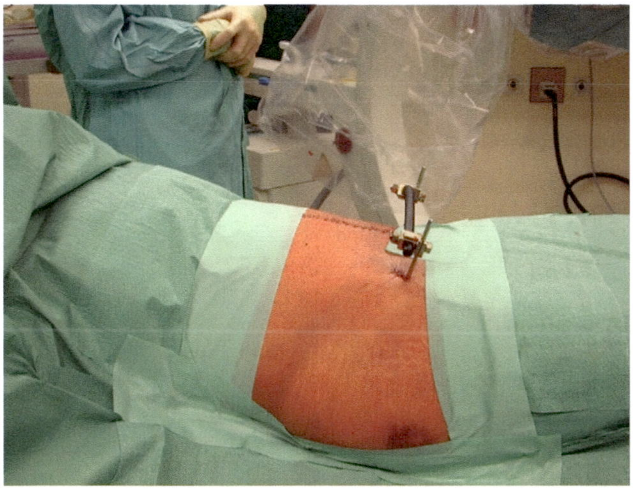

Fig. 31.17 Typical draping of the pelvic region for iliosacral screw fixation

injury [26]. Often, some posterior malreduction is observed, which is best visualized on the pelvic inlet view.

If closed reduction maneuvers fail, open reduction should be considered [26].

31.7.6 Skin Incision

For SI joint injuries, after closed reduction, the entry point is located approximately 2 cm posterior to the intersection point of the femoral shaft axis line and a vertical line from the ASIS to the OR table (Fig. 31.21) [26].

31.7.7 Confirmation of the Wire/Drill Position

Several intraoperative x-rays are necessary to confirm the correct wire/drill position during insertion to avoid extraos-

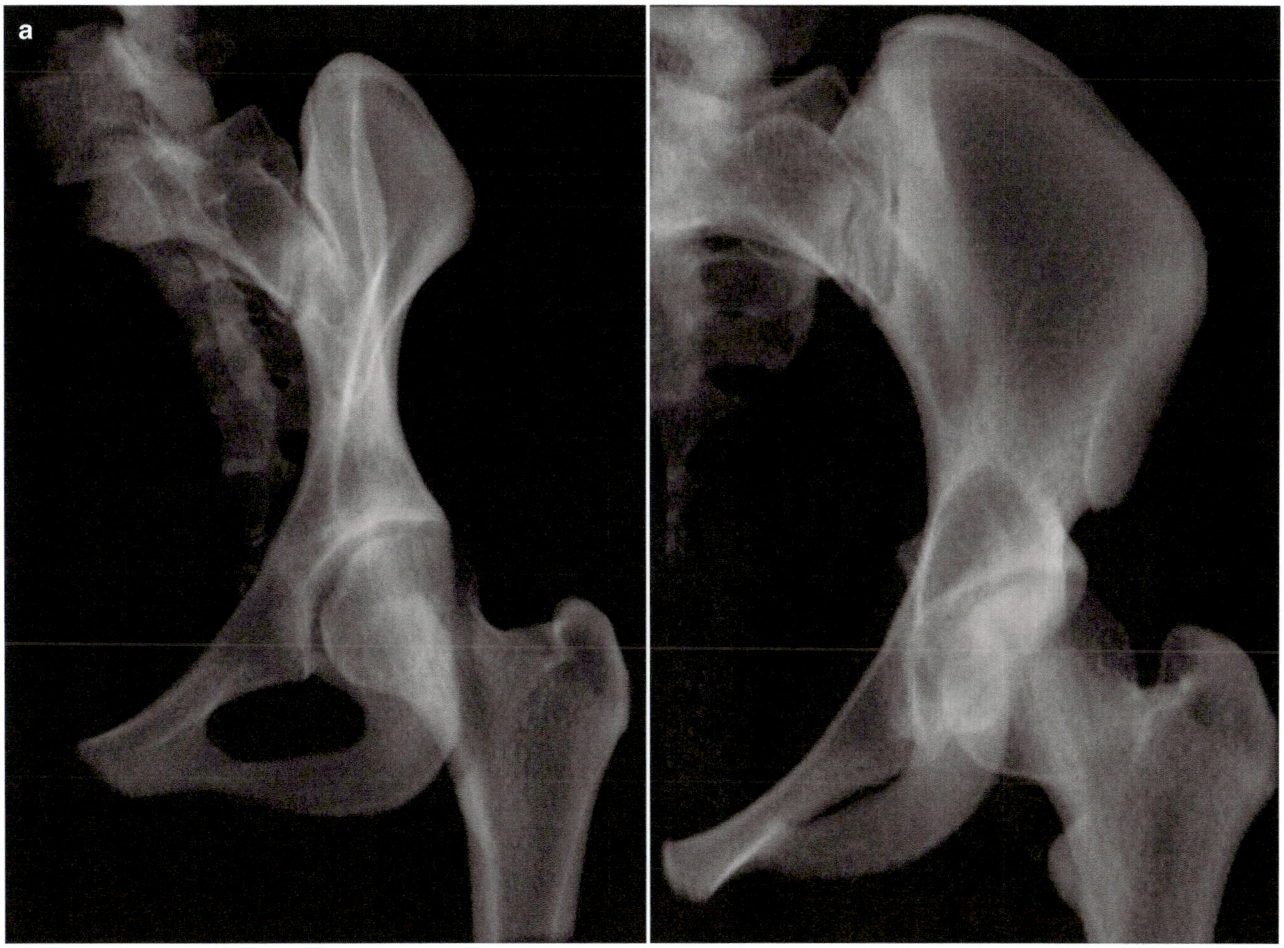

Fig. 31.18 (**a**) Obturator oblique view and pelvic Inlet view for analysis of the quality of reduction of the SI joint. (**b**) Intraoperative Inlet and Outlet views after closed reduction of temporary fixation of the disrupted SI joint with a K-wire, which is slightly placed superior and posterior to the suspected screw pathway

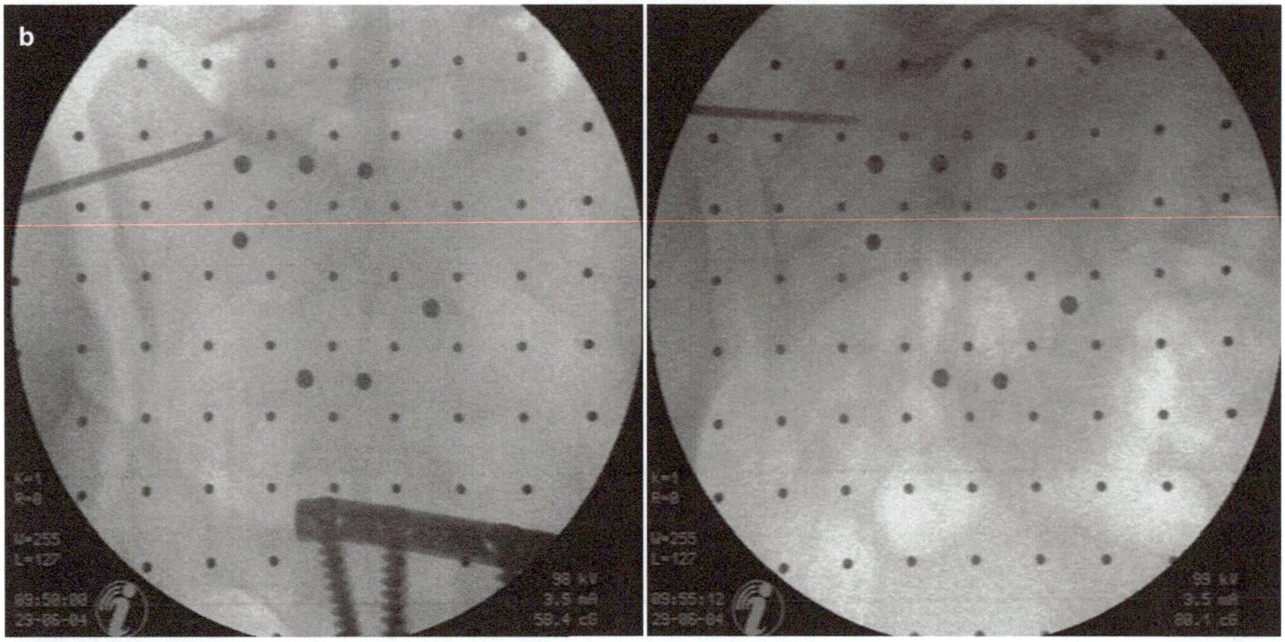

Fig. 31.18 (continued)

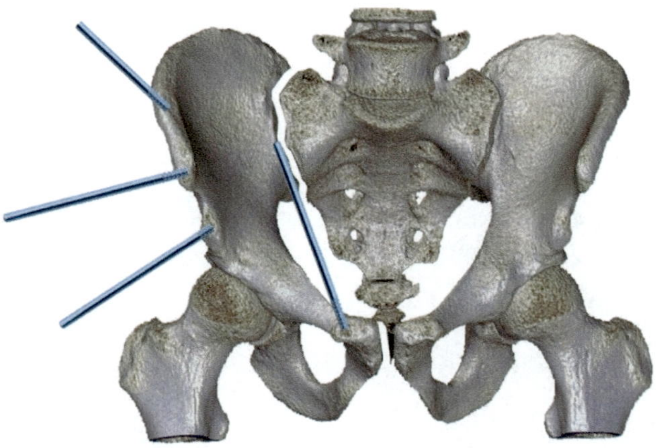

Fig. 31.19 Schematic drawing of possible Schanz screw insertion sites for closed (percutaneous) manipulation of the right hemipelvis for reduction of the SI joint

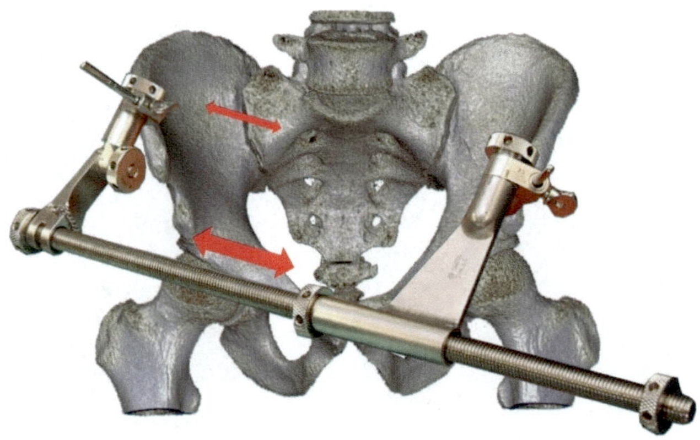

Fig. 31.20 Schematic drawing of reduction of the SI joint using a distractor

seous placement. Starting with true lateral sacral x-rays, inlet and outlet views are analyzed followed by an additional lateral sacral x-ray.

31.7.7.1 True Lateral Sacral X-Ray

Identification of the entry point is performed using the true lateral x-ray of the sacrum (Fig. 31.22) with the x-ray beam centered on the S1 body [26, 78]. The tip of an instrument guides to the optimal starting point (Fig. 31.23).

After skin incision, blunt dissection is performed down to the bone [58, 66]. Here, the guide pin or drill bit is used to "palpate" the change of orientation at the outer ilium at the

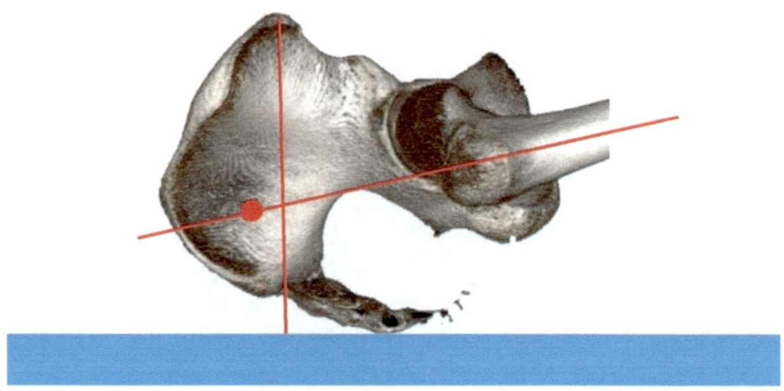

Fig. 31.21 Skin Incision for optimal insertion point according to Routt: approximately 2 cm posterior to the intersection point of the femoral shaft axis line and a vertical line from the ASIS to the OR table

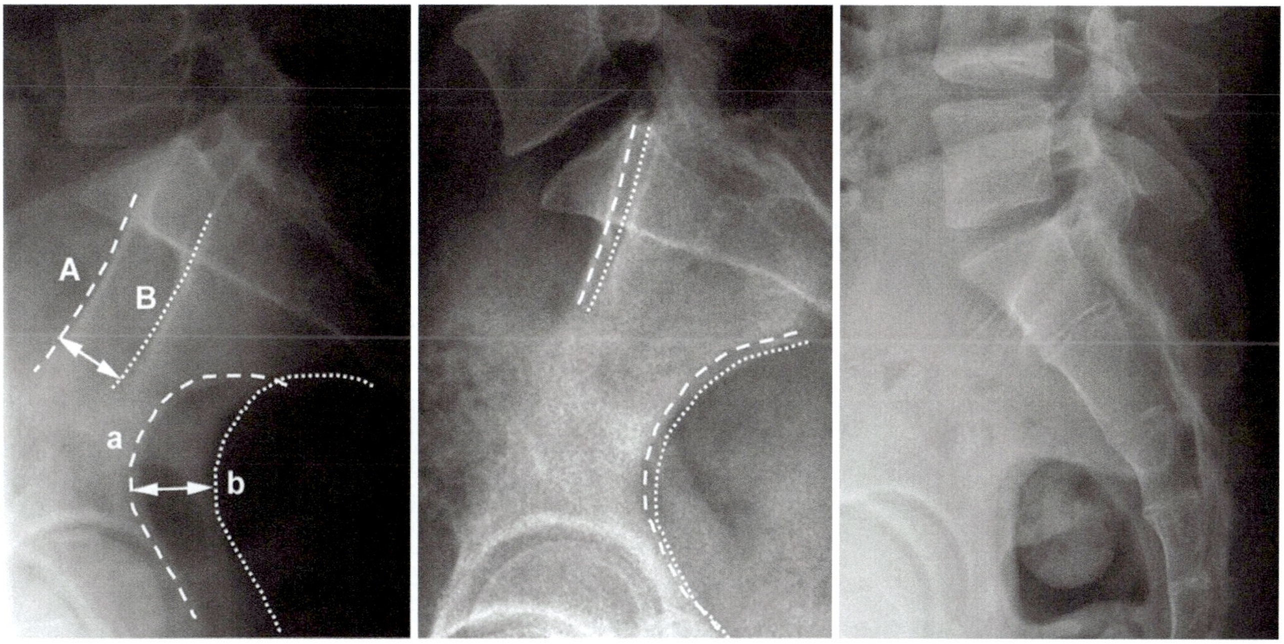

Fig. 31.22 A true lateral sacral view is mandatory to identify the optimal entry point

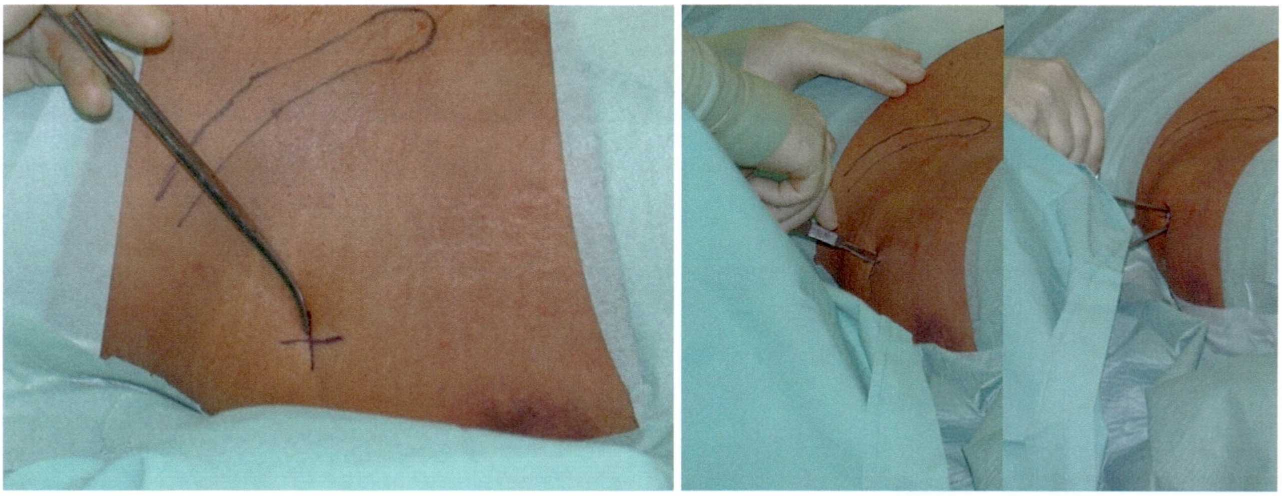

Fig. 31.23 The tip of an instrument guides to the optimal starting point and after skin incision, blunt dissection is performed down to the bone

SI joint level in two planes. A resulting "groove" can be felt to aid orientation (Fig. 31.24). A blunt cannulated instrument such as a clamp is favored.

Matta and Saucedo proposed screw direction toward the S1 body. The starting point at the outer ilium is located 15 mm anterior to the gluteal crest at the midpoint between the iliac crest and the sciatic notch, perpendicular to the ilium [79], which is only possible to identify during open posterior access.

On the true lateral sacral view, the optimal entry point is located in a caudal-cranial direction, starting at the posterior center of the S1 body, few millimeters posterior of the posterior S1 body border (Fig. 31.25). The wire tip is projected on the sacral canal. Drilling of the K-wire into the bone is performed for 2–3 mm, penetrating only the outer cortex of the ilium [31, 58, 66, 78].

The guided direction is controlled with the individual inlet and outlet views. Here, the K-wire should start posterior-lateral at the ilium to run perpendicular to the SI joint. The pin orientation should be guided cephalad to the superior border of the S1 foramen and caudal to the L5/S1 disc space [26].

With only penetrating the first millimeters of the iliac bone, the optimal guide wire direction can be manipulated using the inlet and outlet views [78].

31.7.7.2 Inlet View

The guide wire/drill bit should be orientated into the S1 vertebral body between the spinal canal posterior and the anterior S1 border. The potential end point should be located 1–1.5 cm posterior of the anterior sacral border, exactly ending at the sacral midline [78, 80].

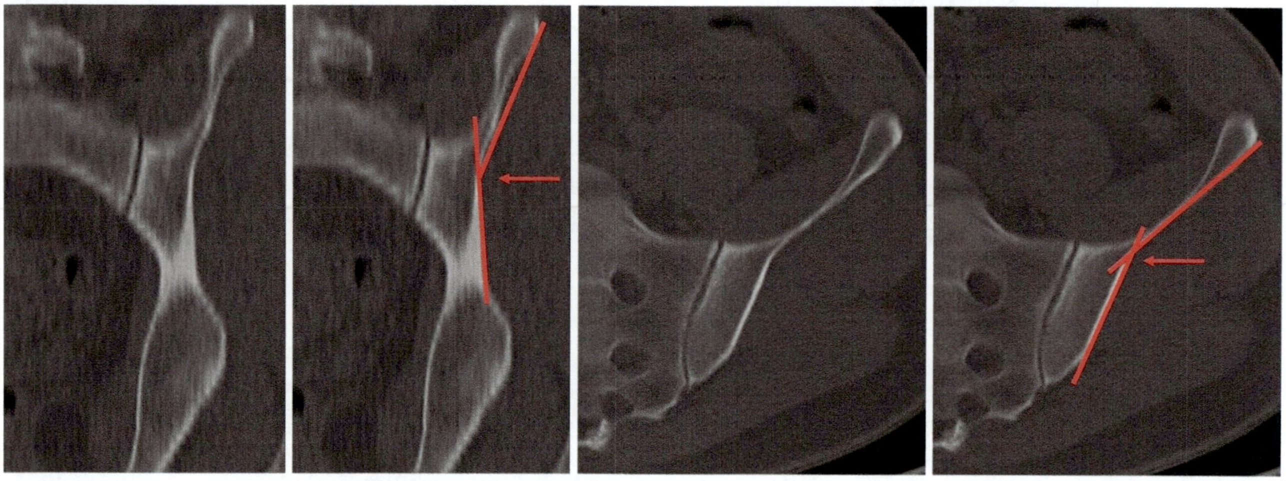

Fig. 31.24 Change of surface orientation on the outer iliac bone in two different planes creating a groove, which can be palpated using a blunt instrument

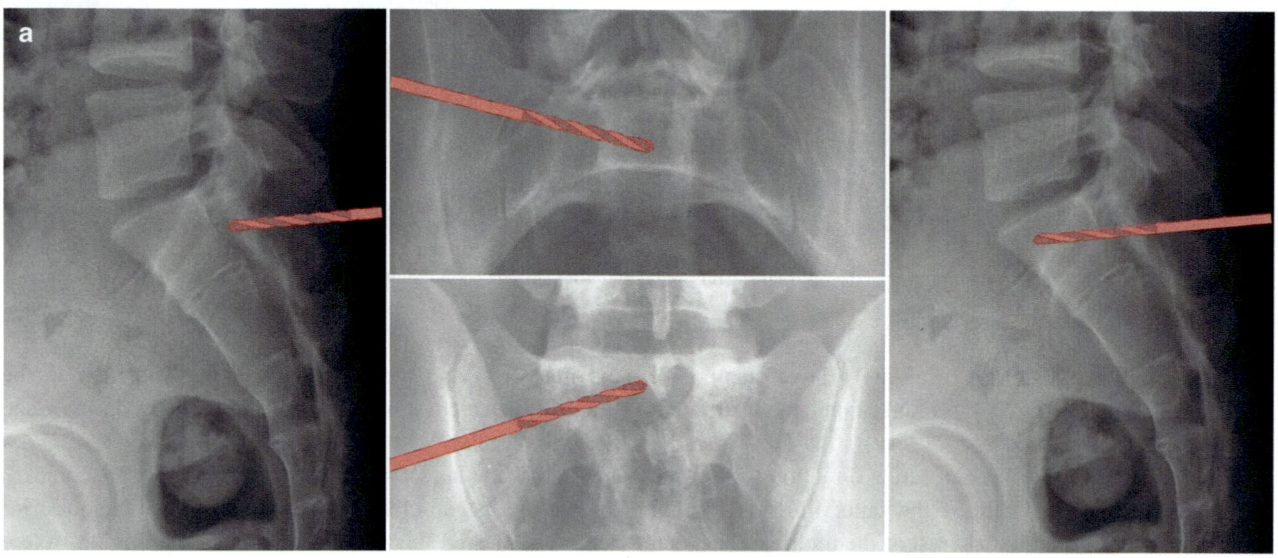

Fig. 31.25 (**a**) Drill bit orientation and potential end point for iliosacral screws in SI joint injuries: the starting point is located a few millimeters posterior of the posterior S1 body border; drilling should end near the anterior S1 cortex and approximately 1 cm inferior to the sacral promontory and 1 cm posterior to the anterior sacral cortex. (**b**) Navigation-assisted iliosacral screw insertion into S1 and S2 showing the intraoperative screw trajectories

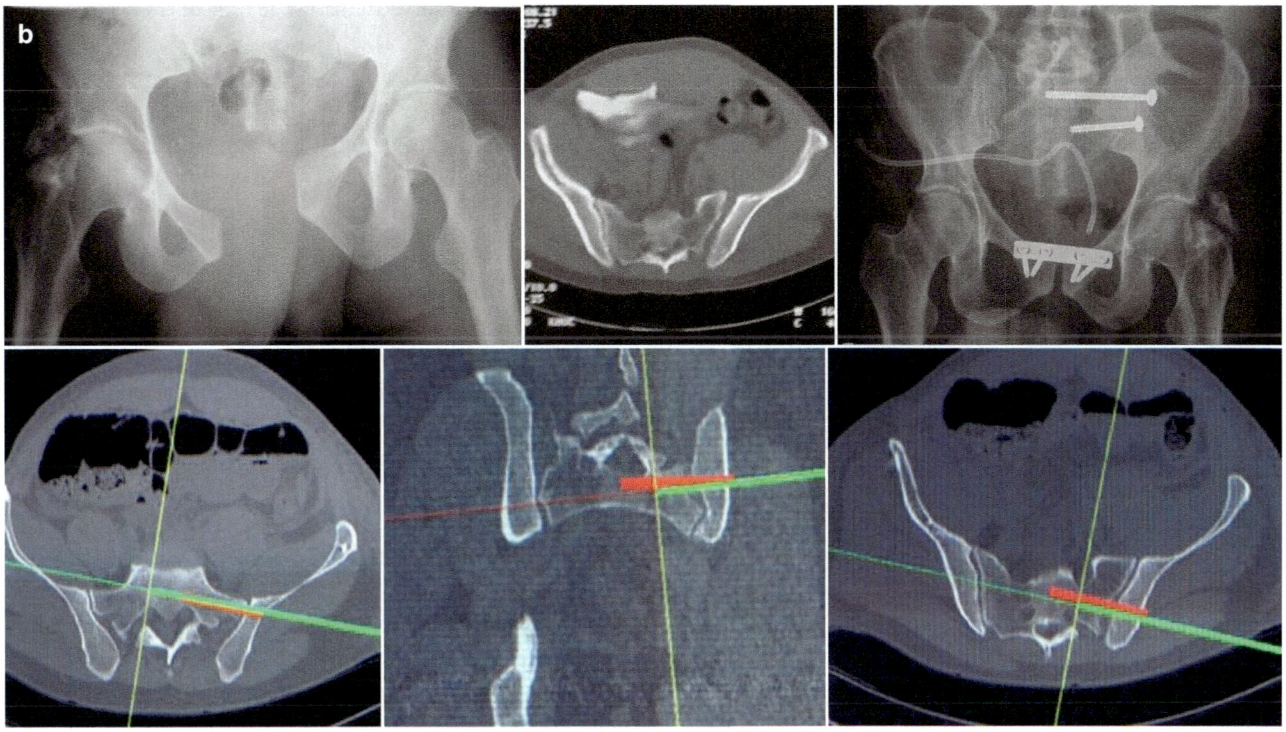

Fig. 31.25 (continued)

31.7.7.3 Outlet View

The guide wire/drill bit path should be orientated between the S1 neuroforamen inferior and the L5/S1 disc space superior. A high orientated drill tip position near the superior S1 body border can indicate anterior drill penetration, especially if combined with a far anterior position of the drill tip on the inlet view. The ideal drill direction is parallel to the superior S1 endplate. Tactile feeling of penetration of exclusively three cortices is safe.

The starting point is located at the level of the first sacral foramen and directed toward the opposite upper corner of first sacral body [32].

In SI joint disruptions the screw should be placed perpendicular to the joint plane and tilted slightly upward in the frontal plane of the sacral bone (Outlet view) and with a slight posteroanterior screw angulation in the horizontal plane (Inlet view) [28].

31.7.7.4 True Lateral Sacral X-Ray

The imaginary potential endpoint of the wire/drill should be orientated approximately 1 cm inferior to the sacral promontory and 1 cm posterior to the anterior sacral cortex (Fig. 31.11) [78].

31.7.8 Screw Orientation

Several data exist regarding optimal screw angulation relative to the inlet and outlet planes [8, 11, 15, 19, 21, 32, 36, 81]. Depending on the different anatomical sacral shape, no universal angles (superior inclination in the outlet plane, anterior inclination in the inlet plane) can be proposed.

In normal nondysmorphic sacra, the following angulations are reported:

- Superior inclination (outlet): 20–30° inclination can be expected (16° [81], 21° [11], 22° [15], 31° [36], 19–45° [8], 32° [19])
- Anterior inclination (inlet): 10–15° inclination can be expected (4° [11], 7° [19], 11° [15], 14° [36], 0–25° [8], 28° [81])

In dysmorphic sacra, lower angulations were reported [11]:

- Superior inclination (outlet): 30° inclination can be expected
- Anterior inclination (inlet): 15° inclination can be expected

31.7.9 Wire Placement

The threaded wire is inserted into the S1 body using a hammer or by oscillation drilling.

Following optimum guide wire/drill positioning, the length is measured.

Now the cannulated drill is passed over the threaded wire and the hole is drilled. In order to avoid opposite wire penetration, drilling should stop approximately 1 cm lateral to the end of the wire (Fig. 31.26).

31.7.10 Screw Type

Different screws are available for iliosacral screw stabilization. 6.5–7.3 mm cannulated screws, fully or partially threaded are recommended [31, 58, 62, 66, 68, 70, 78, 82].

In general, screws with a short thread are recommended for screw fixation of the SI joint, while for sacral fractures fully threaded screws may be used in order to avoid overcompression [83].

Screws with a short thread should be used in SI joint injuries to allow adequate joint compression. Two screws are recommended routinely [80]. Alternatively, two screws are inserted into S1 or one screw into S1 and another screw into S2 [68].

Additional washers reduce the risk of iliac bone penetration. An obturator oblique inlet or outlet view can confirm the adequate washer position at the outer iliac surface.

31.7.11 Expected Screw Length

Some data exist regarding the expected screw length:

- Gardner et al. reported an iliosacral screw length of at least 75 mm [11].
- Conflitti et al. reported a mean screw length of 100.8 mm (87.1–114.4 mm) [43].
- Wendt et al. analyzed female and male sacra with an expected screw length of 84.5 mm and 81.6 mm, respectively [19].
- Chon et al. observed a screw length of 98.8 mm (range 82.4–132.2 mm) [32].

> The expected screw length for oblique iliosacral screws is approximately 85 mm.

31.7.12 Radiographs

Finally, standard intraoperative radiographs are taken: true lateral sacral view, pelvic inlet and outlet projections, and an obturator oblique inlet view, which enables good recognition of the lateral boundary of the cortex of the ilium.

31.7.13 Postoperative Course

It is unclear whether to perform anterior ring stabilization first or after posterior stabilization [58, 66].

Following wound irrigation, the skin is closed using standard techniques.

Partial weight bearing of the injured side with 15 kg BW for maximum 6 weeks using two crutches is recommended. A pelvic anteroposterior radiograph and a posterior CT scan of the pelvis are typically performed to verify the screw position.

31.7.14 Complications

Several potential complications are associated with this technique:

- There is a potential risk of injury to the gluteal vessel and nerve bundle if screws enter too far toward a posteroinferior screw insertion site [23]
- Iatrogenic nerve damage
- Screw loosening
- Incorrect screw position (Fig. 31.27)
- Loss of reduction

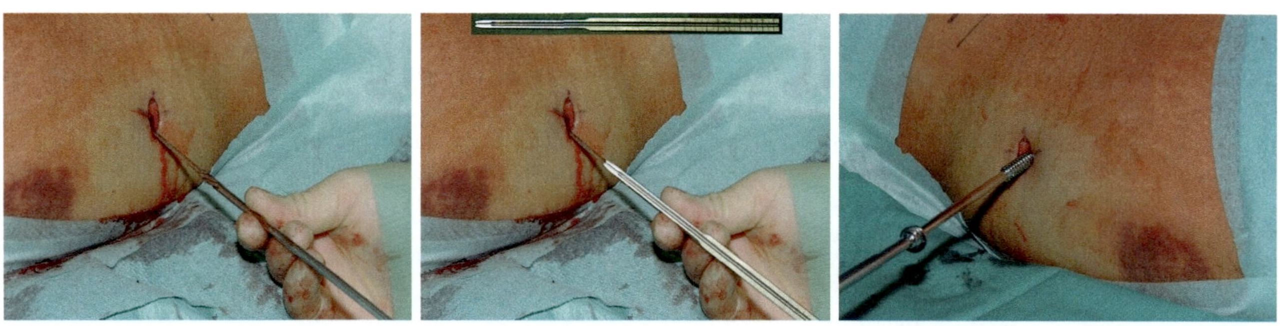

Fig. 31.26 After insertion of the guide wire, drilling is performed using the oscillating technique and after length measurement, the screw is inserted (always using a washer). A short threaded screw is used

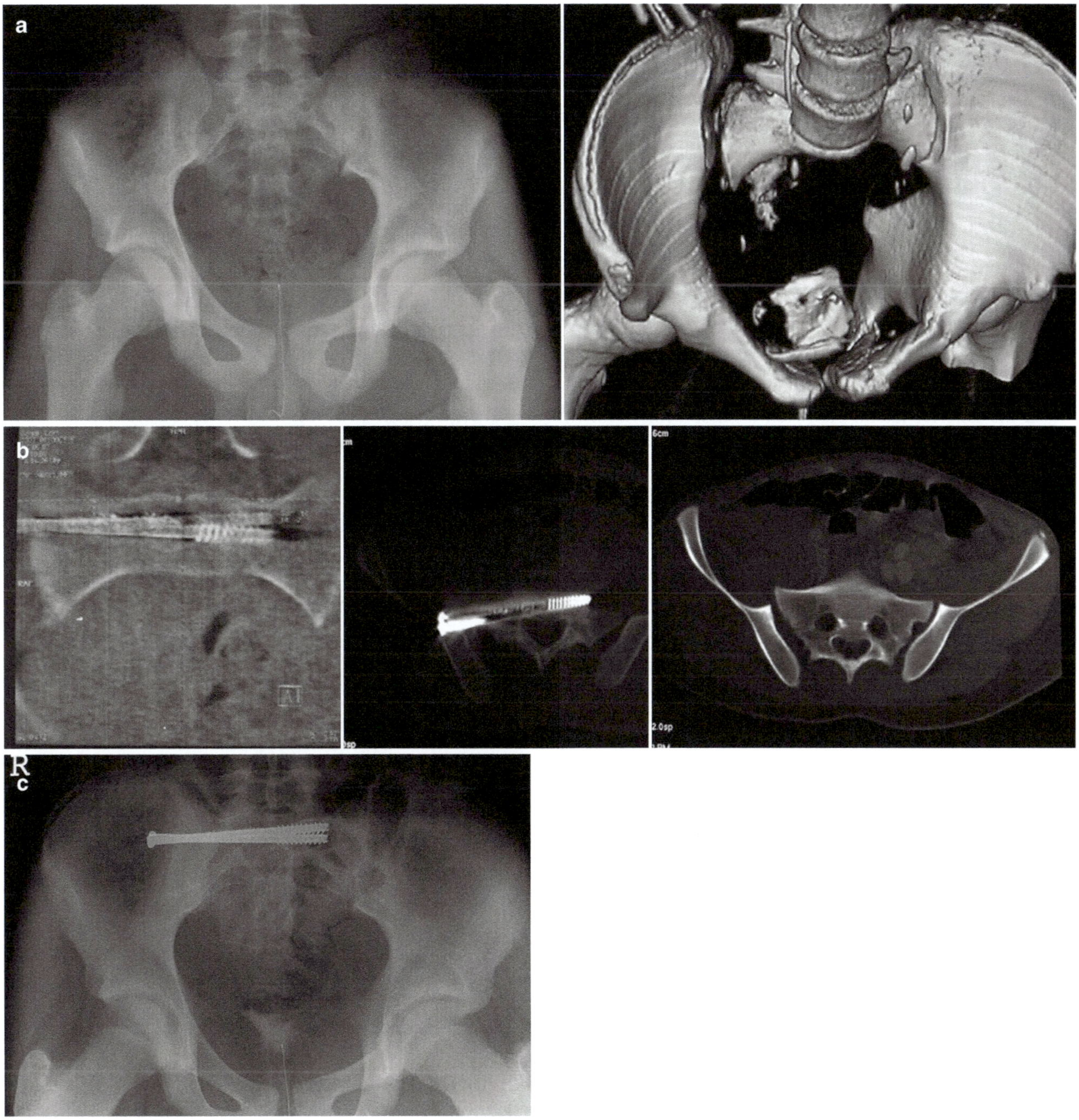

Fig. 31.27 (**a**) Case example of a malpositioned screw: 16-year-old male after roll-over injury with a type C injury (right SI joint dislocation, left pubic rami fractures). (**b**) The intraoperative view shows a too posterior positioned screw. The postoperative CT indicates a too long screw and a malreduced SI joint. (**c**) The postoperative x-ray shows too cranially positioned screws

31.8 Transverse Iliosacral Screw Fixation of Unstable Sacrum Fractures

After initiation of iliosacral screw fixation of sacral fractures by Ebraheim et al. [58, 67] and Duwelius et al. [66, 84], it was the merit of Chip Routt to describe the anatomical basis and the operative technique in detail [18, 85].

31.8.1 Indications

The classical indications for transverse iliosacral screw fixation of sacral fractures include:

- Sacral fractures without concomitant nerve damage in type C pelvic injuries, which can be reduced anatomically using a closed technique [31]

- (Bilateral) U-shaped sacral fractures [33, 86]
- Minimally displaced spinopelvic dissociation injuries [87–89]
- Incomplete sacral fractures [90]

31.8.2 Patient Positioning

Prone, (semi-)lateral, and supine positioning can be performed (Fig. 31.14) [62, 66–70].

The patient is usually placed on a radiolucent OR table in the supine position (Fig. 31.14) [26]. A lumbopelvic support is advised to enable sufficient posterior access (Fig. 31.15) [31].

Positioning must allow pelvic inlet and outlet views, and the true lateral sacral x-ray. Historically, the angulation of pelvic inlet and outlet views in relation to the anterior-posterior plane of the pelvis were described as being 40° in each plane [71].

An optimal inlet angulation for the S1 body of approximately 25° and a corresponding outlet angle of approximately 50° are recommended [72–75]. Sacral dysmorphism lead to an increase of the outlet angle of 5° (Fig. 31.16) [73].

From a clinical perspective, the optimum pelvic inlet view is achieved when the first and second sacral bodies directly overlap, while an optimal pelvic outlet view is achieved when the upper border of the pubic symphysis/pubic rami is projected on the second sacral vertebra (Fig. 31.16).

31.8.3 Anesthesiology

General anesthesia is routinely recommended [26]. But even local anesthesia or epidural anesthesia is possible [58, 62, 66, 68, 70]. Somatosensory-evoked potential monitoring [26, 76, 77] is not routinely used.

31.8.4 Draping

The lower abdomen and the affected half of the pelvis are draped (Fig. 31.17). Depending on the amount of displacement and the necessity of reduction, the leg is mobile draped.

31.8.5 Closed Reduction

The already described reduction maneuvers are performed when necessary (Figs. 31.19 and 31.20).

The true inlet view is used to analyze the anterior reduction, while the outlet view confirms craniocaudal reduction.

If closed reduction maneuvers fail, open reduction should be considered [31, 90, 91].

Reilly et al. performed an anatomical analysis of sacral fracture malreduction [10]. With cranial displacements of 5, 10, 15, and 20 mm, the resultant bone contact area decreased by 30%, 56%, 81%, and 90%, respectively.

> The maximum accepted malreduction should be <5 mm for safe intraosseous screw insertion.

Thus, slightly displaced sacral fractures can be fixed in situ. In displaced fractures, anterior pelvic fixation is usually performed first [92] as limited posterior reduction is thus often already achieved.

The exact vector of the reduction is not known. Reduction, and, in particular, retention of the reduction are of critical importance.

It is imperative that the reduction be checked using the image intensifier in order to avoid incorrect screw positioning [31].

31.8.6 Skin Incision

The entry point is located approximately 2 cm posterior to the intersection point of the femoral shaft axis line and a vertical line from the ASIS to the OR table (Fig. 31.21) [31, 91].

31.8.7 Confirmation of the Wire/Drill Position

Several intraoperative x-rays are necessary to confirm the correct wire/drill position during insertion to avoid extraosseous placement. Starting with true lateral sacral x-ray, inlet and outlet views are analyzed followed by an additional lateral sacral x-ray.

31.8.8 Radiographs

31.8.8.1 True Lateral Sacral X-Ray

Identification of the entry point is performed using the true lateral x-ray of the sacrum (Fig. 31.28) with the x-ray beam centered on the S1 body [26, 78]. The tip of an instrument guides to the optimal starting point (Fig. 31.29).

After skin incision, blunt dissection is performed down to the bone [58, 66]. Here, the guide pin or drill bit is used to "palpate" the change of orientation at the outer ilium at the SI joint level in two planes. A resulting "groove" can be felt to aid orientation (Fig. 31.24). A blunt cannulated instrument such as a clamp is favored.

After identification of the target area below the level of the sacral alar slope and between the anterior and posterior border of the sacral cortex (Fig. 31.30), the guide wire is hammered approximately 2–3 mm into the bone, thus penetrating only the outer iliac cortex (Fig. 31.31) [31, 91]. This

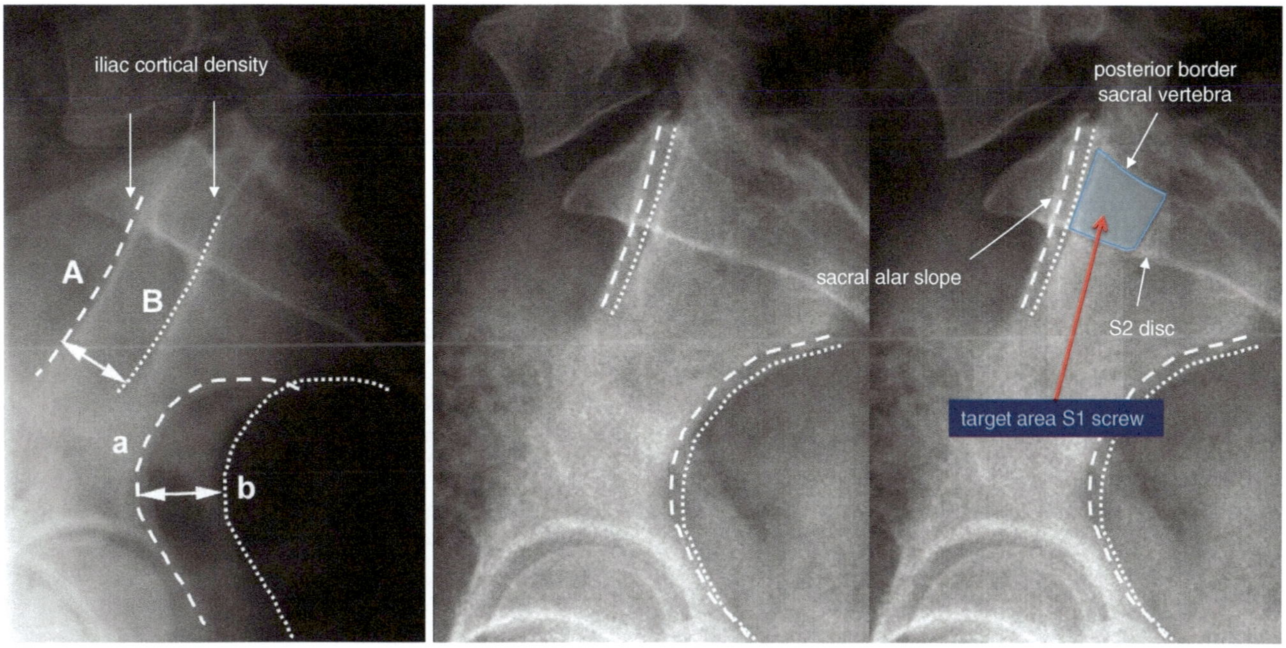

Fig. 31.28 The postoperative x-ray shows too cranially positioned screws

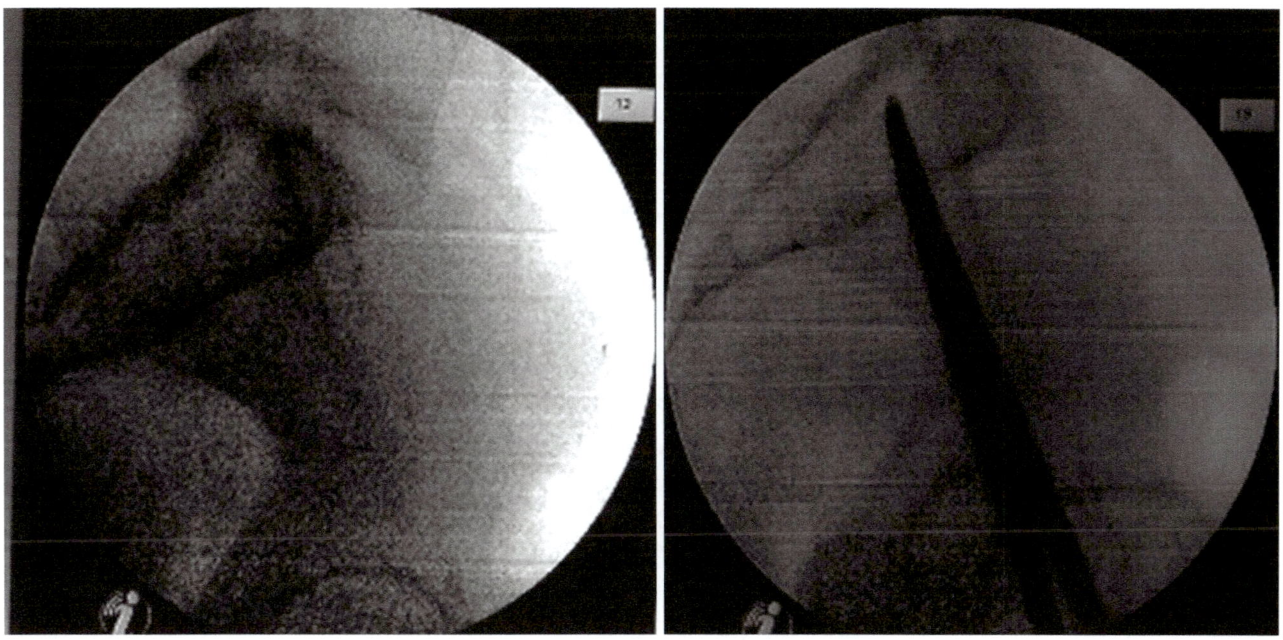

Fig. 31.29 The tip of an instrument guides to the optimal starting point on the true lateral x-ray

allows for manipulation of the wire direction on the inlet and outlet views to be safely within the bone corridor.

The guided direction is controlled with the individual inlet and outlet views. Here, the K-wire should start in the middle of the S1 bone corridor in both planes. The pin orientation should be guided horizontally (Fig. 31.32) [31, 91].

31.8.8.2 Inlet View

The guide wire/drill bit should be orientated horizontal through the complete S1 sacral bone corridor. The anterior and posterior border of the bone corridor can be usually clearly identified (Fig. 31.32).

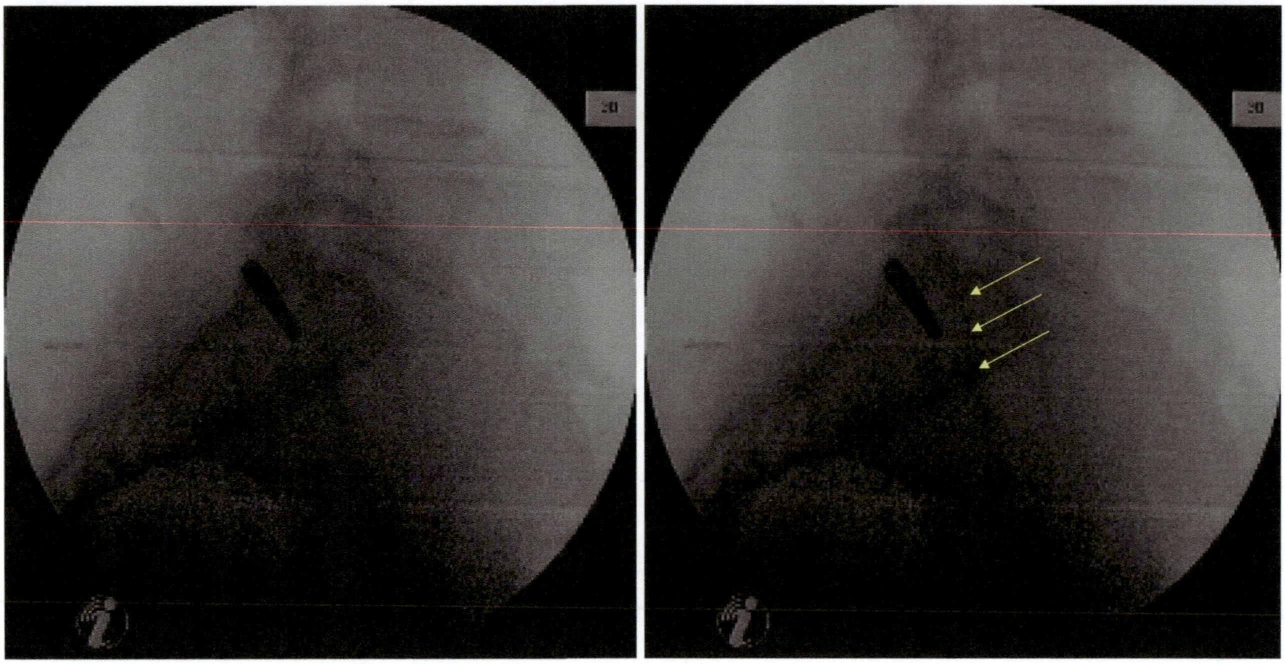

Fig. 31.30 Marking of the bony entry point with the inserted guide wire

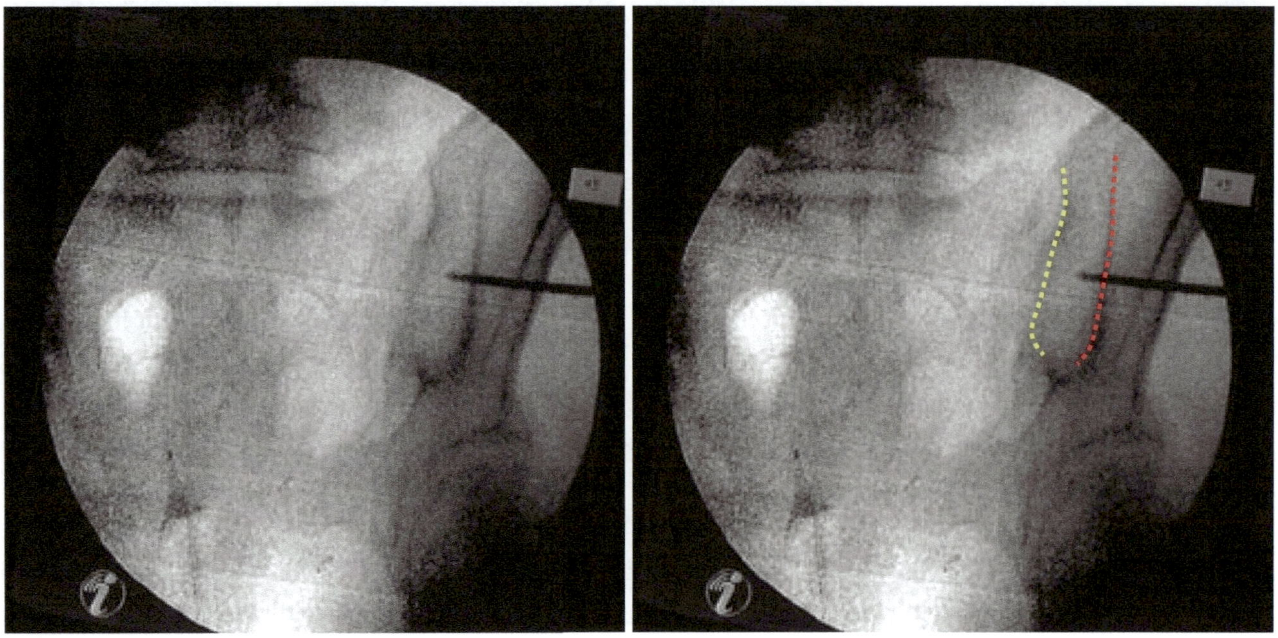

Fig. 31.31 Insertion of the guide wire into the bone, only penetrating the outer iliac cortex (red dotted line); yellow line: inner iliac cortex

31.8.8.3 Outlet View

On the outlet view, the superior tangent to the S1 sacral foramen should be identified. The superior border of the sacrum is identified (Fig. 31.32).

Using both views, the guide wire can be guided through the whole sacrum (Fig. 31.32).

By palpation of both feet, while hammering or drilling the guide wire into the bone, any motoric reaction implies inadequate wire placement and should lead to correction of the wire position.

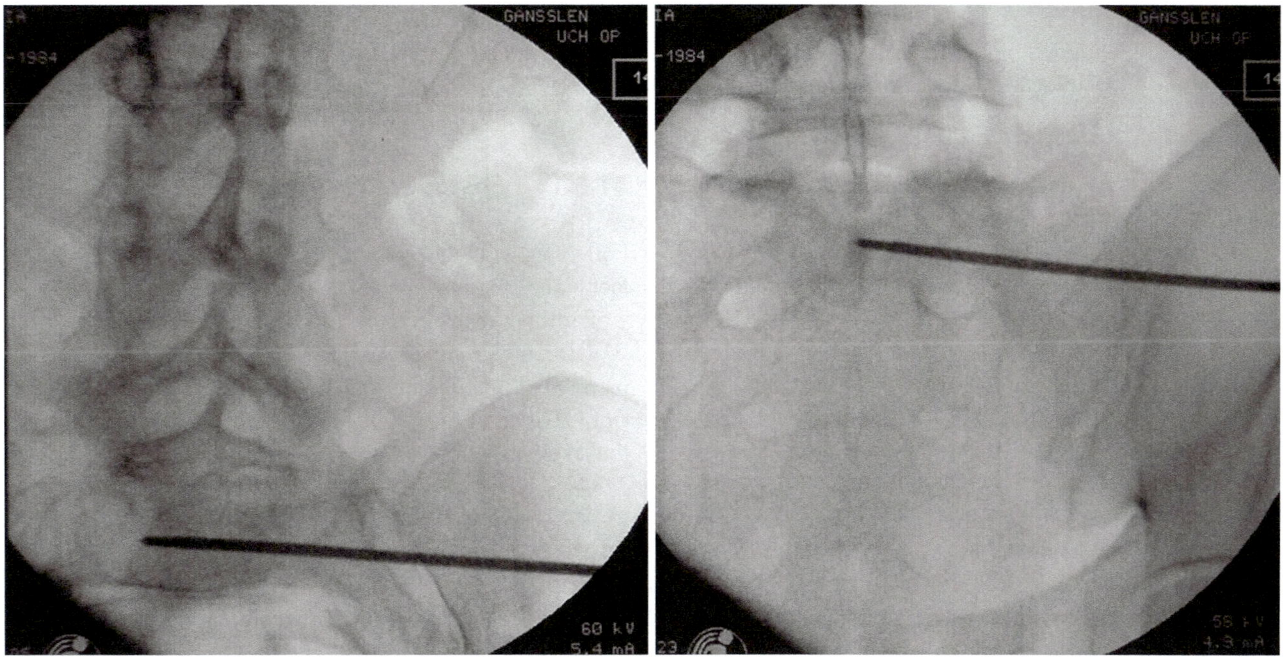

Fig. 31.32 Near horizontal/transverse orientation of the guide wire in the Inlet and Outlet view

31.8.9 Screw Orientation

A pure horizontal/transverse screw orientation is usually possible. Three screw positions are possible:

- Screw tip ending in the middle of the sacrum (transalar, Denis type I fractures [93])
- Screw tip ending near the opposite SI joint in the sacrum (transforaminal/central, Denis type II or III fractures [93])
- Screw bridging both SI joints (complete intraosseous iliosacral screw, bilateral sacral fractures [94, 95])

31.8.10 Wire Placement

The threaded wire is inserted into the S1 body using a hammer or by oscillation drilling.

Following optimum guide wire/drill positioning, the length is measured (Fig. 31.33).

Now the cannulated drill is passed over the threaded wire and the hole is drilled (Fig. 31.34). In order avoid opposite wire penetration, drilling should stop approximately 1 cm lateral to the end of the wire.

> Again, by palpation of both feet, while hammering or drilling the guide wire into the bone, any motoric reaction implies inadequate wire placement and should lead to correction of the wire position.

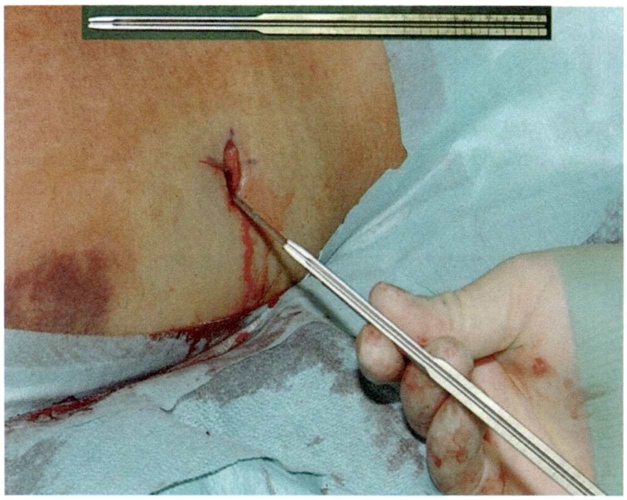

Fig. 31.33 Length measurement

31.8.11 Screw Type

Different screws are available for iliosacral screw stabilization. 6.5–7.3 mm cannulated screws, fully or partially threaded are recommended [31, 58, 62, 66, 68, 70, 78, 82].

In general, screws with a short thread are recommended for screw fixation of the SI joint while for sacral fractures fully threaded screws may be used in order to avoid overcompression [83].

> As fracture compression can be harmful due to comminution, fully threaded screws are recommended in sacral fractures.

31.8.12 Expected Screw Length

The expected screw length depends on the fracture type and the resulting treatment concept:

- Denis type I fractures: 60–80 mm screw length
- Denis type II/III fractures: 120–130 mm screw length
- Fully bridging: 160 ± 10 mm screw length

31.8.13 Screw Insertion

The screw is inserted with a washer. Again, both feet are palpated for any motoric reaction. Both the inlet and outlet views allow for optimal screw path and position of the washer (Fig. 31.35).

31.8.14 Radiographs

Finally, standard intraoperative radiographs are taken: true lateral sacral view (Fig. 31.35), pelvic inlet and outlet projections, and an obturator oblique inlet view, which enables good recognition of the lateral boundary of the cortex of the ilium (Figs. 31.36, 31.37, 31.38, 31.39, and 31.40).

31.8.15 Postoperative Course

Following wound irrigation, the skin is closed using standard techniques.

Partial weight bearing of the injured side with 15 kg BW for maximum 6 weeks with two crutches is recommended. A pelvic anteroposterior radiograph and a posterior CT scan of the pelvis are typically performed to verify the screw position.

31.8.16 Complications

Several potential complications are associated with this technique:

- There is a potential risk of injury to the gluteal vessel and nerve bundle, if screws enter too far toward a posteroinferior screw insertion site [23]
- Iatrogenic nerve damage
- Screw loosening
- Incorrect screw position (Fig. 31.41)
- Loss of reduction

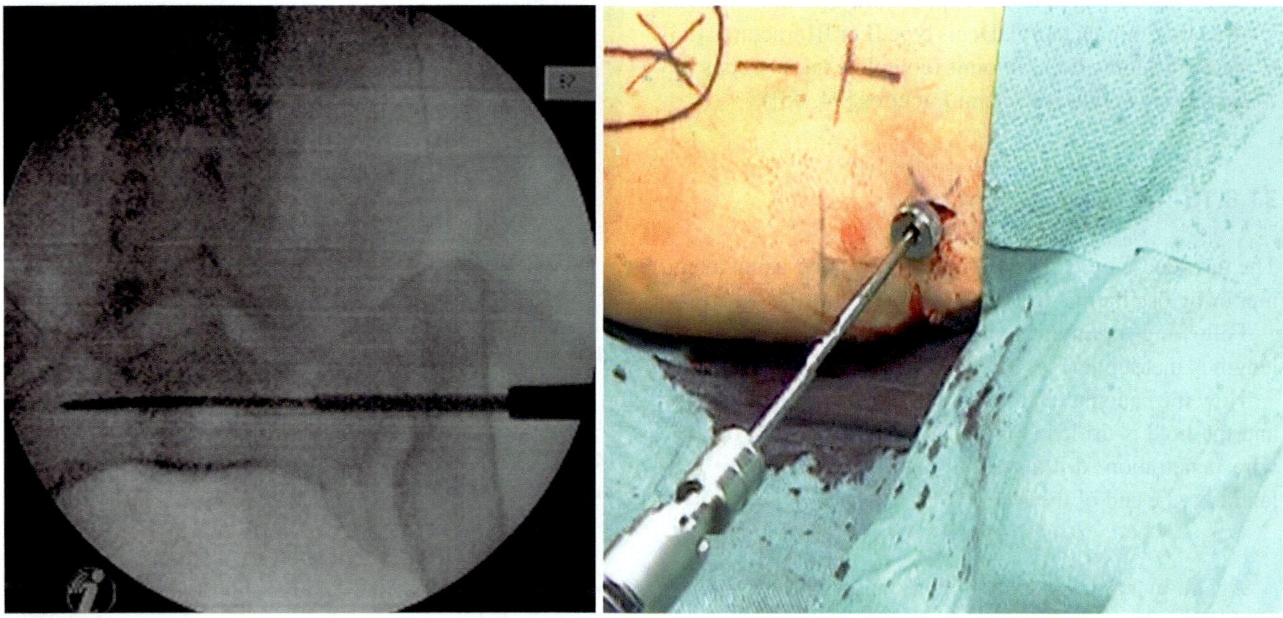

Fig. 31.34 Drilling process

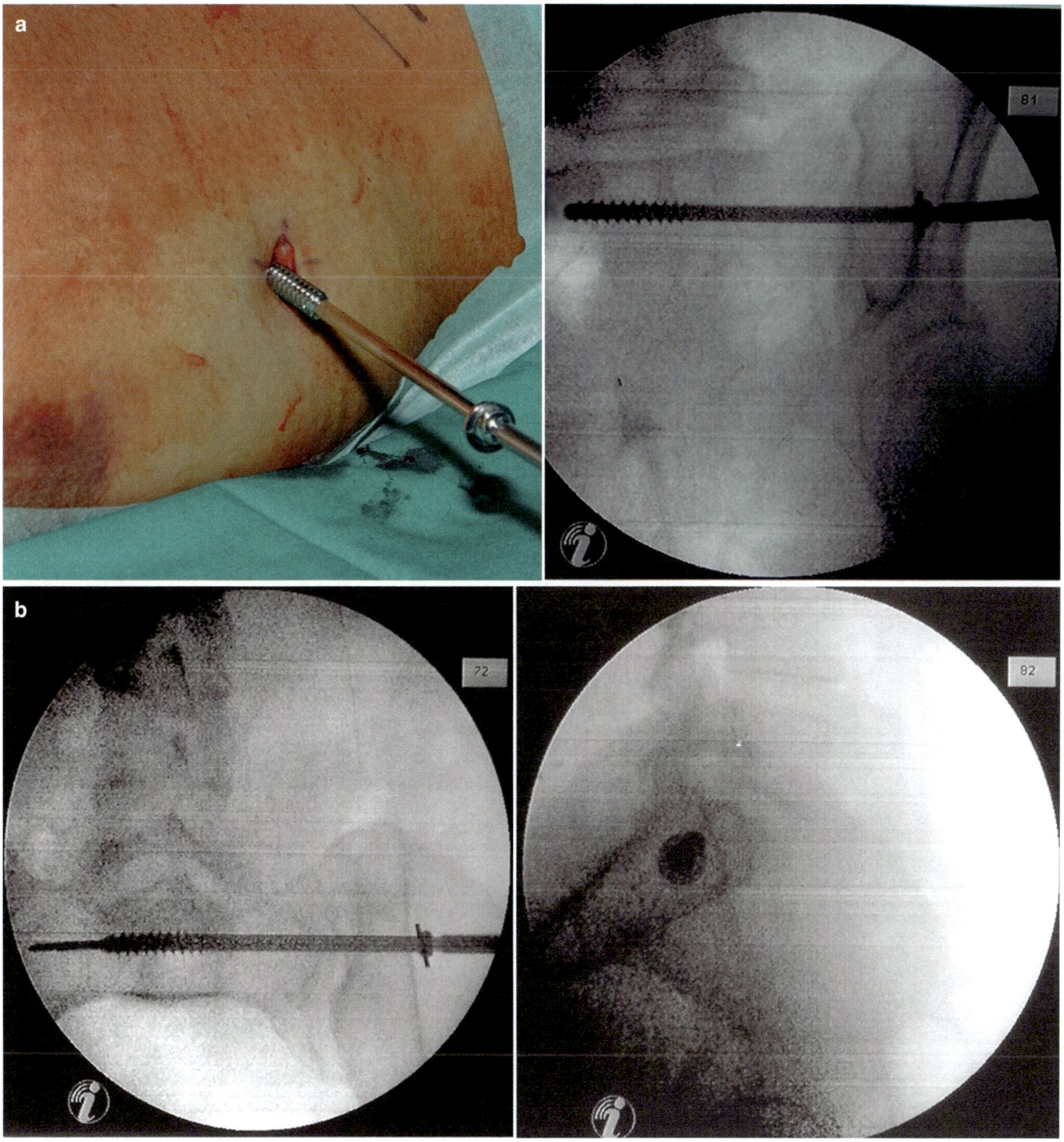

Fig. 31.35 (**a**) Screw insertion. The washer stops at the outer iliac cortex. Here, a partially threaded screw is used. (**b**) Confirmation of the screw path on the Inlet view and true lateral sacral view. Note: the position of the washer at the outer iliac surface

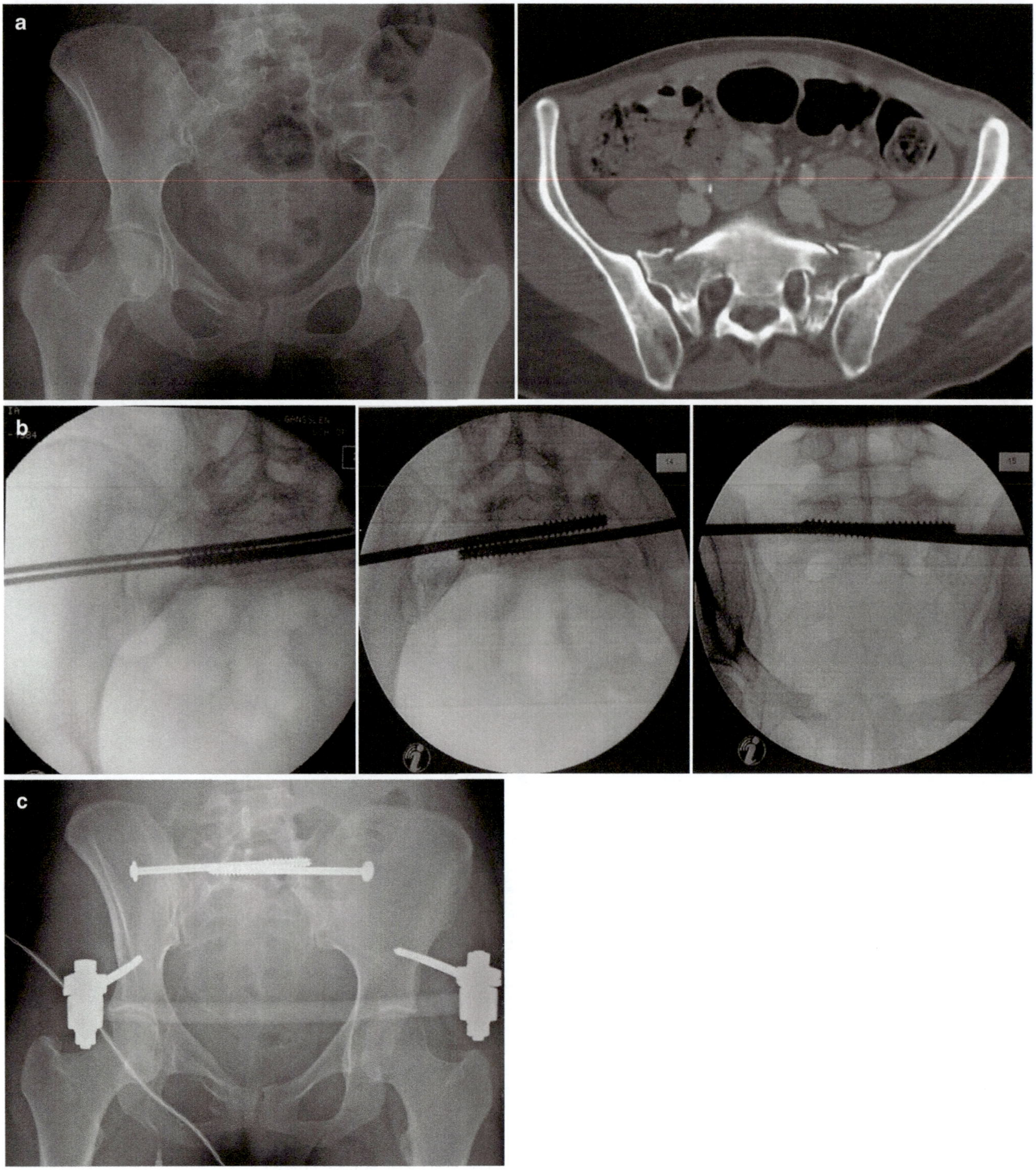

Fig. 31.36 (**a**) Dysmorphic sacrum with bilateral foraminal sacrum fractures and an undisplaced transverse fracture component (U-shaped fracture>). (**b**) Bilateral iliosacral screw stabilization: after insertion of the first screw on the left side, the guide is drilled through the screw from left to right until skin penetration is visible. Then, a second guide is inserted from right to left parallel to the first guide and a second screw is inserted. (**c**) Postoperative x-ray, confirming adequate screw position

31.9 Implant Removal

For a long time, several authors recommended routine implant removal of joint bridging implants, e.g., iliosacral screws [31, 96–98]. In contrast, others recommended implant removal only in cases with implant failure or infection [99, 100] and a routine removal was considered unusual [101].

Stuby et al. analyzed 35 of 80 surgically treated cases with implant removal after type B and -C injuries between 2003 and 2010, representing an implant removal rate of 44% [102]. Overall, at the posterior pelvis 24 iliosacral screws and 1 spinopelvic implant were removed after a mean of 14.6 months. Indications included subjective posterior pelvic pain in 46%, 33% recommended decision of the treating surgeon, and due to patient's desire in 40%. Twenty-eight percent of the iliosacral screws showed slight signs of implant loosening (11/39). An overall complication rate of 20% was observed, including the anterior pelvis ring, and only 3/11 patients after posterior pelvic ring implant removal reported a clinical benefit.

Routt et al. already stated that iliosacral screw removal is controversial. Potential advantages include posterior pelvic ring pain relief and remobilization of the (uninjured) fixed SI joint, especially in younger patients. Potential disadvantages include the potential surgical difficulty due to relevant scar

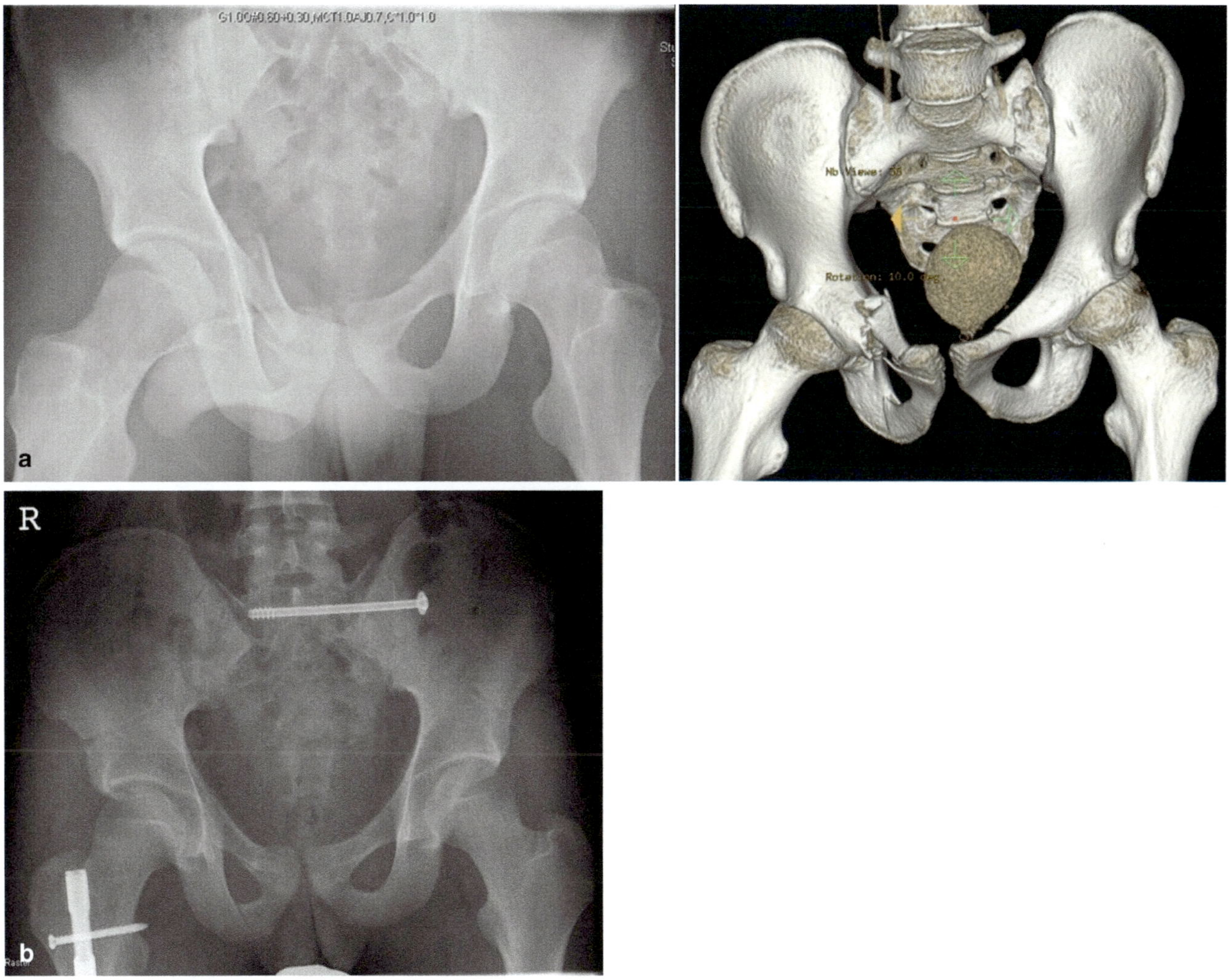

Fig. 31.37 (**a**) Left foraminal sacrum fracture in a dysmorphic sacrum. (**b**) Postoperative x-ray (the screw seems to be relatively cranially placed). (**c**) Postoperative CT reveals adequate, intraosseous screw position. Due to the dysmorphy, a different, non-horizontal screw path was performed

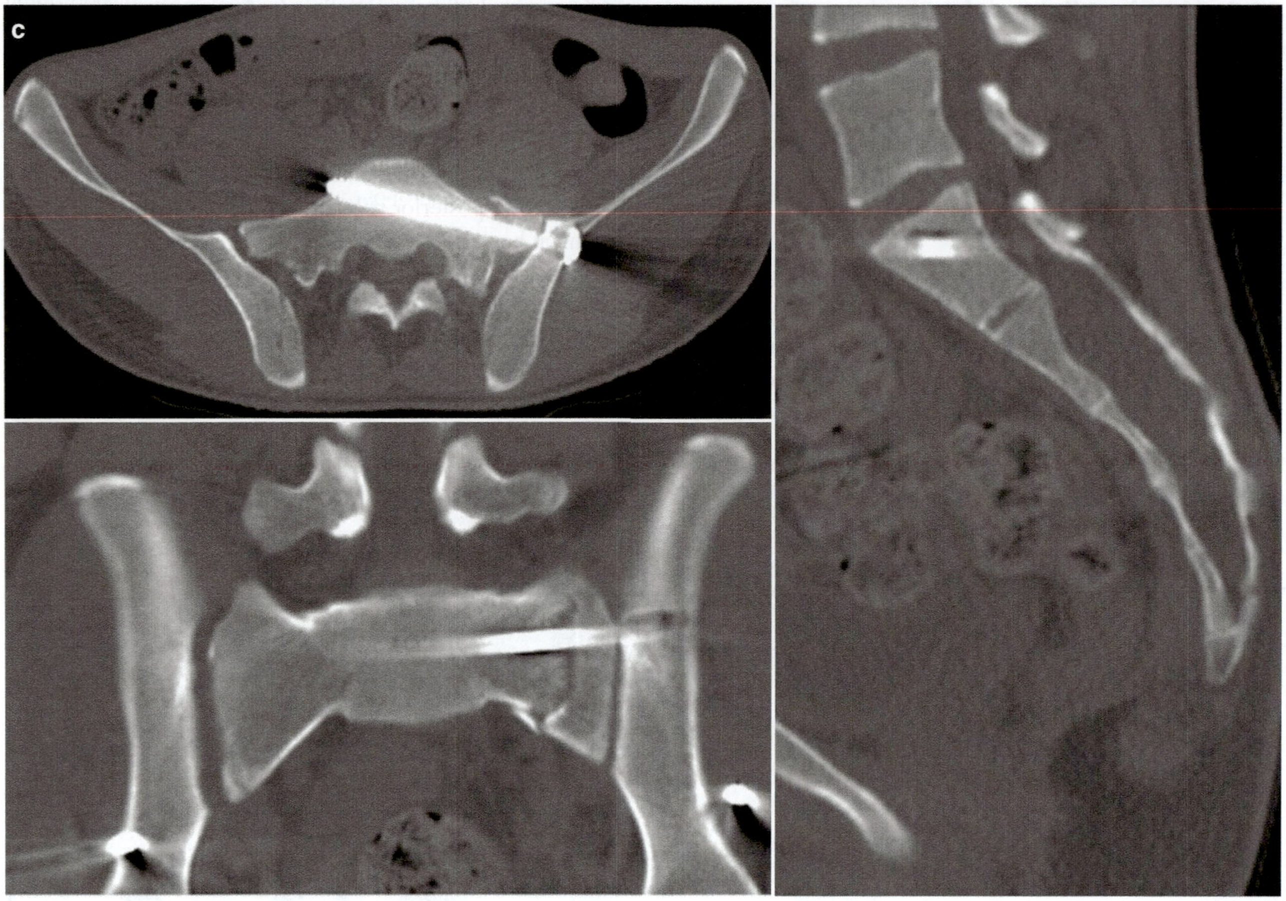

Fig. 31.37 (continued)

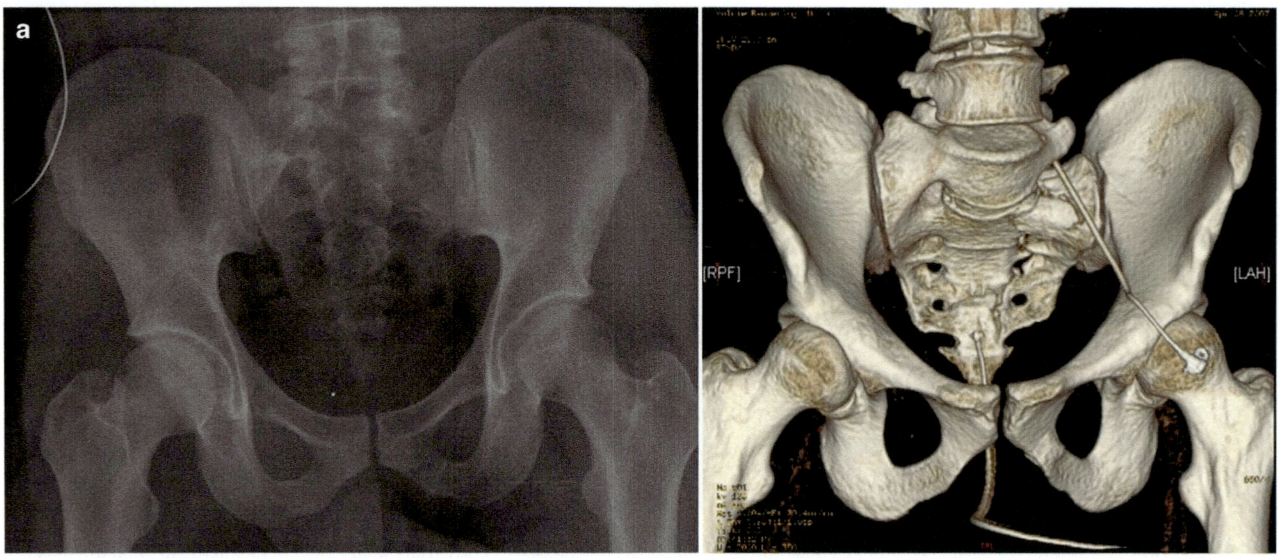

Fig. 31.38 (a) Left foraminal sacrum fracture in a hemi-sacralized fifth lumbar spine. (b) Postoperative x-ray and CT evaluation of the correct screw path

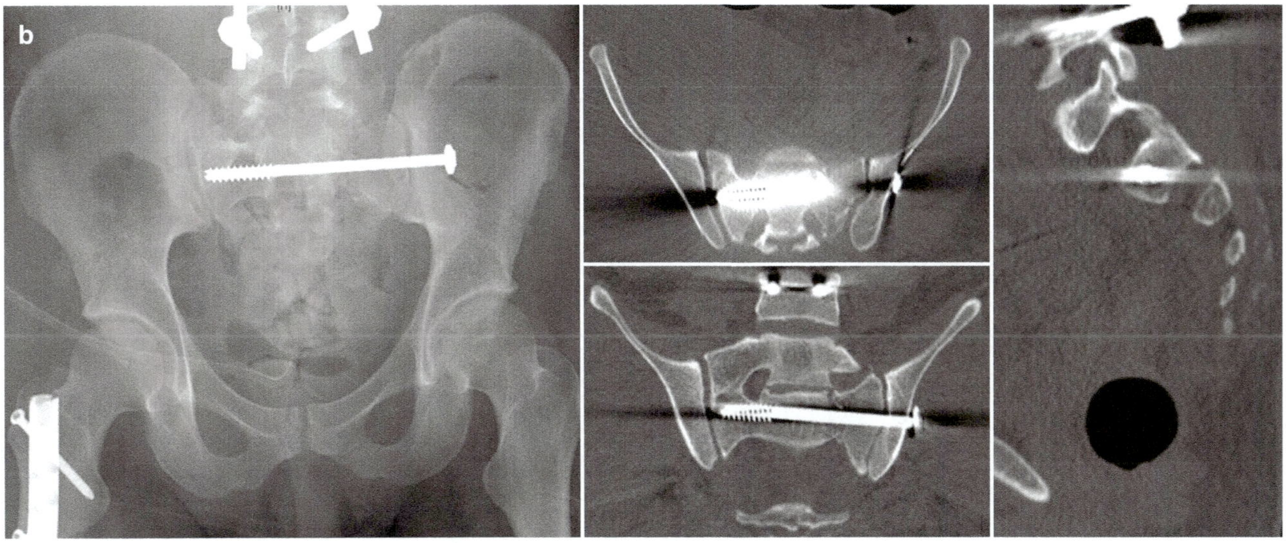

Fig. 31.38 (continued)

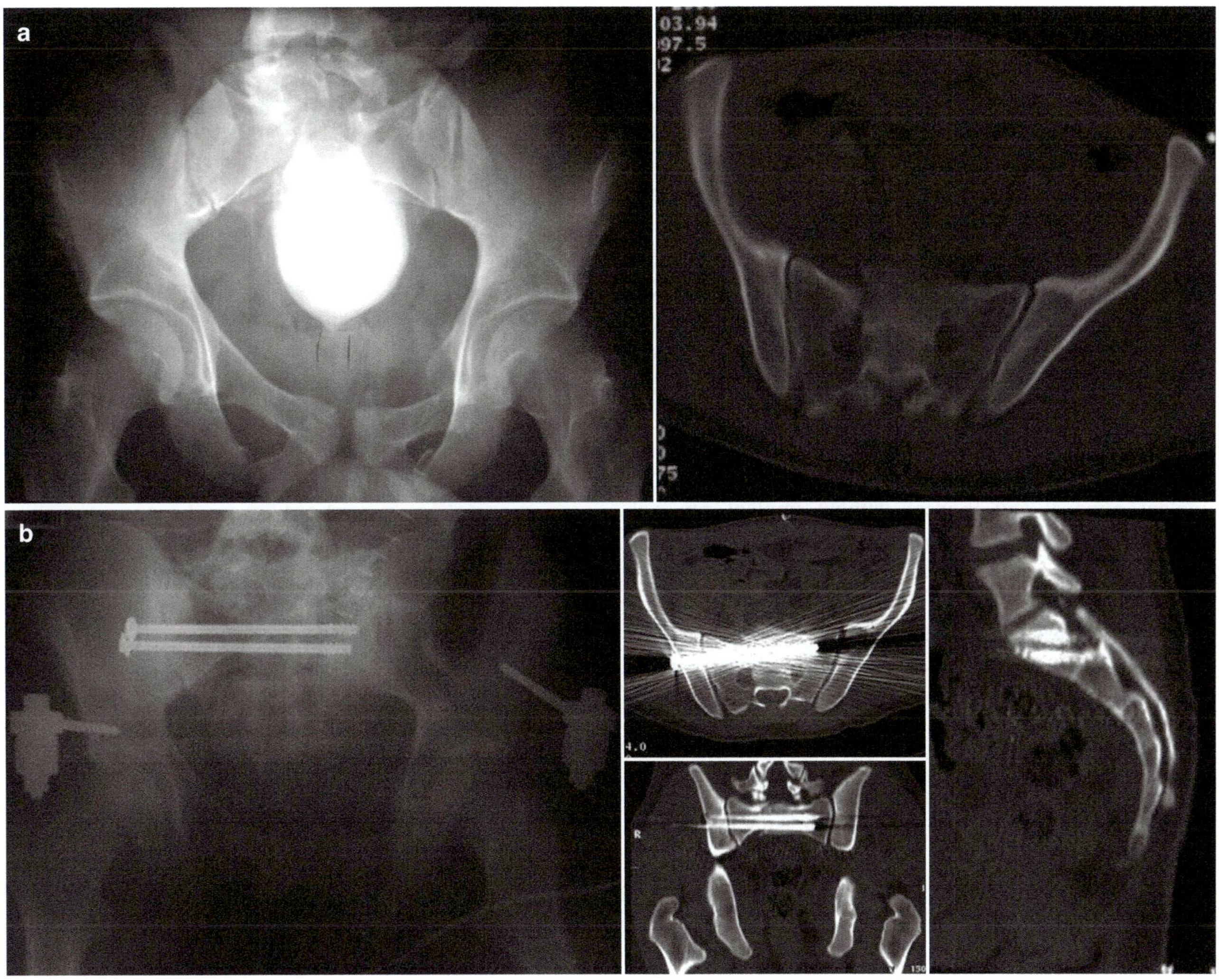

Fig. 31.39 (a) Right displaced foraminal sacrum fracture. (b) Stabilization with two screws inserted into the S1 transverse corridor. (c) Follow-up result after 1 year with uneventful healing

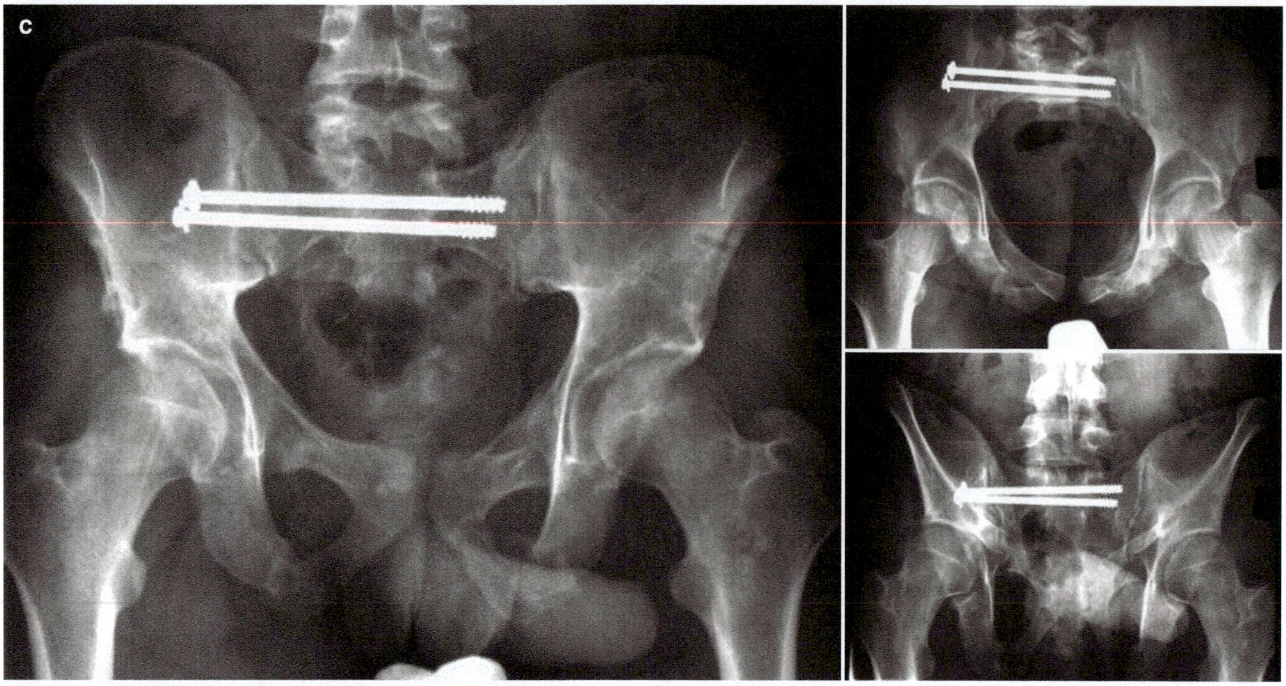

Fig. 31.39 (continued)

formation around the screw head and the additional washer, the need for a new/different/longer incision, potential risk of screw breakage, and the potential necessity for an open removal technique [103].

Recent analyses stated that bridging the contralateral uninjured SI joint with a transverse transsacral-transiliac screw or bar resulted in no differences regarding pain and function compared to the affected SI joint 1 year after surgery [94, 95].

The only larger series dealing with the clinical effect of iliosacral screw removal was performed by Yücel et al. in 2004 [104]. In 21 patients with type C injuries, 12 had implant removal and 9 were without implant removal. Indications for implant removal were based on clinical signs in eight cases and in four a planned removal was performed. Overall, 83.3% showed clinical improvement [104].

Recently, Pieske et al. reported a rate of 46.5% implant removal after a mean of 11 months, but no data regarding type and clinical effect were reported [69].

> Implant removal is not routinely performed after iliosacral screw fixation. A clinical benefit cannot clearly be expected. Bridging an uninjured SI joint seems to have no negative clinical effect.

31.10 Results

31.10.1 CT-Guided Percutaneous Iliosacral Screw Placement

In 1987, Ebraheim et al. first reported on CT-guided percutaneous iliosacral screw fixation in three patients after procedure testing in eight cadaver specimens [58] followed by a clinical analysis of 21 patients [67].

Indications included SI joint dislocations, sacral fractures, and even ilium fractures. Epidural or local anesthesia in the prone or lateral decubitus position was performed and one or two 6.5 mm cannulated screws, in some cases supported by a transsacral bar and inserted.

Nelson et al. and Duwelius et al. reported on a first larger clinical series of 13 patients with SI joint dislocations or unstable sacral fractures, posteriorly stabilized with 7.0 mm cannulated screws under CT guidance under epidural or general anesthesia (3× bilaterally = 16 screws) [66, 84].

The procedure time exceeded 90 min in the majority of cases with minimal blood loss. Neurological injury due to the procedure was not reported. One of these patients developed a superficial wound infection. The quality of reduction was not clearly defined, but the majority had a reduced posterior pelvis of <5 mm. It was noted that severe preoperative

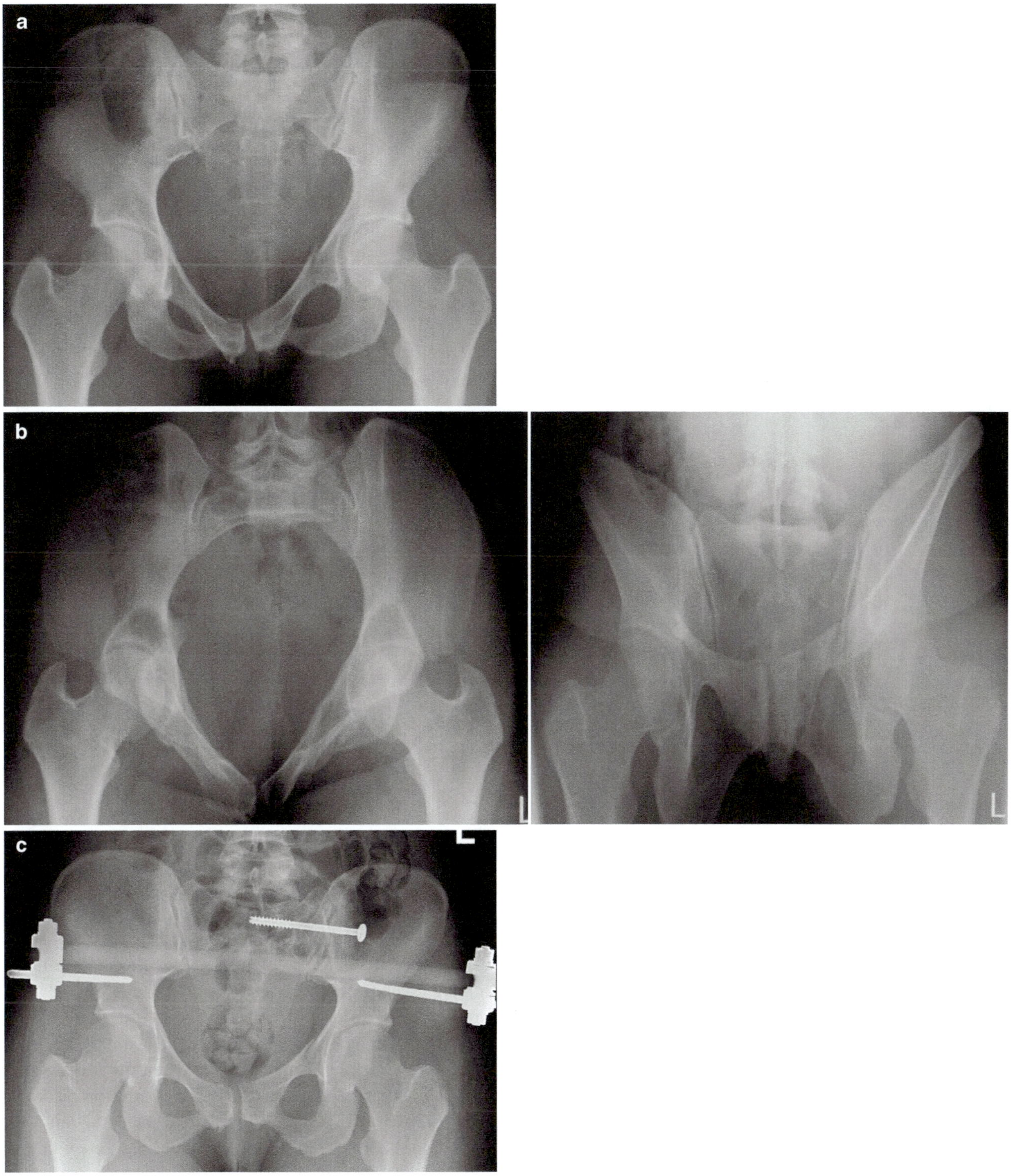

Fig. 31.40 (**a**) Left undisplaced sacrum fracture. (**b**) Corresponding Inlet and Outlet views. (**c**) Unilateral iliosacral screw stabilization of the sacrum. (**d**) Intra- and postoperative confirmation of the correct screw path. (**e**) Follow-up result after 1 year with anatomic healing

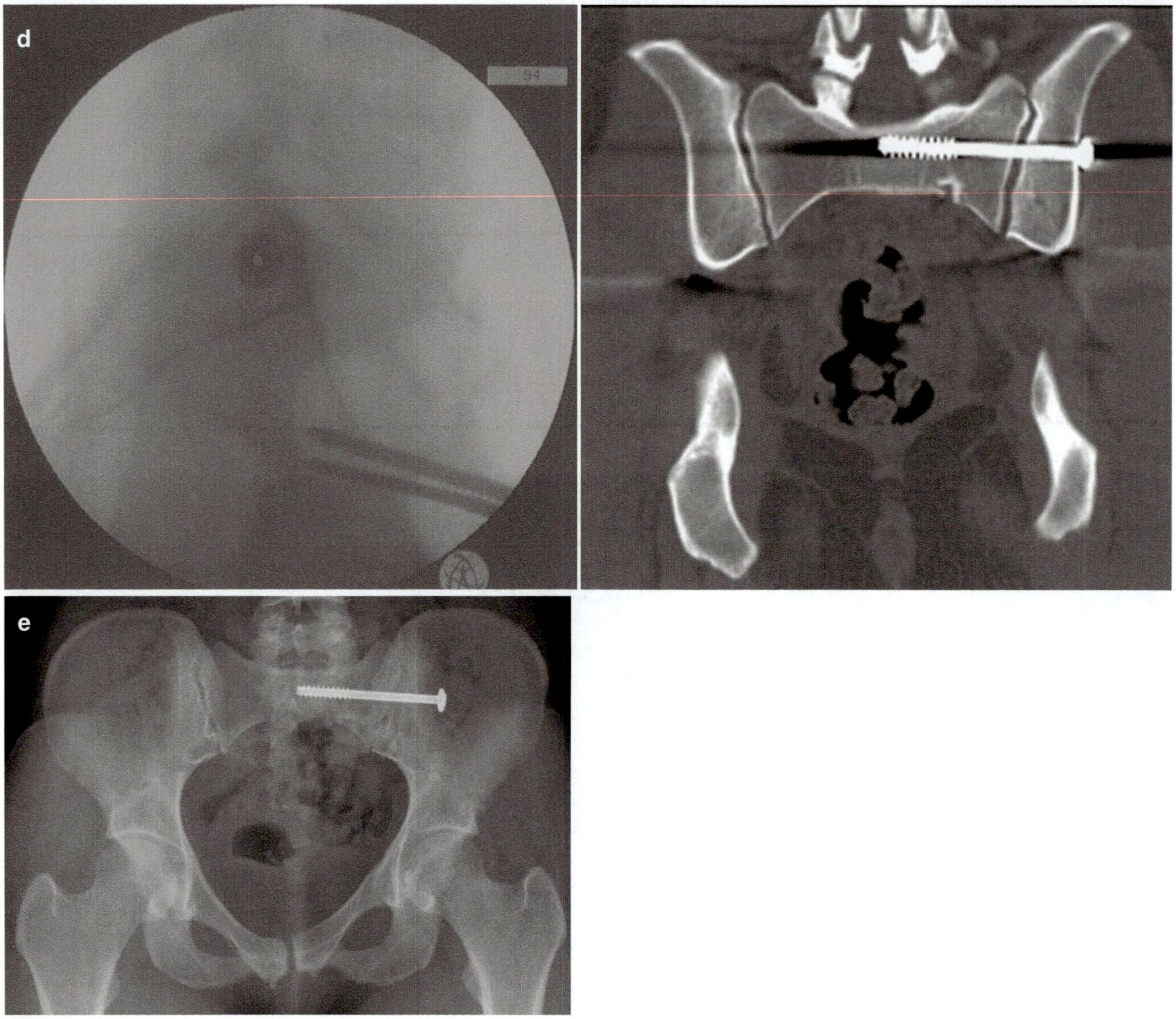

Fig. 31.40 (continued)

displacement could usually not be reduced anatomically. No long-term complications at latest follow-up were observed.

Jakob et al. performed CT-guided fixation in 13 patients with 15 posterior type C injuries using overall 27 screws [68].

In four cases, a type C disrupted SI joint was stabilized. Only two of these patients had anatomic reductions (mean preintervention displacement: 15.3 mm, mean postintervention displacement: 9.6 mm). In nine cases, a type C sacral fracture was stabilized. The mean preintervention craniocaudal displacement was 6.9 mm and could be reduced to 5.7 mm, while the dorsoventral displacement was reduced from 4.6 mm to 1.9 mm. In 93%, the screw position was rated perfect. Eighty percent of the patients showed bony healing. One case of nonunion after a sacral fracture was reported (7%). In three cases, implant related complications were observed: 1× screw breakage, 2× screw dislocations. Implant related complications were observed when only one screw was inserted.

Blake-Toker et al. analyzed 20 patients with SI joint injuries treated with 22 CT-guided percutaneous iliosacral screw fixation under general anesthesia in the oblique prone or lateral position [62]. The procedure time averaged 82 min with a minimal blood loss of <10 mL. Except one screw migration, no complications occurred.

Ziran et al. reported on 66 patients with different posterior injuries. Several fractures and SI joint dislocations were stabilized, without reporting on the fracture type [70].

Baskin et al. published on three pediatric patients with a C1.2. injury (according to Tile), stabilized by CT-guided percutaneous 7.3 mm cannulated screw insertion [61]. In one case, slight secondary migration was reported, while no relevant complications occurred. Reduction was rated near anatomic.

Sciulli et al. used CT guidance in 21 patients with APC, LC, and VS injuries according to Young and Burgess. The procedure time was reported to be 80 min/screw [105]. One screw was too short, while in another case, secondary displacement was observed. Blood loss was rated minimal (<30 mL).

Hong et al. inserted 17 iliosacral screws in 11 patients under local anesthesia [82]. The average insertion time was 30 min. During insertion, two patients suffered from some radicular pain, which resolved after some screw loosening. The average dose-length product was 105.86 mGy * cm/screw.

Pieske et al. recently reported a large series of 136 iliosacral stabilizations in 71 patients in the lateral decubitus position [69]. The mean time for each screw as 88.6 min, which could be reduced to 56.3 min after increased experience. The majority of screws (97.1%) was placed in the correct bone corridor. Reduction was rated nearly anatomic with persistent displacement of 1.3 mm and 1.5 mm in the anterior-posterior and craniocaudal directions, respectively. No complications were observed. The mean effective radiation dose was 5.9 mSv in male patients and 8.7 mSv in female patients.

In a 5-year follow-up analysis, Falzarano et al. reported on 96 polytraumatized patients with Tile type C SI joint injuries treated with 6.0 mm screws, inserted perpendicular to

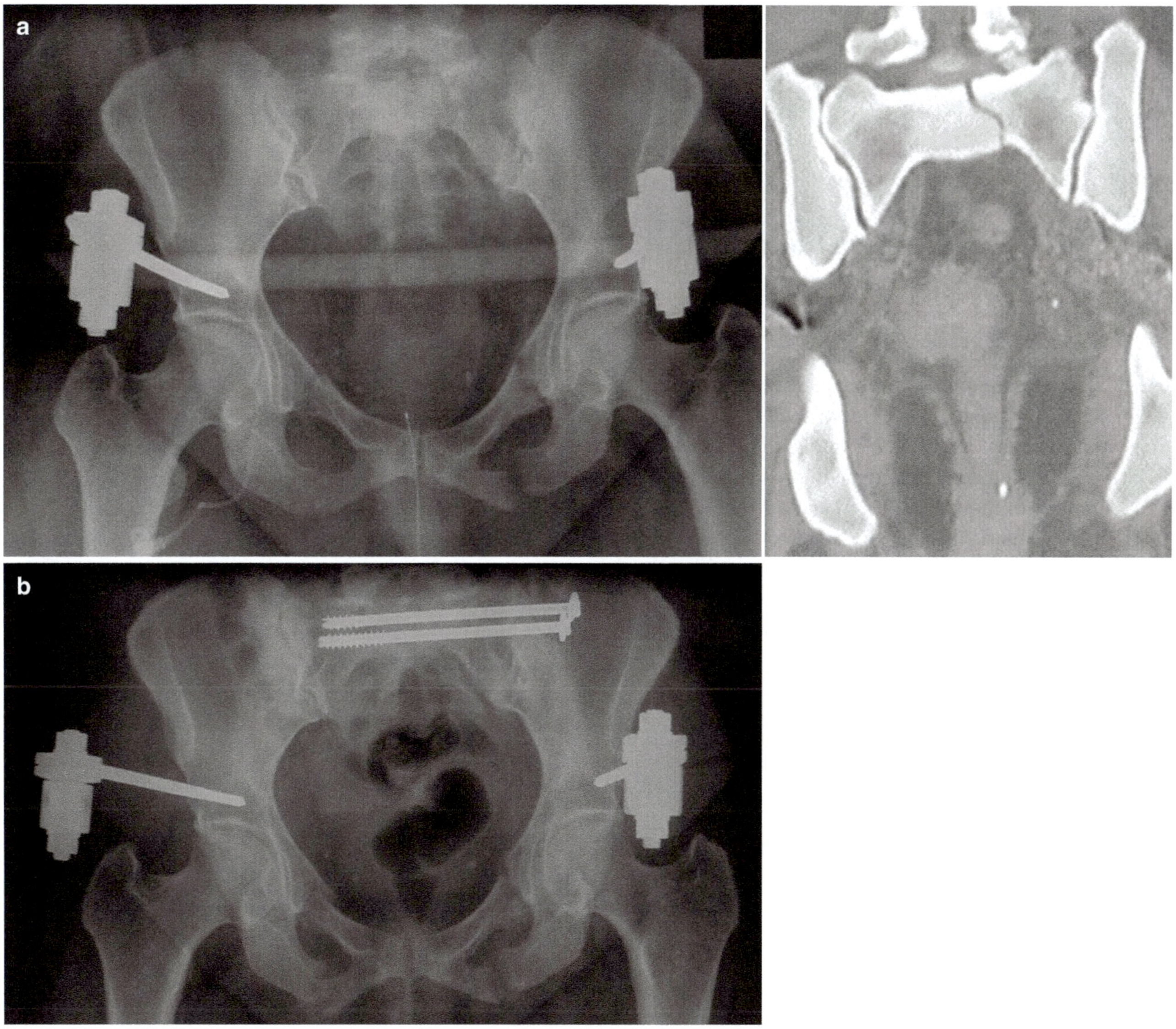

Fig. 31.41 (**a**) Left central sacrum fracture, nearly undisplaced. (**b**) Sacrum stabilization with two S1 screws. (**c**) Postoperative CT reveals malposition of the screws

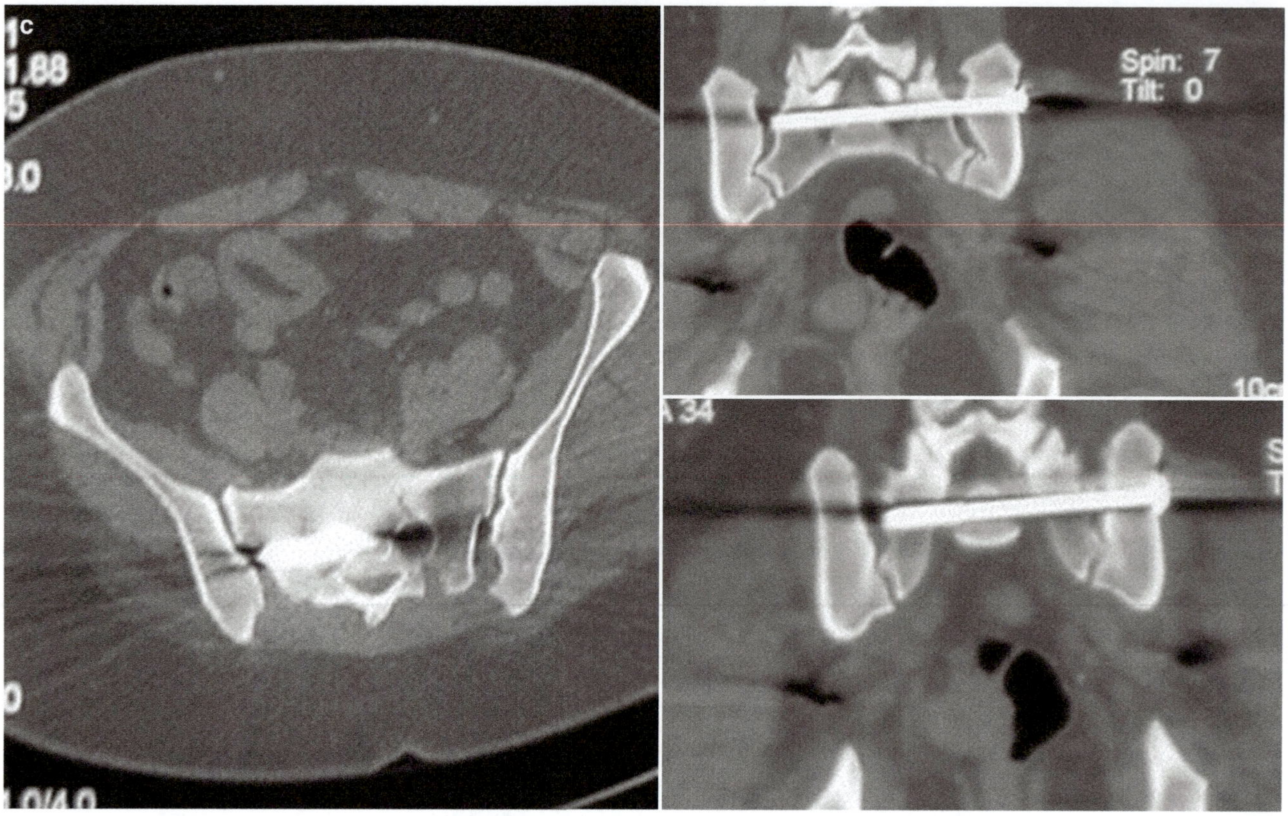

Fig. 31.41 (continued)

the SI joint under CT guidance [106]. The average screw length was 70 mm. 11.3% developed deep vein thrombosis within the first 3 months; 12.5% developed superficial infections at the skin insertion site. No implant failures occurred. Follow-up revealed good functional improvement.

A summary of these data is presented in Table 31.1.

Even in pediatric patients, CT-guided iliosacral screw fixation resulted in good postoperative results without complications [61].

Overall, CT-guided iliosacral fixation shows encouraging results:

- Insertion times 1–2 h
- Minimal blood loss
- Low risk of complications
- High rates of adequate screw positioning
- Acceptable radiation dose

31.10.2 Fluoroscopy-Based Screw Insertion

In 1995 Routt et al. described the technique of fluoroscopic-based application of percutaneous iliosacral screws to fix the disrupted SI joint or sacral fractures and reported on first clinical results of 103 screws [26, 60].

Except two patients, all screws were inserted percutaneously in the supine position after primary anterior pelvic ring fixation. The average procedure time was 29 min, with a mean blood loss of 10.2 mL and a mean fluoroscopy time of 2.1 min. Malreduction was defined as a persistent displacement of >1 cm, which was present in 11.6%. No nonunions or infections were reported.

- Routt et al. reported on 60 patients with sacral fractures (25× type B, 35× type C) treated by iliosacral screw fixation [85]. The mean time for screw application was 28 min, and a fluoroscopy time of 2.3 min was reported. Blood loss was minimal (9 mL in average). Complications included two nonunions, two screw breakages, and fixation failure in five cases (8.3%). No infections were

Table 31.1 Data on CT-guided percutaneous iliosacral screw placement

Author	Year	No.	OR time	Blood loss	f/u[a]	Complications
Duwelius	1992	16	144 min	Minimal	12.6 m	1× screw migration, 2× LLD (1 cm)
Ebraheim	1994	21	125 min	<25 mL	24 m	1× superficial infection, 2× 20° rotational deformity, 21% LBP
Jakob	1997	13	86 min	n.r.	13 m	1× superficial infection, 1× screw breakage, 2× screw migrations
Blake-Toker	2001	22	82 min	<10 mL		1× screw migration
Ziran	2003	66	26 min			1× screw breakage
Sciulli	2007	23	80 min	<30 mL	n.r.	1× screw too short, 1× s displacement
Hong	2010	11	30 min	n.r.	n.r.	1× malreduction
Pieske	2015	71	56 min	n.r.	n.r.	None
Falzarano	2018	96	n.r.	n.r.	60 m	11.3% DVT, 12.5% superficial wound infections, 1× screw breakage, 1× screw loosening

[a](<1 cm); *LBP* low back pain

observed. Reductions <1 cm were gained in 57 patients, while three malreductions with a mean displacement of 1.6 cm were reported.

- Shuler et al. reported on 20 consecutive patients with 5 type B and 15 type C injuries treated by percutaneous fixation under fluoroscopic guidance. The mean operative time was 52 min. No loss of fixation or wound complications were observed [107].
- Keating et al. reported their results of 38 patients with sacral fractures. Screw misplacement occurred in five patients (13.2%). Malunion was observed in 44.1%. 26 patients had long-term follow-up with only 4 (15.4%) reported no pain [108].
- Nork et al. reported on 13 patients with U-shaped sacral fractures treated by in situ fixation using bilateral fully threaded cancellous 7.0-mm cannulated screws in 11 cases. Operative time was 48 min with a radiation exposure of 2.1 min per screw. One patient presented with screw loosening. All fractures healed uneventful [33].
- van den Bosch et al. analyzed 33 screws in 22 patients. CT analysis revealed more malpositions than conventional x-rays [54].
- Hilgert et al. analyzed 12 patients with 24 screws (11 patients with two unilateral screws). The mean surgical time was 55 min; the mean x-ray exposure was 1.6 min per screw [78].
- Gänsslen et al. performed stabilization of minor displaced transforaminal sacral fractures (<5 mm) using a single horizontal screw in 20 patients. The average preoperative displacement of 3.8 mm was decreased by closed reduction to 1.6 mm postoperatively. The average operating time was 5 min; the average x-ray screening time was 2.22 min. Incorrect screw position was observed in three patients (15%). Iatrogenic nerve injury was not observed. All fractures healed within 3 months [31].
- Rysavi et al. reported their results of 102 unstable pelvic ring injuries. The majority of patients had additional anterior ring stabilization (80%). Screw misplacement was observed in 6.9% resulting in neurological impairment in 85.7% of these patients. No fixation failure was observed but eight patients (7.8%) presented with loss of reduction. In one case, intraoperative injury to the superior gluteal artery occurred. 88% showed an anatomic or near to anatomic reduction, while 12% had a persistent displacement >1 cm. Two infections were reported [109].
- Hong et al. reported on 17 screws in 11 patients with sacral fractures. All screws were sufficiently placed intraosseously and a mean procedure time of 30 min/screw as stated. Two patients suffered from temporary radicular pain. 10/11 patients healed without redisplacement [82].
- Zwingman et al. compared computer navigation with conventional screw insertion and reported 42% intraosseous screw pathway in 87 patients with 131 screws. In 19% surgical revision of the screws was necessary. Overall, with computer navigation better results were obtained [110].
- Osterhoff et al. treated 25 lateral compression type B injuries with iliosacral screws (14 bilateral, 11 unilateral screws) (injury 2011). An 8% revision rate was reported due to nerve injury and further two had secondary displacement/implant failure. Neither nonunion nor wound infections were noted [111].
- In a meta-analysis from 2013, Zwingman et al. compared computer navigation with conventional screw application [112]. Analyzing 2353 percutaneous screw implantations in 1731 patients, the malposition rate was 0.1% vs. 2.6%. The revision rate was found to be 1.3% vs. 2.7%.

- In an analysis of 15 patients, the preoperative displacement of 4.13 mm could be reduced to 3.63 mm [65]. The Majeed score at 1 year was graded good to excellent in 80%.
- Using 3D fluoroscopy, Kim et al. performed iliosacral screw fixation in 29 patients (14× type B, 15× type C). The mean operation time was 35.6 min; the mean radiation exposure was 84.0 s. 22.6% screw perforations were observed (extraosseous screw path) with no malposition >2 mm. No other complications were observed [113].
- Elzohairy et al. compared 35 patients with ORIF and 35 patients with CRIF in different type B and -C injuries. The rate of good or excellent results was comparable. No intraoperative complications were observed after ORIF, while two guide wire breakages were observed. One patient in the CRIF group sustained an L5 radiculopathy. Wound complications were more common after ORIF [114].
- Griffin et al. analyzed 30 patients with vertical sacral fractures treated with percutaneous partially threaded iliosacral screw fixation. Different screw configurations were used (isolated S1 screw, two S2 screws, S1 and S2 screws). In four cases (13.3%) secondary displacement with screw failure was observed, all with anterior pelvic ring stabilization [115].
- Hermann et al. retrospectively analyzed the result in 90 patients with foraminal sacral fractures treated with partially threaded screws and observed no nonunions. Of these patients, 60% were treated with one isolated screw and the remaining patients with at least two screws [116].
- Griffin et al. analyzed 32 patients with SI joint (fracture) dislocations treated with percutaneous partially threaded iliosacral screw fixation. Different screw configurations were used (isolated S1 screw, two S2 screws, S1 and S2 screws). No posterior failure occurred [115].

> Fluoroscopy-based iliosacral screw insertion allows for sufficient screw position and adequate clinical results.

31.10.3 Navigation-Assisted Iliosacral Screw Stabilization

Due to the complex pelvic anatomy, high malposition rates and, therefore, optimization of screw placement using navigation-assisted screw insertion was proposed. After extensive scientific work, this concept is now frequently available in clinical practice.

31.10.3.1 Experimental Data

Tonetti et al. were one of the first groups presenting a computer-assisted technique of iliosacral screw placement to increase the accuracy of screw placement using generated 3D CT data in a cadaver model in 1998 [117]. Using an ultrasound-based registration, the screw trajectories were planned, and screws were inserted using the classical surgical technique. Verification of the screw pathway was checked with a CT scan. Only slight differences between the planned entry point and screw depth were found and were 1.9 mm and 0.81 mm, respectively. All screws were intraosseous without penetration of the bone.

Barrick et al. using cadaver pelvic specimens inserted eight S1 and S2 screws supported by computed navigation. All S1 screws were completely intraosseous, while three of the S2 screws showed some signs of cortical penetration [42].

Several further studies confirmed this increase of accuracy in percutaneous screw application around the pelvis [118].

Gautier et al. inserted bilateral iliosacral screws (SI joint trajectories) into the S1 and S2 bodies using a surface-matching algorithm in six plastic pelves [119]. Postoperative CT revealed adequate intraosseous screw path in all screws with only a slight difference between planning and definitive screw course: 2.7 mm for the entry point, 3.5 mm for the target point, and 2° for angular deviation, respectively.

Collinge et al. performed standard and virtual fluoroscopy for iliosacral screw insertion into S1 in 29 pelvic cadavers [120]. The majority of screws (96.5%) of each procedure was completely intraosseous. No injury to neurovascular structures was found during postsurgical cadaver dissection. Virtual fluoroscopy was associated with reduced imaging times.

Briem et al. compared conventional fluoroscopy with fluoroscopy-based 2D and 3D navigation, and CT navigation [63]:

- Conventional screw insertion was found to be the fasted procedure but was associated with two- to threefold imaging time and 20% screw malplacement.
- 2D navigation showed better surgical time but also 20% screw malpositioning.
- CT navigation was associated with two- to threefold increase of the procedure time but less fluoroscopic time and without malposition of screws.
- 3D navigation was found have a short procedure time with the least fluoroscopy time and with 100% adequate screw positions.

Takao et al. could show that even less experienced surgeons show a high rate of adequate guide wire positions using a CT-3D-fluoroscopy matching navigation system [121]. In eight cadaver pelves, correct wire placement was achieved in 100% compared to 50% using conventional techniques or 3D-fluoroscopic navigation. Navigation also reduced the resulting radiation time.

31.10.3.2 Clinical Data

In a first clinical analysis, Tonetti et al. compared ultrasound-assisted computer-assisted surgery (CAS) with percutaneous fluoroscopy-based screw insertion. The CAS system was used in 4 patients and 10 screws were inserted compared to 30 patients with 51 screws using the conventional technique.

Despite a slightly longer surgical time (50 vs. 35 min), CAS allowed for safer screw placement (100% intraosseous vs. 60% intraosseous pathways; 0% vs. 23.3% neurological deficits) and less radiation exposure (0.35 vs. 1.03 min per patient; 0.14 vs. 0.6 min per screw) [122].

Grützner et al. reported their early experience in seven patients with posterior pelvic ring instability CAS percutaneous iliosacral screw osteosynthesis using two cannulated 7.3 mm titanium screws. Screw position was evaluated by a postoperative CT scan. Except for a slight screw thread penetration at the anterior sacral cortex in two patients, no further complications were observed [123].

Several reports confirmed safe application of computer-assisted screw insertion in the pelvic area [124–126].

Arand et al. used an optoelectronic navigation system for iliosacral screw fixation in eight disrupted SI joints and one patient with SI joint degeneration. Complete intraosseous screw placement was found in 21 of 22 screws, while 1 screw showed anterior sacral cortex perforation [127].

Briem et al. performed a clinical case series of 35 screws inserted in 20 patients. The mean procedure time was 36.2 min, and the fluoroscopy time was 0.9 min per screw. Compared to historical conventional data, a significant increase in procedure time and a significant decrease of radiation exposure time were observed [64].

Zwingmann et al. performed a 3D navigation study in 54 patients with 63 iliosacral screws and compared these results with a group of 87 patients (131 screws) after conventional fluoroscopic-guided insertion [110]. Postoperative CT examination found a perfect intraosseous screw course in 81% vs. 42%, resulting in revision rates of 1.6% vs. 19%.

Grossterlinden et al. analyzed 82 patients with 147 iliosacral screws and reported a misplacement rate of 8% [128]. Risk factors for screw malplacement were two unilateral screws inserted into the S1 vertebra and SI joint dislocations. Navigation assistance reduced the misplacement rate from 15% (conventional fluoroscopy) to 3% as well as surgical experience (20% vs. 3.9%).

Peng et al. performed iliosacral screw fixation in different posterior pelvic ring injuries using a CT navigation system in 13 patients [129]. The mean navigation time was 21.2 min, and a radiation exposure of 26.4 mGy was recorded. No screw malpositions nor neurovascular injuries were reported.

In a meta-analysis from 2013, Zwingman et al. reported a malposition rate of 0.1% vs. and a revision rate of 1.3% after navigation-assisted procedures [112].

Zwingmann et al. also reported on complications rates after navigated and conventional iliosacral screw fixations [130]. The intraoperative complication rate was 8.8% vs. 5.9%, respectively.

Takao et al. inserted S1 and S2 screws in six patients with three type B and three type C pelvic ring fractures using CT-3D-fluoroscopy matching navigation. All screws could be inserted properly with no malpositions or neurovascular complications. The difference between the planned and real screw position was 2.5 mm at the entry point and 2.2 mm at the screw tip [121].

In a recent multicenter study, it was found that iliosacral screw application in dysmorphic sacral bones was associated with a significantly higher rate of screw malposition compared to the normal sacrum. 3D navigation could adequately reduce this risk [131].

> Results of experimental and clinical studies indicate that fluoroscopy-based navigation is associated with a lower radiation dose and lower rate of screw malpositioning compared to conventional screw application [132].

31.10.4 Comparable Analyses: Plate vs. Screw for SI Joint Dislocations

There are two studies comparing anterior plating or iliosacral screw fixation of the disrupted SI joint.

Zhang et al. analyzed 38 patients with unilateral sacroiliac screw stabilization and 32 patients with anterior plating [133]. Despite statistical significance, the surgical time was comparable with 113.42 min vs. 123.44 min while the average blood loss was smaller after iliosacral screw fixation (287 mL vs. 426.56 mL). Intraoperative imaging was increased during iliosacral screw fixation. The quality of reduction analyzed with postoperative CT evaluation was rated satisfactory in 86.84% vs. 78.13%, while satisfactory functional results were slightly better after anterior plating (84.21% vs. 87.50%). Potentially, this was due to a lesser complication rate: 15.79% vs. 9.38%.

Only after iliosacral screw fixation, three patients (7.9%) developed iatrogenic lumbosacral trunk injury, while one patient after anterior plating presented with a temporary LCFN lesion.

Overall, despite being less invasive, iliosacral screw fixation was associated with more x-ray exposure and permanent neurologic damage.

In contrast, Li et al. compared 32 patients with anterior plate fixation with 32 patients with percutaneous iliosacral screw fixation and reported longer operation time, higher blood loss, and a higher complication rate. The functional result was also better after iliosacral screw fixation [134].

Gu et al. compared 26 patients with anterior SI joint plate fixation and 26 patients with percutaneous sacroiliac screw fixation. As expected, the procedure time and blood loss were less after iliosacral screw fixation, and, additionally, the long-term result was superior [135].

As a main restriction of these studies, no data were available regarding primary displacement, which can significantly influence the results.

31.11 Conclusion

If the anatomy of the sacrum is respected, iliosacral screw fixation is an adequate stabilization method, which leads to sufficient stability and a high rate of good/excellent clinical results.

References

1. Ebraheim N, Sabry F, Nadim Y, Xu R, Yeasting R. Internal architecture of the sacrum in the elderly. An anatomic and radiographic study. Spine. 2000;25:292–7.
2. Wagner D, Kamer L, Rommens P, Sawaguchi T, Richards R, Noser H. 3D statistical modeling techniques to investigate the anatomy of the sacrum, its bone mass distribution, and the trans-sacral corridors. J Orthop Res. 2014;32:1543–8.
3. Wagner D, Kamer L, Sawaguchi T, Richards R, Noser H, Rommens P. Sacral bone mass distribution assessed by averaged three-dimensional CT models: implications for pathogenesis and treatment of fragility fractures of the sacrum. J Bone Joint Surg Am. 2016;98:584–90.
4. Zheng Y, Lu W, Zhu Q, Qin L, Zhong S, Leong J. Variation in bone mineral density of the sacrum in young adults and its significance for sacral fixation. Spine. 2000;25:353–7.
5. Richards A, Coleman N, Knight T, Belkoff S, Mears S. Bone density and cortical thickness in normal, osteopenic, and osteoporotic sacra. J Osteoporos. 2010;2010:504078. https://doi.org/10.4061/2010/504078.
6. Waites M, Mears S, Mathis J, Belkoff S. The strength of the osteoporotic sacrum. Spine. 2007;32:E652–5.
7. Pal G. Weight transmission through the sacrum in man. J Anat. 1989;162:9–17.
8. Carlson DA, Scheid DK, Maar DC, Baele JR, Kaehr DM. Safe placement of S1 and S2 iliosacral screws: the "vestibule" concept. J Orthop Trauma. 2000;14(4):264–9.
9. Gardner M, Farrell E, Nork S, Segina D, Chip Routt MJ. Percutaneous placement of iliosacral screws without electrodiagnostic monitoring. J Trauma. 2009;66:1411–5.
10. Reilly M, Bono C, Litkouhi B, Sirkin M, Behrens F. The effect of sacral fracture malreduction on the safe placement of iliosacral screws. J Orthop Trauma. 2003;17:88–94.
11. Gardner M, Morshed S, Nork S, Ricci W, Chip Routt MJ. Quantification of the upper and second sacral segment safe zones in normal and dysmorphic sacra. J Orthop Trauma. 2010;24:622–9.
12. Noojin F, Malkani A, Haikal L, Lundquist C, Voor M. Cross-sectional geometry of the sacral ala for safe insertion of iliosacral lag screws: a computed tomography model. J Orthop Trauma. 2000;14:31–5.
13. Eastman J, Adams M, Frisoli K, Chip Routt MJ. Is S3 a viable osseous fixation pathway? J Orthop Trauma. 2018;32:93–9.
14. Hasenboehler E, Stahel P, Williams A, Smith W, Newman J, Symonds D, Morgan S. Prevalence of sacral dysmorphia in a prospective trauma population: implications for a "safe" surgical corridor for sacro-iliac screw placement. Patient Saf Surg. 2011;5(1):8. https://doi.org/10.1186/1754-9493-5-8.
15. Kaiser S, Gardner M, Liu J, Routt MJ, Morshed S. Anatomic determinants of sacral dysmorphism and implications for safe Iliosacral screw placement. J Bone Joint Surg Am. 2014;96(14):e120.
16. Kim J, Jung C, Eastman J, Oh H. Measurement of optimal insertion angle for iliosacral screw fixation using three-dimensional computed tomography scans. Clin Orthop Surg. 2016;8:133–9.
17. Miller A, Chip Routt MJ. Variations in sacral morphology and implications for iliosacral screw fixation. J Am Acad Orthop Surg. 2012;20:8–16.
18. Routt M, Simonian P, Agnew A, Mann F. Radiographic recognition of the sacral alar slope for optimal placement of iliosacral screws: a cadaveric and clinical study. J Orthop Trauma. 1996;10(3):171–7.
19. Wendt H, Gottschling H, Schröder M, Marintschev I, Hofmann G, Burgkart R, Gras F. Recommendations for iliosacral screw placement in dysmorphic sacrum based on modified in-out-in corridors. J Orthop Res. 2018;37(1):689–96. https://doi.org/10.1002/jor.24199.
20. Mendel T, Noser H, Wohlrab D, Stock K, Radetzki F. The lateral sacral triangle—a decision support for secure transverse sacroiliac screw insertion. Injury. 2011;42:1164–70.
21. Mendel T, Radetzki F, Wohlrab D, Stock K, Hofmann G, Noser H. CT-based 3-D visualisation of secure bone corridors and optimal trajectories for sacroiliac screws. Injury. 2013;44:957–63.
22. Goetzen M, Ortner K, Lindtner R, Schmid R, Blauth M, Krappinger D. A simple approach for the preoperative assessment of sacral morphology for percutaneous SI screw fixation. Arch Orthop Trauma Surg. 2016;136:1251–7.
23. Collinge C, Coons D, Aschenbrenner J. Risks to the superior gluteal neurovascular bundle during percutaneous iliosacral screw insertion: an anatomical cadaver study. J Orthop Trauma. 2005;19:96–101.
24. Zhao Y, You L, Lian W, Zou D, Dong S, Sun T, Zhang S, Wang D, Li J, Li W, Zhao Y. Anatomical relation between S1 sacroiliac screws' entrance points and superior gluteal artery. J Orthop Surg Res. 2018;13(1):15. https://doi.org/10.1186/s13018-018-0713-5.
25. Maslow J, Collinge C. Risks to the superior gluteal neurovascular bundle during iliosacral and transsacral screw fixation: a computed tomogram arteriography study. J Orthop Trauma. 2017;31:640–3.
26. Routt M, Simonian P, Inaba J. Iliosacral screw fixation of the disrupted sacroiliac joint. Tech Orthop. 1995;9(4):300–14.
27. Templeman D, Schmidt A, Freese J, Weismann I. Proximity of iliosacral screws to neurovascular structures after internal fixation. Clin Orthop. 1996;329:194–8.
28. Ebraheim N, Xu R, Biyani A, Nadaud M. Morphologic considerations of the first sacral pedicle for iliosacral screw placement. Spine. 1997;22(8):841–6.
29. Day CS, Prayson MJ, Shuler TE, Towers J, Gruen GS. Transsacral versus modified pelvic landmarks for percutaneous iliosacral

screw placement—a computed tomographic analysis and cadaveric study. Am J Orthop. 2000;29(9 Suppl):16–21.
30. Okutan O, Kaptanoglu E, Solaroglu I, Beskonakli E, Tekdemir I. Pedicle morphology of the first sacral vertebra. Neuroanatomy. 2003;2:16–9.
31. Gänsslen A, Hüfner T, Krettek C. Percutaneous iliosacral screw fixation of unstable pelvic injuries by conventional fluoroscopy. Oper Orthop Traumatol. 2006;18:225–44.
32. Chon C, Jeong J, Kang B, Kim H, Jung G. Computational simulation study on ilio-sacral screw fixations for pelvic ring injuries and implications in Asian sacrum. Eur J Orthop Surg Traumatol. 2018;28:439–44.
33. Nork SE, Jones CB, Harding SP, Mirza SK, Routt ML Jr. Percutaneous stabilization of U-shaped sacral fractures using iliosacral screws: technique and early results. J Orthop Trauma. 2001;15(4):238–46.
34. Arman C, Naderi S, Kiray A, Aksu F, Yilmaz H, Tetik S, Korman E. The human sacrum and safe approaches for screw placement. J Clin Neurosci. 2009;16:1046–9.
35. Saluja S, Agarwalwal S, Tuli A, Raheja S, Tigga S, Paul S. Morphometric analysis of the sacrum and its surgical implications. J Clin Diagn Res. 2018;12:AC01–6.
36. Dong Q, Tian W, Ma B. Evaluation and clinical application of sacral S1 vestibule measurements in Chinese adults. Int J Morphol. 2014;32:202–7.
37. Jeong J, Jin J, Kang B, Jung G. Can the possibility of transverse iliosacral screw fixation for first sacral segment be predicted preoperatively? Results of a computational cadaveric study. Injury. 2017;48:2074–9.
38. Mendel T, Noser H, Kuervers J, Goehre F, Hofmann G, Radetzki F. The influence of sacral morphology on the existence of secure S1 and S2 transverse bone corridors for iliosacroiliac screw fixation. Injury. 2013;44:1773–9.
39. König M, Sundaram R, Saville P, Jehan S, Boszczyk B. Anatomical considerations for percutaneous trans ilio-sacroiliac S1 and S2 screw placement. Eur Spine J. 2016;25:1800–5.
40. Gras F, Hillmann S, Rausch S, Klos K, Hofmann G, Marintschev I. Biomorphometric analysis of ilio-sacro-iliacal corridors for an intra-osseous implant to fix posterior pelvic ring fractures. J Orthop Res. 2015;33:254–60.
41. Gras F, Gottschling H, Schröder M, Marintschev I, Hofmann G, Burgkart R. Transsacral osseous corridor anatomy is more amenable to screw insertion in males: a biomorphometric analysis of 280 pelves. Clin Orthop Relat Res. 2016;474:2304–11.
42. Barrick EF, O'Mara JW, Lane HE 3rd. Iliosacral screw insertion using computer-assisted CT image guidance: a laboratory study. Comput Aided Surg. 1998;3(6):289–96.
43. Conflitti J, Graves M, Chip Routt MJ. Radiographic quantification and analysis of dysmorphic upper sacral osseous anatomy and associated iliosacral screw insertions. J Orthop Trauma. 2010;24:630–6.
44. Dilogo I, Fiolin J. Surgical technique of percutaneous iliosacral screw fixation in S3 level in unstable pelvic fracture with closed degloving injury and morrell lavallee lesion: two case reports. Int J Surg Case Rep. 2017;38:43–9.
45. Radetzki F, Wohlrab D, Goehre F, Noser H, Delank K, Mendel T. Anatomical conditions of the posterior pelvic ring regarding bisegmental transverse sacroiliac screw fixation: a 3D morphometric study of 125 pelvic CT datasets. Arch Orthop Trauma Surg. 2014;134:1115–20.
46. Wagner D, Kamer L, Sawaguchi T, Geoff Richards R, Noser H, Uesugi M, Ossendorf C, Rommens P. Critical dimensions of trans-sacral corridors assessed by 3D CT models: relevance for implant positioning in fractures of the sacrum. J Orthop Res. 2017;35:2577–84.
47. Hwang J, Reilly M, Shaath M, Changoor S, Eastman J, Routt M, Sirkin M, Adams M. Safe zone quantification of the third sacral segment in normal and dysmorphic sacra. J Orthop Trauma. 2018;32:178–82.
48. Gorczyca J, Varga E, Woodside T, Hearn T, Powell J, Tile M. The strength of iliosacral lag screw and transiliac bars in the fixation of vertically unstable pelvic injuries with sacral fractures. Injury. 1996;27(8):561–4.
49. Culemann U, Pohlemann T, Hufner T, Gansslen A. 3-dimensional movement analysis after internal fixation of pelvic ring fractures. A computer simulation. Unfallchirurg. 2000;103(11):965–71.
50. Sagi H, Ordway N. and T, D., Biomechanical analysis of fixation of vertically unstable sacroiliac dislocations with iliosacral screws and symphyseal plating. J Orthop Trauma. 2004;18(3):138–43.
51. van Swienen C, van den Bosch E, Snijders C, Kleinrensink G, van Vugt A. Biomechanical comparison of sacroiliac screw techniques for unstable pelvic ring fractures. J Orthop Trauma. 2004;18(9):589–95.
52. Tabaie S, Bledsoe J, Moed B. Biomechanical comparison of standard iliosacral screw fixation to transsacral locked screw fixation in a type C zone II pelvic fracture model. J Orthop Trauma. 2013;27:521–6.
53. Dilogo I, Satria O, Fiolin J. Internal fixation of S1-S3 iliosacral screws and pubic screw as the best configuration for unstable pelvic fracture with unilateral vertical sacral fracture (AO type C1.3). J Orthop Surg (Hong Kong). 2017;25(1):2309499017690985. https://doi.org/10.1177/2309499017690985.
54. van den Bosch E, Zwienen C, van Dijke H, Snijders C, van Vugt A. Sacroiliac screw fixation for Tile B fractures. J Trauma. 2003;55(5):962–5.
55. Lehmann J. Luxation einer Beckenhälfte. Zentralbl Chir. 1934;37:2149–52.
56. Meyer-Burgdorff G. Über Beckenbrüche. Zentralbl Chir. 1936;63:1016.
57. Letournel E. Pelvic fractures. Injury. 1978;10:145–8.
58. Ebraheim N, Rusin J, Coombs R, Jackson W, Holiday B. Percutaneous computed-tomography-stabilization of pelvic fractures: preliminary report. J Orthop Trauma. 1987;1:197–204.
59. Routt M, Kregor P, Mayo K. 103 supine percutaneous iliosacral screws for fixation of the disrupted posterior pelvic ring after indirect reduction: indications, techniques, errors and results. In: Annual meeting OTA, October 1–3, Mineapolis, Minnesota. 1992.
60. Routt M, Kregor P, Simonian P, Mayo K. Early results of percutaneous iliosacral screws placed with the patient in the supine position. J Orthop Trauma. 1995;9(3):207–14.
61. Baskin K, Cahill A, Kaye R, Born C, Grudziak J, Towbin R. Closed reduction with CT-guided screw fixation for unstable sacroiliac joint fracture-dislocation. Pediatr Radiol. 2004;34:963–9.
62. Blake-Toker AM, Hawkins L, Nadalo L, Howard D, Arazoza A, Koonsman M, Dunn E. CT guided percutaneous fixation of sacroiliac fractures in trauma patients. J Trauma. 2001;51(6):1117–21.
63. Briem D, Rueger J, Begemann P, Halata Z, Bock T, Linhart W, Windolf J. [Computer-assisted screw placement into the posterior pelvic ring: assessment of different navigated procedures in a cadaver trial]. Unfallchirurg. 2006;109:640–6.
64. Briem D, Windolf J, Rueger J. [Percutaneous, 2D-fluoroscopic navigated iliosacral screw placement in the supine position: technique, possibilities, and limits]. Unfallchirurg. 2007;110:393–401.
65. Chen P, Hsu W, Li Y, Huang T, Huang T, Peng K. Outcome analysis of unstable posterior ring injury of the pelvis: comparison between percutaneous iliosacral screw fixation and conservative treatment. Biom J. 2013;36:289–94.
66. Duwelius P, Van Allen M, Bray T, Nelson D. Computed tomography-guided fixation of unstable posterior pelvic ring disruptions. J Orthop Trauma. 1992;6(4):420–6.

67. Ebraheim N, Coombs R, Jackson W, Rusin J. Percutaneous computed tomography-guided stabilization of posterior pelvic fractures. Clin Orthop. 1994;307:222–8.
68. Jacob A, Messmer P, Stock K, Suhm N, Baumann B, Regazzoni P, Steinbrich W. Posterior pelvic ring fractures: closed reduction and percutaneous CT-guided sacroiliac screw fixation. Cardiovasc Intervent Radiol. 1997;20:285–94.
69. Pieske O, Landersdorfer C, Trumm C, Greiner A, Wallmichrath J, Gottschalk O, Rubenbauer B. CT-guided sacroiliac percutaneous screw placement in unstable posterior pelvic ring injuries: accuracy of screw position, injury reduction and complications in 71 patients with 136 screws. Injury. 2015;46:333–9.
70. Ziran B, Smith W, Towers J, Morgan S. Iliosacral screw fixation of the posterior pelvic ring using local anaesthesia and computerised tomography. J Bone Joint Surg Br. 2003;85:411–8.
71. Pennal G, Tile M, Waddell J, Garside H. Pelvic disruption: assessment and classification. Clin Orthop. 1980;151:12–21.
72. Gusic N, Grgorinic I, Fedel I, Lemac D, Bukvic N, Gusic M, Cicvaric T, Lovric Z. Fluoroscopic iliosacral screw placement made safe. Injury. 2017;48:S70–2.
73. Pekmezci M, Rotter P, Toogood P, Morshed S, Kandemir U. Reexamination of pelvic inlet and outlet images using 3-dimensional computed tomography reconstructions. J Orthop Trauma. 2014;28:324–9.
74. Ricci W, Mamczak C, Tynan M, Streubel P, Gardner M. Pelvic inlet and outlet radiographs redefined. J Bone Joint Surg. 2010;92-A:1947–53.
75. Young P, Ho K, Nair S, Yeon W. Optimal pelvic inlet and outlet radiograph angles in Korean patients. J Korean Orthop Assoc. 2012;47:9–14.
76. Moed B, Ahmad B, Craig J, Jacobson G, Anders M. Intraoperative monitoring with stimulus-evoked electromyography during placement of iliosacral screws. J Bone Joint Surg. 1998;80-A(4):537–46.
77. Ricci WM, Padberg AM, Borrelli J. The significance of anode location for stimulus-evoked electromyography during iliosacral screw placement. J Orthop Trauma. 2003;17(2):95–9.
78. Hilgert R, Finn J, Egbers H. Technik der perkutanen SI-Verschraubung mit Unterstützung durch konventionellen C-Bogen. Unfallchirurg. 2005;108:954–60.
79. Matta J, Saucedo T. Internal fixation of pelvic ring fractures. Clin Orthop. 1989;242:83–97.
80. French B, Tornetta P. Transiliosakrale Osteosynthese bei instabilen Verletzungen des hinteren Beckenringes. Oper Orthop Traumatol. 2002;14:29–49.
81. Sun X, Li S, Qiu Y, Chen Z, Chen X, Xu L, Zhu Z. Anatomical study of a novel iliosacral screw placement for sacrum-pelvis in adult via computed tomography reconstruction. Spine. 2018;43:E740–5.
82. Hong H, Hong Z, Chen H, Lin L, Zhu Z. Iliosacral screw fixation of transforaminal sacral fractures using local anesthesia and CT. J Am Coll Surg. 2010;211:e7–12.
83. Routt M, Simonian P. Posterior pelvic ring disruptions: iliosacral screws. In: Wiss DA, Editor. Master Techniqes in Orthopaedics: Fractures. Raven Press, New York 1998. p. 595–612.
84. Nelson D, Duwelius P. CT-guided fixation of sacral fractures and sacroiliacal joint disruptions. Radiology. 1991;180:527–32.
85. Routt M, Simonian P. Closed reduction and percutaneous skeletal fixation of sacral fractures. Clin Orthop. 1996;329:121–8.
86. Ruatti S, Kerschbaumer G, Gay E, Milaire M, Merloz P, Tonetti J. Technique for reduction and percutaneous fixation of U- and H-shaped sacral fractures. Orthop Traumatol Surg Res. 2013;99:625–9.
87. Rommens P, Arand C, Thomczyk S, Handrich K, Wagner D, Hofmann A. [Fragility fractures of the pelvis]. Unfallchirurg. 2019;122:469–82.
88. Rommens P, Dietz S, Ossendorf C, Pairon P, Wagner D, Hofmann A. Fragility fractures of the pelvis: should they be fixed? Acta Chir Orthop Traumatol Cechoslov. 2015;82:101–12.
89. Rommens P, Hofmann A, editors. Fragility fractures of the pelvis. Cham: Springer International Publishing AG; 2017. p. 2017.
90. Iorio J, Jakoi A, Rehman S. Percutaneous sacroiliac screw fixation of the posterior pelvic ring. Orthop Clin North Am. 2015;46:511–21.
91. Tonetti J, van Overschelde J, Sadok B, Vouaillat H, Eid A. Percutaneous ilio-sacral screw insertion. Fluoroscopic techniques. Orthop Traumatol Surg Res. 2013;99:965–72.
92. Lindahl J. Management of pelvic ring injuries. Thesis. University of Helsinki, Finland. 2015.
93. Denis F, Steven D, Comfort T. Sacral fractures: an important problem, retrospective analysis of 236 cases. Clin Orthop. 1988;227:67–81.
94. Heydemann J, Hartline B, Gibson M, Ambrose C, Munz J, Galpin M, Achor T, Gary J. Do transsacral-transiliac screws across uninjured sacroiliac joints affect pain and functional outcomes in trauma patients? Clin Orthop. 2016;474:1417–21.
95. Mardam-Bey S, Beebe M, Black J, Chang E, Kubiak E, Bishop J, McAndrew C, Ricci W, Gardner M. The effect of transiliac-transsacral screw fixation for pelvic ring injuries on the uninjured sacroiliac joint. J Orthop Trauma. 2016;30:463–8.
96. Culemann U, Tosounidis G, Reilmann H. [Injury to the pelvic ring. Diagnosis and current possibilities for treatment]. Unfallchirurg. 2004;107:1169–81.
97. Scharf M, Krieg B, Dengler M, Füchtmeier B. Die Implantatentfernung—eine Risiko-Nutzen-Abwägung? OP J. 2016;32:80–8.
98. Tscherne H, Pohlemann T. Tscherne Unfallchirurgie: Becken und Acetabulum. Berlin, Heidelberg, New York: Springer; 1998.
99. Abumi K, Saita M, Iida T. Reduction and fixation of sacroiliac joint dislocation by the combined use of S1 pedicle screws and the Galveston technique. Spine. 2000;25:1977–83.
100. Routt M, Simonian P, Mills W. Iliosacral screw fixation: early complications of the percutaneous technique. J Orthop Trauma. 1997;11(8):584–9.
101. Remiger A, Engelhardt P. Die perkutane iliosakrale Verschraubung von vertikal instabilen Beckenringfrakturen. Swiss Surg. 1996;2:259–63.
102. Stuby F, Gonser C, Baron H, Stöckle U, Badke A, Ochs B. Implantatentfernung nach Beckenringfraktur. OP J. 2016;32:130–7.
103. Routt M, Simonian P, Inaba J. Iliosacral screw complications. Oper Tech Orthop. 1997;7(3):206–20.
104. Yücel N, Lefering R, Tjardes T, Korenkov M, Schierholz J, Tiling T, Bouillon B, Rixen D. [Is implant removal after percutaneous iliosacral screw fixation of unstable posterior pelvic ring disruptions indicated?]. Unfallchirurg. 2004;107:468–74.
105. Sciulli R, Daffner R, Altman D, Altman G, Sewecke J. CT-guided iliosacral screw placement: technique and clinical experience. AJR Am J Roentgenol. 2007;188:181–92.
106. Falzarano G, Rollo G, Bisaccia M, Pace V, Lanzetti R, Garcia-Prieto E, Pichierri P, Meccariello L. Percutaneous screws CT guided to fix sacroiliac joint in tile C pelvic injury. Outcomes at 5 years of follow-up. SICOT J. 2018;4:52. https://doi.org/10.1051/sicotj/2018047.
107. Shuler T, Boone D, Gruen G, Peitzman A. Percutaneous iliosacral screw fixation: early treatment for unstable posterior pelvic ring disruptions. J Trauma. 1995;38(3):453–8.
108. Keating JF, Werier J, Blachut P, Broekhuyse H, Meek RN, O'Brien PJ. Early fixation of the vertically unstable pelvis: the role of iliosacral screw fixation of the posterior lesion. J Orthop Trauma. 1999;13(2):107–13.

109. Rysavý M, Pavelka T, Khayarin M, Dzupa V. Iliosacral screw fixation of the unstable pelvic ring injuries. Acta Chir Orthop Traumatol Cechoslov. 2010;77:209–14.
110. Zwingmann J, Konrad G, Mehlhorn A, Südkamp N, Oberst M. Percutaneous iliosacral screw insertion: malpositioning and revision rate of screws with regards to application technique (navigated vs. conventional). J Trauma. 2010;69:1501–6.
111. Osterhoff G, Ossendorf C, Wanner G, Simmen H, Werner C. Posterior screw fixation in rotationally unstable pelvic ring injuries. Injury. 2011;42:992–6.
112. Zwingmann J, Hauschild O, Bode G, Südkamp N, Schmal H. Malposition and revision rates of different imaging modalities for percutaneous iliosacral screw fixation following pelvic fractures: a systematic review and meta-analysis. Arch Orthop Trauma Surg. 2013;133:1257–65.
113. Kim J, Oh C, Oh J, Lee H, Min W, Kyung H, Yoon S, Mun J. Percutaneous iliosacral screwing in pelvic ring injury using three-dimensional fluoroscopy. J Orthop Sci. 2013;18:87–92.
114. Elzohairy M, Salama A. Open reduction internal fixation versus percutaneous iliosacral screw fixation for unstable posterior pelvic ring disruptions. Orthop Traumatol Surg Res. 2017;103:223–7.
115. Griffin D, Starr A, Reinert C, Jones A, Whitlock S. Vertically unstable pelvic fractures fixed with percutaneous iliosacral screws: does posterior injury pattern predict fixation failure? J Orthop Trauma. 2003;17(6):399–405.
116. Herman A, Keener E, Dubose C, Lowe J. Zone 2 sacral fractures managed with partially-threaded screws result in low risk of neurologic injury. Injury. 2016;47:1569–73.
117. Tonetti J, Carrat L, Lavallee S, Pittet L, Merloz P, Chirossel JP. Percutaneous iliosacral screw placement using image guided techniques. Clin Orthop. 1998;354:103–10.
118. Stockle U, Konig B, Hofstetter R, Nolte L, Haas N. Bildwandler-gestützte Navigation. Eine experimentelle Studie zu Beckenverschraubungen. Unfallchirurg. 2001;104:215–20.
119. Gautier E, Bächler R, Heini P, Nolte L. Accuracy of computer-guided screw fixation of the sacroiliac joint. Clin Orthop. 2001;393:310–7.
120. Collinge C, Coons D, Tornetta P, Aschenbrenner J. Standard multiplanar fluoroscopy versus a fluoroscopically based navigation system for the percutaneous insertion of iliosacral screws. A cadaver model. J Orthop Trauma. 2005;19(4):254–8.
121. Takao M, Nishii T, Sakai T, Sugano N. CT-3D-fluoroscopy matching navigation can reduce the malposition rate of iliosacral screw insertion for less-experienced surgeons. J Orthop Trauma. 2013;27:716–21.
122. Tonetti J, Carrat L, Blendea S, Merloz P, Troccaz J, Lavallée S, Chirossel J. Clinical results of percutaneous pelvic surgery. Computer assisted surgery using ultrasound compared to standard fluoroscopy. Comput Aided Surg. 2001;6:204–11.
123. Grützner P, Rose E, Vock B, Holz F, Nolte L, Wentzensen A. Computer-assistierte perkutane Verschraubung des hinteren Beckenrings. Unfallchirurg. 2002;105:254–60.
124. Hüfner T, Geerling J, Gänsslen A, Kendoff D, Citak C, Grützner P, Krettek C. [Computer-assisted surgery for pelvic injuries]. Chirurg. 2004;75:961–6.
125. Stockle U, Konig B, Dahne M, Raschke M, Haas NP. Navigationsverfahren in der Becken und Azetabulumchirurgie. Klinische Erfahrungen, Indikationen und Grenzen. Unfallchirurg. 2002;105(10):886–92.
126. Stöckle U, Krettek C, Pohlemann T, Messmer P. Clinical applications—pelvis. Injury. 2004;35(Suppl 1):46–56.
127. Arand M, Kinzl L, Gebhard F. Computer-guidance in percutaneous screw stabilization of the iliosacral joint. Clin Orthop. 2004;422:201–7.
128. Grossterlinden L, Rueger J, Catala-Lehnen P, Rupprecht M, Lehmann W, Rücker A, Briem D. Factors influencing the accuracy of iliosacral screw placement in trauma patients. Int Orthop. 2011;35:1391–6.
129. Peng K, Li Y, Hsu W, Wu M, Yang J, Hsu C, Huang T. Intraoperative computed tomography with integrated navigation in percutaneous iliosacral screwing. Injury. 2013;44:203–8.
130. Zwingmann J, Südkamp N, König B, Culemann U, Pohlemann T, Aghayev E, Schmal H. Intra- and postoperative complications of navigated and conventional techniques in percutaneous iliosacral screw fixation after pelvic fractures: results from the German Pelvic Trauma Registry. Injury. 2013;44:1765–72.
131. Matityahu A, Kahler D, Krettek C, Stöckle U, Grutzner P, Messmer P, Ljungqvist J, Gebhard F. Three-dimensional navigation is more accurate than two-dimensional navigation or conventional fluoroscopy for percutaneous sacroiliac screw fixation in the dysmorphic sacrum: a randomized multicenter study. J Orthop Trauma. 2014;28:707–10.
132. Thakkar S, Thakkar R, Sirisreetreerux N, Carrino J, Shafiq B, Hasenboehler E. 2D versus 3D fluoroscopy-based navigation in posterior pelvic fixation: review of the literature on current technology. Int J Comput Assist Radiol Surg. 2017;12:69–76.
133. Zhang R, Yin Y, Li S, Hou Z, Jin L, Zhang Y. Percutaneous sacroiliac screw versus anterior plating for sacroiliac joint disruption: a retrospective cohort study. Int J Surg Case Rep. 2018;50:11–6.
134. Li C. Clinical comparative analysis on unstable pelvic fractures in the treatment with percutaneous sacroiliac screws and sacroiliac joint anterior plate fixation. Eur Rev Med Pharmacol Sci. 2014;18:2704–8.
135. Gu R, Huang W, Yang L, Liu H, Xie K, Huang Z. Comparisons of front plate, percutaneous sacroiliac screws, and sacroiliac anterior papilionaceous plate in fixation of unstable pelvic fractures. Medicine (Baltimore). 2017;96(36):e7775. https://doi.org/10.1097/MD.0000000000007775.

Local Sacral Plating

32

Axel Gänsslen and Jan Lindahl

In the 1980s, many sacrum fractures were missed due to poor image quality, limited use of CT, lack of clinical signs, and common unconsciousness in polytraumatized patients. A treatment concept for these injuries was therefore missing.

In the early 1990s, increasing understanding of fracture morphology and development of several treatment modalities for unstable pelvic injuries led to more precise understanding of treatment of unstable sacral fractures.

The prognostic importance of sacrum fractures has been shown in several studies. A correlation between the fracture course and the probability of fracture-associated neurological damage was identified [1–3].

Denis et al. established a detailed classification of sacrum fractures [1], which was integrated into the current AO/OTA classification [4, 5]. A correlation between fracture localization and incidence of concomitant nerve damage was found. As a consequence, surgical decompression of the spinal canal was recommended.

Nevertheless, until the early 1990s, predominantly nonsurgical treatment of sacrum fractures was performed [6, 7], despite its important biomechanical function. The sacrum transmits the load from the lower extremities to the trunk of the body and is thereby subjected to translational and rotational forces. By tensioning the posterior sacroiliac ligaments, the sacrum is compressed and stabilized between the iliac bones [8–10]. The resulting nutation movement is limited by the pelvic floor ligaments [11, 12].

Since the early 1990s, treatment focused on surgical treatment. Various external and internal osteosynthesis procedures have been reported to stabilize sacral fractures [3, 13–23].

Pohlemann developed the concept of direct sacral plating [19, 20], which led to good posterior pelvic reconstructions, acceptable complication rates, and good to excellent midterm outcomes [24].

There are only few indications for direct sacral plating based on the AO/OTA fracture classification.

Sacral fractures involving the pelvic ring can be divided into stable fractures not disrupting the pelvic ring structure (type A) and vertical fractures with resulting pelvic instability.

According to the AO/OTA classification [4], sacral fractures are classified as:

- OTA A 3.1: coccyx fractures/coccyx dislocations
- OTA A 3.2: undisplaced transverse fractures below S2 without pelvic ring disruption
- OTA A 3.3: dislocated transverse fractures below S2 without pelvic ring disruption
- OTA B 1.2: unilateral open-book sacral fractures
- OTA B 2.1: unilateral lateral compression fractures of the sacrum
- OTA B 3.1: bilateral open-book sacrum fractures
- OTA B 3.3: bilateral lateral compression fractures of the sacrum
- OTA C 1.3: unilateral complete unstable sacrum fracture
- OTA C 2.3: unilateral complete unstable sacrum fracture, contralateral type B injury
- OTA C 3.3: bilateral complete unstable sacrum fractures

The predominant criteria for surgical sacral fracture stabilization include

- Instability
- (Severe) displacement
- Concomitant fracture-related nerve injury

Accordingly, some type A injuries can be treated by direct sacral plating, especially in severely displaced fractures or concomitant sacral nerve root lesions in transverse sacral fractures.

Sacral fractures as part of a pelvic ring type B injury are most commonly lateral compression fractures [25] and do

A. Gänsslen (✉)
Department of Trauma Surgery, Orthopedics and Hand Surgery, Hospital Wolfsburg, Wolfsburg, Germany

J. Lindahl
Orthopaedics and Trauma Surgery, Helsinki University Hospital, Helsinki, Finland

A. Gänsslen et al. (eds.), *Pelvic Ring Fractures*, https://doi.org/10.1007/978-3-030-54730-1_32

not require specific treatment for predominantly minor displacement and instability. Pelvic ring anatomy is adequately reconstructed by using anterior pelvic ring osteosynthesis (e.g., symphyseal plating, external fixator). In case of extremely rare neurological damage of this type of fracture, surgical decompression of the sacral nerve roots can be an option. Osteosynthesis of the sacrum is usually unnecessary.

Sacral fractures as part of pelvic ring type C injuries should be surgically stabilized. The type of osteosynthesis depends on the presence of fracture-associated nerve damage. In the case of relevant or suspected nerve damage, an open procedure is usually used to enable decompression, since a 40% probability of at least partial recovery can be expected immediately postoperatively [24].

The classical indication for direct sacral plating are transforaminal or central sacral fractures, whereas "suicidal jumper fractures" [26] with spino-pelvic dissociation are best treated by lumbo-pelvic fixation.

32.1 Anatomic Basis of Direct Osteosynthesis

When considering direct sacral osteosynthesis, the sacral anatomy is of crucial importance, e.g., localization of the central sacral canal, the sacral foramina, and neurovascular structures.

"Safe zones" for implant placement have been identified in anatomical studies [27, 28]. The sacral neuroforamina gradually increase in their size from S1 to S4. This leads to a reduced "filling" with nerve roots: 1/3–1/4 at the level of S1/S2, 1/6 at the level of S4 [1]. CT morphological studies and studies dealing with geriatric trauma patients confirmed that the densest bone is expected close to the SI joints and at the central sacrum. The lowest bone density was observed paraforaminal and lateral from S1 to S3 and between S1 and S2 [29–31]. This human bone density distribution explains typical fracture patterns observed especially in elderly patients. The optimal bone density is observed directly parallel to the SI joint, and a moderate bone density is observed at the sacral bodies [29–31].

The distal central canal is filled with fat and connecting tissue, approximately 70%, reducing the risk of iatrogenic damage of nerve roots [1, 27].

There two potential main sacral fracture lines, where direct osteosynthesis is possible:

- Transverse fracture line—vertical (along the sacral length) plate or screw application
- Longitudinal fracture line—horizontal (transverse) plate or screw application

Pohlemann analyzed the possibility of screw application in different sacral regions regarding screw orientation and anatomic safety [3, 19, 20]. Lateral, interforaminal, and medial screw orientations were distinguished (Fig. 32.1). In general, perpendicular drill orientation in relation to the posterior sacral surface is always recommended:

- Lateral screw position (longitudinal fracture line): screw placed lateral to the foraminal zone can safely be placed without affecting the foraminal zone or the central canal; the screw direction should be parallel to the SI joint plane and perpendicular to the posterior sacral surface; a K-wire inserted into the SI joint can guide the drill; to avoid injury to neurovascular structures at the anterior sacrum (internal iliac vessels, lumbosacral trunk), oscillation drilling is generally recommended.
- Lateral screw position (transverse fracture line): in transverse fractures, screw orientation can be guided from distal to proximal, as the kyphosis of the sacrum allows placement of one lateral screw parallel to the anterior/posterior cortex; the screw should be directed toward the sacral promontory, resulting in screw lengths of 50–80 mm.
- Medial screw position S1: the optimal starting point is at the distal border of the L5/S1 facet joint; screw orientation can be guided direct perpendicular to the posterior sacral surface or even in a slightly lateral orientation.
- Medial screw position S2–S4: at the imaginary interforaminal line (between the posterior sacral foramina), screws can be safely inserted at the midpoint between two foramina; perforation of the central canal should be avoided.

The classical indications for direct sacral plating include vertical, transforaminal fractures, as relevant bony space is available lateral to the fracture line. More lateral, transalar fractures can also be fixed, depending on the fracture morphology. If these fractures are running too far laterally, plate extension to the iliac crest is optional [19, 20].

For increased safety, the use of a three-fluted drill together with the oscillating drill attachment is generally recommended at the sacrum.

32.1.1 Longitudinal Sacral Fractures

Longitudinal sacral fractures are classified into lateral (transalar), foraminal, and central (medial to the foraminal line) fractures according to Denis [1].

A correlation between the zone of the fracture line (I = transalar, II = transforaminal, III = central) and the rate of neurological deficits could be demonstrated

(I = 5.8%, II = 28.3%, III = 64.0%) [1]. These findings were confirmed by Gibbons et al. [2]. Both groups concluded that a surgical decompression of the central canal may be beneficial for neurologic recovery. Pohlemann et al. observed even higher rates of nerve root injury. After type C injuries the observed rate of neurological deficits was 32.6% in zone I, 42.9% in zone II, and 63.6% in zone III [3, 32].

Pohlemann developed the concept of direct sacral plating ("local osteosynthesis") in the early 1990s. Transverse plating or plating using specially designed plates were recommended [19, 20].

32.2 Operative Technique

A standardized operative technique is recommended.

32.2.1 Positioning

Standard prone position on a radiolucent operating table is performed, allowing intraoperative fluoroscopic standard projections (AP true lateral sacral view, inlet-, and outlet views).

32.2.2 Landmarks

The following landmarks are identified (Fig. 32.2):

- Both posterior iliac crests
- Both PSIS
- Spinal processes of L4 and L5
- Sacral midline
- Upper end of the rima ani

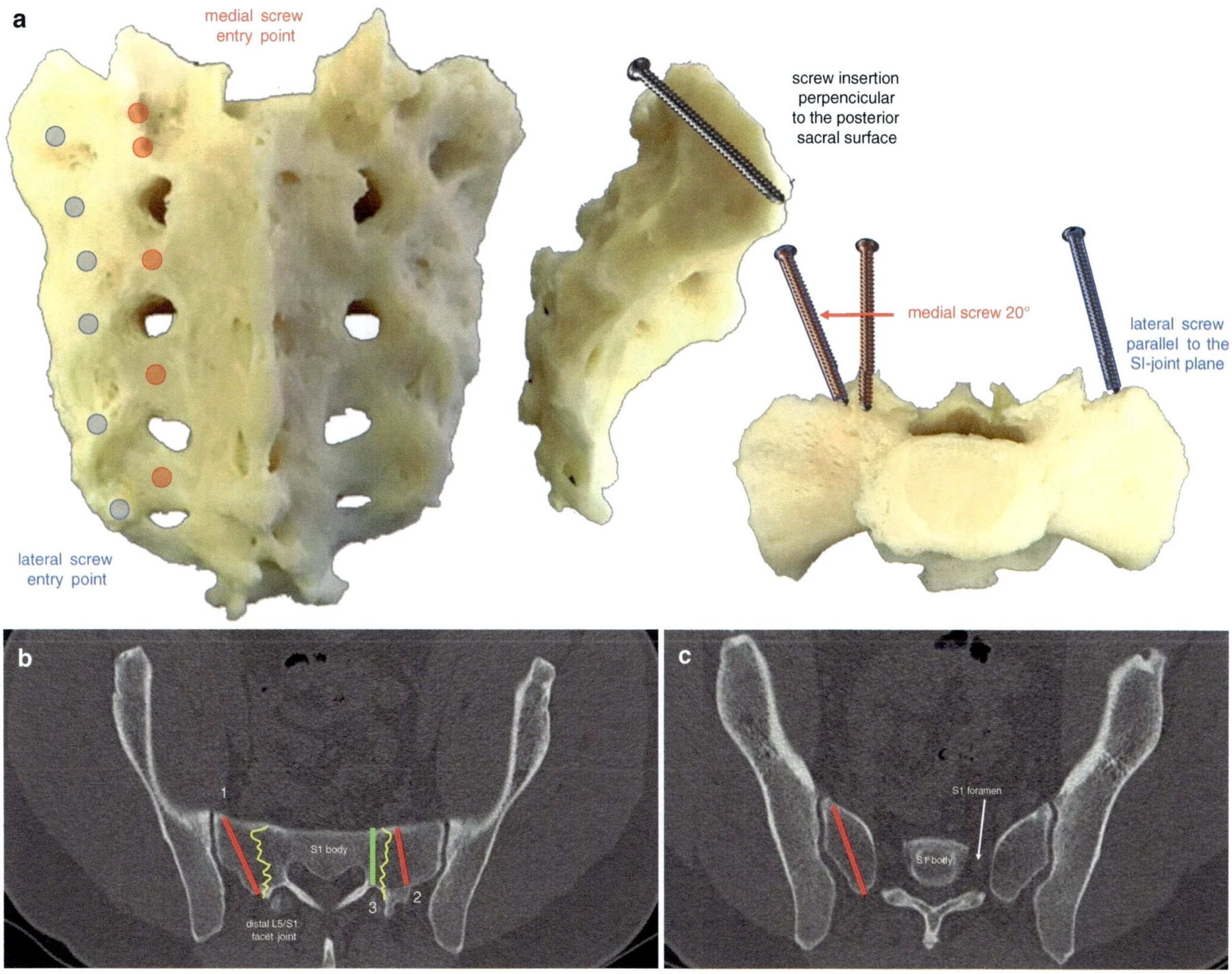

Fig. 32.1 (**a**) Possible application areas and screw angulations for plate fixation at the sacral bone. (**b**) Screw orientation at the level of S1: screws can be placed slightly lateral to the foraminal zone parallel to the SI joint (1). Alternatively, a more straight screw orientation can be used, directly below the level of the L5/S1 facet joint (2) or in a slight medial direction, starting lateral (3). (**c**) At the level of the S1 foramen, only parallel lateral screws can be inserted. (**d**) At the level of the S2 body, a parallel screw to the SI joint level (1) and a straight screw orientation (2) can be used. (**e**) Additionally, very long screws can be guided from distal to proximal parallel to the SI joint. Proximal cortical penetration should be avoided!

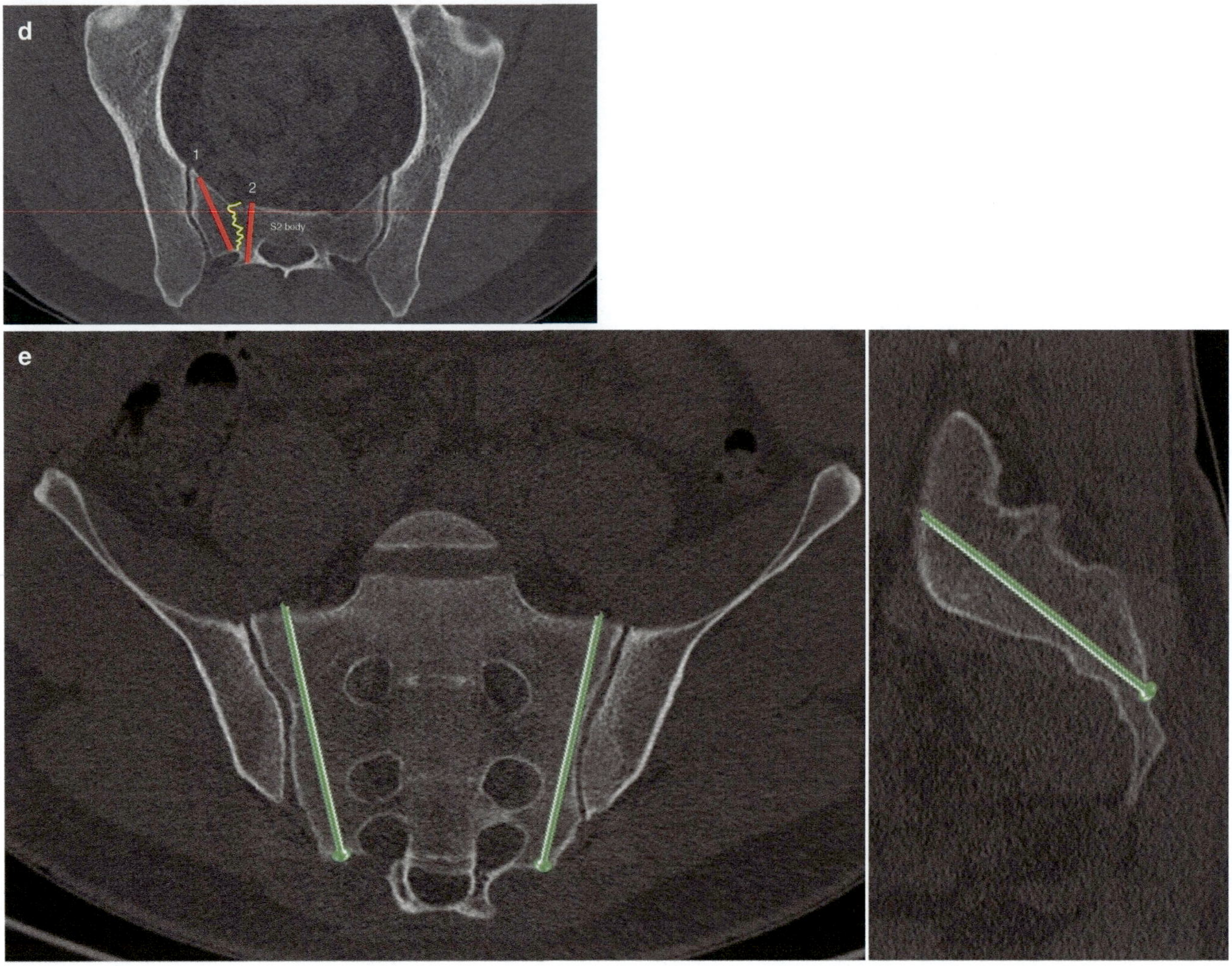

Fig. 32.1 (continued)

32.2.3 Draping

Draping is performed with access to the recommended landmarks. The thoraco-lumbar junction should be included into draping. It is usually not necessary to freely drape the leg on the fractured side, as reduction can be performed exclusively at the sacrum.

32.2.4 Incision

The skin incision varies depending on the fracture pattern (Fig. 32.2):

- Unilateral transforaminal and transalar fractures: longitudinal incision in the midline between the posterior iliac crest and the medial sacral crest
- Central and bilateral sacrum fractures: longitudinal midline incision close to the central sacral crest, slightly lateral to the midline

32.2.5 Dissection

The lumbosacral fascia is incised close to its origin at the spinal processes of L4 and L5 and along the medial sacral crest as in spinal surgery (Fig. 32.2). Using a sharp dissector or a cautery knife, the erector trunci muscle is elevated from the posterior sacral surface as far lateral and proximal as necessary. Mobilization of the muscle is possible up to the posterior SI joint ligaments. A distal detachment of the muscle, creating a "muscle flap," is avoided as this led to an inacceptable higher rate of soft-tissue problems [24]. If more mobility of the muscle is needed, a second fascial incision close to

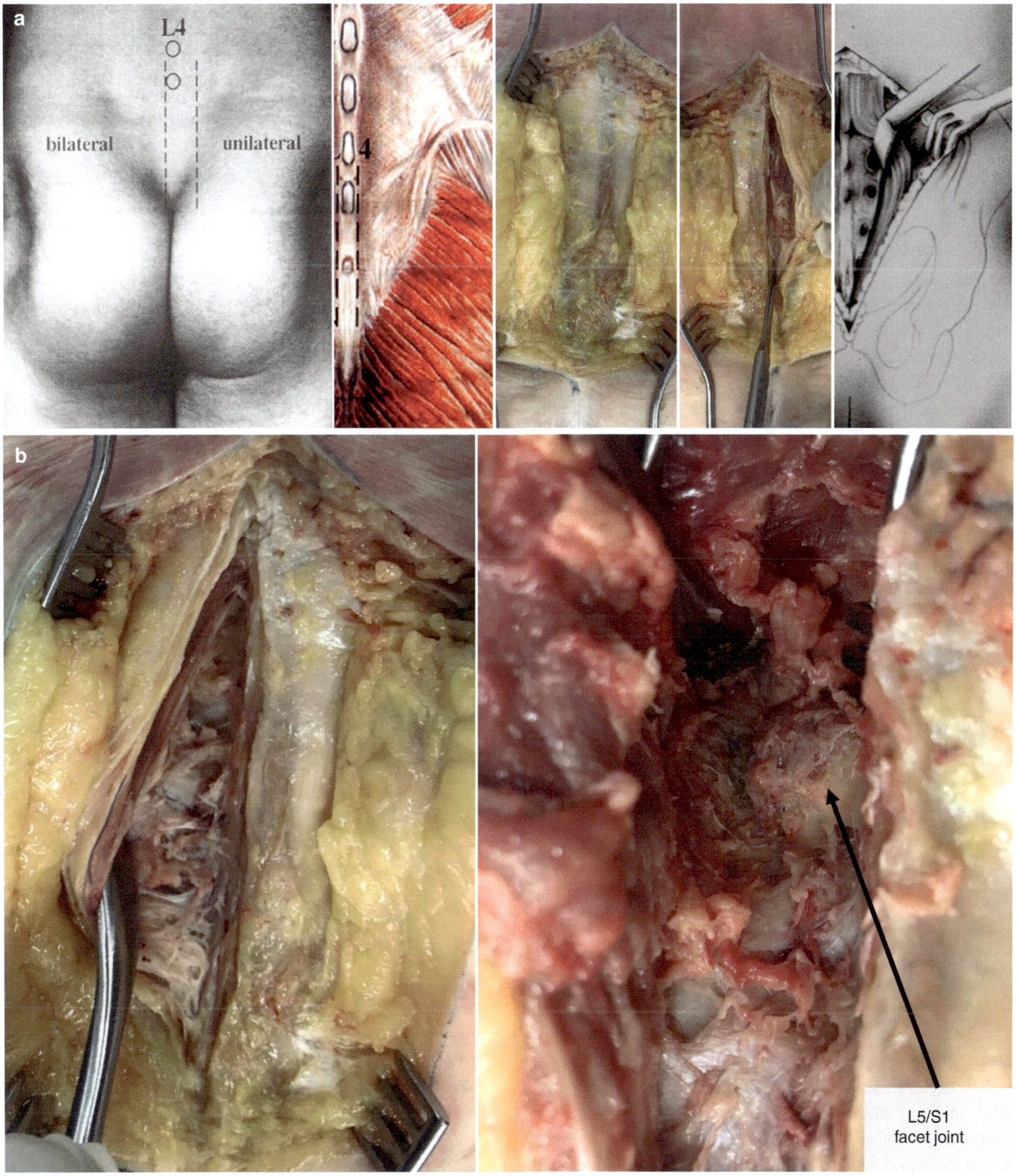

Fig. 32.2 (**a**) Two possible incisions for direct posterior approach to the sacrum. Fascial dissection should avoid complete elevation of the erector trunci muscle, as this was found to be associated with wound problems. (**b**) Latertal mobilization of the erector trunci muscle (left) and proximal extension until identification of the L5/S1 facet joint

the SI joint is performed to mobilize the muscle either medial or lateral. In bilateral or central fractures, bilateral fascial and muscular dissection should be considered. Thus, the complete posterior aspect of the sacrum can be exposed, and the foraminal area can sufficiently be visualized for control of reduction or even posterior sacral decompression (Fig. 32.2).

32.3 Reduction

Before starting reduction maneuvers, the fracture line is completely cleaned and inspected (Fig. 32.3). After disimpaction (Fig. 32.4), a lamina spreader is inserted for fracture line debridement (Fig. 32.5). Free fragments should be removed or if possible reduced. If such fragments compromise the sacral nerve roots, careful extraction under direct visualization is performed (Fig. 32.6).

Typically, depending on the injury mechanism, transforaminal fractures show a vertical displacement, some lateral widening or lateral compression deformity, and/or anterior-posterior displacement. These displacements have to be analyzed preoperatively and addressed intraoperatively:

- Lateral compression: disimpaction can be achieved by insertion of a lamina spreader and careful lateral distraction (Fig. 32.7); alternatively or additionally, a standard distractor is applied to both posterior iliac crests and distraction is performed by careful fracture line widening (Fig. 32.8); care has to be taken to avoid sacral nerve root stretching; thus, direct visualization can protect the nerve roots during manipulation.
- Vertical displacement: application of an oblique orientated distractor can improve reduction of cranio-caudal deformities (Fig. 32.8); complete mobilization of the vertical fracture line from posterior, additional disimpaction by using chisels or raspatories up to the anterior cortex and further careful fracture mobilization in a Kapandji-type technique under direct visualization into the fracture zone leads to optimal reduction; care has to be taken to avoid an iatrogenic injury to the presacral venous plexus
- lateral widening: pointed reduction forceps are used to compress the fracture sites (Fig. 32.9); their tips are positioned lateral onto the iliac crest or on the outer side of the ilium and the opposite tip is placed at the central sacral spine
- anterior-posterior displacement: reduction can be achieved by slight manual elevation of the patient using the distractor or by insertion of a Hohmann retractor or raspatory; the latter should be inserted between the two posterior cortices; after insertion of the tip of these instruments, the instrument is turned and the cortex is levered to reduce the deformity [33]

Control of reduction is easy by inspecting the specific fracture pattern at the interforaminal region (Fig. 32.9).

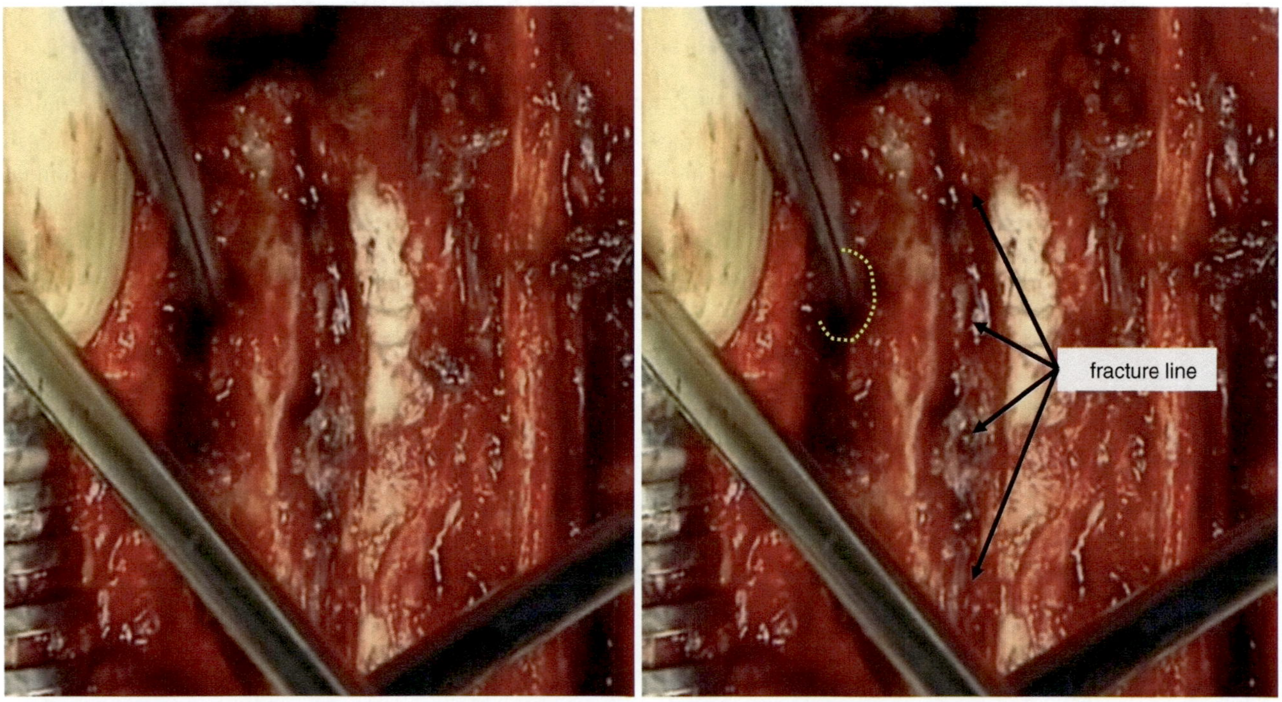

Fig. 32.3 Longitudinal transforaminal fracture line. The S2 foramen is marked with a tweezers

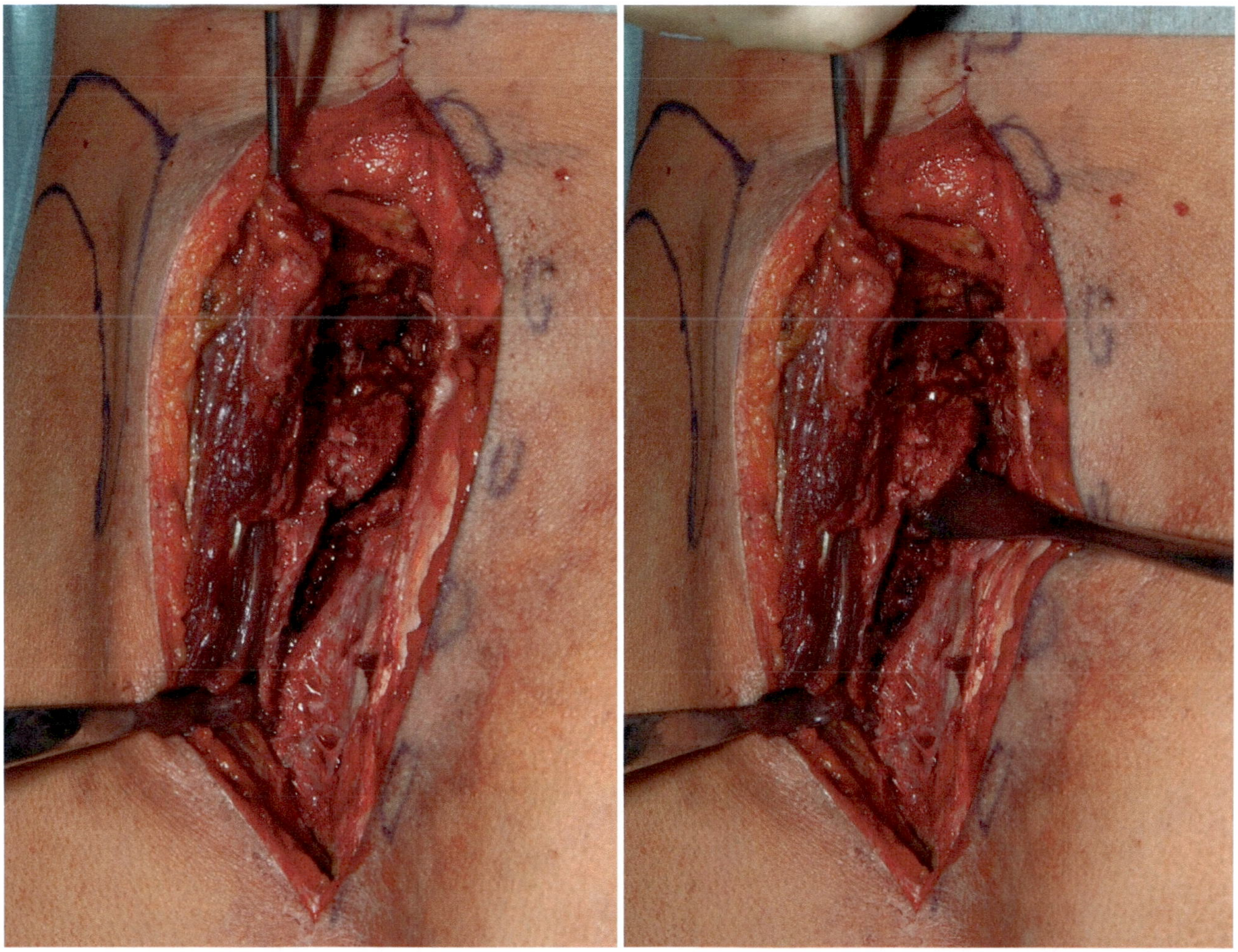

Fig. 32.4 Fracture opening by insertion and tilting using a Cobb elevator

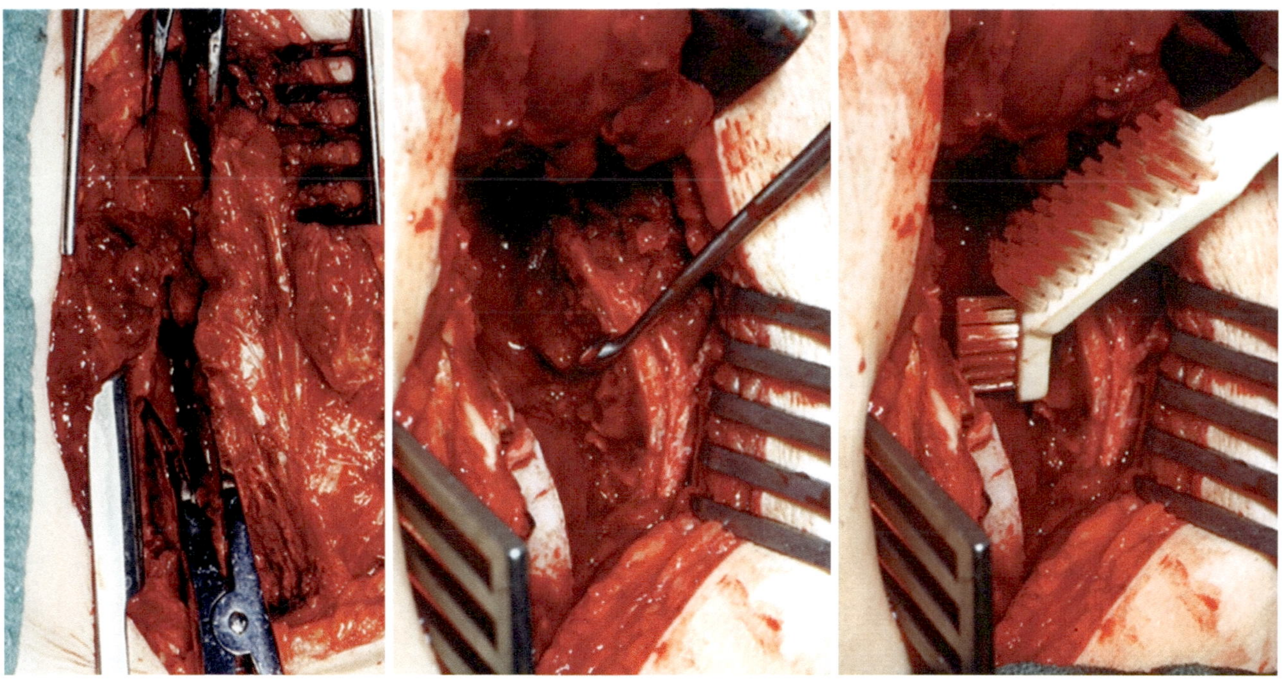

Fig. 32.5 Debridement of the sacral fracture line. Opening of the fracture by insertion of a laminar spreader, cleaning with a brush

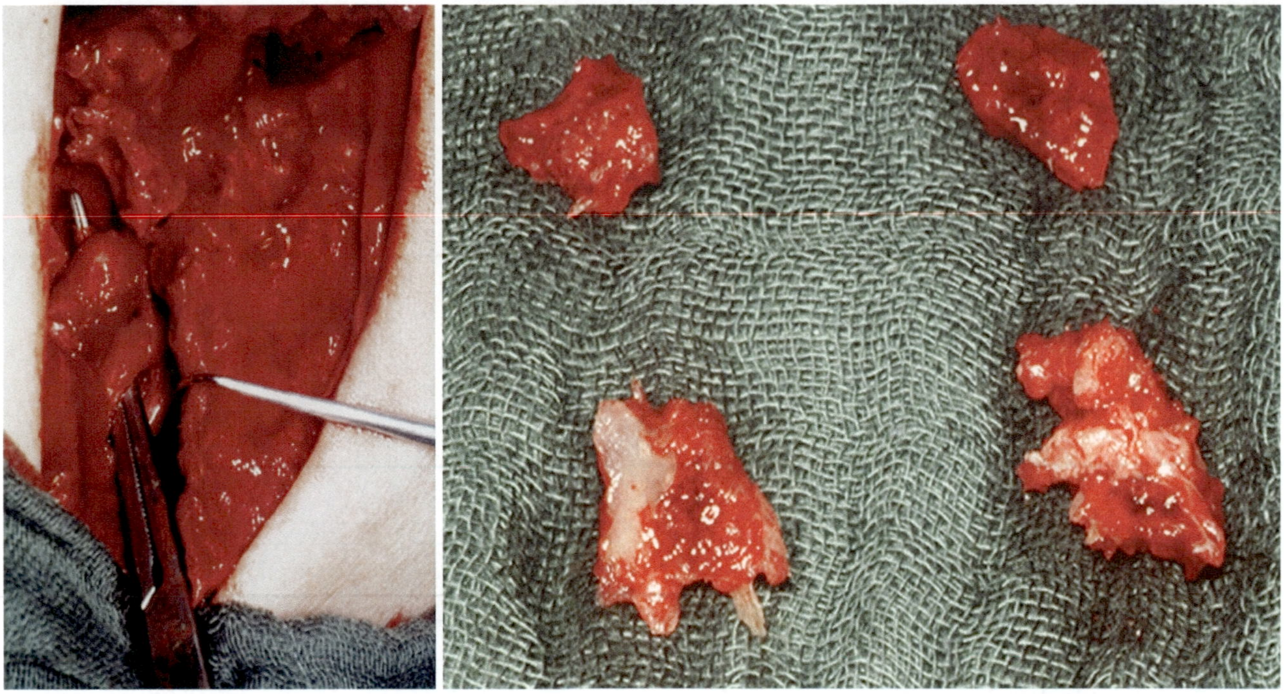

Fig. 32.6 Sacral nerve root decompression (neurolysis) and removal of several fragments

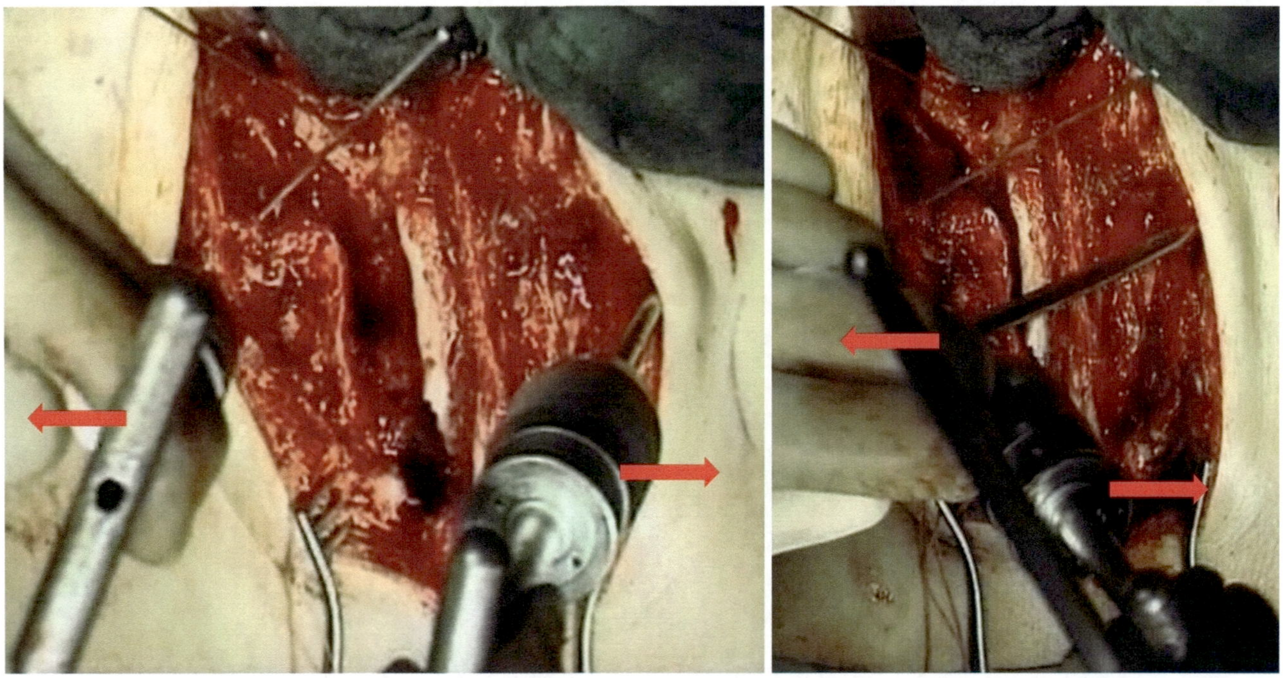

Fig. 32.7 Fracture reduction with Schanz screws inserted on each side of the posterior iliac crest by tilting and compression

32.4 Decompression

Early decompression of sacral nerve roots was advocated by several authors [1–3, 19, 20, 32, 34]. Here, posterior laminectomy was favored.

With increasing experience in treating unstable sacral fractures, relevant data are today available to deal with sacral nerve root injury.

Three types of sacral nerve root injury are possible, and the effect of decompressions was analyzed [35–37]:

- Neuropraxia (= stretching injury of nerve roots) typically recovers over time without intervention.
- Nerve root compression (by fragments or deformity) may improve with decompression or fracture reduction.
- Neurotmesis (= transection of nerve roots) is not expected to recover.

Recently, a literature analysis found no benefit of formal laminectomy and indirect decompression with respect to neurologic recovery [38].

> The best decompression maneuver seems to be adequate/anatomic reduction of the fracture.

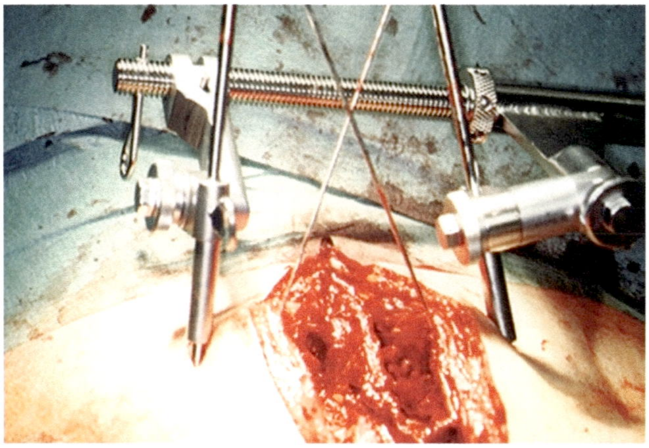

Fig. 32.8 Fracture reduction support using a distractor: the K-wires mark the orientation of the SI joints

32.5 Choice of Implants

Implants which can be used for stabilization include standard small fragment DC plates, 3.5 mm reconstruction plates, H plates which are cut to the required length, and flat 1/3 tubular plates, respectively. The position of the implants is determined by the specific fracture pattern. In general, two plates at different sacral levels are used:

- Transalar fractures (zone I): if enough space is available lateral to the fracture line, a H plate at the level of S1 and additionally at the S3 and/or S4 level is applied; the distal fracture line can also be stabilized by 1/3 tubular plates; if medial screw fixation cannot be realized, the midline has to be crossed and a DC- or reconstruction plate is used, a

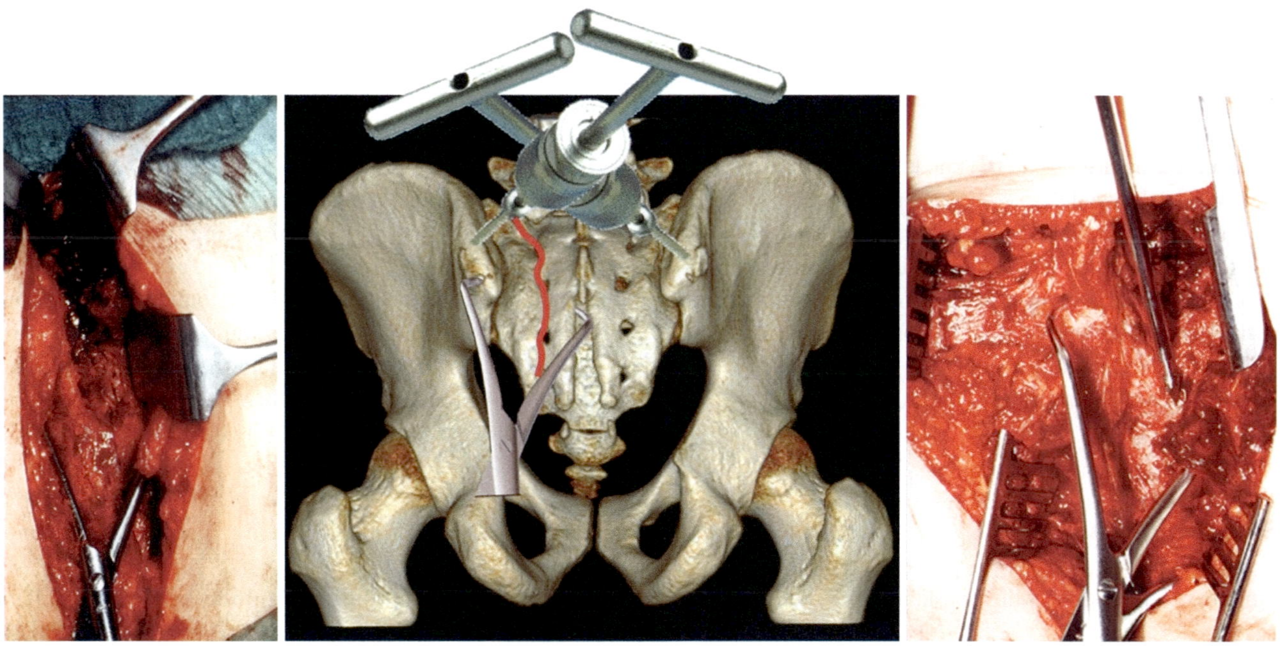

Fig. 32.9 Fracture reduction using a pointed reduction forceps

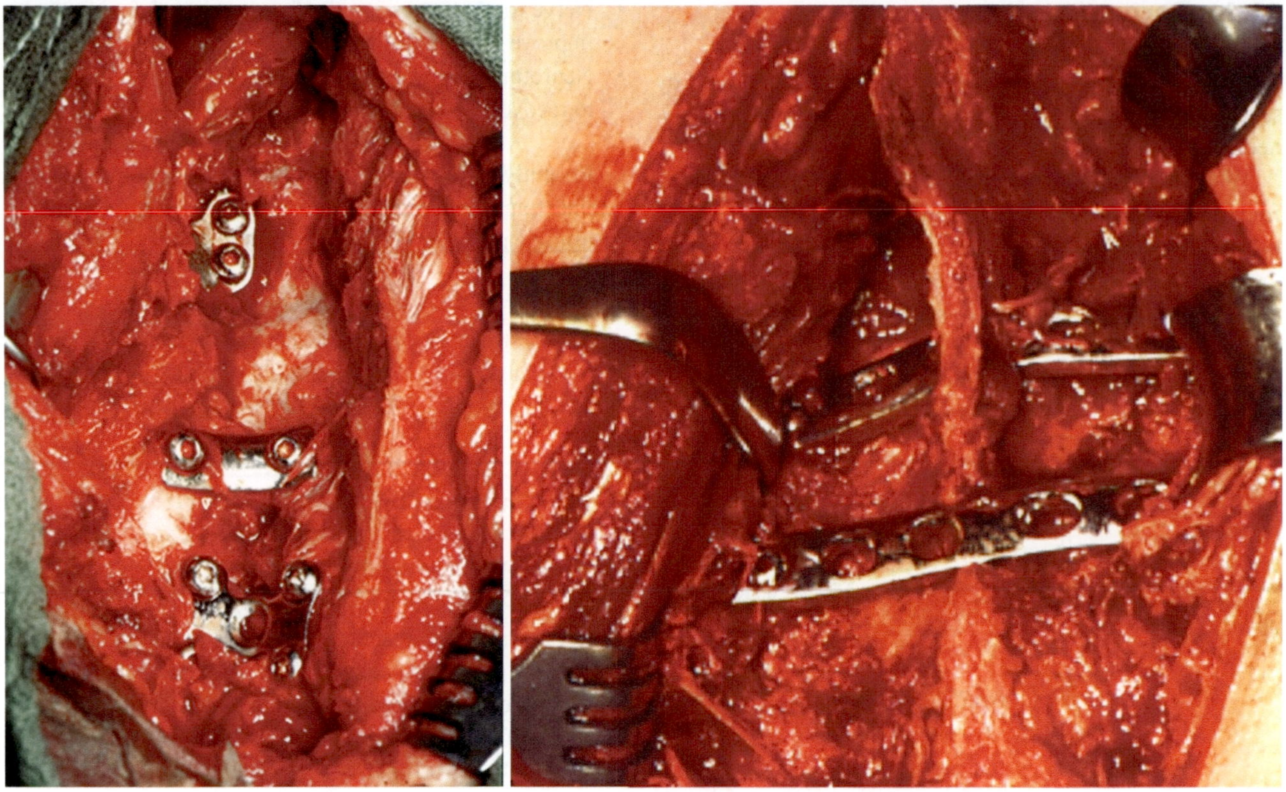

Fig. 32.10 Plate stabilization using small plates (left) or transverse sacral plates (right)

second distal plate can be added; in comminuted fractures lateral fixation must include the ilium.

- Transforaminal fractures (zone II): this is the classical indication for localized plating techniques (Fig. 32.10); standard or modified small fragment plates (H plates, flat 1/3 tubular plates or specially designed plates) can be used [19, 20]; again, the distal fracture line is stabilized by additional H plates or 1/3 tubular plates at the level S3 and/or S4.
- Central fractures (zone III) and bilateral fractures are stabilized by two DC- or reconstruction plates which are positioned parallel to each other at the level S1 and S3 (Fig. 32.10); the plate is fixed with one lateral screw parallel to the SI joint on each side; to increase stability, additional medial screws can be inserted; in comminuted fractures over-compression must be avoided; the plates then act as "neutralization" plates.

32.6 Results

Only two studies dealt with this stabilization concept.

- Gänsslen et al. reported on 32 patients using different "local" stabilization methods [24]. Primary neurologic evaluation revealed eight patients with fracture-related nerve deficits (25%), six after transforaminal fractures, and one after a lateral and one after a central fracture.

  Internal stabilization was performed in average 8 days. The mean operation time was 151 min and blood loss of 770 mL was recorded. In all patients with nerve deficits, intraoperative inspection of the nerve roots and fragment extraction/decompression was performed. Of these, 50% had recovery (1× complete, 3× partial) during further course. Stabilization included 24 direct platings, 6 had ilio-sacral plate stabilization (bridging of one SI joint), and 2 had ilio-iliacal plating (bridging of both SI joints).

  The quality of reduction was anatomic in 26 cases, in 5 cases a maximum of 5 mm cranial displacement persisted, and in 1 case of a comminuted transforaminal fracture during pregnancy a persistent 10 mm distraction of the fracture side was accepted (Figs. 32.11, 32.12, 32.13, and 32.14).

  In one patient, loss of reduction with implant failure was observed. Three patients had local wound complications.
- Recently, Acklin et al. reported their results of parallel, double locking plate fixation of type C injuries in 27 patients [39]. Eight patients had neurological deficits (29.6%). Despite 83% excellent and 17% good functional

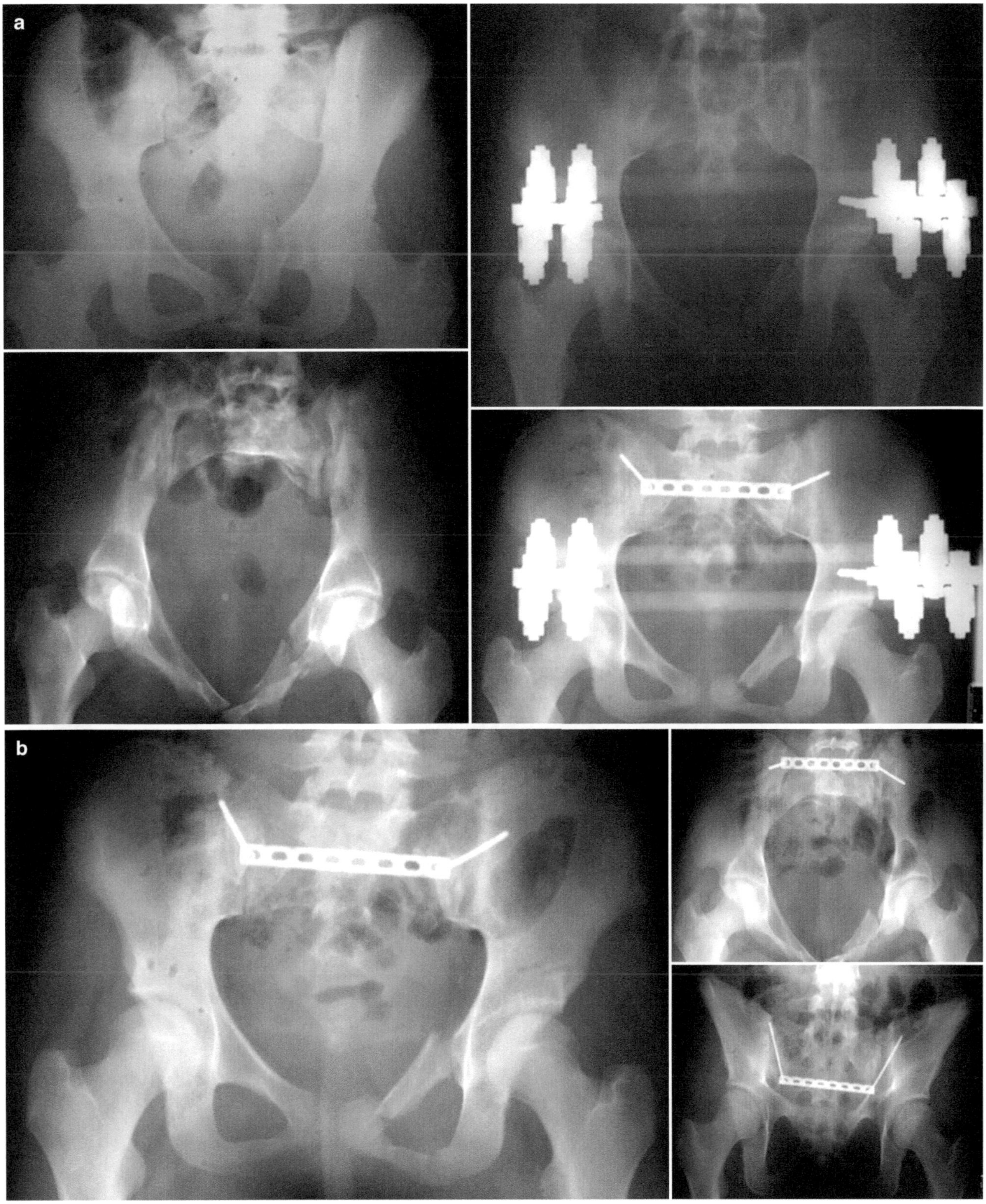

Fig. 32.11 (**a**) Left transforaminal sacral fracture. Primary external fixation followed by posterior plate fixation in both posterior iliac areas. Note: the SI joint widening results from anterior compression injury of the sacrum. (**b**) Follow-up x-rays after 3 months

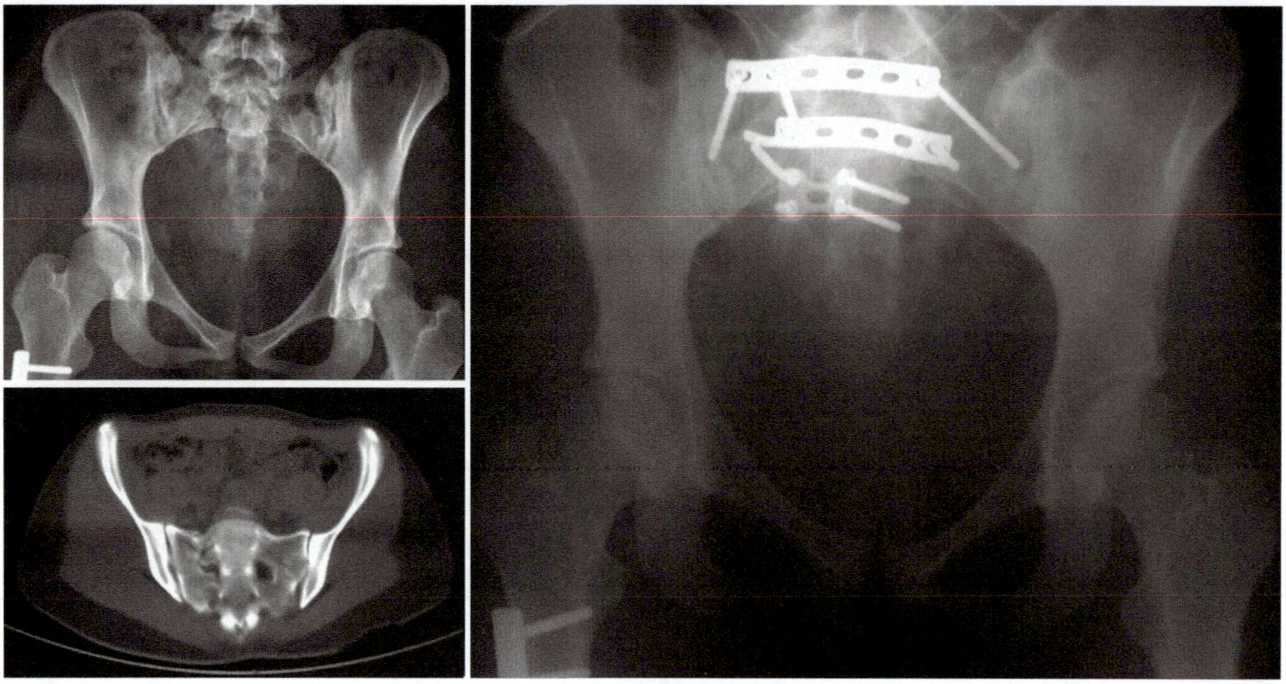

Fig. 32.12 Right foraminal sacral fracture. Stabilization with three plates, fixed only in the sacral bone

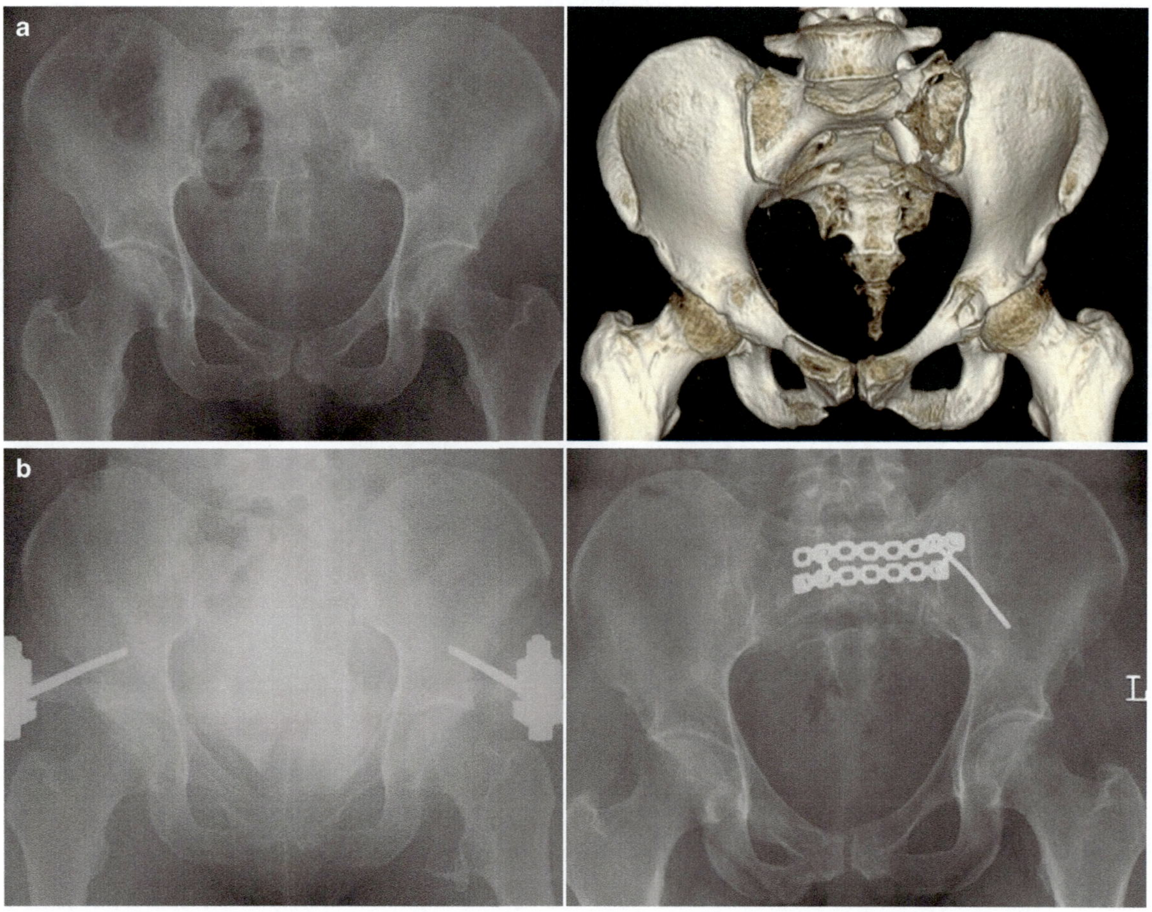

Fig. 32.13 (**a**) Left foraminal sacral fracture. (**b**) Emergency stabilization with a supraacetabular external fixator. Definitive sacral stabilization with two plates. (**c**) Postop CT shows adequate sacral reconstruction

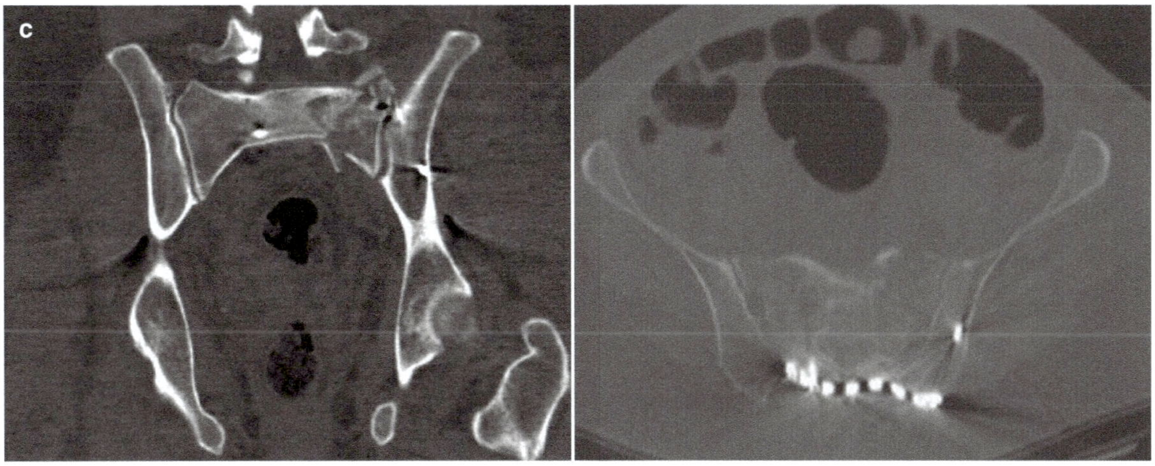

Fig. 32.13 (continued)

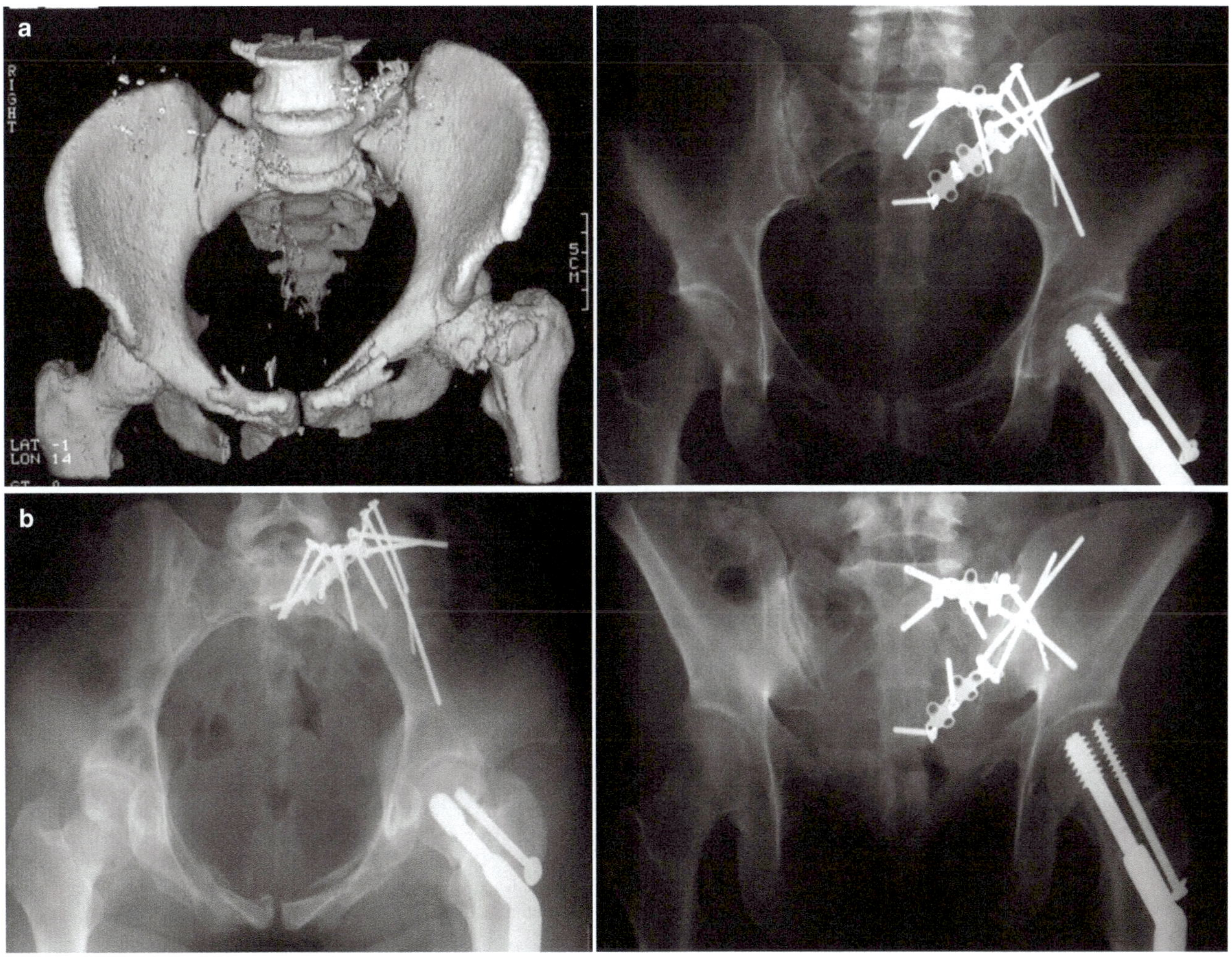

Fig. 32.14 (**a**) Severely displaced lateral sacral fracture, treated with sacro-iliacal plate stabilization. (**b**) Inlet and Outlet views confirm adequate reconstruction

results, one nonunion, five infections, and in 5 patients local discomfort due to plate prominence were reported.

Overall, the concept of direct plating is feasible with high rates of anatomic reconstructions. Local soft-tissue problems have to be considered.

References

1. Denis F, Steven D, Comfort T. Sacral fractures: an important problem, retrospective analysis of 236 cases. Clin Orthop. 1988;227:67–81.
2. Gibbons K, Soloniuk D, Razack N. Neurological injury and patterns of sacral fractures. J Neurosurg. 1990;72:889–93.
3. Pohlemann T, Gänsslen A, Tscherne H. Die Problematik der Sakrumfraktur, klinische Analyse von 377 Fällen. Orthopade. 1992;21:400–12.
4. AO Foundation. Fracture and dislocation classification compendium—2018: pelvic ring. J Orthop Trauma. 2018;32(Suppl 1):S71–6.
5. AO Spine. Sacral spine fractures classification system. 2017. https://aospine.aofoundation.org/-/media/project/aocmf/aospine/documents/clinical-library-andtools/classifications/aos_injury_classification_pocket_card_20200331_sacral.pdf?la=en&hash=2F044D9684DA5735F10B284259509EDC5E9D43BD.
6. Sabiston C, Wing P. Sacral fractures: classification and neurologic implications. J Trauma. 1986;26(12):1113–5.
7. Wörsdörfer O, Magerl F. Sacrumfrakturen. Hefte Unfallheilk. 1980;149:203–14.
8. Albee F. A study of the anatomy and the clinical importance of the sacroiliac joint. JAMA. 1909;53:1273–6.
9. Meyer G. Der Mechanismus der Symphysis sacro-iliaca. Arch Anat Physiol. 1878;2:1–19.
10. Rauber-Kopsch. Lehrbuch und Atlas der Anatomie des Menschen. Leipzig: Georg Thieme; 1940.
11. Berner W. Biomechanische Untersuchungen am Sakroiliakalgelenk, Topographie, Beanspruchung und operative Stabilisierung. Habilitationsschrift. Hannover. 1986.
12. Kapandji I. Funktionelle Anatomie der Gelenke. Bd.III: Rumpf und Wirbelsäule. Enke, Stuttgart. 1985.
13. Egbers H, Draijer F, Havemann D, Zenker W. Stabilisierung des Beckenrings mit Fixatuer externe: biomechanische Untersuchungen und klinische Erfahrungen. Orthopade. 1992;21:363–72.
14. Josten C, Schildhauer T, Muhr G. Therapie instabiler Sacrumfrakturen bei Beckenringbrüchen. Chirurg. 1994;65:970–5.
15. Käch K, Trentz O. Distraktionsspondylodese des Sakrums bei "Vertical-shear-Läsionen" des Beckens. Unfallchirurg. 1994;97(1):28–38.
16. Levine A. Fixation of fractures of the sacrum. Oper Tech Orthop. 1997;7(3):221–31.
17. Nelson D, Duwelius P. CT-guided fixation of sacral fractures and sacroiliac joint disruptions. Radiology. 1991;180:527–32.
18. Norris B, Bosse M, Kellam J, Sims S. Pelvic fractures: sacral fixation. In: Wiss DA, editor. Master techniqes in orthopaedics: fractures. 1998. p. 613–30.
19. Pohlemann T, Tscherne H. Fixation of sacral fractures. Tech Orthop. 1995;9(4):315–26.
20. Pohlemann T, Tscherne H. Die operative Therapie von Sakrumfrakturen. Oper Orthop Traumatol. 1996;8(1):55–72.
21. Routt M, Simonian P. Closed reduction and percutaneous skeletal fixation of sacral fractures. Clin Orthop. 1996;329:121–8.
22. Schildhauer T, Josten C, Muhr G. Triangular osteosynthesis of vertically unstable sacrum fractures: a new concept allowing early weight bearing. J Orthop Trauma. 1998;12(5):307–14.
23. Templeman D, Goulet J, Duwelius P, Olson S, Davidson M. Internal fixation of displaced fractures of the sacrum. Clin Orthop. 1996;329:180–5.
24. Gänsslen A, Pape HC, Lehmann U, Lange U, Krettek C, Pohlemann T. Open reduction and internal fixation of unstable sacral fractures. Zentralbl Chir. 2003;128(1):40–5.
25. Pohlemann T, Gänsslen A, Hartung S, für die Arbeitsgruppe Becken, H.T., H., Beckenverletzungen/Pelvic Injuries. Hefte zu "Der Unfallchirurg". Heft 266. 1998.
26. Roy-Camille R, Saillant G, Gagana G, Mazel C. Transverse fracture of the upper sacrum: suicidal jumper's fracture. Spine. 1985;10(9):838–45.
27. Asher M, Strippgen W. Anthropometric studies of the human sacrum related to dorsal transsacral implant design. Clin Orthop. 1985;203:58–62.
28. Mirkovic S, Abitol J, Steinmann J, Edwards C, Schaffler M, Massie J, Garfin S. Anatomic consideration for sacral screw placement. Spine. 1991;16(6):289–94.
29. Wagner D, Kamer L, Rommens P, Sawaguchi T, Richards R, Noser H. 3D statistical modeling techniques to investigate the anatomy of the sacrum, its bone mass distribution, and the trans-sacral corridors. J Orthop Res. 2014;32:1543–8.
30. Wagner D, Kamer L, Sawaguchi T, Richards R, Noser H, Hofmann A, Rommens P. Morphometry of the sacrum and its implication on trans-sacral corridors using a computed tomography data-based three-dimensional statistical model. Spine J. 2017;17:1141–7.
31. Wagner D, Kamer L, Sawaguchi T, Richards R, Noser H, Rommens P. Sacral bone mass distribution assessed by averaged three-dimensional CT models: implications for pathogenesis and treatment of fragility fractures of the sacrum. J Bone Joint Surg Am. 2016;98:584–90.
32. Pohlemann T, Tscherne H. Indikationen zur chirurgischen Therapie von Sacrumfrakturen. Chirurg. 1992;63(11):884–96.
33. Mast J, Jakob R, Ganz R. Planning and reduction techniques in fracture surgery. Berlin, Heidelberg, New York: Springer; 1989.
34. Schmidek H, Schmith D, Kristiansen D. Sacral fractures. Neurosurgery. 1984;15:735–46.
35. Bodkin P, Choksey M. Management of a sacral fracture with neurological injury. J Orthop Sci. 2006;11:524–8.
36. Tötterman A, Glott T, Madsen J, Roise O. Unstable sacral fractures: associated injuries and morbidity at 1 year. Spine. 2006;31:E628–35.
37. Zelle B, Gruen G, Hunt T, Spoeth S. Sacral fractures with neurological injury: is early decompression beneficial? Int Orthop. 2004;28:244–51.
38. Kepler C, Schroeder G, Hollern D, Chgapman J, Fehlings M, Dvorak M, Bellabarba C, Vaccaro A. Do formal laminectomy and timing of decompression for patients with sacral fracture and neurologic deficit affect outcome? J Orthop Trauma. 2017;31:S75–80.
39. Acklin Y, Germann M, Sommer C. Double locking plate fixation of sacral fractures in unstable pelvic ring C-type injuries. Oper Orthop Traumatol. 2015;27:74–9.

Lower Transverse Sacral Fractures

33

Axel Gänsslen and Jan Lindahl

Lambotte in 1913 first described the morphology and a treatment concept for transverse sacral fractures [1]. He already stated that lower transverse sacral fractures are extremely rare lesions, most often as a result of a violent direct blow (fall on the seat). The fragment, detached by a transverse line passing through sacred foramina, displaces anteriorly into the pelvis. Problems with compression of pelvic organs can be a consequence. He already recommended an osteosynthesis technique. Using a median incision, fracture debridement is performed, followed by vertical screw osteosynthesis (Fig. 33.1). Additionally, a paraosseous metal suture can be inserted.

Westerborn stated that the transverse fracture line is usually located at the level of S4. A transverse and slightly oblique fracture orientation is commonly seen, with the anterior fracture starting at the level of the S3 foramina ending posterior at the S4 foramina [2].

The first small series on four cases was described by Wakeley [3]. The fractures were always due to severe local direct violence, due to a kick from a horse, a fall onto the edge of the pavement, or due to a kick during a game of football. Some irrelevant anterior displacement was seen. In female patients, the fractures presented with signs of neuralgia of the fourth sacral nerve. No accompanying rectal injury was observed.

Hallgrimsson reported on three cases, presented delayed after injury without any additional nerve deficit, and all sustaining a direct injury to the sacrum [4].

The first excellent overview on this fracture type was reported by Rowell [5].

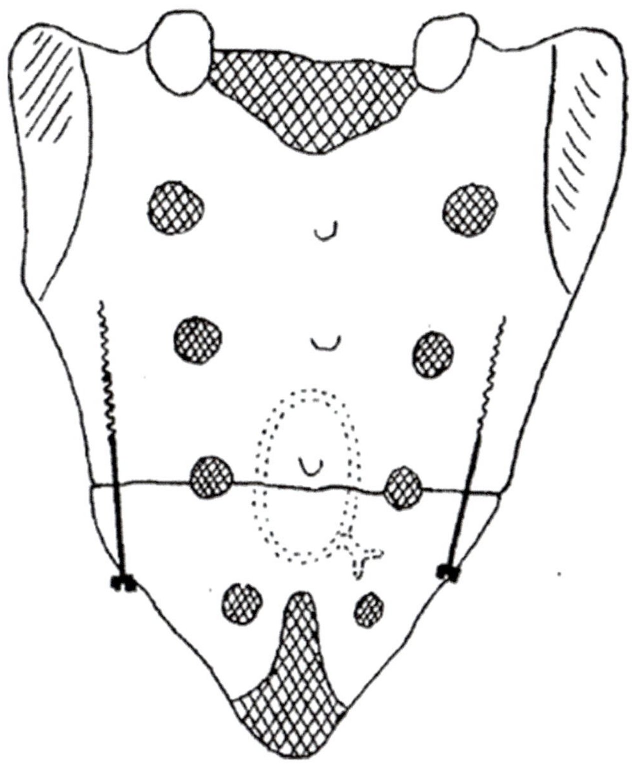

Fig. 33.1 Lambotte's concept of stabilization of transverse sacral fractures

33.1 Classification

Bonin in 1945 integrated transverse fractures of the sacrum at the level of the third sacral foramen into his sacral fracture classification [6]. Based on the injury mechanism, Schmidek et al. divided transverse sacral fracture into the direct trauma group [7], which was additionally performed by Gibbons [8].

According to the current most accepted classification of sacral fractures by Denis et al., these specific fractures are included into the group involving the region of the central spinal canal (zone III fractures) [9]. A correlation between the zone of the fracture line and the rate of neurological

A. Gänsslen (✉)
Department of Trauma Surgery, Orthopedics and Hand Surgery, Hospital Wolfsburg, Wolfsburg, Germany

J. Lindahl
Orthopaedics and Trauma Surgery, Helsinki University Hospital, Helsinki, Finland

A. Gänsslen et al. (eds.), *Pelvic Ring Fractures*, https://doi.org/10.1007/978-3-030-54730-1_33

deficits could be demonstrated with an increasing rate of nerve injury from lateral to medial. They concluded that a surgical decompression of the central canal and the region of the foramina may have a beneficial effect to the neurologic situation. These findings were confirmed by other authors [8, 10].

According to the AO/OTA classification, this injury type was classified as a stable A3 injury not involving the biomechanical ring structure of the pelvis [11–13]. Thus, these injuries represent transverse fractures below the level of S2.

Recently, isolated transverse sacral fractures were classified as type A fractures into the new spinal classification scheme and were further subdivided into [14]:

- A2 injuries: nondisplaced transverse fractures
- A3 injuries: displaced transverse fractures

33.2 Epidemiology

No clear data exist concerning incidence, classification, treatment, and results. Transverse sacral fractures are extremely rare [1–6, 8, 15–17]. Pohlemann et al. observed this fracture type in 3.7% of cases [10, 16].

In the German Multicenter Study Pelvis, transverse fractures of the sacrum were observed in 21 patients within the group of 728 type A injuries (2.9%) [15]. In the group of pelvic ring injuries (n = 1356), this fracture type represents 1.5% of injuries.

33.3 Mechanism of Injury

Rowell distinguished between a direct and indirect mechanism. Transverse fractures were supposed to be a result of an indirect force acting on the coccyx or lower end of the sacrum working like a lever near the convexity of the sacral curve, while direct injuries are less common [5]. In contrast, Schmidek et al. stated a more common direct force transmission to the buttock [7].

> Transverse fractures of the sacrum below the level of the sacroiliac joints are believed to be the result of a direct blow against the sacrum, e.g., after a simple fall or a kick [5, 7, 18].

The fourth sacral vertebra is the most commonly involved [5, 7]. A force acting on the distal sacrum or the coccyx acts as a lever arm resulting in fatigue fracture at the convexity of the distal sacrum. Higher fractures at the level above S3 are the result of indirect forces as the upper two sacral segments resist more energy against direct forces [5].

These fractures are most commonly undisplaced, but some anterior angulation can be possible, while lateral displacement is extremely rare. The more anterior displacement, more the lesions of the cauda equina were observed [5].

> Transverse sacral fractures are commonly seen at the fourth sacral body, as here the sacral kyphosis has its largest angle [5, 7, 9, 18].

33.4 Concomitant Injuries

Local complications occur with unknown frequency. Potential local injuries include:

- Vascular injury to the middle sacral artery and, more common to the extensive sacral venous plexus, can result in a presacral hematoma [5]
- Cauda equina lesions due to compression from the upper margin of the anteriorly displaced lower fragment [5]
- Sacral nerve root injury, despite minimal displacement [6]
- Significant soft-tissue injury (e.g. open fractures) [5]
- Rectum injury [5, 17]
- Cerebrospinal fluid leakage [5]

Rowell stated that "additional nerve root injuries are often missed, as the patients do not draw attention to them" [5].

33.5 Clinical Examination

Typical clinical signs include localized pain, often with radiation to the perianal region, occasionally to the gluteal or lumbar region [5]. Additionally, local bruising and local tenderness can be observed [4, 5].

Clinically, pain is the most common complaint [15], local tenderness or local bruising is also reported. Lying in the supine position or sitting increases pain, sometimes pain worsened with walking.

Rectal examination is recommended to detect presacral hematoma and to analyze potential instability as well as confirmation of rectal injury.

Neurological examination should focus on complete or partial saddle anesthesia, with or without sphincter disturbances. In males, impotence can occasionally be the result of this injury [5].

- Gibbons et al. reported on seven patients, four of them with isolated injuries [8]. Fractures below the level of S4 showed no neurological deficit, while fractures above that level presented often with bowel and bladder incontinence. In the latter cases, it remained unclear, if these injuries involved the upper sacral segments, e.g., S1 and S2.
- Pohlemann et al. analyzed 14 patients (3.7% of all sacral fractures) of which 1 patient presented with a combined L5/S1 and cauda lesion [10]. In five of these patients, no information regarding potential nerve deficits were stated in the patient report.

Overall, neurological deficits seem to be uncommon. Several studies reported only minor incidence of concomitant nerve damage in this subgroup [10, 19–21] and fracture instability was not a problem [20]. Neurologic sequelae can be present, especially bladder dysfunctions and fecal incontinence were reported [9, 18].

33.6 Radiography

Traditionally, anterior-posterior radiographs were associated with a high rate of overlooked injuries [3–5, 17].

These fractures are most commonly undisplaced, but some anterior angulation can be possible, while lateral displacement is extremely rare.

Thus, a true lateral radiograph of the sacrum can detect these injuries (Fig. 33.2).

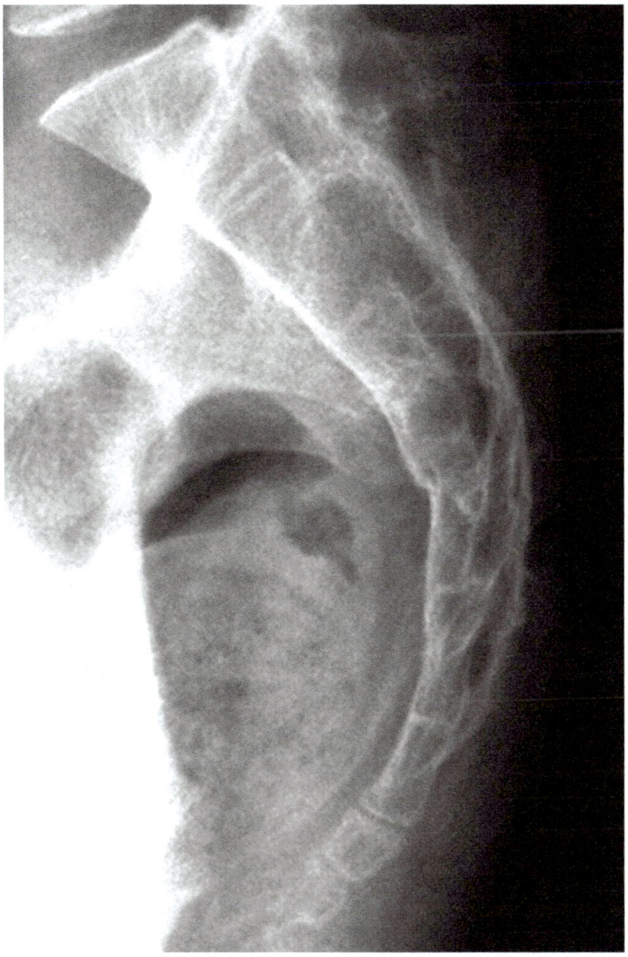

Fig. 33.2 Lateral sacral x-ray to detect transverse sacral fractures

The gold standard of diagnosis of these fractures after performing a pelvic AP view to exclude accompanying pelvic injuries is the computed tomography (Fig. 33.3), probably with multiplanar reconstructions [17, 22].

> A low-dose CT scan for investigation of lower transverse sacral fractures represents the gold standard.

33.7 Treatment

Lambotte already described open reduction and internal fixation with cerclage and/or screw osteosynthesis as a treatment option [1].

Fractures without significant displacement can sufficiently be treated, pain dependent, with simple bed rest [5].

Rowell recommended fracture manipulation through the rectum in more displaced fractures and also stated to consider operative reduction [5]. Gibbons et al. stated that operative reduction and decompression could lead to nerve injury recovery [8].

Overall, laminectomy and sacral decompression are proposed in displaced transverse fractures with an additional neurological deficit [5, 9, 17, 23]; no clear data exist regarding operative fixation of these fractures.

For optimizing postoperative rehabilitation, distal sacral plate stabilization after open decompression of the central sacral canal has to be considered. As reduction of the displaced fractures is proposed to be the primary mechanism of neurological recovery, stable fixation minimizes the risk of secondary redisplacement. Closed reduction techniques were seen to be ineffective [5].

Recently, osteosynthesis in two age extremes were reported. Garnon et al. described a screw osteosynthesis with cement augmentation in a 57 year old osteoporotic woman [24], and Baba-Rasul et al. performed a K-wire fixation in a 12 year old girl [25].

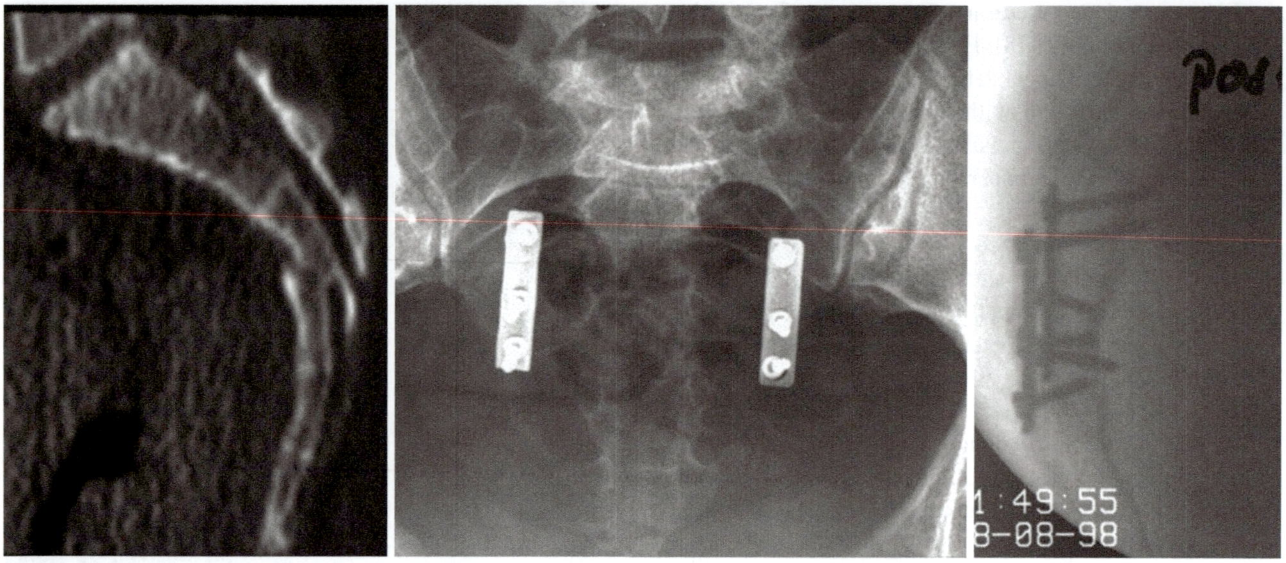

Fig. 33.3 Gold standard in radiography for sacral transverse fractures: sagittal CT reconstruction. Treatment with ORIF and bilateral longitudinal plate osteosynthesis in a patient with severe pain and incomplete cauda syndrome

Open reduction and stabilization of displaced fracture should be considered optional (Fig. 33.3).

In conclusion, whereas undisplaced lower transverse fractures of the sacrum have a low incidence of additional local complications, displaced fractures have a special risk of concomitant sacral nerve root lesions. In these rare cases, early open reduction with posterior sacral decompression of the nerve roots and sacral plate stabilization are recommended.

References

1. Lambotte A. Chirurgie opératoire des fractures. répité, vol. 1913. Bruxelles: Société Franco-Belge D'Editions Scientifiques; 1948. p. 126–44.
2. Westerborn A. Beiträge zur Kenntnis der der Beckenbrüche und Beckenluxationen. Acta Chir Scand Suppl. 1928;8:10–375.
3. Wakeley C. Fractures of the pelvis: an analysis of 100 cases. Br J Surg. 1930;17:22–29.
4. Hallgrimsson S. Three cases of fractures of the sacrum. Acta Orthop Scand. 1938;9:100–14.
5. Rowell C. Fracture of the sacrum with hemisaddle anaesthesia and cerebrospinal fluid leak. Med J Aust. 1965;1:16–9.
6. Bonnin J. Sacral fractures and injuries to the cauda equina. J Bone Joint Surg. 1945;27:113–27.
7. Schmidek H, Schmith D, Kristiansen D. Sacral fractures. Neurosurgery. 1984;15:735–46.
8. Gibbons K, Soloniuk D, Razack N. Neurological injury and patterns of sacral fractures. J Neurosurg. 1990;72:889–93.
9. Denis F, Steven D, Comfort T. Sacral fractures: an important problem, retrospective analysis of 236 cases. Clin Orthop. 1988;227:67–81.
10. Pohlemann T, Gänsslen A, Tscherne H. Die Problematik der Sakrumfraktur, klinische Analyse von 377 Fällen. Orthopade. 1992;21:400–12.
11. Kellam J, Meinberg E, Agel J, Karam M, Roberts C. Pelvic ring. In: Fracture and dislocation classification compendium-2018: international comprehensive classification of fractures and dislocations committee. J Orthop Trauma. 2018;32:S71–6.
12. Müller M. The comprehensive classification of fractures: pelvis. Müller Institute, Berne, Switzerland; 1996.
13. OTA. Fracture and dislocation compendium. J Orthop Trauma. 1996;10(Suppl. 1):71–5.
14. Kellam J, Meinberg E, Agel J, Karam M, Roberts C. Spine. In: Fracture and dislocation classification compendium-2018: international comprehensive classification of fractures and dislocations committee. J Orthop Trauma. 2018;32:S145–60.
15. Pohlemann T, Gänsslen A, Hartung S, für die Arbeitsgruppe Becken, H.T., H., Beckenverletzungen/Pelvic Injuries. Hefte zu "Der Unfallchirurg". Heft 266. 1998.
16. Pohlemann T, Gänsslen A, Tscherne H. Die Sakrumfraktur. Unfallchirurg. 2000;103:769–86.
17. Weaver E, England G, Richardson D. Sacral fracture: case presentation and review. Neurosurgery. 1981;9(6):725–8.
18. Chiaruttini M. Transverse sacral fracture with transient neurologic complication. Ann Emerg Med. 1987;16(1):111–3.
19. Borelli J, Helfet D. Pelvic and acetabular trauma. Curr Opin Orthop. 1992;3(5):592–8.
20. Bottini A, Seljeskog E. Fractures of the sacrum. In: Doty JR, Rengachary SS, editors. Surgical disorders of the sacrum. New York: Thieme, Medical Puplishers Inc.; 1994. p. 133–42.

21. Hofmann G. Spätfolgen und Begutachtung nach Beckenfrakturen und -luxationen. Hefte zur Unfallheilkunde. Heft 164. 1984. p. 251–4.
22. Whelan M, Gold R. Computed tomography of the sacrum: 1. Normal anatomy. AJR. 1982;139:1183–90.
23. Fardon D. Displaced transverse fracture of the sacrum with nerve root injury: report of a case with successful operative management. J Trauma. 1979;192:119.
24. Garnon J, Koch G, Ramamurthy N, Bauones S, Caudrelier J, Tsoumakidou G, Cazzato R, Gangi A. Percutaneous imaging-guided screw fixation of osteoporotic transverse fractures of the lower sacrum with cement augmentation: report of 2 cases. Cardiovasc Intervent Radiol. 2017;40:1105–11.
25. Baba-Rasul I, Hama Ameen H, Khazendar A, Hasan S. A rare case of isolated lower segment transverse sacral fracture in a 12-year-old girl and its management by fixation with K-wire. World Neurosurg. 2017;97:758.

Ilio-Iliacal Osteosynthesis

34

Bernd Füchtmeier, Franz Müller, and Axel Gänsslen

Bridging the sacrum is an additional option in treating posterior pelvic type C sacral fractures, described in the 1980s in North America by experienced pelvic surgeons [1–7].

This concept was already proposed by Albin Labotte in his monograph in 1913 [8].

Several types of osteosyntheses were reported in the literature. The main indications were bilateral injuries, especially bilateral sacroiliac dislocations or comminuted sacral fractures.

Beside sacral bars, 3.5 mm plate fixation and the so-called double cobra plate were introduced as stabilization techniques.

Mears favored the double cobra plate in bilateral unstable sacroiliac dislocations or comminuted sacral fractures [4, 5] as it is more effective than previous stabilization techniques, e.g., threaded sacral bars with/without supplementary cancellous lag screws. In smaller patients, already a 4.5 mm reconstruction plate was advised. Mears had already recommended osteotomy of the posterior superior iliac spines for insertion of the plate [5].

Matta additionally recommended such a construct [3]. The main disadvantage was the extensive soft-tissue stripping at the posterior pelvis.

Presently, five different ilio-iliacal techniques are described:

- Transiliacal internal fixator (TIFI)
- Ilio-iliacal plate osteosynthesis
- Posterior sacral bar stabilization
- Intraosseous sacral bar stabilization (transiliac-sacral-iliac bar stabilization)
- Locked transsacral screw fixation

34.1 Transiliacal Internal Fixator (TIFI) Osteosynthesis

Füchtmeier et al. introduced the concept of a transiliacal internal fixator (TIFI) bridging both the sacroiliac joint and the whole sacrum (Fig. 34.1) [9].

It is a minimally invasive stabilization technique for treating complete SI joint disruptions or Denis type I or II injuries of the posterior pelvic ring.

7.0 mm pedicle screws were inserted 1–2 cm at the superior border of the PSIS, parallel to the superior gluteal line. These were connected by a subfascial inserted bar which was fixed with the locking head pedicle screws to form an locked construct.

34.1.1 Experimental Data

In a cadaveric analysis on five pelves, a C1.2 injury was created with dissection of the symphyseal and sacroiliac ligaments. The symphysis was fixed with a locking plate and the posterior pelvis was fixed with the TIFI construct. TIFI and iliosacral screw fixation led to comparable three-dimensional stability [10].

Salášek et al. performed an additional analysis in type C sacral fractures comparing TIFI with two iliosacral screws in a finite element model resulting in a significant higher stiffness and lower stress using TIFI [11]. TIFI, therefore, was recommended in transforaminal sacral fractures with or without comminution zones.

B. Füchtmeier
Krankenhaus Barmherzige Brüder, Klinik für Unfallchirurgie, Regensburg, Germany
e-mail: Bernd.Fuechtmeier@barmherzige-regensburg.de

F. Müller
Department of Trauma Surgery, Orthopaedics and Sports Medicine, Hospital Barmherzige Brüder Regensburg, Regensburg, Germany

A. Gänsslen (✉)
Department of Trauma Surgery, Orthopedics and Hand Surgery, Hospital Wolfsburg, Wolfsburg, Germany

A. Gänsslen et al. (eds.), *Pelvic Ring Fractures*, https://doi.org/10.1007/978-3-030-54730-1_34

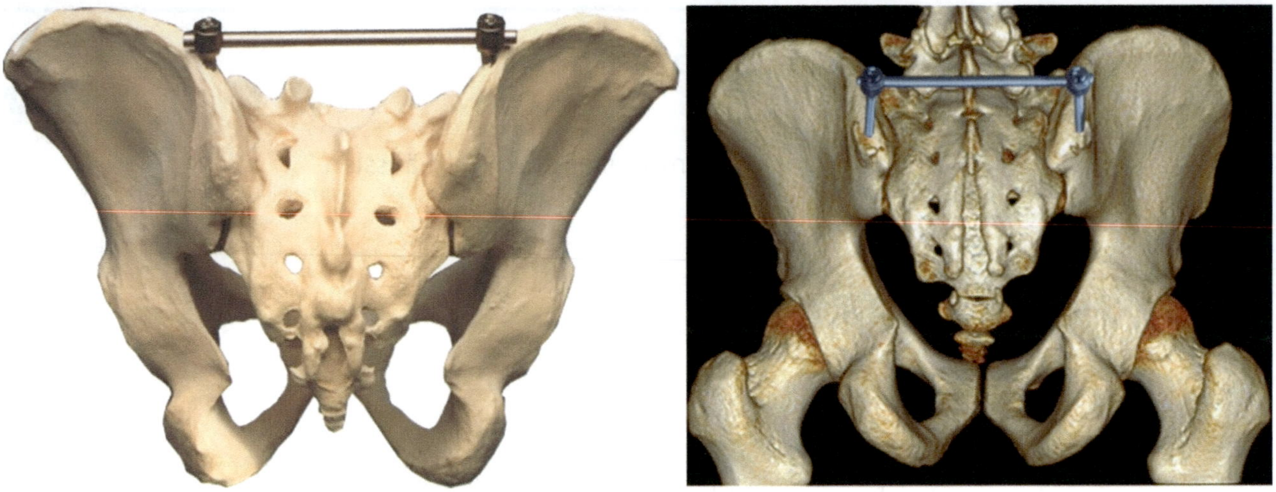

Fig. 34.1 TIFI construct

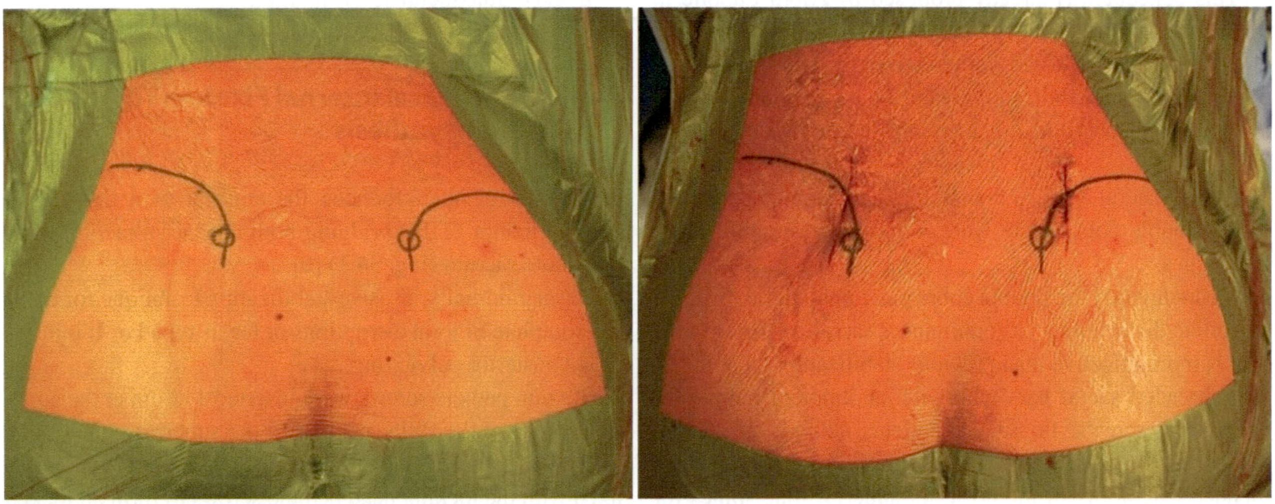

Fig. 34.2 Skin incision for TIFI and ilio-iliacal tension band plate insertion slightly lateral to the PSIS

34.1.2 Operative Technique

Posterior inspection of the soft-tissue envelope and searching for degloving injuries (Morel-Levallée lesion) are crucial before starting the procedure.

Beside an anterior-posterior view of the whole pelvis, a CT scan of the pelvis is mandatory, as it allows clear identification of the fracture pathology and prior planning of the length of the plate. Additionally, oblique views can be helpful.

Like in other treatment concepts of pelvic stabilization, in type C injuries, often the anterior pelvis is fixed first.

34.1.2.1 Positioning

Surgery is performed under general anesthesia and after antibiotic single-shot prophylaxis (second-generation cephalosporin).

The patient is placed symmetrical in the standard prone position, allowing intraoperative standard x-rays: AP pelvis, inlet-, and outlet views. The pelvis can be supported by a towel roll or comparable positioning aids to get full access to both the outer sides of the ilium.

34.1.2.2 Incision and Dissection

A 3–4 cm long incision is made 1 cm lateral to the PSIS (Fig. 34.2). The pedicle screw insertion point is identified at the posterior iliac crest, approximately 1–2 cm cranial to the PSIS. The ilium is opened using the pedicle opening awl, parallel to the posterior gluteal line.

34.1.2.3 Implant Introduction

The pedicle screws are inserted (Fig. 34.3). Screw lengths of 50–60 mm are typically possible. In the sagittal plane, screw

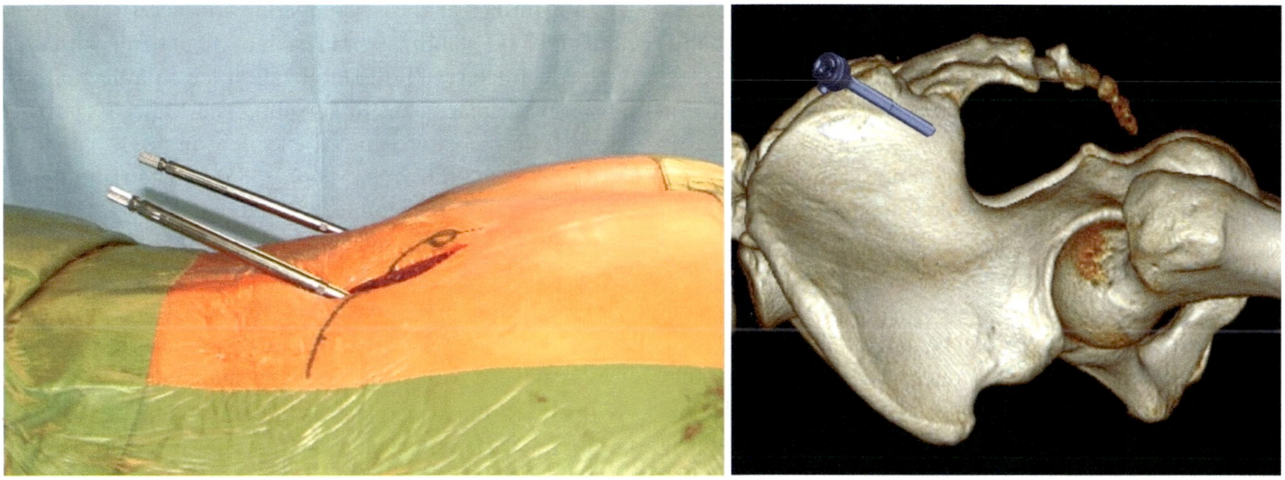

Fig. 34.3 The pedicle screws are inserted with an angle <30° to the longitudinal axis of the lumbar spine to avoid implant-related soft-tissue prominence

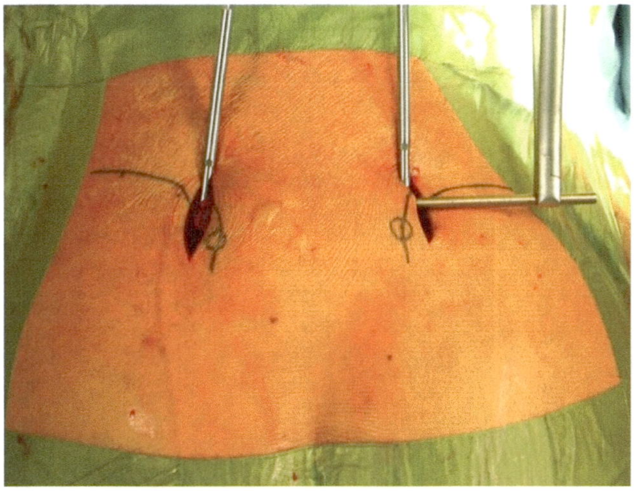

Fig. 34.4 Insertion of the connecting rod

orientation should be as "flat" as possible, representing an angle <30° to the longitudinal axis of the lumbar spine to avoid implant-related soft-tissue prominence.

The pedicle screws are connected with a subfascially inserted transverse orientated connecting rod (Fig. 34.4). Depending on the local anatomy, it may be necessary to bend the lateral parts of this rod.

34.1.2.4 Reduction

Depending on the fracture pattern, fracture distraction or compression is performed. In severely displaced fractures, percutaneous inserted Schanz screws can support the reduction maneuver using the "joystick technique.".

In a few cases, temporary K-wire fixation of the reduction is considered an option. Reduction should not be performed by manipulating the pedicle screws to avoid screw loosening.

Control of reduction is performed by standard intraoperative imaging techniques, including AP pelvic and oblique views (e.g., inlet and outlet views). Intraoperative 3D imaging can be an option.

34.1.3 After Treatment

Partial weight bearing on the affected side with 15 kg body weight for 6 weeks is recommended, with full weight bearing on the opposite side.

34.1.4 Clinical Results

Füchtmeier et al. reported on their initial experience on 31 patients with pelvic ring type C injuries (23 sacral fractures, 8 sacroiliac dislocations) with TIFI stabilization [9]. Posterior pelvic ring stabilization was performed on average after 4.7 days. The mean surgery time was 28.4 min, and the intraoperative blood loss was calculated to be <50 mL. The average fluoroscopy time was 0.3 (±0.2) min. Displacement could be reduced from a mean of 8.7 mm preoperatively to 2.5 mm. Procedure-related complications were observed in three patients: one implant loosening without loss of reduction, two local infections. Implant removal was performed on average after 1 year.

Of these, 28 patients could be followed-up after 2 years. The clinical result was graded excellent in 8, good in 10, fair in 9, and poor in 1 patient. The latter suffered from permanent pain with impairment of the bladder and rectal function.

The radiological result was graded anatomic in 11, 16 had malhealing <5 mm, and only 1 patient healed in >5 mm displacement.

The same group reported their long-term results in overall 67 patients at least 3 years after trauma (mean 37 months) [12]. The long-term clinical result was graded excellent in 23 (37.1%), good in 19 (30.6%), fair in 15 (24.2%), and poor in 5 patients after complex pelvic trauma using the POS. Of these, 45 (72.6%) healed with posterior anatomical healing, 16 healed in slight posterior malposition with displacement <5 mm at the posterior pelvis, and 1 had displacement >5 mm. Overall, 56% had a good to excellent pelvic outcome score (Figs. 34.5 and 34.6).

Salášek et al. evaluated 27 patients after TIFI stabilization of type C injuries [13]. All fractures healed within 6 months. One loss of reduction was observed. The functional long-term result after a mean of 16 months was graded excellent in 9 patients (33.3%), good in 14 patients (51.9%), and satisfactory in 4 (14.8%) using Majeed's score.

In a further analysis, comparing iliosacral screw fixation and TIFI stabilization in each of 32 patients with type C sacral fractures, TIFI stabilization led to a decrease of posterior displacement to 2.2 mm. The Majeed scores at latest follow-up were graded excellent in 56.0%, good in 16.0%, fair in 20.0%, and poor in 8.0%. The radiological result was graded anatomic in 17 patients (53.1%), 10 had malhealing <5 mm, and 5 patients healed with >5 mm displacement.

Overall, TIFI implantation was preferred in transforaminal and central sacral fractures as iliosacral screw fixation was associated with a higher complication rate [14].

With increasing experience in geriatric patients, Schmitz et al. could show that the TIFI concept even led to good results in elderly patients with osteoporosis [15].

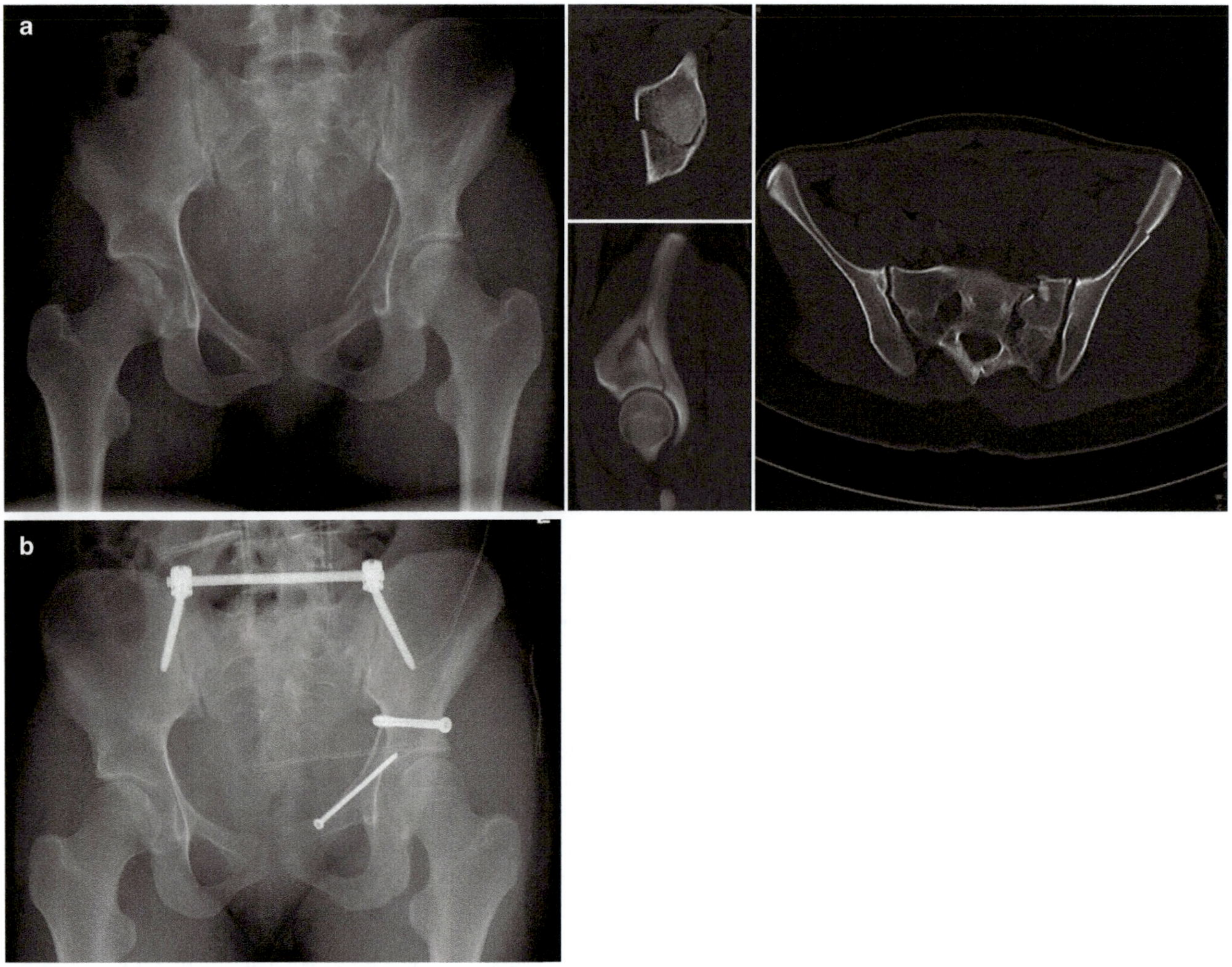

Fig. 34.5 (**a**) 18-year-old woman after MVA with left sacral fracture, left acetabular fracture (anterior column), and right pubic ram fracture. (**b**) After percutaneous fixation of the acetabulum, TIFI stabilization was performed

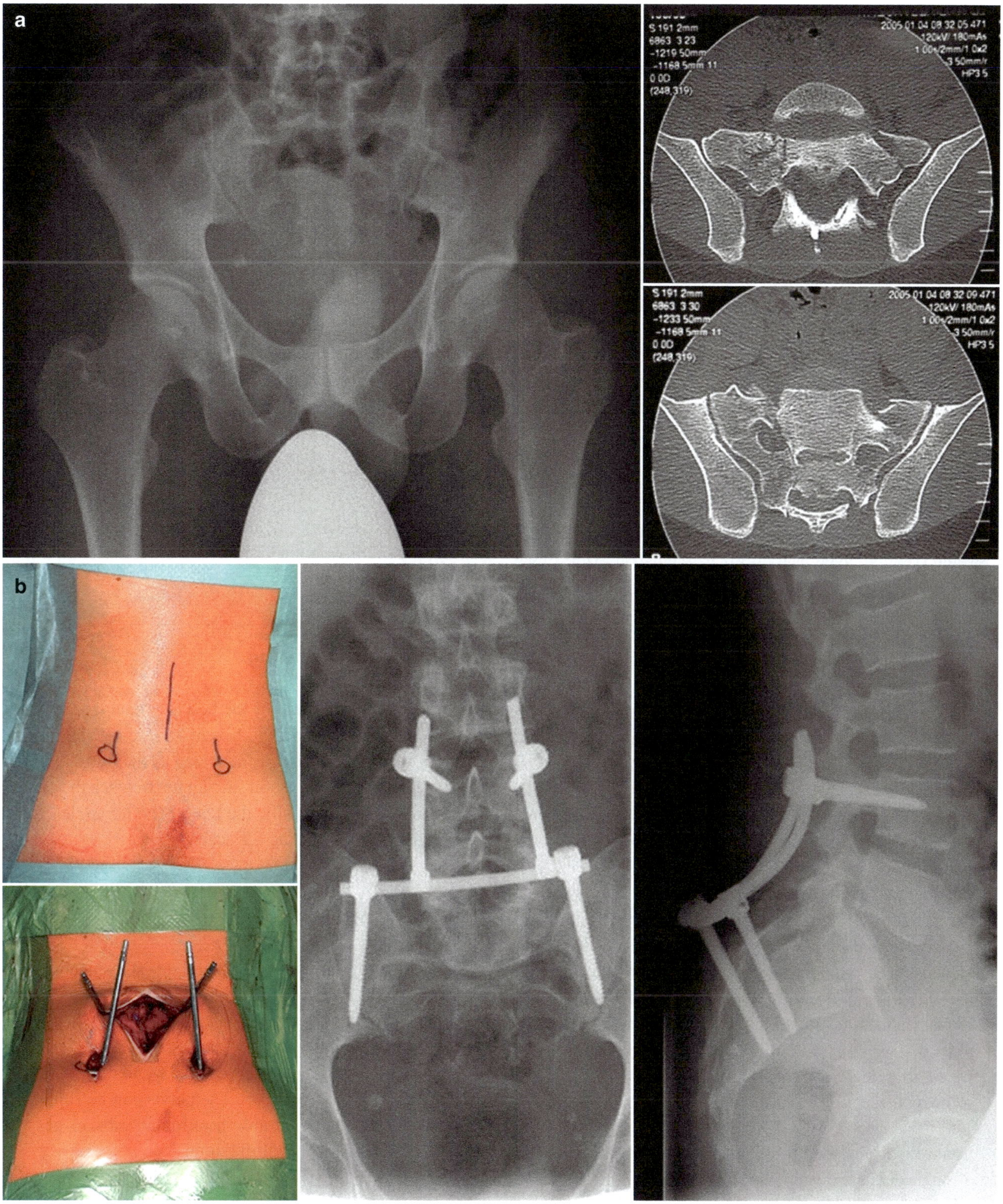

Fig. 34.6 (**a**) Bilateral sacral fractures with a transverse fracture component (lumbopelvic dissociation injury) after a fall from 4 m. (**b**) Lumbopelvic stabilization using the TIFI

34.2 Ilio-Iliacal Tension Band Plate Osteosynthesis

Ilio-iliacal osteosynthesis is an option for minimally invasive stabilization of unilateral or even bilateral posterior pelvic ring type C injuries.

Technically, it is a simple procedure with a low risk for iatrogenic nerve injuries, but soft-tissue problems have to be considered [16]. The potential disadvantage of bridging an uninjured sacroiliac joint is refuted in the meantime [17, 18].

Due to close relationship of the plate to the soft-tissue envelope, implant removal has to be considered, if these are subjectively disturbing.

Biomechanical data indicate that ilio-iliacal plates osteosynthesis is an adequate stabilization method:

- Rubash et al. confirmed that in type C pelvic injuries (bilateral sacroiliac disruptions, type C3) anterior external fixation supplemented with the double cobra plate at the posterior pelvis led to near physiological loads [19].
- Albert et al. tested the 4.5 mm reconstruction plate in a cadaveric biomechanical model with anterior symphyseal plating (type C1.2); the fixation strength was comparable to other posterior stabilization techniques [20].
- Yinger et al. performed a comparable biomechanical analysis on a plastic bone model using several posterior stabilization methods including a posterior 3.5 mm reconstruction tension band plate ± one 6.5 mm iliosacral screw [21]; in contrast, these osteosyntheses resulted in less stiffness than isolated iliosacral screw fixation of the disrupted SI joint.
- Wu et al. tested a type C1.3 injury with a transforaminal sacral fracture and a symphyseal disruption [22]; the pubic symphysis was fixed with a plate and posterior fixation included fixation with two iliosacral screws, a tension band plate (TBP), and the newly developed minimally invasive adjustable plate (MIAP); the classical TBP was weakest with 4 mm displacement under 500 N loads compared to 2.4 mm (sacroiliac screws) and 2.8 mm (MIAP).
- Biomechanical testing of the 4.5 mm locked compression plate in a sacral fracture plastic model revealed that compared to spinal instrumentation posterior tension band osteosynthesis was biomechanically less strong [23].

Theoretical analyses using finite element models could also show adequate posterior stability:

- In a type C1.3 model with symphyseal plating and posterior narrow DC-tension band plate osteosynthesis, sufficient stability could be found, which was comparable to cadaver analyses [24].
- Chen et al. analyzed Denis type I, II, and III vertical sacral fractures with ipsilateral superior and inferior pubic ramus fractures [25]; posterior tension band plating was sufficient for all three posterior ring lesions, while in Denis type III sacral fractures the plate was superior to iliosacral screws.

34.3 Operative Technique

34.3.1 Indications

Classical indications are unstable unilateral or bilateral type C injuries with sacral or sacroiliac instability, especially with minor displacement, as closed reduction can be difficult using the minimally invasive procedure. In contrast, comminuted ilium fractures and poor conditioned skin and soft-tissues can lead to complications and, therefore, are stated as contraindications.

34.3.2 Preoperative Work-Up

The preoperative work-up, implant planning, patient positioning, preoperative reduction, and draping are comparable to the TIFI technique.

34.3.3 Implant Planning

The preoperative CT scan of the pelvis is analyzed to identify the plate length and the potential screw lengths. The length of the lateral screws is analyzed as they bridge the SI joints and penetrate the lateral sacrum not to reach the medial foraminal line. Additionally, the plate bending angle can be measured bilaterally on the CT scan.

34.3.4 Positioning

Surgery is performed under general anesthesia and after antibiotic single-shot prophylaxis (second-generation cephalosporin).

The patient is then placed symmetrical in the standard prone position, allowing intraoperative standard x-rays: AP pelvis, inlet-, and outlet views. The pelvis can be supported by a towel roll or comparable positioning aids to get full access to both outer sides of the ilium.

34.3.5 Reduction

Reduction can be performed by leg traction or intraoperatively by using a distractor. Additionally, manipulation of the hemipelvis can be performed using the joy stick technique via stab incisions.

34.3.6 Draping

It is most often only necessary to drape the area of the pelvis. In severely displaced fractures, depending on the fracture configuration, one or both legs can be draped to allow intraoperative manipulation (reduction).

34.3.7 Incision

After identification of the landmarks by palpation or under an image intensifier, both the posterior superior iliac spines and the posterior iliac crests are marked with a pen. Additionally, the potential skin incision is marked.

A skin incision is made of approximately 4–6 cm length over the PSIS and the posterior-inferior iliac crest (Fig. 34.7). After subcutaneous dissection, the gluteal fascia and the PSIS are identified.

34.3.8 Deep Dissection

Fascial incision is performed on both sides of the iliac crest at the level of the PSIS to fully expose the PSIS. Bleeding on the outer side of the ilium is managed by local compression and/or electrocoagulation.

In the majority of cases, bilateral osteotomy of the posterior crest is necessary to avoid skin and subcutaneous pressure by the plate (Fig. 34.8). A cubiform bone block is removed for optimal fitting of the plate. The osteotomy should not exceed a depth of more than 1.5–2 cm. Otherwise, it is difficult to position the plate on the posterior sacral surface.

Using a long raspatory, the erector trunci muscles on the posterior sacral surface back are tunneled. A chisel can be necessary to fracture the sacral spine at the median sacral crest.

34.3.9 Plate Introduction

There are several options for posterior plate stabilization.

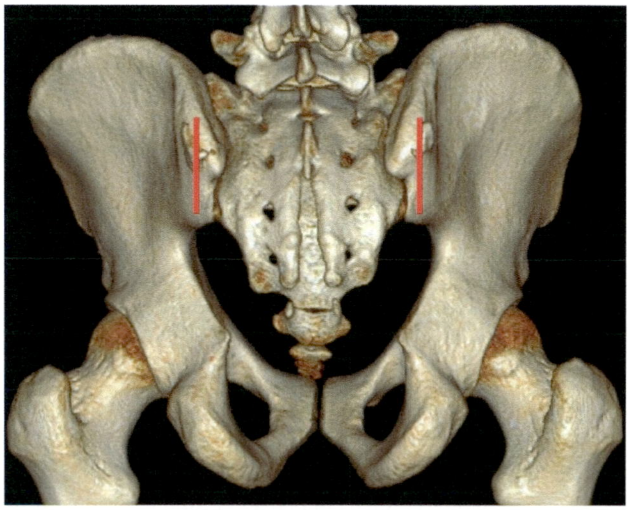

Fig. 34.7 Bilateral skin incision for ilio-iliacal tension band plate stabilization

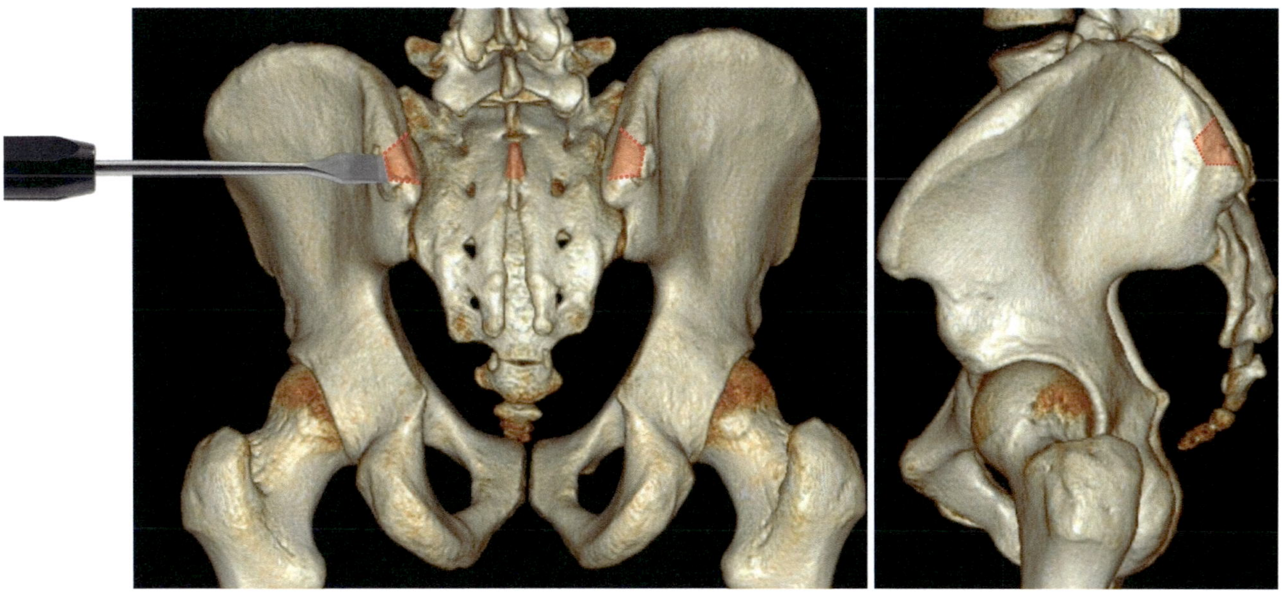

Fig. 34.8 Using a chisel, part of the posterior iliac crest and from the median sacral spine is often removed to allow insertion of the plate without harming the soft-tissue envelope

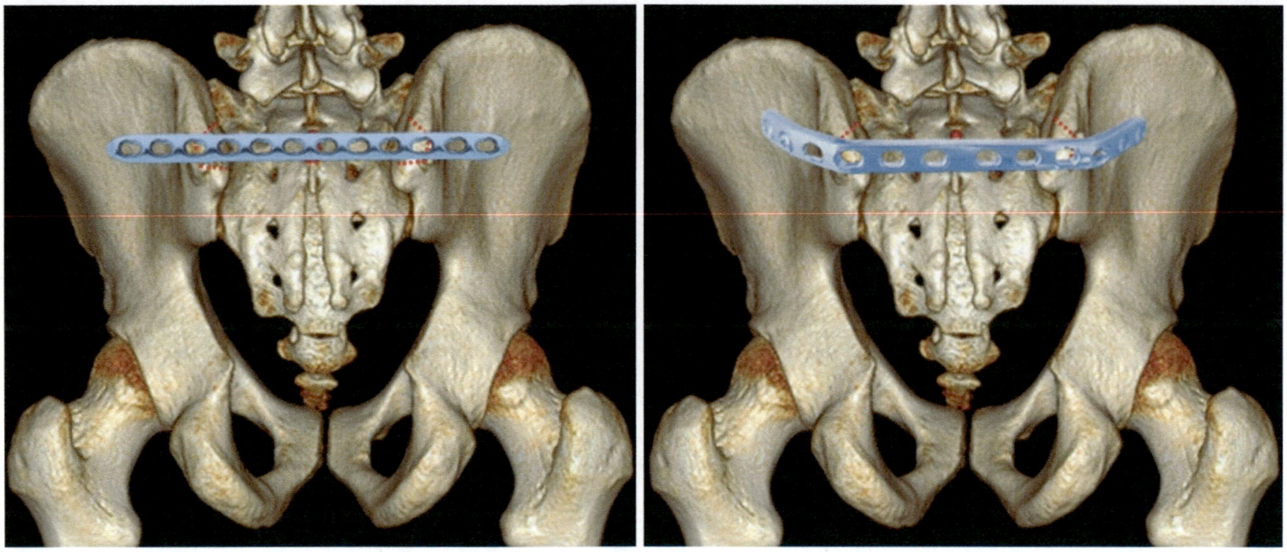

Fig. 34.9 The chosen plate is bilaterally bended according to the posterior pelvic anatomy

The gold standard is use of a 4.5 mm pelvis reconstruction plate (11–15 hole), which is inserted through the tunnel (Fig. 34.9). Correct plate length is crucial, which is measured preoperatively using the CT. If too long a plate is chosen, it is more difficult to adapt the plate to the lateral iliac bone structures through a minimally invasive approach [16]. Too short a plate does not allow adequate fixation with three screws on each side.

The chosen plate is then bended according to preoperative bending angles, typically approximately 70°. Dolati proposed a sequential bending, with first bending one side, then introduction of the plate through the tunnel to the opposite side followed by in situ bending of the contralateral side [16]. We prefer a bilateral initial bending [26].

The plate is then inserted through the tunnel until reaching the opposite side and then turned axially 180° that the bending edges fit with the outer iliac surface.

Depending on the chosen plate two possible fixation concepts are possible:

- 4.5 mm reconstruction plate: screw fixation of the plate on both sides from medial to lateral with three to four screws on each side fixed within the ilium [16]; the estimated screw lengths are 30–45 mm; large-fragment, fully threaded, cancellous bone screws are preferred; refixation of the osteotomized bone blocks with a small-fragment cancellous bone screw is performed at the end of the procedure.
- 4.5 mm locking compression plate: after contouring and positioning of the plate, first the plate is fixed at the hole positioned directly above the posterior iliac crest with a 4.5 mm cortical screw in each iliac wing. Thereafter, lateral locking screws are inserted perpendicular to the outer iliac surface (Fig. 34.10); these screws can bridge the sacroiliac joints, depending on which stability of the construct should be achieved [26].

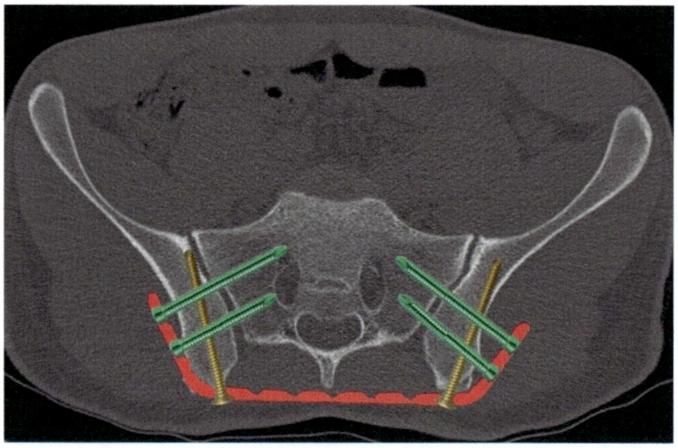

Fig. 34.10 Standard screws are usually inserted into the supraacetabular bone corridor, and locking head screws are inserted from lateral to medial into the sacrum

34.3.10 After Treatment

To avoid soft-tissue pressure complications, the patient should not lie on hard surfaces directly postoperative. Mobilization is performed on day 1 using partial weight bearing for 4 weeks, followed by pain-adapted weight bearing. Implant removal is only necessary if local implant-related disturbances are reported.

Table 34.1 Perioperative results after ilio-iliacal tension band plating

Author	Plate	*n*	Male	Type C*	Day	Blood loss	OR time	Preoperative displacement	Postoperative displacement
Krappinger	4.5 reco	31	24	31	10	n.a.	82	16.1	6.1
Suzuki	4.5 reco	19	12	19	6.4	1053	243	n.a.	5.0
Kobbe	4.5 reco	23	13	23	4.9	n.a.	101	n.a.	n.a.
Hao	4.5 reco	21	16	5	5	50–150	60	n.a.	n.a.
Ayoub	3.5 reco	42	27	42	n.a.	181.4	43.3	7.8	2.0
Dienstknecht	TIFI	67	38	67	1–12	50	n.a.	8.7	n.a.
Salášek	TIFI	27	15	27	6		29		
Salášek	TIFI	32	16	32	5.5		48.2		

*number of type C injuries
reco reconstruction plate

34.3.11 Errors, Hazards, and Complications

There are several potential complications associated with this treatment construct:

- Incomplete reduction
- Sacral nerve root damage due to overcompression or during closed reduction
- Loss of reduction, especially in osteoporotic fractures

34.4 Clinical Results

Several analyses are available with clinical results using this technique (Tables 34.1 and 34.2, Figs. 34.11 and 34.12).

- In 1993, Albert et al. analyzed 15 patients with posterior pelvic fixation using a 4.5 mm reconstruction plate in 11 type C and 4 type B injuries with sacral fractures [20]. For plate insertion, three incisions were made: one 6 cm midline incision to control the plate course and two 8 cm oblique incisions at the level of posterior superior iliac spine (PSIS), both directed inferior and lateral. Transosseous insertions at both PSIS were the main steps during application. Both ends of the plate were contoured against the outer surface of the ilium and fixed with two 6.5 mm cancellous screws.

  The radiological results were excellent with no loss of reduction and fracture healing in all patients. No implant-related complications were observed and no hardware removal was clinically necessary. Persistent posterior pelvic discomfort was reported in 57%.
- A comparable percutaneous technique with subfascial ilio-iliacal plate osteosynthesis technique was analyzed in 25 with different posterior pelvic ring injuries after a mean of 17 months. Radiological analysis using the outcome instrument of the German Multicenter Study Group Pelvis (POS) revealed 64% posterior anatomic reconstructions (maximal displacement <5 mm). Thirty-two percent had slight displacement (5–10 mm) [16].

Table 34.2 Intermediate-term results after ilio-iliacal tension band plating

					Clinical result				
Author	Plate	*n*	No f/u	Impl compl	*e*	*g*	*f*	*p*	Outcome Score
Krappinger	4.5 reco	31	23	5	8	9	4	2	POS
Suzuki	4.5 reco	19	18	2	5	8	4	1	Majeed
Kobbe	4.5 reco	23	21	3	11	4	6	0	POS
Hao	4.5 reco	21	20	0	17		3		Lindahl
Ayoub	3.5 reco	42	42	5	14	16	6	6	POS
Dienstknecht	TIFI	67	62						POS
Salášek	TIFI	27	27	1	9	14	4		Majeed
Salášek	TIFI	32		2	17	5	6	8	Majeed

Impl compl imüplant complications

- The same group reported on clinical results and social reintegration after an average of 20 months in 23 patients with unstable pelvic injuries [27]. The clinical outcome (POS) was graded excellent or good in 73.9%. Social reintegration was recorded complete in 39.1% and incomplete in 43.5%. There was a trend for better clinical results with anatomic reconstructions. Negative prognostic factors influencing the long-term result were the presence of a lumbosacral plexus lesions and permanent urogenital complaints. Patients with multiple traumas (polytrauma) led to worse social integration.
- In a further analysis, 18 patients with comminuted sacral fractures were stabilized with an ilio-iliacal plate osteosynthesis. Using the Majeed score 72.2% of patients were graded excellent or good with a mean score of 78.5 points. Radiographic healing with persistent displacement <5 mm was only observed in 50%, and 38.9% healed in 5–10 mm displacement. A persistent neurological deficit lead to significant lower scores [28].
- Hao reported follow-up results in 20 patients with locked 4.5 mm plate stabilization in 16 type B and 5 type C injuries [29]; 85% excellent or good radiological results (dis-

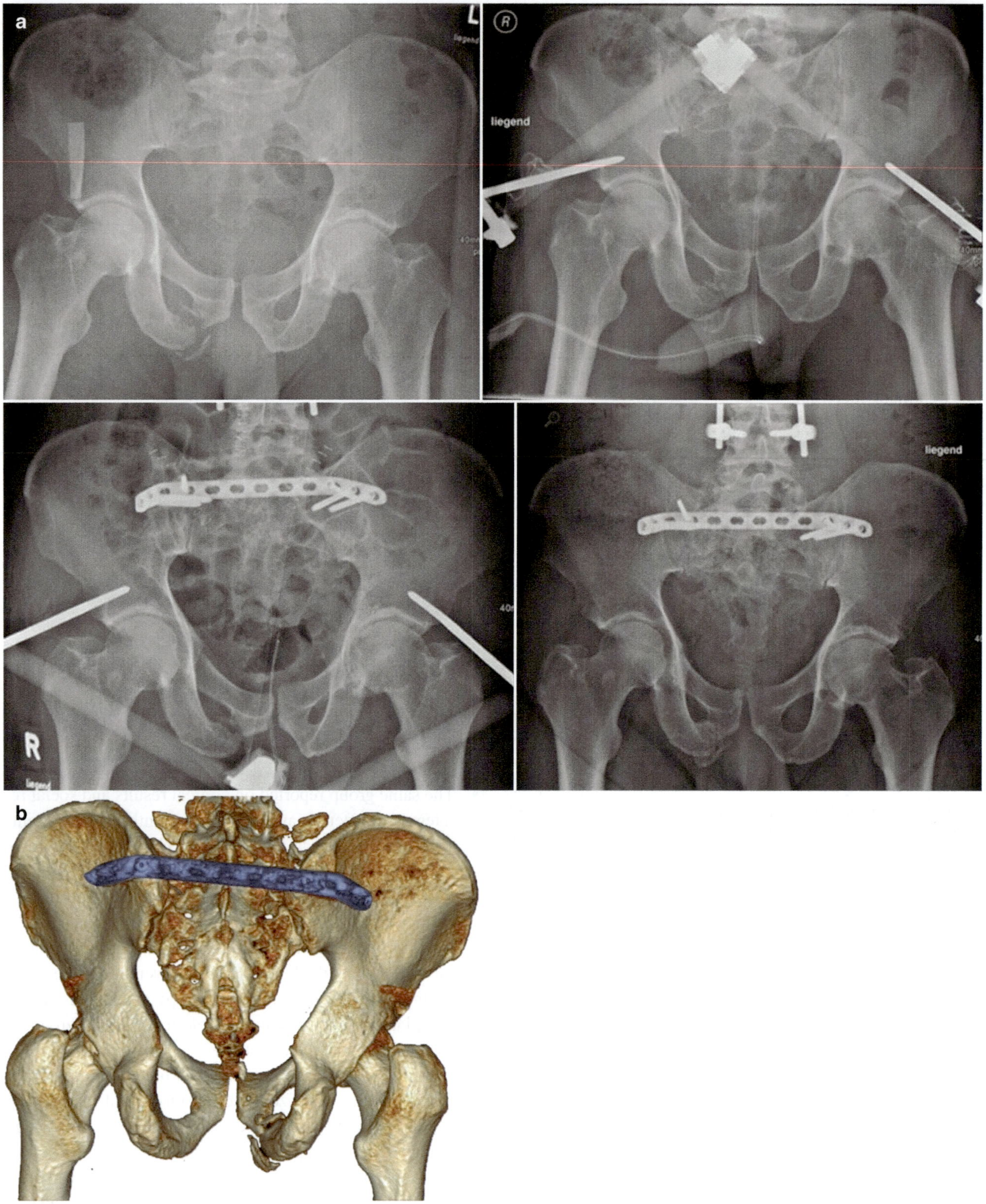

Fig. 34.11 (**a**) Right C1.3 injury, stabilized using an ilio-iliacal plate. (**b**) Postop CT shows the plate position

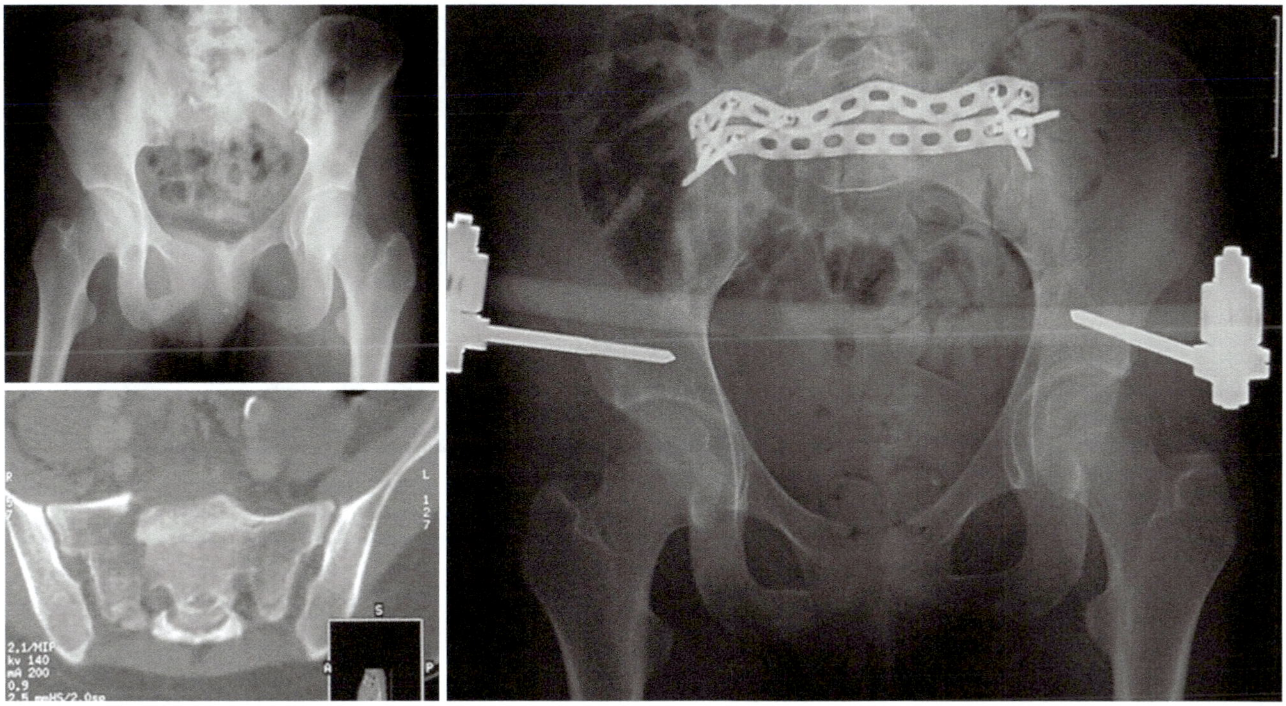

Fig. 34.12 Right C1.3.2 injury (transforaminal sacral fracture), stabilized using two ilio-iliacal plates

placement <10 mm) were recorded; the functional outcome was excellent or good in 90%.

- Kobbe et al. performed locked ilio-iliacal plate osteosynthesis in 23 patients with type C injuries [26]. Of these, 21 patients had follow-up after a mean of 30 months. Stabilization-related complications were observed with one superficial wound infection and six minor implant-related discomforts. No loss of reduction was observed. The long-term clinical result was graded excellent in 52.4%, good in 19% and fair in 28.6% using POS. Eighty-one percent healed with posterior anatomical healing and the remaining 19% with displacement <5 mm at the posterior pelvis. Overall, 2/3 had a good to excellent pelvic outcome score. 71.4% had full social re-integration and 90.5% had an unchanged social status.
- Chen et al. developed a comparable implant, the minimally invasive adjustable plate, which allows even distraction of lateral compression fractures or compression [30]. Sixteen patients with 6 type B and 10 type C injuries were treated with this plate. The average preoperative displacement of 23.6 mm could be adequately reduced. Duration of surgery was 49 min with an intraoperative blood loss of 80 mL. No surgery-related complications were observed. At latest follow-up (mean 30 months) 15 of 16 patients achieved osseous. No loss of reduction or implant-associated problems was recorded. The functional outcome was graded excellent in 10, good in 4, and fair in 2 patients.
- In a recent analysis of 42 type C sacral fractures, stabilization was performed using a subcutaneous 3.5 mm reconstruction plate through vertical or transverse incisions [31]; after a mean of 22 months 14 patients had excellent scores, 16 had good, 6 had fair, and 6 had poor scores according to the POS.

34.5 Sacral Bar Fixation

Lambotte in 1913 described the techniques of extraosseous sacral bar stabilization [8].

Recently, two different concepts have been available for sacral bar fixation: intraosseous application, especially in geriatric patients, and the classical extraosseous posterior procedure.

34.5.1 Extraosseous Sacral Bar Fixation

Shaw et al. first introduced the concept of posterior extraosseous sacral bar fixation [32]. Data on biomechanical testing

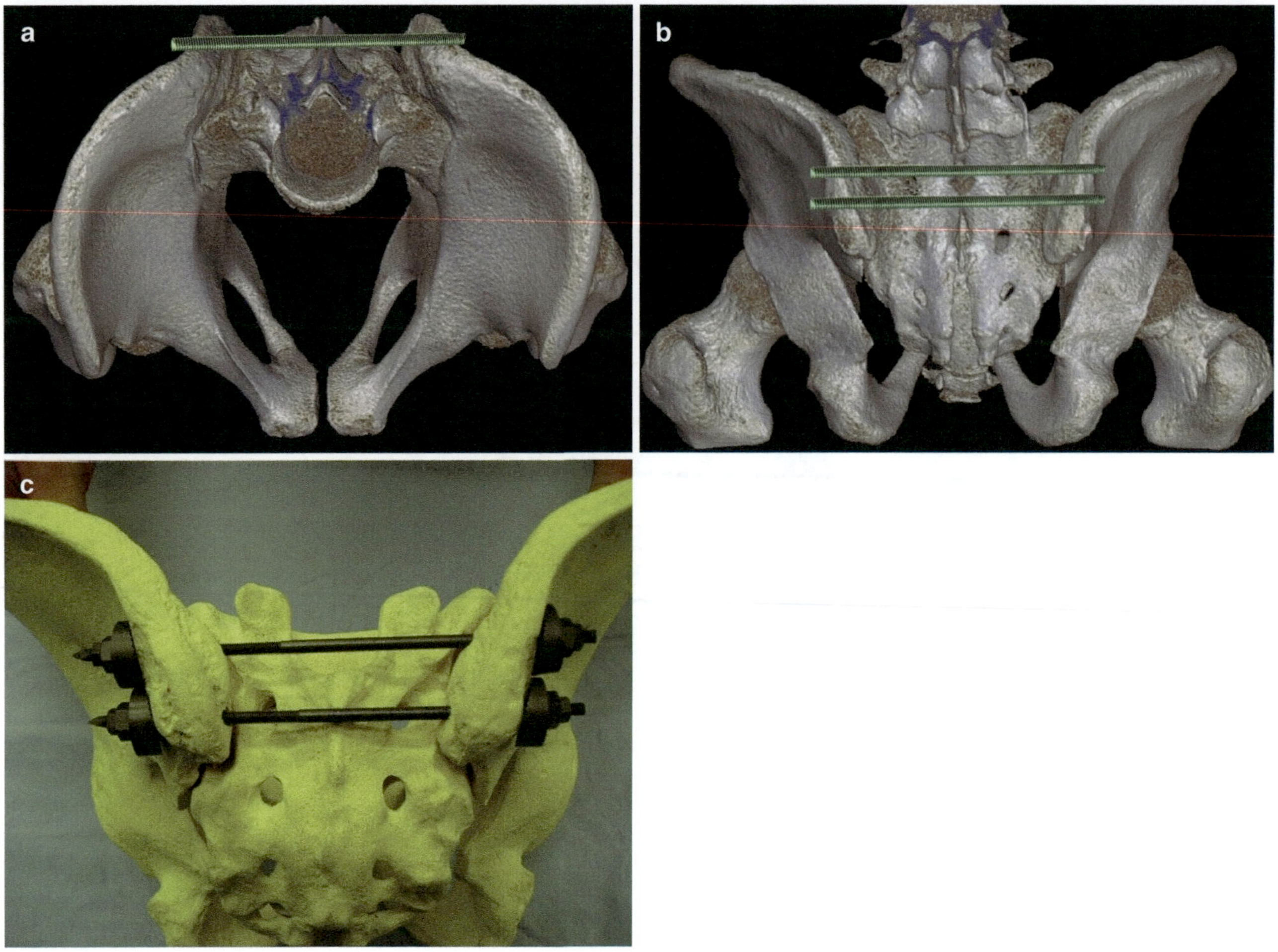

Fig. 34.13 (**a**) Position of the sacral rods, posterior to the sacrum. (**b**) Usually, two sacral rods are inserted at the level of the PSIS. (**c**) Model with attached sacral bars

were reported, together with clinical cases. Two threaded compression rods were placed between both PSIS (Fig. 34.13).

Surgical indications include bilateral sacroiliac disruptions or fracture-dislocations, unilateral sacroiliac disruptions or fracture-dislocations, fractures with gross displacement of the hemipelvis with bony or soft-tissue interposition, and patients who cannot tolerate prolonged bed rest [32].

The technique described by Shaw includes the following steps [32]:

- Prone positioning between two operating tables to hang the first applied anterior frame free between the tables
- Curved skin incisions over both PSIS
- Exposure of both sacroiliac joints and both lateral iliac wings
- Elevation of the gluteal muscles
- Debridement of the disrupted sacroiliac joint
- Two threaded compression rods are drilled between both PSIS placed posterior to the sacrum
- Two-hole dynamic compression plates used as washers

With increasing experience of treating unstable pelvic injuries, the concepts of anterior and posterior stabilization were favored in the mid1980s.

Interestingly, extensive experimental research was conducted on biomechanical studies [21, 32–35] and on the anatomic basis [36] for sacral bar application, whereas clinical results are missing (Fig. 34.14).

34.5.2 Experimental Data

In the biomechanical analysis by Shaw, testing anterior external frames and internal fixation of the symphysis with addition to sacral bar stabilization at the posterior pelvis, the combined anterior and posterior fixation was adequate, especially when anterior internal fixation methods were used. Even in bilateral sacroiliac joint disruptions (dislocation plus fracture-dislocation), little displacement occurred [32].

Stocks et al. analyzed three constructs in a unilateral vertical shear sacral fracture model: isolated anterior external frame ± sacral bars, or sacral bars with one or two symphy-

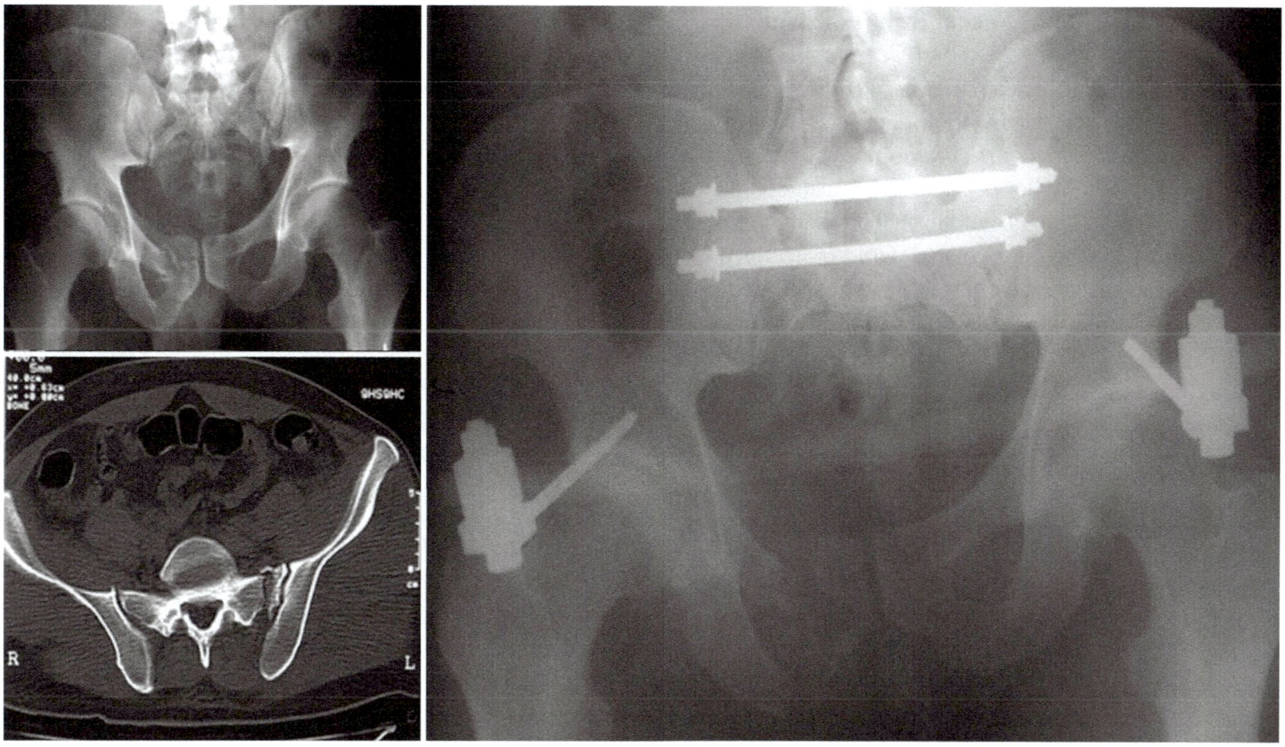

Fig. 34.14 Left C1.3.1 injury (transalar sacral fracture), stabilized using sacral bars

seal plates. Posterior stabilization increased the strength and rigidity of any anterior fixation. Anterior internal osteosynthesis in combination with sacral bars led to two-thirds strength of the intact pelvis [32].

Pohlemann et al. used a single-leg stance model and tested different stabilization methods in transforaminal sacral fractures [35]. Sacral bars were associated with highest loads of failure compared to local osteosynthesis or an internal sacral fixator. The mode of failure for sacral bars was shearing with compression at the cranial-posterior fracture zone [37].

Additionally, Comstock et al. compared four different stabilization constructs in a C1.2 unstable pelvic cadaver analysis with a sacroiliac dislocation in conjunction with ipsilateral rami fractures [33]. Posterior fixation included sacroiliac screws, anterior SI plates, sacral bars, and a combination of SI screws and sacral bars. The combined posterior fixation with sacroiliac screws and sacral bars without anterior fixation restored 90% of the intact pelvic stability.

Kraus analyzed several stabilization constructs in synthetic molded pelvic models with a C1.2 injury. Additionally, highest strengths were reached with combined iliosacral screw fixation and sacral bars [34].

Yinger et al. performed a comparable biomechanical analysis on a plastic bone model using several posterior stabilization methods including sacral bar fixation with or without additional iliosacral screws [21]; a moderate stability could be conformed for fixation of the disrupted SI joint, when one sacral bar was combined with one iliosacral screw. A second sacral bar could not significantly increase the overall stability.

34.5.3 Intraosseous Sacral Bar Fixation

Intraosseous sacral bar fixation was proposed for geriatric trauma patients as an alternative to iliosacral screw fixation, especially in the common bilateral sacral insufficiency fracture lesions.

Vanderschot et al. performed a feasibility study on CT data and reported on four patients where the bar was correctly inserted [38]. The safe area was defined at the level of S1 and S2. The bony channel was larger in male than in female patients. An iliac-sacral-iliac bar (>4 mm) could be inserted in all men, but in only 50% at the S1 level and in 80% at the S2 level in women.

Mehling et al. reported on 11 geriatric patients with a mean age of 73 years and intraosseous sacral bar insertion into S1 [39]. One patient developed a temporary L5 nerve lesion. At latest follow-up all fractures healed and all patients had clinical improvement.

34.6 Technique of Sacral Bar Fixation

Indications for sacral bar fixation are identical to all other posterior pelvic ring stabilization concepts. Thus, typical indications are type C injuries with either complete sacral fractures (Denis I, II, III) or sacroiliac (fracture-) dislocations. Potential contraindications include sacral fractures with a risk of compression-related nerve root injury (e.g., intra-foraminal fragments) or far posterior located ilium fractures [40, 41]. Anterior fixation of the pelvis should be first performed [41].

34.6.1 Landmarks

In the prone position, after sterile draping, the landmarks of the posterior-lateral iliac crest parallel to the SI joint and the PSIS are marked.

34.6.2 Incision

The skin incision starts at the PSIS and is orientated cranially along the posterior iliac crest approximately 5 cm.

34.6.3 Dissection

After identification of the gluteal fascia on the fractures side, the fascia is dissected at the lateral border of the iliac crest and the gluteal muscles are epifascially dissected from the underlying bone. Dissection is maximally performed until reaching the posterior gluteal line on the outer ilium surface.

34.6.4 Reduction

Classical reduction techniques are used. In rotational deformities, a Schanz screw, inserted into the posterior iliac crest can be used to manipulate the hemipelvis using the "joystick technique."

Alternatively, insertion of a pointed reduction forceps, placed at the posterior sacral spine and at the iliac crest or at the outer side of the ilium, can support reduction.

Insertion of K-wires from lateral to central allow to hold the reduction, until definitive fixation is performed.

34.6.5 Sacral Rod Application

Application of typically two sacral bars can be performed free hand or using an aiming device [40, 41].

A true lateral view of the sacrum or a hyperinlet view can be helpful to guide the drill bit. The drill should be placed directly posterior to the sacral cortex. It can be helpful to start with the more inferior bar. One drill should be at the level of both PSIS and the second approximately 2 cm cranially.

34.6.6 Fixation

After inserting one sacral bar, sacral washers and nuts are fixed to the bar. Under continuous image intensification, the final check avoiding overcompression of the sacrum is made. Two bars are always recommended to avoid rotation.

34.7 Locked Transsacral Screw Fixation

As an alternative, locked transsacral screw fixation is based on the same concepts as intraosseous sacral bar fixation.

Moed and Whiting proposed a modification of an iliosacral screw fixation where a fully or partially threaded screw is inserted over a washer from one side of the pelvis, bridging both sacroiliac joints and fixed outside the opposite iliac cortex with a self-locking nut [42]. They noted no implant- and treatment-related complications. This technique was considered an alternative in unstable bilateral posterior ring lesions.

Bridging unaffected sacroiliac joints did not influence the clinical long-term result [18].

In geriatric patients, often a fully threaded long iliosacral screw is increasingly inserted in minimal displaced bilateral sacral insufficiency fractures (Fig. 34.15).

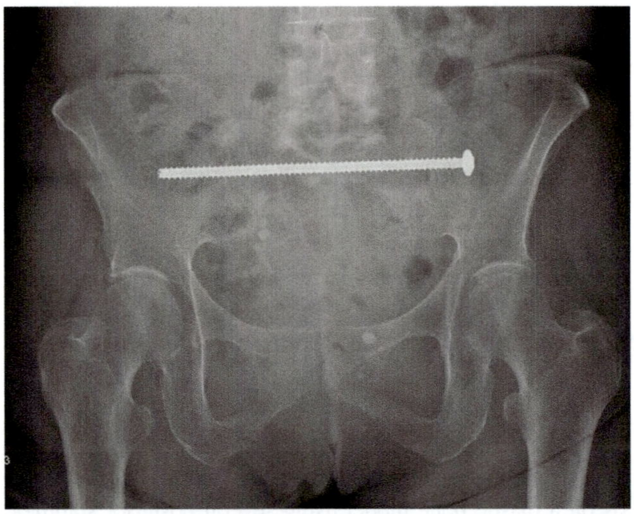

Fig. 34.15 Fully threaded (intraosseous) iliosacral screw stabilization is frequently performed in geriatric with bilateral sacral insufficiency fractures of the sacrum

34.8 Summary

Ilio-iliacal osteosynthesis is a sufficient technique for posterior pelvic ring stabilization with adequate clinical and radiological results. Angular stability leads to adequate stiffness with a low rate of secondary displacement. The complication rate is low.

Ilio-iliacal techniques have some disadvantages, including limited reduction possibilities, bilateral bridging of the SI joint in the unilateral injury pattern, difficulty in precontouring the plate, and a higher rate of symptomatic implants [27, 28].

References

1. Kellam J, Browner B. Fractures of the pelvic ring. in: skeletal trauma, Chapter 31. Philadelphia: WB Saunders Company; 1992. p. 849–97.
2. Kellam JF, McMurtry RY, Paley D, Tile M. The unstable pelvic fracture—operative treatment. Orthop Clin North Am. 1987;18(1):25–41.
3. Matta J, Saucedo T. Internal fixation of pelvic ring fractures. Clin Orthop. 1989;242:83–97.
4. Mears D, Rubash H. External and internal fixation of the pelvic ring. AAOS Instr Course Lect. 1984;33:144–58.
5. Mears D, Rubash H. Pelvic and acetabular fractures. Thorofare, New Jersey: Slack; 1986.
6. Tile M. Fractures of the pelvis and acetabulum. Baltimore: Williams & Wilkins; 1984.
7. Tile M. Pelvic ring fractures: should they be fixed? J Bone Joint Surg. 1988;70-B:1–12.
8. Lambotte A. Chirurgie opératoire des fractures. répité, vol. 1913. Bruxelles: Société Franco-Belge D'Editions Scientifiques; 1948. p. 126–44.
9. Füchtmeier B, Maghsudi M, Neumann C, Hente R, Roll C, Nerlich M. [The minimally invasive stabilization of the dorsal pelvic ring with the transiliacal internal fixator (TIFI)—surgical technique and first clinical findings]. Unfallchirurg. 2004;107:1142–52.
10. Anderson C, Chong A, Pence C, Dart B, Wooley P. Minimally invasive posterior pelvic bridging osteosynthesis for type C injuries: biomechanical evaluation. Poster No. 1427 • ORS 2012 Annual Meeting. 2012.
11. Salášek M, Jansová M, Kren J, Pavelka T, Weisová D. Biomechanical comparison of a transiliac internal fixator and two iliosacral screws in transforaminal sacral fractures: a finite element analysis. Acta Bioeng Biomech. 2015;17:39–49.
12. Dienstknecht T, Berner A, Lenich A, Nerlich M, Fuechtmeier B. A minimally invasive stabilizing system for dorsal pelvic ring injuries. Clin Orthop. 2011;469:3209–17.
13. Salášek M, Pavelka T. [Minimally invasive fixation of the pelvic ring with a transiliacal internal fixator]. Acta Chir Orthop Traumatol Cechoslov. 2012;79:335–40.
14. Salášek M, Pavelka T, Křen J, Weisová D, Jansová M. [Minimally invasive stabilization of posterior pelvic ring injuries with a transiliac internal fixator and two iliosacral screws: comparison of outcome]. Acta Chir Orthop Traumatol Cechoslov. 2015;82:41–7.
15. Schmitz P, Baumann F, Grechenig S, Gaensslen A, Nerlich M, Müller M. The cement-augmented transiliacal internal fixator (caT-IFI): an innovative surgical technique for stabilization of fragility fractures of the pelvis. Injury. 2015;46(Suppl 4):S114–20.
16. Dolati B, Larndorfer R, Krappinger D, Rosenberger R. Stabilization of the posterior pelvic ring with a slide-insertion plate. Oper Orthop Traumatol. 2007;19:16–31.
17. Heydemann J, Hartline B, Gibson M, Ambrose C, Munz J, Galpin M, Achor T, Gary J. Do transsacral-transiliac screws across uninjured sacroiliac joints affect pain and functional outcomes in trauma patients? Clin Orthop. 2016;474:1417–21.
18. Mardam-Bey S, Beebe M, Black J, Chang E, Kubiak E, Bishop J, McAndrew C, Ricci W, Gardner M. The effect of transiliac-transsacral screw fixation for pelvic ring injuries on the uninjured sacroiliac joint. J Orthop Trauma. 2016;30:463–8.
19. Rubash H, Brown T, Nelson D, Mears D. Comparative mechanical performance of some new devices for fixation of unstable pelvic ring fractures. Med Biol Eng Comput. 1983;21:657–63.
20. Albert M, Miller M, MacNaughton M, Hutton W. Posterior pelvic fixation using a transiliac 4.5-mm reconstruction plate: a clinical and biomechanical study. J Orthop Trauma. 1993;7(3):226–32.
21. Yinger K, Scalise J, Olson SA, Bay BK, Finkemeier CG. Biomechanical comparison of posterior pelvic ring fixation. J Orthop Trauma. 2003;17(7):481–7.
22. Wu T, Chen W, Li X, Zhang Q, Lv H, Zhang Y. Biomechanical comparison of three types of internal fixation in a type C zone II pelvic fracture model. Int J Clin Exp Med. 2015;8:1853–61.
23. Shinohara K, Takigawa T, Tanaka M, Sugimoto Y, Arataki S, Ito Y, Ozaki T. Biomechanical comparison of posterior fixation using spinal instrumentation and conventional posterior plate fixation in unstable vertical sacral fracture. Acta Med Okayama. 2016;70:97–102.
24. Bodzay T, Burján T, Bagdi C, Flóris I, Vendégh Z, Váradi K. Evaluation of stabilization methods of pelvic ring injuries by finite element modeling. Joint Dis Relat Surg. 2007;18:108–15.
25. Chen H, Wu L, Zheng R, Liu Y, Li Y, Ding Z. Parallel analysis of finite element model controlled trial and retrospective case control study on percutaneous internal fixation for vertical sacral fractures. BMC Musculoskelet Disord. 2013;14:217. https://doi.org/10.1186/1471-2474-14-217.
26. Kobbe P, Hockertz I, Sellei R, Reilmann H, Hockertz T. Minimally invasive stabilisation of posterior pelvic-ring instabilities with a transiliac locked compression plate. Int Orthop. 2012;36:159–64.
27. Krappinger D, Larndorfer R, Struve P, Rosenberger R, Arora R, Blauth M. Minimally invasive transiliac plate osteosynthesis for type C injuries of the pelvic ring: a clinical and radiological follow-up. J Orthop Trauma. 2007;21:595–602.
28. Suzuki T, Hak D, Ziran B, Adams S, Stahel P, Morgan S, Smith W. Outcome and complications of posterior transiliac plating for vertically unstable sacral fractures. Injury. 2009;40:405–9.
29. Hao T, Changwei Y, Qiulin Z. Treatment of posterior pelvic ring injuries with minimally invasive percutaneous plate osteosynthesis. Int Orthop. 2009;33:1435–9.
30. Chen W, Hou Z, Su Y, Smith W, Liporace F, Zhang Y. Treatment of posterior pelvic ring disruptions using a minimally invasive adjustable plate. Injury. 2013;44:975–80.
31. Ayoub M, Gad H, Seleem O. Standalone percutaneous transiliac plating of vertically unstable sacral fractures: outcomes, complications, and recommendations. Eur Spine J. 2016;25:1153–62.
32. Stocks G, Gablel D, Noble P, Hanson G, Tullos H. Anterior and posterior internal fixation of vertical shear fractures of the pelvis. J Orthop Res. 1991;9:237–45.
33. Comstock C, van der Meulen M, Goodman S. Biomechanical comparison of posterior internal fixation techniques for unstable pelvic fractures. J Orthop Trauma. 1994;10:517–22.
34. Kraus E, Schlickewei W, Cordey J, Wahl D, Kuner E, Perren S. Methode zur vergleichenden Messung der Stabilität von Osteosynthesen am dorsalen Beckenring. Unfallchirurgie. 1998;24(1):25–31.

35. Pohlemann T, Angst M, Schneider E, Ganz R, Tscherne H. Fixation of transforaminal sacrum fractures: a biomechanical study. J Orthop Trauma. 1993;7(2):107–17.
36. Ebraheim N, Coombs R, Hoeflinger M, Zeman C, Jackson W. Anatomical and radiological considerations in compressive bar technique for posterior pelvic disruptions. J Orthop Trauma. 1991;5(4):434–8.
37. Culemann U, Pohlemann T, Hufner T, Gansslen A. 3-dimensional movement analysis after internal fixation of pelvic ring fractures. A computer simulation. Unfallchirurg. 2000;103(11):965–71.
38. Vanderschot P, Meuleman C, Lefèvre A, Broos P. Trans iliac-sacral-iliac bar stabilisation to treat bilateral lesions of the sacro-iliac joint or sacrum: anatomical considerations and clinical experience. Injury. 2001;32:587–92.
39. Mehling I, Hessmann M, Rommens P. Stabilization of fatigue fractures of the dorsal pelvis with a trans-sacral bar. Operative technique and outcome. Injury. 2012;43:446–51.
40. Depuy-Synthes, Sacral Bar Kit—Surgical Technique. 2017. http://synthes.vo.llnwd.net/o16/LLNWMB8/US%20Mobile/Synthes%20North%20America/Product%20Support%20Materials/Technique%20Guides/DSUSTRM09161022_Sacral_Bar_Kit_TG_150dpi.pdf.
41. ITS, Sacral Rods—Sakralstäbe. 2010. http://www.its.med-hold.com/attachments/066_SR_de.pdf.
42. Moed B, Whiting D. Locked transsacral screw fixation of bilateral injuries of the posterior pelvic ring: initial clinical series. J Orthop Trauma. 2010;24:616–21.

Lumbopelvic Fixation

35

Jan Lindahl and Axel Gänsslen

The sacrum is a median triangular bone, connecting the two innominate bones to the lumbar spine. The three pelvic bones are held together by extremely strong ligaments. Sacrum is a kyphotic structure consisting of five fused sacral vertebrae and coccygeal bones. The lumbosacral area has the highest degree of numerical variation in the axial skeleton.

Major traumatic forces on the pelvis are needed to cause significant disruptions. Because the lumbosacral junction is located anterior to the SI joint, the body weight transmitted to the superior surface of the sacrum acts as a rotary force, with an axis centered on S2; this force causes the sacral promontory to tilt forward and the apex to tilt backward [1].

Fracture patterns in the sacrum range from crush lesions in the lateral sacrum to spinopelvic dissociations.

The spinopelvic dissociation is a rare, high-energy injury pattern located in the sacrum. It is characterized by bilateral vertical sacral fractures in conjunction with a transverse sacral fracture. Denis's classification system of sacral fractures does not recognize the combination of bilateral vertical and transverse fracture lines that cause spinopelvic dissociation [2]. Spinopelvic dissociation injury causes the spine and upper central segment of the sacrum to dissociate from the pelvic ring and caudal sacral segments [3, 4]. This pattern results in discontinuity between the spine and pelvis, leading to instability in all three planes.

During the past few decades, the rate of osteoporotic pelvic fractures in the older population has increased consistently [5, 6]. Low-energy fractures in osteoporotic patients are defined as fragility fractures of the pelvis (FFP). The term "fragility fracture" is used instead of stress, fatigue, or insufficiency fracture to describe osteoporosis-associated fractures due to a minor trauma or with no obvious trauma history [7–11].

Fragility fractures of the sacrum (FFS) might also have combined vertical and transverse fracture elements with spinopelvic dissociation. FFS are often combined with a fracture of the anterior pelvic ring; hence, they are classified as a part of fragility fractures of the pelvis (FFP) [7, 8].

35.1 Historical Experience

Early reports on lumbopelvic dissociation injuries were predominantly case reports, analyzing the injury mechanism, the neurological deficit, and the clinical course.

In 1969, Purser described a case of a spinopelvic dissociation injury without neurological impairment after a lateral side impact MVA crash in a 19-year-old woman [12]. Eight weeks of traction resulted in acceptable reduction with only slight flexion deformity. A U-shaped injury (S1 transverse component) was confirmed by lateral sacral view and tomography with bilateral L5 transverse process injuries.

Fardon et al. described a case of a 41 year old man with a flexion deformity of the first sacral vertebra with secondary L5/S1 nerve deficit (developed on day 2) [13]. Posterior sacral nerve root decompression was performed on day 38 using a posterior approach. A bony fragment compressed the S1 nerve roots, and posterolateral spondylodesis was performed using local bone. A partial neurological recovery was observed within 6 months (right > left). The patient developed erectile dysfunction and had permanent nerve dysfunction below the knee level on the left side. Bone healing was stated at a follow-up after 2.5 years. Fardon recommended that "early closed or open reduction is theoretically ideal."

Bucknill et al. reported on three cases with U-shaped S1 injuries [14]. In all three cases, secondary nerve deficits developed due to inadequate early mobilization and conservative treatment was performed. Neurological function at least partially recovered after several months.

J. Lindahl
Orthopaedics and Trauma Surgery, Helsinki University Hospital, Helsinki, Finland

A. Gänsslen (✉)
Department of Trauma Surgery, Orthopedics and Hand Surgery, Hospital Wolfsburg, Wolfsburg, Germany

A. Gänsslen et al. (eds.), *Pelvic Ring Fractures*, https://doi.org/10.1007/978-3-030-54730-1_35

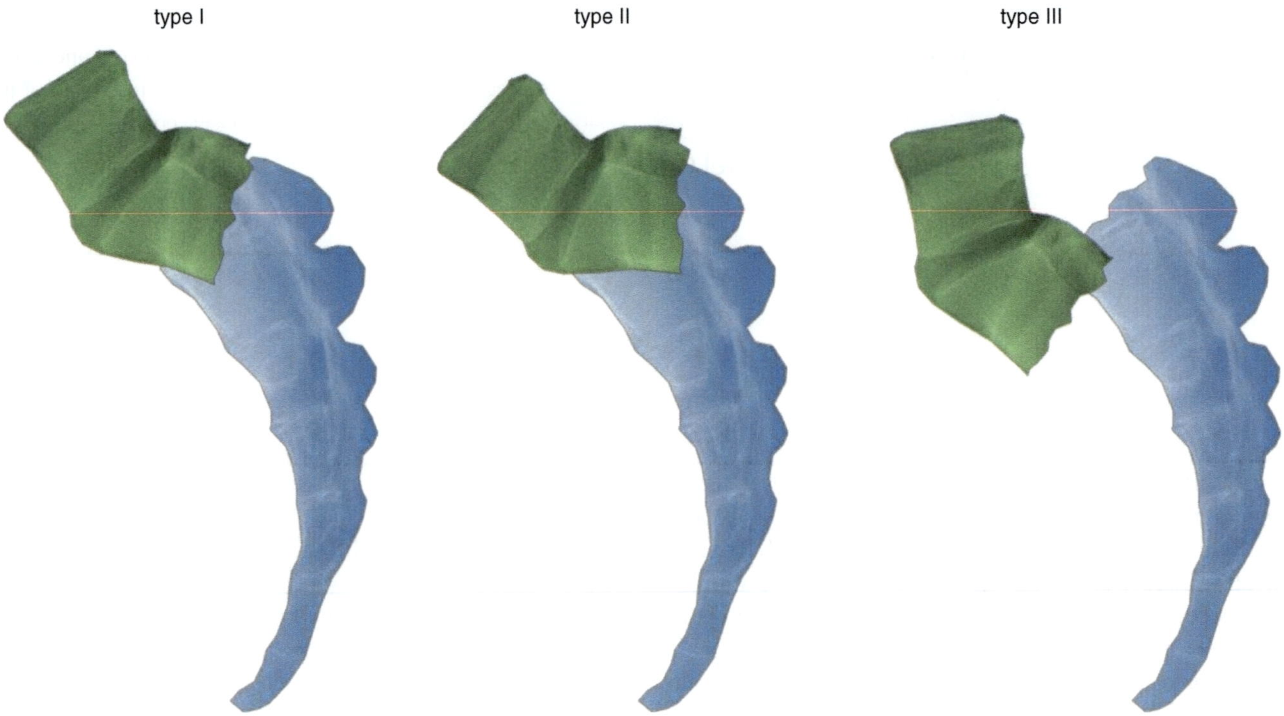

Fig. 35.1 Roy-Camille classification of lumbopelvic injuries (details: see text)

Das De et al. identified a hyperflexion with compression as a main injury mechanism, which can be accompanied with a rotational instability, when the L5/S1 facet joint is involved [15]. Posterior sacral nerve root decompression and spondylodesis were recommended. In one case an additional stabilization was performed using an interspinous wiring. No neurological deterioration was related to surgery. Comparable reports were published by Dowling et al. and Fisher et al. [16, 17].

In 1985, Roy-Camille et al. were the first to present a larger series on these injuries, and a first attempt of a fracture classification was recommended [9]. A detailed analysis of the injury biomechanics and mechanism, the fracture course, and clinical course was reported. Additionally, results of an experimental study were presented.

In summary, the following findings were presented:

- A fall from great height is a common injury mechanism ("suicidal jumper's fracture," observed in 11 of 13 cases).
- Kyphosis with leg flexion or lordosis with leg extension often results in these injuries.
- Bilateral longitudinal sacral fractures (alar region) are combined with a horizontal fracture line at the level of S2/3 or less common at the level of S1/2 with/without an intermediate fragment.
- Biomechanical experiments confirmed clinical morphological findings.

These findings led to the Roy-Camille classification of lumbopelvic injuries (Fig. 35.1):

- Type 1 injury: flexion fracture with simple anterior bending of the upper sacrum
- Type 2 injury: flexion fracture with posterior displacement of the upper fragment presenting in a horizontal shape
- Type 3 injuries: extension fracture with anterior displacement of a vertically orientated upper fragment slipping downward

Treatment consisted of surgery in 10 of 13 cases. A midline posterior approach was favored to fully observe the transverse fracture component and the involved nerve roots. The fracture zone was opened and reduction was performed using intraoperative traction, distracting forceps, or using a distracting Harrington rod. Sagittal reduction was performed using a lever maneuver. In the last two cases, plate or Harrington rod stabilization was performed.

In seven cases, neurological recovery was reported, while perineal recovery was observed in only one case.

In 1991, Strange-Vognsen et al. added a fourth fracture type to the Roy-Camille classification [18]. An undisplaced sagittal S1/2 injury with severe comminution of the U-shaped fragment, treated nonoperatively, was presented.

Since the early 1990s, several authors presented cases treated operatively using different techniques [6, 19–24].

In the late 1990s, Schildhauer et al. proposed a standardized treatment concept for vertically unstable sacral fractures, including bilateral complete posterior instabilities. A triangular concept with stabilization between the L4 and L5 pedicles and the posterior aspect of the iliac bone or the sacral wing lateral to the sacral fracture was combined with iliosacral screw fixation in unilateral or ilio-iliacal plate fixation in bilateral fractures or unilateral fractures with marked displacement [25].

35.2 Biomechanics of Lumbopelvic Fixation

Few studies analyzed lumbopelvic fixation concepts.

Schildhauer et al. analyzed the triangular concept of sacral fracture osteosynthesis and compared these results to iliosacral screw and pubic screw fixations in a C1.3.2 c1 injury model in a single leg stance simulation. Lumbopelvic fixation with an additional iliosacral screw resulted in significant lower displacements with higher overall stability [26].

Zheng et al. analyzed the effect of two different iliac screw lengths on overall stability in a lumbosacral instability model [27]. No difference between 70 mm screws and 138 mm screws was observed.

Min et al. compared triangular osteosynthesis with two iliosacral screws inserted into S1 [28]. Despite a greater stiffness of two screws, the ultimate load and rotational stiffness was comparable.

Song et al. performed a finite element analysis comparing unilateral lumbopelvic fixation, bilateral lumbopelvic fixation, and unilateral iliac fixation with bilateral lumbar pedicle screws in an unilateral sacral fracture model [29]. Bilateral lumbopelvic fixation resulted in highest stiffness. Unilateral fixation led to lumbopelvic imbalance.

Recently, Jazini et al. analyzed minimally and severely displaced foraminal sacral fractures. Lumbopelvic fixation resulted in least instability of all tested constructs [30]. Adding an iliosacral screw and extension to L4 were associated with optimal results, proposing the latter concept for highly comminuted fractures.

> Spinopelvic stabilization concepts are biomechanically sufficient to stabilize highly unstable sacral fracture situations.

35.3 Classification of Spinopelvic Dissociations

In general, high-energy injuries can be distinguished from low-energy (geriatric) injuries.

35.3.1 High-Energy Injuries

Roy-Camille et al. described spinopelvic dissociation injury, but they classified only transverse sacral fracture and not bilateral vertical fracture components [9].

Later, Strange-Vognsen and Lebech added a fourth type, which is an axial loading injury with a segmentally comminuted S1 body [18]. However, this type 4 fracture is a burst fracture of S1–S2 with bone retropulsion, not a true transverse sacral fracture [31].

The outcome study of H-shaped sacral fracture with spinopelvic dissociation by Lindahl et al. showed that the Roy-Camille classification is not prognostic of neurological impairment after operative treatment [3]. They found out that neurological recovery and clinical outcome were associated with the degree of initial translational displacement of the transverse sacral fracture. Therefore, it is useful to subcategorize transverse sacral fractures, as partially displaced or completely displaced, and add these subcategories to the original Roy-Camille type 2 and three sacral fractures. According to this modified classification system, the transverse sacral fractures are divided into five types (Fig. 35.2) [3]:

- Type 1: Flexion injury without translational displacement
- Type 2a: Flexion injury with partial anterior translational displacement
- Type 2b: Flexion injury with complete anterior displacement of the distal sacral segment
- Type 3a: Extension injury with partial posterior translational displacement
- Type 3b: Extension injury with complete posterior displacement of the distal sacral segment

35.3.2 Low-Energy Injuries

The Rommens and Hofmann classification system of fragility fractures of the pelvis (FFP) differentiate isolated anterior lesions (type I) and posterior pelvic injuries as well as a combinations of these including the degree of displacement and hence the degree of pelvic instability (types II, III, and IV, see Chap. 4) [32]. FFP IV injuries are defined as displaced bilateral posterior pelvic ring injuries. Three subgroups are distinguished:

- Type IVa: bilateral ilium fractures or bilateral SI joint disruptions
- Type IVb: spinopelvic dissociation with a bilateral sacral fracture connected with a transverse fracture line (H- or U-type sacral fractures)

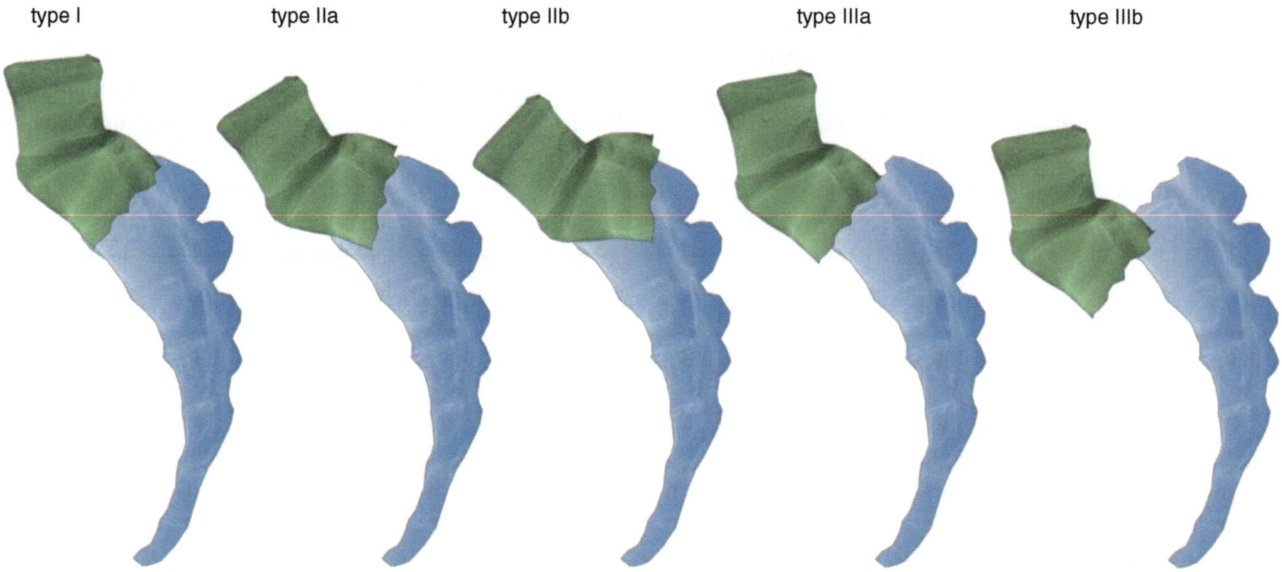

Fig. 35.2 Lindahl classification of lumbopelvic injuries (details: see text)

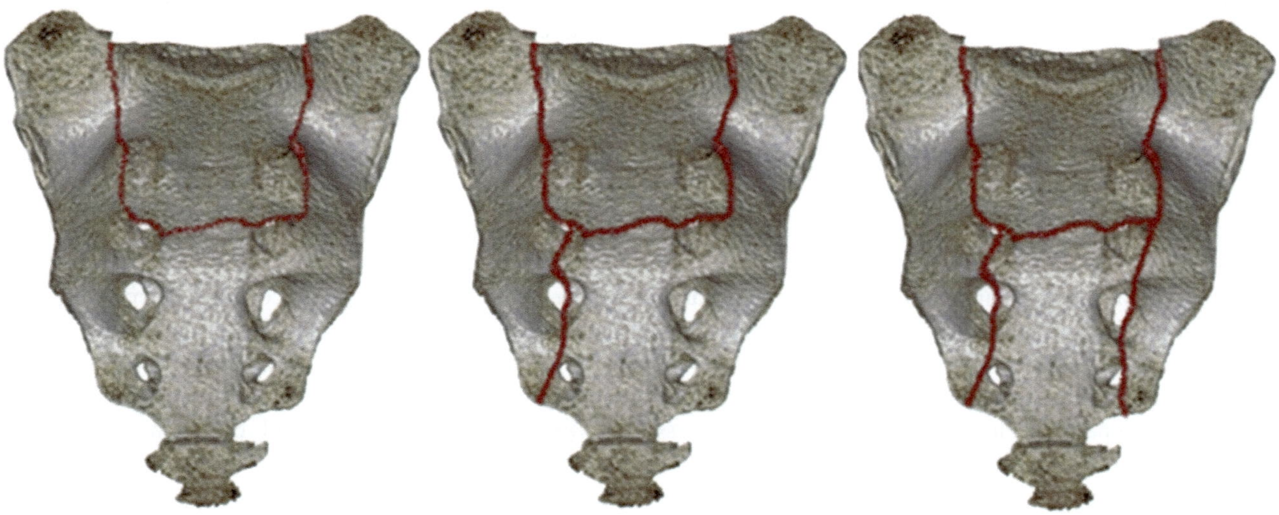

Fig. 35.3 Fracture morphology of different spinosacral dissociation injuries

- Type IVc: combination of bilateral posterior pelvic disruptions including a sacral fracture and an anterior pelvic ring injury

Lumbopelvic dissociation injuries are included in FFP type IVb and IVc.

35.4 Fracture Morphology

Most commonly spinopelvic dissociations are described by their fracture morphology (Fig. 35.3). Bilateral vertical sacral fractures associated with a transverse fracture might form the following fracture patterns [9, 31, 33–36]:

- H-type
- U-type
- T-type
- Y-type (or Lambda-type)

Gupta et al. analyzed the fracture morphology in 21 patients [37]. CT analysis confirmed five (24%) U-shaped, six (29%) H-shaped, four (19%) Y-shaped, and six (29%) burst fractures, respectively. In 16 patients (76%) the transverse fracture component was at the level of S2 and in the remaining patients at the level of S2/S3. In 73% a Denis zone II vertical fracture was present, and in 24% a zone III configuration. 43% present with sacral spinal canal stenosis and 90% had sacral foraminal narrowing.

The mean kyphotic angulation was 17.4° and a mean translation of 2.5 mm was observed, most frequently with anterior translation.

Lindahl et al. analyzed the morphology of H-shaped sacral fractures in 36 patients [3]. The transverse sacral fracture in the Roy-Camille type 2 fractures was at S2 level in 11 of 15 cases (73%), whereas the Roy-Camille type 3 transverse fractures were between the S1 and S2 vertebral bodies in 14 of 21 cases (67%). No burst fractures of S1 [18] were observed.

35.5 Neurologic Injury

AO/OTA type C1.3 fractures of the sacrum may result in a neurologic injury in up to 40% of cases [38] and H-shaped sacral fractures with spinopelvic dissociation in up to 100% of cases [3, 4, 39].

The nerve injury may involve more than one nerve root and can be unilateral or bilateral depending on the fracture pattern and location. The injury can range from a neuropraxic injury due to nerve contusion or shearing injury, to transection of nerve roots.

In H-shaped sacral fractures with spinopelvic dissociation, transverse fractures are often angled, and they undergo translational displacement or even complete fracture displacement. This condition results in gross spinopelvic instability and neurological deficits in the cauda equina.

Another common presentation is an injury to the L5 and S1 nerve roots associated with vertical sacral fracture lines. The L5 nerve root can be injured as a result of vertical shear displacement of the sacrum and is often accompanied by a fracture of the transverse process of L5. A S1 nerve root injury is associated with transforaminal (zone II) sacral fractures [2]. Neurologic deficits range from bowel or bladder dysfunction to complete cauda equina syndrome, and from L5 or/and S1 paresthesia to total footdrop [40, 41].

Sacral fractures that only cause injuries to the nerve roots from S2 to S5 (without S1 nerve root involvement) might be overlooked due to the lack of motor or sensory deficits in the lower leg. Urinary and anal continences and sexual function require at least unilateral preservation of the S2 and S3 nerve roots [42].

Therefore, clinical examination of trauma patients sustaining sacral fractures requires both examination of lower extremity sensory and motor function and examination to identify injuries to the lower sacral plexus. A rectal examination is performed to evaluate sphincter contraction and to exclude possible rectal injury as a sign of an open pelvic fracture. Light touch and pinprick sensation should be assessed for the perianal dermatomes of S2 to S5.

The Gibbons classification is most often used to classify the neurological deficit (Fig. 35.4).

35.6 Management

Initial management is directed at restoring hemodynamic stability. Associated head, thoracic, abdominal, pelvic, musculoskeletal, or soft tissue injuries should be promptly assessed and addressed.

Treatment for H-shaped sacral fracture with spinopelvic dissociation has evolved from a nonoperative approach to open or closed reduction and segmental lumbopelvic fixation [3, 4, 9, 43–45].

> The goals of treatment are realignment of the sacrum and pelvic ring, restoration of spinopelvic stability, and decompression of the neural injury indirectly with fracture reduction and/or directly with a sacral laminectomy.

H-shaped sacral fractures are the most difficult to reduce and stabilize because they potentially allow both hemipelves to displace cranially, anteriorly, and rotationally in the sagittal plane (flexion) and also rotationally in the horizontal plane (internal or external rotation), with respect to the upper central sacral segment and the lumbar spine.

U-shaped sacral fractures with spinopelvic dissociations [31, 46] are more stable and less complicated. Many of

Grade	Criteria
Grade 1	No neurologic deficit
Grade 2	Paraesthesias/sensory changes only
Grade 3	Motor weakness or loss but bowel/bladder control intact
Grade 4	Motor and/or sensory deficits associated with loss of bowel/bladder control

Fig. 35.4 Gibbons classification of neurological impairments after sacrum fractures

these injuries, especially minimally displaced U-shaped sacral fractures, can be treated with percutaneous iliosacral screw fixation [34, 35], posterior ilio-iliacal (transsacral) plate fixation [33], or with triangular osteosynthesis [33, 34]. However, depending on the degree of fracture comminution, fracture displacement, and fracture complexity, U-shaped sacral fractures might also be very challenging to reduce and stabilize.

The deformity of the entire pelvic ring increases in complexity with the addition of an injury in the anterior pelvic ring. The frequency of an injury to the anterior part of the pelvic ring varies between 52 and 78% [3, 4, 46].

35.7 Internal Fixation Techniques

The concept of lumbopelvic fixation is well established for the treatment of unilateral unstable and displaced sacral fractures.

After the initiation of the concept of triangular osteosynthesis (Fig. 35.5) by Schildhauer et al., several authors reported on adequate results of unilateral sacral fractures with a high rate of good and excellent clinical results, a high bone healing rate, and a low rate of secondary displacements. Even soft tissue complications were infrequently observed [47–50].

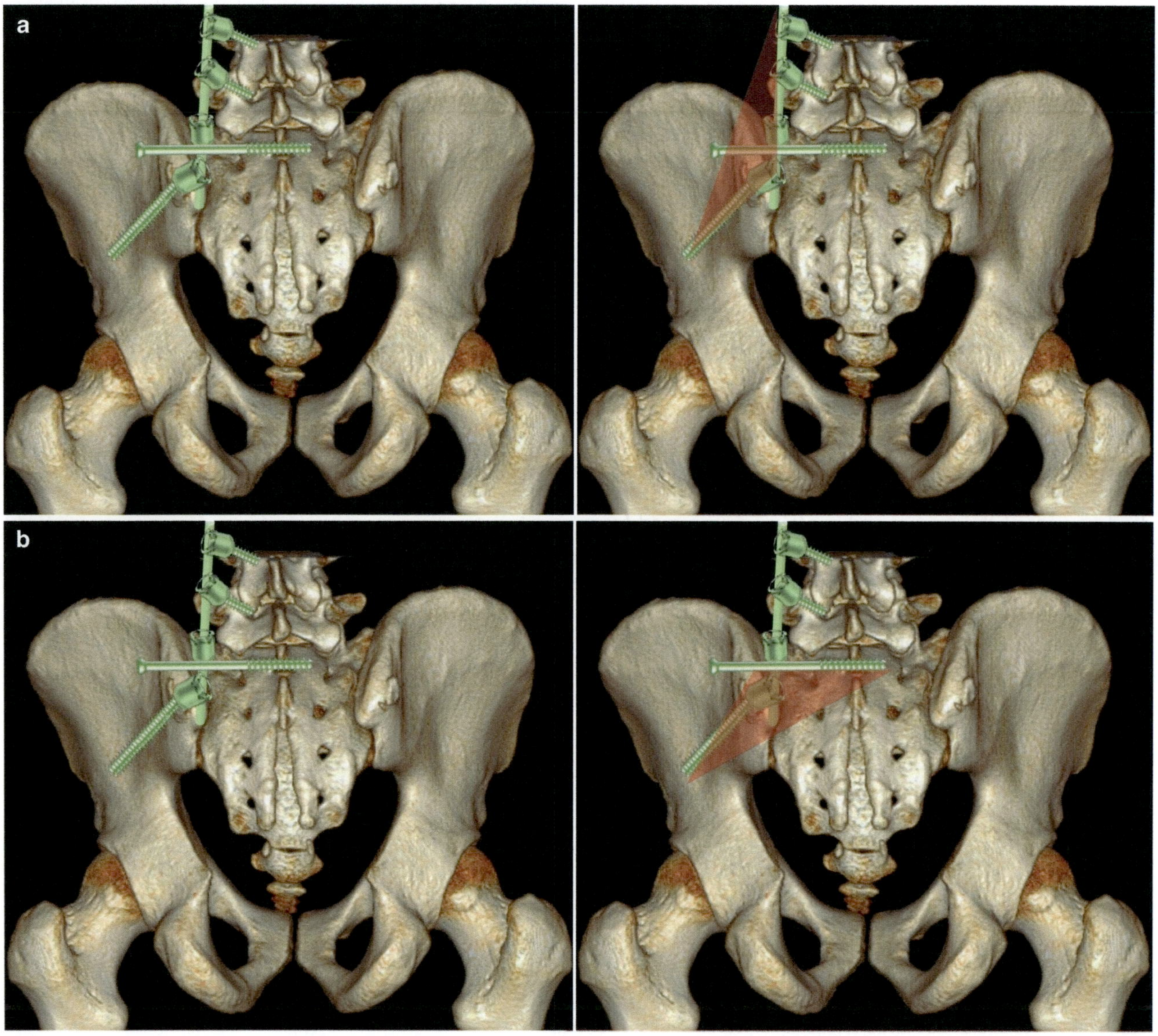

Fig. 35.5 (**a**) Concept of triangular osteosynthesis initiated by Schildhauer et al. (**b**) Concept of triangular osteosynthesis initiated by Schildhauer et al.

Roy-Camille et al. presented first three different types of fixation techniques for spinopelvic dissociations, including lumboiliac plates, lumbosacral plates, and Harrington rods connected to a transverse bi-iliac bar [9]. In all these techniques, proximal stability was achieved at the L4 and L5 laminae or pedicles, and distal stability was achieved at the upper central segment of the sacrum or the iliac wings.

Lumbopelvic fixation of H-shaped sacral fractures is achieved by connecting the lumbar spine to the ilium with segmental spinal fixation system. Allen and Ferguson were the first to report on their experience with the Galveston technique where the distal fixation points are located on the posterior part of the iliac wings, above the sciatic notch and between the laminas [51]. The proximal stability is achieved at the L4 and L5 pedicles.

In the lumbopelvic technique, pedicle screws are inserted in the pedicles of L4 and L5, and the caudal screws are inserted into the iliac bones (and into the S1 body). Following fracture reduction, the alignment and rotational stability are maintained by locking the pedicle screws and iliac screws using contoured spinal rods. Lumbopelvic fixation has been demonstrated to provide substantially better stiffness to other techniques [25, 26].

Very few studies have been published on the use of segmental lumbopelvic fixation in the management of H-shaped sacral fractures with spinopelvic dissociation [3, 4, 39, 44, 45]. However, more clinical studies have been published on U-shaped sacral fractures with minimal invasive reduction and fixation techniques [33–35, 46, 52].

Lumbopelvic fixation seems to be a reliable treatment method for H-shaped sacral fracture with spinopelvic dissociation, and it provides sufficient stability for fracture union with a relative low rate of complications and long-term sequelae [3, 4, 39, 44, 45].

Lumbopelvic fixation is also the treatment of choice for displaced T- and Y-shaped sacral fractures. However, most of U-shaped sacral fractures are suitable for minimally invasive or limited access surgery. Open reconstruction could be a salvage option for fractures with massive displacement of the bony elements.

35.8 H-Shaped Sacral Fracture with an Anterior Pelvic Ring Injury

The question of whether the anterior pelvic ring injury requires internal fixation when lumbopelvic fixation is performed posteriorly remains to be discussed.

Nondisplaced and stable fractures of the pubic rami can be treated nonoperatively. However, disruptions of the symphysis pubis and displaced unstable pubic rami fractures should be realigned and stabilized through an anterior approach [3]. Frequently, the anterior pelvic ring injury can be realigned and stabilized through limited measures such as anterior plate fixation or the use of retrograde pubic rami screws.

A staged reconstruction is performed when a combined H-shaped sacral fracture and an additional unstable anterior pelvic ring injury is present. The unstable injuries of the anterior part of the pelvic ring are most commonly operated on first [3, 4]. Anterior stabilization provides protection for the pelvic ring during a procedure performed with the patient prone and will aid in reduction of the posterior part of the pelvic ring [3].

> Anterior stabilization is recommended first for easier posterior reconstruction in displaced injuries [3, 53].

35.9 Preoperative Planning

The classification and detailed analyses of the sacral fracture and other fracture patterns are based on the pelvic plain radiographs and CT scans.

Three-dimensional image reconstructions based on CT scans of the pelvis provide considerable information on the location and stability of pelvic fractures. 3D CT enhances the understanding of each fracture lines and the separate fragments by simulating the gross anatomy of the injured pelvis. In particular, rotational deformities and displacements of the pelvis are best visualized with 3D CT. Pelvic AP radiography and CT with 3D image reconstructions will confirm the type of pelvic injury, the presence or absence of instability, and the degree of each displacements. It is necessary to acquire 3D CT images prior to a definitive surgical treatment of an unstable pelvic fracture. 3D CT facilities are currently available in most trauma centers; therefore, oblique pelvic inlet and outlet views are no longer essential for diagnostics or for preoperative planning. L5 transverse process fractures with the fracture line into the pedicle should be noted as they may compromise the ability to safely insert L5 pedicle screws. The overall morphology of the sacrum and sacral ala is also evaluated to determine the presence of sacral dysmorphism.

35.10 Surgical Approach

The patient is positioned prone on a standard radiolucent operating table (Fig. 35.6). Intraoperative image intensification control with AP, inlet, outlet, and true lateral views should be possible for the procedure. Longitudinal leg traction with a post between the legs against the perineum should be avoided because it will prevent the reduction of the distal

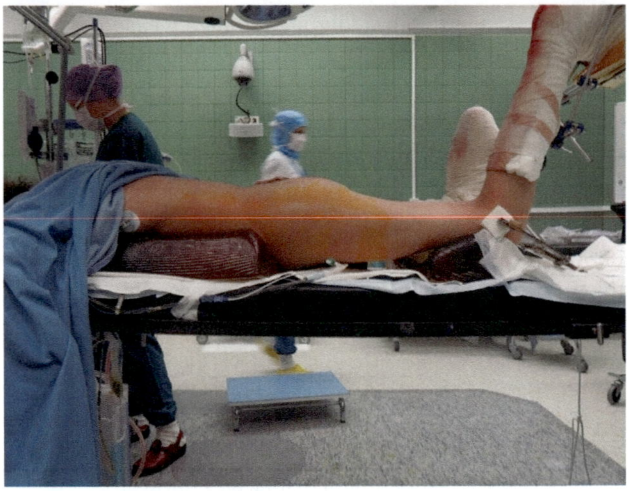

Fig. 35.6 Lumbopelvic fixation of an H-shaped sacral fracture. Patient is on prone position on a radiolucent trauma table with the hips in slight extension

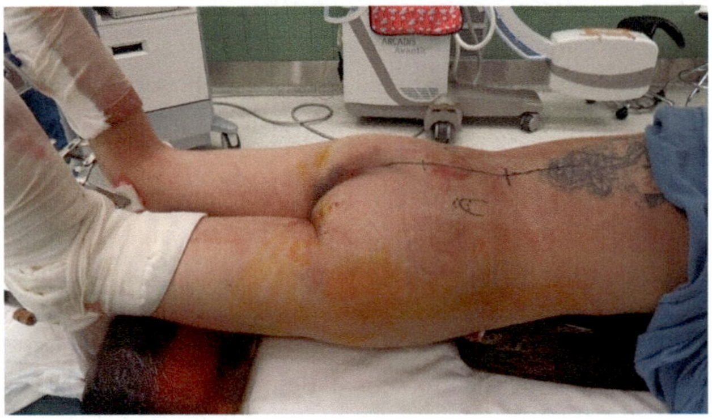

Fig. 35.7 Posterior midline incision

caudal sacral segment into the caudal direction, and also correction of vertical displacements and sagittal plane flexion deformity of the sacral fracture components.

Positioning should allow internal and external rotation of the hemipelves and even adduction and adduction of the lower extremities and hip hyperextension [54]. As an adjunct, a pelvic skeletal stabilization frame as proposed by Matta [55] can support the reduction and mobilization of the fracture against a fixed hemipelvis [54].

Draping should include the entire lumbopelvic region down to the natal cleft and should be extended laterally to allow iliosacral screw insertion.

A posterior midline approach is commonly used to expose the lower lumbar spinal segments, posterior sacral injury, and medial aspect of posterior iliac wings (Fig. 35.7). A midline skin incision is made from L3–L4 to S3. The dissection is carried down to the thoracolumbar fascia, which is incised close to the spinous processes.

Dissection is performed into the intermuscular plane between the multifidus and erector spinae muscles.

The dissection at the cephalad portion of the incision is continued down onto the transverse processes of L4 and L5. The caudal portion of the incision is continued onto posterior superior iliac spine (PSIS). The paraspinal muscles are detached from the posterior aspect of the sacrum, exposing the sacral fracture lines. The sacrospinalis muscle can be mobilized laterally without distal transection to allow medial visualization for pedicle screw placement. The caudal part of the sacrospinalis muscle can be mobilized either medially or laterally for the placement of iliac screws. The entry points for the iliac screws are located on the medial aspect of the posterior superior and posterior inferior iliac spines (PSIS and PIIS).

35.11 Lumbopelvic Reduction and Fixation Techniques

The authors' preferred technique in reducing and stabilizing H-shaped sacral fractures is described in the following section.

35.11.1 Instrumentation

The method for lumbopelvic fixation includes two pairs of 6 mm lumbar pedicle screws, bilateral 6 mm longitudinal rods, one (or two) transverse connector, and two pairs of 8 mm iliac screws.

Additionally, the complete set of pelvic reduction forceps should be available, especially a large laminar spreader, large pelvic reduction forceps (pointed reduction forceps, Weber, Verbrugge, and angled jaw clamps), and a laminectomy tray and setup for potential sacral nerve root decompression.

A cell saver should be considered [54].

35.11.2 Lumbar Pedicle Screw Placement

The L4 and L5 pedicle screws are inserted. Techniques for pedicle screw placement in the lumbar spine are well described. The L5 pedicle access point is identified directly lateral to the L4/5 facet joint. A free hand technique is commonly used. 3D computer-assisted navigation might facilitate screw placement (see Chap. 39). Typical screw sizes range from 6 to 7.5 mm in diameter (6 mm most often used) and 40–55 mm in length in the lower lumbar spine. A pilot hole is placed at the junction of the pars interarticularis with the transverse process and the superior articular process of the segment of interest.

35.11.3 Longitudinal Rods

Longitudinal rods are secured to L4 and L5 pedicle screws after having been contoured to accommodate the lumbosacral lordosis and to lie close to the posterior lamina of the

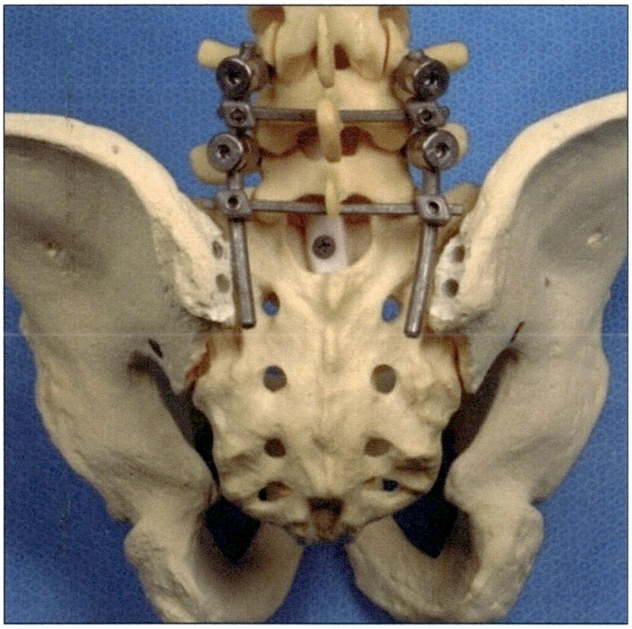

Fig. 35.8 Two pairs of lumbar pedicle screws are inserted into L4-L5. Longitudinal rods are secured to L4 and L5 pedicle screws after having been contoured to accommodate the lumbosacral lordosis. One transverse connecting rod between longitudinal rods is used to secure the fixation

sacrum and medial to the PSISs, and, therefore, adjacent to the intended starting point for the iliac screws (Fig. 35.8).

The authors' preferred technique is to fix the rods to lumbar pedicle screws before final fracture reduction. The rods should be long enough to reach down to at least the PIIS level after reduction. The initial vertical displacement of both hemipelves should be taken into account when measuring the length of the rods.

35.11.4 Connecting Rod

One transverse connecting rod between longitudinal rods is used to secure the fixation. In some rare cases, two rods might be used to increase the stability of lumbopelvic fixation (Fig. 35.8).

35.11.5 Fracture Reduction

Several concepts for reduction of the spinopelvic deformity are presented in the literature.

Ruatti et al. recommended initial closed reduction with bilateral transcondylar traction (15% of BW) in the supine position on a slightly Trendelenburg-like inclined table, especially in multiple injured patients, where no primary definitive treatment is possible [10]. Additional hyperlordosis using padding of the lumbosacral junction can support the reduction maneuver. Feeling of hearing of a cracking sound indicates reduction [10].

Plitz et al. performed intraoperative reduction with elevating the entire trunk by inflating an air bag, positioned under the chest, for kyphosis compensation [56].

Williams et al. recommend traction as the first reduction maneuver in the prone position, which is performed under fluoroscopic visualization. With the iliac and lumbar screws in place, manipulation is also possible by inserting the corresponding screw drivers to manipulate the pelvis against the spine. Longitudinal traction and kyphosis reduction are possible by additionally using a distraction instrument [53].

Starantzis et al. proposed a further step-by-step reduction concept [57]:

- Ipsilateral insertion of the L4 pedicle screw and the iliac screw
- Ipsilateral rod connection to the pedicle and iliac screw performing ipsilateral distraction and some sagittal alignment
- Contralateral L4 and L5 pedicle screw and iliac screw insertion
- Contralateral rod connection to the iliac screw
- Simultaneous and alternate tightening of the pedicle screws (bilaterally) for definitive sagittal reduction
- Final contralateral screw tightening and ipsilateral rod exchange for L5 pedicle screw insertion

We propose operative reduction and correction of displacements and rotational deformities of both hemipelves and the caudal segment of the sacrum using two pairs of pointed reduction clamps and caudal distraction of the distal part of the sacrum [3, 44, 45]:

- The distal end of the longitudinal rods and the superior aspect of the posterior iliac crests are the insertion points for the first pair of pointed reduction forceps bilaterally.
- The longitudinal rods fixed to pedicle screws act as a counter force for the final vertical correction of the sacral fracture components.
- Reduction of the hemipelves into a dorsal direction by traction is performed by the second pair of pointed reduction forceps (Fig. 35.9).
- Simultaneous longitudinal femoral traction (manual) and hyperextension of both hip joints facilitate reduction of vertical translation and sagittal plane flexion deformity [3, 44, 45, 54]; a distractor can additionally be used (Fig. 35.10).
- Reduction of lateral translation (diastasis, when present) in vertical fracture lines using pelvic reduction forceps placed on the outer surface of the PSIS and the longitudinal rod [3, 44, 45].
- Insertion of two pairs of 8 mm iliac screws adjacent to the prepositioned rod into the iliac bones with the Galveston technique [51].

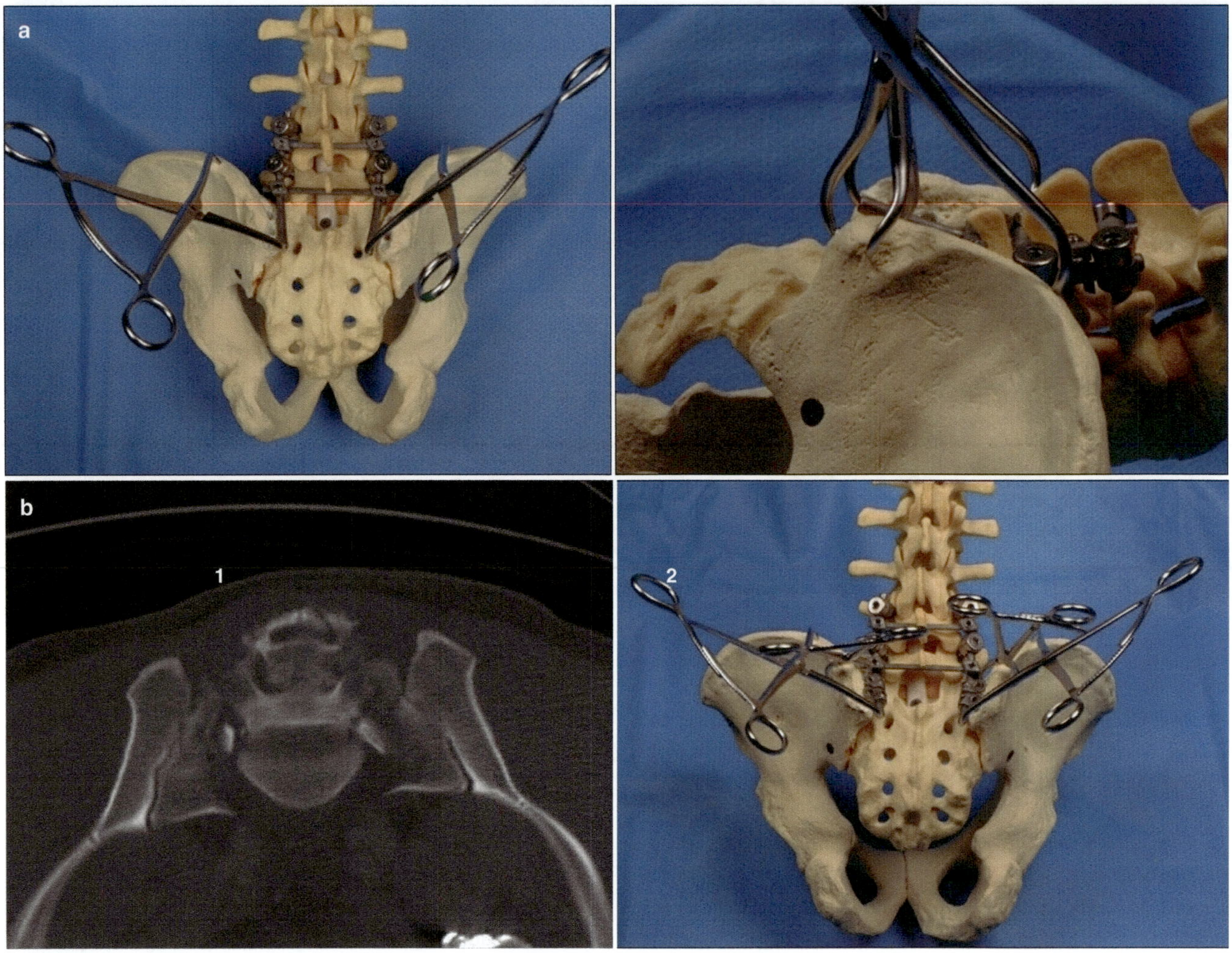

Fig. 35.9 (**a**) The operative reduction of cranial displacement in the vertical fracture lines is performed with reduction clamps and caudal distraction of the distal part of the sacrum. The longitudinal rods fixed to pedicle screws act as a counterforce for the final vertical correction of both hemipelvis. (**b**) Simultaneous reduction of the hemipelvis into a dorsal direction by traction is performed by the second pair of reduction clamps. Simultaneous bilateral manual femoral traction and hyperextension of both hip joints are also used

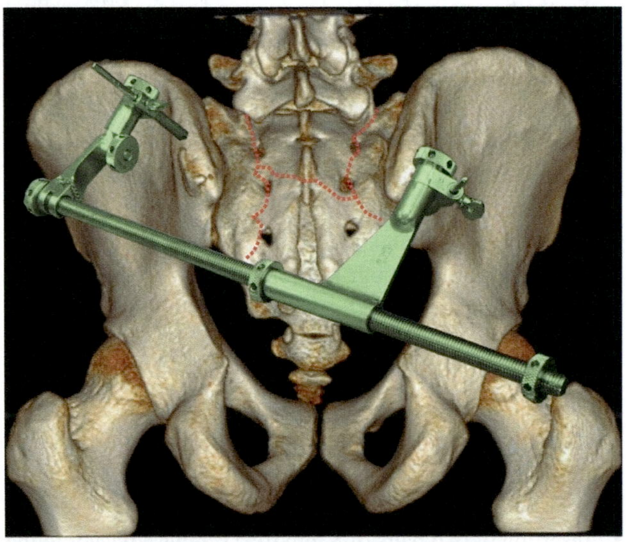

Fig. 35.10 Fracture disimpaction and longitudinal traction can be performed using a distractor

- Image intensification control with pelvic AP, inlet, outlet, and true lateral views.
- When accurate reduction is obtained, iliac screws are connected to the longitudinal rods with offset connectors.
- Fine tuning of reduction of vertical displacement might be performed with a spinal distraction instrument by temporarily loosening offset connectors for the iliac screws, producing distraction between the iliac screws and the transverse connector or the lowest pedicle screw with specific distractor, and retightening the offset connectors.

If anterior pelvic ring injury is not reduced and fixed first, additional reduction maneuvers might be needed:

- External rotation deformity—reduction of external hemipelvic rotation deformity using a laterally applied ball spike pusher pushing on the outer table of the ilium or using a “joystick” screw [54] (Fig. 35.11).

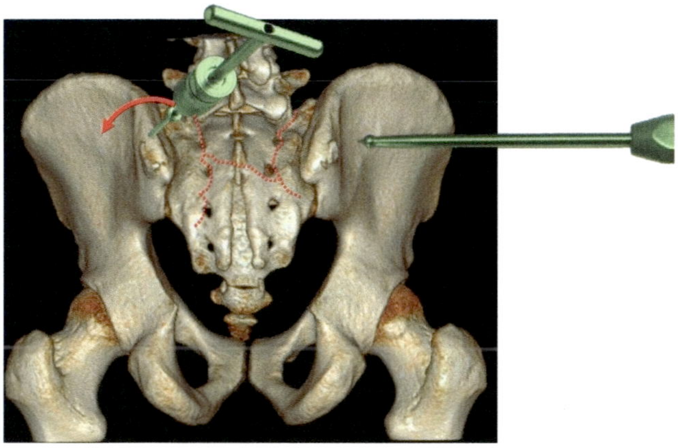

Fig. 35.11 Reduction of external hemipelvic rotation deformity can be controlled by lateral application of a ball spike pusher or using a "joystick" screw

- Transverse component—Kapandji-like reduction maneuver using an elevator (Fig. 35.12).

35.11.6 Iliac Screw Placement

Placement of the iliac screws adjacent to the precontoured and prepositioned rod eliminate the more difficult rod-contouring required when pedicle screws and iliac screws are placed independently before rod application. The entry point for iliac screw placement is located in the cleft between the posterior cortex of the sacrum and the PSIS. This essentially promotes a direct pathway into the bone corridor between the PSIS and anterior inferior iliac spine (AIIS). This technique allows for a lower profile construct and less muscle detachment from the PSISs (Fig. 35.13). The pathway is located by directing a pedicle probe 15° laterally and about 30° caudally. The second iliac screw can be positioned either in parallel, adjacent to the first screw, or is started at a point cephalad to the optimal PSIS-AIIS path and aimed from the iliac tubercle to the AIIS, yielding a triangular configuration (Fig. 35.14).

Alternatively, direct iliac screw placement can be performed by removal of some of bone at the level of the PSIS and then introduction of the screw between the inner and outer tables of the iliac bone.

Visualization of the bone trajectory cephalad to the sciatic notch is performed using the obturator oblique outlet ("teardrop") view (Fig. 35.15) [58–60].

35.11.7 Supplemental Fixation

In patients with a sacral fracture combined with an anterior pelvic injury, a staged reconstruction is performed.

A reconstruction of the anterior part of the pelvic ring is recommended to be performed first, and this is followed by posterior lumbopelvic fixation.

Supplemental internal fixation can be achieved with sacroiliac screws (Figs. 35.5 and 35.16) or posterior sacral or ilio-iliacal plates to maintain fracture reduction while the lumbopelvic fixation is applied or to secure the lumbopelvic fixation.

35.12 Nerve Root Decompression

Laminotomy and foraminotomy, anterior bone disimpaction, and lumbosacral plexus neurolysis can result in sacral nerve root decompression [36].

Lumbopelvic (lumboiliac) fixation allows complete neurological decompression through sacral laminectomy as needed and can enhance the surgeon's ability to perform an open reduction of a displaced sacral vertebral body.

Decompressing a neural injury indirectly with fracture reduction and/or directly with a sacral laminectomy remains controversial [36, 61]. The indications for sacral laminectomy are variable, and no clinical consensus exists [3, 4, 36, 39, 41, 46].

If performed early within the first 24–72 h following injury, a beneficial effect can be expected [62]. However, early surgical decompression may be associated with an increased risk of hemorrhage, wound healing complications due to soft tissue injuries, and possibly to cerebrospinal fluid leak from dural tears [36]. Isolated surgical decompression is rarely indicated [36].

Decompressing a neural injury indirectly with fracture reduction and/or directly with a sacral laminectomy remains controversial. The indications for sacral laminectomy are variable, and no clinical consensus exists [3, 4, 36, 39, 41, 46].

Some authors advocate routine sacral nerve root decompression when a neurological deficit is present or expected [2, 5, 9, 62, 63], while others avoid decompression as irreparable nerve injuries were expected [64–67] and partial or even full recovery is possible without decompression [35, 46, 68, 69].

Neural recovery of transected or avulsed sacral nerve roots is unlikely [36]. Traumatically transected sacral nerve roots are commonly associated with Roy-Camille and Lindahl et al. type 2b and type 3b transverse sacral fracture types (Denis zone III injuries). Avulsions of the lumbopelvic plexus are associated with severely displaced transforaminal vertical sacral fractures (Denis zone II injuries). Surgical decompression may be less useful in these patients with transected lumbosacral nerve roots. Huittinen observed nerve root transection in 35% after transverse sacral fractures [70].

There is only one study comparing patients with or without sacral nerve root decompression in unstable sacral fracture with a neurological deficit. Zelle et al. analyzed the results of six patients with surgical decompression and seven patients without surgical decompression. At an average follow-up of 27.1 months, surgical decompression resulted in

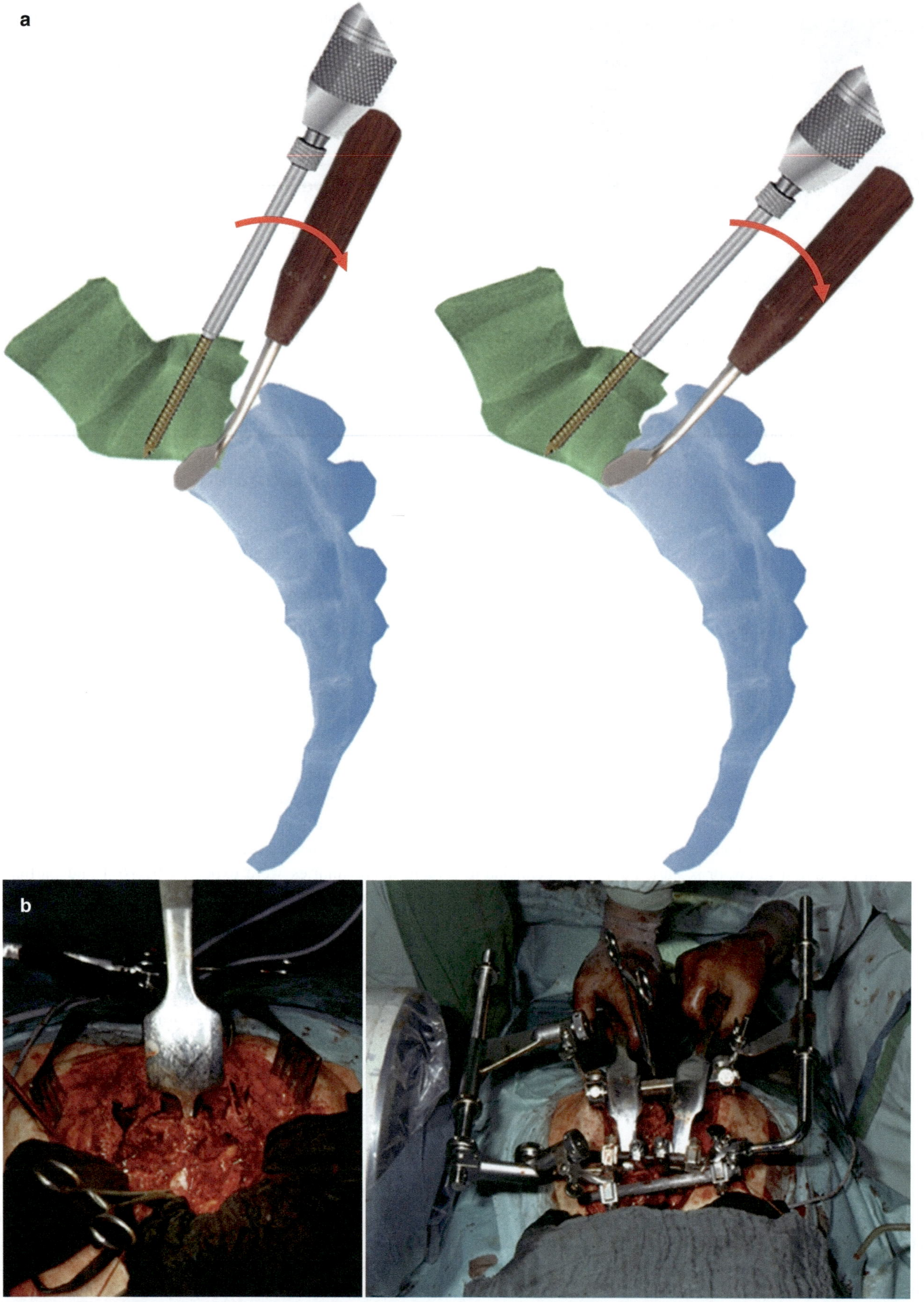

Fig. 35.12 (a) Kapandji-like reduction of the transverse fracture component and intraoperative view using two blunt elevators. (b) Intraoperative Kapandji-like reduction of the transverse fracture component and intraoperative view using one or two blunt elevators

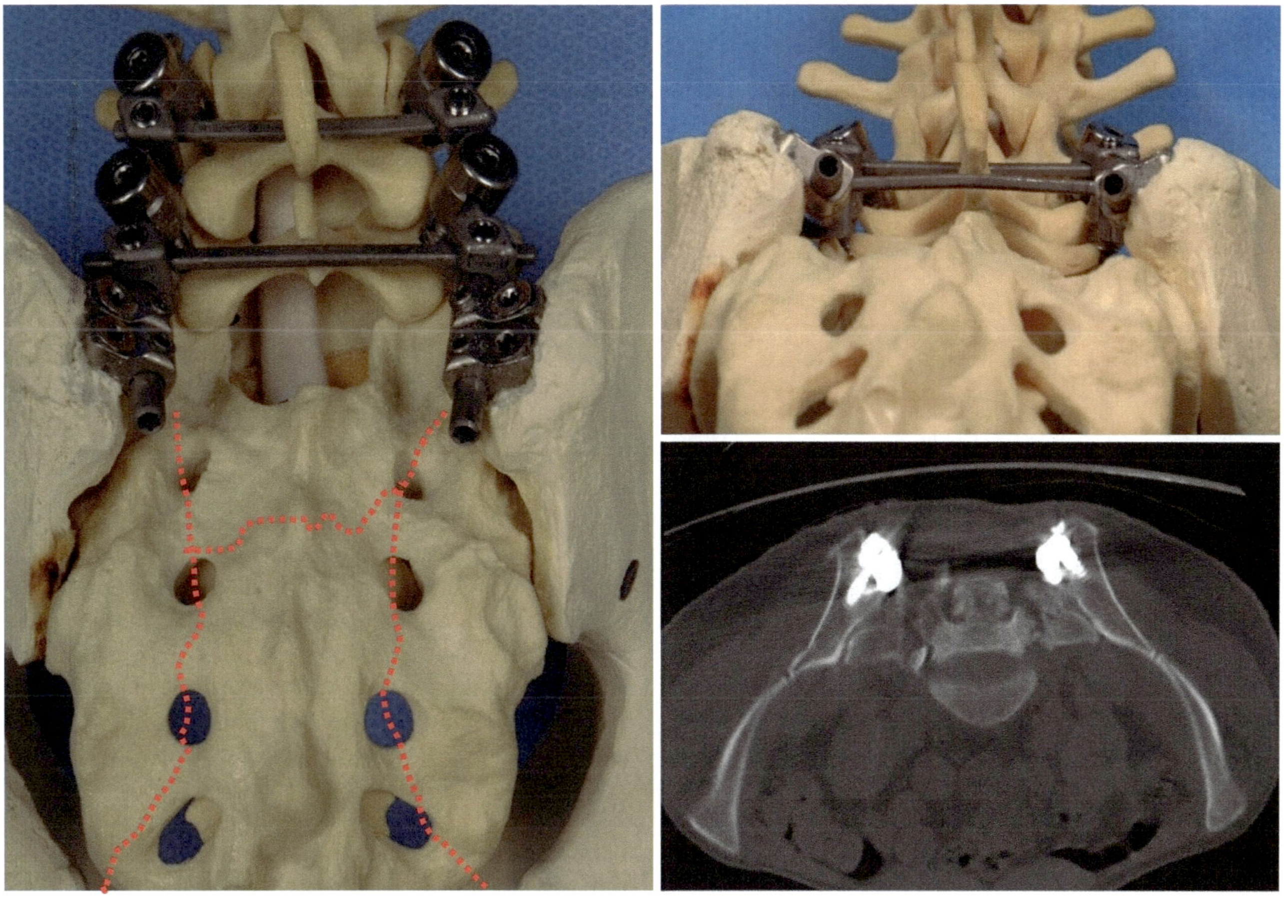

Fig. 35.13 When accurate reduction is obtained, the lumbar spine and central upper sacral segment is fixed to the pelvic ring by placing two pairs of 8 mm iliac screws into the iliac bones with the Galveston technique and connecting them to the longitudinal rods with offset connectors

optimized neurological improvement and better physical function (SF-36 analysis) [11]. However, this was not a prospective randomized comparative study.

Indirect decompression of the lumbosacral (vertical fracture lines) and sacral neural roots (the transverse fracture line) is achieved through reduction and stable fixation of all the main sacral fracture components.

> Accurate reduction of all sacral fracture components is probably the most important part of the surgical procedure for sacral nerve root decompression.

In the follow-up study by Lindahl et al. [3], all 36 patients with an H-shaped sacral fracture showed some evidence of neurological recovery, except one that had a thoracic spinal fracture and a spinal cord injury. Direct decompression by sacral laminectomy was performed for all completely displaced transverse sacral fracture with occlusion of the central sacral canal and in the patients in which a clear translational displacement remained in the transverse fracture line after the final reduction as assessed by a true lateral sacral fluoroscopic view. In cases with comminuted sacral lamina (floating dorsal sacrum) and/or good sagittal alignment after the final reduction, sacral laminectomy was not performed. Cauda equina syndrome was present in 29 patients (81%). Of these patients, nearly two-thirds experienced full neurological recovery of bladder and bowel functions. One-third of the patients had permanent bladder and bowel impairment, with no recovery, based on the Gibbons criteria [65]. The Gibbons score did not improve in 11 of 16 patients (69%) with complete translational fracture displacements in the transverse sacral fracture. Those results suggested that a shearing injury had transected the sacral nerve roots. For those patients, sacral laminectomy did not improve the outcome of bladder and bowel function. However, in five patients (31%) with complete fracture displacement, the Gibbons score improved, probably due to a less severe neuropraxic type of sacral nerve root injury. In those five cases, a sacral laminectomy most likely had a positive influence on recovery. Of 36 patients, 7 (19%) underwent a full neurological recovery. Eight patients (22%) were left with sensory deficits, while nine patients (25%) had motor and sensory deficits in the lower extremities. Twelve patients (33%) had permanent cauda equina deficits.

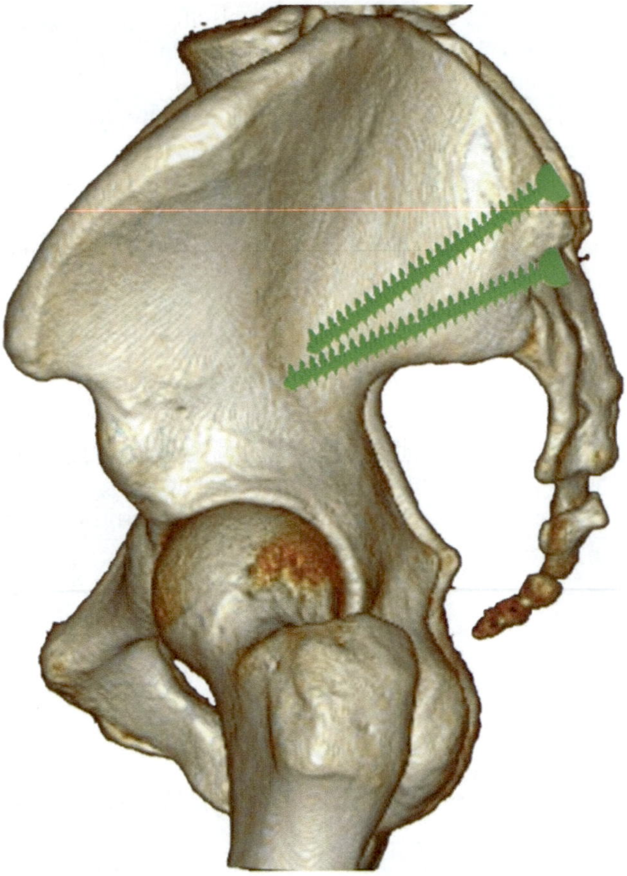

Fig. 35.14 Possible screw trajectories using one or two screws

Consistent with these results, a recent study by Lehman et al. revealed that almost one-third of patients reported residual bladder and bowel dysfunctions [71].

When sacral laminectomy was performed as a standard procedure for all sacral fractures, regardless of the initial degree of fracture displacement, no improvement was observed in the rate of neurological recovery [4]. Therefore, the sacral laminectomy seemed to be indicated in cases of completely displaced transverse sacral fractures due to occlusion of the central sacral canal at the level of the transverse sacral fracture [3]. Although it is difficult to evaluate the effect of surgical decompression on neurological recovery, particular attention should be paid to achieving indirect neural decompression by performing a sacral fracture reduction as accurately as possible.

During sacral laminectomy, an attempt should be made to repair any dural tears that are encountered to minimize the chances of a pseudomeningocele developing [36]. In the presence of satisfactory lumbopelvic stabilization but persistent spinal canal or neuroforaminal compromise, a focal limited decompression may be performed within the first 2 weeks after injury with use of a limited midline exposure and fluoroscopy-guided focal laminectomy [8].

We recommend surgical decompression [3]:

- For all type 2b and 3b transverse sacral fractures
- For type 2a and 3a transverse sacral fractures, when a perioperative true lateral fluoroscopy shows severe nar-

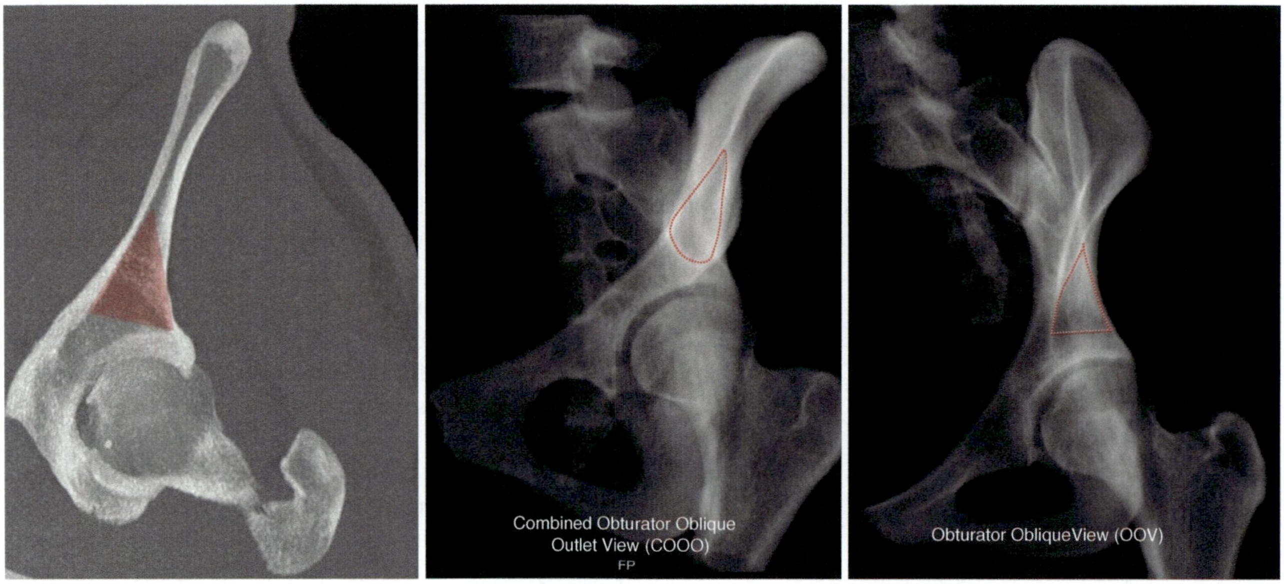

Fig. 35.15 CT-anatomy of the supraacetabular bone corridor for iliac screw placement and recommended intraoperative x-rays to confirm optimal screw placement

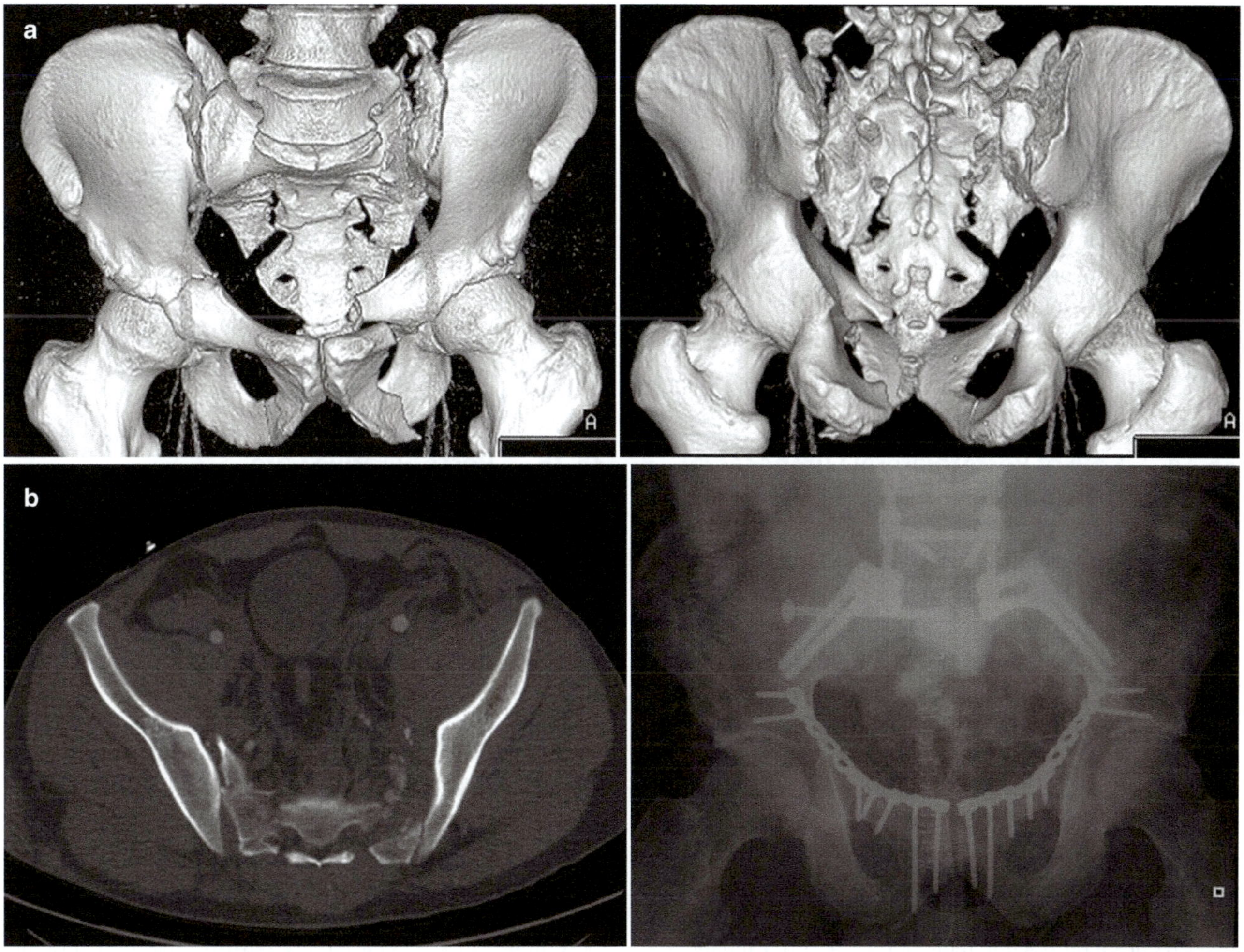

Fig. 35.16 (**a**) Treatment of an H-shaped sacral fracture with spinopelvic dissociation in a 34-year-old male who was run over by a car. Bilateral rami fractures associated with the H-shaped sacral fracture are shown in 3D-reconstructed images of the anterior and the posterior pelvis. (**b**) Contrast-enhanced CT image shows the bilaterally fractured posterior ring structure. X-ray image shows the result of the two-stage pelvic reconstruction. The first stage consisted of anterior pelvic ring fixation; the second stage consisted of a segmental lumbopelvic fixation. An additional iliosacral screw was placed with the percutaneous technique to fix the transiliac fracture dislocation of the right SI joint

rowing of the central sacral canal, following fracture reduction and lumbopelvic fixation

Improvement in neurological impairment can be expected after surgical treatment, but it is not clear whether sacral laminectomy improves neurological recovery compared to indirect decompression with sacral fracture reduction alone [3, 4, 39, 41, 46]. The definitive surgical treatment of spinopelvic dissociation injuries should be performed at the earliest point after emergent treatment of other organ systems has been adequately addressed and the patient is physiologically stable for sacral fracture surgery.

35.13 Timing of Surgery

Early realignment of the sacrum, restoration of spinopelvic stability, and decompression of the nerve roots are thought to provide the best possible environment for neurological recovery. However, several days are often required to optimize patient physiological status after severe blood loss, and hemodynamic instability, or severe concomitant injuries, before it is possible to perform definitive surgical treatment for a spinopelvic dissociation [4, 33].

Schildhauer et al. [4] reported that they did not find any association between the timing of decompression and the degree of neurological recovery. Similarly, in the study by Lindahl et al. [3], the timing of lumbopelvic fixation and neurologic decompression was not associated with neurological recovery or clinical outcome. However, Ayoub reported better neurological recovery when primary decompression was made within 8 days from the trauma [39].

Definitive surgical treatment should be performed only after the patient is stabilized and when they can tolerate a prolonged operation with a potential for marked perioperative blood loss. In addition, it may benefit the outcome to delay treatment until an orthopaedic surgeon with sufficient expertise is available.

35.14 Role of Posterolateral Lumbosacral Arthrodesis

In the series of Schildhauer et al. [4], posterolateral arthrodesis across the instrumented lumbosacral levels was carried out by decorticating the facet joints, lumbar transverse processes and sacral ala, and applying the morcellized laminectomized bone to the lateral gutters bilaterally.

Ayoub made posterolateral arthrodesis across the instrumented levels only in case of direct decompression by sacral laminectomy (50% of patients) [39].

Lindahl et al. performed lumbopelvic fixation without posterolateral arthrodesis at the lumbosacral junction [3].

In all these series, segmental lumbopelvic fixation provided sufficient stability for bony union with no postoperative loss of sacral fracture reduction [3, 4, 39]. Lindahl et al. reported asymptomatic late breakage (fatigue fracture) of components of the lumbopelvic fixator in 33% of patients without any effect on the end radiological or clinical results [3]. This result was consistent with the findings by Bellabarba et al. [40], who reported asymptomatic rod fractures in 31% of patients, even when posterolateral arthrodesis had been performed.

> Based on the current literature, lumbopelvic fixation appears to be sufficiently stable without posterolateral arthrodesis.

35.15 Fragility H-Shaped Sacral Fracture with Spinopelvic Dissociation

Rommens and Hofmann recommend surgical treatment in FFP type 3 and 4 injuries, if the patient is not able to mobilize out of bed during the first 3–5 days despite pain therapy or if increasing dislocation of fracture fragments during the early follow-up period is noticed [32]. FFP type 4b fractures of the sacrum might be treated with minimally invasive fracture fixation, either by transsacral screws or bilateral iliosacral screws [32, 72]. H- or U-type fracture patterns functionally represent spinopelvic dissociation. These injuries are unstable and should be fixed in a minimal invasive way in cases with no or only slight displacement. However, if gross displacement is present, lumbopelvic stabilization is recommended (Fig. 35.17). In FFP with a concomitant displaced anterior pelvic ring injury, anterior fixation is also recommended [73]. However, if FFP is diagnosed with delay and a strong callus formation in the anterior part of the pelvis is visible, the rami fractures can be treated nonoperatively.

35.16 Postoperative Care

Lumbopelvic fixation provides adequate stability to permit early bed-to-chair transfer and sitting. Ambulation and weight bearing after lumbopelvic fixation of spinopelvic dissociations are possible within pain limits and when allowed by the associated lower extremity injuries.

35.17 Long-Term Results of Lumbopelvic Fixation in Spinopelvic Dissociation Injuries

Because of the rarity and heterogeneous nature of sacral fractures with spinopelvic dissociation, published studies of these injuries have been largely retrospective in nature and have involved mostly small treatment groups.

Siebkler et al. analyzed the results of conservative treatment in 11 patients with Denis Zone III injuries consisting of 6 Roy-Camille type I and 5 type II injuries with a mean kyphotic angle of 57°. At a mean of 43 months, all fractures were healed but six patients showed an increased kyphotic angle, without influence on short-term outcome. Two patients presented with early neurological deterioration requiring sacral decompression. Complete bowel and bladder loss improved to voluntary sphincter control in all three cases. Overall, eight patients reported residual bowel, bladder, and/or sexual dysfunction and all had some lower back pain [74].

Additionally, few factors have been identified that are associated with outcomes after operative treatment.

Most of high-energy H-shaped (and T-, and Y-shaped) sacral fractures are stabilized with a lumbopelvic fixation construct. Bilateral iliosacral screw fixation or nonoperative treatment is recommended by some authors but only in nondisplaced or minimally displaced injuries. However, in low-energy fragility fractures of the sacrum with spinopelvic dissociation, minimal invasive fixation techniques are recommended [7, 32, 72].

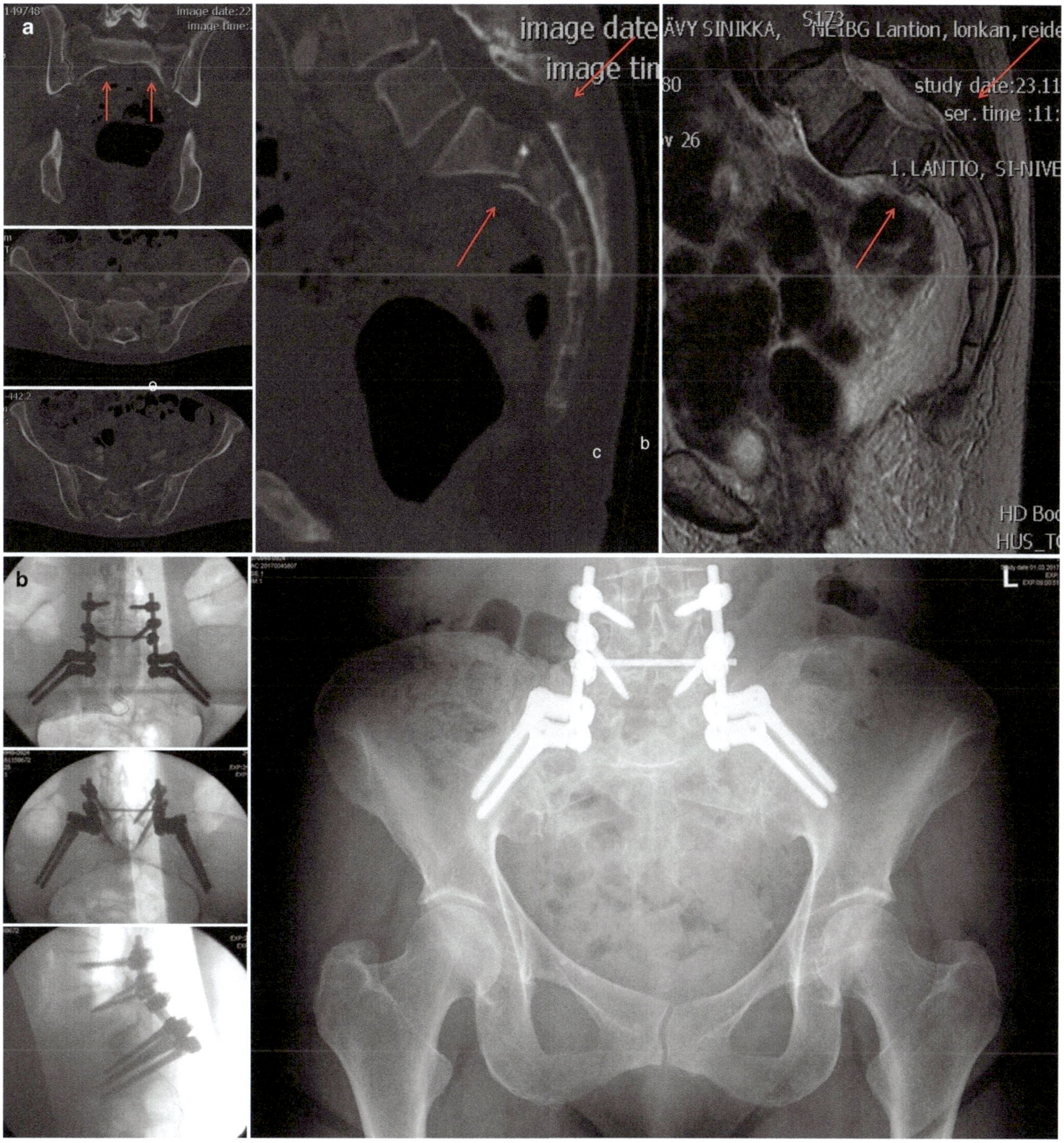

Fig. 35.17 (**a**) Lumbopelvic fixation of an FFS type IVb with spinopelvic dissociation in a 70-year-old female. CT images and sagittal MRI images show the bilaterally fractured sacrum with a type 2a transverse sacral fracture after a falling accident. (**b**) Lumbopelvic fixation was performed due to severe pain problems and inability to walk. Full weight bearing was allowed after surgery and pelvis x-ray 6 months later shows good alignment. (**c**) CT images 2 years postoperatively show good fracture healing. The clinical outcome was good

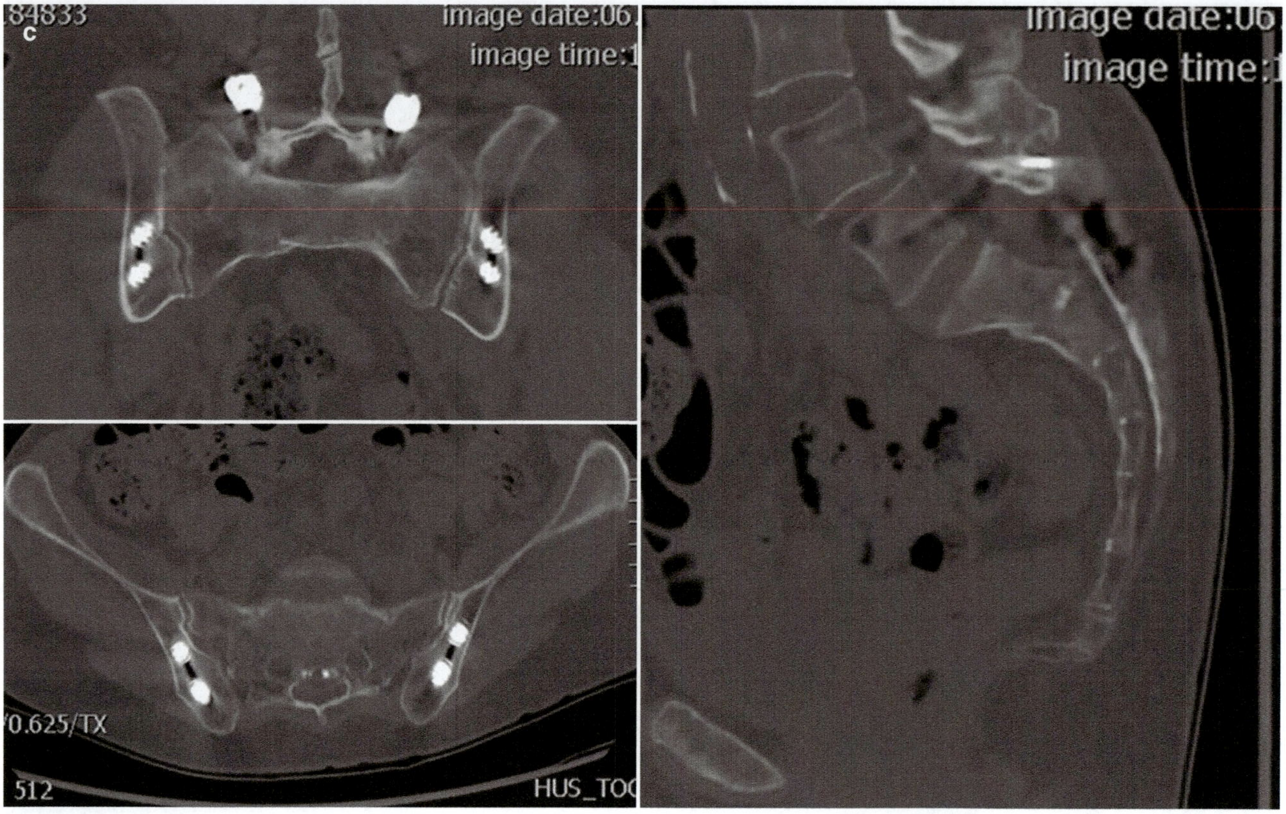

Fig. 35.17 (continued)

- Schildhauer et al. treated 19 patients with open reduction, surgical neural element decompression with sacral laminectomy, segmental lumbopelvic stabilization, and lumbosacral posterolateral arthrodesis [4]. The stabilization construct consisted of a bilateral lumbopelvic (iliac) internal fixator connected with a transverse bar. Fifteen of these patients had an H-shaped sacral fracture, two patients a U-shaped, and two patients a Y-shaped sacral fracture. Seventeen patients were followed up for at least 12 months. Their kyphotic deformity was reduced from an average of 43° to 20°. No loss of reduction was seen at follow-up. Neurological recovery was observed in 83% of patients, with full recovery of bowel and bladder function in 47%.
- In an outcome study of 36 patients with an H-shaped sacral fracture, Lindahl et al. reported excellent (displacement ≤5 mm, 19 patients) or good (displacement ≤10 mm, 17 patients) radiological end results in all cases in the vertical sacral fractures [3]. Postoperatively there was no loss of sacral fracture reduction (Figs. 35.18, 35.19, and 35.20). Kyphosis in the transverse sacral fracture improved from a mean of 38° to 22°, and the translational displacement improved from a mean of 15 to 6 mm. Postoperatively, there was no loss of sacral fracture reduction. They found a significant association between the radiological and clinical outcomes. Patients with anatomical or near-anatomical reductions had a better clinical outcome than those with >5 mm residual displacement in the vertical sacral fracture lines. In addition, both the residual postoperative AP translation and kyphosis of the transverse sacral fracture were smaller in patients with good clinical outcomes than in those with poor outcomes. At least some neurological recovery was observed in 34 out of 35 patients with an associated sacral plexus injury. The only patient without any neurological improvement had the T12 burst fracture with associated paraplegia. Seventeen of 29 patients (59%) with a cauda equina injury (Gibbons grade 4) had full recovery of their bladder and bowel functions. Of 36 patients, 7 (19%) underwent a full neurological recovery, 8 (22%) were left with sensory deficits, while 9 (25%) had motor and sensory deficits in the lower extremities, and 12 (33%) had permanent cauda equina deficits. An accurate reduction of all fracture components was associated with better clinical outcome.
- Sapkas et al. presented long-term results after operative treatment of anterior displaced transverse spinopelvic dissociation sacral fractures in five patients with a minimum follow-up of 5 years (5–24 years) [75]. Four patients had plate or rod stabilization. Neurological recovery was graded almost complete in one patient and incomplete in the remaining patients.

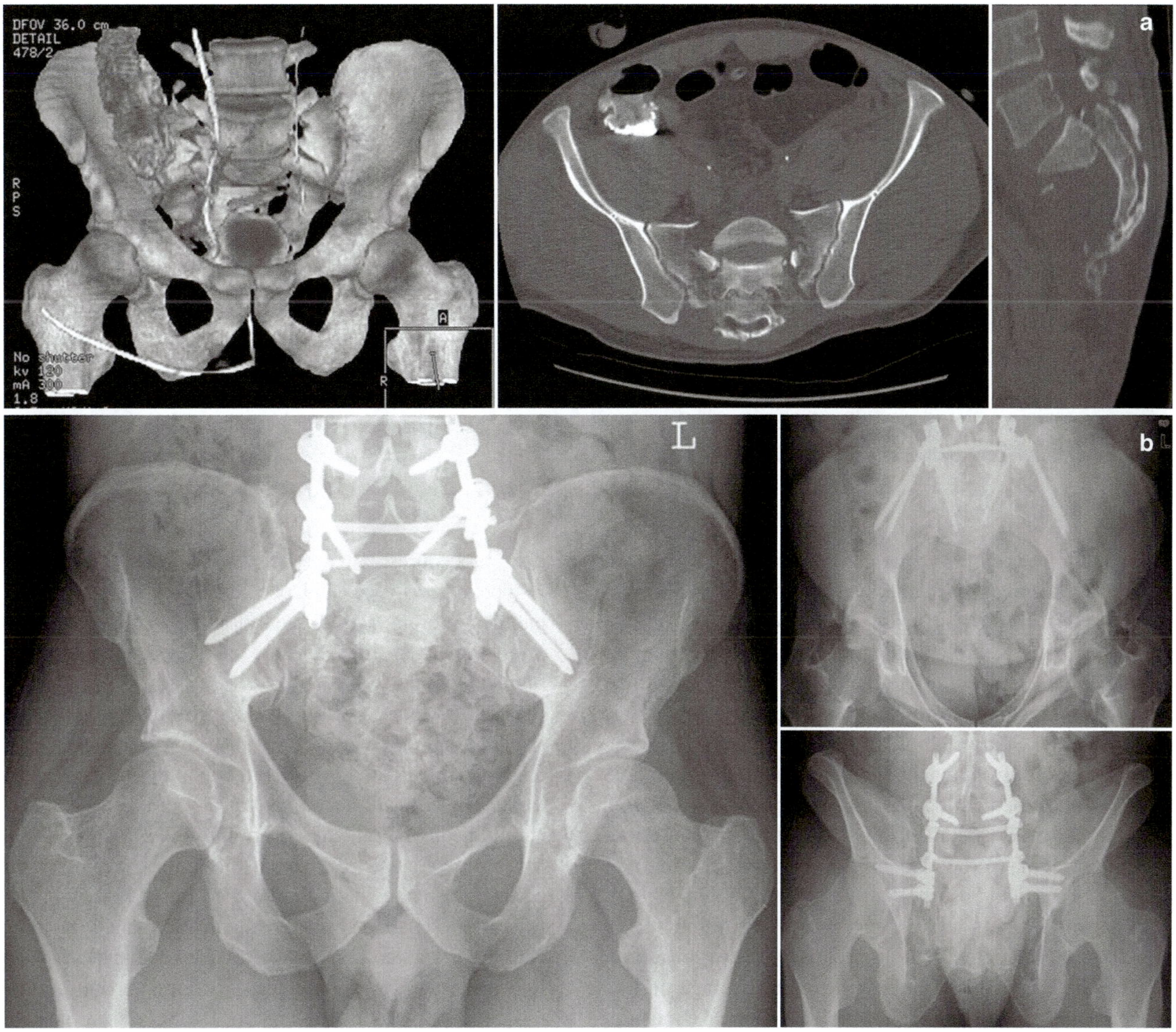

Fig. 35.18 (**a**) Management of an H-shaped sacral fracture with spino-pelvic dissociation without an anterior pelvic ring injury in a 37-year-old male, who fell from the fifth floor. 3D-image reconstruction and CT image show displaced bilateral vertical transforaminal sacral fractures, which caused L5 and S1 nerve root injuries and resulted in severe motor deficiencies of the lower legs. The sagittal CT image shows a type 3b transverse sacral fracture with complete translational fracture displacement between S1 and S2. (**b**) Postoperative AP, Inlet and Outlet x-ray views show the results of pelvic reconstruction. Treatment included an operative reduction and lumbopelvic fixation with sacral laminectomy, performed 5 days later, when the patient was hemodynamically stable. A clear neurological recovery was detected, and after long rehabilitation, the patient was able to return back to work. (**c**) At the end of follow-up, 6 years from the accident, the patient had no pain, but reported deficiencies in micturition and slight bowel incontinence; therefore, the POS clinical outcome was graded fair. CT examination showed healing of the fractures

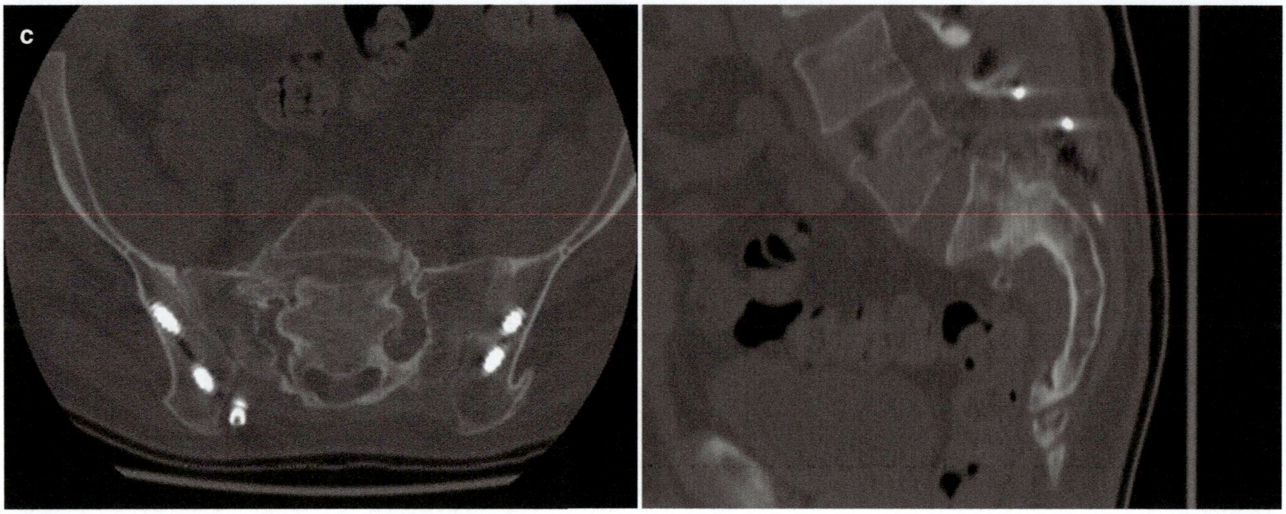

Fig. 35.18 (continued)

- Ayoub followed up 28 patients with spinopelvic dissociation and sacral cauda equina syndrome treated with spinopelvic fixation [39]. In this series, 96% of cases had partial or complete neurological recovery. Nineteen patients (68%) had excellent or good clinical outcome according to the outcome instrument of the German Pelvic Multicenter Study Groups (POS/GSM1 Scale). However, no severe fall from heights injuries were in this material.
- He et al. presented long-term results of 21 patients with lumbopelvic dissociation injuries, all treated with posterior sacral nerve root decompression, lumbopelvic internal fixation, and posterolateral fusion [76]. The mean OR time was 190 min with a mean blood loss of 960 mL. In 12 patients complete neurological recovery was observed. The Gibbons grading improved from an average of 3.43 preoperatively to 1.76 at latest follow-up after a mean of 20 months.
- Adelved et al. analyzed 13 patients (5× operative treatment, 8× nonoperative treatment) after a mean of 7.7 years [77]. Of five patients after lumbopelvic fixation, four had a persistent neurological deficit and a mean pain VAS of 5.2. The primary kyphosis decreased in three patients.
- De Iure et al. analyzed long-term results of ten consecutive patients after lumboiliac fixation [78]. Three patients had significant discomfort.
- Williams et al. presented the results of 17 patients after a mean of 21 months [53]. The mean operative time was 144 min with an average blood loss of 202 mL. Five patients had adequate reduction. One patient developed deep wound infection, requiring several debridements. At follow-up, 14 patients presented with normal bladder function.
- Jazini et al. reported on eight patients with minimally invasive lumbopelvic fixations [79]. The anterior pelvic ring was additionally stabilized in three cases using standard procedures. There were two T-type injuries, four H-type, one U-type, and one lambda-type injury. Four patients presented with neurological deficits and had improvement in three. In four cases, secondary implant removal was performed.
- Tian et al. reported on 18 consecutive patients who sustained a spinopelvic dissociation injury (mean age of 33.1 years) treated with lumbopelvic fixations and depending of an accompanying neurological injury, simultaneous sacral canal decompression (6 cases) [80]. In 16 cases, a fall resulted in this injury, while in two cases a traffic accident caused the injury. Ten U-shaped fractures, 6 H-shaped fractures, and 2 Y-shaped fractures were observed, corresponding to 12 type II and 6 type III injuries of the Roy-Camille classification. At a mean follow-up of 32.4 months all sacral fractures were healed. According to the Majeed score, 12 cases were graded excellent, 4× good, and 2 cases as fair. An anatomical reconstruction was observed in 11 cases, a satisfactory reduction in 6, and an unsatisfactory reduction in 1 case. The average Gibbons score improved from 2.5 to 1.4 at 24 months. There were five cases that had complications. Two wound complications were observed, which healed after local debridement, and one patient presented with deep wound infection. In two cases, implant removal became necessary due to prominent and mechanically disturbing implants.

According to the current literature, the most reliable surgical method for treatment of H-shaped (and T-, and Y-shaped) sacral fractures is segmental lumbopelvic fixation.

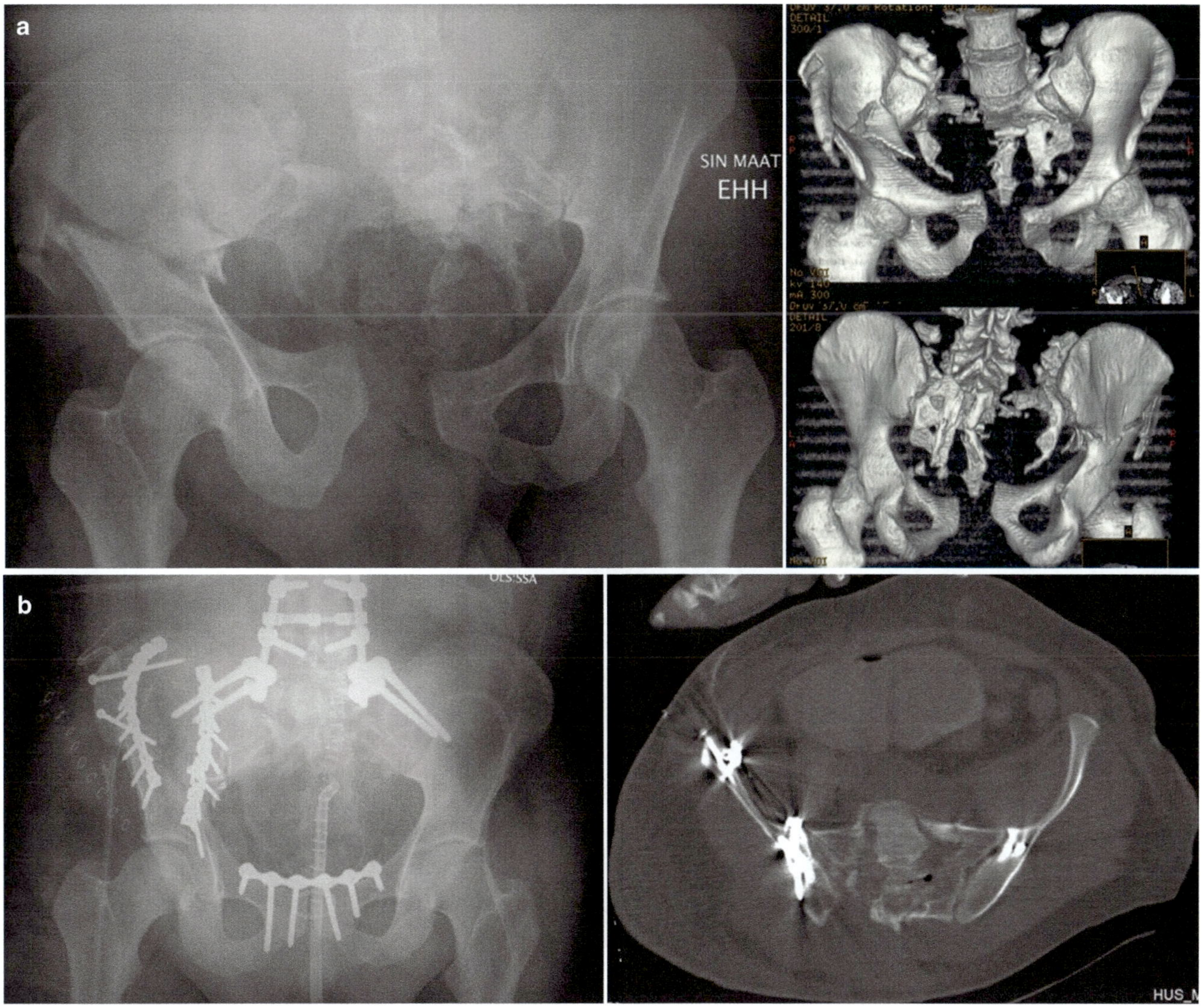

Fig. 35.19 (**a**) Two-stage reconstruction of a comminuted H-shaped sacral fracture with concomitant anterior and posterior pelvic fractures in a 27-year-old male after a jump from the fifth floor. The transverse sacral fracture was segmental with complete fracture displacement at S2 level and cauda equina deficits. (**b**) Concomitant injuries included a transiliac fracture and disruption of the symphysis pubis. A staged reconstruction was carried out; first, the symphysis pubis and the iliac wing were fixed in supine position followed by segmental lumbopelvic fixation and sacral laminectomy in prone position

Due to the limited amount of published cases, an evidence-based treatment strategy cannot be identified. Early realignment of the sacrum, restoration of spinopelvic stability, and decompression of the nerve roots could be a salvage option for displaced sacral fractures with spinopelvic instability and typical deformity of the bony elements.

35.18 Complications

Lumbopelvic fixation was associated with a relative low rate of complications in long-term sequelae [3, 39, 40].

In the study by Lindahl et al., no deep surgical site infection (SSI) with exposure of the hardware was diagnosed [3]. However, two superficial wound infections (6%) occurred after open fractures. These infections were treated with local wound therapy and antibiotics.

In a study of 19 patients with lumbopelvic fixation and sacral laminectomy, 5 patients (26%) developed wound healing problems [40]. Three of these were treated with surgical debridement in the operating room, and two were treated with local wound therapy, including hematoma or seroma evacuation. There were no lasting complications such as chronic osteomyelitis noted.

Ayoub reported wound infections in seven patients (25%) [39]. Three patients, who initially had Morel-Lavallée degloving soft tissue injury, were managed with wound washout and debridement. Hardware prominence

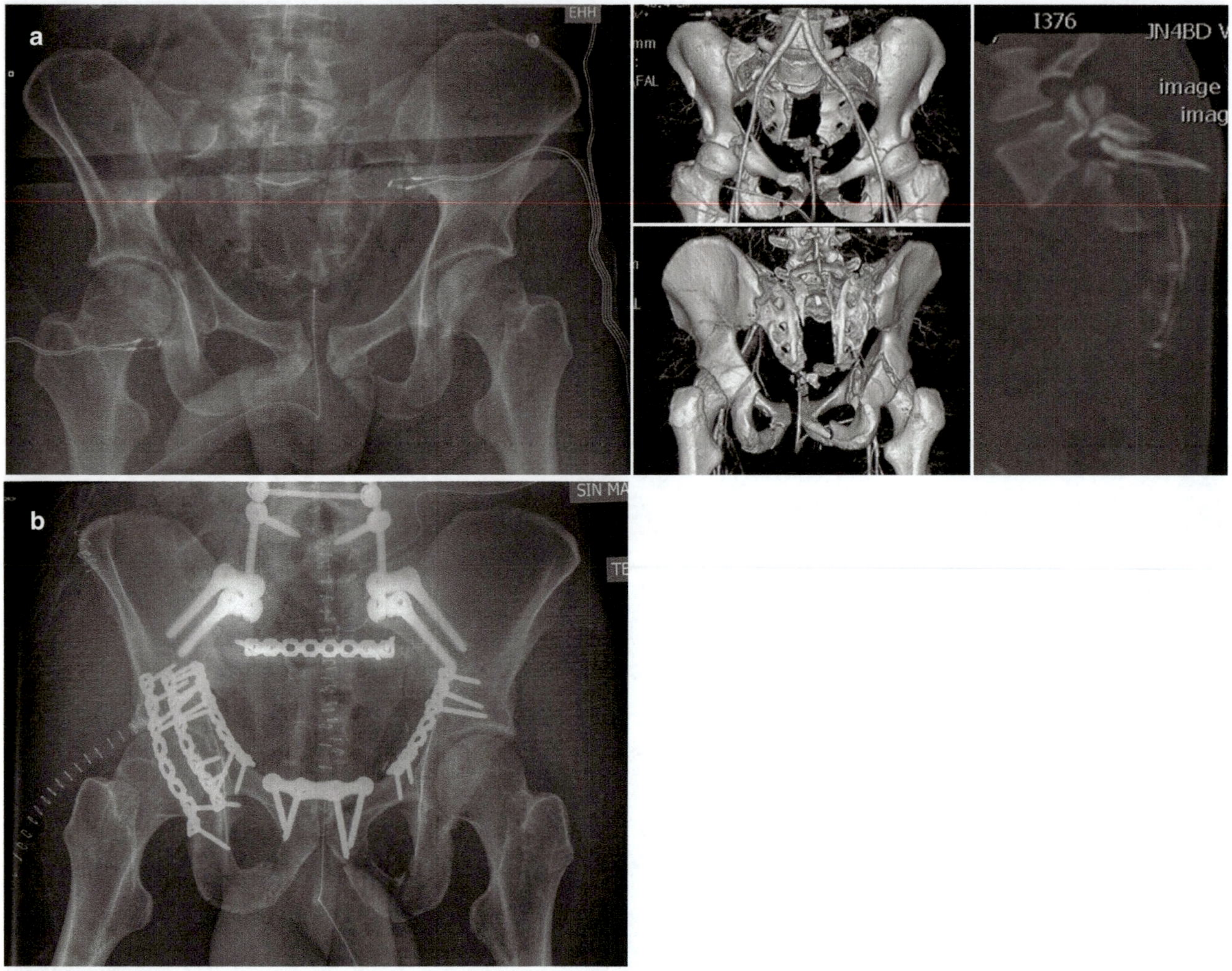

Fig. 35.20 (**a**) Three-stage reconstruction of a T-shaped sacral fracture with three major concomitant pelvic injuries, cauda equina injury, and bilateral L5-S1 nerve roots injuries in a 32-year-old male, who jumped from the fifth floor. Bilateral acetabular fractures, a T-type fracture on the right side, a low anterior column fracture on the left side, and disruption of the symphysis pubis associated with spinopelvic dissociation are shown in pelvis x-ray and 3D-reconstructed images of the anterior and the posterior pelvis. Sagittal CT image shows a comminuted type 3b transverse sacral fracture with complete translational fracture displacement at the level of S2. (**b**) Postoperative pelvic x-ray. The first stage consisted of anterior fixation of both acetabulum fractures and the symphysis pubis; the second stage consisted of a segmental lumbopelvic fixation and a supplemental transverse plate fixation of the sacrum, and the third stage consisted posterior fixation the right acetabulum. (**c**) Pelvis x-ray and lateral x-ray 2.5 years after the operation. The patient was able to walk without aids, had slight pelvic pain at rest (VAS 2-3/10), and reported slight deficiencies in micturition and slight bowel dysfunction

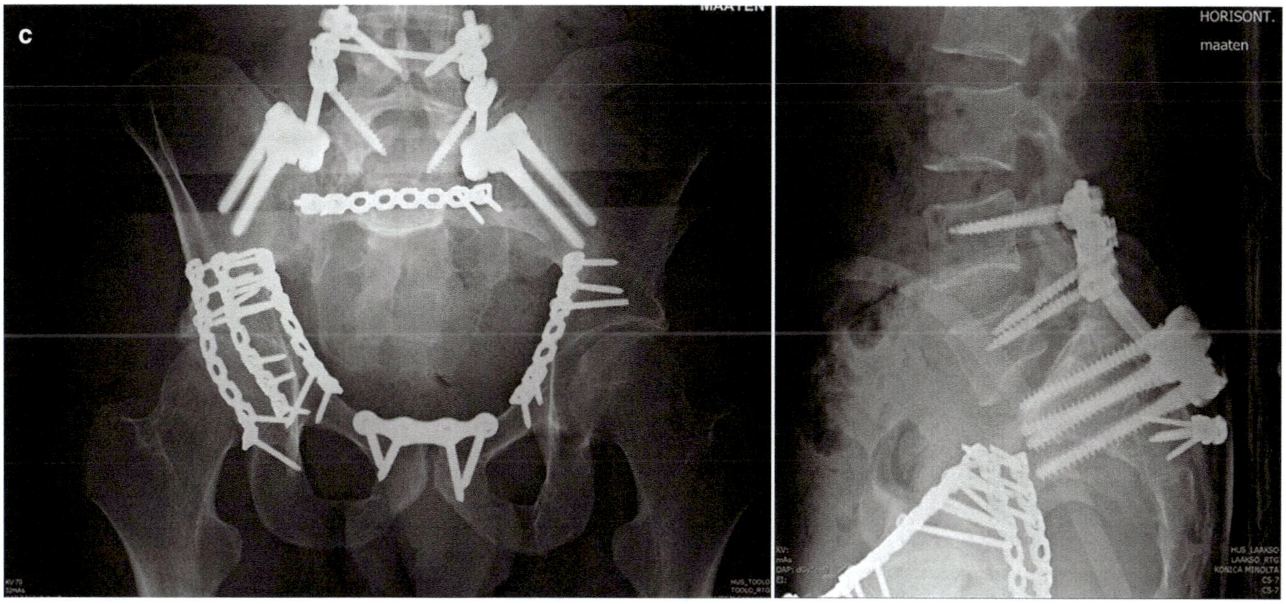

Fig. 35.20 (continued)

was documented in 18% of cases. Implant removal was made after 18 months.

> Posterior prominence of the iliac screws relative to the plane of the PSISs should be avoided.

Special attention should be paid to placing the longitudinal rods as close as possible to the dorsal surface of the sacrum, and medial to, but not posterior to, the PSIS; the starting points should be medialized and the heads of the iliac screws should be countersunk to avoid soft tissue and wound healing problems.

No neurological injuries related to operative treatment were diagnosed. No patients showed deterioration in the Gibbons score when the preoperative score was compared to the final follow-up score [3].

35.19 Late Reconstruction of Spinopelvic Dissociations

The diagnosis of traumatic spinopelvic dissociations is often missed or delayed due to the difficulty in imaging the upper sacrum and the transverse sacral fracture component with AP pelvis radiography. Angulation of a fractured sacral segment can produce a paradoxical inlet view of the upper sacrum on the standard AP pelvic radiograph [35] (Fig. 35.21). Delayed diagnosis is avoided by high clinical suspicion, early lateral sacral radiographs, and pelvic CT-based sagittal image reconstructions.

Even in cases with delay of several weeks from the trauma, surgical treatment should be considered. In the study of Lindahl et al. [3], three (8%) patients had late reconstructions (26, 29, and 34 days after the injury) because of delayed diagnosis ($n = 2$) or severe polytrauma ($n = 1$). In all of these late reconstructions the radiological end result was good (displacement ≤10 mm), and all of them had at least some neurologic recovery (Fig. 35.21).

Recently, Li et al. reported on 12 patients (5× type II, 3× type III, 4× type IV injuries according to Roy-Camille/Strange-Vognsen) with delayed treatment after a mean of 90 days [38]. An isolated posterior sacral canal decompression was performed without osteosynthesis. Nine patients had an additional anterior ring injury. All fractures healed. At the mean follow-up of 18 months, the mean Majeed score was 76 points (2× excellent, 5× good, 3× fair, 1× poor). The Gibbons score improved from an average of 2.8 to 1.9. Full recovery was observed in four patients and three patients had no recovery. The average subjective pain (VAS) value was 2.2. Two patients reported on sexual dysfunction.

35.20 Conclusions

- Sacral fracture with spinopelvic dissociation is a rare injury pattern.
- Neurologic impairments are present in nearly all cases.
- Open reduction along with lumbopelvic fixation (Fig. 35.22) is a reliable treatment method for displaced H-, T, and Y-shaped sacral fractures (Fig. 35.23).

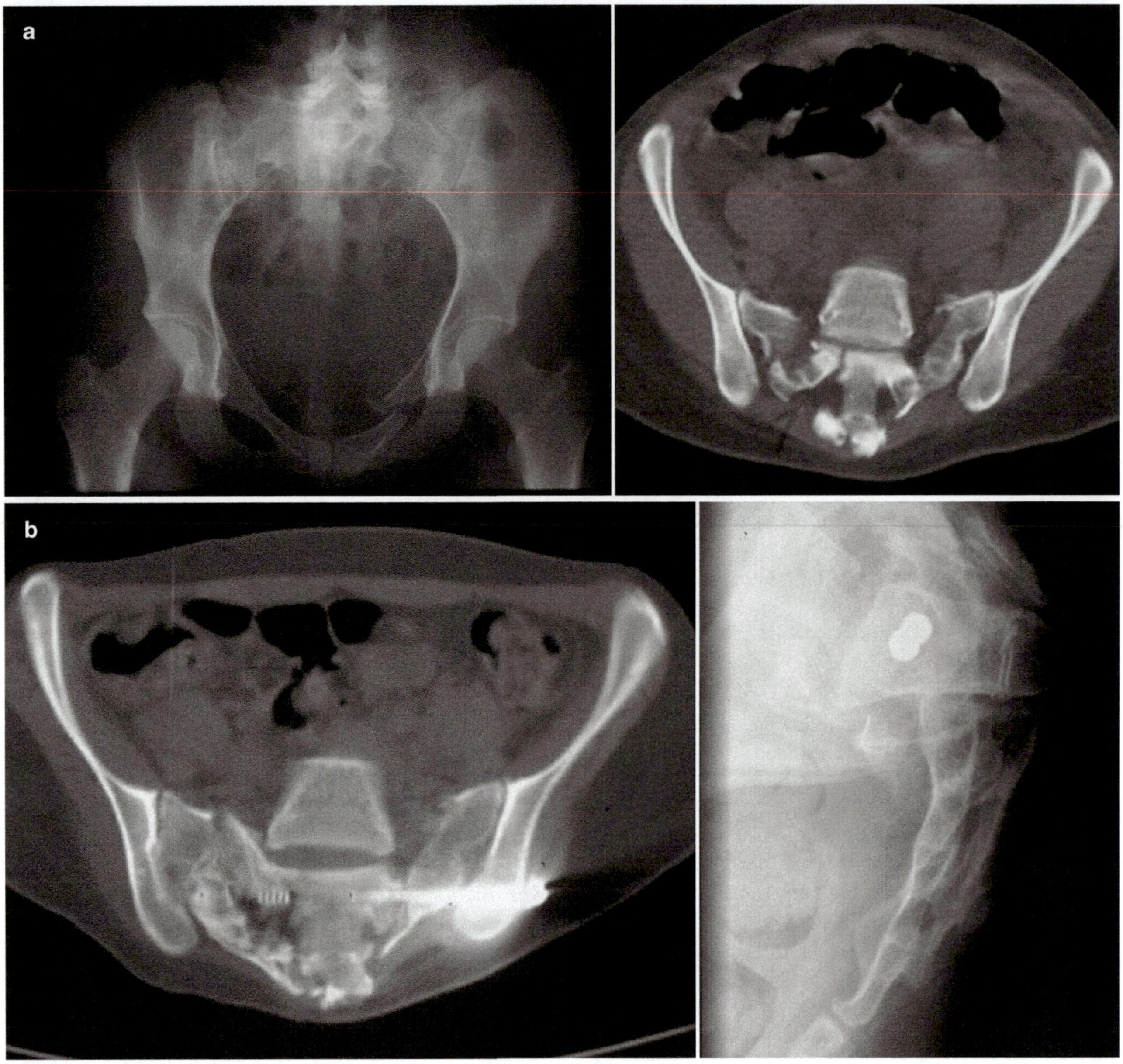

Fig. 35.21 (**a**) Late reconstruction of an initially missed H-shaped sacral fracture with spinopelvic dissociation in a 16-year-old girl, who fell from the roof of a house (9 m). A paradoxical inlet view of the upper sacrum on the standard AP pelvic radiograph, and severe displacements in vertical fracture lines at the axial CT images. (**b**) The first surgery consisted of minimal invasive iliosacral screw fixation without any sacral fracture reduction and pubic rami plate fixation. The right diagnosis was made 5 weeks later. (**c**) Type 2b completely displaced transverse S2 fracture and bilateral transforaminal sacral fractures were opened through the initial fracture lines, surgically reduced and fixed with lumbopelvic construct. Decompressive sacral laminectomy was also performed. The patient had good neurological recovery; after 15 years from the injury she had no bowel or urinary problems or motor deficiencies, but some radicular pain in the lower legs. The patient was working as a cook, was able to wander in Lapland, and to do some sports

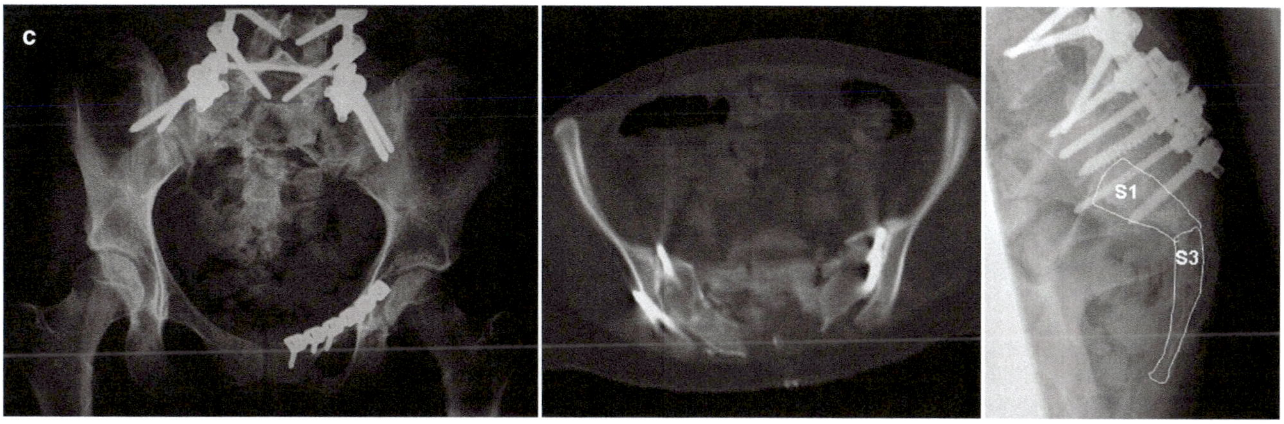

Fig. 35.21 (continued)

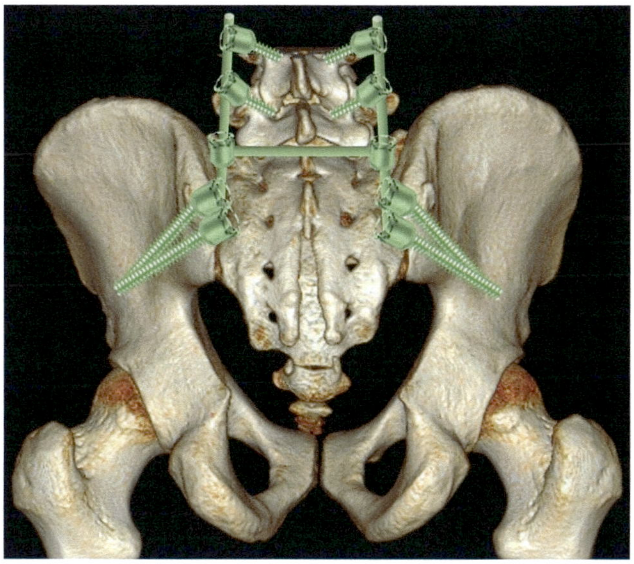

Fig. 35.22 Schematic drawing of the classical lumbopelvic fixation strategy

- Lumbopelvic fixation provides sufficient stability for fracture union with a relatively low rate of complications and long-term sequelae.
- The most common method for treatment of U-shaped sacral fractures is percutaneous iliosacral screw fixation (lumbopelvic fixation for fractures with massive displacement).
- The injuries of the anterior part of the pelvic ring are operated on first, when present.
- Indirect decompression of the lumbosacral (vertical fracture lines) and sacral nerve roots (transverse fracture line) is achieved through reduction and stable fixation of all sacral fracture components (probably the most important part of the surgical procedure).
- Direct nerve root decompression by sacral laminectomy is recommended:
  - For all type 2b and 3b completely displaced transverse sacral fractures
  - For type 2a and 3a transverse sacral fractures with severe narrowing of the central sacral canal after fracture reduction (lateral fluoroscopy).
- In spinopelvic dissociations, quality of reduction in terms of residual postoperative vertical and AP displacements in the vertical sacral fracture lines and translational displacement and kyphosis in the transverse sacral fracture is associated with the clinical outcome.
- Accurate reduction of all sacral fracture components is associated with better clinical outcomes.

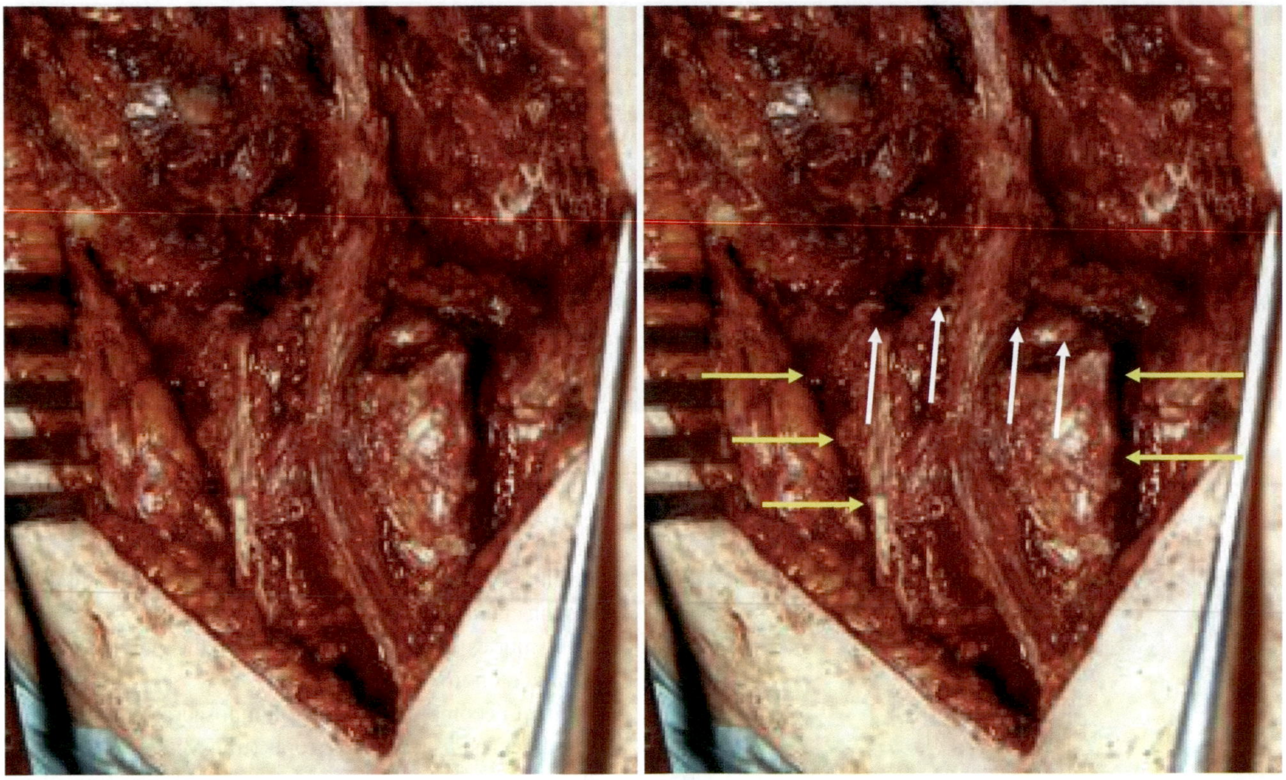

Fig. 35.23 Intraoperative view of a typical lumbopelvic dissociation fracture pattern: vertical fracture lines (yellow arrows) and transverse fracture component (white arrows)

References

1. Rengachary S. Surgical anatomy of the sacrum. In: Doty JR, Rengachary SS, editors. Surgical disorders of the sacrum. New York: Thieme Medical Publishers, Inc.; 1994. p. 21–33.
2. Denis F, Steven D, Comfort T. Sacral fractures: an important problem, retrospective analysis of 236 cases. Clin Orthop. 1988;227:67–81.
3. Lindahl J, Mäkinen T, Koskinen S, Söderlund T. Factors associated with outcome of spinopelvic dissociation treated with lumbopelvic fixation. Injury. 2014;45:1914–20.
4. Schildhauer T, Bellabarba C, Nork S, Barei D, Routt JM, Chapman J. Decompression and lumbopelvic fixation for sacral fracture-dislocations with spino-pelvic dissociation. J Orthop Trauma. 2006;20:447–57.
5. Kim M, Reidy D, Nolan P, Finkelstein J. Transverse sacral fractures: case series and literature review. Can J Surg. 2001;44:359–63.
6. Van Savage J, Dahners L, Renner J, Baker C. Fracture-dislocation of the lumbosacral spine: case report and review of the literature. J Trauma. 1992;33:779–84.
7. Rommens P, Ossendorf C, Pairon P, Dietz S, Wagner D, Hofmann A. Clinical pathways for fragility fractures of the pelvic ring: personal experience and review of the literature. J Orthop Sci. 2015;20:1–11.
8. Routt ML Jr, Simonian P, Swiontkowski M. Stabilization of pelvic ring disruptions. Orthop Clin North Am. 1997;28:369–88.
9. Roy-Camille R, Saillant G, Gagana G, Mazel C. Transverse fracture of the upper sacrum suicidal jumper's fracture. Spine. 1985;10(9):838–45.
10. Ruatti S, Kerschbaumer G, Gay E, Milaire M, Merloz P, Tonetti J. Technique for reduction and percutaneous fixation of U- and H-shaped sacral fractures. Orthop Traumatol Surg Res. 2013;99:625–9.
11. Zelle B, Gruen G, Hunt T, Speth S. Sacral fractures with neurological injury: is early decompression beneficial? Int Orthop. 2004;28:244–51.
12. Purser D. Displaced fracture of the sacrum: report of a case. J Bone Joint Surg. 1969;51-B:346–7.
13. Fardon D. Displaced fracture of the lumbosacral spine with delayed cauda equina deficit. Report of a case and review of the literature. Clin Orthop. 1976;120:155.
14. Bucknill T, Blackburne J. Fracture-dislocation of the sacrum, report of three cases. J Bone Joint Surg. 1976;58-B(4):467–70.
15. Das De S, McCreath S. Lumbosacral fracture-dislocation. JBJS. 1981;63-B(1):58–60.
16. Dowling T, Epstein JA, Epstein NE. S1-S2 sacral fracture involving neural elements of the cauda equina. A case report and review of the literature. Spine. 1985;10(9):851–3.
17. Fisher R. Sacral fracture with compression of cauda equina: surgical treatment. J Trauma. 1988;28(12):1678–80.
18. Strange-Vognsen H, Lebech A. An unusual type of fracture in the upper sacrum. J Orthop Trauma. 1991;5(2):200–3.
19. Giudicelli P, Goubeau J, Chammas M, Ledoux D, Allieu Y. [Transverse fracture of the upper sacrum with major displacement. CT reconstruction: case report]. Rev Chir Orthop Reparatrice Appar Mot. 2000;86:402–6.
20. Hessmann M, Rommens P. Transverse fracture-dislocation of the sacrum: a diagnostic pitfall and a surgical challenge. Acta Chir Belg. 2002;102:46–51.

21. Markel D, Raskas D, Graziano G. Case report: a case of traumatic spino-pelvic dissociation. J Orthop Trauma. 1993;7(6):562–6.
22. Mukundala V, Lim H. Traumatic posterior rotatory fracture-dislocation of lumbo-sacral spine. Singap Med J. 2001;42:82–4.
23. Rodriguez-Fuentes A. Traumatic sacrolisthesis S1-S2: report of a case. Spine. 1993;18(6):768–71.
24. van der Werken C, van Tets W. Intrapelvic intrusion of the lumbosacral spine. Acta Orthop Belg. 1992;58:336–8.
25. Schildhauer T, Josten C, Muhr G. Triangular osteosynthesis of vertically unstable sacrum fractures: a new concept allowing early weight-bearing. J Orthop Trauma. 1998;12:307–14.
26. Schildhauer T, Ledoux W, Chapman J, Henley M, Tencer A, Routt JM. Triangular osteosynthesis and iliosacral screw fixation for unstable sacral fractures: a cadaveric and biomechanical evaluation under cyclic loads. J Orthop Trauma. 2003;17:22–31.
27. Zheng Z, Yu B, Chen H, Aladin D, Zhang K, Zhang J, Liu H, Luk K, Lu W. Effect of iliac screw insertion depth on the stability and strength of lumbo-iliac fixation constructs: an anatomical and biomechanical study. Spine (Phila Pa 1976). 2009;34:565–72.
28. Min K, Zamorano D, Wahba G, Garcia I, Bhatia N, Lee T. Comparison of two-transsacral-screw fixation versus triangular osteosynthesis for transforaminal sacral fractures. Orthopedics. 2014;37:754–60.
29. Song W, Zhou D, He Y. The biomechanical advantages of bilateral lumbo-iliac fixation in unilateral comminuted sacral fractures without sacroiliac screw safe channel: a finite element analysis. Medicine (Baltimore). 2016;95(40):e5026.
30. Jazini E, Klocke N, Tannous O, Johal H, Hao J, Salloum K, Gelb D, Nascone J, Belin E, Hoshino C, Hussain M, O'Toole R, Bucklen B, Ludwig S. Does lumbopelvic fixation add stability? A cadaveric biomechanical analysis of an unstable pelvic fracture model. J Orthop Trauma. 2017;31:37–46.
31. Robles L. Transverse sacral fractures. Spine J. 2009;9:60–9.
32. Rommens P, Hofmann A. Comprehensive classification of fragility fractures of the pelvic ring: recommendations for surgical treatment. Injury. 2013;44:1733–44.
33. Gripnau A, Boele van Hensbroek P, Haverlag R, Ponsen K, Been H, Goslings J. U-shaped sacral fractures: surgical treatment and quality of life. Injury. 2009;40:1040–8.
34. Hunt N, Jennings A, Smith M. Current management of U-shaped sacral fractures or spino-pelvic dissociation. Injury. 2002;33:123–6.
35. Nork S, Jones C, Harding S, Mirza S, Routt JM. Percutaneous stabilization of U-shaped sacral fractures using iliosacral screws: technique and early results. J Orthop Trauma. 2001;15:238–46.
36. Vaccaro A, Kim D, Brodke D, Harris M, Chapman J, Schildhauer T, Routt C, Sasso R. Diagnosis and management of sacral spine fractures. Instr Course Lect. 2004;53:375–85.
37. Gupta P, Barnwell J, Lenchik L, Wuertzer S, Miller A. Spinopelvic dissociation: multidetector computed tomographic evaluation of fracture patterns and associated injuries at a single level 1 trauma center. Emerg Radiol. 2016;23:235–40.
38. Lindahl J, Hirvensalo E. Outcome of operatively treated type-C injuries of the pelvic ring. Acta Orthop. 2005;76:667–78.
39. Ayoub M. Displaced spinopelvic dissociation with sacral cauda equina syndrome: outcome of surgical decompression with a preiliminary management algorithm. Eur Spine J. 2012;21:1815–25.
40. Bellabarba C, Schildhauer T, Vaccaro A, Chapman J. Complications associated with surgical stabilization of high-grade sacral fracture dislocations with spino-pelvic instability. Spine. 2006;31:S80–8.
41. Yi C, Hak D. Traumatic spinopelvic dissociation or U-shaped sacral fracture: a review of the literature. Injury. 2012;43:402–8.
42. Gunterberg B. Effects of major resection of the sacrum. Acta Orthop Scand Suppl. 1976;162:1–38.
43. Chou D, El-Daly I, Ranganathan A, Montgomery A, Culpan P, Bates P. Spinopelvic dissociation: a retrospective case study and review of treatment controversies. J Am Acad Orthop Surg. 2018;26:e302–12.
44. Lindahl J. Operative treatment of severely comminuted sacral fractures. Finn J Orthop Traumatol. 2003;26:42–3.
45. Lindahl J, Hirvensalo E. Pedicle screw spinal fixation system in the treatment of comminuted sacral fractures (Transpedikulaarinen fiksaatiolaite pirstaleisten sakrummurtumien hoidossa). Finn J Orthop Traumatol. 1998;21:219–24.
46. Tan G, He J, Fu B, Li L, Wang B, Zhou D. Lumbopelvic fixation for multiplanar sacral fractures with spinopelvic instability. Injury. 2012;43:1318–25.
47. Hess F, Abu-Tair U, Knoth C, Zettl R. Lumbopelvic stabilisation in patients over 50 with posterior pelvic ring fracture. Ortho Rheum Open Access J. 2016;2(3):OROAJ.MS.ID.55586.
48. Keel M, Benneker L, Siebenrock K, Bastian J. Less invasive lumbopelvic stabilization of posterior pelvic ring instability: technique and preliminary results. J Trauma. 2011;71:62–70.
49. Nothofer W, Thonke N, Neugebauer R [Therapy of unstable sacrum fractures in pelvic ring fractures with dorsal sacrum distraction osteosynthesis]. Unfallchirurg. 2004;107:118–27.
50. Tiemann A, Schmidt C, Josten C. [Triangular vertebropelvine stabilisation of unstable posterior pelvic ring fractures]. Zentralbl Chir. 2003;128:202–8.
51. Allen B, Ferguson R. The Galveston technique for L rod instrumentation of the scoliotic spine. Spine. 1982;7:276–84.
52. König M, Jehan S, Boszczyk A, Boszczyk B. Surgical management of U-shaped sacral fractures: a systematic review of current treatment strategies. Eur Spine J. 2012;21:829–36.
53. Williams S, Quinnan S. Percutaneous lumbopelvic fixation for reduction and stabilization of sacral fractures with spinopelvic dissociation patterns. J Orthop Trauma. 2016;30:e318–24.
54. Sagi H. Technical aspects and recommended treatment algorithms in triangular osteosynthesis and spinopelvic fixation for vertical shear transforaminal sacral fractures. J Orthop Trauma. 2009;23:354–60.
55. Matta J, Yerasimides J. Table-skeletal fixation as an adjunct to pelvic ring reduction. J Orthop Trauma. 2007;21:647–56.
56. Piltz S, Rubenbauer B, Böcker W, Trentzsch H. Reduction and fixation of displaced U-shaped sacral fractures using lumbopelvic fixation: technical recommendations. Eur Spine J. 2018;27:3025–33.
57. Starantzis K, Mirzashahi B, Behrbalk E, Sadat M, Shafafy M. Open reduction and posterior instrumentation of type 3 high transverse sacral fracture-dislocation: technical note. J Neurosurg Spine. 2014;21:286–91.
58. Gänsslen A, Hildebrand F, Klebingat M, Nerlich M, Lindahl J. Chapter 22: Special screws and views. In: Gänsslen, et al., editors. Acetabular fractures: diagnosis, indications, treatment strategies. New York: Thieme; 2017. ISBN-13: 978-3132415607.
59. Gänsslen A, Pohlemann T, Krettek C. Supraacetabular external fixation for pelvic ring fractures. Oper Orthop Traumatol. 2005;17:296–312.
60. Schildhauer T, McCulloch P, Chapman J, Mann F. Anatomic and radiographic considerations for placement of transiliac screws in lumbopelvic fixations. J Spinal Disord Tech. 2002;15:199–205.
61. Schroeder G, Savage J, Patel A, Stover M. Spinopelvic fixation in complex sacral fractures. J Bone Jt Surg Rev. 2015;3(3):e4. https://doi.org/10.2106/JBJS.RVW.N.00007.
62. Schmidek H, Schmith D, Kristiansen D. Sacral fractures. Neurosurgery. 1984;15:735–46.
63. Ebraheim N, Biyani A, Salpietro B. Zone III fractures of the sacrum. Spine. 1996;21(20):2390–6.
64. Fountain S, Hamilton R, Jameson R. Transverse fractures of the sacrum. J Bone Joint Surg. 1977;59-A(4):486–9.
65. Gibbons K, Soloniuk D, Razack N. Neurological injury and patterns of sacral fractures. J Neurosurg. 1990;72:889–93.

66. Phelan S, Jones D, Bishay M. Conservative management of transverse fractures of the sacrum with neurological features. J Bone Joint Surg. 1991;73B:969–71.
67. Sabiston C, Wing P. Sacral fractures: classification and neurologic implications. J Trauma. 1986;26(12):1113–5.
68. Dussa C, Soni B. Influence of type of management of transverse sacral fractures on neurological outcome. A case series and review of literature. Spinal Cord. 2008;46:590–4.
69. Hu X, Pei F, Wang B, He J, Kong Q, Tu C. Application triangular osteosynthesis for vertical unstable sacral fractures. Eur Spine J. 2013;22:503–9.
70. Huittinen V. Lumbosacral nerve injury in fracture of the pelvis. Acta Chir Scand. 1972;(Suppl 429):1–43.
71. Lehman RJ, Kang D, Bellabarba C. A new classification for complex lumbosacral injuries. Spine J. 2012;12:612–28.
72. Sanders D, Fox J, Starr A, Sathy A, Chao J. Transsacral-transiliac screw stabilization: effective for recalcitrant pain due to sacral insufficiency fracture. J Orthop Trauma. 2016;30:469–73.
73. Wagner D, Ossendorf C, Gruszka D, Hofmann A, Rommens P. Fragility fractures of the sacrum: how to identify and when to treat surgically? Eur J Trauma Emerg Surg. 2015;41:349–62.
74. Siebler J, Hasley B, Mormino M. Functional outcomes of Denis zone III sacral fractures treated nonoperatively. J Orthop Trauma. 2010;24:297–302.
75. Sapkas G, Mavrogenis A, Papagelopoulos P. Transverse sacral fractures with anterior displacement. Eur Spine J. 2008;17:342–7.
76. He S, Zhang H, Zhao Q, He B, Guo H, Hao D. Posterior approach in treating sacral fracture combined with lumbopelvic dissociation. Orthopedics. 2014;37:1027–32.
77. Adelved A, Tötterman A, Glott T, Hellund J, Madsen J, Røise O. Long-term functional outcome after traumatic lumbosacral dissociation. A retrospective case series of 13 patients. Injury. 2016;47:1562–8.
78. De Iure F, Cappuccio M, Palmisani M, Pascarella R, Commessatti M. Lumboiliac fixation in lumbosacral dislocation and associated injuries of the pelvis and lumbosacral junction: a long-term radiological and clinical follow-up. Injury. 2016;47:44–8.
79. Jazini E, Weir T, Nwodim E, Tannous O, Saifi C, Caffes N, Costales T, Koh E, Banagan K, Gelb D, Ludwig S. Outcomes of lumbopelvic fixation in the treatment of complex sacral fractures using minimally invasive surgical techniques. Spine J. 2017;17:1238–46.
80. Tian W, Chen W, Jia J. Traumatic spino-pelvic dissociation with bilateral triangular fixation. Orthop Surg. 2018;10:205–11.

Part IV

Special Situations

Pediatric Pelvic Ring Injuries

36

Annelie-Martina Weinberg and Axel Gänsslen

Trauma is still the leading cause of death in children [1]. Morbidity and mortality are a result of concomitant injuries in the majority of cases and not from the pelvic fracture itself. In contrast, postmortem studies showed a high rate of pelvic fracture related deaths and a high incidence of pelvic fractures [2]. Therefore, treatment of pelvic fractures is aimed to either anatomically stabilize the pelvis and to avoid injury-related death.

36.1 Anatomic Characteristics

The growing pelvis differs from that of adults. The pelvic bones are less brittle and are covered with a thick periosteum. In addition, the ligaments are relatively stronger, growth centers and joints, e.g., the sacroiliac joints and the pubic symphysis, are present, which allow for a significant absorption capacity.

Compared to adults, the pediatric pelvis is more elastic and contains more cartilage [3].

This elasticity results primarily in plastic deformity when forces act on the pelvic bone [4] with the possibility of recoiling the deformity but normally not to the preinjury level. Thus, asymmetry can be seen without fracture presence, comparable to bowing of forearm bones. Overall, injuries tend to be more stable as the relatively thick periostium restricts bony displacement.

Due to this elasticity, the intrapelvic viscera are not sufficiently protected, and intrapelvic organ injuries can occur without the presence of pelvic fractures or dislocations [5]. Consequently, more energy is required to produce a fracture [3, 5], and energy can be transferred to the pelvic viscera even after fractures have been sustained. Therefore, even simple or minimal displaced fractures are mainly the result of a high-energy trauma with a significant risk of additional intrapelvic and intraabdominal injuries [5]. This leads to a relatively high incidence of isolated pubic rami fractures or fractures of the iliac wing (Fig. 36.1) [6–17].

In contrast, the presence of a complete disruption of the anterior and posterior pelvis or a complex pelvic injury is, therefore, a high risk factor of morbidity and mortality [18, 19].

> The presence of a pediatric pelvic fracture/injury is a sign of relevant forces acting on the pelvic region and, therefore, a risk factor of morbidity and mortality.

36.2 Epidemiology

Pelvic ring injuries in children are rare with an incidence of 2.7% in the late 1990s [18]. The yearly incidence is expected to be 1.1–8.8/year [4, 19–22]. The incidence of pediatric pelvic fractures within the group of pediatric children is reported to be 49/100000 children [23]. Ten percent of children have unstable immature pelvic fractures [24] and 18.3% incidence of complex pelvic trauma within the group of pediatric pelvic injuries is reported [19].

> A much higher incidence of complex pelvis trauma is observed in (unrestrained) children, increasing the risk of morbidity and mortality.

The incidence of pediatric pelvic fractures in the group of pediatric patients is between 0.3 and 3.5% [8, 16, 25–30].

The main problem in analyzing the literature is the different definition of the upper age level of "pediatric pelvic trauma" with a range between 14 and 20 years.

A.-M. Weinberg
Department of Orthopaedics and Trauma, Medical University of Graz, Graz, Austria
e-mail: anneliemartina.weinberg@medunigraz.at

A. Gänsslen (✉)
Department of Trauma Surgery, Orthopedics and Hand Surgery, Hospital Wolfsburg, Wolfsburg, Germany

A. Gänsslen et al. (eds.), *Pelvic Ring Fractures*, https://doi.org/10.1007/978-3-030-54730-1_36

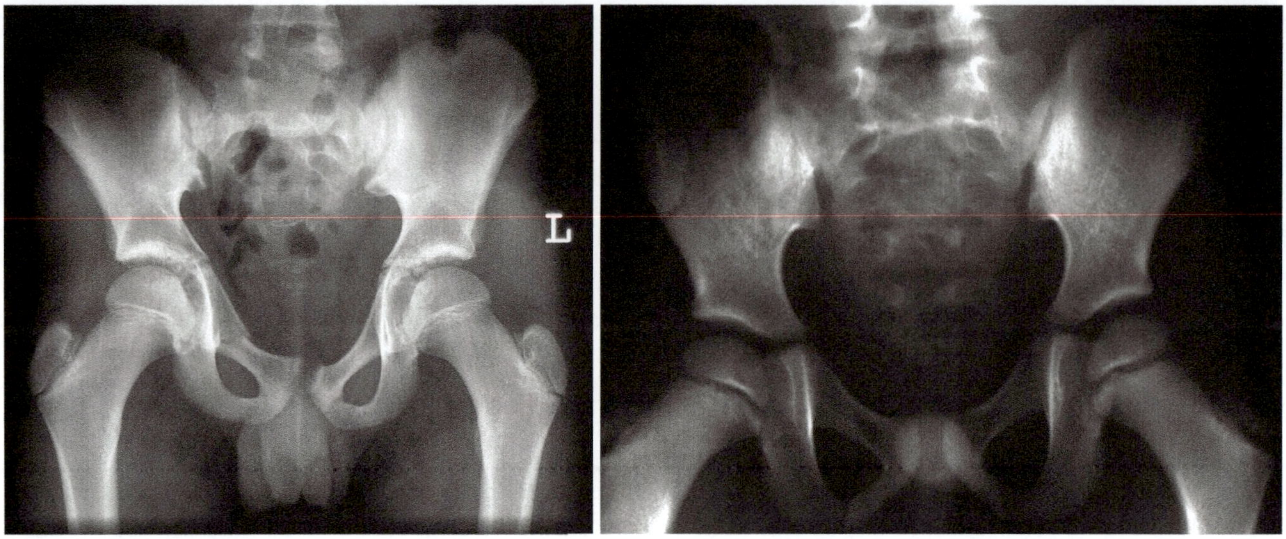

Fig. 36.1 Isolated right upper pubic rami fracture (left) and right iliac wing fracture (right) as typical examples of pediatric pelvic ring fractures

Overall, there is a male predominance resulting in a male/female ratio of approximately 1.4:1. The mean age depends on the age definition of the pediatric group. In the classical immature group of patients ≤14 years of age, the mean age is 8.2 years [4, 11, 12, 21]. Authors reporting on patients up to 16 years of age, a mean age of 9.4 years was stated [2, 7, 8, 13, 16, 20], whereas both groups together showed a mean age of 9 years.

Recently, Zwingmann et al. could show an age-dependent increase of pediatric pelvic fractures [31]:

- Children 1–5 years: 6.6% pelvic fractures within pediatric injuries
- Children 6–10 years: 10.5% pelvic fractures within pediatric injuries
- Children 11–14 years: 15.3% pelvic fractures within pediatric injuries

36.3 Mechanism of Injury

More than 80% of all pelvic injuries are a result of high-energy trauma [7, 8, 15, 20, 28, 30, 32–34].

A pedestrian struck by a car is the most common mechanism in nearly 60%, followed by motor vehicle passengers in approximately 20% and rarely the patients suffer from bicycle and motorcycle accidents.

Pedestrian injuries decrease with increasing age: young children (1–5 years: 50.0%; 6–10 years: 56.3%; and 11–14 years: 31.1%) [31].

A fall from height was responsible to produce a pediatric pelvic fracture in nearly 10%. Crush injuries, injuries sustained during sport activities, and farm accidents are uncommon [35].

An important prognostic mechanism of injury is the history of a rollover or crush mechanism (ISS up to 40 points, 86.6%. associated injuries, 20% mortality rate >70% local complication rate) [36].

> High-energy trauma is the predominant injury mechanism in patients sustaining pelvic ring injuries.

36.4 Associated Injuries

Analysis of the American National Inpatient Pediatric Database revealed that children with pelvic injuries had 5.2 concomitant injuries in average [23], while recently 2.3 concomitant injuries were observed in a small sample of patients [33].

A high injury severity is observed in pediatric patients with pelvic ring injuries, representing a polytrauma group of patients.

> The average ISS value, analyzing 1328 patients, is 21.7 points [7, 13, 15, 30, 31, 34, 37, 38], indicating a polytrauma population.

Recent data confirm the high injury severity. Data from the German Pelvic Trauma Registry reported an ISS of 16.7 points [38]. In contrast, data from Great Britain found a nearly doubled ISS of 31.4 points [34], while data from the

London area reported an ISS of 25 points [33]. The recent German analysis found an identical ISS of approximately 25 points, independent of the age group of the patients [31].

> Pediatric patients presenting with pelvic fractures are at high risk of multiple injuries.

36.4.1 Pelvic Bleeding

Life-threatening bleeding from pediatric pelvic fractures is rarely seen and is reported to range from only 0–2% (Fig. 36.2) [9, 10, 12, 39]. No clear data on transfusion requirements exist. It can be expected that 10–40% of patients need transfusions [10, 17, 34, 37, 39–41]. Approximately 10–31% of the patients are in traumatic-hemorrhagic shock at admission [12, 39].

The source of potentially fatal hemorrhage is commonly secondary to the associated intraabdominal and intrathoracic organ injuries [7, 8, 15–17, 20, 27, 39, 40, 42, 43]. Interventional or surgical pelvic bleeding control is rarely necessary [7, 33, 34, 37].

The rate of additional retroperitoneal hematoma is reported to be between 9 and 46% [7, 13, 39], and hematoma within the true pelvis is found between 9 and 39%. Pelvic vascular lesions are present in 2–8% [19, 39, 44]. This incidence increases in complex pelvic trauma up to 43% [19].

The presence of a posterior pelvic injury was associated with a higher risk of pelvic bleeding [45].

36.4.2 Open Fractures

Patients with open pelvic fractures are severely injured with a mortality rate up to 20%, requiring an aggressive management concept (Fig. 36.2) [19, 36]. Perineal injuries were found in 3.5–7.8% [11, 12, 19, 46]. The reported rate of open fractures is 1.9–12.9% [36, 37, 46].

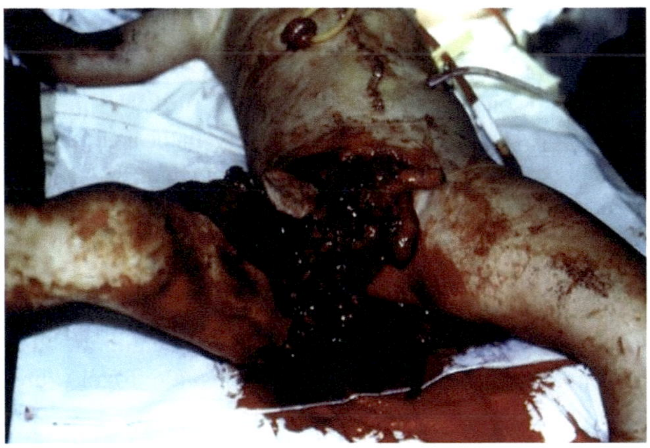

Fig. 36.2 Open pelvic fracture after rollover injury with life-threatening hemorrhage

36.4.3 Truncal Injuries

The main additional truncal injury is head injury in about 40% [7, 8, 15, 16, 20, 33, 34, 37]. One fourth of the patients had concomitant chest and one fifth had additional abdominal injuries. Spinal injuries are less common with an incidence of 7%.

36.4.4 Extremity Injuries

Nineteen percent of the patients had an additional femur fracture and 13% an additional tibia fracture [7, 8, 15, 16, 20, 33, 34, 37]. Humerus fractures are present in 5.5% and forearm fractures in 5% [8, 11, 12, 15, 39, 40, 44]. After complex pelvic trauma, these rates are significantly higher with 9.5% injuries of the upper and 57% of the lower extremities [19].

36.4.5 Nerve Injuries

The rate of additional lumbosacral plexus injury is low ranging from 0.8% to a maximum of 6.1% [4, 11, 13, 19, 39, 40, 46].

36.4.6 Genitourinary Injuries

The incidence of genitourinary injuries is approximately 10% [7, 8, 11, 13, 16, 19, 21, 25, 30, 33, 34, 37, 42, 44, 45]. These rates increase to 40–50% in cases after crush injuries or complex pelvic trauma [19, 36].

10.7% of these injuries were bladder injuries and one fourth of the patients (26.4%) had an additional urethral lesion. Injuries of the kidneys can be observed in 8.3%, vaginal lacerations in 14.9%, and rectal injuries in 10.7% [7, 8, 11, 13, 16, 19, 21, 25, 30, 42, 44, 45]

Macrohematuria is observed in 7–57% [17, 39, 44, 46, 47] and microhematuria in 21–36% [39, 47].

> Concomitant head, chest, and lower extremity injuries are common in nearly every third patient (Table 36.1).

Table 36.1 Number of relevant associated injuries

Author	Year	No.	Head	Chest	Abdominal	Limbs	Femur	Tibia	Spine	GU
Kruppa	2018	90	44	14	34	?	15		7	14
Chotai	2018	53	22	15	12	42	11	7	6	3
Tosounidis	2015	49	33	30	19	?	7	7	7	3
Banerjee	2009	44	5	15	6	?	?	?	6	?
Spiguel	2006	13	4	4	2	?	?	?	0	2
Chia	2004	125	53	33	20	50			?	20
Grisoni	2002	57	15	4	8	?	7	5	?	2
Silber	2001	166	64	33	32	?	39	24	2	15
		597	240	148	133	92/178	64/325	43/325	28/402	59/553
			40.2%	24.8%	22.3%	51.7%	19.7%	13.2%	7%	10.7%

36.5 Clinical Examination

In selected patients, especially in awake patients, pelvic fractures can sufficiently be detected or ruled out by clinical examination alone.

Primary inspection of the undressed patient should focus on pelvic asymmetry, differences in leg length, pelvic soft tissue injury around the complete pelvis including the perineum, search for urethral or vaginal bleeding, and search for differences of the color of the feet, probably indicating vascular impairments.

The ATLS concept proposes digital rectal examination as a standard in the secondary survey to identify certain occult injuries. The value of this examination technique in pediatric patients is still unclear due to high false-positive and -negative rates and poor sensitivity [48, 49].

Overall, clinical examination of the pelvis was associated with a sensitivity of 69% and a specificity of 95%. The positive predictive value was 65% and the negative predictive value was 91% [10]. Pelvic instability is rarely seen in pediatric pelvic fractures (1/33 patients, 3%) [29].

Additional diagnostics, like primary bedside hemoglobinometry, evaluation of the vascular and neurological status is recommended. Early protection against hypothermia should be performed with connective patient warming systems.

36.6 Radiological Examination

The gold standard in pediatric pelvic injury examination still remains the anterior-posterior pelvic x-ray, even when the possibility of the presence of a pelvic fracture is <1% with a negative clinical examination (Fig. 36.3). This is also due to medicolegal aspects as clinical evaluation can be negative while even minor displaced fractures can be present.

Recent data suggest that in the hemodynamically stable patient, who is awake and alert without signs of peripheral nerve lesions and a negative pelvic examination, the standard AP x-ray cannot longer be recommended [50, 51], whereas in unstable pediatric patients an AP x-ray together with an abdominal-pelvic CT scan is mandatory [52].

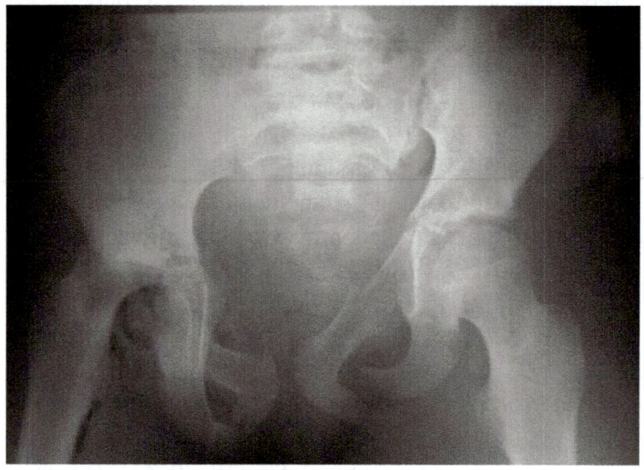

Fig. 36.3 Pelvic a.p. x-ray as the gold standard of radiological evaluation, especially in the unstable pelvis and in patients with hemodynamic instability

> Standard x-rays and CT are recommended in hemodynamically unstable patients or only in selected patients.

Other pelvic views (inlet, outlet, and Judet views) and magnetic resonance imaging (MRI) allow further delineation of the more complex aspects of the injury. In the acute assessment of pelvic fractures there is usually no place for this type of additional diagnostics, while determining the need for elective operative treatment, their value is not definitively stated in the literature.

Comparable to adults, conventional cystography is not further required for the detection and classification of bladder injuries. In suspected urethral lesions, a retrograde urethrogram is still the diagnostic standard.

Computed tomography (CT) has an increasing place in the initial evaluation of the pediatric trauma patient (Fig. 36.4) [53], and there is a potential advantage in pediatric polytrauma patients [46, 53]. Presently, the rate of pri-

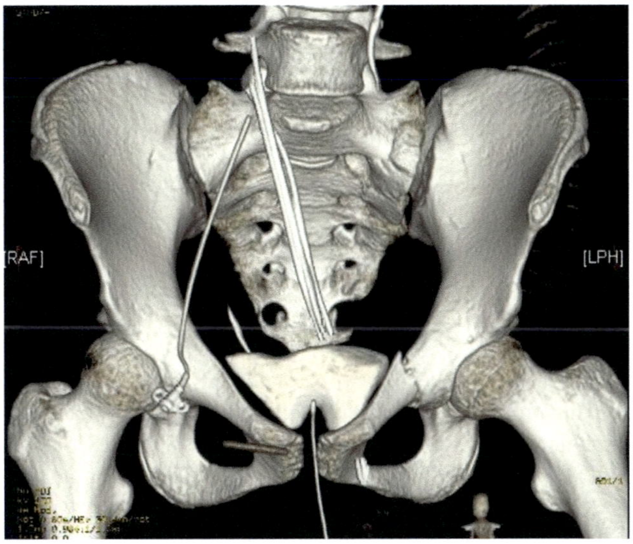

Fig. 36.4 Pelvic CT, to analyze injuries in detail

marily performed CT diagnostic is between 60 and 80% [7, 8, 14, 52]. There is a clear trend of performing CT evaluation even in the pediatric group with a recent CT rate of >90% [33]. Here, CT replaced conventional x-rays. Therefore, if in doubt, additional CT should be obtained [46, 53, 54]. But, despite additional fracture detection, a management change is rarely necessary [8, 14, 52].

> CT is the diagnostic modality of choice, if indicated.

There are some special remarks analyzing pediatric radiographs. The presence of physes and apophyses may make radiographic recognition of fractures difficult. The symphyseal width changes with different ages [55]. Additionally, CT analysis of disrupted SI joints showed typically Salter-Harris type I and II lesions of the joint and normally no pure dislocations [56].

Silber et al. found significant differences comparing pediatric patients with immature and mature pelvic injuries. In the immature pelvic fracture group, significantly more pubic rami fractures and iliac wing fractures were observed, whereas in the mature fracture group significantly more acetabular fractures and fractures with pubic and SI joint diastasis were seen [57].

Kraus in 1930 reported that the symphyseal width decreases continuously from approximately 10 mm in the toddler age to 2 mm in older age of 50 years [58]. Patel and Chapman observed a width of 7.4 mm in the first months of life, which decreases to 5.4 mm at the age of 16 years [55].

Recently, the age-dependent width of the pubic symphysis and the SI joints was analyzed by different groups using especially CT data.

Data for the symphysis width were analyzed:

- McAlister et al. measured symphyseal width using standard radiographs in 316 consecutive pediatric patients (165 boys, 151 girls), which were separated by gender and divided into three age groups: 2–6 years, 7–10 years, and 11–14 years [59]. Normal values between 5.2 and 8.4 mm were observed with an average width of 6.8 mm. Interestingly, a subsequent widening was observed within the three age groups: 6.6 mm, 6.8 mm, 7.2 mm, respectively. It was concluded that a width > 8.4 mm should lead for further evaluation for pathology.
- Bayer et al. analyzed 350 CT scans of children in different age groups: 0–6 years, 7–11 years, 12–15 years, and 16–17 years. The mean width in these age groups was 5.4 mm, 5.3 mm, 4.1 mm, and 3.5 mm in girls, and 5.9 mm, 5.4 mm, 5.2 mm, and 4.0 mm in boys, respectively [60].
- A further CT analysis of 1020 CT axial scans in pediatric patients (2–18 years) revealed an average pubic symphyseal width at 2 years for boys of 6.35 mm and of 5.85 mm in girls. A decrease to 3.68 mm in boys and 3.92 mm in girls at an age of 18 years was observed [61].
- Recently, data on 811 CT measurements of the pubic symphysis were analyzed, stating that from age 2–16 years, the average pubic symphysis width decreased from 5.55 to 3.69 mm [62].

> The width of the pubic symphysis decreases from 5 to 6 mm 2 years after birth to 3–4 mm in early adulthood using CT analyses.
> In pediatric trauma patients <10 years of age, a symphyseal width >10 mm should lead to suspicion of injury [61].

The width of the SI joint was also analyzed using CT data:

- Oetgen et al. reported a decrease of the SI joint width from 3.11 to 1.80 mm in the ages of 2 and 16 years, respectively [62]
- Further CT analysis reported an average width of 4.4–4.5 mm in 2 year old children, which decreases to 2.0–2.3 mm in 18 year old children [61]; girls presented with slightly larger widths with increasing age.

36.7 Clinical Relevance

> In pediatric trauma patients <10 years of age, a width of the SI joint >8 mm should lead to suspicion of sacroiliac injury [61].

36.8 Classification

Several pelvic ring fracture classifications are used in the literature. The most commonly used classifications are the classifications of Key and Conwall [63], Torode and Zieg [17], and the classification of the AO/Orthopaedic Trauma Association [64].

Key and Conwall Classification [63]:

I: No break in the pelvic ring (avulsion, iliac wing, upper, or lower pubic fracture)
II: Single break in the pelvic ring
III: Double break in the pelvic ring (anterior posterior, straddle fracture)
IV: Isolated acetabular fracture

The distribution of the Key and Conwall classification fracture types was analyzed by several authors [7, 10, 12]. In the series by Chia et al. there were 55.8% type I injuries, 27.5% type II injuries, and 11.7% type III injuries. Isolated acetabular fractures were seen in 5% [7].

The two smaller series found an overall frequency of 37.5%, 42.8%, 10.7%, and 8.9%, respectively [10, 12].

The Torode classification also distinguishes four fracture groups [17]:

I: Avulsion fractures
II: Iliac wing fractures
III: Simple pelvic ring fractures (pubic rami fractures, stable symphyseal disruptions)
IV: Ring disruption fractures (unstable pelvic segment, straddle fractures, additional acetabular fractures, anterior + posterior ring fractures)

The minority of fractures belongs to group I and the majority of fractures to group III. Four analyses were presented in the current literature [13–16]. The overall frequency of fracture types showed 3.1% type I, 14.8% type II, 54.5% type III, and 27.6% type IV fractures.

The AO/OTA classification of pelvic injuries is well established in the adult group [64]. This classification analyses the injury pattern depending on specific fracture locations and evaluates the type of pelvic stability. Three different groups of stability/instability are distinguished:

- Type A: stable injuries, the mechanical ring structure of the pelvic ring remains intact
- Type B: partially unstable injuries with partial posterior, rotational instability after antero-posterior or lateral compression
- Type C: unstable injuries with combined anterior and posterior (vertical) instability

Table 36.2 Distribution of AO/OTA fracture types in pediatric pelvic fractures

Author	Year	No.	A (no./%)	B (no./%)	C (no./%)
LaneO'Kelly	1995	68	50 (73.5%)	8 (11.8%)	10 (14.7%)
Grisoni	2002	55	46 (83.7%)	8 (14.5%)	1 (1.8%)
		123	78%	13%	9%
Hauschild	2008	101	58 (57.4%)	27 (26.7%)	16 (15.8%)
Zwingmann	2015	182	93 (51.1%)	55 (30.2%)	34 (18.7%)
Tosounidis	2015	36	15 (41.7%)	20 (55.5%)	1 (2.8%)
Zwingmann	2018	503	266 (52.9%)	175 (34.8%)	62 (12.3%)
Krupp	2018	90	24 (26.7%)	64 (71.1%)	2 (2.2%)
		912	50%	37.4%	12.6%

The proportion of fracture groups in pediatric trauma patients was analyzed by different authors [8, 11, 18, 31, 34, 37, 38] (Table 36.2).

During the last decades, with increasing use of CT diagnostics even in pediatric patients with suspected pelvic ring injuries, a clear trend to more unstable fracture patterns was observed, as posterior lesions were more frequently detected (Table 36.2).

Analyzing patients with complex pelvic trauma, Meyer-Junghänel et al. found less often stable type A injuries (19%), but 28.6% rotationally unstable injuries and 52.4% type C injuries [19].

An overall rate of 50% type A injuries, 40% type B injuries, and 10% type C injuries can be expected (Fig. 36.5).

For emergency classification of these injuries and to facilitate the identification of life-threatening pelvic injuries, the following definitions have been shown to be useful even in the pediatric trauma group, as they are practicable and of relevance regarding prediction of mortality [65]:

- *Simple pelvic fractures* with little soft tissue injury and pure osteoligamentous instability: This group covers about 90% of pelvic fractures
- *Complex pelvic trauma* as a pelvic fracture combined with a serious soft tissue lesion in the pelvic region
- Fractures with *pelvic and hemodynamic instability*: mechanically unstable pelvic fractures (type B or C) combined with hemodynamic instability related to the pelvic injury with a systolic blood pressure of <70 mmHg and/or a hemoglobin concentration of <8 g/dL on admission
- *Traumatic hemipelvectomy*: a total or subtotal dislocation of one or both hemipelvises with complete disruption of the vascular and neural structures of the pelvis

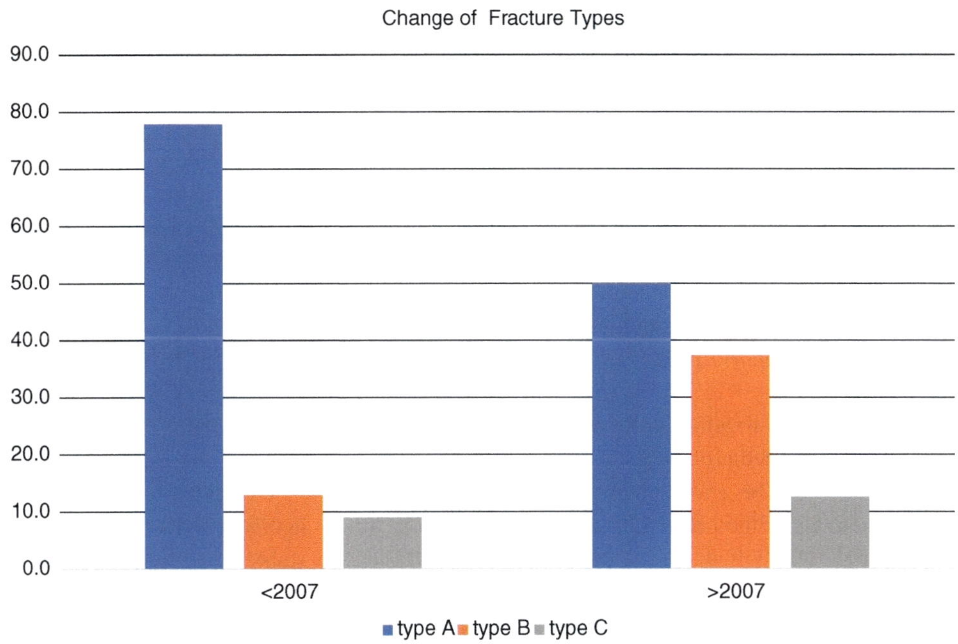

Fig. 36.5 Epidemiology of pelvic ring fracture types

36.9 Emergency Treatment

Emergency treatment in the pediatric trauma patient with a pelvic fracture is orientated to concepts established in adults [66]. The main parameters in decision making are the hemodynamic situation and the grade of potential mechanical instability of the pelvis [65].

It has to be considered that the child has a longer hemodynamic compensation before a severe shock state results in a potential near fatal situation [67].

Hauschild et al. analyzed that in children pelvic emergency measures were performed in 17.9% compared to a rate of 11.1% in adults patients [18].

Due to the anatomical differences of the child's pelvis and the higher risk of injury to the pelvic viscera, it has to be considered that the presence of pelvic and extremity fractures predicts concomitant abdominal and head injuries [15, 40, 68, 69] and, therefore, the overall risk of bleeding complications [17, 27, 45, 68, 69].

Bleeding is commonly secondary to associated solid-organ injuries [15, 17, 27, 39, 40, 42, 47].

Recently, Tosounidis et al. reported a mean transfusion rate of 2.5 PRBC in 12.2% of patients [34]. These patients had a significantly higher ISS compared to nontransfused patients.

> Emergency treatment is more often performed orientated to concepts established in adults.

36.9.1 Pelvic Bleeding Control

To evaluate the hemodynamic situation, a helpful parameter is the initial base deficit, which is a strong prognostic indicator of shock, high injury severity, shock-related complications, and mortality [70].

Pelvic hemorrhage control is performed using angiography/embolization and pelvic packing. Angiography and embolization are rarely necessary [7, 33, 34, 37, 71].

The incidence of angiographic interventions is reported to be maximally 5% [72]. In a recent analysis, of 12.2% hemodynamically unstable patients, none required embolization to control hemorrhage [34], while Kruppa et al. reported a rate of approximately 2% [37].

Direct bleeding control is possible by vascular ligation, vascular clips (clamps), and rarely by vascular reconstruction of major vessels and is the principal aim of every hemostasis in the pelvic region [73]. The more common venous bleedings from large ruptured venous plexus have the disadvantage of a time-consuming bleeding control with sometimes additional blood loss. Therefore, in exsanguinating diffuse pelvic bleeding, pelvic tamponade is proposed under a condition of emergent posterior pelvic ring stabilization [74]. Therefore, angiography/embolization is recommended in patients with moderate hemodynamic instability, whereas pelvic packing is recommended in patients "in extremis" [73, 75].

> Pelvic bleeding control has to be performed in less than 2% of patients. Concepts from adult experience are transferred to the pediatric population.

36.9.2 Pelvic Emergency Fixation

Historically it was stated that operative pelvic stabilization to control bleeding is rarely necessary [12, 39]. Today, several emergency procedures are described to stabilize a mechanical unstable pelvis.

Antishock trousers are no longer routinely used in adults due to their high rate of complications [73]. Prophylactic application of pelvic slings, pelvic bed sheets, or pelvic belts at the scene or in the emergency department has to be considered in pediatric patients with unstable pelvic fractures [76].

Pelvic external fixation is the commonly used stabilization technique in pediatric pelvic fractures [8, 13, 16, 17, 21, 31, 34, 77–81]. The classical external fixator is predominantly used, while the pelvic C-clamp is exceptionally used (Fig. 36.6) [31].

Advantages of the external fixator are its fast and less morbid application even in pediatric patients, compared to other surgical treatments for unstable pelvic fractures, and, therefore, it provides an excellent alternative to pelvic open reduction in the acute treatment of pediatric patients with multisystem injuries.

McIntyre et al. found 60% success rate after external fixator application [45]. Even in children, the pelvic C-clamp can be used to stabilize the posterior pelvic ring [31, 82].

> Emergency stabilization of unstable pelvic ring injuries in children should at least be stabilized by pelvic binding or external fixation.

Definitive reduction and internal fixation in acute management are only recommended when the patient is in a stable condition. Symphyseal plating, anterior plating of the SI joint, and application of iliosacral screws are feasible [33, 83].

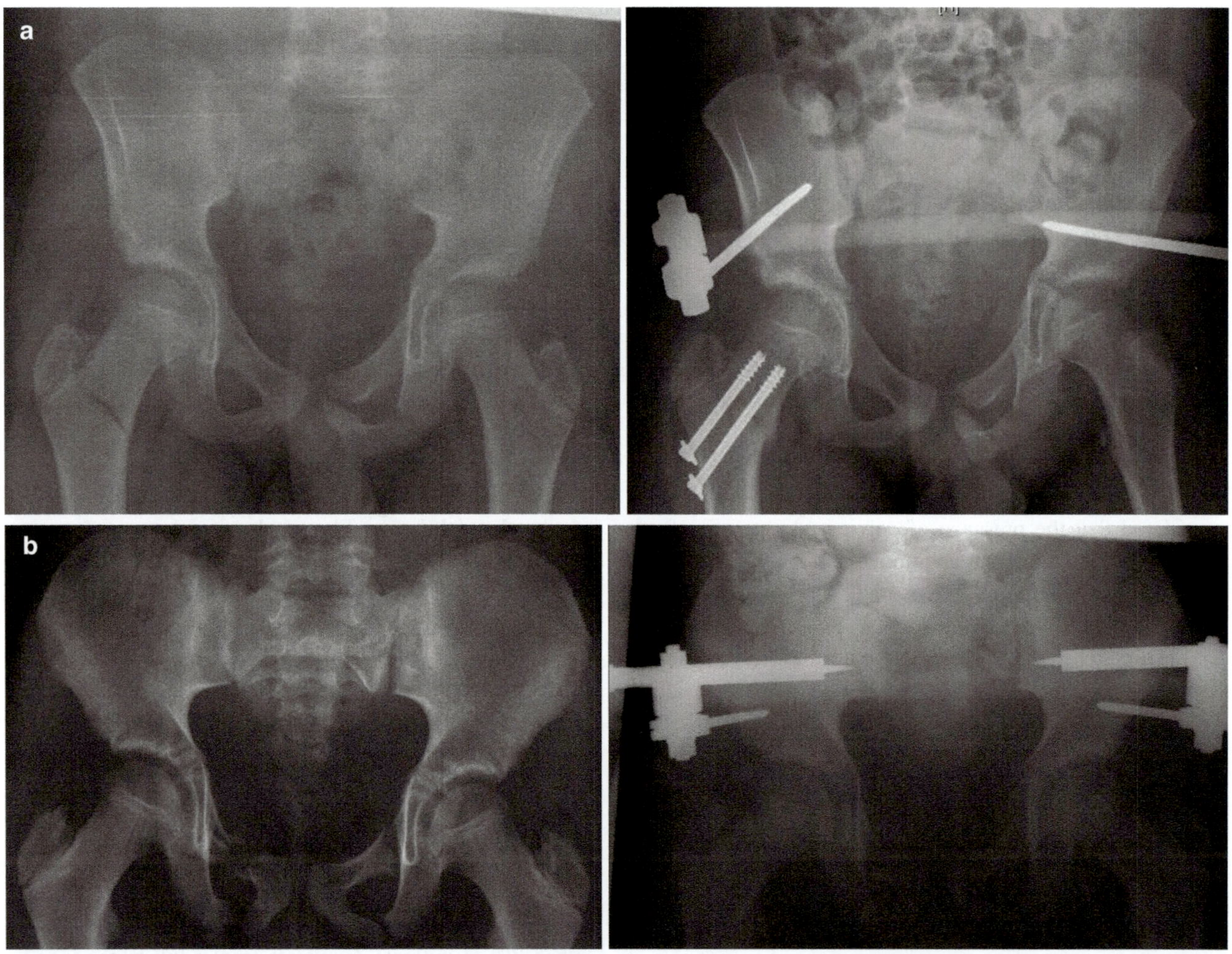

Fig. 36.6 (**a**) Emergency stabilization of the pelvis in children: an external fixator is predominantly used; alternatively the pelvic C-clamp can be used. (**b**) Emergency stabilization of the pelvis in children: an external fixator is predominantly used; alternatively the pelvic C-clamp can be used

36.10 Definitive Treatment

There was a long-term dominance of nonoperative treatment in pediatric pelvic fractures proposing bed-rest, traction, pelvic slings, or hip spica casts [12, 13, 17, 25, 40, 42, 47, 84, 85].

> The primary treatment aim is the anatomic reduction and maintenance of a symmetrical pelvis [40, 86].

This can be achieved in the majority of children by conservative functional treatment.

Recently, operative stabilization of pelvic ring injuries in children plays an increasing role in present management concepts. Several authors report on their experience with closed or open reduction especially in unstable pelvic ring injuries (Table 36.3). Most authors prefer external fixation [17, 31, 33, 34, 78–81].

Today, external fixation is still rarely performed and is stated to be indicated only when pelvic ring displacement is greater than 2 cm to avoid limb length discrepancies [32, 33, 87]. In contrast, Keshishyan et al. reported better results after external fixation compared to conservative treatment [2].

As previous authors have suggested that nonoperative management of displaced pelvic fractures may result in pelvic asymmetry, leading to poor clinical results, several authors focused on operative stabilization of the pelvic ring [13, 17, 77, 88, 89].

Accepted indications for operative fixation include:

- Concomitant treatment when open wound treatment is necessary
- Additional hemorrhage control during resuscitation [6]
- Optimization of patient mobility
- Prevention of deformity in severely displaced fractures [2, 40, 80, 84, 86]
- In special situations to improve patient care (e.g., polytrauma)

Therefore, only displaced fractures require surgical reduction and stabilization [6, 15, 17, 33, 34, 86, 90] and, therefore, only case descriptions are reported in the literature.

- Zimmermann et al. stabilized three children with PDS banding of the pubic symphysis in two and of the SI joint in one case [91].
- Gänsslen et al. reported on symphyseal plating and anterior plating of a disrupted SI joint of a C1.2 injury in a 3 year old child with a good clinical and radiological follow-up result after 17 months [92].
- Stiletto et al. performed open reduction and anterior plate osteosynthesis of a disrupted SI joint without anterior ring stabilization in two patients ≤3 years of age [89].
- Blasier et al. analyzed 43 of 57 patients with unstable Tile type B and C injuries. Thirteen patients were treated operatively. In nine patients, combined anterior plating and posterior iliosacral screw fixation was performed, one patient had an external fixator alone, and in three patients manipulative reduction and application of a spica cast were performed [6].
- Baskin et al. treated SI joint (fracture) dislocations by closed reduction and CT-guided percutaneous iliosacral screw fixation in three children with aged 8, 13, and 14 years [77]. In all three cases an anterior external fixator was additionally applied prior to posterior ring fixation.

Table 36.3 Numbers of type of treatment

Author	Year	Conservative	EF	ORIF	CRIF	ORIF + EF	% osteosynthesis	No.	overall
Kruppa	2018	85					5.6	5	90
Chotai	2018	51	0	0	2	0	3.8	2	53
Zwingmann	2018	429					24.6	140	569
Tosounidis	2015	32	3	0	1	0	11.1	4	36
Zwingmann	2015	170					18.3	38	208
Banerjee	2009	43	1	0	0	0	2.2	1	44
Spiguel	2006	11	2	0	0	0	15.4	2	13
Karunakar	2005	134	0	12	2	0	9.5	14	148
Chia	2004	118	2	5	0	0	5.6	7	125
Grisoni	2002	52	0	0	0	1	1.8	1	57
Silber	2001	165	0	1	0	0	0.6	1	166
Uppermann	2000						9.5	9	95
Rieger	1997	38	6	6	1	0	29.6	16	54
Keshishyan	1995	31	12	0	0	0	27.9	12	43
Rangger	1994	18	1	1	1	0	14.3	3	21
Barabas	1991						5.5	3	55
Stachel	1987						2.8	3	108
Musemeche	1987	51	2	4	0	0	10.5	6	57

EF External fixation, *ORIF* Open reduction internal fixation, *CRIF* Closed reduction internal fixation

All cases showed near-anatomic reduction. Removal of the external fixator was performed after 5–6 weeks postoperatively. At follow-up at least 12 months postinjury, only slight impairments at the posterior pelvis were observed.
- Chotai et al. reported on two iliosacral screw fixations and Tosounidis et al. on one case [33, 34].

Despite these case presentations, especially performed in type C injuries of the pelvis, no clear concept can be guided from the recent literature.

There is still a wide range of operative intervention in pediatric pelvic fractures ranging from 0.6% up to 30% with comparable rates of external fixation and internal fixation [2, 7, 8, 12, 13, 15, 16, 20–22, 25, 30, 88].

The Hannover group developed a concept based on their experience of several long-term sequelae after treating pediatric patients with complex pelvic trauma [19].

Beside the hemodynamic status, treatment considerations depend on the patient's age, fracture type, and the stability of the pelvic ring [65]. A comparable concept was recently reported by Silber and colleagues [57].

36.11 Treatment Options in Pelvic Ring Instability

For pediatric patients with stable hemodynamics and an unstable pelvic ring (type B or -C injuries), anatomic and stable pelvic ring reconstruction is the primary treatment goal.

> The indication and localization of pelvic ring stabilization primarily depend on pelvic stability.

- Type A injuries: surgical stabilization is normally not required, as functional treatment will not lead to further displacement; treatment consists of short time bed-rest and early pain-dependent ambulation; ORIF is only performed in severely displaced or open fractures, e.g., iliac crest fractures, pubic rami fractures with the risk of concomitant bladder lesions, and rarely in avulsion fractures in young athletes.
- Type B injuries: operative stabilization of the anterior pelvic ring provides sufficient stabilization for early ambulation with partial weight bearing; type B injuries with symphyseal disruption should be treated by open reduction and plate stabilization of the pubic symphysis as external fixation alone leads to a high rate of secondary displacement in adults, whereas the more "stable" lateral compression injuries, especially minimally displaced lateral compression sacral fractures, in the majority of cases, can be treated by conservative means; external fixation of these injuries is rarely necessary.
- Type C injuries: treatment consists of combined posterior and anterior stabilization as posterior displacement of >5 mm leads to a high rate of malunion.

> The chosen implant depends on the fracture/injury region and, more importantly, on the patient's age.

In adolescent patients (age 14–18 years), the well-known stabilization concepts can also be applied to the pediatric group [66].

Within the group of immature patients with an open triradiate cartilage, patients with an age ≤10 years and patients between 10–14 years are distinguished.

In patients >10 years of age, standardized implants, comparable to adults, can be used. Alternatively, anatomically adapted implants have to be considered.

In the younger age group (age ≤10 years), the special anatomic situation has to be considered when choosing the type of osteosynthesis:

- *Symphyseal disruption:* screw/cerclage osteosynthesis, possibly with additional transosseous suturing in toddlers, in older children plate osteosynthesis with a two-hole 1/3 tubular plate or a two–four-hole small fragment plate (Figs. 36.7, 36.8, and 36.9)
- *Displaced upper pubic rami fractures:* in risk of bladder laceration: open reduction and stabilization in toddlers with a K-wire, in older children with a 3.5 mm transpubic cortical screw (Fig. 36.10)
- *Unstable transpubic fractures as part of a type B or -C injury:* supraacetabular external fixator (Fig. 36.11)
- *Iliac wing fracture:* in toddlers: K-wire stabilization, in older children screw- and/or plate osteosynthesis (Fig. 36.12)
- *Transiliac fracture dislocation ("crescent fracture"):* posterior screw fixation of the iliac fracture by closed or open reduction (Fig. 36.13)
- *Sacroiliac dislocation:* anterior plate osteosynthesis with "mini-implants" (e.g. small H-plate), in older patients three-hole small fragment plates (Figs. 36.14 and 36.15)
- *Sacral fractures:* minimal invasive stabilization technique with percutaneous iliosacral K-wire fixation or with a 3.5 mm screw

Mobilization with partial weight bearing is started within the first week postoperatively or dependent on associated injuries. A pain-dependent mobilization is favored. Typically, removal of internal implants is recommended after 3–6 month. An external fixator can be replaced 2–3 weeks postoperatively.

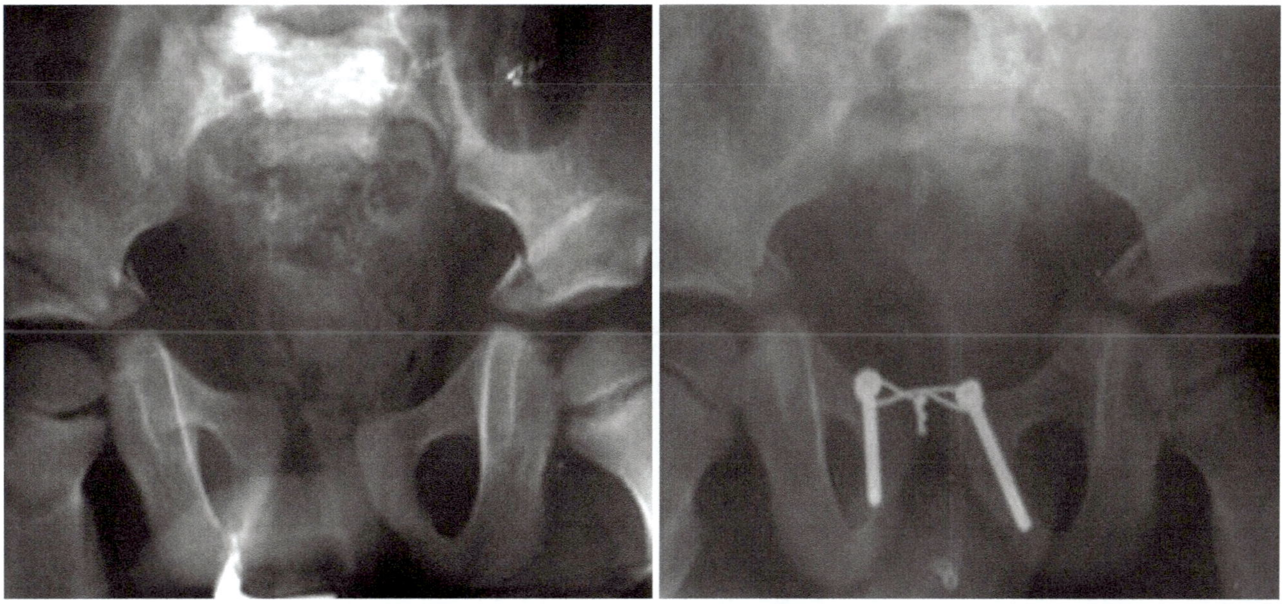

Fig. 36.7 Stabilization of the disrupted pubic symphysis in a young child using dynamic stabilization concepts with screws and wire-fixation

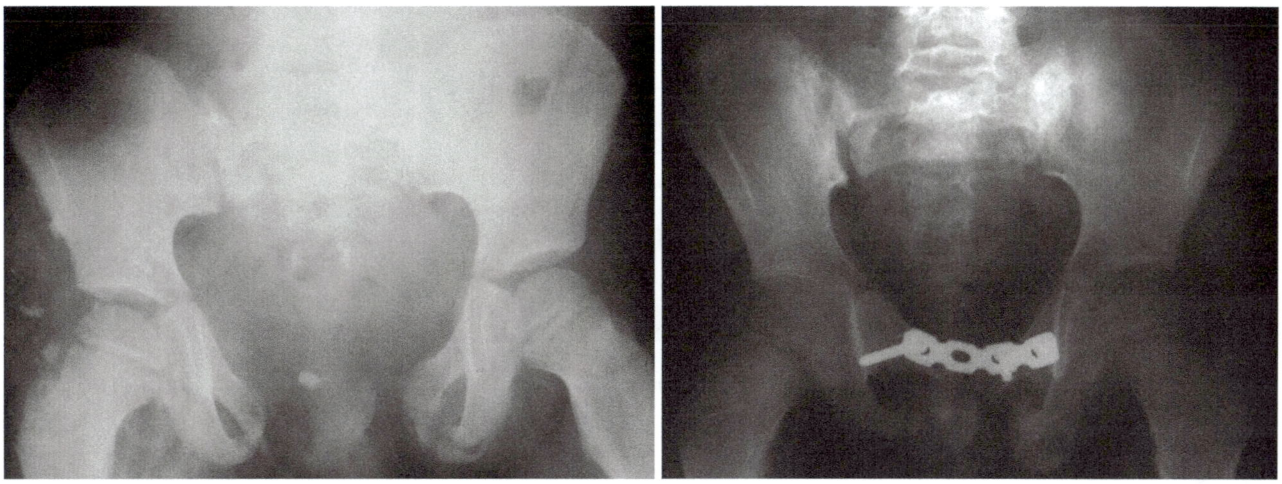

Fig. 36.8 Stabilization of the disrupted pubic symphysis in a middle-aged child using a small three-hole 3.5 mm plate

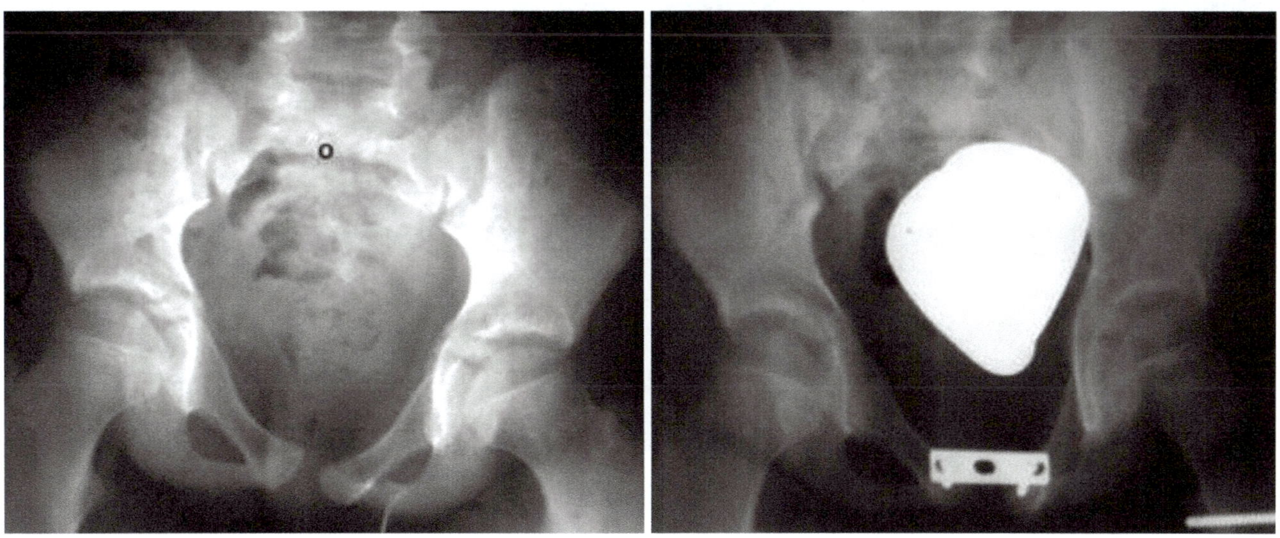

Fig. 36.9 Stabilization of the disrupted pubic symphysis in an older child using a standard plate

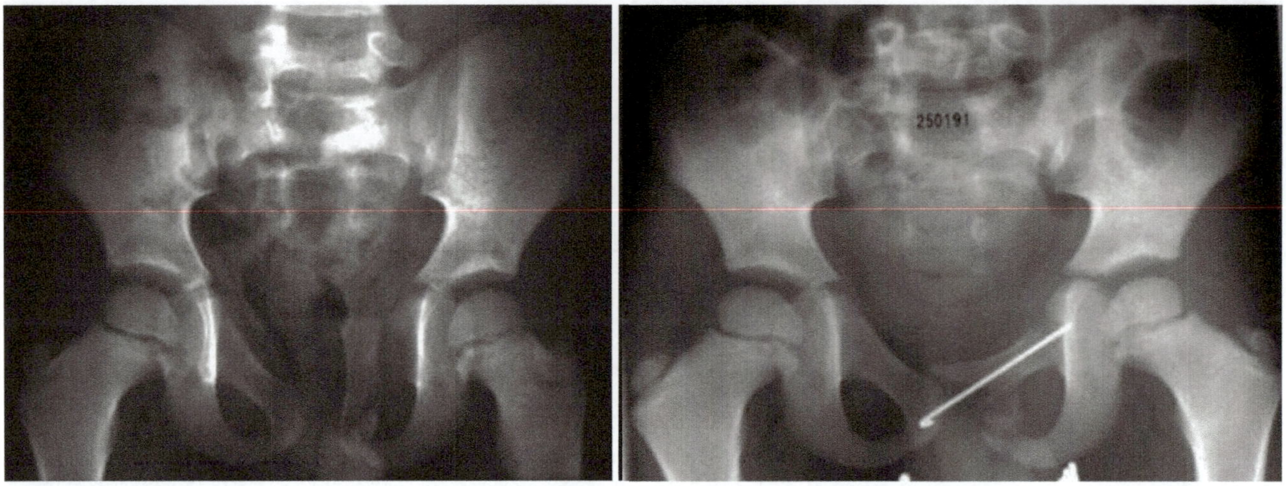

Fig. 36.10 Stabilization of a displaced pubic rami fracture with a K-wire

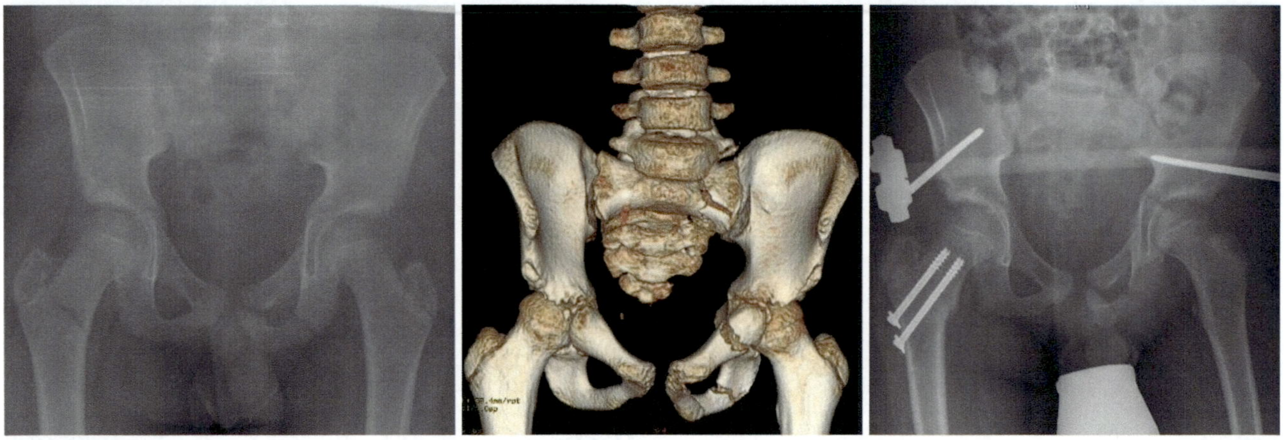

Fig. 36.11 Anterior stabilization of a displaced pubic rami fracture with an external fixator in an unstable type C injury (left sacrum fracture)

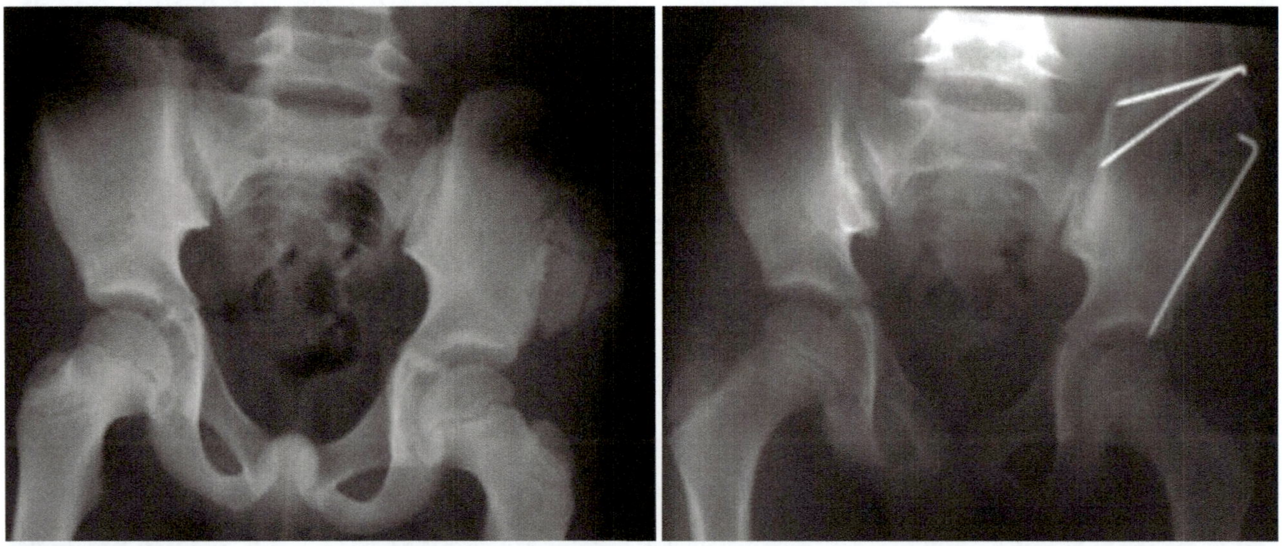

Fig. 36.12 Displaced iliac wing fracture stabilization with K-wires

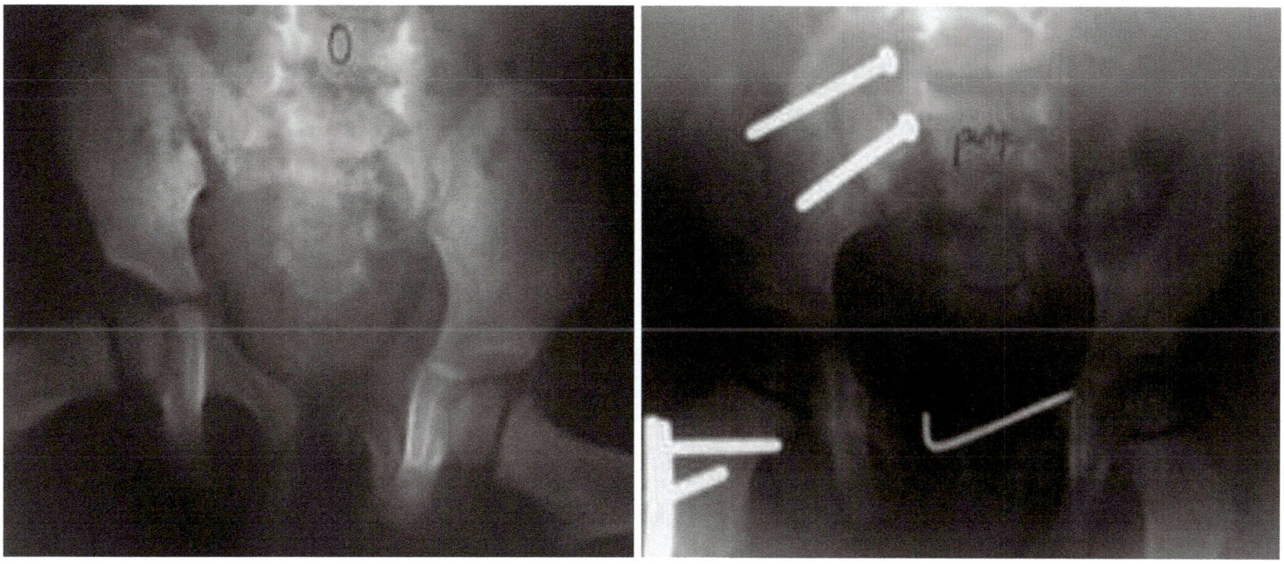

Fig. 36.13 Stabilization of a crescent fracture (iliac SI joint dislocation) with two 3.5 mm screws in a 3-year-old child (conversion of a type C injury into a type B injury)

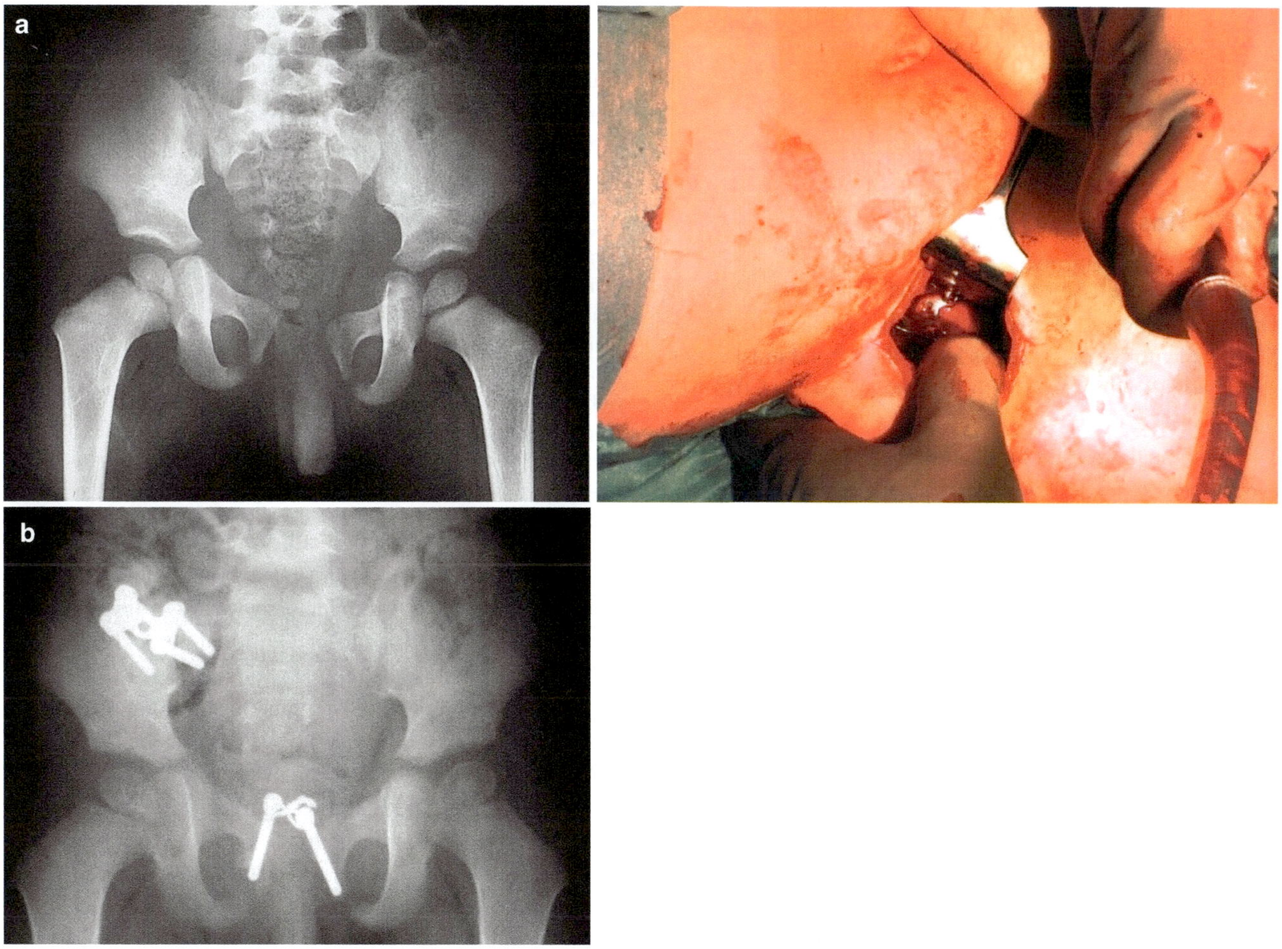

Fig. 36.14 Anterior plate stabilization of the disrupted SI joint in a 3-year-old child. Source: Gänsslen A, Pohlemann T. Kapitel 11.1 Kindliche Beckenringfrakturen, p. 209 (Fig. 11.4 a, b); in: Tscherne H, Pohlemann T (Eds.). Tscherne Unfallchirurgie – Becken und Acetabulum. Springer Verlag Berlin, Heidelberg, New York, 1998

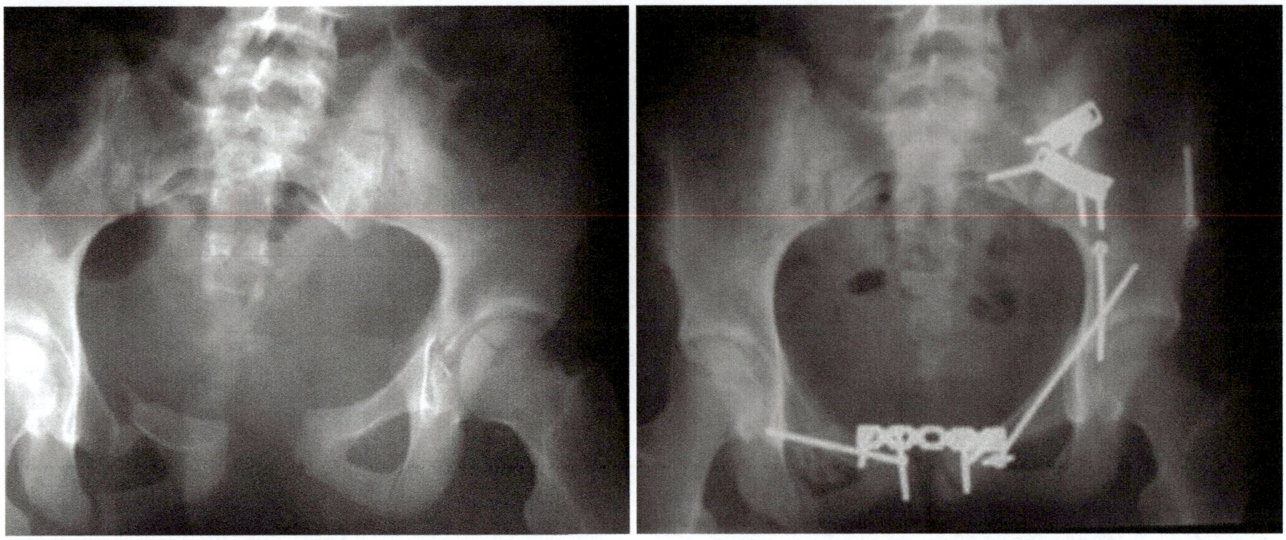

Fig. 36.15 Anterior plate stabilization of the disrupted SI joint in a 14-year-old child. Source: Gänsslen A, Pohlemann T. Kapitel 11.1 Kindliche Beckenringfrakturen, p. 208 (Fig. 11.3 a, c); in: Tscherne H, Pohlemann T (Eds.). Tscherne Unfallchirurgie – Becken und Acetabulum. Springer Verlag Berlin, Heidelberg, New York, 1998

Recent analyses reported a pelvic ring stabilization rate of 22.5% [34], all in unstable type B and -C injuries. External and internal fixation concepts were used. All three patients with type C injuries had internal fixation.

36.12 Hospital Course

Data from the American National Inpatient Pediatric Database showed an average length of hospital stay of 5.2 days, with pelvic fractures being the second most expensive hospitalization cause with an average cost of 15,011.61$/patient [23].

The typical duration of stay in the hospital is reported to range between 1 and 4 weeks, with a median of 8–9 days [7, 9, 16, 20, 31, 34, 37, 93], and the majority of patients can be discharged home (approximately 70%) [16, 20].

Within this time, an average of 1 week is for ICU treatment and observation [7, 15, 20, 31, 34].

36.13 Mortality

Present mortality is reported to between 0 and 16% with an average rate of 6.2% (Table 36.4) [7–9, 15, 16, 20, 30, 33, 34, 37, 38, 52, 93].

Recently, an analysis of 569 pediatric patients (age < 15 years) with at least AIS 2 pelvic injuries showed an overall mortality rate of 6.8% [31].

Some authors state that death from pelvic fractures is rare in children [12, 47, 68]. Analysis of the available data shows an incidence of approximately 1% [13, 15, 18, 40].

Table 36.4 Mortality in pediatric pelvic fractures since the year 2000

Author	Year	No. of patients	Patients died	%
Kruppa	2018	90	2	2.2
Chotai	2018	53	3	5.7
Tosounidis	2015	36	4	11.1
Zwingmann	2015	208	13	6.8
Banerjee	2009	44	7	15.9
Spiguel	2006	13	0	0
Vitale	2005	1190	86	7.2
Chia	2004	125	5	4
Grisoni	2002	57	3	5.3
Guillamondegui	2002	130	3	2.3
Junkins	2001	16	2	12.5
Silber	2001	166	6	3.6
Uppermann	2000	95	4	4.2
		2233	**138**	**6.2**

Analysis of the cause of death showed a significant association with additional severe head injury and the overall injury severity [93]. Further factors which significantly influence mortality were the presence of complex pelvic trauma (19% mortality) [19], the type of pelvic fracture [17, 45], and the presence of an open crush injury, a subgroup of complex pelvic trauma (20% mortality) [36], whereas in the analysis of Subasi et al., no change in overall mortality could be found in unstable type B and -C injuries [94].

Recently, it was confirmed that higher mortality rates of approximately 15% (doubled to that of type A and B injuries) were observed in Tile type C injuries [31].

The overall mortality rate in pediatric patients with pelvic ring injuries is slightly higher than in adults and depends on the instability of the pelvis.

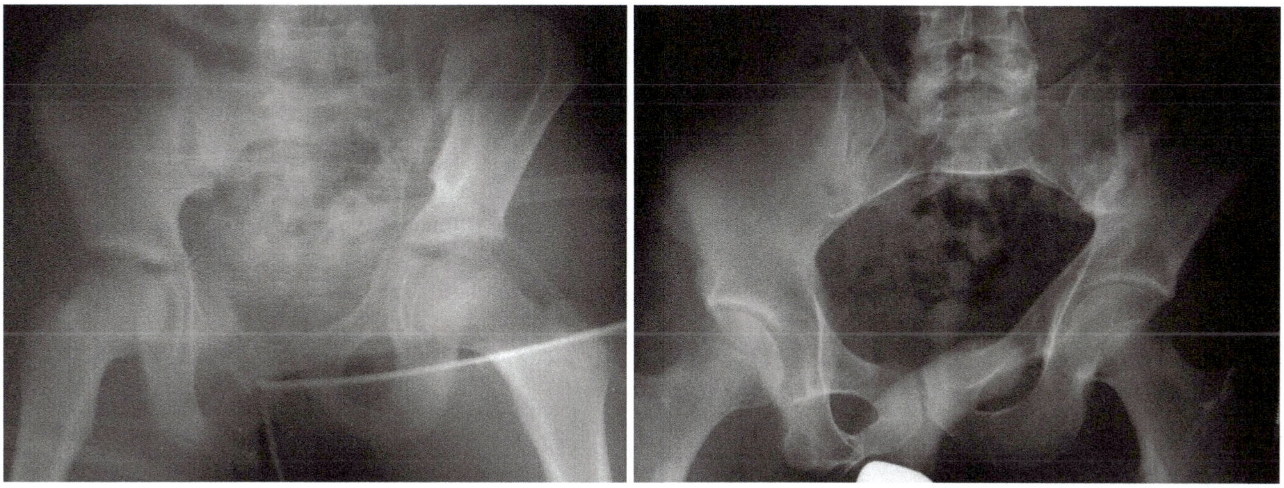

Fig. 36.16 Example of long-term sequelae after conservative treatment of an unstable pediatric pelvic ring injury (left crescent fracture) with hemipelvic malhealing

36.14 Long-Term Results

Several long-term problems are reported in the literature (Fig. 36.16).

Fracture-related sequelae were persistent nerve deficits [7, 78], recto-vaginal fistula [12], dyspareunia or altered vaginal sensation, vaginal obstructive complications [95], and pelvic infection [12].

Especially after complex pelvic trauma, a high rate of local complications was observed. Mosheiff et al. observed 11 wound and septic complications in 15 patients with open crush injuries of the pelvis in 15 patients (73%), 2 cases of recurrent bowel obstructions, and 1 case of a vascular graft failure [36]. Meyer-Junghänel et al. reported 38% complication rate [19]. Two patients had wound complications and three had severe bleeding complications.

The majority of reported complications are due to bony healing. These are leg length discrepancies [7, 78], delayed pubic union [78], fracture nonunion [7, 13, 17, 78, 96], subluxation of an SI joint [7], premature sacroiliac fusion [17, 42, 78, 90], persistent symphyseal diastasis [13, 17, 96], symphyseal ankylosis [22], pelvic asymmetry due to malhealing [22, 78], hemipelvic undergrowth [17, 42, 78, 90], development of lumbar scoliosis [7], and low back pain [42, 78].

Nonunions of the anterior pelvic ring, including diastasis of the pubic symphysis, usually cause no long-term problems and thus do not need specific treatment [13, 17, 78, 96].

Malunion can create leg length discrepancy and may lead to low back pain and spinal deformity [42, 78], but no data on displacement tolerance are available from the literature.

Sacroiliac injury can progress to premature sacroiliac fusion with the development of hemipelvic undergrowth [17, 42, 78, 90].

> Injury-related bone healing problems develop especially in unstable fracture situations.

Several reports focus on long-term results.

One hundred and twenty six children had a follow-up after a mean of 4 years (1–28 years) in the analysis by Richter et al. [81]. Eleven patients had pain, 16 had impairments during sporting activity, and in 14 patients the pelvis showed clinical asymmetry. Bony deformities were present in 29 cases (23%).

Rieger et al. analyzed 35/44 patients after an average of 135 months (18–235) [13]. They found an increase in long-term problems from type A to type C injuries. Eleven of 12 patients after type A injury were without any symptoms; only one patient reported low back pain, probably due to leg length discrepancy after femoral and lower leg fractures. The incidence of long-term problems is, therefore, 8.3%. Of eight type B injuries, in one case a nonunion at the anterior ring together with degenerative changes of the SI joint was observed but with only slight clinical impairments. Another patient showed a symphysiodesis and a third patient developed urethral stenosis resulting in an overall incidence of 37.5% long-term sequelae. Of 11 patients after type C injuries, seven reported on low back pain and two had functional restriction due to pelvic injury related gait abnormalities and nerve injuries. The overall incidence of long-term-sequelae was 63.6%.

Schwarz et al. in a multicenter study had long-term results in 17 of 32 patients (follow-up rate: 53%), which were less than 12 years at the time of injury [86] and found a correlation between healing in malposition and poor results. Follow-up was at least 2 years after the injury ranging from 2 to 25 years. Low back pain was present in six patients (35.3%). This correlated strongly with pelvic asymmetry. Eight patients had lumbar scoliosis and eight had significant radiographic asymmetry (each: 47.1%). Five patients had a leg length discrepancy of >2 cm (29.4%). Overall, five patients complained about chronic back pain (29.4%).

In a former analysis, Schwarz et al. reported on long-term results of 17 children from a multicenter study [97]. Nine patients had type B and eight type C injuries. No nonunions were observed. One patient had hemipelvic asymmetry due to acetabular dysplasia. Two patients had asymptomatic widening of the pubic symphysis and ten patients had scoliosis. Again, there was a correlation between the clinical and radiological results.

Meyer-Junghänel et al. analyzed 16 of 21 (76.2%) patients after complex pelvic trauma [19]. Nine patients were completely pain free at an average follow-up of 9 years. Three had moderate to severe pain. Persistent nerve deficits could not be observed. Four patients had urinary incontinence (25%). The radiological result showed only nine anatomical healings (incidence of radiological abnormalities: 43.7%). Two patients had a malhealing with 10–12 mm displacement. Three patients showed degenerative changes at the SI joint and three patients had an ankylosed SI joint. Two patients developed ankylosis of the pubic symphysis. Reevaluation of the primary and follow-up x-rays found overlooked injuries in eight patients. In the majority of patients, sacral fractures were not diagnosed primarily.

Blasier et al. found no significant difference in subjective scoring between type B and -C injuries for pain at rest, pain with activity, limp, and leg length discrepancy. Overall, there were 92% good or excellent results in the patients who were treated operatively and 80% good or excellent results in the patients who were treated nonoperatively [6].

Subasi et al. followed 55 patients with unstable type B and -C injuries (95% of their series) after a mean of 7.4 years. Gait abnormalities were seen in four patients (7.3%), leg length discrepancies and low back pain each in six patients (10.9%), degenerative SI joint changes and symphyseal sclerosis each in two patients (3.6%), and an ankylotic SI joint in one patient. Additionally, there were 11 urethral strictures (20%), 6 patients suffered from urinary incontinence, and 6 from erectile dysfunctions (10.9%). Fifty-six percent of the patients had long-term psychiatric disorders [94].

Overall, after type C injuries more long-term sequelae were observed.

Smith et al. analyzed 20 patients 3–12 years of age with unstable fractures at an average follow-up of 6.5 years. In patients with primary pelvic asymmetry, no remodeling was observed until the last examination [24]. Overall, 17 of 20 patients showed pelvic asymmetry. There was a 48% vs. 18% reduction of asymmetry after operative vs. conservative treatments. External fixation alone showed more asymmetry than results after anterior + posterior stabilization. After type C injuries, asymmetry was 3.5 cm initially and 3.3 cm at follow-up after external fixation and 3.9 cm and 0.6 cm after posterior internal fixation.

> Long-term sequelae can be observed in several children, especially after unstable injury patterns and complex pelvic trauma.

36.15 Conclusion

Pelvic ring injuries in children ≤14 years are rare. The main injury mechanism is a high-energy trauma resulting in a significant rate of additional truncal injuries. Anatomical differences compared to adults result in larger forces necessary to produce pelvic injuries. The rate of complex pelvic trauma is higher. The mortality rate is comparable to adults with 6.4%. Emergency treatment is orientated to adult standards, whereas definitive treatment is performed by conservative means in the majority of patients.

During the last years, increasing evidence shows that unstable injuries should be treated by external or internal fixation techniques with child-adapted implants. The main treatment modality is the external fixator.

Present data on long-term results after pediatric pelvic trauma indicate several long-term sequelae in unstable pelvic injuries depending on the instability of the child's pelvis at the time of injury. There is good correlation between the clinical and radiological results. Type A injuries normally heal without any problems.

References

1. Snyder C, Jain V, Saltzman D, Strate R, Perry J, Leonard A. Blunt trauma in adults and children: a comparative analysis. J Trauma. 1990;30(10):1239–45.
2. Keshishyan R, Rozinov V, Malakhov O, Kuznetzov L, Strunin E, Cogovadze G, Tsukanov V. Pelvic polyfractures in children. Clin Orthop. 1995;320:28–33.
3. Currey J, Butler G. The mechanical properties of bone tissue in children. J Bone Joint Surg. 1975;57-A(6):810–4.
4. Stuhler T, Stankovic P, Krause P, Koch A. Kindliche Beckenfrakturen: Klinik, Spätergebnisse, Biomechanik. Arch Orthop Unfall-Chir. 1977;90:187–98.
5. Ogden J. Chapter 15: Pelvis. In: Ogden J, editor. Skeletal injury in the child. Philadelphia: Lea & Febiger; 1982. p. 423–46.

6. Blasier RD, McAtee J, White R, Mitchell DT. Disruption of the pelvic ring in pediatric patients. Clin Orthop. 2000;376:87–95.
7. Chia J, JHolland A, Littel D, Cass D. Pelvic fractures and associated injuries in children. J Trauma. 2004;56:83–8.
8. Grisoni N, Connor S, Marsh E, Thompson G, Cooperman D, Blakemore L. Pelvic fractures in a pediatric level I trauma center. J Orthop Trauma. 2002;16(7):458–63.
9. Junkins E, Furnival R, Bolte R. The clinical presentation of pediatric pelvic fractures. Pediatr Emerg Care. 2001;17:15–8.
10. Junkins E, Nelson D, Carroll K, Hansen K, Furnival R. A prospective evaluation of the clinical presentation of pediatric pelvic fractures. J Trauma. 2001;51(1):64–8.
11. Lane-O'Kelly A, Fogarty E, Dowling F. The pelvic fracture in childhood: a report supporting nonoperative management. Injury. 1995;26(5):327–9.
12. Musemeche C, Fischer R, Cotler H, Andrassy R. Selective management of pediatric pelvic fractures: a conservative approach. J Pediatr Surg. 1987;22(6):538–40.
13. Rieger H, Brug E. Fractures of the pelvis in children. Clin Orthop. 1997;336:226–39.
14. Silber JS, Flynn JM, Katz MA, Ganley TJ, Koffler KM, Drummond DS. Role of computed tomography in the classification and management of pediatric pelvic fractures. J Pediatr Orthop. 2001;21(2):148–51.
15. Silber JS, Flynn JM, Koffler KM, Dormans JP, Drummond DS. Analysis of the cause, classification, and associated injuries of 166 consecutive pediatric pelvic fractures. J Pediatr Orthop. 2001;21(4):446–50.
16. Spiguel L, Glynn L, Liu D, Statter M. Pediatric pelvic fractures. A marker for injury severity. Am Surg. 2006;72:481–4.
17. Torode I, Zieg D. Pelvic fractures in children. J Pediatr Orthop. 1985;5(1):76–84.
18. Hauschild O, Strohm P, Culemann U, Pohlemann T, Suedkamp N, Koestler W, Schmal H. Mortality in patients with pelvic fractures. Results from the German pelvic injury register. J Trauma. 2008;64:449–55.
19. Meyer-Junghänel L, Gänsslen A, Pohlemann T, Tscherne H. Behandlungsergebnisse nach komplexem Beckentrauma bei Kindern. Unfallchirurg. 1997;100(3):225–33.
20. Banerjee S, Barry M, Paterson M. Paediatric pelvic fractures. 10 years experience in a trauma centre. Injury. 2009;40:410–3.
21. Rangger C, Gabl M, Dolati B, Spiss R, Beck E. Kindliche Beckenfrakturen. Unfallchirurg. 1994;97(12):649–51.
22. Stachel P, Hoffmann-v. Kap-herr S. Der Stellenwert der Operation bei Beckenfrakturen. In: Hoffmann-v S, editor. Kap-herr: Operationsindikationen bei Frakturen im Kindesalter. Stuttgart, New York: Gustav Fischer Verlag; 1987. p. 126–30.
23. Galano G, Vitale M, Kessler M, Hyman J, Vitale M. The most frequent traumatic orthopaedic injuries from a national pediatric inpatient population. J Pediatr Orthop. 2005;25:39–44.
24. Smith W, Shurnas P, Morgan S, Agudelo J, Luszko G, Knox E, Georgopoulos G. Clinical outcomes of unstable pelvic fractures in skeletally immature patients. J Bone Joint Surg. 2005;87-A(1):2423–31.
25. Barabas Z, Hargitai E, Doczi J, et al. Zentbl Chir. 1991;116(3):215.
26. Hart D, Wang M, Griffith P, McComb J. Pediatric sacral fractures. Spine. 2004;29(6):667–70.
27. Ismail N, Bellemaire J, Mollitt D, DiScala C, Koeppel B, Tepas J. Death from pelvic fracture: children are different. J Pediatr Surg. 1996;31(1):82–5.
28. Nabaweesi R, Arnold M, Chang D, Rossberg M, Ziegfeld S, Sawaya D, Bathurst M, Colombani P, Abdullah F. Prehospital predictors of risk for pelvic fractures in pediatric trauma patients. Pcdiatr Surg Int. 2008;24:1053–6.
29. Ramirez D, Schuette J, Knight V, Johnson E, Denise J, Walker A. Necessity of routine pelvic radiograph in the pediatric blunt trauma patient. Clin Pediatr. 2008;47(9):935–40.
30. Uppermann J, Gardner M, Gaines B, Schall L, Ford H. Early functional outcome in children with pelvic fractures. J Pediatr Surg. 2000;35:1002–5.
31. Zwingmann J, Lefering R, Maier D, Hohloch L, Eberbach H, Neumann M, Strohm P, Südkamp N, Hammer T. Pelvic fractures in severely injured children: results from the TraumaRegister DGU. Medicine. 2018;97:e11955. https://doi.org/10.1097/MD.0000000000011955.
32. Bent M, Hennrikus W, Latorre J, Armstrong D, Shaw B, Jones K, Seagl L. Role of computed tomography in the classification of pediatric pelvic fractures—revisited. J Orthop Trauma. 2017;31:e200–4.
33. Chotai N, Alazzawi S, Zehra S, Barry M. Paediatric pelvic fractures: a review of 2 cohorts over 22 years. Injury. 2018;49:613–7.
34. Tosounidis H, Sheikh H, Giannoudis P. Pelvic fractures in paediatric polytrauma patients: classification, concomitant injuries and early mortality. Open Orthop J. 2015;9:303–12.
35. Gänsslen A, Hildebrand F, Heidari N, Weinberg A. Pelvic ring lnjuries in children. Part l: epidemiology and primary evaluation. A review of the literature. Acta Chir Orthop Traumatol Cechoslov. 2012;79:493–8.
36. Mosheiff R, Suchar A, Porat S, Shmushkevich A, Segal D, Liebergall M. The "crushed open pelvis" in children. Injury. 1999;30(Suppl 2):B14–8.
37. Kruppa C, Khoriaty J, Sietsema D, Dudda M, Schildhauer T, Jones C. Does skeletal maturity affect pediatric pelvic injury patterns, associated injuries and treatment intervention? Injury. 2018;49:1562–7.
38. Zwingmann J, Aghayev E, Südkamp N, Neumann M, Bode G, Stuby F, Schmal H. Pelvic fractures in children results from the german pelvic trauma registry: a cohort study. Medicine. 2015;94:e2325. https://doi.org/10.1097/MD.0000000000002325.
39. Reichard S, Helikson M, Shorter N, White RJ, Shemeta D, Haller JJ. Pelvic fractures in children. J Pediatr Surg. 1980;15:727–34.
40. Bryan W, Tullos H. Pediatric pelvic fractures: review of 52 patients. J Trauma. 1979;19(11):799–805.
41. de la Calva C, Jover N, Alonso J, Salom M. Pediatric pelvic fractures and differences compared with the adult population. Pediatr Emerg Care. 2018. [Epub ahead of print]. https://doi.org/10.1097/PEC.0000000000001411.
42. Garvin KL, McCarthy RE, Barnes CL, Dodge BM. Pediatric pelvic ring fractures. J Pediatr Orthop. 1990;10(5):577–82.
43. Marcus R, Mills M, Thompson G. Multiple injury in children. J Bone Joint Surg. 1983;65-A:1290–4.
44. Sy M, Diouf S, Ndoye M, Mdiaye M, Fall I, Diop E, Diagne B. Les fractures du bassin chez l'enfant. Rev Chir Orthop. 1995;81:538–45.
45. McIntyre R, Bensard D, Moore E, Chambers J, Moore F. Pelvic fracture geometry predicts risk of life-threatening hemorrhage in children. J Trauma. 1993;35(3):423–9.
46. Ducloyer P, Filipe G. Les fractures du bassin de l'enfant à l'exclusion des fractures isolées du cotyle et du sacrum. Chir Pediatr. 1988;29(2–3):72–90.
47. Reed M. Pelvic fractures in children. J Can Assoc Radiol. 1976;27:255–61.
48. Kristinsson G, Wall S, Crain E. The digital rectal examination in pediatric trauma: a pilot study. J Emerg Med. 2007;32(1):59–62.
49. Shlamovitz G, Mower W, Bergman J, Crisp J, DeVore H, Hardy D, Sargent M, Shroff S, Snyder E, Morgan M. Lack of evidence to support routine digital rectal examination in pediatric trauma patients. Pediatr Emerg Care. 2007;23(8):537–43.
50. Kevill K, Wong A, Goldman H, HGershel J. Is a complete trauma series indicated for pediatric trauma victims? Pediatr Emerg Care. 2002;18:75–8.
51. Quick T, Eastwood D. Pediatric fractures and dislocations of thc hip and pelvis. Clin Orthop. 2005;432:87–96.
52. Guillamondegui OD, Pryor JP, Gracias VH, Gupta R, Reilly PM, Schwab CW. Pelvic radiography in blunt trauma resuscitation: a diminishing role. J Trauma. 2002;53(6):1043–7.

53. Fayad L, Corl F, Fishman E. Pediatric skeletal trauma: use of multiplanar reformatted and 3D 64-row multidetector CT in the mergenca department. Radiographics. 2009;29:135–50.
54. McDonald G. Pelvic disruptions in children. Clin Orthop. 1980;151:130–4.
55. Patel K, Chapman S. Normal symphysis width in children. Clin Radiol. 1993;47:56–7.
56. Krajbich J, Daneman A, Smith C, Donoghue V. Sacro-iliac joint injuries in children. J Bone Joint Surg. 1985;67-B(2):333.
57. Silber JS, Flynn JM. Changing patterns of pediatric pelvic fractures with skeletal maturation: implications for classification and management. J Pediatr Orthop. 2002;22(1):22–6.
58. Krauss F. Über Symphysensprengung. Zentbl Chir. 1930;3: 134–5.
59. McAlister D, Webb H, Wheeler P, Shinault K, Teague D, Fish J, Beall D. Pubic symphyseal width in pediatric patients. J Pediatr Orthop. 2005;25:725–7.
60. Bayer J, Neubauer J, Saueressig U, Südkamp N, Reising K. Age- and gender-related characteristics of the pubic symphysis and triradiate cartilage in pediatric computed tomography. Pediatr Radiol. 2016;46:1705–12.
61. Kalenderer Ö, Turgut A, Bacaksız T, Bilgin E, Kumbaracı M, Akkan H. Evaluation of symphysis pubis and sacroiliac joint distances in skeletally immature patients: a computerized tomography study of 1020 individuals. Acta Orthop Traumatol Turc. 2017;51: 150–4.
62. Oetgen M, Andelman S, Martin B. Age-based normative measurements of the pediatric pelvis. J Orthop Trauma. 2017;31:e205–9.
63. Key J, Conwell H. Management of fractures, dislocations and sprains. St. Louis: Mosby; 1951. p. 779–812.
64. OTA. Fracture and dislocation compendium. J Orthop Trauma. 1996;10(Suppl 1):71–5.
65. Pohlemann T, Gänsslen A, Partenheimer A. Becken und Acetabulumverletzungen im Kindesalter, Kapitel 18. In: Weinberg AM, editor. Tscherne Unfallchirurgie, Verletztungen im Kindesalter. Heidelberg, New York: Springer; 2006. p. 577–602.
66. Tscherne H, Pohlemann T. Tscherne Unfallchirurgie: Becken und Acetabulum. Berlin, Heidelberg, New York: Springer; 1998.
67. Advanced Trauma Life Support (ATLS). Student Course Manual. American College of Surgeons. 2018.
68. Bond S, Gotschall C, Eichelberger M. Predictors of abdominal injury in children with pelvic fracture. J Trauma. 1991;31(8):1169–73.
69. Vazquez W, Garcia V. Pediatric pelvic fractures combined with an additional skeletal injury is an indicator of significant injury. Surg Gynecol Obstet. 1993;177:468–72.
70. Jung J, Eo E, Ahn K, Noh H, Cheon Y. Initial base deficit as predictors for mortality and transfusion requirement in the severe pediatric trauma except brain injury. Pediatr Emerg Care. 2009;25(9):579–81.
71. Qasim Z, Massod R, Mateen M. Successful use of angiographic embolization to control hemorrhage from blunt pelvic trauma in a pediatric paients. J Pak Med Assoc. 2004;54(1):32–3.
72. Demetriades D, Karaiskakis M, Velmahos G, Alo K, Murray J, Chan L. Pelvic fractures in pediatric and adult trauma patients. Are they different injuries? J Trauma. 2003;54:1146–51.
73. Gänsslen A, Giannoudis P, Pape HC. Hemorrhage in pelvic fracture: who needs angiography? Curr Opin Crit Care. 2003;9(6):515–23.
74. Pohlemann T, Gänsslen A, Bosch U, Tscherne H. The technique of packing for control of hemorrhage in complex pelvic fractures. Tech Orthop. 1995;9(4):267–70.
75. Gänsslen A, Hildebrand F, Pohlemann T. Management of hemodynamic unstable patients "in extremis" with pelvic ring fractures. Acta Chir Orthop Traumatol Cechoslov. 2012;79:193–202.
76. Simpson T, Krieg JC, Heuer F, Bottlang M. Stabilization of pelvic ring disruptions with a circumferential sheet. J Trauma. 2002;52(1):158–61.
77. Baskin K, Cahill A, Kaye R, Born C, Grudziak J, Towbin R. Closed reduction with CT-guided screw fixation for unstable sacroiliac joint fracture-dislocation. Pediatr Radiol. 2004;34:963–9.
78. Engelhardt P. Die Malgaigne-Beckenringverletzung im Kindesalter. Orthopade. 1992;21:422–6.
79. Gottorf T, Egbers H. Behandlungsergebnisse kindlicher Beckenfrakturen. Zentbl Chir. 1991;116(3):215–6.
80. Reff R. The use of external fixation devices in the management of severe lower-extremity trauma and pelvic injuries in children. Clin Orthop. 1984;188:21–33.
81. Richter H. Beckenfrakturen im Kindesalter. Zentrbl Chir. 1991;116(3):214–5.
82. Holt G, Mencio G. Pelvic C-clamp in a pediatric patient. J Orthop Trauma. 2003;17(7):525–7.
83. Routt ML Jr, Nork SE, Mills WJ. High-energy pelvic ring disruptions. Orthop Clin North Am. 2002;33(1):59–72, viii.
84. Nierenberg G, Voloin G, Bialik V, Stein H. Pelvic fractures in children: a follow-up in 20 children treated conservatively. J Pediatr Orthop. 1993;1:140–2.
85. Quinby W. Fractures of the pelvis and associated injuries in children. J Ped Surg. 1966;1(4):353–64.
86. Schwarz N, Posch E, Mayr J, Fischmeister FM, Schwarz AF, Ohner T. Long-term results of unstable pelvic ring fractures in children. Injury. 1998;29(6):431–3.
87. Holdon C, Holman J, Hermann M. Pediatric pelvic fractures. J Am Acad Orthop Surg. 2007;15:172–7.
88. Karunakar M, Goulet J, Mueller K, Bedi A, Le T. Operative treatment of unstable pediatric pelvis and acetabular fractures. J Pediatr Orthop. 2005;25(1):34–8.
89. Stiletto R, Baacke M, Gotzen L. Comminuted pelvic ring disruption in toddlers. Management of a rare injury. J Trauma. 2000;48:161–4.
90. Heeg M, Klassen H. Long-term outcome of sacroiliac disruptions in children. J Pediatr Orthop. 1997;17:337–41.
91. Zimmermann T, Patzak H, Kelm C, Flechsenhar K, Kune K. Treatment of ruptures of the symphysis and iliosacral joint in pediatric patients. Eur J Pediatr Surg. 1993;2(6):348–51.
92. Gänsslen A, Pohlemann T, Hüfner T, Lobenhoffer P, Tscherne H. Interne Osteosynthese nach instabiler Beckenringfraktur bei einem 3-jährigen Kind. Unfallchirurg. 1998;101(7):570–3.
93. Vitale M, Kessler M, Choe J, Hwang M, Tolo V, Skaggs D. Pelvic fractures in children. An exploration of practice patterns and patient outcomes. J Pediatr Orthop. 2005;25(5):581–7.
94. Subasi M, Arslan H, Necmioglu S, Onen A, Özen S, Kaya M. Long-term outcomes of conservatively treated paediatric pelvic fractures. Injury. 2004;35:771–81.
95. Fowler J, Goodman G, Evans J, Schober J. Long-term vaginal sequelae secondary to pediatric pelvic fracture. J Pediatr Adolesc Gynecol. 2009;22:e15–9.
96. Ganz R, Gerber C. Fehlverheilte kindliche Frakturen im Becken- und Hüftbereich. Orthopade. 1991;20:346–52.
97. Schwarz N, Mayr J, Fischmeister F, Schwarz A, Posch E, Öhner T. 2-Jahres-Ergebnisse der konservativen Therapie instabiler Beckenringfrakturen bei Kindern. Unfallchirurg. 1994;97(9):439–44.

Avulsion Injuries

37

Axel Gänsslen and Annelie-Martina Weinberg

In the developing skeleton, apophyses serve as secondary ossification centers, which develop during the second decade of life. They serve as origin and insertion sites of muscles and tendons.

Thus, in skeletally immature patients, especially in young athletes at the age of 14–17 years, there is a risk of injury to these areas as the physis in this age is the weakest area of the musculotendinous connection to the bone due to perpendicular forces acting on the apophysis.

Histologically, a zonal organization can be observed until definitive apophyseal closure [1]. During growth, excretion of somatotropic hormone increases the columnar cartilage layer in the apophyseal growth zone, which leads to a decrease in tensile strength of the attached muscles connected to the apophysis and, additionally, androgens increases muscle power [2].

The typical apophyses at the pelvis are the anterior superior iliac spine (ASIS) with insertion of the sartorius muscle, the anterior inferior iliac spine (AIIS), origin of the rectus muscle, the ischial tuberosity (IT), origin of the hamstrings, the iliac crest (IC) with insertion of the abdominal wall muscles, and the superior corner of pubic symphysis (SCPS) [3].

Repetitive overuse of the musculotendinous unit can lead to apophysitis, whereas a sudden concentric or eccentric forceful muscular contraction of the attached musculotendinous junction while sprinting, jumping, or in sports, e.g., soccer, is supposed to be the main cause of pelvic avulsion injuries [3–5].

Different data exist regarding age of appearance and age of fusion of the pelvic apophyses [2, 6–9].

A. Gänsslen (✉)
Department of Trauma Surgery, Orthopedics and Hand Surgery, Hospital Wolfsburg, Wolfsburg, Germany

A.-M. Weinberg
Department of Orthopaedics and Trauma, Medical University of Graz, Graz, Austria
e-mail: anneliemartina.weinberg@medunigraz.at

Historical data reported inconsistent results with a wide range regarding appearance and closure [10–14]. A more recent CT analysis found a comparable gender-related appearance and closure of pelvic apophyses, while female apophyses appeared and closed approximately 1–2 years earlier than male apophyses [15] (for details, see subchapters).

37.1 Epidemiology

The first large series on pelvic apophyseal avulsion fractures was published in 2001. Rossi et al. reported on 203 cases with different avulsion injuries in a youth patient group (mean age: 13.8 years): 53.7% ischial tuberosity avulsions, 22.2% anterior inferior iliac spine avulsions, 19.2% anterior superior iliac spine avulsions, 7% avulsions of the superior corner of the pubic symphysis, and 3% iliac crest avulsions [3].

A second large series was published in 2014 by Schuett et al. [16]. Two hundred and twenty eight pelvic avulsion injuries were reported in 225 patients (76% male patients) with a mean age of 14.4 years. In contrast, AIIS avulsions were most common (49%), followed by 30% ASIS avulsions, 11% IT avulsions, and 10% IC avulsions. It was already stated that AIIS avulsion fractures had the worst prognosis with 4.47 times higher rate of chronic pain, whereas 4/5 nonunions developed at the IT. The main risk factor (26-fold higher) for nonunion was fracture displacement >20 mm.

Eberbach et al. analyzed the literature and reported the following frequencies of pelvic avulsion injuries:

- 33.2% anterior inferior iliac spine (AIIS)
- 29.7% ischial tuberosity (IT)
- 27.9% anterior superior iliac spine (ASIS)
- 6.7% iliac crest (IC)
- 1.8% lesser trochanter (LT)
- 1.2% superior corner of the pubic symphysis (SCPS)

A. Gänsslen et al. (eds.), *Pelvic Ring Fractures*, https://doi.org/10.1007/978-3-030-54730-1_37

37.2 Anterior Inferior Iliac Spine Avulsion (AIIS) Injuries

Injury to the rectus femoris muscle origin arises of two possible ways. The rectus femoris has two heads: the straight head originates on the anterior inferior iliac spine and the reflected head at the region above the upper acetabular rim. A third head was described in the literature and was observed in a recent analysis in 83% of the analyzed cases [17]. This third head runs to the iliofemoral ligament and to the tendon of the gluteus minimus muscle.

The straight head is involved in the beginning of hip flexion. Further flexion is then performed by the reflected head [18].

Therefore, two possible bony avulsion injuries are possible when these origins come under tension or excessive contraction.

Contraction or tensioning of the straight head results in strain of the musculotendinous junction of the direct head or avulsion fracture of the anterior inferior iliac spine (AIIS) (Fig. 37.1).

In contrast, the reflected head or even the "third head" can result in superior acetabular rim avulsion (SARA) by direct means or indirectly by tensioning of the iliofemoral ligament (Fig. 37.2) [19, 20].

Historically, only few cases of AIIS avulsion fractures have been reported in the literature. Köhler reported the first case of AIIS avulsion in a 13.5 year old boy, treated in 1926, injured during excessive running [21]. In 1935, Gallagher presented two additional cases, which he termed "sprinter's fracture" [22].

37.2.1 Anatomy

The apophysis of the AIIS normally develops between the 11th and 15th year of age and fuses between the 16th and 18th year of age [19, 23]. The physis is the weakest link of the muscle-tendon-bone connection [24]. Morscher demonstrated the weakness of the apophyses during puberty due to hormonal influence [25].

The AIIS is the origin of the straight head (pars directa) of the rectus femoris muscle, whereas the iliofemoral ligament and the reflected head of this muscle insert on the inferior part of the apophysis or between the AIIS and the acetabular rim [26].

37.2.2 Epidemiology

The majority of reports in the literature are dealing with AIIS avulsions. Lau et al. observed no case of this injury in a 5 year and 7 month period in a children's hospital [27]. In the analysis of Rossi et al. from the Italian Olympic Committee, of all patients with pelvic avulsion fractures, 45 patients had an avulsion fracture of the AIIS (22.7%). Overall, in all 1238 treated athletes during a 22 year period, an incidence of 3.6% was reported. On average, two cases per year were seen in this analysis [3]. Linni et al. observed ten AIIS avulsion fractures in a time period of 22 years (0.45 cases/year). Of all 22 patients this avulsion type had the highest incidence (45.5%) [28]. Fernbach et al. reported on 20% AIIS injuries in a group of 20 patients. All patients were male and sustained their injury during athletics [29]. Kameyama et al. found 240 documented cases of ASIS injury and 150 AIIS injury in Japan [30]. In another study Kameyama et al. analyzed 30 iliac spine injuries during a 7 year period of which 20 had ASIS injury and 10 had AIIS injury. All patients with AIIS injury were male with a mean age of 13.5 years. The side distribution was 1:1 [31].

The documented risk period is reported to be between the 13th and 16th years of age [4, 22, 28, 31–43].

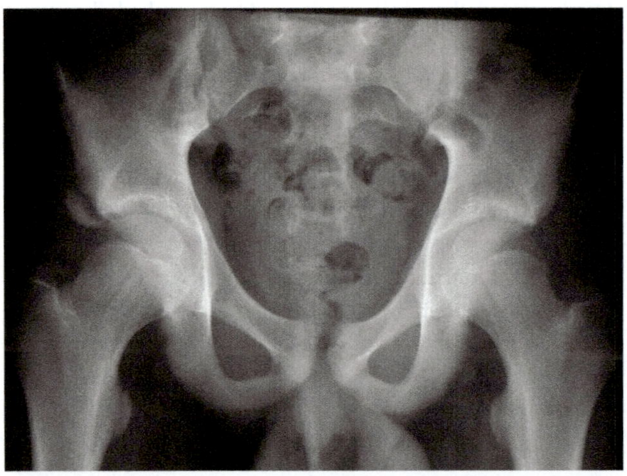

Fig. 37.1 AIIS avulsion (right) sustained during soccer playing (forceful kick)

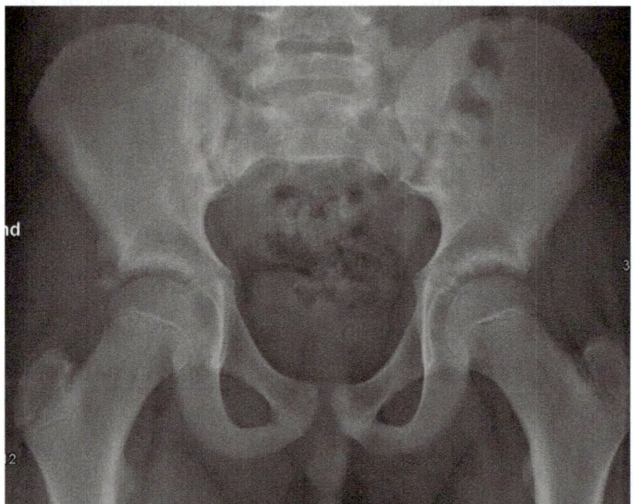

Fig. 37.2 SARA-lesion after running in sports

37.2.3 Mechanism of Injury

The predominant injury mechanism is an indirect mechanism due to excessive contraction or extension of the rectus femoris muscle. Due to the course of the straight head of the rectus muscle, during initial flexion of the hip or excessive contraction of the rectus femoris muscle the straight head is first set under tension and with ongoing flexion it becomes slack, whereas the reflected head then tightens late in the flexion phase [38, 41]. In contrast, avulsion of the AIIS by direct trauma is rare [26].

The principal mechanism resulting in AIIS avulsion is a forceful extension of the hip [44, 45] or excessive flexion of the hip while extending the knee (e.g., "kicking in the air" during soccer) [3]. Alternatively, the pull of the straight head of the rectus femoris muscle, caused by hip hyperextension and knee flexion, is another possible mechanism [44].

Forced hip and knee joint extensions are considered to be the main cause of AIIS avulsion in the starting phase during sprinting in soccer players, field hockey players, runners, tennis players, and hurdlers [3, 4, 16, 22, 28, 31–37, 39–41, 45–50].

Thus, avulsion fractures of the AIIS were called "sprinter's fracture" [22].

Rossi et al. described that soccer, athletics, and tennis are to be the most common causes of avulsion fracture to the AIIS. Soccer was responsible in 40%, athletics and tennis each in 22.2%, gymnastics in 6.7%, and wrestling and fencing each in 4.4% of the cases [3].

Steinbrück et al. reported several injury mechanisms: they stated that this injury can occur due to sudden contraction of the rectus femoris muscle while starting to sprint, a sudden fall during activities, and due to maximum kicking during soccer [23].

Additionally, the main cause of this injury in the study of Linni et al. was soccer in 70% and in one each case of gymnastics, skating, and riding [28].

In the analysis of Kameyama et al. again 70% of the patients sustained their injury during soccer playing, whereas one patient each was performing high jumping, jogging, and sprinting [31].

In rare situations, a combined anterior hip dislocation with avulsion fracture of the AIIS and ASIS due to suspected direct trauma during hip dislocation can result [51, 52].

37.2.4 Symptoms

A good overview of the possible symptoms during examination and history was reported by Steinbrück et al. [23]. Frequently, there is a history of a whip-cracking type noise or an audible "pop" [23, 37, 42, 53].

Overall, there is a wide range of possible symptoms: sharp pain in the hip region [22, 53], local swelling in the inguinal region [44], visible hematoma [23], local tenderness and pain on palpation [22, 33, 38, 44, 45, 53], painful restricted range of motion (flexion, extension) [22, 23, 33, 42, 44, 53], limited (painful) hip abduction [23, 43], weakness of hip flexion and typically weakness in knee extension [53], crepitation [23], and rarely mild vasomotor disturbances [22].

Overall, these injuries are less painful than injuries to the ASIS [29].

37.2.5 Diagnostics

The conventional pelvic anterior-posterior x-ray is the initial gold standard (Fig. 37.1) but can be without signs of injury to the AIIS [3, 24]. In rare situations, contralateral plain x-rays can exclude or confirm the injury [54].

Oblique views (Iliac oblique view) are often necessary and recommended to distinguish between avulsion injuries and a normal apophysis (Fig. 37.3) [3, 23, 45, 49, 55].

The fragment is typically small and crescent-shaped (Fig. 37.4) [4, 21, 53, 56] or triangular [57].

Displacement is usually minor, <3 mm, because the uninjured reflected head of the rectus femoris muscle avoids larger displacement [31, 58, 59].

Maximum displacement is up to 1 cm with inferior displacement [21, 26, 29, 43, 53, 60] just proximally above the rim of the acetabulum. A significantly inferior displaced ASIS avulsion fracture can also mimic this injury [33, 61, 62].

Bilateral AIIS avulsions are rare [43, 53, 63].

The value of ultrasonography and MRI is unclear. Pisacano et al. analyzed MRI and ultrasonography for diagnosing AIIS avulsion fractures [64]. All three cases with AIIS avulsion fractures were identified on MRI and ultrasonography. Sonographical signs of avulsion injury compared with the contralateral side were widening of the physis, displacement of the apophysis, hypoechoic or mixed echogenic edema, hemorrhage in the widened space (Fig. 37.5), and hyperemia in power Doppler sonography [64]. Sonography is considered as an alternative modality when conventional x-rays fail to reveal a suspected avulsion [64].

In contrast, MRI was stated unspecific as low-signal cortical fragments due to missing bone marrow in these fragments can make diagnosis difficult. MRI is more important to exclude relevant musculotendinous injury [65]. Only indirect sings, like hematoma and/or periosteal stripping, waviness, and retraction of the torn tendon with the fragment can be demonstrated [66].

Sanders recommended CT diagnostics [45], but overall ultrasound, CT, and MRI are usually not required in the acute

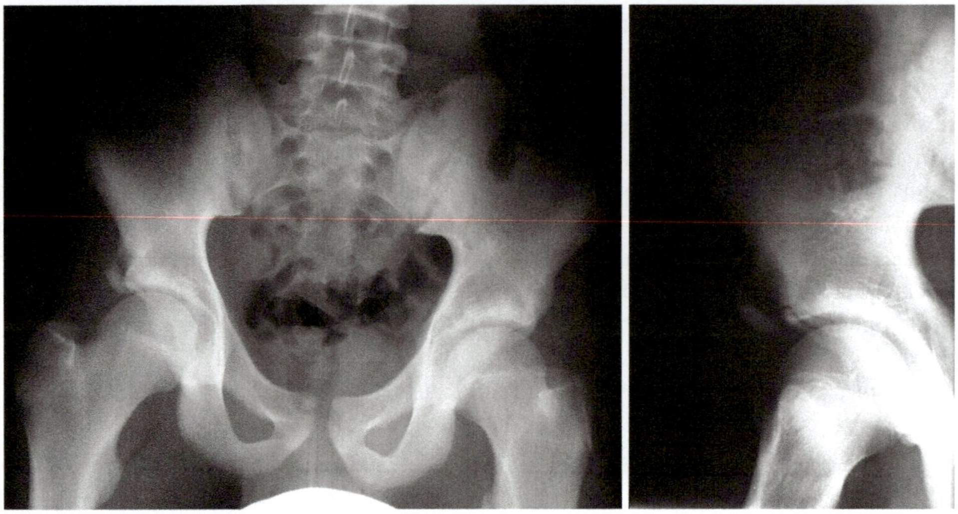

Fig. 37.3 Oblique views (Iliac oblique view) can be helpful to analyze the location and size of the fragment

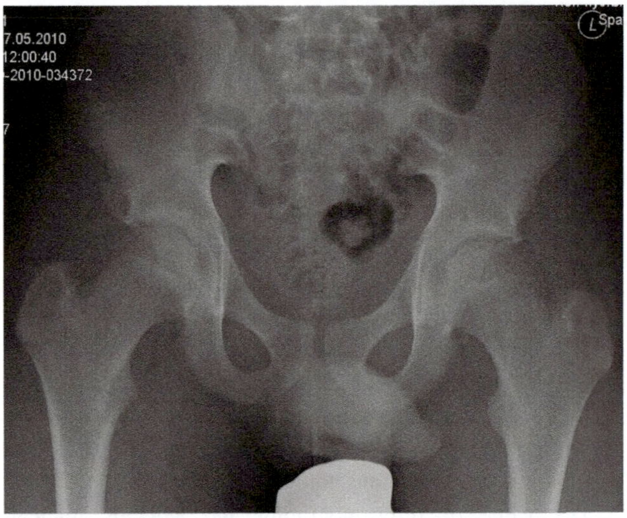

Fig. 37.4 The fragment is typically small and crescent-shaped

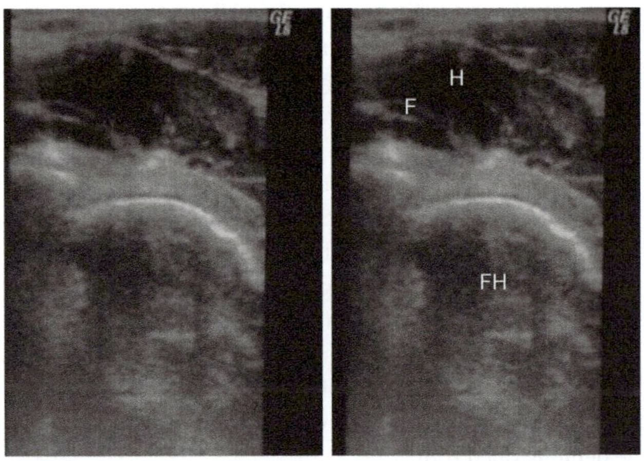

Fig. 37.5 Ultrasonography of an AIIS lesion: the hematoma formation (H) anterior to the upper femoral head (FH) and even the fragment (F) can be visualized

phase. These imaging methods have their main value in undisplaced fractures or nonossified apophyses [50, 65, 67].

The differentiation between the AIIS avulsion fracture and the superior acetabular rim avulsion (SARA) can be made by radiography or CT.

Chronic AIIS avulsion fractures can mimic tumor lesions [34, 35, 41]. Radiologically, they can present as exostosis [34], myositis ossificans [21], tendoligamentous calcifications [26], or tumor-like ossifications of the apophysis [23, 41, 45].

From the differential diagnostic standpoint, an os acetabuli [29, 59] and a neoplasm have to be considered (Fig. 37.6). The latter can be an osteosarcoma [41], Ewing's sarcoma [49], or other tumors. Benign lesions can be osteomyelitis [4]. Rarely, lower quadrant abdominal pain and clinical signs of an ileus can be present [4]. Therefore, biopsy can be an option to exclude tumor lesions [26, 35, 36, 41], but unnecessary biopsy should not be considered [35, 41].

Additionally, hypertrophic bone can develop [47], which can clinically result in femoroacetabular impingement syndrome (Fig. 37.6), especially in late diagnosed patients [39, 68].

A significantly displaced ASIS avulsion fracture can be misinterpreted as an AIIS avulsion [33, 61, 62].

37.2.6 Treatment

Conservative treatment of an avulsed AIIS is performed in the majority of patients leading to excellent clinical results [31, 49, 53, 62]. After conservative treatment no significant migration of the fragment occurred within 36 months postinjury [31].

In the large analysis by Rossi et al. no patient with an injury of the AIIS was treated operatively [3]. Steinbrück treated patients with AIIS injuries conservatively with bed rest in hip flexion for 2–3 weeks [23]. Linni et al. performed conservative treatment in all patients [28]. Kameyama et al. performed con-

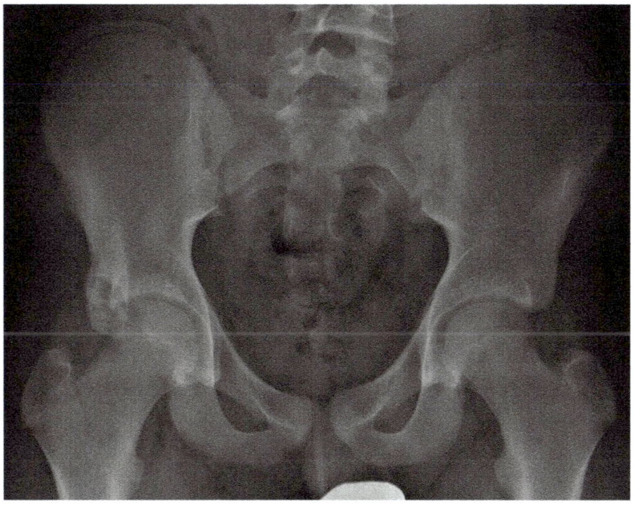

Fig. 37.6 Old AIIS injury with hypertrophic bone formation resulting in clinical signs of femoroacetabular impingement (FAI)

servative treatment in nine and screw fixation of the AIIS in one patient [31]. Even a case with a displacement of 2 cm did well with conservative treatment [69]. Thus, osteosynthesis (screw fixation) is rarely recommended [31, 70].

Conservative treatment consists primarily of ice-therapy, nonsteroidal antiinflammatory drugs (e.g., ibuprofen), limited weight bearing with crutches, and passive-assisted range of motion exercises dependent on the amount of pain [53]. Fixation of the hip in 30° flexion is performed to release tension to the rectus muscle, with or without an additional spica cast [58].

Recently, several authors favor a 4–5-step program of rehabilitation [4, 43]. During the first week initial rest, isometric muscle exercises and weight protection are recommended. In the second to fourth week, passive motion, walking with crutches (no/partial weight bearing), and gentle stretching are allowed. In the fourth to sixth week, active motion and strengthening, isokinetic exercises, and active joint movements are usually possible and thereafter athletic participation can be started [4, 43].

The time to full recovery after AIIS avulsion fracture has been reported to vary from 3 weeks to 4 months [4, 21, 22, 26, 44, 53, 57].

In contrast, Linni et al. reported 30% persisting symptoms after 2–24 months postinjury [28]. This led to defining indications for operative treatment:

- Screw fixation, if displacement is >2.5 cm [39]
- ORIF, if displacement is >3 cm [71]
- Resection, after exostosis formation [39, 72]

> If diagnosed early, conservative treatment leads to good and excellent results in the majority of patients [4].

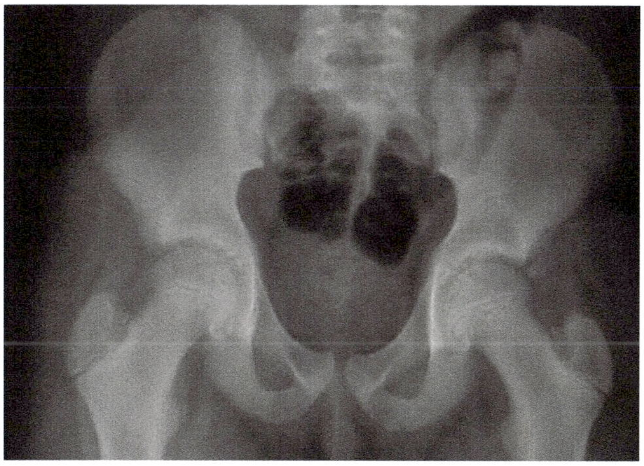

Fig. 37.7 Left SARA avulsion injury

In a comparable analysis (11× operative vs. 4× conservative treatment) of 15 patients with AIIS avulsion fractures, long-term outcomes after 1 year were comparable, but patients after ORIF had faster recovery [48]. Interestingly, in 73% radiological CAM-type femoroacetabular impingement developed.

Sinikumpu et al. analyzed 11 athletic patients with surgical treatment of an avulsed AIIS fracture. The indication for surgery was displacement >20 mm in all cases. Two had fragment resection and nine had anchor fixation or transosseous suturing. At latest follow-up at least 1 year after surgery, 81.8% reported a good outcome [73].

In a meta-analysis by Eberbach et al., highly active patients with >15 mm displacement of any avulsion injuries, including AIIS injuries, profited from surgical treatment [74].

37.3 Superior Acetabular Rim Avulsion

Injury to the reflected head or even the "third head" of the rectus abdominis muscle can result in superior acetabular rim avulsion (SARA) by direct means or indirectly by tensioning of the iliofemoral ligament [19, 20]. These injuries are rare (Fig. 37.7) [32, 38, 75].

37.4 Anterior Superior Iliac Spine Avulsion (ASIS) Injuries

At the anterior iliac crest, at the level of the ASIS, the sartorius muscle and slightly posterior the tensor fasciae latae muscle have their origins. Sudden contraction or hyperextension can cause injury to the physis of the ASIS (Fig. 37.8). Thus, the majority of these injuries occur in the athletes.

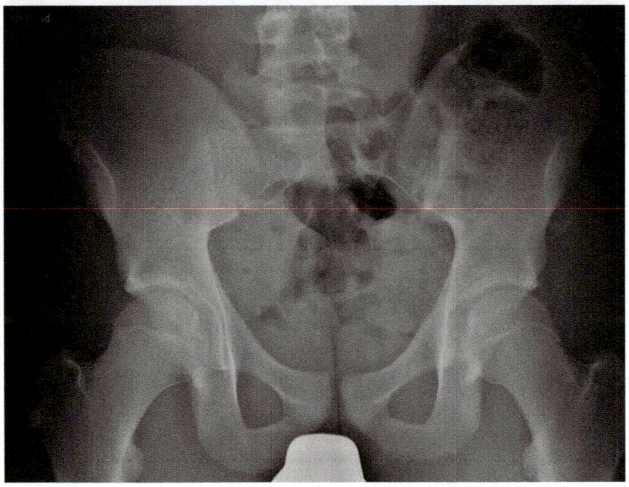

Fig. 37.8 Left ASIS avulsion injury

37.4.1 Anatomy

Parvaresh et al. performed a literature review and stated that the ASIS fragment appears with 16 years (median: males 14 years, females 15 years) and closure is observed at 25 years of age (median: males 18 years, females 15.8 years) [15].

37.4.2 Epidemiology

ASIS avulsions are the third frequent avulsion injury around the pelvis [74].

Lau et al. observed 12 cases of this injury in a 5 year and 7 month period in a children's hospital [27].

In the analysis of Rossi et al. from the Italian Olympic Committee, of all 203 patients with pelvic avulsion fractures, 39 patients had an avulsion fracture of the ASIS (19.2%). Overall, in all 1238 treated athletes during a 22 year period, an incidence of 3.1% was reported. In average, two cases per year were seen in this analysis [3].

Linni et al. observed two ASIS avulsion fractures in a time period of 22 years (0.1 cases/year) [28].

Kameyama et al. found 240 documented cases of ASIS injury and 150 AIIS injury in Japan [30].

In another study Kameyama et al. analyzed 20 ASIS injuries during a 7 year period. Except one, all patients with ASIS injury were male with a mean age of 14.5 years. The side distribution was 3:1 for the right side [31].

The documented risk period is reported to be between 12 and 13 years of age [27].

37.4.3 Mechanism of Injury

The classical mechanism is a sudden contraction of the sartorius muscle with the hip extended and the knee flexed.

Rossi et al. described that soccer, athletics, and gymnastics were to be the most common causes of avulsion fracture to the ASIS [3].

In the analysis of Kameyama et al., the majority of patients (80%) sustained their injury during running or sprinting [31].

In rare situations, a combined anterior hip dislocation with avulsion fracture of the AIIS and ASIS due to suspected direct trauma during hip dislocation can result [51, 52].

Porr et al. observed ASIS avulsion injuries after running and kicking, while the most common injury mechanism was a fracture after iliac crest bone harvesting [76].

Schuett et al. observed predominantly running/sprinting mechanisms (50% of ASIS injuries), while kicking resulted more often in AIIS injuries [16].

37.4.4 Symptoms

Physical evaluation reveals local swelling, a direct pain maximum at the ASIS or over the course of the sartorius muscle. Tenderness and pain during provocative maneuvers are typically positive.

Also, an avulsion can present with signs of meralgia paraesthetica [77].

37.4.5 Diagnostics

The conventional pelvic anterior-posterior x-ray is the initial gold standard (Fig. 37.9). Due to overprojection and the often very small avulsion fragments, diagnosis can be difficult.

An iliac oblique view can be sometimes helpful to detect these injuries (Fig. 37.9) [9]. In delayed cases, an MRI can be useful. Sonography is valuable to detect local hematoma formation [77].

37.4.6 Treatment

In the large analysis by Rossi et al., only two of 39 patients with an injury of the ASIS were treated operatively [3].

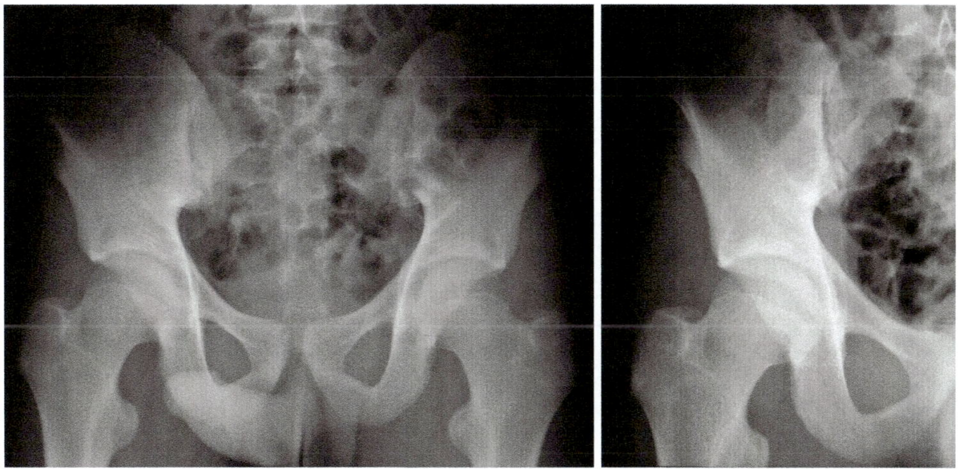

Fig. 37.9 Right ASIS avulsion injury

Steinbrück treated patients with ASIS injuries conservatively with bed rest for 2–3 weeks with the hip joint slightly flexed [23].

Kautzner et al. recommended initial bed rest, hip positioning at 70–90° of flexion for 3 weeks, and local pain treatment for conservative treatment [78]. After 3 weeks, physiotherapy and partial weight bearing were allowed for 3 weeks followed by pain-dependent full weight bearing. After 6 months, standard sporting activities were normally possible. With surgical treatment, sporting activities were already possible after 3 months, but implant removal was considered between 6 and 12 months, requiring further surgery. A comparable concept was proposed by Stancak et al. [48]. After 12 months, all patients, with/without surgery, presented with bone healing, full range of motion, and without local pain [78].

Linni et al. performed a conservative treatment for his two patients [28].

Kameyama et al. performed conservative treatment in ten patients and screw fixation/K-wire fixation in another ten patients [31]. The long-term results were exclusively good and excellent in both groups.

Indications for operative treatment include:

- Screw fixation, if displacement is >2 cm [73]
- ORIF, if displacement is >1 cm [48]
- Resection, after exostosis formation [39, 72]

In a comparable analysis (13× operative vs. 10× conservative treatment) of 23 patients with ASIS avulsion fractures, long-term outcomes after 1 year were comparable, but patients after ORIF had faster recovery [48].

Sinikumpu et al. analyzed four athletic patients after surgical treatment of an avulsed ASIS fracture. The indication for surgery was displacement >20 mm in all cases. Two transosseous sutures were performed; each had resection and screw fixation, respectively. At latest follow-up at least 1 year after surgery, 75% reported a good outcome [73].

Kautzner et al. analyzed 23 patients in a 8-year period (19 male, 4 female patients). The mean age at the time of injury was 15.1 years. Ten patients presented with minimally displaced avulsion fractures and were treated conservatively with bed rest, pain medication, and 70–90° hip flexion for 3 weeks. Thirteen patients sustained displaced injuries and were treated with lag screw fixation with/without an additional K-wire using an anterior approach. Recovery was faster after surgery, but 5 out of 13 patients developed some heterotopic bone formation [78].

37.5 Iliac Crest Avulsion Injuries

There are three possible type of injuries involving the iliac crest apophysis [79]:

- Acute avulsion injury from sudden abdominal wall contraction
- Direct contusion ("hip pointer" injury)
- Overuse and chronic trauma due to repetitive muscle contraction ("apophysitis")

37.5.1 Appearance and Closure

The iliac crest apophysis develops in male patients between 12 and 15 years (median 14 years), and closure is observed between 16 and 23.9 years (median 21.6 years). In females, the apophysis appears between 11.3 and 15.9 years (median 14.4 years) and closure is found at an age of 15.8–25.8 years

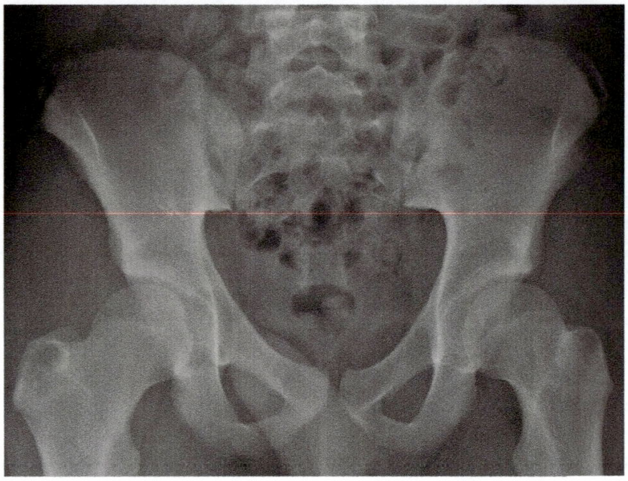

Fig. 37.10 Rare case of a right-sided iliac crest avulsion injury presenting with significant pain

(median 23.3 years) [15]. Ossification typically starts from anterior to posterior [14, 80].

37.5.2 Epidemiology

Injuries to this apophysis are uncommon (Fig. 37.10). In a recent meta-analysis, 6.7% of all pelvic avulsion injuries were IC injuries [74]. In large series, a total of 500 patients could be analyzed [3, 16, 48]. The frequency of iliac crest avulsion injuries was 5.6% (range: 1.5–10.1%).

37.5.3 Injury Mechanism

A forced contraction of the inserting abdominal wall muscles is supposed to be the main cause of iliac crest avulsion injuries, often in tennis, wrestling, and gymnastics [3].

37.5.4 Radiology

In the majority of cases, a standard pelvic AP x-ray is performed for diagnosing this injury.

Lombardo et al. stated that a discontinuity of the anterior part of the iliac apophysis can be physiologically present after even direct contusion (hip pointer injury [81]) in young adults, thus, making the radiological diagnosis difficult [80].

MRI diagnostics show that overuse injuries typically present with increased signal intensity on water-sensitive sequences and only mild physeal widening. Additional bone and/or muscle edema can be present [79].

Avulsion injuries should be diagnosed if there is a definitive displacement at the iliac crest [79, 82–84].

There was a comparable gender distribution in these injuries. The mean radiographic displacement was 6.6 mm, and the involved size at the iliac crest was 45.8 mm [16].

37.5.5 Treatment

Only few case reports dealt with treatment of iliac crest avulsion injuries. Conservative treatment is the treatment of choice in these injuries [16, 48, 82, 84, 85].

In the largest series of 25 cases, no refractures or nonunions were observed at follow-up and one patient had persistent hip pain [16], all after conservative treatment. Pain usually disappears within 3 months [48].

Rarely, open reduction along with screw fixation is performed [73, 83]. As with other pelvic avulsion injuries, displacement determines the need for ORIF. Displacement of >30 mm is a potential indication for operative stabilization [86].

A recent analysis described ten patients with IC avulsion fractures, which were treated by open reduction and screw fixation [87]. Normal activity was reached after 4 weeks, and after a mean of 11.2 months normal individual athletic activity was reached.

37.6 Ischial Tuberosity Avulsion

The IT appears late and fusion is observed between the twentieth and thirtieth year of age.

Parvaresh et al. performed a literature review and stated that the IT fragment appears between the ages of 13–18 years (median: males 14 years, females 12.6 years), and closure is observed between 20 and 25 years of age (median: males 20.6 years, females 20.2 years) [15].

In a detailed forensic analysis, the ischial tuberosity apophysis appeared between the ages of 15.34 and 16.17 years for males, and between 14.39 and 15.64 years for females. Ossification starts between 18.50 and 19.17 years for males, and 18.73 and 19.44 years for females, and full ossification was observed between 22.93 and 23.30 years for males, and 23.62 and 24.07 years for females [88].

37.6.1 Anatomy

The hamstring complex consists of three separate muscles: the semimembranosus (SM), the semitendinosus (ST), and the biceps femoris muscle (BF) originating just underneath the gluteus maximus at the pelvic bone.

Anatomically, there is the common (conjoined) tendon of ST and BF on the ischium, originating medially, while the

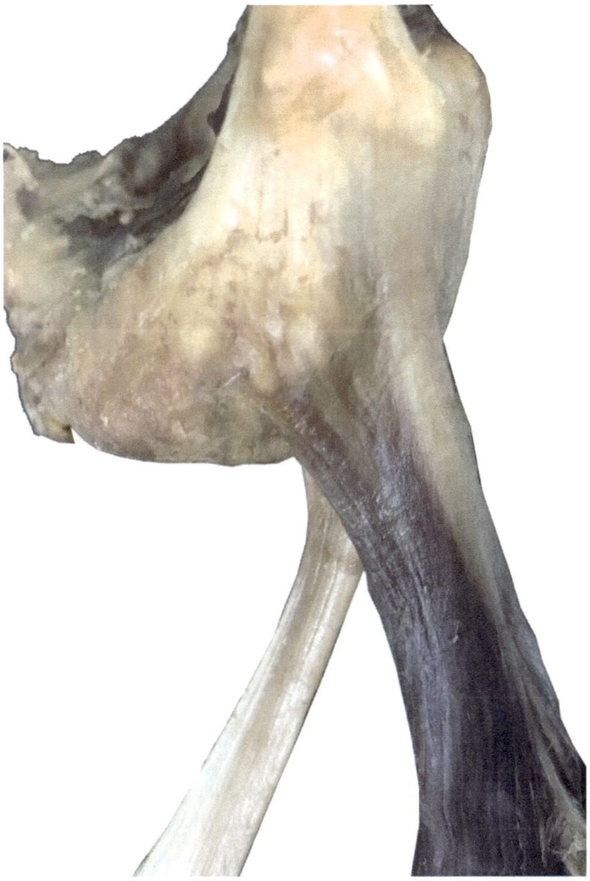

Fig. 37.11 Anatomy of the hamstring origin at the ischial tuberosity

semimembranosus originates more laterally (Fig. 37.11) [89–91].

ST and BF split approximately 9.9 cm from their origins, and the mean distance to the inferior border of the gluteus maximus is approximately 6.3 cm. There is a close relationship to the sciatic nerve, which runs slightly lateral to the ischial tuberosity [90, 91].

The common ST/BF originates from the posteromedial aspect of the ischial tuberosity in an oval of 2.5 × 1.8 cm. More anterior, the smaller SM origin is located with a length of 1.1 cm and a width of 1.3 cm [92].

The hamstring muscles have a broad origin at the lateral ischial tuberosity. Due to their great power, typically, the avulsed part with a larger fragment consists of the whole apophysis, not involving the obturator foramen.

In rare cases, extended avulsion injury of the ischial tuberosity is observed. It can be distinguished from classical avulsion injuries by their involvement of the obturator foramen. Davis reported on such a case with fracture directly below the acetabular level and fracture at the inferior pubic rami, which was fixed by plate osteosynthesis [93]. Often high-energy trauma was responsible for such an injury (Fig. 37.12).

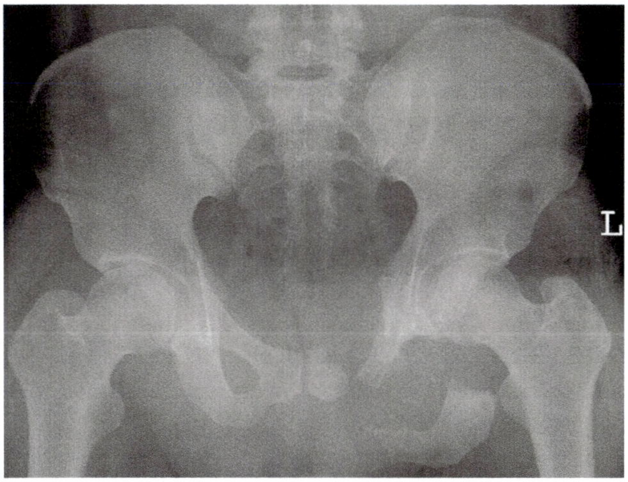

Fig. 37.12 Extended avulsion injury of the complete inferior ischium in a patient with additional bilateral open-book injury

37.6.2 Epidemiology

Hamstring avulsion fractures are rare (2.9%) when considering proximal hamstring injuries [94]. These injuries are typically observed in young male patients.

In the analysis of Rossi et al. from the Italian Olympic Committee, of 203 patients with pelvic avulsion fractures, 109 patients had an avulsion fracture of the IT (53%). Overall, in all 1238 treated athletes during a 22 year period, an incidence of 8.8% was reported. In average, five cases per year were seen in this analysis [3].

Linni et al. observed no ischial tuberosity avulsion in a time period of 22 years [28]. Fernbach et al. reported on 30% AIIS injuries in a group of 20 patients. All patients were male and sustained their injury during athletics [29].

37.6.3 Mechanism of Injury

IT avulsions typically are observed between begin of apophyseal ossification and fusion [95].

The typical mechanism is an extreme contraction of the hamstring complex often during sprinting activities or sudden and excessive lengthening as a result of forced hip flexion, while the knee is extended, when kicking a ball, jumping, figure skating, and performing splits during gymnastics or cheerleading [3, 7, 76, 96].

Additionally, the injury mechanism can be an extreme abduction, even in elderly patients [97].

The most common sports resulting in IT avulsions were soccer and gymnastics in the analysis by Rossi [3], while Schuett et al., besides running/sprinting activities in 36%, observed injury from falling in 12% [16].

37.6.4 Diagnostics

Clinically, pain at the ischial tuberosity and large posterior hematoma formation can be present [98]. Pain in the buttock region and on palpation, antalgic gait, or even inability to walk can be further signs of this injury, but radiographically, musculotendinous injuries have to be distinguished.

The clinical signs are nonspecific. Thus, posterior thigh pain, and even radiation to the groin, can be present [24].

It should be considered that the adductor magnus muscle also originates from the ischial tuberosity, and therefore strain injuries of the adductor can mimic IT avulsion injuries [24].

Radiologically, a typical crescent type fragment can be seen just lateral to the IT with inferior and lateral displacements (Fig. 37.13) [7].

Nonunion or malunion can lead to development of relevant bone masses around the IT, which can be misinterpreted as tumors [9, 99, 100] or even infection.

Typically, large displacements are present with IT avulsion being the most displaced avulsion injuries. Sinikumpu et al. observed a mean displacement of 47.7 mm [73].

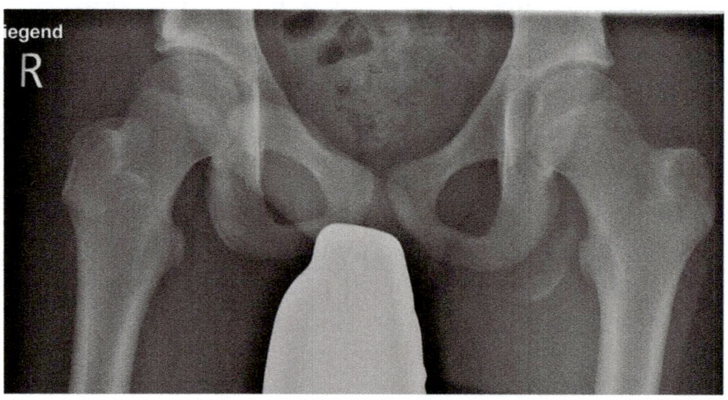

Fig. 37.13 Typical crescent shape of the avulsed fragment

37.6.5 Classification

According to Fetzer et al., bony avulsion injuries are classified as Grade IIIb injuries [101].

37.6.6 Treatment

Proximal osseus avulsion injuries were historically treated nonoperatively [101]. Despite a high nonunion rate (Fig. 37.14) of up to 70% most patients only showed minimal disability [99]. These nonunions present with a potential risk of sciatic nerve entrapment and injury to the inferior gluteal neurovascular bundle after nonoperative treatment [102–104].

During the last years, operative treatment became a consistent treatment option [101].

Indications for surgery included:

- Displacement >3 cm [105]
- Displacement >2 cm [106–109]
- Displacement >1.5 cm [98, 110]
- Symptomatic nonunions

Especially in symptomatic nonunions, good results were reported with plate fixation ± bone grafting via the Kocher-Langenbeck approach or a direct subgluteal crease approach [102, 111].

> Operative treatment is increasingly favored in IT avulsion injuries.

37.6.7 Results

Interestingly, compared to ASIS and AIIS avulsion fractures, no large patient reports dealt with IT avulsion fractures (Fig. 37.15).

Recently, Ferlic et al. reported on the management of 13 patients and their follow-up results at least 24 month postinjury [98].

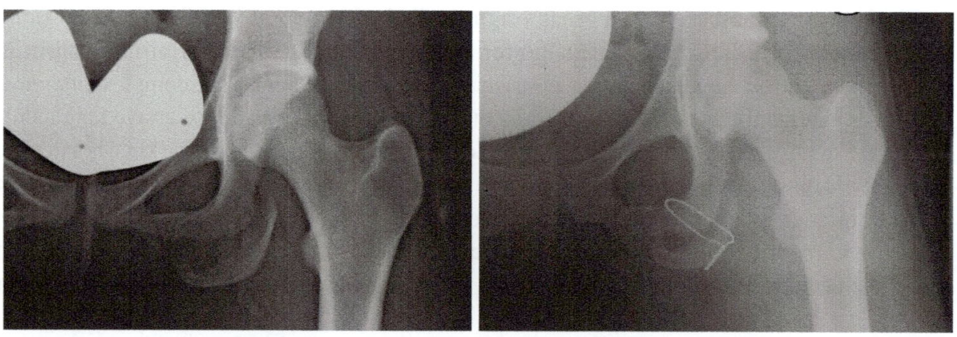

Fig. 37.14 Nonunion of an avulsed IT fragment. Even after surgery, only subjective instability was reduced without adequate reduction of the fragment

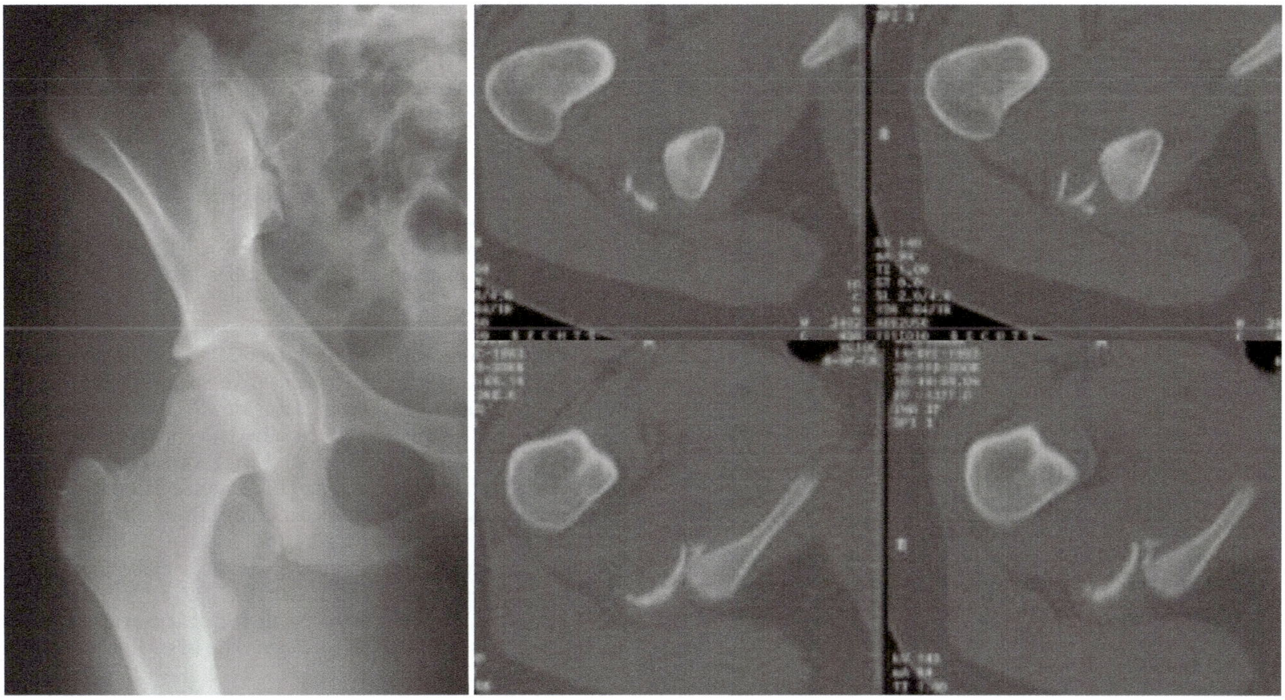

Fig. 37.15 Case of a displaced and rotated IT avulsion, diagnosed with conventional x-ray and CT

Soccer playing was the major cause of injury in 11 patients, while 1 fracture was sustained during volleyball and 1 after a motorcycle accident. Of these, five had operative treatment with screw fixation of the displaced (>15 mm) avulsed fragment. At follow-up, free active and passive ROM was observed, and muscular strength was comparable to the uninjured side.

Of the remaining eight patients with conservative treatment, all had a good functional outcome, despite two patients developing fragment nonunion.

Sinikumpu et al. analyzed 11 athletic patients with surgical treatment of an avulsed IT fracture using different techniques including five fixations. The indication for surgery was displacement >20 mm in nine and 15–120 mm displacement in two patients. At latest follow-up at least 1 year after surgery, 72.7% reported a good outcome [73].

In an analysis by Schuett, 4 of 20 patients (16%) with IT avulsion injuries developed nonunion [16].

Overall, ischial tuberosity avulsion resulted in moderate outcomes in 72.7% of the cases [73].

37.7 Pubic Symphysis Avulsion

At the inferior pubic ramus, the adductor longus, adductor brevis, and gracilis muscles have their origins, while at the superior ramus the distal rectus abdominis muscle is attached. Rarely, sudden contraction or repetitive stress can present with an avulsion injury at these sites.

Sinikumpu et al. analyzed five athletic patients with surgical treatment of an avulsed pubic symphysis fracture. Even patients with displacement <15 mm were treated operatively. Four patients had fixation and one fragment resection was performed. At latest follow-up at least 1 year after surgery, all athletes reported a good outcome [73].

37.8 Lesser Trochanter Avulsion

Avulsion of the lesser trochanter is uncommon during sports and is most often observed in soccer players [62].

Forceful contraction of the iliopsoas muscle with a fixed extended hip joint can lead to this injury.

37.9 Summary

Even today, the primary treatment aim is conservative treatment. Especially in ASIS, AIIS, and IT injuries with significant displacement and in highly active sports patients, surgical treatment should be considered.

References

1. Putz R, Milz S. Makroskopische und funktionelle Anatomie der Apophysenfugen. Orthopade. 2016;45:199–205.
2. Engel A, Siegler H, Kristen K. Chapter: Sportorthopädische Probleme. 16.2 Apophysenschädigungen der Hüfte und des Beckens. aus CJ Wirth, L Zichner (Hrsg), Ch Tschauner (Ed.): Orthopädie und Orthopädische Chirurgie. Stuttgart: Georg Thieme Verlag; 2004. p. 492–4.
3. Rossi F, Dragoni S. Acute avulsion fractures of the pelvis in adolescent competitive athletes: prevalence, location and sports distribution of 203 cases collected. Skelet Radiol. 2001;30:127–31.
4. Metzmaker J, Pappas A. Avulsion fractures of the pelvis. Am J Sports Med. 1985;13:349–57.
5. Waters P, Millis M. Hip and pelvic injuries in the young athlete. Clin Sports Med. 1988;7:513–22.
6. Hösli P, von Laer L. Traumatische Apophysenlösungen im Bereich des Beckens und des koxalen Femurendes. Orthopade. 1995;24:429–35.
7. Paletta GJ, Andrish J. Injuries about the hip and pelvis in the young athlete. Clin Sports Med. 1995;14:591–628.
8. Pohlemann T, Gänsslen A, Partenheimer A. Becken und Acetabulumverletzungen. In: Weinberg A, Tscherne H, Hrsg. Unfallchirurgie im Kindesalter. Berlin, Heidelberg, New York: Springer; 2006. p. 579–602.
9. Wirth T. Avulsionsverletzungen der Hüftregion des Jugendlichen. Orthopade. 2016;45:213–8.
10. Acheson R. The Oxford method of assessing skeletal maturity. Clin Orthop. 1957;10:19–39.
11. Camp J, Cilley E. Diagrammatic chart showing time of appearance of various centers of ossification and period of union. Am J Roentgenol. 1931;26:905–6.
12. Flecker H. Roentgenographic observations of the times of appearance of epiphyses and their fusion with the diaphyses. J Anat. 1932;67:118–64.
13. Kaufmann H. Röntgenbefunde am kindlichen Becken bei angeborenen Skelettaffektionen und chromosomalen Aberrationen. Stuttgart: G. Thieme; 1964.
14. Risser J. The iliac apophysis; an invaluable sign in the management of scoliosis. Clin Orthop. 1958;11:111–9.
15. Parvaresh K, Upasani V, Bomar J, Pennock A. Secondary ossification center appearance and closure in the pelvis and proximal femur. J Pediatr Orthop. 2018;38(8):418–23.
16. Schuett D, Bomar J, Pennock A. Pelvic apophyseal avulsion fractures: a retrospective review of 228 cases. J Pediatr Orthop. 2015;35:617–23.
17. Tubbs R, Stetler W, Savage A, Shoja M, Shakeri A, Loukas M, Salter E, Oakes W. Does a third head of the rectus femoris muscle exist? Folia Morphol (Warsz). 2006;65(4):377–80.
18. Doskocil M, Med M, Vimmer T. Musculus rectus femoris. Acta Chir Orthop Traumatol Czech. 1987;54:99–107.
19. Gray. In: Warwick R, Williams PL, editors. Gray's anatomy. 35th ed. Edinburgh: Longmon; 1973.
20. Tillmanns H. Die Verletzungen und chirurgischen Krankheiten des Beckens. Stuttgart: Deutsche Chirurgie, Verlag Enke; 1905. p. 65.
21. Köhler A. Becken. In: Grenzen des Normalen und Anfänge des Pathologischen im Röntgenbilde. 7. Auflage. Leipzig: Georg Thieme Verlag; 1939. p. 257–8.
22. Gallagher J. Fracture of the anterior inferior spine of the ilium. Ann Surg. 1935;102:86–8.
23. Steinbrück K, Krahl H. Apophysäre Frakturen am Becken beim Jugendlichen. In: Pförringer W, Rosemeyer B, editors. Die Epiphysenfugen. München: perimed Fachbuch-Verlagsgesellschaft mbH Erlangen; 1987. p. 182–94.
24. Morelli V, Weaver V. Groin injuries and groin pain in athletes: part 1. Prim Care. 2005;32(1):163–83.
25. Morscher E, Desaulles P. Die Festigkeit des Wachstumsknorpels in Abhängigkeit von Aler und Geschlecht. Schweiz Med Wschr. 1964;17:582.
26. Lagier R, Jarret G. Apophysiolysis of the anterior inferior iliac spine. A histological, clinical and radiological study. Arch Orthop Unfallchir. 1975;83(1):81–9.
27. Lau L, Mahadev A, Hui J. Common lower limb sports-related overuse injuries in young athletes. Ann Acad Med Singap. 2008;37:315–9.
28. Linni K, Mayr J, Hollwarth ME. [Apophyseal fractures of the pelvis and trochanter minor in 20 adolescents and 2 young children]. Unfallchirurg. 2000;103(11):961–4.
29. Fernbach SK, Wilkinson RH. Avulsion injuries of the pelvis and proximal femur. AJR Am J Roentgenol. 1981;137(3):581–4.
30. Kameyama O, Ogawa R, Kumamoto M. Sports injuries in terms of bi-articular muscle function. Hum Mov Sci. 1994;13:683–95.
31. Kameyama O, Ogawa R. Avulsion fracture of the iliac spine during sporting activity. J Orthop Sci. 1996;1:356–62.
32. Deehan DJ, Beattie TF, Knight D, Jongschaap H. Avulsion fracture of the straight and reflected heads of rectus femoris. Arch Emerg Med. 1992;9(3):310–3.
33. Huang Y, Lien F. Avulsion fracture of the anterior inferior iliac spine. J Emerg Crit Care Med. 2008;19(2):57–8.
34. Irving MH. Exostosis formation after traumatic avulsion of the anterior inferior iliac spine. Report of two cases. J Bone Joint Surg Br. 1964;46:720–2.
35. Karakas HM, Alicioglu B, Erdem G. Bilateral anterior inferior iliac spine avulsion in an adolescent soccer player: a typical imitator of malignant bone lesions. South Med J. 2009;102(7): 758–60.
36. Knobloch K, Kramer R, Sommer K, Gansslen A, Vogt PM. [Avulsion injuries of the anterior inferior iliac spine among soccer players—a differential diagnosis to neoplasm decades following the trauma]. Sportverletz Sportschaden. 2007;21(3):152–6.
37. Mader TJ. Avulsion of the rectus femoris tendon: an unusual type of pelvic fracture. Pediatr Emerg Care. 1990;6(3):198–9.
38. Nanka O, Havranek P, Pesl T, Dutka J. Avulsion fracture of the pelvis: separation of the secondary ossification center in the superior margin of the acetabulum. Clin Anat. 2003;16(5): 458–60.
39. Rajasekhar C, Kumar KS, Bhamra MS. Avulsion fractures of the anterior inferior iliac spine: the case for surgical intervention. Int Orthop. 2001;24(6):364–5.
40. Reina N, Accadbled F, de Gauzy JS. Anterior inferior iliac spine avulsion fracture: a case report in soccer playing adolescent twins. J Pediatr Orthop B. 2010;19(2):158–60.
41. Resnick JM, Carrasco CH, Edeiken J, Yasko AW, Ro JY, Ayala AG. Avulsion fracture of the anterior inferior iliac spine with abundant reactive ossification in the soft tissue. Skelet Radiol. 1996;25(6):580–4.
42. Swischuk LE. Wrestling: pain in the thigh. Avulsion fracture of the anterior inferior iliac spine. Pediatr Emerg Care. 2004;20(4):259–60.
43. Yildiz C, Yildiz Y, Ozdemir MT, Green D, Aydin T. Sequential avulsion of the anterior inferior iliac spine in an adolescent long jumper. Br J Sports Med. 2005;39(7):e31.
44. Atalar H, Kayaoglu E, Yavuz OY, Selek H, Uras I. Avulsion fracture of the anterior inferior iliac spine. Ulus Travma Acil Cerrahi Derg. 2007;13(4):322–5.
45. Sanders TG, Zlatkin MB. Avulsion injuries of the pelvis. Semin Musculoskelet Radiol. 2008;12(1):42–53.
46. Ahmadi A, Kreusch-Brinker R, Mellerowicz H, Wolff R. Apopohysenausriß am becken und der unteren Extremität durch Sport. Sportverletz Sportschaden. 1987;3:113–7.
47. Keats T. The spectrum of musculoskeletal stress injury. Curr Probl Diagn Radiol. 1984;3:7–51.

48. Stancak A, Kautzner J, Trc T, Havlas V. Treatment of pelvic avulsion fractures in children and adolescents. Rozhl Chir. 2017;96:156–65.
49. Sundar M, Carty H. Avulsion fractures of the pelvis in children: a report of 32 fractures and their outcome. Skelet Radiol. 1994;23(2):85–90.
50. Vandervliet EJ, Vanhoenacker FM, Snoeckx A, Gielen JL, Van Dyck P, Parizel PM. Sports-related acute and chronic avulsion injuries in children and adolescents with special emphasis on tennis. Br J Sports Med. 2007;41(11):827–31.
51. Meyer NJ, Schwab JP, Orton D. Traumatic unilateral avulsion of the anterior superior and inferior iliac spines with anterior dislocation of the hip: a case report. J Orthop Trauma. 2001;15(2):137–40.
52. Reggiori A, Brugo G. Traumatic anterior hip dislocation associated with anterior and inferior iliac spines avulsions and a capsular-labral lesion. Strategies Trauma Limb Reconstr. 2008;3(1):39–43.
53. Gomez JE. Bilateral anterior inferior iliac spine avulsion fractures. Med Sci Sports Exerc. 1996;28(2):161–4.
54. Amendola A, Wolcott M. Bony injuries around the hip. Sports Med Arthrosc Rev. 2002;10:163–7.
55. Klümper A. Apophysenverletzungen bei Jugendlichen und Abrißverletzungen. In: Klümper A, editor. Sporttraumatologie. ECOMED-Verlag; 2002. p. III-14, 2–7.
56. Pavlov H. Roentgen examination of groin and hip pain in the athlete. Clin Sports Med. 1987;6:829–43.
57. Weitzner I. Fracture of the anterior superior spine of the ilium in one case, and anterior inferior in another case. AJR Am J Roentgenol. 1935;33:39–40.
58. Bartl R, Bartl-Vischer C, Brauner H. [Apophyseolysis and avulsion fractures of the anterior inferior iliac spine. A case report]. Unfallchirurgie. 1997;23(2):74–7.
59. Canale S, King R. Pelvic and hip fractures. In: Rockwood Jr C, Wilkings K, King R, editors. Fractures in children. Philadelphia: J.B. Lippincott Company; 1991. p. 991–1046.
60. Yildiz C, Aydin T, Yildiz Y, Kalyon TA, Basbozkurt M. Anterior inferior iliac spine apophyseal avulsion fracture. J South Orthop Assoc. 2003;12(1):38–40.
61. Chen L, Chan S. Anterior inferior iliac spine avulsion fracture in an adolescent runner: a case report. J Emerg Crit Care Med. 2008;19(1):35–8.
62. Stevens MA, El-Khoury GY, Kathol MH, Brandser EA, Chow S. Imaging features of avulsion injuries. Radiographics. 1999;19(3):655–72.
63. Bachmann W. Un cas d'arrachment bilateral de l'espine iliaque anteroinferiore. Schweiz Med Wochenschr. 1941;22:721–2.
64. Pisacano RM, Miller TT. Comparing sonography with MR imaging of apophyseal injuries of the pelvis in four boys. AJR Am J Roentgenol. 2003;181(1):223–30.
65. Brittenden J, Robinson P. Imaging of pelvic injuries in athletes. Br J Radiol. 2005;78(929):457–68.
66. Bencardino J, Palmer W. Imaging of hip disorders in athletes. Radiol Clin North Am. 2002;40:267–87.
67. Boutin R, Russell C, Steinbach L. Imaging of sports-related muscle injuries. Radiol Clin North Am. 2002;40:333–62.
68. Pan H, Kawanabe K, Akiyama H, Goto K, Onishi E, Nakamura T. Operative treatment of hip impingement caused by hypertrophy of the anterior inferior iliac spine. J Bone Joint Surg Br. 2008;90(5):677–9.
69. Howard F, Piha R. Fractures of the apophyses in adolescent athletes. JAMA. 1965;192:150–2.
70. Pogliacomi F, Calderazzi F, Paterlini M, Ceccarelli F. Surgical treatment of anterior iliac spines fractures: our experience. Acta Biomed. 2014;85(Suppl 2):52–8.
71. Schwobel MG. [Apophyseal fractures in adolescents]. Chirurg. 1985;56(11):699–704.
72. Ducloyer P, Filipe G. [Apophyseal avulsion of the pelvis in children]. Chir Pediatr. 1988;29(2–3):91–2.
73. Sinikumpu J, Hetsroni I, Schilders E, Lempainen L, Serlo W, Orava S. Operative treatment of pelvic apophyseal avulsions in adolescent and young adult athletes: a follow-up study. Eur J Orthop Surg Traumatol. 2018;28:423–9.
74. Eberbach H, Hohloch L, Feucht M, Konstantinidis L, Südkamp N, Zwingmann J. Operative versus conservative treatment of apophyseal avulsion fractures of the pelvis in the adolescents: a systematical review with meta-analysis of clinical outcome and return to sports. BMC Musculoskelet Disord. 2017;18:162. https://doi.org/10.1186/s12891-017-1527-z.
75. Caudle R, Crawford A. Avulsion fracture of the lateral acetabular margin. A case report. J Bone Joint Surg Am. 1988;70:1568–70.
76. Porr J, Lucaciu C, Birkett S. Avulsion fractures of the pelvis—a qualitative systematic review of the literature. J Can Chiropr Assoc. 2011;55:247–55.
77. Hsu C, Wu C, Lin S, Cheng K. Anterior superior iliac spine avulsion fracture presenting as meralgia paraesthetica in an adolescent sprinter. J Rehabil Med. 2014;46:188–90.
78. Kautzner J, Trc T, Havlas V. Comparison of conservative against surgical treatment of anterior-superior iliac spine avulsion fractures in children and adolescents. Int Orthop. 2014;38:1495–8.
79. Hébert K, Laor T, Divine J, Emery K, Wall E. MRI appearance of chronic stress injury of the iliac crest apophysis in adolescent athletes. Am J Roentgenol. 2008;190:1487–91.
80. Lombardo S, Retting A, Kerlan R. Radiographic abnormalities of the iliac apophysis in adolescent athletes. J Bone Joint Surg Am. 1983;65:444–6.
81. Blazina M. The "hip-pointer", a term to describe a specific kind of athletic injury. Calif Med. 1967;106:450.
82. Aksoy B, Oztürk K, Ensenyel C, Kara A. Avulsion of the iliac crest apophysis. Int J Sports Med. 1998;19:76–8.
83. Casabianca L, Rousseau R, Loriaut P, Massein A, Mirouse G, Gerometta A, Khiami F. Iliac crest avulsion fracture in a young sprinter. Case Rep Orthop. 2015;2015:302503. https://doi.org/10.1155/2015/302503. Epub 2015 Sep 1.
84. Valdés M, Molins J, Acebes O. Avulsion fracture of the iliac crest in a football player. Scand J Med Sci Sports. 2000;10:178–80.
85. Lambert M, Fligner D. Avulsion of the iliac crest apophysis: a rare fracture in adolescent athletes. Ann Emerg Med. 1993;22:1218–20.
86. Singer G, Eberl R, Wegmann H, Marterer R, Kraus T, Sorantin E. Diagnosis and treatment of apophyseal injuries of the pelvis in adolescents. Semin Musculoskelet Radiol. 2014;18:498–504.
87. Li X, Xu S, Lin X, Wang Q, Pan J. Results of operative treatment of avulsion fractures of the iliac crest apophysis in adolescents. Injury. 2014;45:721–4.
88. Zhang K, Dong X, Chen X, Zhang L, Deng Z. The ossification of the ischial tuberosity for forensic age diagnostics in conventional radiography. Aust J Forensic Sci. 2014;46:455–62.
89. Koulouris G, Connell D. Hamstring muscle complex: an imaging review. Radiographics. 2005;25:571–86.
90. Miller S, Gill J, Webb G. The proximal origin of the hamstrings and surrounding anatomy encountered during repair. A cadaveric study. J Bone Joint Surg Am. 2007;89:44–8.
91. Miller S, Webb G. The proximal origin of the hamstrings and surrounding anatomy encountered during repair. Surgical technique. J Bone Joint Surg Am. 2008;90(Suppl 2):108–16.
92. van der Made A, Wieldraaijer T, Kerkhoffs G, Kleipool R, Engebretsen L, van Dijk C, Golanó P. The hamstring muscle complex. Knee Surg Sports Traumatol Arthrosc. 2015;23:2115–22.
93. Davis J, Charalambides C, Bircher M. Avulsion fracture of the ischium. Injury. 1998;29:632–5.
94. Orava S, Ala-Ketola L. Avulsion fractures in athletes. Br J Sports Med. 1977;11:65–71.

95. Davis K. Imaging of the hamstrings. Semin Musculoskelet Radiol. 2008;12:28–41.
96. Tehranzadeh J. The spectrum of avulsion and avulsion-like injuries of the musculoskeletal system. Radiographics. 1987;7(5):945–74.
97. Somville F, Vriends D, Feyen J. Traumatic avulsion fracture of the ischial tuberosity in an elderly patient. Acta Orthop Belg. 2011;77:122–4.
98. Ferlic P, Sadoghi P, Singer G, Kraus T, Eberl R. Treatment for ischial tuberosity avulsion fractures in adolescent athletes. Knee Surg Sports Traumatol Arthrosc. 2014;22:893–7.
99. Barnes S, Hinds R. Pseudotumor of the ischium: a late manifestation of avulsion of the ischial epiphysis. J Bone Joint Surg Am. 1972;54:645–7.
100. Brandser E, el-Khoury G, Kathol M. Adolescent hamstring avulsions that simulate tumors. Emerg Radiol. 1995;2:273–8.
101. Fetzer G, Fischer D. Chapter 18: Hamstring injuries. In: Guanche C, editor. Hip and pelvis injuries in sports medicine. Philadelphia: Wolters Kluwer; 2010. p. 181–91.
102. Gidwani S, Jagiello J, Bircher M. Avulsion fracture of the ischial tuberosity in adolescents—an easily missed diagnosis. BMJ. 2004;329:99–100.
103. Hamada G, Rida A. Ischial apophysiolysis (IAL). Report of a case and review of the literature. Clin Orthop. 1963;31:117–30.
104. Miller A, Stedman G, Beisaw N, Gross P. Sciatica caused by an avulsion fracture of the ischial tuberosity. A case report. J Bone Joint Surg Am. 1987;69:143–5.
105. Colosimo A, Wyatt H, Frank K, Mangine R. Hamstring avulsion injuries. Oper Tech Sports Med. 2005;13:80–8.
106. Bencardino J, Mellado J. Hamstring injuries of the hip. Magn Reson Imaging Clin N Am. 2005;13:677–90.
107. Biedert R. Surgical management of traumatic avulsion of the ischial tuberosity in young athletes. Clin J Sport Med. 2015;25: 67–72.
108. Kujala U, Orava S. Ischial apophysis injuries in athletes. Sports Med. 1993;16:290–4.
109. Servant C, Jones C. Displaced avulsion of the ischial apophysis: a hamstring injury requiring internal fixation. Br J Sports Med. 1998;32:255–7.
110. Gill D, Clark W. Avulsion of the ischial apophysis. Aust N Z J Surg. 1996;66:564–5.
111. Pilichou A, Sekouris N, Nikolaou V, Demetriou E, Angoules A. Missed avulsion fracture of the Ischial tuberosity in an adolescent competitive athlete: case report and literature review. J Trauma Treat. 2014;S2:002. https://doi.org/10.4172/2167-1222.S2-002.

Fragility Fractures

38

Franz Müller, Bernd Füchtmeier, Jan Lindahl, and Axel Gänsslen

Fragility fractures are defined as a result of a force that is not able to fracture healthy bones and are due to a reduced compression and torsional strength of the bone according to the WHO definition [1].

The frequency of fragility fractures of the pelvis (FFP) increases continuously [2–5].

Pelvic fractures in geriatric patients are considerably different to those of younger patients as these are mainly caused by trivial falls to the ground and are often the result of preexisting impairments of bone quality.

Geriatric pelvic fractures usually are not accompanied with hemodynamic instability or concomitant injuries of vessels and nerves [6].

Pol Rommens and coworkers in 2017 published an excellent book, *Fragility Fractures of the Pelvis*, which is still the basis of our understanding of these specific fractures.

It is beyond the scope of this chapter to perform a comparable analysis of the literature.

Therefore, this chapter should guide as a summary of the well-analyzed different treatment options in geriatric pelvic ring fractures.

For detailed information, we point toward this book and the resulting review publications [6–17].

F. Müller
Department of Trauma Surgery, Orthopaedics and Sports Medicine, Hospital Barmherzige Brüder Regensburg, Regensburg, Germany

B. Füchtmeier
Krankenhaus Barmherzige Brüder, Klinik für Unfallchirurgie, Regensburg, Germany
e-mail: Bernd.Fuechtmeier@barmherzige-regensburg.de

J. Lindahl
Orthopaedics and Trauma Surgery, Helsinki University Hospital, Helsinki, Finland

A. Gänsslen (✉)
Department of Trauma Surgery, Orthopedics and Hand Surgery, Hospital Wolfsburg, Wolfsburg, Germany

38.1 Pathophysiology of Fragility Fractures

To understand the different types of FFP, the changes in the anatomy of the pelvis in geriatric patients need to be addressed. Especially at the posterior pelvic ring, significant changes occur during aging.

Aging is often associated with different physiological and pathological changes of the internal structure of the pelvis.

Cortical bone is the solid osseous shell surrounding the bone and is covered by the periosteum, while trabecular bone shows a characteristic network of lamellar bone [18]. Cortical bone is stiffer than trabecular bone and can resist higher stresses, but a low resistance to strain, while trabecular bone is porous with a low resistance to stress and a high resistance to strain [19, 20].

Aging results in different adaptions and modifications of the internal bone structure. Bone strength decreases with age resulting in weak trabecular areas especially in the sacral bone [15–17, 21, 22].

The bone mineral density of the sacrum is physiologically irregular depending on specific bone zones (see Chap. 2).

- Ebraheim et al. reported the weakest bone zones to be in the lateral sacral alar of S1 and at the level of the junction of S2 and S3, while the strongest bone zone was observed between the S1 and S2 foramina [22].
- A CT analysis of the normal sacrum revealed a reduced bone density in typical sacral regions, with lowest bone density paraforaminal lateral and between S1 and S2 [15, 17].
- The mean bone mineral density (BMD) of the S1 was found to be 31.9% higher than that of the sacral alar, and the highest bone mineral density is typically observed near the lateral posterior and lateral anterior part of the S1 body [23].

A. Gänsslen et al. (eds.), *Pelvic Ring Fractures*, https://doi.org/10.1007/978-3-030-54730-1_38

- A DEXA scan analysis found highest cancellous BMD in the anterior two thirds of the S1 body, while the highest cortical BMD was observed anteriorly [24].

Clinical Relevance

The internal bone density can explain specific fracture patterns in traumatic and fragility fractures of the sacrum [25], and, therefore, specific screw pathways can be recommended.

A typical internal trabecular pattern of the upper sacrum was found by Pal et al., which shows strong trabeculae running from the superior surface of the S1 body to the articular surface of the SI joint, from the articular process and the S1 pedicle to the SI joint, from the posterolateral angle of the ala (attachment site of the lumbosacral ligament) to the S1 body, and from the lateral portion of the laminae to the auricular surface [26].

These anatomical and physiological distributions of the bone mineral density (BMD) lead to an ongoing reduction in special areas at the sacrum. In patients with reduced BMD, a so-called alar void can be observed, as in the lateral sacrum which shows the weakest BMD [17, 27].

The lateral sacrum represents a weak area for "development" of insufficiency fractures.

Thus, typical fracture configurations can be observed in geriatric patients. The dynamics of the bone weakness results in an ongoing development of these fractures:

- Anterior sacral compressions injuries
- Uni- and bilateral "transalar" vertical fractures
- Additional horizontal fracture lines between S1 and S2 or S2 and S3 [28]

At the sacrum, typical spinopelvic dissociation fracture lines can be observed, with or without displacement. These fractures are considered clinically mild low-energy resultant "suicidal jumper's fractures" [10] compared to the well-described classical high-energy spinopelvic dissociation injuries [29, 30].

Primary or secondary osteoporosis is often present in the elderly population >65 years of age [31]. Secondary osteoporosis can be a result of vitamin D deficiency, long-term cortisone treatment, immobilization, rheumatoid arthritis, radiotherapy of the pelvic region, etc.

Additionally, age-related loss of function and from preexisting diseases are relevant in the elderly, including peripheral arteriosclerosis (grade IV), coronary heart disease, hepatitis virus infection/cirrhosis, carcinoma/malignant diseases, coagulation disorders, or adipositas, which are observed in one third within this population [32].

Fragility fractures often present first as superior pubic ramus fractures but due to the dynamic instability can result in higher instability grades of the pelvic ring structure. The end result can be a complete collapse of the pelvic ring [9].

It is suspected that the pelvic ligaments remain stronger than the bony structures. This can lead to a restricted displacement with only minor fracture displacement for long times [6, 14].

Fractures of the posterior pelvic ring (sacrum) are usually combined with fractures of the anterior pelvic ring.

Involvement of the pelvic joints, especially the SI joint, indicate a more chronic process of dynamic instability [10].

In adults, typically a relevant force acting on the pelvis results in displaced pelvic ring instability. With nonoperative treatment, there is only a risk of increasing displacement without additional fracture sites. In contrast, in geriatric patients, a more dynamic instability is often observed. It is not unusual that after a simple low-energy mechanism, standard pelvic x-rays and even CT examination fail to detect (cortical) fractures. Radiological reevaluation some weeks later, indicated by persisting pain, then reveals fractures zones at typical localizations (e.g., sacral alar, upper pubic rami), which may increase over time leading to real anterior and posterior complete instability of the pelvis.

This dynamic change with resultant instability does not correspond to clinical instability as these patients often are still able to walk or mobilize (painfully). Additionally, the morphological classification of the injury changes. Rommens et al. compared adult pelvic ring injuries as a high-energy explosion, while fragility fractures more correspond to an implosion as the pelvic ligaments remain intact [10].

FFP corresponds more to a dynamic pathology, while classical pelvic ring fracture in adults present with a more static appearance.

38.2 Radiological Diagnostics

Standard radiographs of the pelvic ring (e.g., anterior-posterior and inlet/outlet views, or even a true lateral sacral view to identify the characteristic kyphotic sacral deformity) should be considered in every patient after low- or high-energy trauma to the pelvis or in patients with relevant pain at the pelvis.

Advanced imaging modalities including CT with axial, sagittal, and coronal reconstructions should be performed in conventionally detected (anterior) pelvic ring fractures for detailed analysis of the bony architecture. Also, MRI or bone scans can be helpful to detect areas of increased stress or pathology [33].

Conventional radiography is often impaired by overlying bowel and bladder content, or rarefication of the bone structure. Thus, posterior pelvic ring fractures are detected initially in only 0–10% and after CT confirmation retrospective diagnosis is possible in 20–34% [34–37].

Lyders et al. could show that FFPs present as transalar vertical dense/sclerotic areas parallel to SI joint, and visible fracture lines are present as sclerotic areas in 57% and true fractures in 12.5% [38]. The development of visible fractures was observed within 1–13 months.

In contrast, CT allows for fracture detection in 75%, with an overall sensitivity of 60–75% [34, 35, 38]. The most common sacral fracture pattern was a bilateral vertical fracture with a single horizontal component ("H"-pattern) [27].

MRI is nearly 100% sensitive with a characteristic bone marrow edema and hypotensive fracture lines [34, 38].

Bone scintigraphy is the most sensitive examination with a Honda sign present in 20–40%. A 96% sensitivity and a 92% positive predictive value are associated with this diagnostic procedure [38].

CT and MRI represent the current gold standard in evaluating FFP.

38.3 Classification of Geriatric Pelvic Fractures

Historically, pelvic ring injuries in the elderly were classified according to the accepted AO/OTA classification scheme.

Based on the fracture types (A, B, and C), clinical data and treatment recommendations could be evaluated. The following analyses did not distinguish between high- and low-energy injuries.

38.3.1 Type A Injuries

Historical data indicated a high incidence (>70%) of type A injuries in elderly patients and a short rehabilitation phase was proposed, as these fractures were stated as benign fractures [39].

In contrast, Gertzbein et al. in 1977 stated that "in isolated anterior pelvic ring fractures in the older age group scintigraphically a posterior injury was detected in most patients" [40].

Koval et al. in 1997 analyzed patients with anterior ring injuries in detail and observed that these patients had a mean length of hospital stay of 14 days, 16% moderate to severe pain at 1 year, and one fourth of patients were still limping. Additionally, a 10% 1-year mortality rate was observed [41].

Simple anterior ring injuries in geriatric patients were not as simple as expected and a misclassification was observed.

38.3.2 Type B Injuries

With increasing use of CT evaluation of pelvic ring injuries, more posterior lesions were detected.

In 15%, classical lateral compression fractures (type B2) were observed, often after a simple fall during walking [42]. Stabilization of these injuries was rarely necessary [43]. It was already noted that especially in patients ≥65 years, mobilization was often impaired due to severe pain [44] and these patients had a mean hospitalization of 3–4 weeks [31].

Pain was identified as a relevant indicator of delayed mobilization.

Gänsslen et al. stabilized patients with ongoing pain with an anterior external fixator to reduce pain using the stabilizing effect [45].

In 25 patients ≥65 years, after external fixator application, pain-dependent mobilization was allowed and a clinical reevaluation was performed after 3 weeks. Here, the transverse bar was removed and if no pain was present, the fixator was removed and mobilization was performed with full weight bearing. If inguinal pain at the fracture site was still present, the transverse bar was reattached for one further week.

Within 4 weeks, an adequate subjective pain control was observed (Fig. 38.1).

Stabilization of unstable pelvic ring injuries leads to adequate pain reduction and allows mobilization.

38.3.3 Type C Injuries

The corresponding incidence of type C injuries was low with <5% but these injuries were associated with a high mortality rate (37%) in patients >60 years of age [46]. Pohlemann et al. stated these injuries as a "one-chance situation" [43, 47].

Mortality correlated with additional hemodynamic instability with a fourfold increase: if >15 PRBC were transfused a mortality rate of 38% was observed, if these patients were hemodynamically unstable at admission [48].

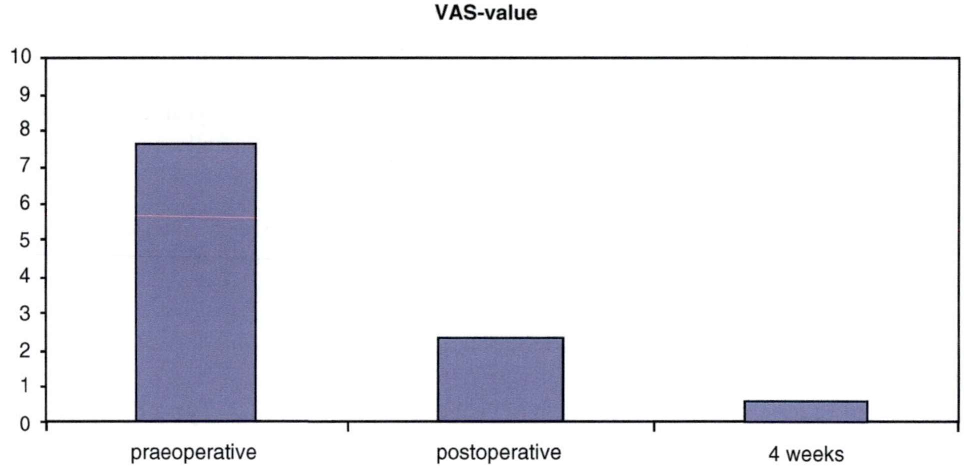

Fig. 38.1 Pain course change from preoperative to postoperative and at early follow-up

38.4 Classification of Fragility Fractures of the Pelvis

With the ongoing demographic change, new pelvic fracture patterns were identified in the elderly population, leading to special treatment considerations [12].

The present well-accepted comprehensive FFP-classification of these geriatric fractures was proposed by Rommens et al., which guided special stabilization techniques [8, 10–14].

FFP type I injuries represent isolated anterior pelvic ring injuries. With increasing use of CT diagnostics in the majority of all suspected pelvic fracture patients, these injuries are expected in low frequencies. Two subgroups were distinguished:

- FFP type Ia: unilateral anterior pelvic ring fracture
- FFP type Ib: bilateral anterior pelvic ring fracture

FFP type II injuries are defined as nondisplaced posterior lesions with or without an additional anterior pelvic ring injury. These injuries account for approximately 50% of all FFP [14].

- FFP type IIa: isolated nondisplaced posterior injury (most commonly an anterior sacral fracture)
- FFP type IIb: sacral crush fracture with a concomitant anterior pelvic ring injury (B2 or LC 1 injury)
- FFP type IIc: nondisplaced sacral, sacroiliac, or iliac fracture with a concomitant anterior pelvic ring injury

FFP type III injuries present with a displaced unilateral posterior injury combined with an anterior pelvic ring lesion, according to a type C injury of the pelvis.

- FFP type IIIa: displaced ilium fracture
- FFP type IIIb: displaced SI joint disruption
- FFP type IIIc: displaced unilateral sacral fracture

FFP type IV injuries are defined as displaced bilateral posterior pelvic ring injuries.

- FFP type IVa: bilateral ilium fractures or bilateral SI joint disruptions
- FFP type IVb: spinopelvic dissociation with a bilateral longitudinal Denis zone I injury and an additional transverse fracture component (H-, U-type injuries)

FFP type IVc: combination of different posterior instabilities

CT or MRI scans are essential for precise diagnosis and, particularly, for the detection/exclusion of posterior pelvic ring involvement.

The main advantages of the FFP-classification include an age-related approach to typical fracture types, allowing for fracture type-dependent treatment recommendations [6, 9–14].

Recently, the reliability of this new classification was analyzed.

Krappinger et al. reported a moderate interobserver reliability with Kappa values ranging from 0.42 to 0.59, representing an overall agreement of 61%, while the intraobserver reliability was substantial with Kappa values ranging from 0.68 to 0.72, indicating a 77% agreement [49]. Lowest reliability was observed for type IIc, IIIc, and IVb injuries.

> The FFP-classification of geriatric pelvic ring injuries is useful.

38.5 Classification-Adapted Treatment

38.5.1 FFP Type I Injuries

These fractures are rare and consist of isolated anterior pelvic ring injuries after CT or MRI diagnostics, excluding posterior ring involvement. Unilateral (FFP type Ia) or bilateral (FFP type Ib) anterior pelvic ring fractures are distinguished. Even this "simple" injury type is associated with a relevant 1-year and 5-year mortality with 13.3% and 45.6%, respectively [44]. In another study, the corresponding mortality rates at 1, 5, and 10 years were 24.7%, 64.4%, and 93.8%, respectively [50]. Additionally, morbidity was increased with a complication rate of 20% during hospital admission, mainly caused by infectious diseases (urinary tract infection, pneumonia). In a recent study on long-term results of 117 patients with anterior ring injuries, relevant morbidity was reported [51].

The predominant treatment recommendation is conservative treatment [6, 9–13, 52].

38.5.1.1 Principles of Conservative Treatment

The main symptom in patients with fragility fractures of the pelvis is pain. Thus, adequate pain therapy to allow adequate and early mobilization is the primary treatment aim. Rommens et al. focused on [14]:

- Pain-dependent mobilization/weight bearing
- Functional status dependent physiotherapy

It has to be considered that a too aggressive mobilization may lead to additional fragility fractures in the pelvic ring with enhanced instability [14].

When the patients cannot be adequately mobilized, the outcome of conservative treatment is often poor with loss of social and physical independence and autonomy [53].

Therefore, Rommens et al. recommend extended radiographic diagnostics for detection of dynamic posterior pelvic ring involvement, if pain reduction and mobilization are unsuccessful after 1 week, resulting in a change of the fracture type and which potentially leads to operative treatment [9, 10].

Additional pharmacotherapy should be initiated with vitamin D supplementation if necessary, recombinant parathyroid hormone, and or bisphosphonates [13].

Wagner et al. analyzed the midterm effects of conservative treatment and reported on several risks [52]:

- Bed rest results in 12 days to 8 weeks treatment duration
- Symptom improvement/full mobilization: 4 weeks to 3.3 months
- 20–52% complication rate
- 10–45 days length of hospital stay
- 3–10% in-hospital mortality
- 11–19% 1-year mortality
- 16–18% independent life (after 1 year)
- Up to 50% loss of independence

> Conservative treatment is the first line of treatment in FFP type I injuries. Rarely, surgical stabilization should be considered.

38.5.2 FFP Type II Injuries

These fracture types are associated with a nondisplaced posterior lesion with or without an additional anterior pelvic ring injury. These injuries account for approximately 50% of all FFP [14] and are moderately unstable. The fracture types include isolated nondisplaced posterior (most commonly an anterior sacral fracture) injury (FFP type IIa), a sacral crush fracture with a concomitant anterior pelvic ring injury (FFP type IIb), or a nondisplaced sacral, sacroiliac or iliac fracture with a concomitant anterior pelvic ring injury (FFP type IIc).

It should be considered that these fractures can dynamically end in unstable fracture situations.

FFP type IIa injuries are uncommon, and Rommens recommended conservative/functional treatment as the first treatment option. As in FFP type I injuries, if this treatment fails, early radiographic diagnostics is clearly recommended [6, 9–14, 52].

In contrast to type I injuries, a prolonged remodeling and convalescence time is observed, and early mobilization can lead to dynamic instability and even nonunions. Therefore, minimally invasive fixation techniques (e.g., sacroplasty) should be considered.

Frey et al. recommended isolated sacroplasty in such minor unstable fractures and reported excellent and fast pain relief in the majority of patients with a low complication rate. Comparable results were reported by Andresen et al., with significant pain reduction on the second postoperative day, which persisted up to 12 months [21].

In FFP type IIb and IIc injuries, primary conservative and functional treatment is recommended [6, 9–14, 52].

If these treatment options fail, a more aggressive approach is favored using percutaneous techniques [12]. Rommens et al. recommended percutaneous iliosacral screw fixation (two screws into S1 or one screw each into S1, S2) combined with a retrograde anterior column screw [12]. Technically, the screw thread should be placed into the central sacral areas, and the use of washers is recommended [12, 54].

Possibly, additional cement augmentation (sacroplasty) should be considered as experimentally a better fixation strength was observed [55].

Höch et al. analyzed the outcome and survival rate of nonoperative versus operative treatment for lateral compression fractures in a retrospective study of 128 patients (aged ≥65 years) [56]. Higher complications rates were observed after operative treatment 18% vs. 8%), but 18% of primarily conservatively treated patients needed operative treatment after discharge due to worsening pain and mobilization. Despite an overall high mortality rate at the 2-year follow-up (30%), patients with operative treatment had a significant higher survival rate (82% vs 61%), while no difference was found regarding pain and quality of life.

In a further study, Höch et al. compared 35 nonoperatively treated patients with type B 2.1 injuries and 36 operatively treated patients using the SF-36 and the EQ5D after at least 1 year following trauma [57]. At a follow-up after a mean of 47 months, the mean VAC pain value was 2.8 and 2.6 after nonoperative vs. operative treatments, respectively. The mean SF-36 PCS was 44.8 points and the mean SF-36 MCS was 52.6 points, both lower than the normal German population. The EQ-5D was 89.5 and 91.8, and its mean VAS was 75.5 and 79.7, respectively. Operatively treated patients had a significantly higher complication rate (18% vs. 8%). Thus, nonoperative treatment was recommended especially for younger patients.

The aim of this study was to identify potential risk factors for pelvic insufficiency fractures and to collect information on their short- and long-term outcomes.

Maier et al. reported a relevant loss of autonomy in these fracture types after conservative treatment, often requiring nearly doubled daily assistance compared to patients without fractures [53].

> In FFP type II fractures, a slightly more aggressive approach for surgical stabilization should be considered, especially when clinical complaints persist for 2–4 weeks with conservative treatment.

38.5.3 FFP Type III Injuries

FFP type III injuries are unstable and posterior displacement is likely. Therefore, a clear indication for surgery is recommended [6, 9–14]. Additionally, a concomitant anterior pelvic ring injury should be addressed. A minimally invasive stabilization concept is favored.

Anterior techniques include:

- Percutaneous retrograde superior ramus screw
- Plating for symphysis disruption
- Supraacetabular internal fixator (INFIX)

Posterior stabilization techniques include:

- Open reduction and plate osteosynthesis of ilium fractures
- Open/closed reduction and iliac lag screw fixation
- Posterior ilioiliacal fixation strategies (e.g., transiliac internal fixator (TIFI), ilioiliacal minimal-invasive plate stabilization, intra-/extraosseous sacral bar fixation) with or without cement augmentation
- Open reduction, anterior plating of SI joint injuries
- Percutaneous iliosacral screw fixation of SI joint disruption or sacrum fractures with or without cement augmentation
- Sacroplasty

> In FFP type III fractures, closed reduction along with internal fixation is recommended.

38.5.4 FFP Type IV Injuries

FFP type IV lesions are associated with the most relevant mechanical pelvic ring instability. A complete spinopelvic dissociation with or without uni- or bilateral anterior disruption is observed.

FFP type IVa lesion with bilateral iliac fractures are rare. Stabilization is performed using standard stabilization concepts of ilium fractures, which need most often open reduction and internal fixation.

FFP type IVb lesions present as classical lumbopelvic dissociation injuries (see Chap. 35). Thus the concept of lumbopelvic stabilization allows adequate stability with immediate full weight bearing. In undisplaced H-type injuries, bilateral iliosacral screw fixation or unilateral complete bilateral iliosacral screw fixation and the options of ilioiliacal fixation concepts can be performed.

> In FFP type IV fractures, closed or open reduction and internal fixation are recommended. Type IV b injuries should be treated by lumbopelvic fixation concepts.

38.6 Relevance of Augmentation

Biomechanical analyses clearly proposed cement augmentation to increase the stiffness of osteosynthesis techniques around the pelvis.

Hack et al. evaluated the primary stability of cement augmentation of cannulated and perforated iliosacral screws under cyclic loading. No significant difference was observed [58]. In contrast, Grechenig et al. observed a higher stiffness and pullout forces with augmentation [55].

This is supported by recent clinical analyses.

Schmitz et al. performed cement-augmented posterior screw fixation in 15 patients with different FFP [59]. The average age of the patients was 79.9 years. Four patients were treated using a cement-augmented transiliac internal fixation method (TIFI), and seven patients received a cement-augmented iliolumbar fixation. No adverse effects were observed, and adequate stability allowing early full weight bearing was possible.

Höch et al. performed cement augmentation of sacroiliac screw fixation in 34 patients. Screw-related complications occurred with two screws but were not related to cement augmentation. Pain was significantly reduced [56].

In contrast, Eckardt et al. observed 18% rate of screw loosening without augmentation [60].

Augmentation should be considered optional to support standard stabilization techniques at the posterior pelvic in patients with FFP.

38.7 Summary

- FFPs present as a dynamic problem with an increase of pelvic ring instability and resultant clinical impairment, when treated insufficiently.
- A stability-based concept is favored in FFP based on the FFP classification according to Pol Rommens.
- Osteosynthesis concepts should be as minimally invasive as possible.
- Standardized techniques can be used to stabilize the whole pelvic ring.
- Augmentation is a potential option to increase construct stability.

References

1. WHO. Guidelines for preclinical evaluation and clinical trials in osteoporosis. Geneva: World Health Organization; 1998. p. 59.
2. Andrich S, Haastert B, Neuhaus E, Neidert K, Arend W, Ohmann C, Grebe J, Vogt A, Jungbluth P, Rösler G, Windolf J, Icks A. Epidemiology of pelvic fractures in Germany: considerably high incidence rates among older people. PLoS One. 2015;10(9):e139078.
3. Buller T, Best M, Quinnan S. A nationwide analysis of pelvic ring fractures: incidence and trends in treatment, length of stay, and mortality. Geriatr Orthop Surg Rehabil. 2016;7:9–17.
4. Kannus P, Parkkari J, Niemi S, Sievänen H. Low-trauma pelvic fractures in elderly Finns in 1970–2013. Calcif Tissue Int. 2015;97:577–80.
5. Sullivan M, Baldwin K, Donegan D, Metha S, Ahn J. Geriatric fractures about the hip: divergent patterns in the proximal femur, acetabulum, and pelvis. Orthopedics. 2014;37:151–7.
6. Rommens P, Wagner D, Hofmann A. Fragility fractures of the pelvis. JBJS Rev. 2017;5(3). pii: 01874474-201703000-00004. https://doi.org/10.2106/JBJS.RVW.16.00057.
7. Dietz S, Hofmann A, Rommens P. Haemorrhage in fragility fractures of the pelvis. Eur J Trauma Emerg Surg. 2015;41:363–7.
8. Oberkircher L, Ruchholtz S, Rommens P, Hofmann A, Bücking B, Krüger A. Osteoporotic pelvic fractures. Dtsch Arztebl Int. 2018;115:70–80.
9. Rommens P, Arand C, Hofmann A, Wagner D. When and how to operate fragility fractures of the pelvis? Indian J Orthop. 2019;53:128–37.
10. Rommens P, Arand C, Thomczyk S, Handrich K, Wagner D, Hofmann A. [Fragility fractures of the pelvis]. Unfallchirurg. 2019;122:469–82.
11. Rommens P, Dietz S, Ossendorf C, Pairon P, Wagner D, Hofmann A. Fragility fractures of the pelvis: should they be fixed? Acta Chir Orthop Traumatol Cechoslov. 2015;82:101–12.
12. Rommens P, Hofmann A. Comprehensive classification of fragility fractures of the pelvic ring: recommendations for surgical treatment. Injury. 2013;44:1733–44.
13. Rommens P, Hofmann A, editors. Fragility fractures of the pelvis. Cham: Springer International Publishing AG; 2017.
14. Rommens P, Ossendorf C, Pairon P, Dietz S, Wagner D, Hofmann A. Clinical pathways for fragility fractures of the pelvic ring: personal experience and review of the literature. J Orthop Sci. 2015;20:1–11.
15. Wagner D, Kamer L, Rommens P, Sawaguchi T, Richards R, Noser H. 3D statistical modeling techniques to investigate the anatomy of the sacrum, its bone mass distribution, and the trans-sacral corridors. J Orthop Res. 2014;32:1543–8.
16. Wagner D, Kamer L, Sawaguchi T, Richards R, Noser H, Hofmann A, Rommens P. Morphometry of the sacrum and its implication on trans-sacral corridors using a computed tomography data-based three-dimensional statistical model. Spine J. 2017;17:1141–7.
17. Wagner D, Kamer L, Sawaguchi T, Richards R, Noser H, Rommens P. Sacral bone mass distribution assessed by averaged three-dimensional CT models: implications for pathogenesis and treatment of fragility fractures of the sacrum. J Bone Joint Surg Am. 2016;98:584–90.
18. Osterhoff G, Morgan E, Shefelbine S, Karim L, McNamara L, Augat P. Bone mechanical properties and changes with osteoporosis. Injury. 2016;47(Suppl 2):11–20.
19. Keaveny T, Hayes W. Mechanical properties of cortical and trabecular bone. In: Bone mechanics handbooks. 1st ed. Boca Raton: CRC Press; 1993. p. 285–344.
20. Nordin M, Frankel V. Basic biomechanics of the musculoskeletal system. 4th ed. Baltimore: Lippincott Williams & Wilkins; 2012.
21. Andresen R, Radmer S, Kamusella P, Wissgott C, Banzer J, Schober H. Treatment of Denis 1, 2 and 3 insufficiency fracture zones of the os sacrum. Individual approaches adapted to the course of the fracture in CT-assisted balloon sacroplasty. Osteology. 2012;21:168–73.
22. Ebraheim N, Sabry F, Nadim Y, Xu R, Yeasting R. Internal architecture of the sacrum in the elderly. An anatomic and radiographic study. Spine. 2000;25:292–7.
23. Zheng Y, Lu W, Zhu Q, Qin L, Zhong S, Leong J. Variation in bone mineral density of the sacrum in young adults and its significance for sacral fixation. Spine. 2000;25:353–7.
24. Richards A, Coleman N, Knight T, Belkoff S, Mears S. Bone density and cortical thickness in normal, osteopenic, and osteoporotic sacra. J Osteoporos. 2010. https://doi.org/10.4061/2010/504078.
25. Waites M, Mears S, Mathis J, Belkoff S. The strength of the osteoporotic sacrum. Spine. 2007;32:E652–5.
26. Pal G. Weight transmission through the sacrum in man. J Anat. 1989;162:9–17.
27. Linstrom N, Heiserman J, Kortman K, Crawford N, Baek S, Anderson R, Pitt A, Karis J, Ross J, Lekovic G, Dean B. Anatomical and biomechanical analyses of the unique and consistent locations of sacral insufficiency fractures. Spine. 2009;34:309–15.
28. Wagner D, Hofmann A, Kamer L, Sawaguchi T, Richards R, Noser H, Gruszka D, Rommens P. Fragility fractures of the sacrum occur in elderly patients with severe loss of sacral bone mass. Arch Orthop Trauma Surg. 2018;138:971–7.
29. Lindahl J, Mäkinen T, Koskinen S, Söderlund T. Factors associated with outcome of spinopelvic dissociation treated with lumbopelvic fixation. Injury. 2014;45:1914–20.

30. Roy-Camille R, Saillant G, Gagana G, Mazel C. Transverse fracture of the upper sacrum suicidal jumper's fracture. Spine. 1985;10(9):838–45.
31. Morris R, Sonibare A, Green D, Masud T. Closed pelvic fractures: characteristics and outcomes in older patients admitted to medical and geriatric wards. Postgrad Med J. 2000;76:646–50.
32. Makary M, Segev D, Pronovost P, Syin D, Bandeen-Roche K, Patel P, Takenaga R, Devgan L, Holzmueller C, Tian J, Fried L. Frailty as a predictor of surgical outcomes in older patients. J Am Coll Surg. 2010;210:901–8.
33. Scolaro J, Zamorano D. Diagnosis and management of sacral insufficiency fractures. Curr Orthop Pract. 2016;27:36–40.
34. Cabarrus M, Ambekar A, Lu Y, Link T. MRI and CT of insufficiency fractures of the pelvis and the proximal femur. AJR Am J Roentgenol. 2008;191:995–1001.
35. Gotis-Graham I, McGuigan L, Diamond T, Portek I, Quinn R, Sturgess A, Tulloch R. Sacral insufficiency fractures in the elderly. J Bone Joint Surg. 1994;76-B:882–6.
36. Leroux J, Denat B, Thomas E, Blotman F, Bonnel F. Sacral insufficiency fractures presenting as acute low-back pain. Biomechanical aspects. Spine. 1993;18:2502–6.
37. Schicho A, Schmidt S, Seeber K, Olivier A, Richter P, Gebhard F. Pelvic X-ray misses out on detecting sacral fractures in the elderly—importance of CT imaging in blunt pelvic trauma. Injury. 2016;47:707–10.
38. Lyders E, Whitlow C, Baker M, Morris P. Imaging and treatment of sacral insufficiency fractures. AJNR Am J Neuroradiol. 2010;31:201–10.
39. Zuckerman JE. Comprehensive care of orthopaedic injuries in the elderly. Baltimore: Urban & Schwarzenberg; 1990.
40. Gertzbein S, Chenoweth D. Occult injuries of the pelvic ring. Clin Orthop. 1977;128:202–7.
41. Koval K, Aharonoff G, Schwartz M, Alpert S, Cohen G, McShinawy A, Zuckerman J. Pubic rami fracture: a benign pelvic injury? J Orthop Trauma. 1997;11(1):7–9.
42. Henry SM, Pollak AN, Jones AL, Boswell S, Scalea TM. Pelvic fracture in geriatric patients: a distinct clinical entity. J Trauma. 2002;53(1):15–20.
43. Pohlemann T, Gänsslen A, Hartung S, für die Arbeitsgruppe Becken, H.T., H., Beckenverletzungen/Pelvic Injuries. Hefte zu "Der Unfallchirurg". Heft 266. 1998.
44. Hill R, Robinson C, Keating J. Fractures of the pubic rami. Epidemiology and five-year survival. J Bone Joint Surg. 2001;83-B:1141–4.
45. Gänsslen A, Hildebrand F, Krettek C. Supraacetabular external fixation for pain control in geriatric type B pelvic injuries. Acta Chir Orthop Traumatol Cechoslov. 2013;80:101–5.
46. Chong K, DeCoster T, Osler T, Robinson B. Pelvic fractures and mortality. Iowa Orthop J. 1997;17:110–4.
47. Tscherne H, Pohlemann T. Tscherne Unfallchirurgie: Becken und Acetabulum. Berlin, Heidelberg, New York: Springer; 1998.
48. Naam N, Brown W, Hurd R, Burdge R, Kaminski D. Major pelvic fractures. Arch Surg. 1983;118:610–7.
49. Krappinger D, Kaser V, Kammerlander C, Neuerburg C, Merkel A, Lindtner R. Inter- and intraobserver reliability and critical analysis of the FFP classification of osteoporotic pelvic injuries. Injury. 2018;50:337. https://doi.org/10.1016/j.injury.2018.11.027.
50. van Dijk W, Poeze M, van Helden S, Brink P, Verbruggen J. Ten-year mortality among hospitalised patients with fractures of the pubic rami. Injury. 2010;41:411–4.
51. Loggers S, Joosse P, Jan Ponsen K. Outcome of pubic rami fractures with or without concomitant involvement of the posterior ring in elderly patients. Eur J Trauma Emerg Surg. 2019;45:1021. https://doi.org/10.1007/s00068-018-0971-2.
52. Wagner D, Ossendorf C, Gruszka D, Hofmann A, Rommens P. Fragility fractures of the sacrum: how to identify and when to treat surgically? Eur J Trauma Emerg Surg. 2015;41:349–62.
53. Maier G, Kolbow K, Lazovic D, Horas K, Roth K, Seeger J, Maus U. Risk factors for pelvic insufficiency fractures and outcome after conservative therapy. Arch Gerontol Geriatr. 2016;67:80–5.
54. Bishop J, Behn A, Castillo T. The biomechanical significance of washer use with screw fixation. J Orthop Trauma. 2014;28:114–7.
55. Grechenig S, Gänsslen A, Gueorguiev B, Berner A, Müller M, Nerlich M, Schmitz P. PMMA-augmented SI screw: a biomechanical analysis of stiffness and pull-out force in a matched paired human cadaveric model. Injury. 2015;46(Suppl 4):125–8.
56. Höch A, Pieroh P, Henkelmann R, Josten C, Böhme J. In-screw polymethymethacrylate-augmented sacroiliac screw for the treatment of fragility fractures of the pelvis: a prospective, observational study with 1-year follow-up. BMC Surg. 2017;17(1):132. https://doi.org/10.1186/s12893-017-0330-y.
57. Höch A, Schneider I, Todd J, Josten C, Böhme J. Lateral compression type B 2-1 pelvic ring fractures in young patients do not require surgery. Eur J Trauma Emerg Surg. 2018;44:171–7.
58. Hack J, Krüger A, Masaeli A, Aigner R, Ruchholtz S, Oberkircher L. Cement-augmented sacroiliac screw fixation with cannulated versus perforated screws—a biomechanical study in an osteoporotic hemipelvis model. Injury. 2018;49:1520–5.
59. Schmitz P, Baumann F, Grechenig S, Gaensslen A, Nerlich M, Müller M. The cement-augmented transiliacal internal fixator (caT-IFI): an innovative surgical technique for stabilization of fragility fractures of the pelvis. Injury. 2015;46(Suppl 4):114–20.
60. Eckardt H, Egger A, Hasler R, Zech C, Vach W, Suhm N, Morgenstern M, Saxer F. Good functional outcome in patients suffering fragility fractures of the pelvis treated with percutaneous screw stabilisation: assessment of complications and factors influencing failure. Injury. 2017;48:2717–23.

Intraoperative 3D Imaging of the Pelvic Ring

39

Benedict Swartman, Jochen Franke, Paul Alfred Grützner, Holger Keil, and Axel Gänsslen

39.1 Technology

Due to the complex anatomy of the pelvis, 3D imaging is very useful for both diagnostics and intraoperative control. The primary benefit of intraoperative imaging lies in the possibility of carrying out a reduction and position check of the implants during the procedure. This has been shown to avoid revision operations later [1, 2]. In addition, an intraoperatively generated 3D data set can be used as a basis for 3D navigation.

Three different techniques are currently available intraoperatively: mobile 3D C-arms, floor- or ceiling-mounted hybrid C-arms, and intraoperative CTs (sliding gantry/mobile CT). The advantages and disadvantages result from the comprehension of the respective technique. The following description is aimed at the clinical user and is intended to assist in the selection of the appropriate system.

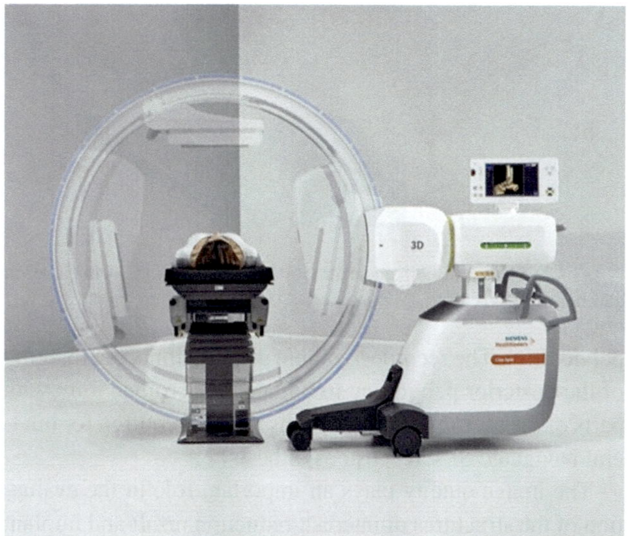

Fig. 39.1 Example of a mobile 3D C-arm

39.1.1 Mobile C-Arms

The mobile C-arm combines an x-ray unit with a mobile base. It delivers projection images in real time on a connected monitor trolley. The x-ray unit consists of a radiation source and an image intensifier or, alternatively, a digital detector, each of which is mounted at one end of the "C." A prerequisite for the acquisition of 3D information is the capturing of the same object from different directions. Therefore, 3D-capable C-arms are equipped with a motor that moves the "C" at a defined speed. Similar to CT technology, a rotation around the object takes place in which images are automatically generated at intervals of a few degrees of angle (Fig. 39.1). The individual images are then processed by an integrated computer into a 3D data set within a few seconds. In case of a so-called isocentric C-arm, the point around which the radiation source and detector moves is called the "isocenter." A C-arm is considered isocentric when the C forms a complete semicircle. In C-arms without generating a semicircle, an additional translational movement of the C by another motor is required (Fig. 39.2).

Conventional image intensifiers allow, limited by detector size and gantry opening, the 3D data acquisition of a cube volume of approximately 12 cm edge length. It should be ensured that the anatomical region to be imaged is located in the center of rotation. A corresponding central positioning of the patient to prevent a collision of the patient or the table with the device is, therefore, a prerequisite. Limitations may, therefore, occur depending on the soft tissue mantle of the patient and the anatomical region of interest (e.g., posterior

B. Swartman · J. Franke · P. A. Grützner · H. Keil
Department for Orthopedics and Orthopedic Trauma, BG-Klinik Ludwigshafen, Ludwigshafen am Rhein, Germany
e-mail: benedict.swartman@bgu-ludwigshafen.de; jochen.franke@bgu-ludwigshafen.de; aed@bgu-ludwigshafen.de; holger.keil@bgu-ludwigshafen.de

A. Gänsslen (✉)
Department of Trauma Surgery, Orthopedics and Hand Surgery, Hospital Wolfsburg, Wolfsburg, Germany

A. Gänsslen et al. (eds.), *Pelvic Ring Fractures*, https://doi.org/10.1007/978-3-030-54730-1_39

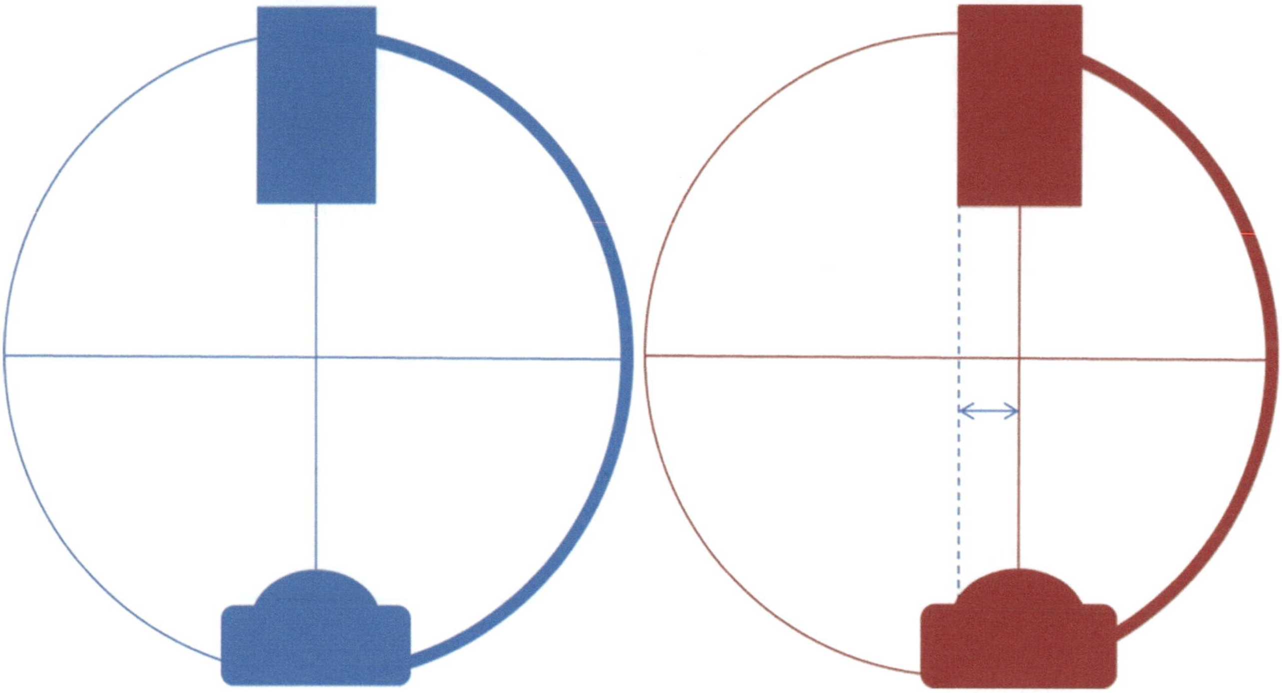

Fig. 39.2 Concept of a standard mobile isocentric 3D C-arm (blue) and a non-isocentric C-arm, requiring translational movement of the "C" by another motor (red)

pelvic ring). The recorded volume usually limits the imaging of the posterior pelvic ring to unilateral sacroiliac joint with parts of the sacrum (e.g., two scans may be required for bilateral navigated SI screw osteosynthesis).

The image quality plays an important role in the evaluation of the structures of interest: reduction result and implant position. In general, a better image quality is accompanied by an increased radiation dose. An obese habitus of the patient, relevant differences in density (air, table parts), but above all metal implants in the immediate vicinity significantly reduce the image quality in terms of resolution and contrast. In the area of metal implants, star-shaped artifacts are formed which have a partly outshining, partly extinguishing character (Fig. 39.3). They are caused by the orbital rotation of the C-arm and simultaneous radiation at specific intervals. The radiation is absorbed or deflected by the metal, and the information beyond the metal is lost. Software solutions are now available for artifact reduction, but these can also be accompanied by a loss of bony image information.

Due to its mobility, the C-arm is versatile. It is not limited to one operating room and is, therefore, an advantage in a facility with several operating rooms and a high volume of operations requiring 3D imaging. The control area is usually approximately 4 m. This allows the staff involved to leave the control area during the scan without leaving the room or taking off their sterile scrubs. The normal OR walls completely shield the scattered radiation and, thus, ensure the protection of the neighboring rooms. Mobility also allows the greatest possible flexibility in patient positioning and operating setup (see below).

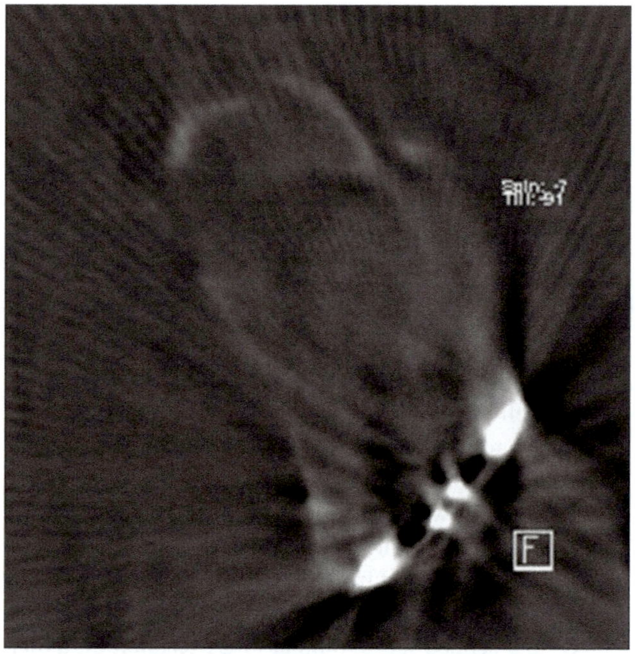

Fig. 39.3 Example of star-shaped artifacts in a 3D scan of a calcaneus osteosynthesis

39.1.2 O-Arm

The O-arm combines an x-ray-tube with a detector in a covered full ring. The advantage compared to the standard C-arm is better image quality due to 360° versus 190° rotation. It is a mobile system, and the control area resembles

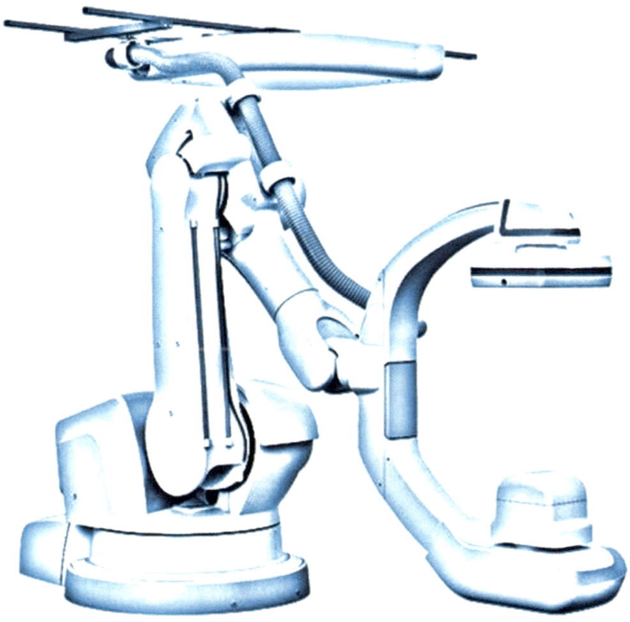

Fig. 39.4 Drawing of a Hybrid-OR, floor/ceiling-mounted C-arm

that of a C-arm. The O-arm provides a retractable section in the ring to allow easier patient positioning. A limited gantry opening of about 70 cm has to be considered. The O-arm is widely use, especially in North American hospitals.

39.1.3 Hybrid-OR, Floor/Ceiling-Mounted C-Arm

Ground- or ceiling-mounted C-arm differs from mobile C-arms in being stationary. Although the devices were equipped with digital flat-panel detectors earlier, the technology and construction of the actual C-arm hardly differ.

The C-arm is mounted on a robot arm or on rails in the floor or ceiling, which allow all directions of movement (Fig. 39.4). The robot arm is based on arms used in automatic production in the automotive industry. The joints of the robot arm allow all degrees of motion in guiding the C-arm and thus make motorization of the C-arm for rotation around the object unnecessary.

Due to the flat detector, the detector size is larger (30 × 40 cm) compared to the conventional image intensifier, which leads to an increased 3D volume of about 23 × 23 × 23 cm. The limitations in image quality correspond to the mobile C-arm. The control zone requires that the OR team leaves the room but is uncritical with regard to the constructional requirements.

A major advantage is the navigation and referencing of the image to the patient. As the robot forms a unit with the table via its floor mounting, it knows at all times the physical relation to the table and can automatically adapt to changes

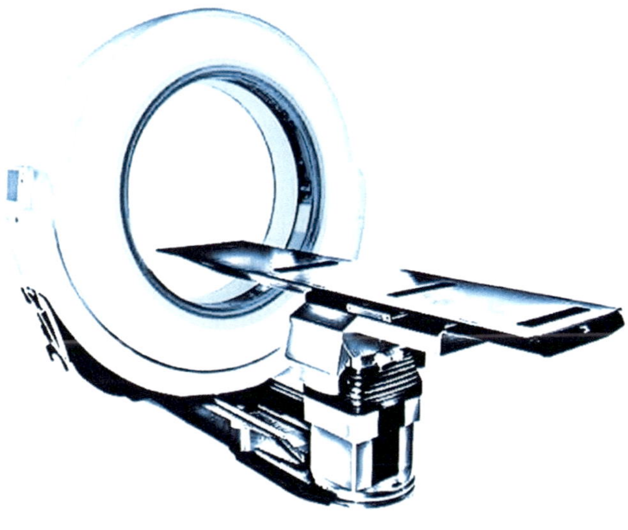

Fig. 39.5 Drawing of a mobile CT

of the table position. A disadvantage is its limitation to one operating room in terms of limited planning of surgical teams and interventions.

39.1.4 Intraoperative CT (iCT)

Due to its high resolution and maximum image quality, computed tomography (CT) continues to be the gold standard for assessing reduction and implant position as well as for preoperative planning and navigation.

Two types of systems are available for the realization of an iCT.

- The "sliding gantry" describes a device, which is mounted stationary, but which can be moved on rails to and from the operating area, thus leaving the space required for surgery. As with the conventional CT known from the x-ray department, a closed ring forms the gantry, the opening of which is limited for the patient, table, and any instruments. As with an external CT, the control area is approximately 6 m and requires the corresponding constructional requirements with leaded walls, an outer room for the staff, signal lamps, information signs, and an appropriate high power supply.
- The second possibility is a mobile CT, which combines the image quality of a CT with the mobility of a classical mobile C-arm (Fig. 39.5). The ring-shaped closed gantry with the table and the column forms a mobile unit on wheels. The original operating column cannot be used. The mobile unit can theoretically be changed between different operating rooms. Advantages are the flexible positioning of the patient in the room and the relative positioning of CT, instrument tables, navigation equip-

ment, and respirator. Sometimes, it makes sense to position the CT at the foot or head end, but in others also at the side in order to rotate the table 90° in the direction of the gantry before the scan. When changing the device between different rooms, some restrictions have to be considered: the mentioned constructional prerequisites for radiation protection and power supply have to be maintained. For flexible use in different rooms, before purchase, necessary building modifications should be considered. Due to its mobility, the mobile CT is slightly smaller than the "sliding gantry" for weight saving and better handling. However, the image quality is slightly inferior to the external CT [3].

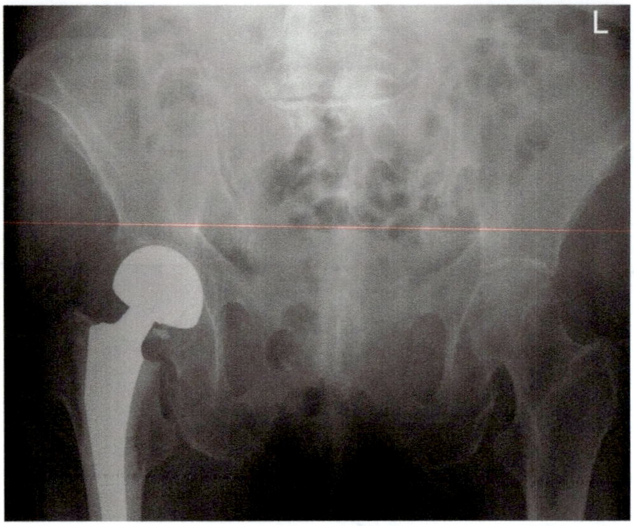

Fig. 39.6 Outlet view in geriatric patient: the optimal bone corridor for safe iliosacral screw insertion can be difficult to identify due to bowel gas overlay

39.2 Indications

The indications for intraoperative 3D imaging combine a complex anatomical region with difficult accessibility and close location between risk structures and safe corridors for the implants to be placed. Especially at the pelvis, safe screw placement plays a decisive role due to the proximity to lumbar and sacral nerve roots, large vessels, and joints. The increasing age of patients causes an increase in osteoporotic insufficiency fractures that require surgical stabilization and multimorbid patients, which require short operating times and small approaches. Due to the increasing use of minimally invasive techniques, 3D imaging is also helpful in combination with navigation.

39.2.1 Iliosacral Screw Fixation

In unstable fractures of the posterior pelvic ring (type B or C injuries), surgical stabilization is indicated. Depending on the biomechanical treatment goal, the technique involves fixation of the SI joint with fully or partially threaded iliosacral screws placed into the vertebral body of S1 or S2. The corresponding corridors are narrow depending on the individual anatomy and the number of desired screws.

Depending on bone quality and soft tissue mantle, the assessment of anatomical structures in 2D fluoroscopy can be limited. The sacral neuroforamina in the outlet projection are partially difficult to recognize due to the possible intestinal gas overlay (Fig. 39.6). Since visualization of these structures is essential to prevent neurostructural damage, 3D imaging is particularly suitable in these cases. The possibility of 3D navigation is also beneficial for the safe placement of SI screws. Another indication for 3D imaging is the intraoperative control of reduction and implant position. This may save the patient for further potential revision procedures.

In unilateral fixation, it is important to ensure that the scanned area includes the corridors for the planned screws or already inserted screws. It can be helpful to position the patient more at the lateral border of the table to place the field of view and the isocenter of the C-arm near the midline of the table to avoid collisions during scanning. In bilateral stabilizations, two separate scans are usually required when using the mobile C-arm because the depicted volume is too small. For bilateral navigation, it is typical to attach only one reference base to one side of the iliac crest. However, the reference array must be aligned in such a way that it does not touch the C-arm or the CT gantry during the scan and can be detected by the infrared camera at any time. In addition, it can be challenging to bring the instruments into the field of view of the infrared camera with the reference base simultaneously. In the case of isolated treatment of the posterior pelvic ring, prone positioning may be particularly helpful in obese patients.

39.2.2 Lumbopelvic Stabilization

Lumbopelvic stabilization is often performed in severely displaced type C injuries. It utilizes pedicle screw instrumentation as commonly used in spinal surgery. Lumbar pedicle screws are connected to ilium screws by bended longitudinal rods.

Lumbar pedicle screw placement does not necessarily require 3D imaging since the pedicles are large and can usually be well visualized using 2D fluoroscopy. The iliac screw corridors are also relatively large. In case of limited image quality or uncertainty regarding the position of the screws, 3D imaging is recommended.

3D imaging also allows immediate intraoperative quality control of screw insertion and corresponding documentation.

39.2.3 Sacral Bar Stabilization

Sacral bar treatment plays a particularly important role in bilateral insufficiency fractures of the posterior pelvic ring. A solid steel threaded rod is passed intraosseous from one side through S1 to the other side and fixed at both ends with washers, nuts, and locking nuts. Biomechanically, axial load transfer occurs through the sacral vertebrae to the strong medial cortices of the ilium [4]. Due to the comparable iliosacral bone corridor, sacral bar application also benefits from 3D imaging and navigation for the abovementioned reasons.

39.2.4 Superior Ramus Screw

Intramedullary screws at the anterior pelvic ring are suitable for the stabilization of acetabular anterior column fractures and superior ramus fractures as part of pelvic ring injuries (see Chap. 24).

During insertion, a flexible titanium screw of sufficient length is guided through the strong cortex of the upper pubic ramus. Usually, the position of the screw can be adequately assessed using inlet-, outlet-, and Judet projections. In poor bone quality, however, the cortex may be too weak for easy guidance with a risk of cortical penetration. In these cases, navigation of the screw corridor and thus 3D imaging may become necessary. Depending on the fracture extent, reduction control may only be possible using 3D imaging (Fig. 39.7).

In conclusion, 3D imaging may be necessary for

- Iliosacral osteosyntheses (e.g., iliosacral screw, sacral bar) depending on bone quality and imaging conditions, especially in the context of 3D navigation
- Lumbopelvic stabilization, when intraoperative 2D fluoroscopy results in inadequate visualization
- Intramedullary ramus screws in fractures close to the acetabulum and in cases of poor bone quality

3D imaging and 3D navigation can improve the quality of treatment in the abovementioned indications, avoid revision operations, and facilitate the procedure for the surgeon [5]. However, it is always advisable to also be familiar with 2D techniques if there is a system error or 3D imaging is not possible due to problems with patient positioning or anatomical understanding.

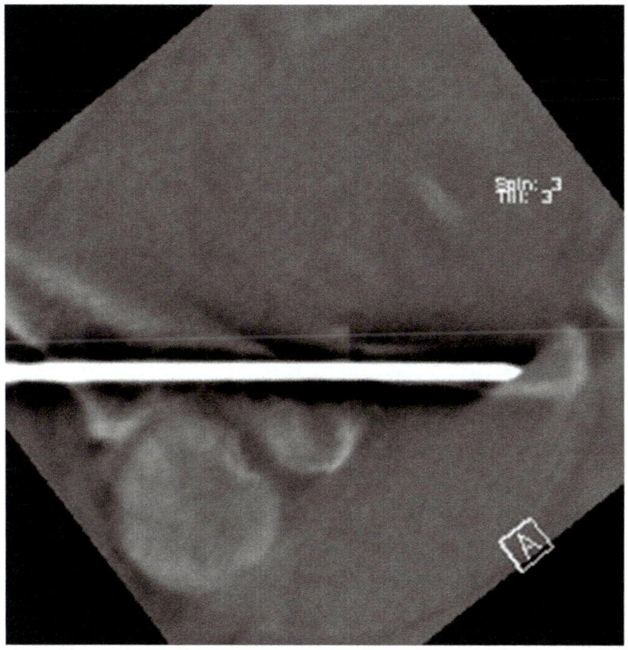

Fig. 39.7 Intraoperative view of an antegrade wire insertion into the upper pubic ramus

39.3 Practice of Intraoperative 3D Imaging

The use of devices for intraoperative 3D imaging urges the surgical team to think about the setup of the OR in advance.

Depending on the selected/available imaging device, special draping, patient positioning, and necessary hardware, the surgery should be planned to avoid hustling during surgery.

A 3D C-arm, mobile or fixed, can be used like a conventional C-arm to continuously verify distinct steps of the surgical procedure by 2D images; thus an additional C-arm is not needed.

In contrast, an intraoperative CT scanner is not capable of acquiring fluoroscopic images, so the surgeon needs to decide if an additional 2D C-arm is needed for the procedure. Navigation is recommended, when fracture reduction maneuvers are performed requiring radiographic control.

39.3.1 Patient Positioning

Several aspects have to be respected regarding positioning and hardware use.

Using 3D C-arms, radiopaque positioning materials have to be outside the scanning area. Therefore, a radiolucent OR table is strongly recommended. Using a partial radiolucent OR table, the field of interest pelvis should be placed on carbon parts and away from the table column.

In the lateral position, radiolucent props are useful or standard props have to be placed outside the scanning field. Although CT scanners are less susceptible to metal artifacts, these aspects have to be observed as the image quality decreases significantly with radiopaque materials in the scanning field. The use of a vacuum mattress in contrast to metal side props in case of lateral positioning can help avoid these issues.

39.3.2 Draping

During draping, the potential risk of surgical field or equipment contamination should be considered.

Using a 3D C-arm, this can be achieved by using larger drapes on the lateral side of the patient, while C-arm draping is performed in a standard way.

Using a CT scanner, a detailed planning of the draping considering the dimensions of the scanner have to be respected. While some devices offer a large gantry opening that allows performing the scan without draping the scanner itself (Fig. 39.8), other devices need to be draped separately before the patient can be transferred into the scanner. It is strongly recommended to try different scenarios and define standard procedures for positioning and draping before an actual surgical procedure is performed.

39.3.3 Setup

The setup of the OR should be defined in advance and kept constant for similar procedures.

Moving of the patient or equipment should be avoided as possible. Usually, the C-arm is positioned opposite to the position of the surgeon to allow free view into the surgical field for the surgeon.

In bilateral procedures, changing of the C-arm position should be avoided.

Using an intraoperative CT scanner, an additional C-arm can become necessary, especially if navigation is not possible or desired. In these cases, additional efforts are planned to allow intraoperative 2D- and CT imaging without the need of hustling with the equipment (Fig. 39.9).

3D imaging can be time consuming and exposes the patient to additional radiation; so it is reasonable to use 3D imaging on distinct key sections during the procedure. The corresponding flowcharts to procedures with and without navigation are shown in Figs. 39.10 and 39.11.

The conduct of the procedure of 3D imaging itself depends on the selected machine and will be described on the basis of an isocentric flat-panel device (Siemens Cios Spin/Erlangen/Germany), which shows only little differences on other machines:

1. The C-arm has to be positioned orthogonally to the patient.
2. The region of interest (e.g., the left SI joint) has to be positioned centrally in the anteroposterior and lateral views.
3. The scan parameters need to be defined and a collision test has to be done.

If everything is correct, the staff leaves the C-arm control area and the scan is conducted.

After acquiring of the images, the device calculates a 3D volume that is presented on the screen. The postprocessing of the scan is crucial. As the relative orientation of the region of interest toward the C-arm is not synchronized, the volume is initially aligned not in a standardized way and needs to be adjusted in all three standard planes to allow reliable assessment.

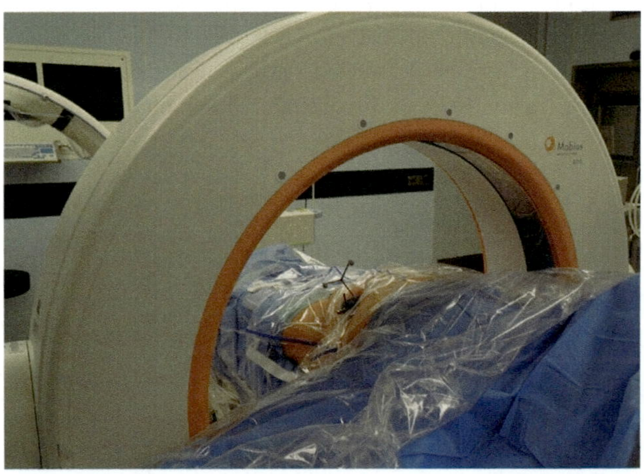

Fig. 39.8 Draping-free CT scanner

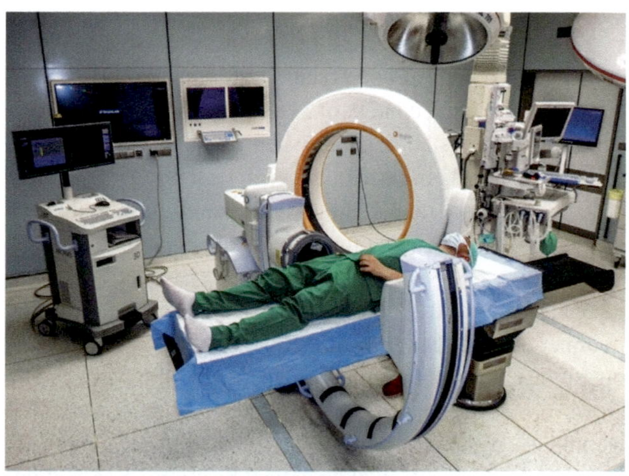

Fig. 39.9 Positioning during combined use of an intraoperative CT scanner and a mobile C-arm

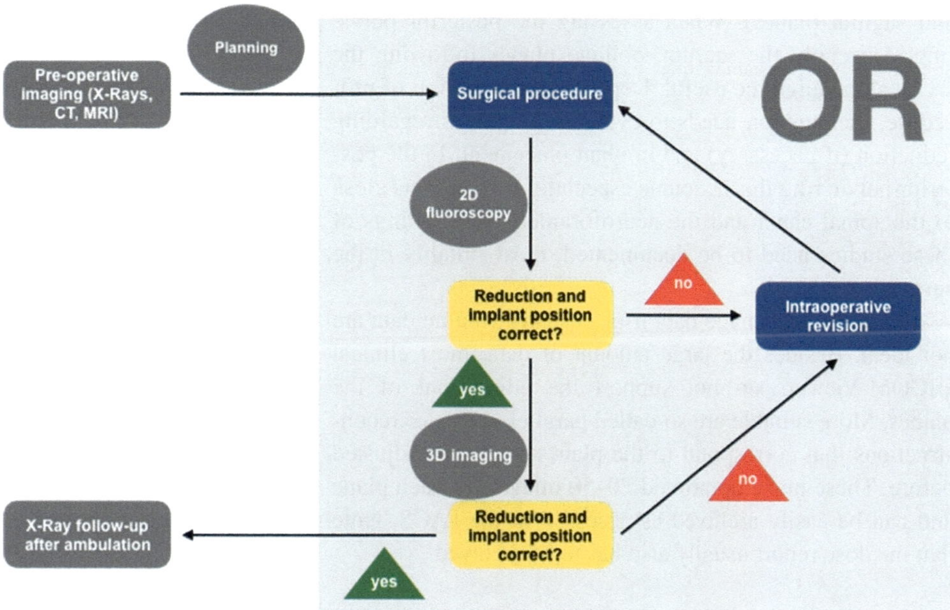

Fig. 39.10 Flowchart of planning and intraoperative use of 2D fluoroscopy and 3D imaging *without* navigation

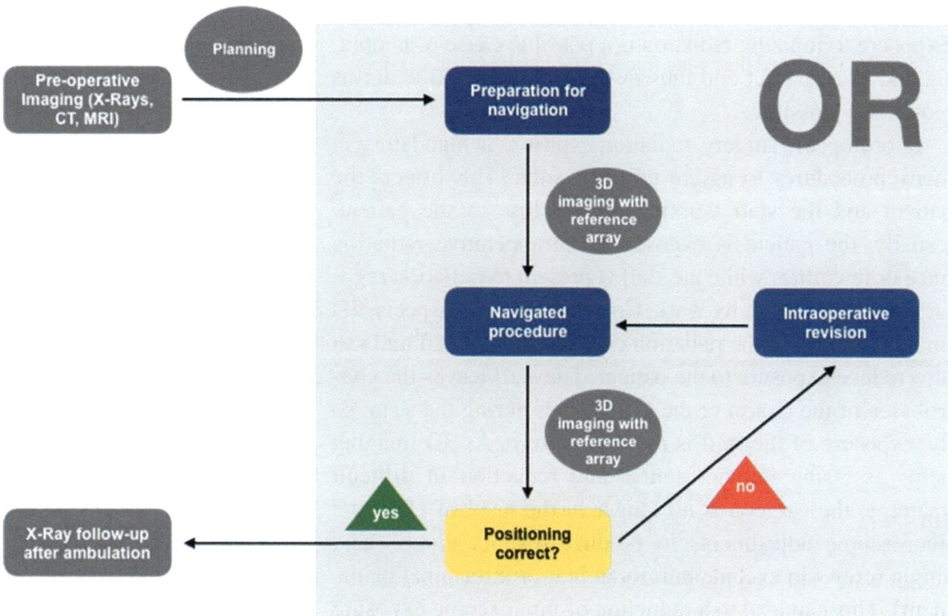

Fig. 39.11 Flowchart of planning and intraoperative use of 2D fluoroscopy and 3D imaging *with* navigation

Using intraoperative CT imaging, the procedure is slightly different. First, the patient needs to be placed within the gantry of the scanner (see Fig. 39.8). Depending on the size of the gantry and local preferences, special draping needs to be attached in advance. To define the scan field, a so-called scout scan is performed, which generates a 2D image in an anteroposterior or lateral view. Then, the area of the actual scan can be defined and the scan itself is performed. From the medico-legal point, a CT scanner belongs to a different class of imaging devices compared to standard C-arms; local regulations might necessitate the device to be operated by the radiological department. After acquiring of the images, postprocessing has to be done according to the abovementioned.

Advanced imaging and navigation is teamwork.

39.3.4 Assessment and Documentation

The 3D volume data needs to be formatted according to standard planes during radiological assessment. Usually, these planes are perpendicular to each other (coronal, axial, and sagittal planes). When assessing the posterior pelvic ring, especially the sacrum, oblique planes following the sacral slope might be useful. Depending on the kind of procedure, the surgeon needs to evaluate all planes regarding reduction (if necessary) and implant placement. In the posterior pelvic ring this accounts especially for implants close to the spinal canal and the neuroforamen. The findings of these studies need to be documented, most suitably in the surgery report.

To archive the image data itself, usually volume data are not ideal. Besides the large amount of data, most clinical DICOM-Viewers do not support the adjustment of the planes. More suitable are so-called parallel ranges or reconstructions that correspond to the planes that were adjusted before. These make up around 20–50 images for each plane and can be easily archived as accessed in the PACS. Note that the dose report usually also has to be archived.

39.3.5 Radiation Protection

Exposure to ionizing radiation is a possible cause of neoplasia and eye cataract and thus needs to be reduced as far as reasonably possible.

In orthopedic surgery, radiation exposure is mandatory in many procedures to assure proper results. This affects the patient and the staff working on or close to the patient. Usually, the patient is exposed to intraoperative radiation once or few times while the staff is present to radiation regularly as part of the daily work. Considering these aspects, 3D imaging improves the radiation exposure to the staff and can also reduce exposure to the patient. The staff leaves the control area of the C-arm or the CT scanner during the scan; so the exposure of the staff is reduced to zero. As 3D imaging helps assessing implant course and reduction in difficult anatomy, the surgeon is no longer in the need of elaborate fluoroscopic adjustments to produce distinct views (e.g., single screws to exclude intraforaminal or intraspinal placement). This can lead to a reduction of fluoroscopic exposure to the patient and, thus, radiation dose. If a navigation procedure is performed, there is less radiation exposure to the staff and the patient compared to standard 3D imaging (registration and verification).

Nonetheless, standard radiation exposure reduction measures should be applied when working with imaging devices [6].

> Radiation exposure to the staff can be significantly reduced by leaving the control area during imaging procedures.

39.4 Navigation

Navigation describes technical solutions to visualize to position of instruments or implants in imaging data of the operative field. Early concepts were developed during the 1980s that lead to the development of several commercially available products today [7]. Basically, these systems connect imaging data with a live tracking of instruments; so the position of instruments can be shown within image data.

39.4.1 Indication and Benefits

Navigation is of major advantage, where the anatomy of the patients remains constant to a wide extent during surgery.

> Navigation is static!

Once the system has been registered with an image data set, it does not recognize changes of the actual anatomy.

The essential benefit of navigation is the visualization of instruments or trajectories in anatomic regions where visualization by fluoroscopy is difficult or even impossible and proper implant placement relies on the experience of the surgeon. This has been shown to significantly improve safety of implant placement in the posterior pelvic ring [5]. Another benefit is the possibility to reduce radiation exposure during navigation as usually no further imaging is necessary.

Therefore, indications, ideal for navigation, include implant placements in non- or minor displaced fractures. Most commonly, iliosacral screw placement in SI joint disruptions or sacral fractures are selected indications. If these injuries are displaced, reduction is performed using the screws; so the change of the actual anatomy does not affect the implant placement (Fig. 39.12 shows a navigated placement of an iliosacral SI joint screw).

Lumbopelvic instrumentation can also benefit from navigation. If a data set of an appropriate volume is available, it is possible to place the pedicle screws as well as the pelvic screws with only one registration process. This facilitates the procedure significantly and reduces radiation dose to the patient, especially if intraoperative image data are used.

> Good results in navigated procedures depend on proper preparation and a possibly constant anatomy.

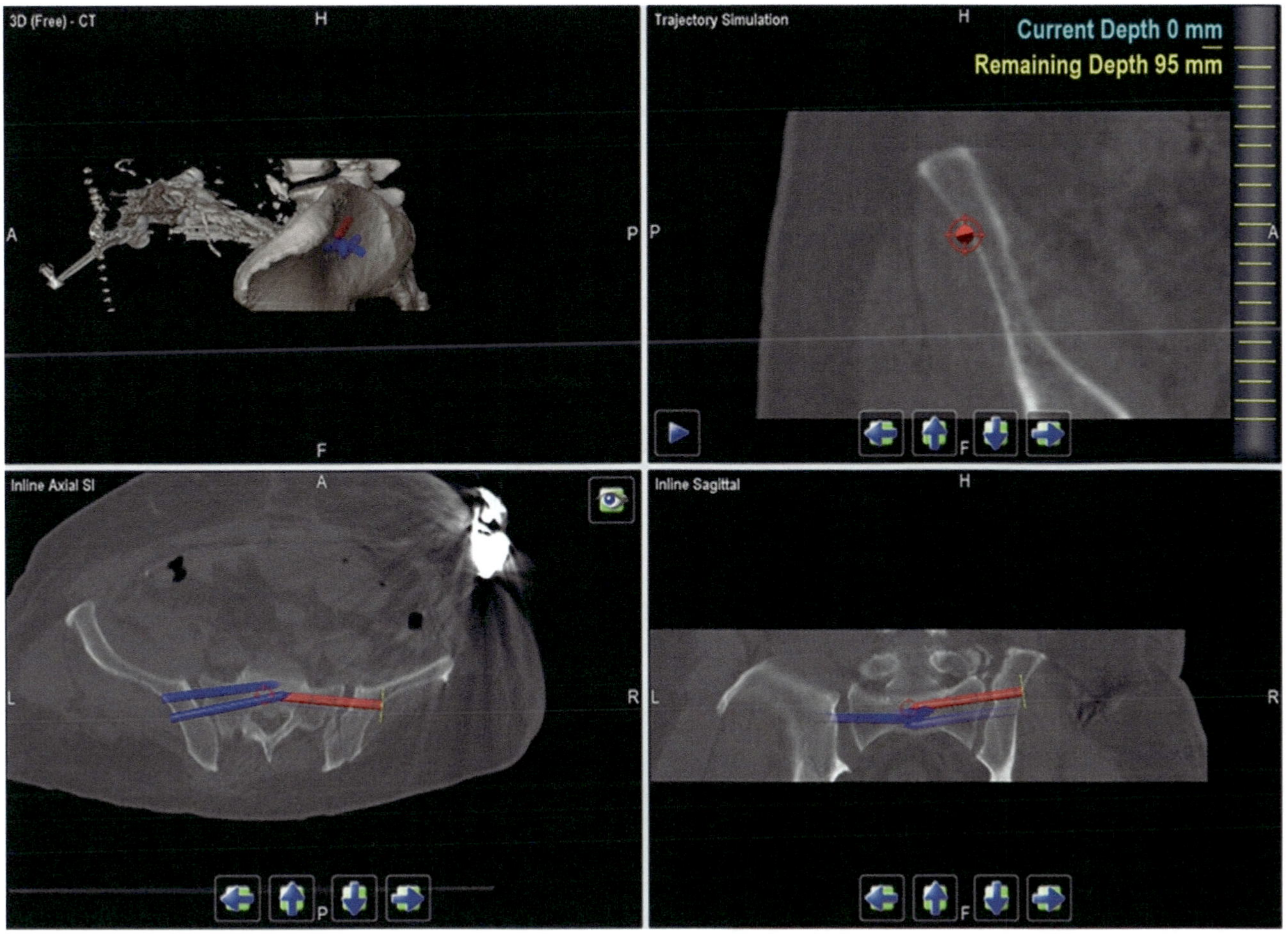

Fig. 39.12 Navigated placement of iliosacral SI joint screws showing the planned screw trajectories

39.4.2 Technical Aspects

Navigation is in widespread use in joint replacement surgery where usually image-free navigation is used. No image data of the actual patient but rather a generic model of the particular joint is available and anatomical landmarks are registered to the actual patient. This concept is suitable especially for prosthetic implantation as alignment is more crucial than exact placement. In contrast, this concept cannot be used for stabilization of the fractured pelvic ring, as exact hardware placement has priority.

Projection of instruments or their trajectories into 2D images of the actual anatomy is as well a form of appearance of navigation. Although in these cases, the problems of 2D imaging regarding the pelvic ring have to be considered.

Most common (and reasonable) is the use of 3D navigation in pelvic surgery. Using this technique, the position of implants is projected live onto a 3D image data set and allows the surgeon to ensure proper implant placement.

Tracking of the instruments is realized either by an optical system with a stereo camera system that emits infrared light reflected by geometrically arranged markers on the instruments. The reflected signals are again registered by the camera (Fig. 39.13). There are also systems available that realize tracking by electromagnetic fields that are created close to the surgical area. With specially designed instruments or implants, the system registers the changes in the field by the instruments and calculates their position.

As these systems are more vulnerable to distortions, most common optical systems are used. The main issues related to this are the necessity of a direct line of sight from the reference array and the instruments to the camera. Depending on the situs, sometimes it is difficult to have all arrays in the optimal visual area. As for all of these aspects relating to advanced intraoperative imaging and additional devices, this requires proper planning and a deep understanding of the procedure by the whole surgical team.

There are several options to create a navigable image data set. Intraoperative image sets that are acquired by a 3D C-arm or intraoperative CT are commonly used. All modern navigation solutions allow for direct and automatic registration of these data sets. The position of the imaging device is

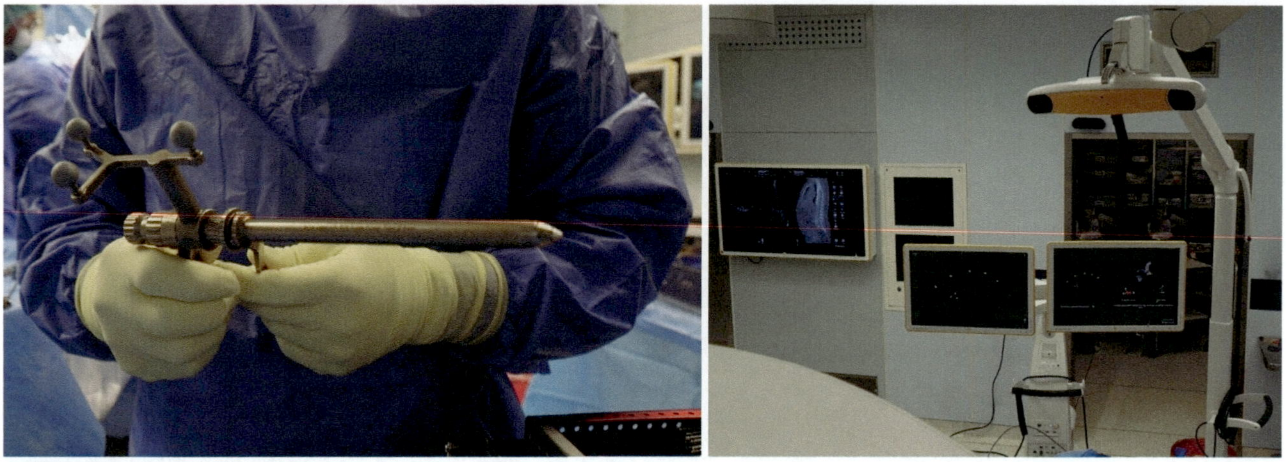

Fig. 39.13 Calibration of a drill guide and appearance on the stereo camera and the monitor cart where the surgeon can view the resultant navigation

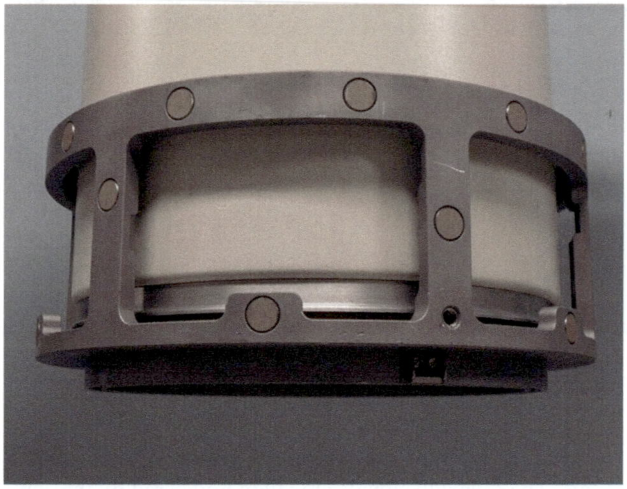

Fig. 39.14 A marker array on a 3D C-arm to allow intraoperative detection of the C-arm by the navigation camera

also captured by the navigation camera by special markers (Fig. 39.14).

This results in an automatic registration of the image volume to the actual spatial dimensions and no further registration is necessary to navigate within the image set. Another significant advantage for the use of intraoperative data is the possibility of acquisition after positioning of the patient and after possible reduction maneuvers resulting in most accurate imaging data respecting the actual situation.

Disadvantages include the reduced image quality, especially of 3D C-arms compared to stationary CT scanners, and the limited field of view. Additionally, devices for intraoperative 3D imaging are cost intensive.

Additionally, it is possible to use preoperative CT or MRI data sets for navigation. Then, the CT data set has to be registered with the reference arrays of the navigation system to connect the dimensions of the image data to the actual spatial relations. Several solutions exist:

- A navigated pointer can be placed to distinct anatomical landmarks in the operative field that are given by the navigation system; an open exposure of bony structures used as landmarks are required, which limits the possibilities of minimally invasive surgery.
- 2D/3D registration: several (at least two) fluoroscopic views of the anatomic region with a specific marker array in place are captured; using this information, registration of the CT data set to the marker arrays can be computed.
- 3D/3D registration is another method to use a preoperative CT data set (if a high-contrast navigation data set with a large field of view is needed); an automatically registered intraoperative 3D data set is created by a 3D C-arm and matched to a preoperative CT that includes the volume of the intraoperative data; the navigation can so be extended to the whole volume of the CT.

Besides the increased efforts that are needed for all manual registration procedures, one intrinsic disadvantage is the change between the anatomy during CT aquisition and the real situation on the operating table. This can only be partly compensated by the registration process; so a certain inaccuracy needs to be anticipated.

When using an intraoperative data volume, an accuracy of about 1 mm can be achieved.

39.5 Summary

Navigation enables the surgeon to use more minimally invasive approaches and to place implants precisely and safe (Figs. 39.15 and 39.16). Patient safety is enhanced by

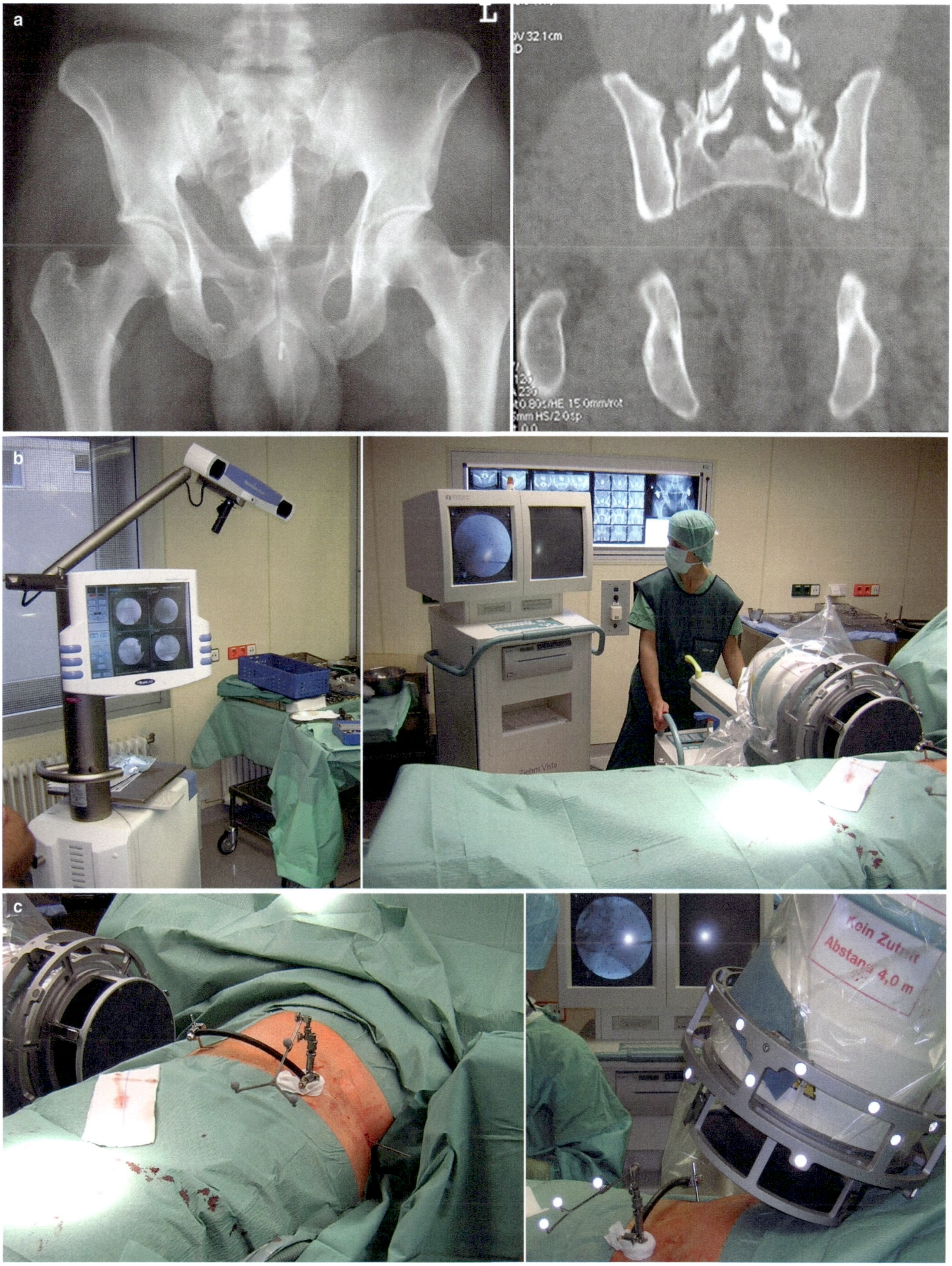

Fig. 39.15 (**a**) Pelvic ring type C injury with bilateral pubic rami fractures and a complete left sacrum fracture. (**b**) Intraoperative navigation setup: lateral sacrum view. (**c**) Optical markers attached to the applied external fixator. (**d**) Calibration of the drill bit and navigation of the drilling process. (**e**) Intraoperative views after screw insertion. (**f**) Postoperative view showing the well-placed iliosacral screw in a dysmorphic sacrum. Courtesy by Axel Gänsslen

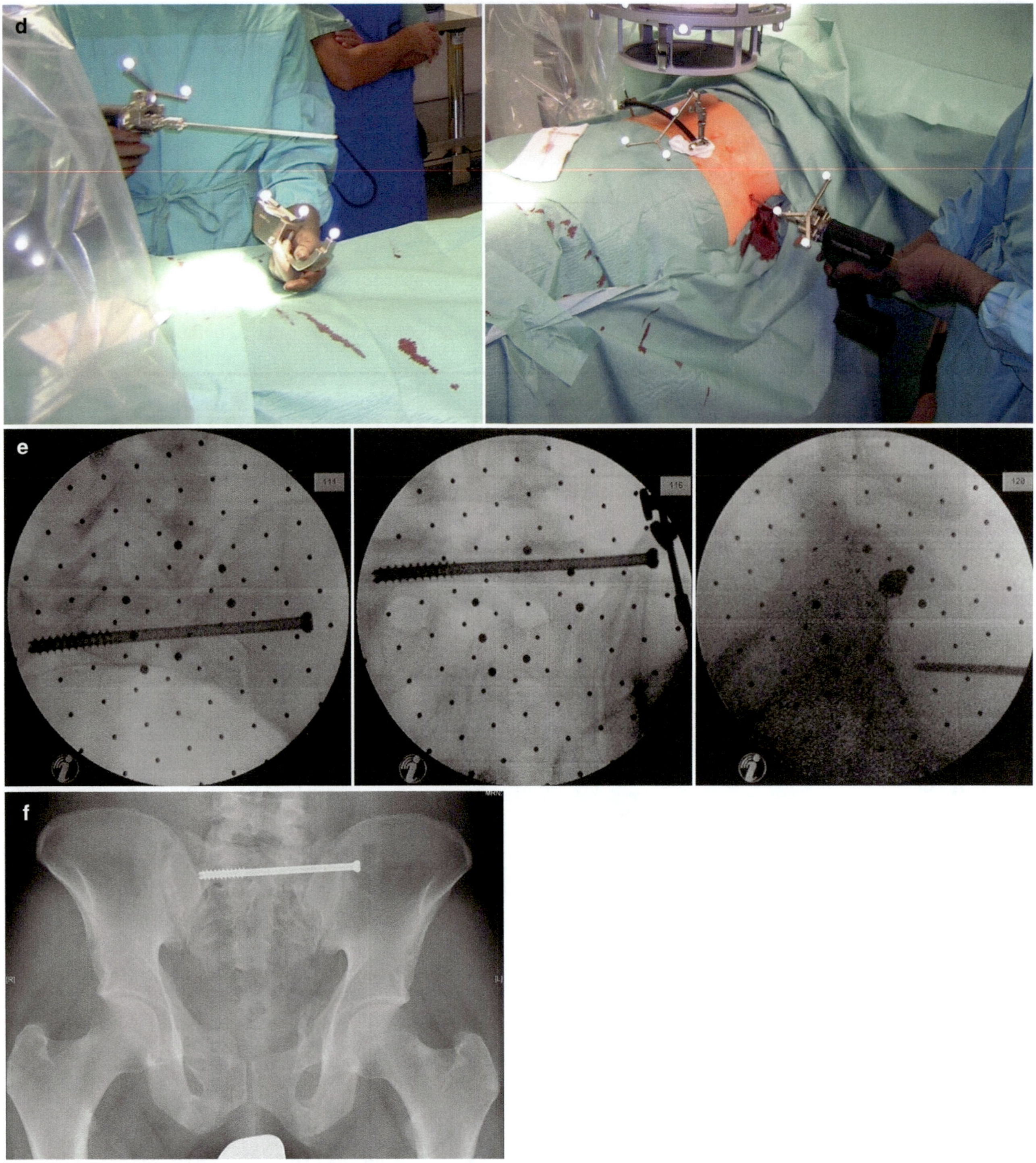

Fig. 39.15 (continued)

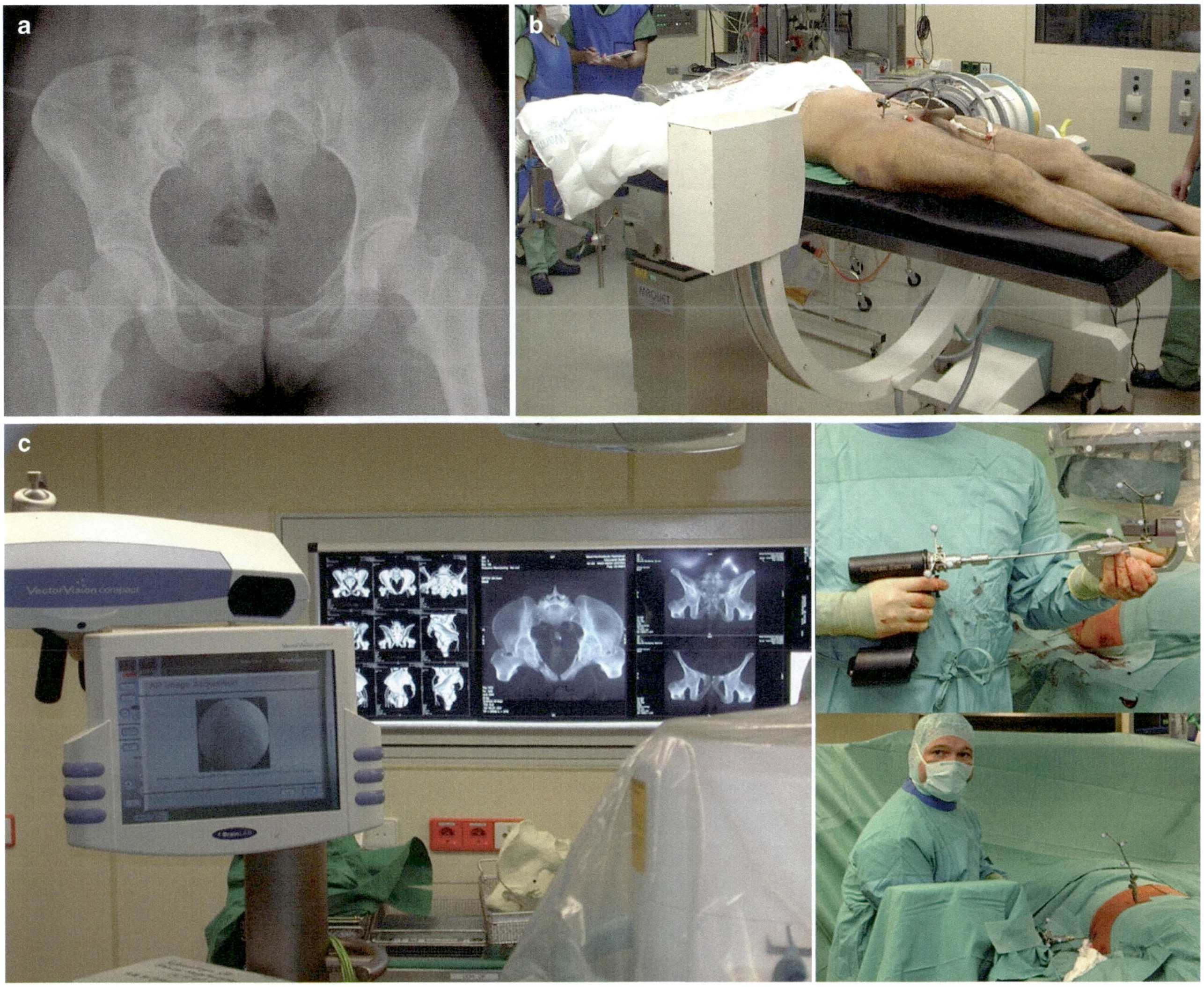

Fig. 39.16 (**a**) Pelvic ring type C injury with bilateral pubic rami fractures and a complete left sacrum fracture in a dysmorphic sacrum. (**b**) Standard supine positioning with lumbosacral support on a radiolucent OR table. (**c**) Intraoperative setup : drill calibration and drilling process under navigation assistance. (**d**) Monitor detail: drill calibration. (**e**) Drilling with optical markers attached to the drilling machine. (**f**) Fluoroscopic view of the planned (red) and present position (incl. the expected position) of the drill (yellow). (**g**) Intraoperative views after screw insertion. (**h**) Postoperative view with the well-located screw. Courtesy by Axel Gänsslen

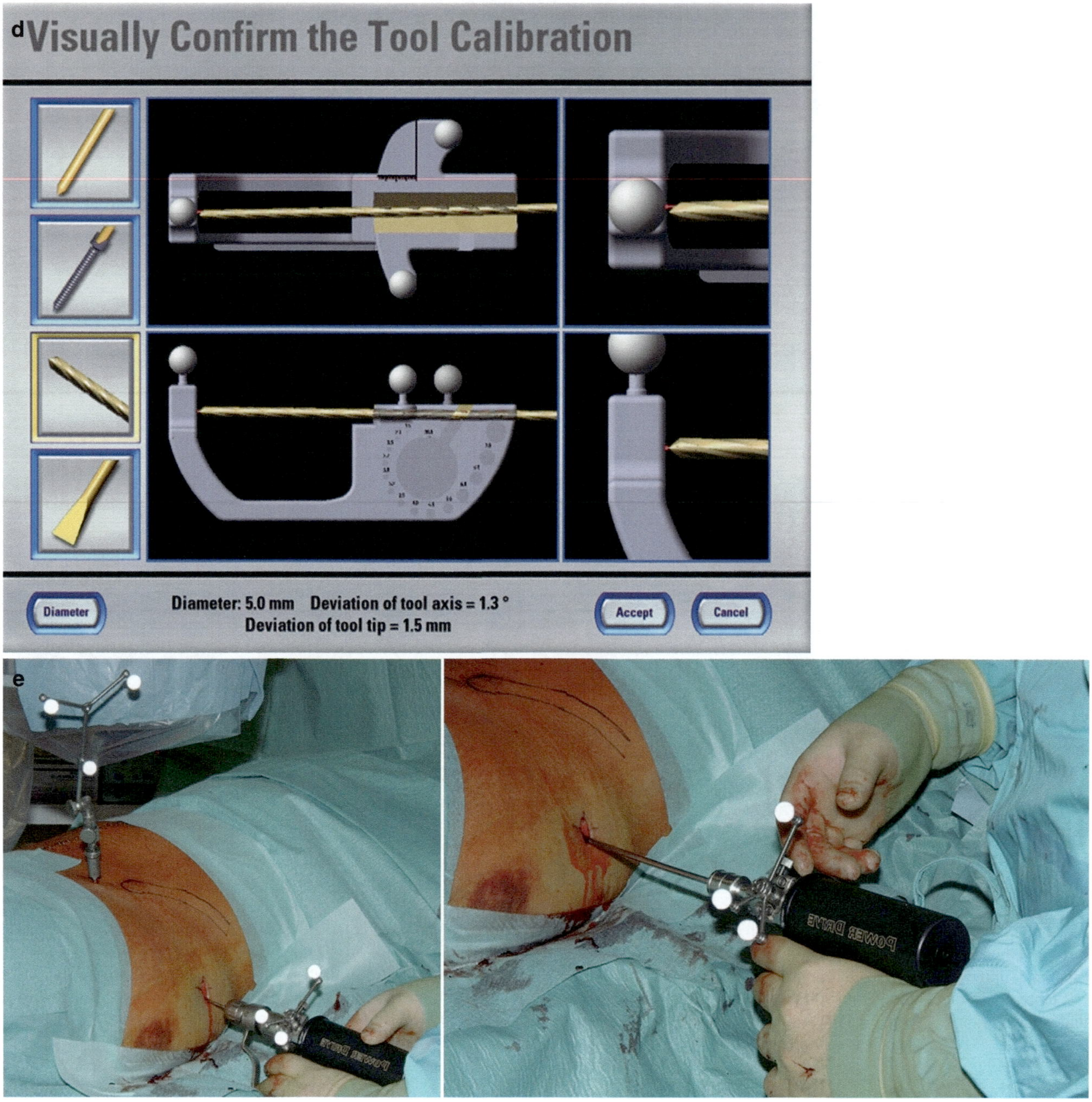

Fig. 39.16 (continued)

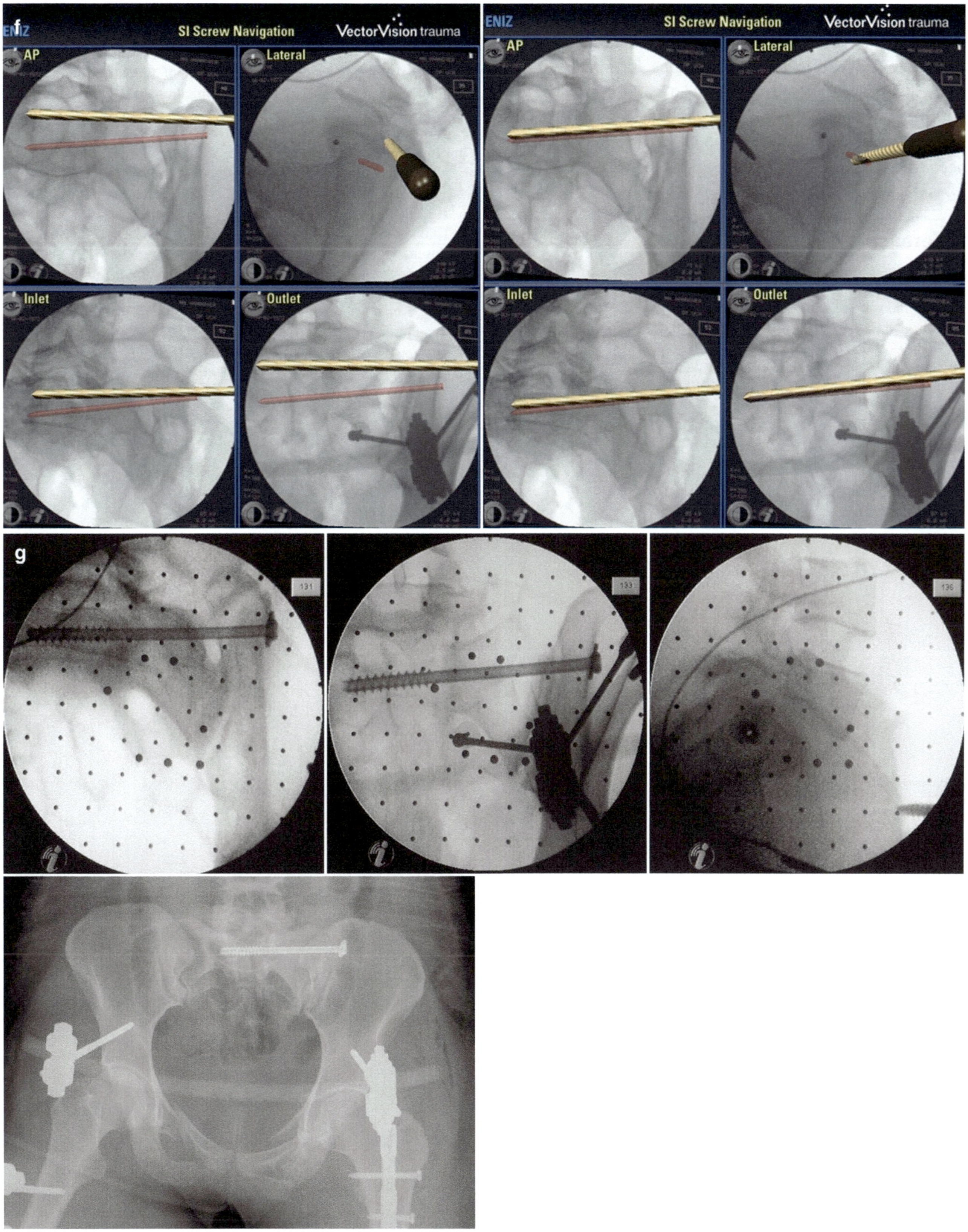

Fig. 39.16 (continued)

increased certainty in instrument and implant handling as well as radiation exposure can be reduced substantially. As procedures have to be adapted to the use of navigation, the surgical team needs to be trained and a learning curve to benefit from the technical possibilities is considered. The aspect of increased hardware and additional sterile equipment costs need to be evaluated.

References

1. Franke J, Wendl K, Suda A, Giese T, Grützner P, von Recum J. Intraoperative three-dimensional imaging in the treatment of calcaneal fractures. J Bone Joint Surg Am. 2014;96:e72. https://doi.org/10.2106/JBJS.L.01220.
2. Vetter S, Euler F, von Recum J, Wendl K, Grützner P, Franke J. Impact of intraoperative cone beam computed tomography on reduction quality and implant position in treatment of tibial plafond fractures. Foot Ankle Int. 2016;37:977–82.
3. Keil H, Beisemann N, Schnetzke M, Vetter S, Swartman B, Grützner P, Franke J. Intraoperative assessment of reduction and implant placement in acetabular fractures-limitations of 3D-imaging compared to computed tomography. J Orthop Surg Res. 2018;13:78. https://doi.org/10.1186/s13018-018-0780-7.
4. Rommens P, Ossendorf C, Pairon P, Dietz S, Wagner D, Hofmann A. Clinical pathways for fragility fractures of the pelvic ring: personal experience and review of the literature. J Orthop Sci. 2015;20:1–11.
5. Thakkar S, Thakkar R, Sirisreetreerux N, Carrino J, Shafiq B, Hasenboehler E. 2D versus 3D fluoroscopy-based navigation in posterior pelvic fixation: review of the literature on current technology. Int J Comput Assist Radiol Surg. 2016;12:69–76.
6. Singer G. Occupational radiation exposure to the surgeon. J Am Acad Orthop Surg. 2005;13:69–76.
7. Mezger U, Jendrewski C, Bartels M. Navigation in surgery. Langenbecks Arch Surg. 2013;398:501. https://doi.org/10.1007/s00423-013-1059-4.

Implant Removal

40

Christian Pfeifer and Axel Gänsslen

40.1 General Indications

Beside a clear indication regarding all external fixation devices [1] (external fixator, pelvic C-clamp), recommended general criteria for implant removal at the pelvis include:

- Infection [2, 3]
- Allergic implant-related reactions or allergy to metal components [2, 4]
- Epiphyseal-bridging implants
- Temporary joint arthrodesis
- Intraarticular hardware/screw misplacements [5]
- Critical soft-tissue status related to implants [1, 2]
- Development of non-unions
- Secondary implant loosening/breakage with resulting soft-tissue compromise or infection
- Potential risk of corrosion, carcinogenesis, and osteopenia
- Wires
- Subjective disturbing implants
- Risk of implant-related tendon injuries
- Biomechanical causes

Implant removal was proposed only in symptomatic patients [6, 7].

40.2 Pelvic Indications

Clear recommendations regarding implant removal are missing in the existing literature [2, 8–14].

For a long time, several authors recommended routine implant removal of joint-bridging implants, e.g., iliosacral screws [8, 9, 13, 15]. In contrast, others recommended implant removal only in cases with implant failure or infection [16, 17], and a routine removal was considered unusual [18].

In contrast, for implants at the iliac crest or superior pubic rami screws, the benefit of implant removal has to be related to the surgical risk [2, 8, 13].

It is often difficult to distinguish implant-related complaints from degenerative complaints [19]. Data from the German Multicenter Study Group showed that after type C injuries, approximately 20% of patients persistently suffer from some posterior pelvic pain, despite anatomical healing, indicating the relevance of the initial soft-tissue injury [20].

Additionally, it has to be considered that with increasing time from primary surgery, implant removal can be technically demanding due to extensive scar formation or osseous coverage of implants [19].

Scharf et al. recommended routine pelvic implant removal when implants are bridging joints, e.g., symphysis plate, iliosacral screws, TIFI (transiliac internal fixator), lumbopelvic stabilization constructs, and anterior SI joint plates, and thus a potential risk of implant loosening or implant failure could be expected. Joint-bridging reconstruction plates should be removed after 9–12 months (symphyseal plate), while implants located deep in the pelvis should be left in place due to the potential risk of surgery-related morbidity [15].

Stuby et al. analyzed 35 of 80 surgically treated cases with implant removal after type B and C injuries between 2003 and 2010, representing an implant removal rate of 44% [19, 21]. The following implants were removed:

- 15 symphyseal plates
- 24 iliosacral screws
- 1× spinopelvic implant

On average, implant removal was performed after 14.6 months at the posterior pelvic ring and after 20.2 months

C. Pfeifer
Department of Trauma Surgery, University Hospital Regensburg, Regensburg, Germany
e-mail: christian.pfeifer@ukr.de

A. Gänsslen (✉)
Department of Trauma Surgery, Orthopedics and Hand Surgery, Hospital Wolfsburg, Wolfsburg, Germany

A. Gänsslen et al. (eds.), *Pelvic Ring Fractures*, https://doi.org/10.1007/978-3-030-54730-1_40

at the anterior pelvic ring. Only 3/11 patients after posterior pelvic ring implant removal reported a clinical benefit.

Before implant removal, 79% (n = 11) of symphyseal plates showed signs of implant loosening (n = 5) or breakage (n = 6). Iliosacral screws showed slight implant loosening in 28% (11/39).

> Therefore, in general, an individual approach to implant removal is recommended [19].

40.3 Iliosacral Screws

Routt et al. developed the concept of percutaneous iliosacral screw fixation based on a detailed understanding of the surgical and radiographic anatomy of the sacrum [22–24].

This group already stated that iliosacral screw removal is controversial. Potential advantages include posterior pelvic ring pain relief and remobilization of the (uninjured) fixed SI joint, especially in younger patients. Potential disadvantages include the potential surgical difficulty due to relevant scar formation around the screw head and the additional washer, the need for a new/different/longer incision, the potential risk of screw breakage, and the potential necessity for an open removal technique [24].

In several reports, dealing with iliosacral screw fixation, only selected implant removal was recorded:

- Nork et al. reported on one case with clinical benefit after screw removal due to local pain [25].
- French et al. recommended implant removal in cases with infection after open posterior approach and screw fixation [26].
- Tsukushi et al. removed two iliosacral screws after SI joint fixation after 6 months [27].
- Baskin reported on one case of screw removal due to posterior complaints after 2 mm screw migration with optimization of the clinical disturbances [28].
- Osterhoff et al. reported one case with iliosacral screw removal in a pregnant patient [29].

The only larger series dealing with the clinical effect of iliosacral screw removal was performed by Yücel et al. in 2004. In 21 patients with type C injuries, 12 had implant removal and 9 were without implant removal. Indication for implant removal was based on clinical signs in eight cases and in four a planned removal was performed. Overall, 83.3% showed clinical improvement after 1 year [14].

Gänsslen et al. generally recommended implant removal 6–12 months after percutaneous iliosacral screw fixation of sacral fractures, as the uninjured SI joint was bridged to allow physiological SI joint mobility [9].

Pieske et al. reported a rate of 46.5% implant removal after a mean of 11 months, but no data regarding indication, complications, or clinical effect were reported [30].

Stuby et al. analyzed 35 of 80 surgically treated cases with implant removal after type B and C injuries of the pelvis between 2003 and 2010, representing an overall implant removal rate of 44% [19, 21]. At the posterior pelvis, as part of this analysis, 24 iliosacral screws and 1 spinopelvic implant were removed after a mean of 14.6 months. Indications included subjective posterior pelvic pain in 46%; 33% were removed based on the decision of the treating surgeon and due to patients' desire in 40%. Twenty-eight percent of the iliosacral screws showed slight signs of implant loosening (11/39). An overall complication rate of 20% was observed (including anterior pelvic ring implant removal), and only 3/11 patients after posterior pelvic ring implant removal reported some clinical benefit.

Recent analyses stated that bridging the contralateral, uninjured SI joint with a transverse transsacral-transiliac stabilization method resulted in no differences regarding pain and function compared to the affected SI joint 1 year after surgery [31, 32].

> Implant removal is not routinely performed after iliosacral screw fixation. A clinical benefit cannot clearly be expected from present data (Fig. 40.1). Bridging an uninjured SI joint seems to have no negative clinical effect.

40.4 Ilioiliacal Stabilization

Several technical options exist for posterior ilioiliacal stabilization of type C injuries of the pelvic ring. These include posterior plate stabilization, the TIFI concept, and sacral bar stabilization. Only data for posterior plating and TIFI can be analyzed from the existing literature.

40.4.1 Plate Stabilization

Albert et al. stated that none of the 14 patients required implant removal [33].

In the analysis of Kobbe et al., 3 of 21 patients required plate removal for minor discomfort after 6, 12, and 14 months, respectively [34].

Dolati et al. analyzed 34 patients with 29.4% with secondary implant removal, which was partially or completely

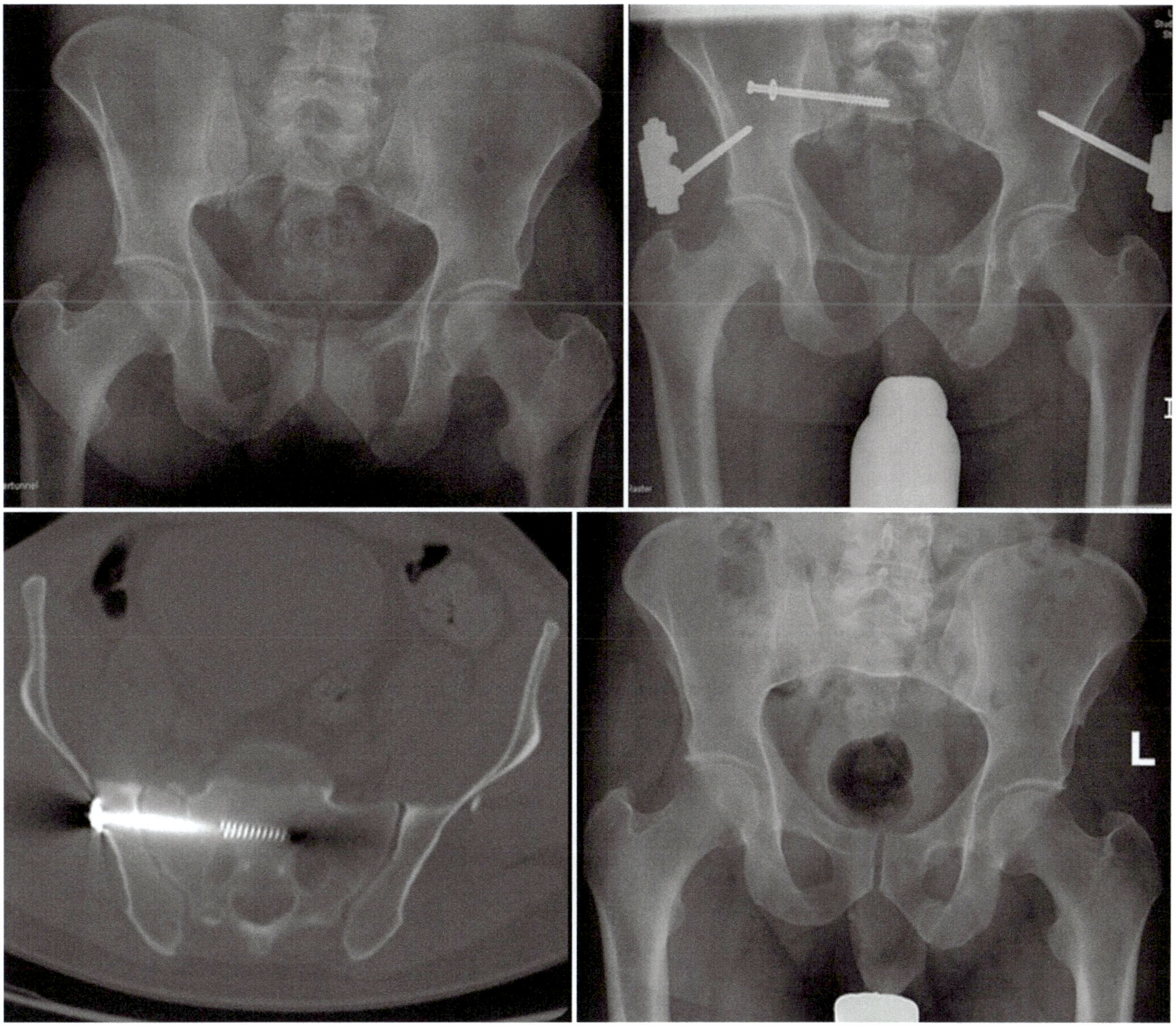

Fig. 40.1 Iliosacral screw stabilization of a sacral fracture resulted in early (2 weeks) implant mobility. Implant removal was performed after 3 months, due to local discomfort

removed. Indications for implant removal included 1× infection, 2× prominent and disturbing screw heads, 4× local discomfort, and 3× elective removal without clinical complaints [35, 36].

Suzuki et al. removed 2 of 19 plates due to infectious complications [37].

Ayoub et al. recently reported on 3 out of 42 patients with implant removal after a mean of 11.7 months as a result of posterior discomfort or pain [38].

Ilioiliacal plate stabilization resulted in a low rate of implant removal. Subjective discomfort or local infection is the main indication for this stabilization concept.

40.4.2 TIFI

In the original description of the TIFI technique (transiliacal internal fixator), Füchtmeier et al. removed all internal fixators after a mean of 11.8 months in two cases early after 4 weeks due to deep wound infection [39]. In an on-going analysis of 67 patients, all implants were removed. In 13 patients implant removal was performed due to local discomfort [40].

Salášek et al. removed the TIFI in 46.9% after a mean of 15.3 months [41]. No surgery-related complications were observed.

The posterior transiliacal internal fixator (TIFI) is removed in at least 50% of cases most often based on the surgeon's recommendation.

40.5 Pubic Symphysis Plate

Historically, implant removal was frequently performed after plate osteosynthesis of the disrupted pubic symphysis.

Weber et al. analyzed 22 patients with pubic symphysis disruption, treated with combined reconstruction plate osteosynthesis and tension band wiring. In 45.5% implant removal was performed after an average of 15.7 months (3–42 months) [42]. Metal removal had no influence on the clinical and radiological long-term result.

Pohlemann et al. recommended implant removal after 6–12 months in all cases to allow physiological movements of the symphysis (Fig. 40.1) [43].

Raman et al. performed a literature review on 482 patients with symphyseal internal stabilization on implant removal and stated that no consensus could be derived for routine implant removal [12]. A 7.5% complication rate was observed with implant removal, with infection being the most common complication.

Giannoudis et al. analyzed 74 patients after symphyseal plating. Implant removal was performed in only four patients (5.4%) in an observational period of 41 months [10]. It was stated that routine removal of the plate is not essential, while in women of childbearing age no clear data were available.

Collinge et al. retrospectively reviewed 126 patients with type B and C injuries treated with anterior plate fixation using a four- or six-hole 3.5 mm plate without locking screws [44]. All type C injuries additionally had posterior stabilization, while type B injuries were fixed posteriorly in 30%. In 75%, radiographic hardware failure was detected at an average follow-up of 12.2 months, including screw loosening/breakage (71% screw loosening, 5% screw breakage, 7% plate breakage, 17% combined screw loosening/breakage). Even in type B injuries, 74% implant failure rate was observed. After type C injuries this rate was 77%. During follow-up of these patients, the symphyseal gap increased from 4.9 to 8.5 mm.

Morris et al. retrospectively reviewed 148 patients with symphyseal disruption, which were fixed with plates, treated using three different plating systems. In three cases double plating was performed [45]. After a minimum follow-up of 12 months, implant breakage was observed in 43%. Of these patients, 96.8% were asymptomatic. In only 3% of patients, revision surgery was indicated.

There is often some secondary widening of the symphyseal space after osteosynthesis of a symphyseal disruption. Lybrand et al. observed 1–2 mm increase until union occurred, also after disk removal or disk retaining procedures [46].

Late fixation failure, e.g., symphyseal widening ± fixation failure is considered a benign condition as few patients need revision surgery [44, 45].

In a series of 37 patients with symphyseal plating (3× type A, 24× type B, 10× type C injuries, 76% posterior fixation), 29.7% rate of symphyseal implant failure was detected [47]. The quality of the reduction was good in 38% (≤5 mm), good in 27% (6–10 mm), and insufficient in 36% (>10 mm) according to Lindahl [48]. The SF-36 score was not significantly affected by implant failure while the Majeed score showed a tendency of better results after implant failure (83 vs. 72 points).

There is no indication for routine implant removal of symphysis bridging implants (Fig. 40.2). Physiological implant mobilization is frequently observed. A high rate of infectious complications has to be considered.

40.6 Retrograde Ramus Screw

No data are available regarding implant removal of retrograde superior ramus screws.

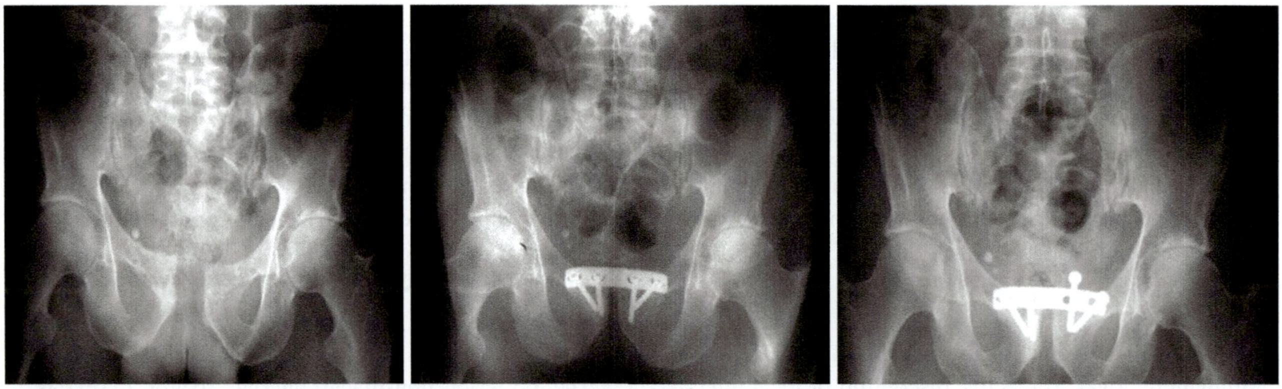

Fig. 40.2 Open book injury, treated with symphyseal plate stabilization. After 6 months screw loosening occurred, without clinical impairments. Implant removal was performed due to patient's wish

40.7 Anterior SI Plate

Several reports dealt with anterior plate stabilization of the disrupted SI joint. Only two reports gave conflicting statements regarding implant removal.

Ragnarsson et al. reported no implant removal after anterior SI joint plating [49].

Gänsslen generally recommended implant removal after approximately 6–12 months to prevent a "spontaneous" fusion of the SI joint to allow physiologic joint movements at the SI joint. Removal is generally recommended in young patients, while in radiographic detected ankyloses, no implant removal is performed [50].

Recent analyses of the effect of bridging the contralateral, uninjured SI joint with a transverse transsacral-transiliac screw resulted in no differences regarding pain and function compared to the involved SI joint 1 year after surgery [31, 32].

There is no clear indication for routine implant removal after anterior SI joint plating.

40.8 Lumbopelvic Fixation

Lumbopelvic fixation strategies, either using open reduction internal fixation or a percutaneous approach, are becoming more and more popular.

In the early years after the introduction of these procedures, implant removal was not generally recommended:

- Schildhauer et al. initially reported one case with implant removal due to deep infection; in an on-going analysis, the osteosynthesis material was removed in 23/48 patients (48%), in one patient for deep wound infection, and in 22 patients routinely, after fracture healing [3].
- Nothofer generally recommended implant removal after 6–9 months due to the bridging of intact motion segments (SI joint, L4/L5 and/or L5/S1 intervertebral disk segment) [51].
- Mouhsine et al. routinely removed metalwork in all seven cases after healing of the fracture, at a mean time of 4.3 months after surgery [52].

In contrast, Bellabarba et al. stated that no clinical benefit exists to electively remove these implants [53].

Indications for implant removal exist in prominent and locally disturbing implants after radiological bone healing after 6–12 months [53].

Radiologically, distal rod breakage can occur due to SI joint motions, which was documented in 10.7%. This finding led many authors to recommend elective removal of the lumbopelvic instrumentation fracture union 6–12 months postoperatively [53–55].

With increasing popularity, newer data from the last 5–6 years are available. The frequency of implant removal of lumbopelvic stabilizations increased:

- 50% implant removal was performed at a median of 8 months after stabilization to prevent sacroiliac arthrodesis or to mobilize the lumbar spine after unilateral lumbopelvic stabilization; the main indication was not related to wound disorders [54]
- 72.7% implant removal after 6–8 months after fracture healing [56]
- 77.8% implant removal after an average of 26 months (13–66 months) [57]
- 95% implant removal, due to pain, resulting in complete pain relief [58]
- 42.8% implant removal due to material prominence and pain [59]
- General implant removal 4–6 months postoperatively, if no spinal fusion was performed [60]
- 27.3% implant removal because of deep infection (after 1 year), implant breakage (after 9 years), and screw loosening (after 7 years) [61]
- 100% implant removal in 3/3 cases [62]
- 29% elective metal removal [63]

Presently, approximately 70–90% of implants are routinely removed.

To minimize complaints of low back and buttock pain, arguments for lumbopelvic fixation removal include [58, 64]:

- Local posterior pelvic pain
- Symptomatic overloading of the contralateral lumbolumbal or lumbosacral articulations due to asymmetric, unilateral, rigid immobilization of the L5/S1 junction
- Painful ipsilateral SI joint
- Prominent hardware
- Wound breakdown

40.9 Anterior External Fixation

Classical external fixators, e.g., anterior supraacetabular and iliac external fixators, are removed after clinical fracture healing.

Newer systems include the subcutaneous fixator and the subcutaneous plate.

The main conclusions from the literature using the subcutaneous anterior pelvic internal fixator fixation are [65–88]:

- Implant removal is recommended at 3–6 months postoperatively
- Irritation of the LCFN is common and resolves latest after implant removal

For subcutaneous anterior pelvic internal plate fixation, implant removal is routinely performed [89].

External and subcutaneous internal fixation devices are routinely removed.

40.10 Implant Removal and Pregnancy

During pregnancy, some relaxation of the pelvic ligaments occurs, which can be disturbed as a result of former anterior or posterior fracture/joint osteosynthesis.

Effects of retained pelvic implants on vaginal delivery are insufficiently stated in the orthopedic and gynecological literatures [90].

The rate of posttraumatic cesarean section is significantly higher than in women without former pelvic fractures [91, 92].

Many obstetricians belief that women after sustaining a pelvic fracture cannot deliver vaginally [92]. The effect of residual pelvic deformity may influence pregnancy outcomes. Thus, routine pelvic implant removal was advocated [93]. The high cesarean section rate is, therefore, explained due to suspected difficulty of vaginal delivery.

The presently sparse literature presents the following statements:

- In near anatomically healed pelves, no routine indication for implant removal exists [91, 93].
- Patients with an initial fracture displacement of >5 mm had 80% cesarean section rate, which was 5.3-fold of the rate of displacements <5 mm [92].
- Pelvic implants justify no indication for cesarean delivery as fixation devices do not preclude successful vaginal delivery [93].

40.11 Summary

Routine removal of pelvic implants is not supported by the recent literature. Joint-bridging implants become loose or even break, which is most often only a radiological phenomenon, with a low clinical consequence.

Some implants present with high local impairments, and, therefore, implant removal should be considered, e.g., lumbopelvic fixation devices, subcutaneous anterior plate, or fixator devices.

References

1. Müller-Färber J. [Removal of metal in traumatology]. Unfallchirurg. 2003;106:653–68.
2. AWMF, Leitlinie der Deutschen Gesellschaft für Unfallchirurgie: Implantatentfernung. AWMF-Leitlinien-Register Nr. 012/004. 2008.
3. Schildhauer T, Josten C, Muhr G. Triangular osteosynthesis of vertically unstable sacrum fractures: a new concept allowing early weight bearing. J Orthop Trauma. 1998;12(5):307–14.
4. Duchna H, Nowack U, Merget R. [Prospective study of the significance of contact sensitization caused by metal implants]. Zentralbl Chir. 1998;123:1271–6.
5. Keating J, Werier J, Blachut P. Early fixation of the vertically unstable pelvis: the role of iliosacral screw fixation of the posterior lesion. J Orthop Trauma. 1999;13:107–13.
6. Brown R, Wheelwright E, Chalmers J. Removal of metal implants after fracture surgery—indications and complications. J R Coll Surg Edinb. 1993;38:96–100.
7. Gösling T, Hüfner T, Hankemeier S. Femoral nail removal should be restricted in asymptomatic patients. Clin Orthop Relat Res. 2004;423:222–6.
8. Culemann U, Tosounidis G, Reilmann H. [Injury to the pelvic ring. Diagnosis and current possibilities for treatment]. Unfallchirurg. 2004;107:1169–81.
9. Gänsslen A, Hüfner T, Krettek C. Percutaneous iliosacral screw fixation of unstable pelvic injuries by conventional fluoroscopy. Oper Orthop Traumatol. 2006;18:225–44.
10. Giannoudis P, Chalidis B, Roberts C. Internal fixation of traumatic diastasis of pubic symphysis: is plate removal essential? Arch Orthop Trauma Surg. 2008;128:325–31.
11. Putnis S, Pearce R, Wali U, Bircher M, Rickman M. Open reduction and internal fixation of a traumatic diastasis of the pubic symphysis. J Bone Joint Surg Br. 2011;93:78–84.
12. Raman R, Roberts C, Pape H, Giannoudis P. Implant retention and removal after internal fixation of the symphysis pubis. Injury. 2005;36:827–31.
13. Tscherne H, Pohlemann T. Tscherne Unfallchirurgie: Becken und Acetabulum. Berlin, Heidelberg, New York: Springer; 1998.
14. Yücel N, Lefering R, Tjardes T, Korenkov M, Schierholz J, Tiling T, Bouillon B, Rixen D. [Is implant removal after percutaneous iliosacral screw fixation of unstable posterior pelvic ring disruptions indicated?]. Unfallchirurg. 2004;107:468–74.
15. Scharf M, Krieg B, Dengler M, Füchtmeier B. Die Implantatentfernung—eine Risiko-Nutzen-Abwägung? OP J. 2016;32:80–8.
16. Abumi K, Saita M, Iida T. Reduction and fixation of sacroiliac joint dislocation by the combined use of S1 pedicle screws and the Galveston technique. Spine. 2000;25:1977–83.
17. Routt M, Simonian P, Mills W. Iliosacral screw fixation: early complications of the percutaneous technique. J Orthop Trauma. 1997;11(8):584–9.
18. Remiger A, Engelhardt P. Die perkutane iliosakrale Verschraubung von vertikal instabilen Beckenringfrakturen. Swiss Surg. 1996;2:259–63.
19. Stuby F, Gonser C, Baron H, Stöckle U, Badke A, Ochs B. Implantatentfernung nach Beckenringfraktur. OP J. 2016;32:130–7.

20. Pohlemann T, Gänsslen A, Hartung S, für die Arbeitsgruppe Becken, H.T., H., Beckenverletzungen/Pelvic Injuries. Hefte zu "Der Unfallchirurg". Heft 266. 1998.
21. Stuby F, Gonser C, Baron H, Stöckle U, Badke A, Ochs G. Implantatentfernung nach Beckenringfraktur. Unfallchirurg. 2012;115:330–8.
22. Routt M, Kregor P, Simonian P, Mayo K. Early results of percutaneous iliosacral screws placed with the patient in the supine position. J Orthop Trauma. 1995;9(3):207–14.
23. Routt M, Simonian P, Inaba J. Iliosacral screw fixation of the disrupted sacroiliac joint. Tech Orthop. 1995;9(4):300–14.
24. Routt M, Simonian P, Inaba J. Iliosacral screw complications. Oper Tech Orthop. 1997;7(3):206–20.
25. Nork SE, Jones CB, Harding SP, Mirza SK, Routt ML Jr. Percutaneous stabilization of U-shaped sacral fractures using iliosacral screws: technique and early results. J Orthop Trauma. 2001;15(4):238–46.
26. French B, Tornetta P. Transiliosakrale Osteosynthese bei instabilen Verletzungen des hinteren Beckenringes. Oper Orthop Traumatol. 2002;14:29–49.
27. Tsukushi S, Katagiri H, Nakashima H, Shido Y, Wasa J. Computed tomography-guided screw fixation of a sacroiliac joint dislocation fracture: a case report. J Orthop Sci. 2003;8:729–32.
28. Baskin K, Cahill A, Kaye R, Born C, Grudziak J, Towbin R. Closed reduction with CT-guided screw fixation for unstable sacroiliac joint fracture-dislocation. Pediatr Radiol. 2004;34:963–9.
29. Osterhoff G, Ossendorf C, Wanner G, Simmen H, Werner C. Posterior screw fixation in rotationally unstable pelvic ring injuries. Injury. 2011;42:992–6.
30. Pieske O, Landersdorfer C, Trumm C, Greiner A, Wallmichrath J, Gottschalk O, Rubenbauer B. CT-guided sacroiliac percutaneous screw placement in unstable posterior pelvic ring injuries: accuracy of screw position, injury reduction and complications in 71 patients with 136 screws. Injury. 2015;46:333–9.
31. Heydemann J, Hartline B, Gibson M, Ambrose C, Munz J, Galpin M, Achor T, Gary J. Do transsacral-transiliac screws across uninjured sacroiliac joints affect pain and functional outcomes in trauma patients? Clin Orthop. 2016;474:1417–21.
32. Mardam-Bey S, Beebe M, Black J, Chang E, Kubiak E, Bishop J, McAndrew C, Ricci W, Gardner M. The effect of transiliac-transsacral screw fixation for pelvic ring injuries on the uninjured sacroiliac joint. J Orthop Trauma. 2016;30:463–8.
33. Albert M, Miller M, MacNaughton M, Hutton W. Posterior pelvic fixation using a transiliac 4.5-mm reconstruction plate: a clinical and biomechanical study. J Orthop Trauma. 1993;7(3):226–32.
34. Kobbe P, Hockertz I, Sellei R, Reilmann H, Hockertz T. Minimally invasive stabilisation of posterior pelvic-ring instabilities with a transiliac locked compression plate. Int Orthop. 2012;36:159–64.
35. Dolati B, Larndorfer R, Krappinger D, Rosenberger R. Stabilization of the posterior pelvic ring with a slide-insertion plate. Oper Orthop Traumatol. 2007;19:16–31.
36. Krappinger D, Larndorfer R, Struve P, Rosenberger R, Arora R, Blauth M. Minimally invasive transiliac plate osteosynthesis for type C injuries of the pelvic ring: a clinical and radiological follow-up. J Orthop Trauma. 2007;21:595–602.
37. Suzuki T, Hak D, Ziran B, Adams S, Stahel P, Morgan S, Smith W. Outcome and complications of posterior transiliac plating for vertically unstable sacral fractures. Injury. 2009;40:405–9.
38. Ayoub M, Gad H, Seleem O. Standalone percutaneous transiliac plating of vertically unstable sacral fractures: outcomes, complications, and recommendations. Eur Spine J. 2016;25:1153–62.
39. Füchtmeier B, Maghsudi M, Neumann C, Hente R, Roll C, Nerlich M. [The minimally invasive stabilization of the dorsal pelvic ring with the transiliacal internal fixator (TIFI)—surgical technique and first clinical findings]. Unfallchirurg. 2004;107:1142–52.
40. Dienstknecht T, Berner A, Lenich A, Nerlich M, Fuechtmeier B. A minimally invasive stabilizing system for dorsal pelvic ring injuries. Clin Orthop. 2011;469:3209–17.
41. Salášek M, Pavelka T. [Minimally invasive fixation of the pelvic ring with a transiliacal internal fixator]. Acta Chir Orthop Traumatol Cechoslov. 2012;79:335–40.
42. Weber K, Vock B, Müller W, Wentzensen A. Rupture of the pubic symphysis: diagnosis, treatment and clinical outcome. Ann Saudi Med. 1999;19:544–6.
43. Pohlemann T, Gänsslen A. Die Operation der Symphysensprengung. Oper Orthop Traumatol. 1999;11:149–59.
44. Collinge C, Archdeacon M, Dulaney-Cripe E, Moed B. Radiographic changes of implant failure after plating for pubic symphysis diastasis: an underappreciated reality? Clin Orthop. 2012;470:2148–53.
45. Morris S, Loveridge J, Smart D, Ward A, Chesser T. Is fixation failure after plate fixation of the symphysis pubis clinically important? Clin Orthop. 2012;470:2154–60.
46. Lybrand K, Kurylo J, Gross J, Templeman D, Tornetta PR. Does removal of the symphyseal cartilage in symphyseal dislocations have any effect on final alignment and implant failure? J Orthop Trauma. 2015;29:470–4.
47. Frietman B, Verbeek J, Biert J, Frölke J. The effect of implant failure after symphyseal plating on functional outcome and general health. J Orthop Trauma. 2016;30:336–9.
48. Lindahl J, Hirvensalo E, Bostman O, Santavirta S. Failure of reduction with an external fixator in the management of injuries of the pelvic ring. Long-term evaluation of 110 patients. J Bone Joint Surg Br. 1999;81(6):955–62.
49. Ragnarsson B, Olerud C, Olerud S. Anterior square-plate fixation of sacroiliac disruption. Acta Orthop Scand. 1993;64(2):138–42.
50. Gänsslen A, Pohlemann T, Krettek C. [Internal fixation of sacroiliac joint disruption]. Oper Orthop Traumatol. 2005;17:281–95.
51. Nothofer W, Thonke N, Neugebauer R. [Therapy of unstable sacrum fractures in pelvic ring fractures with dorsal sacrum distraction osteosynthesis]. Unfallchirurg. 2004;107:118–27.
52. Mouhsine E, Wettstein M, Schizas C, Borens O, Blanc C, Leyvraz P, Theumann N, Garofalo R. Modified triangular posterior osteosynthesis of unstable sacrum fracture. Eur Spine J. 2006;15:857–63.
53. Bellabarba C, Schildhauer T, Vaccaro A, Chapman J. Complications associated with surgical stabilization of high-grade sacral fracture dislocations with spino-pelvic instability. Spine (Phila Pa 1976). 2006;31:S80–8.
54. Keel M, Benneker L, Siebenrock K, Bastian J. Less invasive lumbopelvic stabilization of posterior pelvic ring instability: technique and preliminary results. J Trauma. 2011;71:E62–70.
55. Schildhauer T, Ledoux W, Chapman J, Henley M, Tencer A, Routt MJ. Triangular osteosynthesis and iliosacral screw fixation for unstable sacral fractures: a cadaveric and biomechanical evaluation under cyclic loads. J Orthop Trauma. 2003;17:22–31.
56. Hu X, Pei F, Wang G, He J, Kong Q, Tu C. Application triangular osteosynthesis for vertical unstable sacral fractures. Eur Spine J. 2013;22:503–9.
57. Lindahl J, Mäkinen T, Koskinen S, Söderlund T. Factors associated with outcome of spinopelvic dissociation treated with lumbopelvic fixation. Injury. 2014;45:1914–20.
58. Sagi H, Militano U, Caron T, Lindvall E. A comprehensive analysis with minimum 1-year follow-up of vertically unstable transforaminal sacral fractures treated with triangular osteosynthesis. J Orthop Trauma. 2009;23:313–9.
59. Sobhan M, Abrisham S, Vakili M, Shirdel S. Spinopelvic fixation of sacroiliac joint fractures and fracture-dislocations: a clinical 8 years follow-up study. Arch Bone Jt Surg. 2016;4:381–6.
60. Williams S, Quinnan S. Percutaneous lumbopelvic fixation for reduction and stabilization of sacral fractures with spinopelvic dissociation patterns. J Orthop Trauma. 2016;30:18–24.

61. De Iure F, Cappuccio M, Palmisani M, Pascarella R, Commessatti M. Lumboiliac fixation in lumbosacral dislocation and associated injuries of the pelvis and lumbosacral junction: a long-term radiological and clinical follow-up. Injury. 2016;47:S44–8.
62. Piltz S, Rubenbauer B, Böcker W, Trentzsch H. Reduction and fixation of displaced U-shaped sacral fractures using lumbopelvic fixation: technical recommendations. Eur Spine J. 2018;27:3025–33.
63. Jazini E, Weir T, Nwodim E, Tannous O, Saifi C, Caffes N, Costales T, Koh E, Banagan K, Gelb D, Ludwig S. Outcomes of lumbopelvic fixation in the treatment of complex sacral fractures using minimally invasive surgical techniques. Spine J. 2017;17:1238–46.
64. Kleweno C, Bellabarba C. Lumbopelvic fixation for pelvic fractures. Oper Tech Orthop. 2015;25:270–81.
65. Apivatthakakul T, Rujiwattanapong N. "Anterior subcutaneous pelvic internal fixator (INFIX), is it safe?" A cadaveric study. Injury. 2016;47(10):2077–80.
66. Dahill M, McArthur J, Roberts G, Acharya M, Ward A, Chesser T. The use of an anterior pelvic internal fixator to treat disruptions of the anterior pelvic ring: a report of technique, indications and complications. Bone Joint J. 2017;99-B:1232–6.
67. Eagan M, Kim H, Manson T, Gary J, Russell J, Hsieh A, O'Toole R, Boulton C. Internal anterior fixators for pelvic ring injuries: do monaxial pedicle screws provide more stiffness than polyaxial pedicle screws? Injury. 2015;46(6):996–1000.
68. Fang C, Alabdulrahman H, Pape H. Complications after percutaneous internal fixator for anterior pelvic ring injuries. Int Orthop. 2017;41:1785–90.
69. Gardner M, Mehta S, Mirza A, Ricci W. Anterior pelvic reduction and fixation using a subcutaneous internal fixator. J Orthop Trauma. 2012;26(5):314–21.
70. Hesse D, Kandmir U, Solberg B, Stroh A, Osgood G, Sems S, Collinge C. Femoral nerve palsy after pelvic fracture treated with INFIX: a case series. J Orthop Trauma. 2015;29(3):138–43.
71. Hoskins W, Bucknill A, Wong J, Britton E, Judson R, Gumm K, Santos R, Sheehy R, Griffin X. A prospective case series for a minimally invasive internal fixation device for anterior pelvic ring fractures. J Orthop Surg Res. 2016;11(1):135.
72. Kuttner M, Klaiber A, Lorenz T, Fuchtmeier B, Neugebauer R. [The pelvic subcutaneous cross-over internal fixator]. Unfallchirurg. 2009;112(7):661–9.
73. McDonald E, Theologis A, Horst P, Kandemir U, Pekmezci M. When do anterior external or internal fixators provide additional stability in an unstable (Tile C) pelvic fracture? A biomechanical study. Eur J Trauma Emerg Surg. 2015;41(6):665–71.
74. Merriman D, Ricci W, McAndrew C, Gardner M. Is application of an internal anterior pelvic fixator anatomically feasible? Clin Orthop Relat Res. 2012;470(8):2111–5.
75. Muller F, Stosiek W, Zellner M, Neugebauer R, Fuchtmeier B. The anterior subcutaneous internal fixator (ASIF) for unstable pelvic ring fractures: clinical and radiological mid-term results. Int Orthop. 2013;37(11):2239–45.
76. Osterhoff G, Aichner E, Scherer J, Simmen H, Werner C, Feigl G. Anterior subcutaneous internal fixation of the pelvis—what rod-to-bone distance is anatomically optimal? Injury. 2017;48(10):2162–8.
77. Osterhoff G, Tiziani S, Ferguson S, Spreiter G, Scheyerer M, Spinas G, Wanner G, Simmen H, Werner C. Mechanical testing of a device for subcutaneous internal anterior pelvic ring fixation versus external pelvic ring fixation. BMC Musculoskelet Disord. 2014;15:111.
78. Owen M, Tinkler B, Stewart R. Failure and salvage of "INFIX" instrumentation for pelvic ring disruption in a morbidly obese patient. J Orthop Trauma. 2013;27(10):e243–6.
79. Scheyerer M, Zimmermann S, Osterhoff G, Tiziani S, Simmen H, Wanner G, Werner C. Anterior subcutaneous internal fixation for treatment of unstable pelvic fractures. BMC Res Notes. 2014;7:133.
80. Smith A, Malek I, Lewis J, Mohanty K. Vascular occlusion following application of subcutaneous anterior pelvic fixation (INFIX) technique. J Orthop Surg (Hong Kong). 2017;25(1): 2309499016684994.
81. Vaidya R, Colen R, Vigdorchik J, Tonnos F, Sethi A. Treatment of unstable pelvic ring injuries with an internal anterior fixator and posterior fixation: initial clinical series. J Orthop Trauma. 2012;26(1):1–8.
82. Vaidya R, Kubiak E, Bergin P, Dombroski D, Critchlow R, Sethi A, Starr A. Complications of anterior subcutaneous internal fixation for unstable pelvis fractures: a multicenter study. Clin Orthop Relat Res. 2012;470(8):2124–31.
83. Vaidya R, Martin A, Roth M, Nasr K, Gheraibeh P, Tonnos F. INFIX versus plating for pelvic fractures with disruption of the symphysis pubis. Int Orthop. 2017;41(8):1671–8.
84. Vaidya R, Martin A, Roth M, Tonnos F, Oliphant B, Carlson J. Midterm radiographic and functional outcomes of the anterior subcutaneous internal pelvic fixator (INFIX) for pelvic ring injuries. J Orthop Trauma. 2017;31(5):252–9.
85. Vaidya R, Oliphant B, Jain R, Nasr K, Siwiec R, Onwudiwe N, Sethi A. The bikini area and bikini line as a location for anterior subcutaneous pelvic fixation: an anatomic and clinical investigation. Clin Anat. 2013;26(3):392–9.
86. Vaidya R, Tonnos F, Nasr K, Kanneganti P, Curtis G. The anterior subcutaneous pelvic fixator (INFIX) in an anterior posterior compression type 3 pelvic fracture. J Orthop Trauma. 2016;30(Suppl 2):S21–2.
87. Vigdorchik J, Esquivel A, Jin X, Yang K, Onwudiwe N, Vaidya R. Biomechanical stability of a supra-acetabular pedicle screw internal fixation device (INFIX) vs external fixation and plates for vertically unstable pelvic fractures. J Orthop Surg Res. 2012;7:31.
88. Wang Q, Wang Q, Wang J. Treatment of type B pelvic fracture using anterior subcutaneous internal fixator with triple pedicle screws: a new surgical technique. Arch Orthop Trauma Surg. 2017;137(7):887–93.
89. Hiesterman T, Hill B, Cole P. Surgical technique: a percutaneous method of subcutaneous fixation for the anterior pelvic ring: the pelvic bridge. Clin Orthop Relat Res. 2012;470:2116–23.
90. Riehl J. Caesarean section rates following pelvic fracture: a systematic review. Injury. 2014;45:1516–21.
91. Cannada L, Pan P, Casey B, McIntire D, Shafi S, Leveno K. Pregnancy outcomes after orthopedic trauma. J Trauma. 2010;69:694–8.
92. Copeland C, Bosse M, McCarthy M, MacKenzie E, Guzinski G, Hash C, Burghess A. Effect of trauma and pelvic fracture on female genitourinary, sexual and reproductive function. J Orthop Trauma. 1997;11(2):73–81.
93. Vallier H, Cureton B, Schubeck D. Pregnancy outcomes after pelvic ring injury. J Orthop Trauma. 2012;26:302–7.

41 Infectious Complications After Pelvic Ring Surgery

Gloria Hohenberger, Axel Gänsslen, Mario Staresinic, and Jan Lindahl

Posttraumatic and postsurgical infection of the pelvic ring can be associated with relevant morbidity, extending the hospital stay and leading to several additional surgical procedures.

In general, it is well known that staphylococci represent the most common prevalent species, which account for 20–30% of infection after fracture fixation [1–3].

In the presence of implant-associated infection, even at the pelvic region, primary treatment aims include fracture consolidation and prevention of osteomyelitis, and definite eradication of microorganisms, which is always performed by surgery as antibiotics alone are not capable of safely eradicating biofilm infections [2]. The operative approach for infection control depends on the grade of fracture healing. Additionally, systemic and local antibiotics are proposed to support healing [2, 4, 5].

Only few epidemiological data on postoperative infection after pelvic ring injuries are reported.

Buller et al. analyzed the National Hospital Discharge Survey in a cohort of 1,464,458 patients with pelvic ring injuries from the years 1990–2007 [6]. The reported acute postoperative infection rate was 0.3%, and the rate of wound complications was 0.2%.

Ochenjele et al. analyzed the medical records of 913 patients with different pelvic ring stabilization methods. Of these, 8% of patients required reoperation due to infections, which occurred within 1 month after the index procedure [7]. During the analyzed time frame (2003–2015), this rate did not change significantly.

> A high variability of reported postsurgical infections is stated in the literature.

Overall, postsurgical infections after pelvic ring stabilizations are rare.

In historical analyses, infection rates up to 27% were reported either after external or internal fixation [8–10]; while using percutaneous techniques infection was reported to be negligible [11].

Pavelka et al. reported on 7 postoperative hematomas (5%) in 141 patients treated operatively [12]. Six patients (4%) developed infection treated by surgical revision with implant retention, while in two patients implant removal was additionally necessary.

In patients with internal posterior pelvic ring stabilization, median infection rate of 5.5% was reported in a literature review [13]. The overall rate of pin track infections was 22.9% after isolated anterior external fixation and 20.6% after combined anterior external and posterior internal fixations [13].

Gruen et al. analyzed 54 of 230 consecutive patients with a pelvic ring fracture treated with ORIF using different stabilization techniques and reported 0% infections related to surgery [14].

Pohlemann et al. analyzed 21 patients with open book type B1 injuries where ORIF with a four-hole plate was performed [15]. In one patient (4.8%) deep infection developed and was treated with debridement and screw change.

Van Loon et al. reported on 38 patients with open book type B1 injuries treated with plate osteosynthesis in 37 patients. In three patients early wound healing disturbances required revision (7.9%) and two local hematomas were removed [16].

G. Hohenberger
Department of Orthopaedics and Trauma, Medical University of Graz, Graz, Austria
e-mail: gloria.hohenberger@medunigraz.at

A. Gänsslen (✉)
Department of Trauma Surgery, Orthopedics and Hand Surgery, Hospital Wolfsburg, Wolfsburg, Germany

M. Staresinic
General and Sports Trauma Department, University Hospital Merkur Zagreb, Zagreb, Croatia

J. Lindahl
Orthopaedics and Trauma Surgery, Helsinki University Hospital, Helsinki, Finland

A. Gänsslen et al. (eds.), *Pelvic Ring Fractures*, https://doi.org/10.1007/978-3-030-54730-1_41

Mardanpour et al. analyzed 38 patients with type B and C injures after ORIF and reported on 10.5% deep wound and 10.5% superficial wound infections [17].

Borg et al. analyzed 54 patients with type B and C injures treated with ORIF and percutaneous stabilization techniques. Two deep wound infections were observed (5%) treated with debridement and systemic antibiotics [18].

Lindahl reported a low infection rate of 2% in 101 consecutive patients with type C1-C3 pelvic ring injuries treated with internal fixation techniques [19].

After pelvic ring stabilizations, infection rate of 4–5% can be expected.

Detailed descriptions of these complications are sparsely reported.

Weber et al. were the first to describe a retrospective case series in 2008 [20]. They presented five cases with postoperative infections:

- A 25 year old patient developed chronic osteomyelitis with fistula of the ilia wing after an open pelvic ring injury and stabilization with an external fixator; the pelvic ring was considered stable during fistula revision and sequestrectomy; the identified pathogen was an oxacillin-resistant *S. aureus*.
- A 46-year-old patient developed stable chronic superior rami osteomyelitis as a result of an infected nonunion; fistula revision and resection of the nonunion were performed; the identified pathogen was an oxacillin-resistant *S. aureus*.
- A 35-year-old patient developed acute infection after plate osteosynthesis of an open symphyseal disruption; septic implant removal and fistula debridement resulted in an unstable anterior ring segment, which was fixed with an external fixator; the identified pathogen was an oxacillin-sensitive *S. aureus*.
- A 40-year-old patient with an open pelvic injury with open scrotal laceration and primary plate osteosynthesis of the pubic symphysis was treated with septic implant removal due to local instability and secondary fixation with an external fixator; the identified pathogen was an oxacillin-sensitive *S. aureus*.
- A 28-year-old patient sustained an open pelvic injury with a groin wound and symphyseal disruption; infection was observed after primary symphyseal internal stabilization; treatment consisted of fistula debridement and septic implant removal; the anterior ring segment was considered stable; the identified pathogen was an oxacillin-sensitive *S. aureus*.

An associated literature review identified several cases with infection-related, nontraumatic pelvic ring instabilities. These complications were treated with symphyseal resection. Posterior pelvic ring stabilization is recommended in secondary ring instabilities.

In a Mexican analysis, 5 of 49 patients developed infectious complications after operative stabilization of the pelvic ring [21]:

- A 58-year-old male patient sustained a Tile type C1 fracture (left fracture dislocation of the SI joint, symphyseal disruption + right pubic rami fractures), which was treated with symphyseal double plate osteosynthesis (Pfannenstiel approach) with an additional ramus screw and iliosacral plate osteosynthesis via the first window of the ilioinguinal approach; after 2 years the patients developed local fistula at the symphyseal incision with *S. epidermidis*, which was treated with implant removal and local debridement.
- A 39-year-old male patient sustained a Tile type A2.1 fracture with superior involvement of the acetabulum, treated by ORIF via the first ilioinguinal window; 4 days after stabilization, deep infection developed as a result of a forgotten compress; pathogens found were *E. coli*, *E. faecalis*, and *B. fragilis*; surgical revision resulted in uneventful healing.
- A 39-year-old male sustained both column fracture, treated with supraacetabular external fixation on the day of admission; definitive fixation was started on day 8; here, exudate on pin was observed, which was removed but did not interfere with the resulting ilioinguinal approach; pathogens were *E. cloacae* and *S. pneumoniae*.
- A 28 year old male patient sustained polytrauma with Tile type C1 pelvic ring injury, which initially stabilized by external fixation and nonselective embolization of gluteal artery branches; a seroma was noticed after 3 days as a result of an accompanying Morel-Lavallée lesion; surgical revision revealed gluteal muscle necrosis, which was extensively debrided and covered with a rotational flap; pathogens were *E. coli*, *P. aeruginosa*, *E. faecalis*, *S. viridans*, and *P. fluorescens*.
- A 29-year-old female patient was polytraumatized with an open C3 pelvic ring injury with vaginal and bladder lacerations and traumatic occlusion of the right common femoral artery; emergency stabilization was performed with a supraacetabular external fixator; infection developed from the vaginal injury, which required several revisions; pathogens were *C. freundii*, *S. viridans*, *B. fragilis*, *P. aeruginosa*, and *E. cloacae*.

Analyzing these cases, the following recommendations can be proposed:

- Risk factors of secondary infections include the presence of open fractures and Morel-Lavallée lesions.
- If the pelvis is stable → local debridement, implant retention is favored.
- If the pelvis is mechanically unstable → local debridement, implant removal, and conversion to an external fixator should be considered.
- Adequate soft-tissue management is mandatory to reduce the frequency of surgical revisions.

41.1 Risk Factors

Sems et al. retrospectively analyzed the association of an increased body mass index (>30 kg/m^2) and early postoperative complications (within 3 months) after pelvic ring stabilization in 182 patients [22]. The rate of superficial wound infections was comparable with 2.2% vs. 2.1% in nonobese vs. obese patients, while the rate of deep wound infections was significantly higher in obese patients (22.9% vs. 3.7%).

An open posterior pelvic approach resulted in deep infections in 33.3% in obese vs. 8.7% in nonobese patients.

In obese patients, symphyseal plating (14.3% vs. 1.4%), a posterior open approach (30.8% vs. 7.9%), an anterior approach to the posterior ring (25% vs. 20%), and a combined anterior and posterior approach to the posterior pelvic ring (100% vs. 0%) resulted in higher deep infection rates, whereas after external fixation and percutaneous iliosacral screw fixation, no deep infections were observed.

Overall, a high BMI was associated with a significant increase of postoperative complications requiring surgical revisions [22].

This was confirmed in a recent analysis of the National Trauma Databank by Carson et al. who found a higher association of a BMI ≥30 with higher rates of wound infections and wound dehiscence [23].

Obesity is a well-known risk factor of surgical site infection in orthopedics [24].

The relevance of the posterior pelvic approach regarding postoperative infection was retrospectively analyzed by Stover et al. in 236 patients with 268 performed direct posterior approaches. Eight patients developed surgical site infection (3.4%), treated with local surgical debridement, wound closure, and antibiotics. In five patients, reosteosynthesis was performed [25].

In a modification of this approach, Fowler et al. reported a comparable deep infection rate (2.94%) [26]. The patient was treated with two debridements and antibiotics. Open injuries or an associated Morel-Lavallée lesion was not associated with deep wound infection.

After the classical posterior approach to the posterior iliac crest area and the posterior sacrum, an infection rate of approximately 3% can be expected.

Sagi et al. analyzed 170 pelvic and 74 combined pelvic and acetabular stabilizations. The rates of deep infections were 2.9% and 5.4%, respectively. In a matched-pair analysis, the following risk factors could be identified [27]:

- Higher BMI
- Higher ISS
- Preoperative angioembolization
- Preoperative leukocytosis + obesity
- Blood transfusion

The infection rate for combined approaches resulted in a higher infection rate compared to isolated acetabular or pelvic ring surgery.

Risk factors for postsurgical infections include obesity (BMI > 30 kg/m^2), high injury severity, necessity of preoperative angioembolization, combined preoperative leukocytosis + obesity, relevant blood transfusion, and posterior pelvic approaches.

41.2 Stabilization-Associated Complications

Postoperative infectious complications can additionally be analyzed, depending on the chosen stabilization method.

41.3 Symphyseal Plating

Historical results stated an infection rate after symphyseal stabilization between 2 and 3.5% ([28, 29] and unpublished data from the German Multicenter Study Group II).

More recent analyses of the literature indicate an infection rate after symphyseal plating of 4.1% [15, 30–41] (Table 41.1).

A 4% infection rate is observed after symphyseal plate stabilization

Table 41.1 Infection rates after plate stabilization of the disrupted pubic symphysis

Year	Author	No.	Type of osteosynthesis	Infections	Rate (%)
1996	Matta	72	Plate	1/72	1.4
1999	Pohlemann	21	Four-hole DCP	1/21	4.8
1999	Weber	22	Reconstruction plate + tension band	1/22	4.5
2005	Spagnolo	16	Two 90° plates (3.5 mm, 4.5 mm)	0/16	0
2011	Aggarwal	18	Single or double plates	2/18	11.1
2011	Putnis	49	Four-, six-, eight-hole, double plate	0/49	0
2012	Chen	42	Reconstruction plate	8/42	19
2012	Chen	41	Percutaneous 7.3 mm screw	2/41	4.9
2012	Collinge	165	4- or 6-hole Matta plate	2/165	1.2
2014	Adams	25	3.5-mm pelvic reconstruction plate	1/25	4
2015	Yu	27	3.5 mm reconstruction plate	1/27	3.7
2016	Jain	15	Reconstruction plate	2/15	13.3
2017	Park	39	Single six- or four-hole plate	0/39	0
2017	Park	25	Plate + tension band	0/25	0
2017	Vaidya	28	Different plates	4/28	14.3
		605		**25**	**4.1**

41.4 External Fixation

Old data reported high rates of pin tract infection after external fixation. Majeed reported on 30% pin tract infection after percutaneous pinning and 40% after incisional techniques [42].

With increasing knowledge of the application technique, this rate could be reduced. Data from the first German Multicenter Pelvis Study Group observed a pin infection rate of 5,3% (1991–1993) [29], which could be reduced to 0,7% in the second analysis between 1998 and 2000 (unpublished data).

Tucker reported a rate of 2.4% [43] and Gänsslen et al. a rate of 4% [44].

A higher rate was observed by Lindahl et al. [45] who analyzed 110 patients with 70 type B and 40 type C injuries. All patients were treated with an anterior external fixator. Superficial pin infection was observed in 20.9% and deep infection in 2.7%. Treatment consisted of pin removal in one case, while the others were treated by local debridement and antibiotics. This higher rate can be explained due to the remaining overall pelvic ring instability [42], especially in type C injuries.

In 2004, Arazi et al. reported on 41 patients after external fixations and observed 19.5% pin tract infections sufficiently treated with antibiotics and local wound care. Obesity and local skin irritation were present in all of these patients [46].

Comparing iliac crest and supraacetabular pin placement, different pin infection rates can be calculated.

After iliac crest external fixation (Table 41.2), in a literature review of 433 patients [47–50], overall 96 infections were reported (22.17%). In contrast, after 136 supraacetabular fixations (Table 41.3), an infection rate of 11.7% was observed [44, 51–53].

Table 41.2 Results after iliac crest external fixation

Author	Year	No.	Type B	Type C	Poststabilization	Pin site infection
Lindahl	1999	110	70	40	0	26
Tucker	2000	40	15	26	32	1
Arazi	2000	41	24	17	0	8
Mason	2005	52	24	28	0	26
Scaglione	2010	41	35	6	4	13
Vecsei	2010	28	10	18	4	2/20
Mitchell	2013	129	?	?	0	20

Table 41.3 Results after supraacetabular external fixation

Author	Year	No.	Type B	Type C	Poststabilization	Pin site infection
Bellabarba	2001	14			0	4
Gänsslen	2005	20	20	0	0	0
Gänsslen	2005	25	0	25	21	0
Gänsslen	2013	25	25	0	0	2
McDonald	2017	52				10

After external fixation, pin site infection is a common observation. Higher rates are observed with iliac crest application compared to supraacetabular insertion

41.5 Internal Subcutaneous Fixation

Results after internal subcutaneous fixation reported an infection rate of 7.4% in an analysis of 363 patients [39, 54–62] (Table 41.4).

Table 41.4 Results after internal subcutaneous fixation

Author	Year	No.	OTA	Poststabilization	Pin site infection
Kuttner	2009	22	21×C	21	1
Gardner	2012	24	24×C	24	1
Vaidya	2012	24	16×C	16	0
Vaidya	2012	96	?	n.a.	3
Müller	2013	36	36	36	2
Hoskins	2016	21	n.a.	19	3
Wang	2016	26	26×B	0	0
Dahill	2017	47	n.a.	n.a.	2
Fang	2017	43	n.a.	n.a.	14
Vaidya	2017	24	9×C	n.a.	1

41.6 Anterior Plate Osteosynthesis of the SI Joint

Regarding anterior plating of the SI joint (first window of the ilioinguinal approach), little data are available.

Ragnarsson et al. reported a rate of 4.3% [63], while Gänsslen et al. observed 3.7% infections [64]. Data from the German Multicenter Pelvis Study Group observed 2.9% infections between 1991 and 1993, while unpublished data from 1998 to 2000 observed a rate of 4.2%.

After anterior plate osteosynthesis in type C SI joint dislocations, an infection rate of 3–4% can be expected.

41.7 Ilioiliacal Osteosynthesis

Open ilioiliacal techniques include ilioiliacal plate osteosynthesis and the transiliacal internal fixator (TIFI).

Posterior tension band ilioiliacal plate stabilization is often performed. Analyzing reported results from several studies, an infection rate of 3.6% was calculated in 193 patients [65–71].

- Krappinger removed the plate after local debridement 11 weeks after the index procedure [70].
- Suzuki et al. reported two postoperative surgical wound infections after accompanying local Morel-Lavallée lesions [71]. One patient with infection on day 3 was treated with multiple irrigations, debridement, and a rotational gluteal flap without hardware removal. The other patient was treated with several rounds of irrigation and debridement and secondary implant removal after bone healing.
- Kobbe et al. sufficiently treated one superficial wound infection with local debridement [69].
- Ayoub et al. reported on two superficial and one case of deep infections: the former were treated with local dressing change and antibiotics, while the case with deep infection required surgical debridement and intravenous antibiotics [66].

Posterior, less invasive bridging plate stabilization results in an infection rate of 3.6%.

Using the transiliacal internal fixator (TIFI) in 31 cases, two wound infections were reported in the first Regensburg analysis [72]. Both required implant removal. In an ongoing analysis of 67 patients [73], four infections were observed (6%). Schmitz et al. observed 2 superficial wound infections in 15 geriatric patients with cement-augmented TIFI fixation (13.3%) [74]. Salášek and Pavelka reported one case of infection (3.1%), treated with implant removal and local debridement [75].

Overall, the infection rate after TIFI was 6.1%.

41.8 Posterior ORIF of Sacral Fractures

Gänsslen et al. reported a rate of 6.9% of local wound complications (Fig. 41.1) in 32 patients with different "local" sacral stabilization methods [76].

Recently, Acklin et al. reported their results of parallel, double locking plate fixation of sacral type C injuries in 27 patients and observed 18.5% early deep infections [77].

Data from the German Multicenter Pelvis Study Group observed 5.7% infections between 1991 and 1993 [29], while unpublished data from 1998 to 2000 observed a rate of 2.8%.

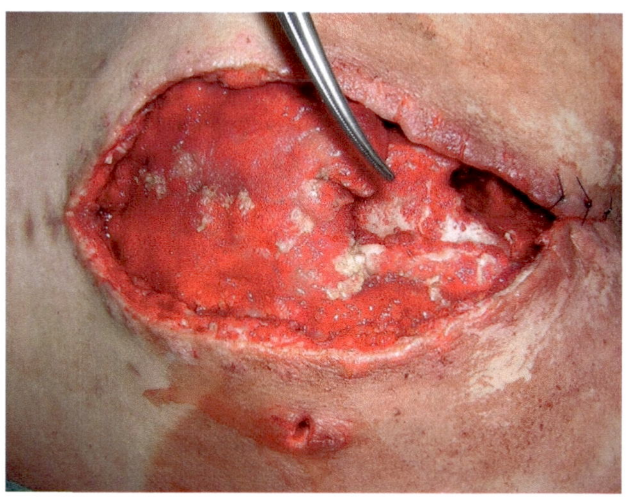

Fig. 41.1 Secondary wound healing requiring flap closure after infection and skin necrosis after a sacral osteosynthesis

The direct posterior midline/paramedian approach to the sacrum is associated with an infection rate of 5–10%. Often muscle flap necrosis was responsible for secondary infection. Therefore, creating a muscular flap with complete distal detachment from the sacrum should be avoided.

41.9 Lumbopelvic Fixations

Schildhauer et al. introduced the concept of lumbopelvic fixation of highly unstable sacral fractures and fracture dislocations [78, 79]. In the treatment of 48 cases, 3 patients (6.25%) developed local infection at the prominent pedicle screw. Despite debridement and irrigation, implant removal became necessary.

A further analysis of this group observed an infection rate of 16% in 19 patients with highly displaced sacral fractures [78, 80].

Further results are presented in Table 41.5 [81–93]:

Overall, the infection rate after lumbopelvic stabilization can be expected to be approximately 10% independent of the type of approach (open versus less/minimal invasive)

Table 41.5 Infection rates after lumbopelvic fixation

Author	Year	No.	Infection	Rate	Treatment
Thiemann	2003	22	3[a]	13.6	Revision
Nothofer	2004	35	3	8.6	Several revisions
Mouhsine	2006	7	1	14.3	Several revisions including debridement, lavage, antibiotic beads, implant removal
Keel	2011	10[b]	0	0	
Jones	2012	15	2	13.3	Debridement
Ayoub	2012	28	7	25	Antibiotics
Hu	2013	22	2	9.1	Debridement and antibiotics
He	2014	21	2	9.5	Debridement, irrigation, antibiotics
Lindahl	2014	36	0	0	
Williams	2016	17[c]	1	5.9	Serial debridements
Sobhan	2016	14	3	21.4	Not recorded
Hess	2016	14	0	0	
Jazini	2018	24[b]	2	8.3	Debridement, irrigation

[a]Wound healing disturbances requiring revision
[b]Less invasive technique
[c]Percutaneous

A recent study compared patients with open and minimally invasive lumbopelvic fixations [94]. No relevant differences regarding infection rates were found. No surgical site infections were seen after percutaneous lumbopelvic stabilization (0%). In the open approach group, 1/16 patients developed infection (6.25%).

41.10 Treatment Concepts

In general, treatment of implant-related infections depends on the amount of fracture healing. Particularly at the pelvis, the stability of the pelvic ring additionally has to be considered.

There is consensus that three conditions should be distinguished regrading treatment [2, 4, 5]:

- Early infection (within 2 weeks after osteosynthesis)
- Delayed infection (approximately 2–10 weeks after osteosynthesis, when there is still potential for further bone/joint healing)
- Late infection/after fracture union

Especially regarding the pelvic ring, additional factors to be considered include:

- Amount of fracture consolidation: fracture consolidation leads to stability or still persistent instability, which influences the decision of implant retention or removal.
- Gross pelvic instability can worsen infection.
- The main primary treatment aim of complete eradication of the infection has to be discussed in relation to fracture consolidation; debridement should remove all infected tissues, including bone to avoid secondary osteomyelitis or joint infection; implant retention/removal has to be discussed by evaluation of pelvic ring stability; thus, partial or suppressive eradiation can be optional, when fracture healing is not yet finished.
- Healing of the soft-tissue envelope.
- Prevention of chronic osteomyelitis: aggressive (bone) debridement is mandatory to avoid infection to surrounding organs and neurovascular structures.

41.10.1 Acute Infection

In the majority of cases, an acute infection (<2 weeks) is detected.

In unequivocal superficial infections, daily wound cleaning and intravenous antibiotic treatment can be considered.

In any deep infection entering the true pelvis, surgical debridement and irrigation, with sparse excision of skin margins and dead space management, are performed until clinical and laboratory parameters confirm healing. During the first debridement, implant stability should be analyzed.

If the implant is stable, it should be retained. In unstable situations, the implant should be removed (reduction of biofilm burden), which leads to pelvic ring instability. Therefore, adding mechanical stability is necessary as instability increases the risk of ongoing infection. According to the ring structure of the pelvis, a potential stable ring is distinguished from rotational and vertical instability according to the AO/OTA classification:

- Type A (in)stability: often an isolated fracture of the anterior ring is present; here, radical debridement of even the bone can be necessary; application of an external fixator to get the pelvis as stable as possible should be considered.
- Type B (rotational) instability: the unstable area is the anterior ring region; a fixation of the anterior ring segment is crucial to control infection; if the pubic symphysis is unstable due to implant removal, restabilization of the symphysis should be considered after plate removal by conversion to an external fixator; due to the extended soft-tissue envelope, supraacetabular pin placement is favored; persistent instability of the whole ring structure can lead to additional iliosacral screw fixation of the affected posterior injury; alternatively a new (titanium) short plate can inserted (two-hole plate to get sufficient stability).
- Type C (vertical) instability: if implant removal is necessary (unstable, loose implants), it is mandatory to address the ring stability by anterior and posterior stabilization of the pelvic ring; in anterior ring fractures, conversion to an external fixator is considered, while at the posterior pelvis, at least an iliosacral K-wire stabilization (2.8 mm/3.0 mm) or an (temporary) iliosacral screw should be inserted; for joint injuries (symphysis, SI joint), stable fixation is advised with less and adequate implants as possible.

41.10.2 Delayed Infection

Delayed infection is present, when there is still the possibility of incomplete fracture/joint healing. The minimal time for joint healing is around 6 weeks after primary treatment. At the anterior ring, typically superior ramus fractures heal within 3–4 weeks after injury, even when no radiological signs of healing are visible and at the posterior pelvic ring, complete ilium fractures typically heal within 6 weeks, as both areas are surrounded by adequate muscles: obturator ring: obturator internus et externus muscles, ilium: iliopsoas and gluteal muscles. In contrast, complete sacral fractures typically present with longer healing times. CT analysis of the whole pelvis is recommended for healing analysis.

In delayed infections, some stability can be expected. Treatment, therefore, consists of adequate debridement and irrigation, systemic antibiotics, and implant retention. In the presence of loose or unstable implants, implant removal and conversion to minimally invasive stabilization concepts (e.g., external fixator, iliosacral screws) is advised. As mentioned, implant removal is often possible after 6 weeks. Debridement should include excision of potentially infected nonunions and excision of a sequestrum (CT analysis).

Dead Space Management

Local antibiotics are considered an option for dead space management. Usually, PMMA bone cement (gentamicin, tobramycin, vancomycin, or cephalosporins) is used. At the pubic symphysis and the SI joint, cement spacers can be inserted in additional minimally invasive stabilization techniques or even during implant retention.

It has to be considered that PMMA may serve as an additional surface for bacteria and only <10% of antibiotics are normally released from PMMA. By mixing different antibiotics (vancomycin + tobramycin) and increasing the porosity of the cement, higher elution doses can be reached.

41.10.3 Late Infection

In the presence of late infection, per definition, the pelvic ring is already healed and, therefore, considered stable. The only exception is an infected nonunion.

In the latter situation, adequate stability is additionally mandatory in combination with standard infection control by adequate debridement and implant removal. Typically, symphyseal excision or ramus excision is without effect on overall pelvic stability. In doubtful cases, anterior external fixation and/or iliosacral screw fixation should be considered.

41.11 Adjuncts of Infection Control

Several adjuncts can be considered when dealing with pelvic soft-tissue infections and true pelvis space infections.

Diabetes is identified as a relevant perioperative risk factor for surgical site infection (SSI) [95].

In spinal surgery, even postoperative elevated glucose levels were identified as independent risk factors of surgical site infection [96]. In orthopedic surgery, hyperglycemia was even associated with the 30-day SSI rate in patients without a history of diabetes [97].

Additionally, malnutrition should be corrected as it is associated with SSI [98].

Coagulation factor XIII may have potential benefit in patients with invasive infections as activated FXIII influences wound healing, tissue repair, and tissue regeneration [99, 100]. No evidence is available to support infection treatment at the pelvis using FXIII, but in geriatric patients with subcutaneous infection, FXIII treatment can be an option.

41.12 Summary

No clear data are available regarding postsurgical infections in pelvic ring injuries. A high variability of reported postsurgical infection rates is reported, ranging from 0.2 to 8%.

Beside standard debridement, irrigation, and systemic/local antibiotic treatment addressing the reduction of the number of pathogens, the stability of the pelvis is essential regarding the decision of implant retention or implant removal. In unstable injury situations, conversion to external fixation or minimally invasive stabilization methods offers an alternative. Bone excision depends on pelvic ring stability and fracture consolidation. Normalization of glucose levels and the nutritional status are prerequisites for adequate treatment.

References

1. Montanaro L, Speziale P, Campoccia D, Ravaioli S, Cangini I, Pietrocola G, Giannini S, Arciola C. Scenery of Staphylococcus implant infections in orthopedics. Future Microbiol. 2011;6: 1329–49.
2. Moriarty T, Kuehl R, Coenye T, Metsemakers W, Morgenstern M, Schwarz E, Riool M, Zaat S, Khana N, Kates S, Richards R. Orthopaedic device-related infection: current and future interventions for improved prevention and treatment. EFORT Open Rev. 2017;1:89–99. https://doi.org/10.1302/2058-5241.1.000037.
3. Trampuz A, Zimmerli W. Diagnosis and treatment of infections associated with fracture-fixation devices. Injury. 2006;37:S59–66.
4. Fang C, Wong T, To K, Wong S, Lau T, Leung F. Infection after fracture osteosynthesis—part II. J Orthop Surg (Hong Kong). 2017;25:2309499017692714. https://doi.org/10.1177/2309499017692714.
5. Metsemakers W, Kuehl R, Moriarty T, Richards R, Verhofstad M, Borens O, Kates S, Morgenstern M. Infection after fracture fixation: current surgical and microbiological concepts. Injury. 2018;49:511–22.
6. Buller L, Best M, Quinnan S. A nationwide analysis of pelvic ring fractures: incidence and trends in treatment, length of stay, and mortality. Geriatr Orthop Surg Rehabil. 2016;7:9–17.
7. Ochenjele G, Reid K, Castillo R, Schoonover C, Montalvo R, Manson T, Sciadini M, Nascone J, Carlini A, O'Toole R. Predictors of unplanned reoperation after operative treatment of pelvic ring injuries. J Orthop Trauma. 2018;32:245–50.
8. Goldstein A, Phillips T, Sclafani S, Scalea T, Duncan A, Goldstein J, Panetta T, Shaftan G. Early open reduction and internal fixation of the disrupted pelvic ring. J Trauma. 1986;26(4):325–33.
9. Kellam J. The role of external fixation in pelvic disruptions. Clin Orthop. 1989;241:66–82.
10. Kellam JF, McMurtry RY, Paley D, Tile M. The unstable pelvic fracture—operative treatment. Orthop Clin North Am. 1987;18(1):25–41.
11. Routt M, Kregor P, Simonian P, Mayo K. Early results of percutaneous iliosacral screws placed with the patient in the supine position. J Orthop Trauma. 1995;9(3):207–14.
12. Pavelka T, Dzupa V, Stulík J, Grill R, Báca V, Skála-Rosenbaum J. [Our results of surgical management of unstable pelvic ring injuries]. Acta Chir Orthop Traumatol Cechoslov. 2007;74:19–28.
13. Papakostidis C, Kanakaris N, Kontakis G, Giannoudis P. Pelvic ring disruptions: treatment modalities and analysis of outcomes. Int Orthop. 2009;33:329–38.
14. Gruen G, Leit M, Gruen R, Garrison H, Auble T, Peitzman A. Functional outcome of patients with unstable pelvic ring fractures stabilized with open reduction and internal fixation. J Trauma. 1995;39(5):838–44.
15. Pohlemann T, Gänsslen A. Die Operation der Symphysensprengung. Oper Orthop Traumatol. 1999;11:149–59.
16. Van Loon P, Kuhn S, Hofmann A, Hessmann M, Rommens P. Radiological analysis, operative management and functional outcome of open book pelvic lesions: a 13-year cohort study. Injury. 2011;42:1012–9.
17. Mardanpour K, Rahbar M. The functional outcome of surgically treated unstable pelvic ring fractures by open reduction, internal fixation. Med J Islam Repub Iran. 2011;25:87–93.
18. Borg T, Berg P, Fugl-Meyer K, Larsson S. Health-related quality of life and life satisfaction in patients following surgically treated pelvic ring fractures. A prospective observational study with two years follow-up. Injury. 2010;41:400–4.
19. Lindahl J, Hirvensalo E. Outcome of operatively treated type-C injuries of the pelvic ring. Acta Orthop. 2005;76:667–78.
20. Weber O, Gravius S, Henkel S, Berdel P, Burger C, Wirtz D. [Pelvic osseous infections: clinical outcome and surgical treatment]. Z Orthop Unfall. 2008;146:510–9.
21. Chana Rodríguez F, Villanueva Martínez M, Ortiz Espada A, Calvo Haro J, Pérez Mañanes R, Vaquero Martín J. [Infections in the surgical management of pelvic ring fractures]. Acta Ortop Mex. 2010;24:163–8.
22. Sems S, Johnson M, Cole P, Byrd C, Templeman D, Minnesota Orthopaedic Trauma Group. Elevated body mass index increases early complications of surgical treatment of pelvic ring injuries. J Orthop Trauma. 2010;24:309–14.
23. Carson J, Shah S, Ortega G, Thamyongkit S, Hasenboehler E, Shafiq B. Complications of pelvic and acetabular fractures in 1331 morbidly obese patients (BMI ≥ 40): a retrospective observational study from the National Trauma Data Bank. Patient Saf Surg. 2018;12:26. https://doi.org/10.1186/s13037-018-0172-2.
24. Morris B, Richards J, Guillamondegui O, Sweeney K, Mir H, Obremskey W, Kregor P. Obesity increases early complications after high-energy pelvic and acetabular fractures. Orthopedics. 2015;38:881–7.
25. Stover M, Sims S, Matta J. What is the infection rate of the posterior approach to type C pelvic injuries? Clin Orthop Relat Res. 2012;470:2142–7.
26. Fowler T, Bishop J, Bellino M. The posterior approach to pelvic ring injuries: a technique for minimizing soft tissue complications. Injury. 2013;44:1780–6.

27. Sagi H, Dziadosz D, Mir H, Virani N, Olson C. Obesity, leukocytosis, embolization, and injury severity increase the risk for deep postoperative wound infection after pelvic and acetabular surgery. J Orthop Trauma. 2013;27:6–10.
28. Kinzl L, Burri C, Wörsdörfer O. Operative Therapie bei Beckenfugenzerreißungen. Hefte zur Unfallheilkunde. Heft 164. 1984. p. 222–3.
29. Pohlemann T, Gänsslen A, Hartung S, für die Arbeitsgruppe Becken, H.T., H., Beckenverletzungen/Pelvic Injuries. Hefte zu "Der Unfallchirurg". Heft 266. 1998.
30. Adams M, Scolaro J, Routt M. The pubic midline exposure for symphyseal open reduction and plate fixation. J Orthop Traumatol. 2014;15:195. https://doi.org/10.1007/s10195-014-0296-9.
31. Aggarwal S, Bali K, Krishnan V, Kumar V, Meena D, Sen R. Management outcomes in pubic diastasis: our experience with 19 patients. J Orthop Surg. 2011;6:21.
32. Chen L, Zhang G, Song D, Guo X, Yuan W. A comparison of percutaneous reduction and screw fixation versus open reduction and plate fixation of traumatic symphysis pubis diastasis. Arch Orthop Trauma Surg. 2012;132:265–70.
33. Collinge C, Archdeacon M, Dulaney-Cripe E, Moed B. Radiographic changes of implant failure after plating for pubic symphysis diastasis: an underappreciated reality? Clin Orthop. 2012;470: 2148–53.
34. Jain M, Runu R, Kumar S, Kumar M. Outcome of plate osteosynthesis in pubic diastasis: an experience of teritiary care centre. Indian J Orthop Surg. 2016;2:326–30.
35. Matta J. Indications for anterior fixation of pelvic fractures. Clin Orthop. 1996;329:88–96.
36. Park M, Yoon S, Choi S, Lee K. Is there a clinical benefit of additional tension band wiring in plate fixation of the symphysis? BMC Musculoskelet Disord. 2017;18:40. https://doi.org/10.1186/s12891-017-1418-3.
37. Putnis S, Pearce R, Wali U, Bircher M, Rickman M. Open reduction and internal fixation of a traumatic diastasis of the pubic symphysis. J Bone Joint Surg Br. 2011;93:78–84.
38. Spagnolo R, Pace F, Bonalumi M, Capitani D. Anterior pelvic ring fractures: a proposal of a variant of osteosynthesis of the pubic symphysis. Eur J Orthop Surg Traumatol. 2010;21:33. https://doi.org/10.1007/s00590-010-0651-3.
39. Vaidya R, Martin A, Roth M, Nasr K, Gheraibeh P, Tonnos F. INFIX versus plating for pelvic fractures with disruption of the symphysis pubis. Int Orthop. 2017;41:1671–8.
40. Weber K, Vock B, Müller W, Wentzensen A. Rupture of the pubic symphysis: diagnosis, treatment and clinical outcome. Ann Saudi Med. 1999;19:544–6.
41. Yu K, Hong J, Guo X, Zhou D. Comparison of reconstruction plate screw fixation and percutaneous cannulated screw fixation in treatment of Tile B1 type pubic symphysis diastasis: a finite element analysis and 10-year clinical experience. J Orthop Surg Res. 2015;10:151.
42. Majeed SA. External fixation of the injured pelvis—the functional outcome. J Bone Joint Surg Br. 1990;72(4):612–4.
43. Tucker MC, Nork SE, Simonian PT, Routt ML Jr. Simple anterior pelvic external fixation. J Trauma. 2000;49(6):989–94.
44. Gänsslen A, Pohlemann T, Krettek C. Supraacetabular external fixation for pelvic ring fractures. Oper Orthop Traumatol. 2005;17:296–312.
45. Lindahl J, Hirvensalo E, Bostman O, Santavirta S. Failure of reduction with an external fixator in the management of injuries of the pelvic ring. Long-term evaluation of 110 patients. J Bone Joint Surg Br. 1999;81(6):955–62.
46. Arazi M, Kutlu A, Mutlu M, Yel M, Kapiciglu M. The pelvic external fixation: the mid-term results of 41 patients treated with a newly designed fixator. Arch Orthop Trauma Surg. 2000;120(10):584–6.
47. Mason W, Khan S, James C, Chesser T, Ward A. Complications of temporary and definitive external fixation of pelvic ring injuries. Injury. 2005;36:599–604.
48. Mitchell P, Corrigan C, Patel N, Silverberg A, Greenberg S, Thakore R, Obremskey W, Ehrenfeld J, Evans J, Sethi M. 13-Year experience in external fixation of the pelvis: complications, reduction and removal. Eur J Trauma Emerg Surg. 2016;42:91–6.
49. Scaglione M, Parchi P, Digrandi G, Latessa M, Guido G. External fixation in pelvic fractures. Musculoskelet Surg. 2010;94:63–70.
50. Vécsei V, Negrin L, Hajdu S. Today's role of external fixation in unstable and complex pelvic fractures. Eur J Trauma Emerg Surg. 2010;36:100–6.
51. Bellabarba C, Ricci W, Bolhofner B. Distraction external fixation in lateral compression pelvic fractures. J Orthop Trauma. 2000;14(7):475–82.
52. Gänsslen A, Hildebrand F, Krettek C. Supraacetabular external fixation for pain control in geriatric type B pelvic injuries. Acta Chir Orthop Traumatol Cechoslov. 2013;80:101–5.
53. McDonald C, Firoozabadi R, Routt ML Jr, Kleweno C. Complications associated with pelvic external fixation. Orthopedics. 2017;40:959–63.
54. Dahill M, McArthur J, Roberts G, Acharya M, Ward A, Chesser T. The use of an anterior pelvic internal fixator to treat disruptions of the anterior pelvic ring: a report of technique, indications and complications. Bone Joint J. 2017;99-B:1232–6.
55. Fang C, Alabdulrahman H, Pape H. Complications after percutaneous internal fixator for anterior pelvic ring injuries. Int Orthop. 2017;41:1785–90.
56. Gardner M, Mehta S, Mirza A, Ricci W. Anterior pelvic reduction and fixation using a subcutaneous internal fixator. J Orthop Trauma. 2012;26(5):314–21.
57. Hoskins W, Bucknill A, Wong J, Britton E, Judson R, Gumm K, Santos R, Sheehy R, Griffin X. A prospective case series for a minimally invasive internal fixation device for anterior pelvic ring fractures. J Orthop Surg Res. 2016;11:135.
58. Kuttner M, Klaiber A, Lorenz T, Fuchtmeier B, Neugebauer R. [The pelvic subcutaneous cross-over internal fixator]. Unfallchirurg. 2009;112(7):661–9.
59. Muller F, Stosiek W, Zellner M, Neugebauer R, Fuchtmeier B. The anterior subcutaneous internal fixator (ASIF) for unstable pelvic ring fractures: clinical and radiological mid-term results. Int Orthop. 2013;37(11):2239–45.
60. Vaidya R, Colen R, Vigdorchik J, Tonnos F, Sethi A. Treatment of unstable pelvic ring injuries with an internal anterior fixator and posterior fixation: initial clinical series. J Orthop Trauma. 2012;26(1):1–8.
61. Vaidya R, Kubiak E, Bergin P, Dombroski D, Critchlow R, Sethi A, Starr A. Complications of anterior subcutaneous internal fixation for unstable pelvis fractures: a multicenter study. Clin Orthop Relat Res. 2012;470(8):2124–31.
62. Wang Q, Wang Q, Wang J. Treatment of type B pelvic fracture using anterior subcutaneous internal fixator with triple pedicle screws: a new surgical technique. Arch Orthop Trauma Surg. 2017;137(7):887–93.
63. Ragnarsson B, Olerud C, Olerud S. Anterior square-plate fixation of sacroiliac disruption. Acta Orthop Scand. 1993;64(2):138–42.
64. Gänsslen A, Pohlemann T, Krettek C. Internal fixation of sacroiliac joint disruption. Oper Orthop Traumatol. 2005;17:281–195.
65. Albert M, Miller M, MacNaughton M, Hutton W. Posterior pelvic fixation using a transiliac 4.5-mm reconstruction plate: a clinical and biomechanical study. J Orthop Trauma. 1993;7(3):226–32.
66. Ayoub M, Gad H, Seleem O. Standalone percutaneous transiliac plating of vertically unstable sacral fractures: outcomes, complications, and recommendations. Eur Spine J. 2016;25:1153–62.

67. Chen W, Hou Z, Su Y, Smith W, Liporace F, Zhang Y. Treatment of posterior pelvic ring disruptions using a minimally invasive adjustable plate. Injury. 2013;44:975–80.
68. Hao T, Changwei Y, Qiulin Z. Treatment of posterior pelvic ring injuries with minimally invasive percutaneous plate osteosynthesis. Int Orthop. 2009;33:1435–9.
69. Kobbe P, Hockertz I, Sellei R, Reilmann H, Hockertz T. Minimally invasive stabilisation of posterior pelvic-ring instabilities with a transiliac locked compression plate. Int Orthop. 2012;36:159–64.
70. Krappinger D, Larndorfer R, Struve P, Rosenberger R, Arora R, Blauth M. Minimally invasive transiliac plate osteosynthesis for type C injuries of the pelvic ring: a clinical and radiological follow-up. J Orthop Trauma. 2007;21:595–602.
71. Suzuki T, Hak D, Ziran B, Adams S, Stahel P, Morgan S, Smith W. Outcome and complications of posterior transiliac plating for vertically unstable sacral fractures. Injury. 2009;40:405–9.
72. Füchtmeier B, Maghsudi M, Neumann C, Hente R, Roll C, Nerlich M. [The minimally invasive stabilization of the dorsal pelvic ring with the transiliacal internal fixator (TIFI)—surgical technique and first clinical findings]. Unfallchirurg. 2004;107:1142–52.
73. Dienstknecht T, Berner A, Lenich A, Nerlich M, Fuechtmeier B. A minimally invasive stabilizing system for dorsal pelvic ring injuries. Clin Orthop. 2011;469:3209–17.
74. Schmitz P, Baumann F, Grechenig S, Gaensslen A, Nerlich M, Müller M. The cement-augmented transiliacal internal fixator (caT-IFI): an innovative surgical technique for stabilization of fragility fractures of the pelvis. Injury. 2015;46(Suppl 4):S114–20.
75. Salášek M, Pavelka T. [Minimally invasive fixation of the pelvic ring with a transiliacal internal fixator]. Acta Chir Orthop Traumatol Cechoslov. 2012;79:335–40.
76. Gänsslen A, Pape HC, Lehmann U, Lange U, Krettek C, Pohlemann T. Open reduction and internal fixation of unstable sacral fractures. Zentralbl Chir. 2003;128(1):40–5.
77. Acklin Y, Germann M, Sommer C. Double locking plate fixation of sacral fractures in unstable pelvic ring C-type injuries. Oper Orthop Traumatol. 2015;27:74–9.
78. Schildhauer T, Josten C, Muhr G. Triangular osteosynthesis of vertically unstable sacrum fractures: a new concept allowing early weight bearing. J Orthop Trauma. 1998;12(5):307–14.
79. Schildhauer T, Josten C, Muhr G. Die trianguläre Osteosynthese instabiler Sakrumfrakturen. Oper Orthop Traumatol. 2001;13:27–42.
80. Bellabarba C, Schildhauer T, Vaccaro A, Chapman J. Complications associated with surgical stabilization of high-grade sacral fracture dislocations with spino-pelvic instability. Spine (Phila Pa 1976). 2006;31:S80–8.
81. Ayoub M. Displaced spinopelvic dissociation with sacral cauda equina syndrome: outcome of surgical decompression with a preliminary management algorithm. Eur Spine J. 2012;21:1815–25.
82. He S, Zhang H, Zhao Q, He B, Guo H, Hao D. Posterior approach in treating sacral fracture combined with lumbopelvic dissociation. Orthopedics. 2014;37:1027–32.
83. Hess F, Abu-Tair U, Knoth C, Zettl R. Lumbopelvic stabilisation in patients over 50 with posterior pelvic ring fracture. Ortho Rheum Open Access. 2016;2:OROAJ.MS.ID.55586.
84. Hu X, Pei F, Wang G, He J, Kong Q, Tu C. Application triangular osteosynthesis for vertical unstable sacral fractures. Eur Spine J. 2013;22:503–9.
85. Jazini E, Weir T, Nwodim E, Tannous O, Saifi C, Caffes N, Costales T, Koh E, Banagan K, Gelb D, Ludwig S. Outcomes of lumbopelvic fixation in the treatment of complex sacral fractures using minimally invasive surgical techniques. Spine J. 2017;17:1238–46.
86. Jones C, Sietsema D, Hoffmann M. Can lumbopelvic fixation salvage unstable complex sacral fractures? Clin Orthop. 2012;470:2132–41.
87. Keel M, Benneker L, Siebenrock K, Bastian J. Less invasive lumbopelvic stabilization of posterior pelvic ring instability: technique and preliminary results. J Trauma. 2011;71:62–70.
88. Lindahl J, Mäkinen T, Koskinen S, Söderlund T. Factors associated with outcome of spinopelvic dissociation treated with lumbopelvic fixation. Injury. 2014;45:1914–20.
89. Mouhsine E, Wettstein M, Schizas C, Borens O, Blanc C, Leyvraz P, Theumann N, Garofalo R. Modified triangular posterior osteosynthesis of unstable sacrum fracture. Eur Spine J. 2006;15:857–63.
90. Nothofer W, Thonke N, Neugebauer R. [Therapy of unstable sacrum fractures in pelvic ring fractures with dorsal sacrum distraction osteosynthesis]. Unfallchirurg. 2004;107:118–27.
91. Sobhan M, Abrisham S, Vakili M, Shirdel S. Spinopelvic fixation of sacroiliac joint fractures and fracture-dislocations: a clinical 8 years follow-up study. Arch Bone Jt Surg. 2016;4:381–6.
92. Tiemann A, Schmidt C, Josten C. [Triangular vertebropelvine stabilisation of unstable posterior pelvic ring fractures]. Zentralbl Chir. 2003;128:202–8.
93. Williams S, Quinnan S. Percutaneous lumbopelvic fixation for reduction and stabilization of sacral fractures with spinopelvic dissociation patterns. J Orthop Trauma. 2016;30:318–24.
94. Pearson J, Niemeier T, McGwin G, Rajaram Manoharan S. Spinopelvic dissociation: comparison of outcomes of percutaneous versus open fixation strategies. Adv Orthop. 2018;2018:5023908. https://doi.org/10.1155/2018/5023908.
95. Martin E, Kaye K, Knott C, Nguyen H, Santarossa M, Evans R, Bertran E, Jaber L. Diabetes and risk of surgical site infection: a systematic review and meta-analysis. Infect Control Hosp Epidemiol. 2016;37:88–9.
96. Olsen M, Nepple J, Riew K, Lenke L, Bridwell K, Mayfield J, Fraser V. Risk factors for surgical site infection following orthopaedic spinal operations. J Bone Joint Surg Am. 2008;90:62–9.
97. Richards J, Kauffmann R, Zuckerman S, Obremskey W, May A. Relationship of hyperglycemia and surgical-site infection in orthopaedic surgery. J Bone Joint Surg Am. 2012;94:1181–6.
98. Skeie E, Koch A, Harthug S, Fosse U, Sygnestveit K, Nilsen R, Tangvik R. A positive association between nutritional risk and the incidence of surgical site infections: a hospital-based register study. PLoS One. 2018;13(5):e0197344. https://doi.org/10.1371/journal.pone.0197344.
99. Dickneite G, Herwald H, Korte W, Allanore Y, Denton C, Matucci Cerinic M. Coagulation factor XIII: a multifunctional transglutaminase with clinical potential in a range of conditions. Thromb Haemost. 2015;113:686–97.
100. Soendergaard C, Kvist P, Seidelin J, Nielsen O. Tissue-regenerating functions of coagulation factor XIII. J Thromb Haemost. 2013;11:806–16.

42 Pelvic Malunion and Nonunion

Jan Lindahl and Axel Gänsslen

Treatment of pelvic malunion (MU) and nonunion (NU) is challenging and often requires extensive surgery with increased morbidity.

> Prevention of pelvic MU or NU is the generally accepted primary treatment aim in treating pelvic ring fractures.

The majority of MUs or NUs is the result of inadequate primary treatment, including lack of proper planning, conservative treatment in unstable fracture patterns, isolated external fixation and/or single anterior fixation of posterior unstable injuries, initial malreduction, or failure of fixation resulting in chronic pain, deformity, gait impairment, and functional disability [1–7].

In a literature review, Kanakaris et al. stated that nonoperative treatment was by far the most common primary treatment modality that led to malalignment, delayed union, or nonunion [8].

Historical data indicate that after conservative treatment of type C pelvic ring injuries, nonunion and malalignment can be expected between 55 and 75% of cases [9–11].

With the ongoing development of standardized treatment concepts, these rates were significantly reduced to only few cases, and, therefore, the individual experience is minor.

Pennal et al. first reported on the management of a large group of 34 pelvic NUs and MUs [12]. Anterior and posterior pain, Trendelenburg limping, clinical instability, and deformity were the most common clinical signs. In the sacroiliac area, a more atrophic appearance of NU was observed, while at the pubic rami area, atrophic and hypertrophic NU were found in comparable rates. Nonoperative treatment led to unfavorable results compared to surgical treatment. The latter included bone grafting and/or stable osteosynthesis. Nearly all patients treated with bone grafting showed bone healing, even after isolated grafting.

NU or MU treatment are demanding treatments but can be associated with good results in experienced hands [13]:

- 50% anatomical reduction
- 35% satisfactory reduction
- 69% no or only slight pain
- 92% satisfaction with result after sitting imbalance

Extensive diagnostics and an adequate morphological analysis have to be performed to develop a detailed treatment plan.

42.1 Clinical Evaluation

Preoperative evaluation should include a detailed history on subjective symptoms, a complete functional lumbopelvic evaluation including analysis of both hip joints, an instability evaluation, analysis of neurological sequelae, urogenital and functional impairments, including sitting imbalance, walking disturbances, necessity of walking supports, sportive dysfunctions, and a complete radiological evaluation of the lumbopelvic region.

42.1.1 Pain Analysis

The most commonly reported symptom in pelvic NU or MU is pain [12], although not all deformities are necessarily painful. The severity of pain often depends on the degree of instability or hemipelvic malposition and is usually located at the posterior sacroiliac region [1, 11, 13]. Additionally, pain can worsen with weight bearing and improve with rest [14].

J. Lindahl
Orthopaedics and Trauma Surgery, Helsinki University Hospital, Helsinki, Finland

A. Gänsslen (✉)
Department of Trauma Surgery, Orthopedics and Hand Surgery, Hospital Wolfsburg, Wolfsburg, Germany

A. Gänsslen et al. (eds.), *Pelvic Ring Fractures*, https://doi.org/10.1007/978-3-030-54730-1_42

Disabling pelvic pain is defined as pain, which is inadequately controlled by classical analgesics and pain management.

The patient is asked for pain maxima, severity of pain (visual analog scale), and localization of pain.

Anterior ring deformities can result in subclinical disturbance, while posterior instability, MU, or NU more frequently presents with (posterior) pain [8, 11, 13, 15, 16]. Pain in the anterior region can be a sign of pelvic instability, especially after anterior-posterior compression injuries [17].

Posterior pelvic pain is difficult to analyze due to the complex anatomy of the posterior pelvic region, especially in malhealed situations. Posterior pelvic pain may result from osteoarthritic changes of the SI joint [18] and can be analyzed by intra- or periarticular injection of local anesthesia, fluoroscopy, or CT. Additionally, a technetium bone scan can be useful [13]. Overall, pain is more common after SI joint injuries than after sacral MU [14].

Occasionally, pain can be located at the lumbar spine, which can be related to pelvic deformity. Therefore, it is important to distinguish pelvic pain from low back pain and from neuropathic pain due to compression or distraction injuries of the lumbosacral plexus. The latter will not improve with surgical treatment of pelvic MU or NU [5, 8, 16]. Significant pelvic obliquity can additionally lead to low back pain [14]. Injuries to the L5/S1 facet joint can also result in posterior pelvic pain [14, 19].

A detailed analysis of the localization and severity of pelvic pain and its correlation to functions/daily activities are, therefore, the basis to get information regarding instability and functional impairments.

In summary, causes of pelvic pain related to MU or NU include [20]:

- Incongruity and instability of the SI joint
- Nonunion of the posterior pelvic ring
- Pressure effect from malaligned bony structures
- Neurogenic type of pain due to nerve root compression in lumbosacral plexus injuries
- Associated trauma to the hip joint
- Persistent low back pain

Additionally, the presence and localization of pain should be correlated to pelvic instability, sitting imbalance, and/or neurological injuries.

Mears et al. analyzed clinical and radiological signs, dependent on the fracture type according to the Tile classification [13]:

- Type A fractures: exclusively anterior pelvic pain
- Type B injuries: pain, pelvic instability, simple rotational deformity, kinked urethra
- Type C injuries: pain, pelvic instability, sitting imbalance, leg length discrepancy

42.1.2 Sitting Imbalance

Symptomatic sitting imbalance (Fig. 42.1) can be a sign of hemipelvic asymmetry. Asymmetry of the ischial tuberosities due to vertical shear malhealing or rotational malalignment can result in impairments.

Cranial hemipelvic displacement can additionally cause leg length discrepancy, sitting imbalance, and standing imbalance. A prominent posterior ilium, resulting from posterior hemipelvic displacement or sagittal malrotation, can impress as discomfort while sitting on a chair or lying in the supine position (Fig. 42.2).

Overall, symptoms related to sitting imbalance are caused by [20]:

- Pressure from a prominent bony projection
- Asymmetry of the ischial tuberosities

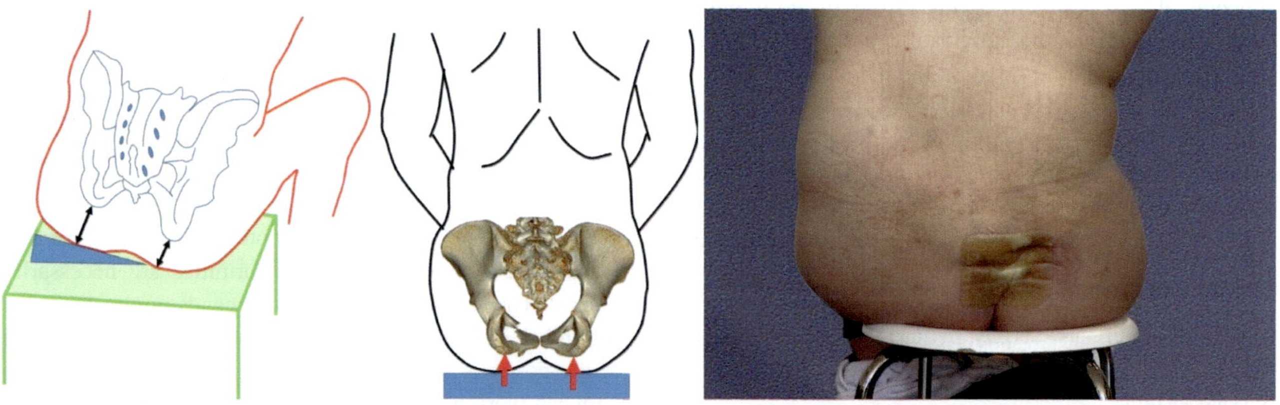

Fig. 42.1 Sitting imbalance: unilateral support can correct the deformity; additionally, posttraumatic scoliosis can mimic sitting imbalance

- Vertical displacement
- Hemipelvic malrotation
- Posterior hemipelvic displacement
- Prominence of the sacrum or the coccyx [13]

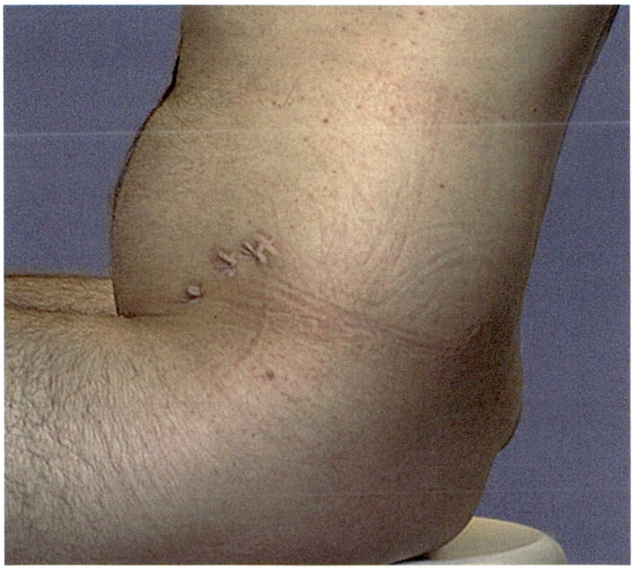

Fig. 42.2 Posterior bone prominence due to sacral fracture malhealing (posterior displacement)

42.1.3 Leg Length Discrepancy

Leg length discrepancy (LLD) can result from vertically unstable fracture patterns or sagittal malrotation. Routine testing of leg length discrepancy, using small wooden boards, should be performed in every patient. Nonoperative measures should have been tested for at least 3 months, e.g., shoe raise and pelvic padding for sitting imbalance [20].

A detailed CT analysis of the "true" leg length difference is considered the gold standard (see below).

42.1.4 Gait Abnormalities

Gait abnormalities can be the result of malhealing. Cranial displacement can lead to relative leg shortening. After unstable type C fractures, average leg length differences of more than 3–6 cm were measured [21].

Rotational malalignment also can alter gait due to the change of the hip joint orientation [14]. Additionally, reduced abductor muscle strength can result in hip joint alterations [1] and posttraumatic femoroacetabular impingement. Accompanying acetabular fractures can result in a femoral anteversion increase [11]. Especially lateral compression injuries can lead to significant internal rotational deformities (Fig. 42.3) [14].

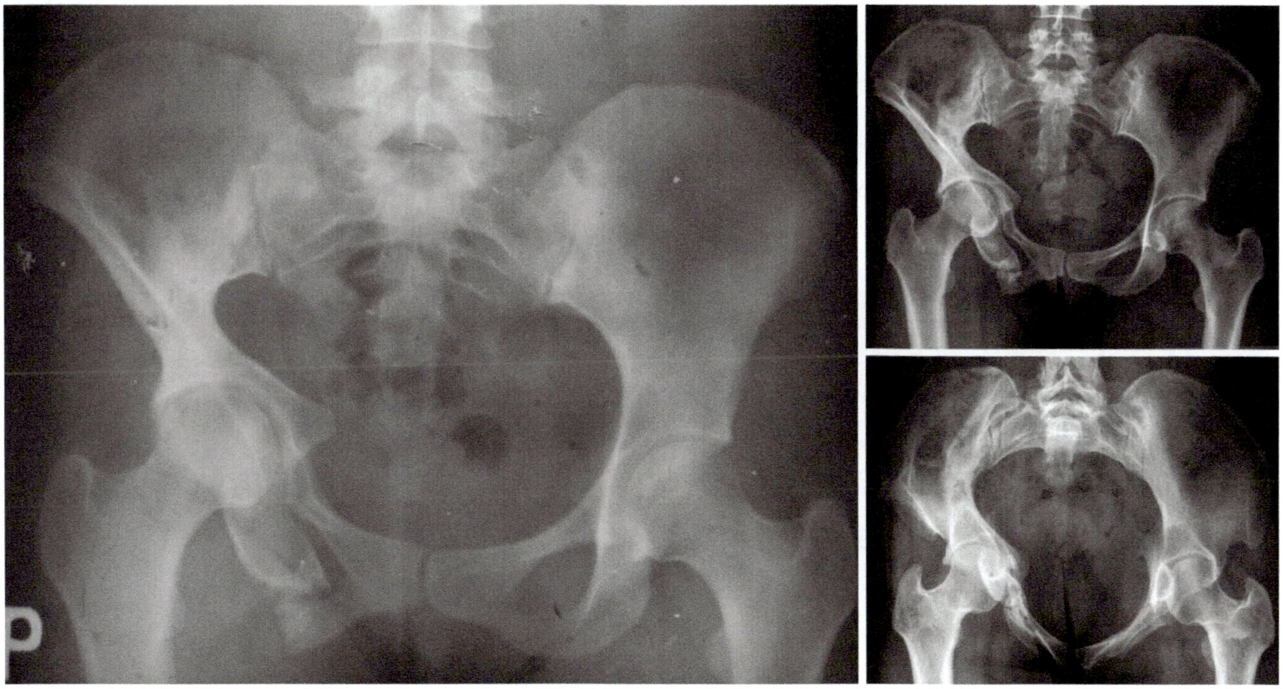

Fig. 42.3 Severe internal rotation deformity after nonoperative treatment of a type C injury (C1.1 injury with a complete ilium fracture)

42.1.5 Instability Analysis

Subjective pelvic instability is a common symptom [8, 11, 13, 15, 16]. Clinical signs of instability can be present as awakening at night or complaints during daily activities [13]. Instability can be static or dynamic. Dynamic instability can be tested using fluoroscopy [13].

Longitudinal traction can be performed for the analysis of vertical (walking) instability and analysis of rotational instability is performed by special tests. Additionally, placing the patient on a fracture table allows performing a continuous traction increase in defined positions of the hip joint for defining instability vectors.

Sagi et al. described radiographic tests for occult instability analysis (Fig. 42.4) [22]:

- External rotation/anteroposterior compression stress examination of the pelvis
- Push–pull stress examination of the pelvis for vertical instability: one extremity is pushed cranially while the other is pulled caudally

These examinations can exclude relevant pelvic instability [23].

42.1.6 Aesthetic Analysis

Aesthetic analysis, especially of the posterior pelvis (bony prominence of the sacrum (Fig. 42.2) or coccyx) and the ischial tuberosities, can confirm pelvic deformities due to cranial or rotational displacement of the injured hemipelvis.

Sacral deformity can be severe in bilateral injuries, which was observed in female patients and those with a low BMI [5, 8, 11, 13, 16, 24].

42.1.7 Urogenital Complaints

Urogenital complaints can be caused by initial pelvic floor injury, urogenital prolapse, or neurological injury [1, 25, 26].

Marked hemipelvic internal rotation (Fig. 42.3) can result in bladder compression which can be accentuated by malhealed or displaced fragments of the upper pubic rami. Symptoms include increased urinary frequency due to bladder impingement and prolonged voiding [14].

Additionally, deformities of the true pelvis can lead to obstetric problems [27]. Medial displacement of the ischial tuberosities can compress the vaginal wall (Fig. 42.5) and produce dyspareunia, causing pain during sexual intercourse [20].

Bucket handle injuries can lead to bladder impingement, and locked pubic symphysis injuries can lead to perineal impingements [14].

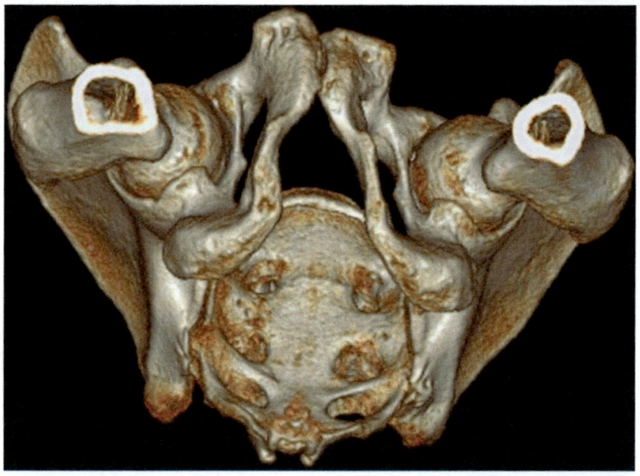

Fig. 42.5 Internal rotation deformity, which led to vaginal impingement

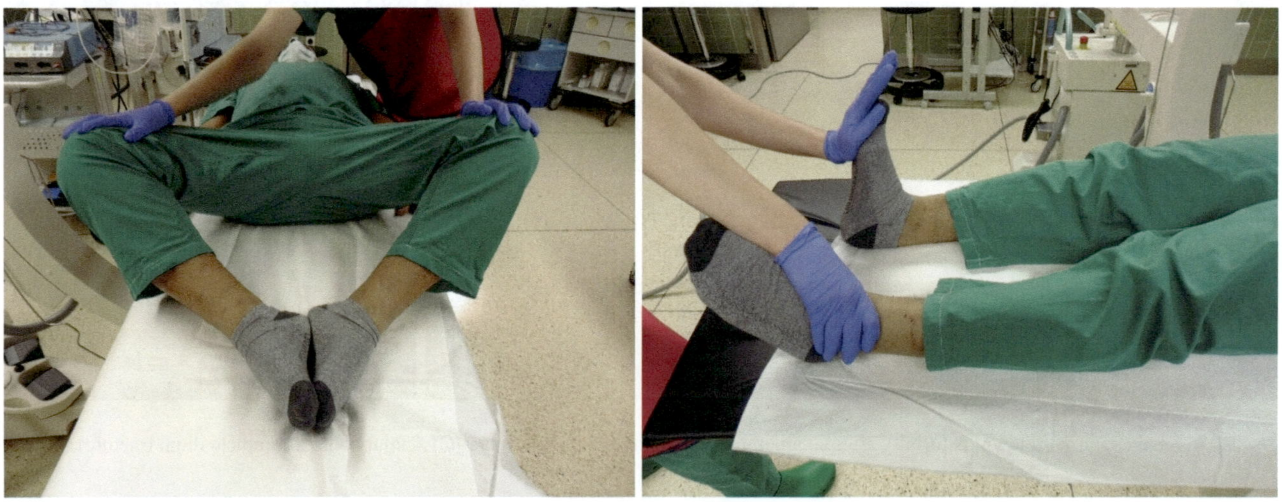

Fig. 42.4 Instability testing by external rotational stress examination and push-and-pull examination acc. to Sagi

Wright et al. observed sexual dysfunctions, depending on special injury locations [28]:

- Fourfold higher risk of sexual and excretory dysfunction in males with SI joint injuries
- 4.8% higher risk of sexual dysfunction in females after symphyseal diastasis
- 12% higher risk of excretory dysfunction in females after symphyseal diastasis

Fracture patterns, minor malalignments, and internal fixation hardware are not indications for cesarean delivery [29].

42.1.8 Neurological Analysis

A detailed neurological evaluation is recommended to identify typical lesions associated with long-term disability after pelvic fractures. The ASIA scheme is recommended (see Chap. 6). Lumbosacral plexus traction lesions most frequently involve the L4 and L5 roots, followed by the superior gluteal nerve [8, 16] and the LCFN [20].

42.2 Radiological Assessment

A detailed radiological deformity and NU analyses of the whole pelvic ring is mandatory.

Beside classical conventional x-rays for analysis of pelvic ring deformity, including pelvic AP x-ray, inlet,- and outlet views, oblique acetabular views, e.g., iliac and obturator oblique views if necessary, and a conventional CT with multiplanar reconstructions are mandatory. A 3D reconstruction can be helpful for better understanding of rotational and translational deformity analyses (Fig. 42.6).

In unilateral deformities, the uninjured hemipelvis can act as a template (Fig. 42.7). Special anatomical landmarks can be compared with the corresponding landmarks on the affected side in all planes [30].

The CT scan is used to clearly define the MU or NU deformity and localization, while the 3D CT scan is useful to develop the treatment plan [4, 25, 31]. Linear, rotational, and vertical displacements can be analyzed.

Mears et al. proposed to use a normal pelvic CT scan and inlet and outlet views for comparison, the latter especially for intraoperative analysis [13].

Leg length discrepancy is determined by measuring the cranial displacement of special landmarks in the anteroposterior pelvic or outlet projection.

New tools include computer-assisted planning programs, which allow manipulation of hemipelvic fragments, and 3D-printing technologies [32].

3D printing allows to define the release and osteotomy areas, implant length, and plate preshaping and placement areas [1]. Additionally, the size of the autografts can be determined. Urological and pelvic floor studies can complement radiological analysis [25, 26].

Preoperatively, an instability analysis can be performed by using single leg stance imaging for detecting symphyseal or even SI joint or nonunion instability.

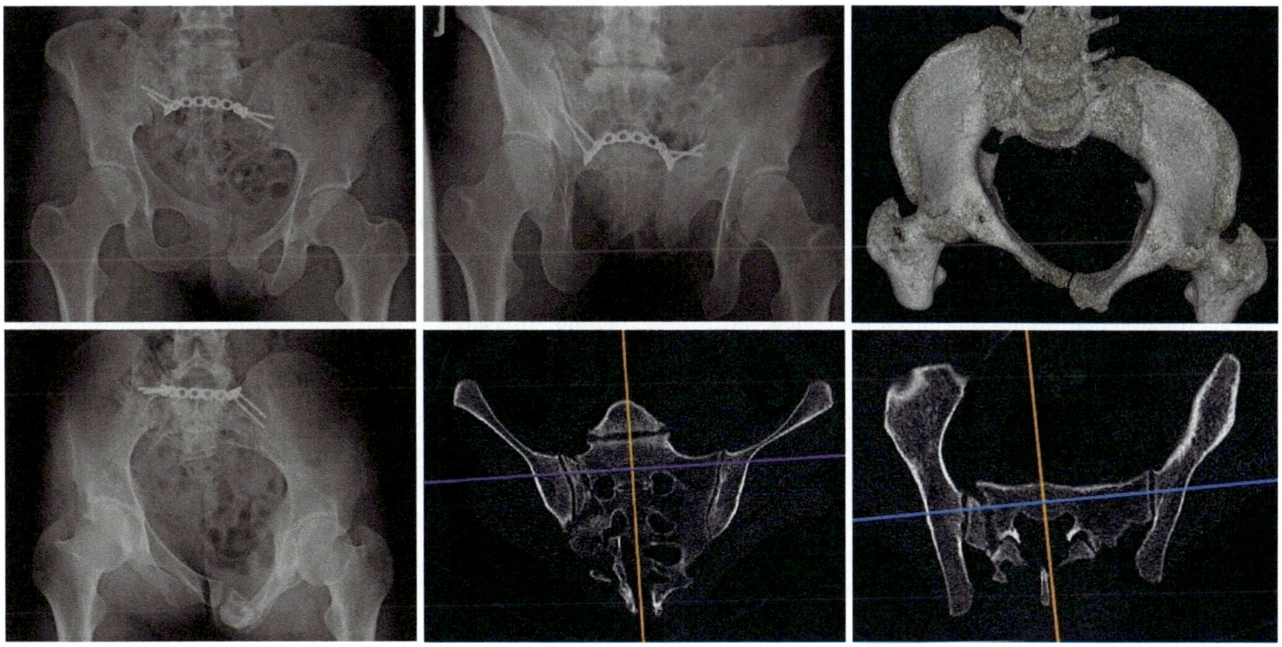

Fig. 42.6 Basic set of x-ray and CT-slices for NU or MU analysis

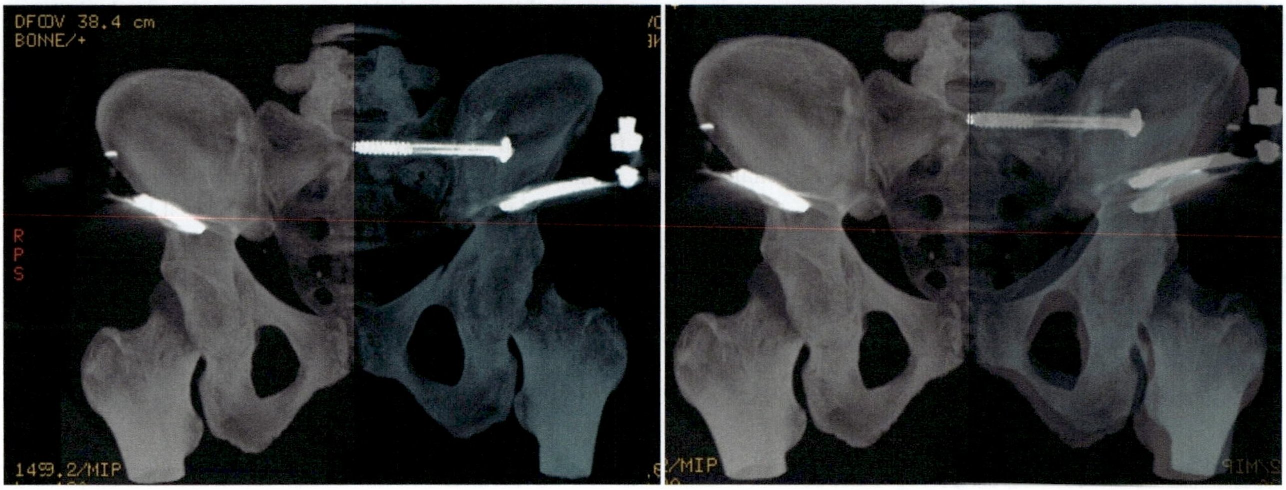

Fig. 42.7 Unilateral left malreduction; using the contralateral side as a template allows for clear identification of the deformity

Manual stress testing in traction and under rotational compression can be performed under image intensifier control [13].

Depending on the rotational axes, flexion/extension, internal/external rotation, and abduction/adduction deformities can be present.

Dickson and Matta first gave recommendations of radiological deformity signs [33].

Flexion and extension deformities are defined as rotations around a horizontal axis through the supraacetabular region [33], best visualized on 3D images. Signs of flexion deformities on conventional views are:

- A cranial crossing of the obturator-acetabular line to the teardrop figure
- An increased and elongated shape of the obturator foramen on the outlet or AP view
- A more caudal ilioischial line relative to the obturator foramen on the outlet view

Internal and external rotational deformities are defined as rotations around a vertical axis through the quadrilateral plate [33], best visualized on standard CT images. Signs of internal rotation deformities on conventional views are:

- A "wider" ischium
- Smaller iliac fossa
- A more lateral ilioischial line in relation to the tear drop figure

Abduction and adduction deformities are defined as rotations around a sagittal axis through each central acetabulum, which has the advantage of not affecting rotational deformities. Pure abduction/adduction deformities are rare and are most often combined with rotational malalignment. The degree of abduction-adduction malalignment is determined by an angle formed between a line from the posterior superior iliac spine to the symphysis and a line in the plane of the sacrum. This angle can be verified using CT images by measuring the distance from the center of the quadrilateral plate to the midline.

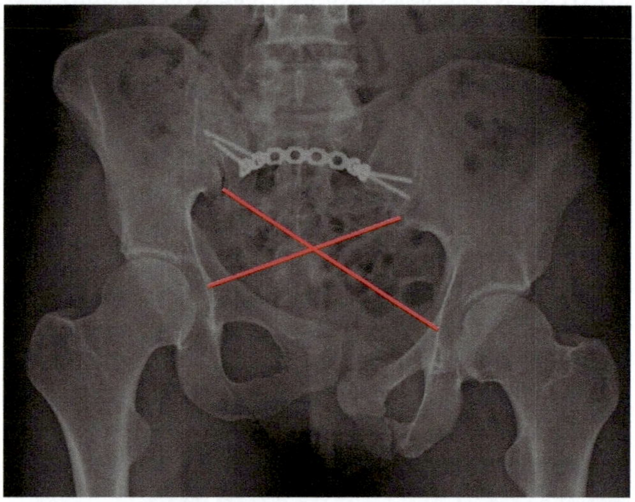

Fig. 42.8 Keshishyan method of deformity analysis; the distance from the lower border of the SI joint to the middle of the internal contour of the contralateral acetabulum

The AP view was used to determine pelvic obliquity.

Sponseller et al. measured the distance from the anterior superior iliac spine to the posterior superior iliac spine, which can be compared to the unaffected hemipelvis [34].

A comparable measurement was introduced by Keshishyan et al. [35]. A quantitative deformity analysis was performed by comparative measurement of diagonal lines of the true pelvis (Fig. 42.8). Keshishyan method of deformity analysis: comparison of the distance from the lower border of the SI joint to the middle of the internal contour of the contralateral acetabulum. A deformity index was calculated as a quotient of difference between both diagonal sizes and the sum of diagonal sizes.

However, these measurements involve a combination of internal/external rotations and abduction/adduction components [33].

Stover et al. proposed a different measurement strategy [36, 37]. Several displacements were analyzed using the AP view of the pelvis, the inlet view, and a true lateral view.

On the AP view (measurement can also be performed using corresponding 3D CT scans), leg length inequality, abduction/adduction deformities, and rotational deformities can be identified (Fig. 42.9a–d):

- Leg length inequality: a horizontal, tangential line to the most upper margin of both acetabula is drawn perpendicular to a vertical line through the middle of the sacrum (a standing radiograph should be used to get the functional LLD)
- Abduction/adduction deformities can be measured by a line starting from the midpoint of the SI joint to specific anterior ring landmarks (e.g., inferior symphyseal point, most prominent point of ischial tuberosity, etc.)
- Medial/lateral displacement: a horizontal line to the anterior superior iliac spine perpendicular to a vertical line through the middle of the sacrum on each side (a difference on length of these line indicate rotational deformity)

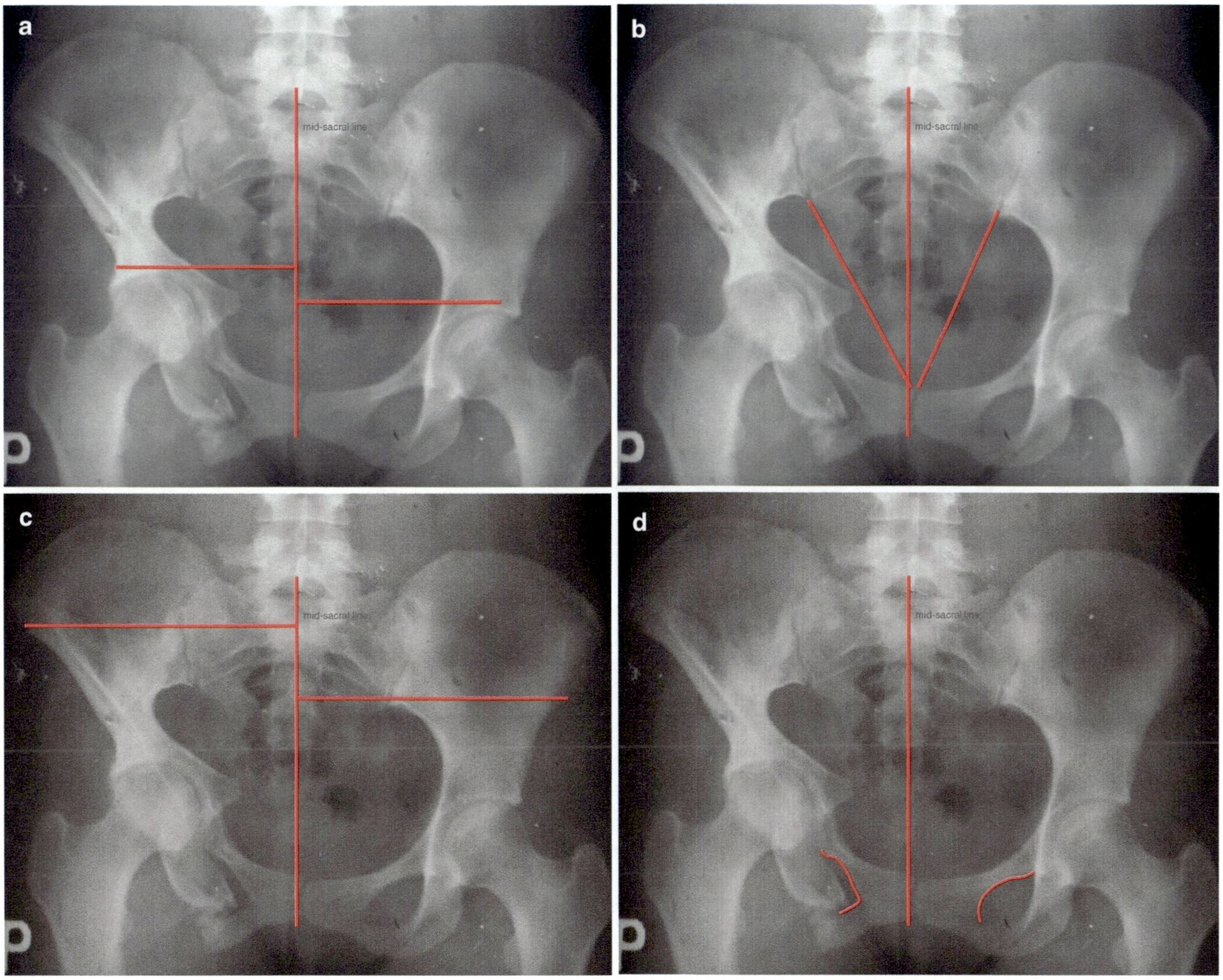

Fig. 42.9 (**a**) Measurement of Leg Length Inequality on the a.p. x-ray: a horizontal, tangential line to the most upper margin of both acetabula is drawn perpendicular to a vertical line through the middle of the sacrum; 2 cm right leg shortening. (**b**) Measurement of ab-/adduction deformities on the a.p. x-ray; a line, starting from the midpoint of the SI joint is drawn to a defined anterior ring landmark point (e.g., inferior symphyseal point, most prominent point of ischial tuberosity, etc.); slight right adduction deformity. (**c**) Measurement of medial/lateral displacement on the a.p. x-ray; a horizontal line to the anterior superior iliac spine perpendicular to a vertical line through the middle of the sacrum on each side (a difference on length of these line indicate rotational deformity); no relevant medial/lateral displecement. (**d**) Measurement of rotational malalignment on the a.p. x-ray; comparable analysis of the shape of the obturator foramen indicated rotational deformity when the midline of the sacrum runs through the pubic symphysis; right internal rotation deformity

- Rotational malalignment: comparable analysis of the shape of the obturator foramen indicated rotational deformity when the midline of the sacrum runs through the pubic symphysis

On the inlet view (measurement can also be performed using corresponding 2D CT scans), rotational deformities and sagittal displacements can be analyzed (Fig. 42.10a–c):

- Rotational malalignment: a line starting from the posterior aspect of the SI joint to specific anterior ring landmarks (e.g., inferior symphyseal point, most prominent point of ischial tuberosity etc.) is compared with the healthy side
- Anterior/posterior displacement: comparable measurement of the posterior symphyseal border (Caution: the physiological pelvic tilt influences this measurement; CT measurement is considered optimal!)
- Medial/lateral displacement: a horizontal line to the anterior superior iliac spine perpendicular to a vertical line through the middle of the sacrum on each side (a difference in length of these lines indicates rotational and medial/lateral displacement/deformity)

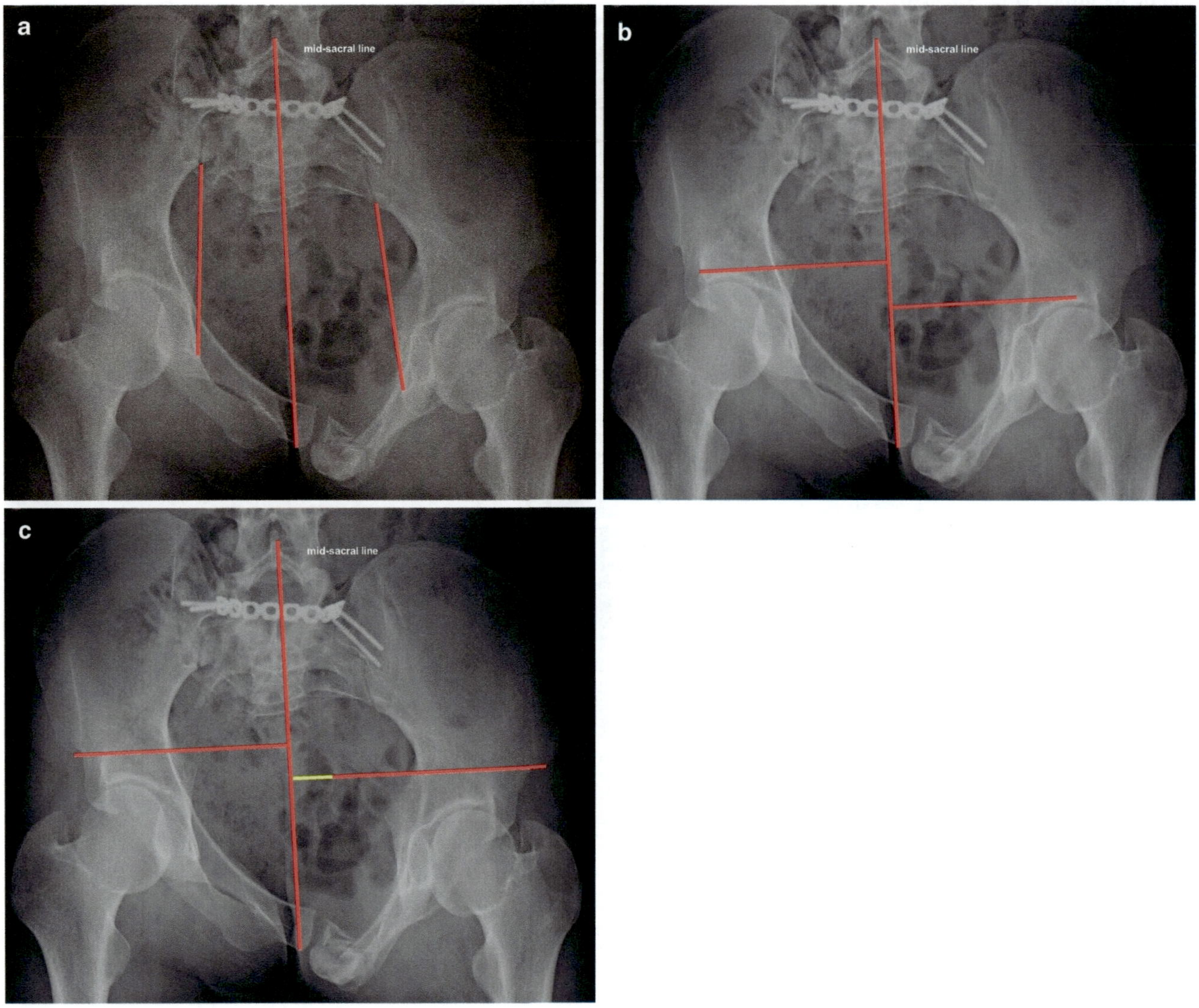

Fig. 42.10 (**a**) Measurement of rotational malalignment on the Inlet view; rotational malalignment; comparison of lines starting from the posterior aspect of the SI joint to specific anterior ring landmark; slight right internal rotation deformity. (**b**) Measurement of anterior/posterior displacement on the Inlet view; comparable measurement of the posterior symphyseal border (in fracture situation, another landmark should be chosen (here: acetabular margin)); right hemipelvic displacement of approximately 2 cm. (**c**) Measurement of medial/lateral displacement on the Inlet view; a horizontal line to the anterior superior iliac spine perpendicular to a vertical line through the middle of the sacrum on each side is drawn; approximately 2.5 cm right medial displacement

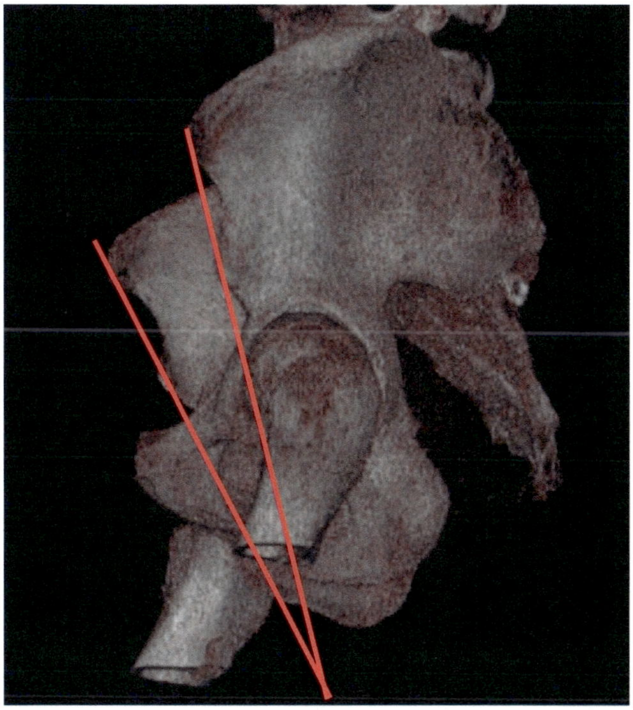

Fig. 42.11 Measurement of flexion/extension deformities; overlapping at the posterior pelvis indicates flexion deformity on the right hemipelvis by measuring the angle between tangential lines on both sides to the AIIS and ASIS

On the true lateral view (measurement can also be performed using corresponding 3D CT scans), flexion/extension deformities can be verified and the resulting relative leg length deformities (Fig. 42.11):

- Flexion/extension deformities: after exact overlapping at the posterior pelvis, the anterior ring is analyzed for differences in shape; a line starting at the SI joint center relative to the anterior tangential border of the anterior ramus indicates flexion deformity.

Sagi et al. presented the concept of inlet and outlet ratios for analyzing displacements [38]. The inlet and outlet views are used:

- Inlet ratio (Fig. 42.12): a line is drawn tangential to the anterior sacral border, perpendicular to the spinous processes and the distance from this line to the subchondral acetabular bone is determined; the ratio is calculated with the affected side being the numerator; identical hemipelvic position has a ratio of 1; posterior translation presents with a ratio <1 and anterior translation with a ratio >1.
- Outlet ratio (Fig. 42.13): a line parallel to the superior endplate of S1 and perpendicular to the spinous processes is drawn; the distance from this line to the subchondral acetabular bone is determined; the ratio is calculated with the affected side being the numerator; identical hemipelvic position has a ratio of 1; superior translation presents with a ratio <1 and inferior translation with a ratio >1.

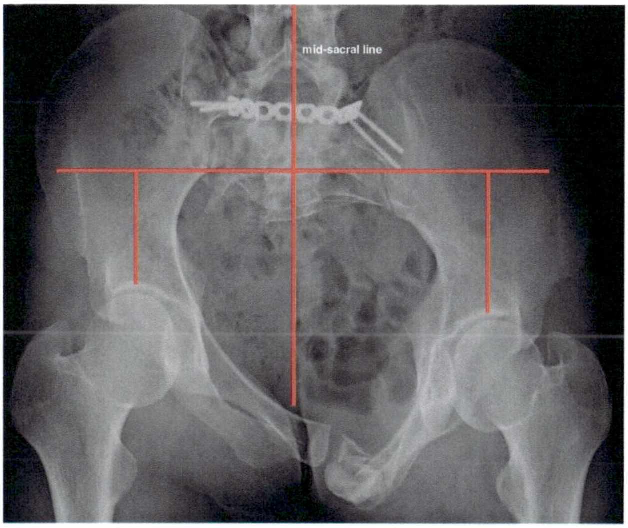

Fig. 42.12 Inlet ratio acc. to Sagi: a line is drawn tangential to the anterior sacral border, perpendicular to the spinous processes and the distance from this line to the subchondral acetabular bone is determined; the ratio is calculated with the affected side being the numerator: 0.8 = 80% indicating posterior translation

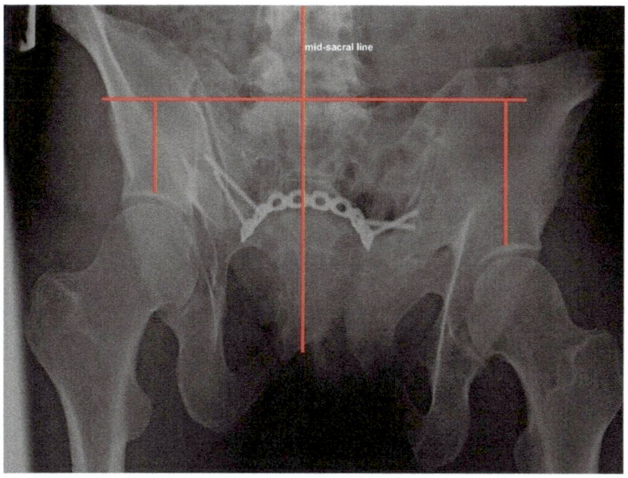

Fig. 42.13 Outlet ratio acc. to Sagi: a line parallel to the superior endplate of S1 and perpendicular to the spinous processes is drawn; the distance from this line to the subchondral acetabular bone is determined; the ratio is calculated with the affected side being the numerator: 0.85 = 85% indicating superior translation

Lefaivre et al. analyzed the Sagi-, Keshishyan, and Lefaivre methods and stated, that overall these measurements show poor reliability. The Sagi method allows only relevant information in displaced deformities, while the best method is that by Keshishyan, but this was difficult to interpret [39].

Nystrom et al. stated that vertical translation of the AP view by measuring the difference in height of the iliac wings in relation to perpendicular lines to the sacral midline and even CT measurement of the anterior SI joint displacement were unreliable [40]. In contrast, Boontanapibul et al. could show an adequate correlation between cadaver displacement and actual radiographic displacement on the pelvic outlet radiograph with two times of actual displacement [41].

In a further analysis by Nystrom et al., a new radiographic technique was presented for measuring axial and sagittal rotational deformities using CT-based reconstruction of standardized pelvic planes [42]:

- Axial rotation: axial reconstructions in the inlet plane; angle between a midsacral line and a line connecting the anterior superior iliac spine and posterior superior iliac spine
- Sagittal rotation: sagittal reconstructions; angle between a line connecting the posterior superior iliac spine, the pubic tubercle, and the superior sacral endplate
- Axial rotational displacement (Fig. 42.14): inlet view; two circles are drawn, which best fit on the iliac wing and acetabulum; the angle between a line connecting the circle centers and the midsacral line is measured
- Sagittal rotational displacement (Fig. 42.15): inlet and outlet views; sagittal rotation represents the arctangent of (o/i)
  - Inlet view: distance from the sacral promontory to the most posterior aspect of the disrupted pubic structure (i)
  - Outlet view: distance between both most superior aspects of the disrupted pubic structure (o)

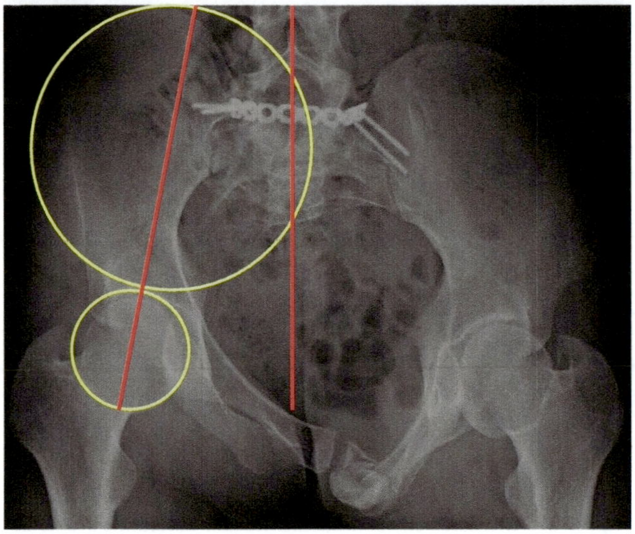

Fig. 42.14 Axial rotational displacement measurement acc. to Nystrom: on the Inlet view two circles are drawn, which best fit on the iliac wing and acetabulum; the angle between a line connecting the circle centers and the midsacral line is measured

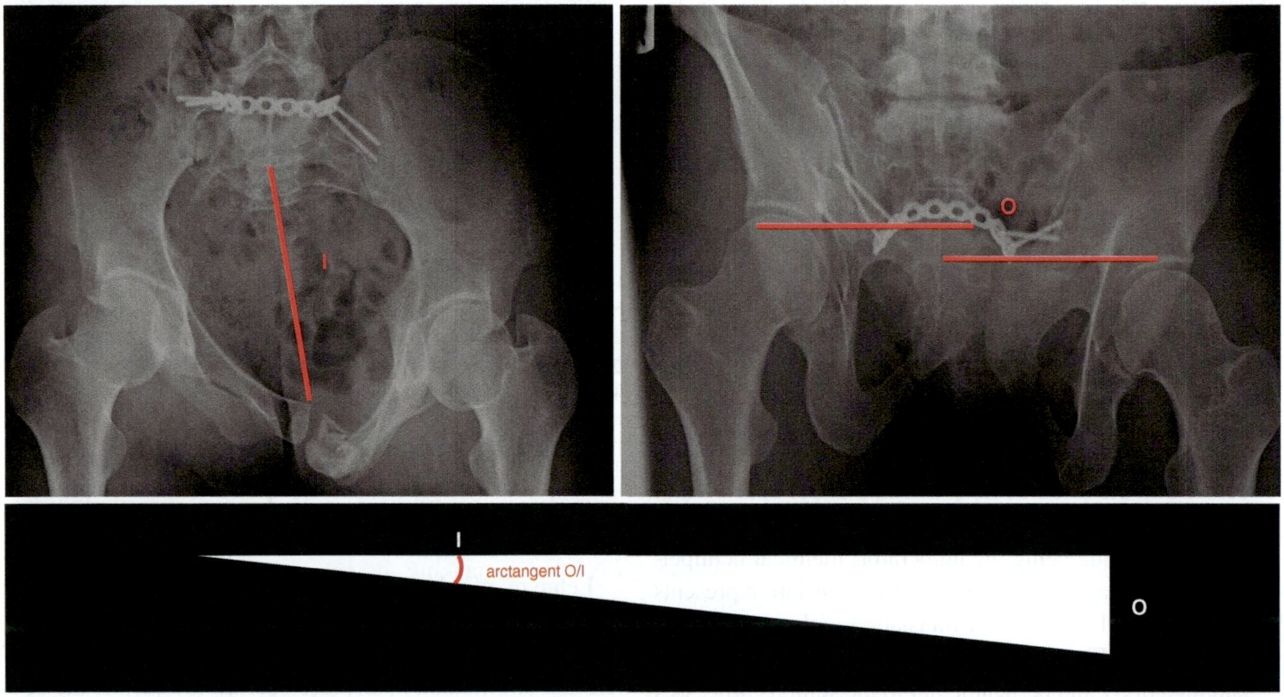

Fig. 42.15 Sagittal rotation measurement acc. to Nystrom: on the Inlet view the distance from the sacral promontory to the most posterior aspect of the disrupted pubic structure (i) is measured and on the Outet view the distance between both most superior aspects of the disrupted pubic structure (o) is measured. The arctangent of O/I represents rotational deformity

Overall, an excellent interobserver reliability and good validity was observed.

Zhao et al. used the uninjured hemipelvis as a template and measured lines between special anatomical landmarks on the AP view, and the inlet and outlet views, reconstructed from CT DICOM data [30]:

- AP view: sagittal rotational displacement: comparing the length between ASIS and ischial tubercle; smaller length = hemipelvic flexion, greater length = hemipelvic extension
- Inlet view: rotational displacement: transverse distance between ASIS and the anterior iliac part of the SI joint; smaller length = internal rotation, longer length = external rotation
- Outlet view: varus and valgus deformity: transverse distance between ASIS and the ischial tubercle; small distance = valgus, longer distance = varus

42.3 Classification

Mears et al. introduced a classification of nonunion and malalignment [13]:

- Type I: undisplaced nonunion
- Type II: stable malalignment
- Type III: unstable, nonunited malalignment
- Type IV: partially stable malalignment with incomplete stabilization by callus and heterotopic bone

Cano-Luís et al. reported a new classification based on residual or complex instability, which also guides to a clear treatment concept. Parameters include pelvic ring deformity, pain localization, leg length discrepancy, sitting imbalance, and a stability test [1].

Residual instability is defined as a missing pelvic ring deformity, while complex instability is associated with some pelvic ring deformity. Thus, the first evaluation consists always of a deformity analysis.

Options for instability testing include:

- Monopedal stance x-rays for detecting anterior instability
- External rotation stress views for detecting anterior instability
- Fluoroscopy-based dynamic stability testing for detecting anterior and posterior instabilities
- Dynamic lumbar spine radiographs to confirm lumbosacral instability (lumbofacet joint instability)

42.3.1 Residual Instability

Per definition, in residual instability, no pelvic deformity, leg length inequalities, or (resulting) sitting imbalance is present [1]. Parameters to be analyzed include only the localization of pain, while in all patients an additional instability testing should be performed.

Based on pain localization, three subtypes are distinguished:

- Type I (anterior injury): anterior pain, no postural instability
- Type II (anterior healed pelvic ring; posterior injury, including external rotation instability with degenerative SI joint changes or vertical instabilities with sacral nonunion; nonunion of the articular pedicle L5/S1 (dynamic x-ray evaluation)): posterior (lumbar) pain
- Type III (combined anterior + posterior injury): type II injury without anterior healing (anterior instability); anterior and posterior pain, instability during walking

42.3.2 Complex Instability

Patients with complex instability always show pelvic deformity due to:

- Type I: malunion
- Type II: nonunion

Depending on the amount of leg length discrepancy (≥3 cm or <3 cm), these types are further subdivided [1].

Typical clinical signs include anterior and posterior pelvic pain, low back pain, claudication and gait instability, sitting imbalance, and neurological and genitourinary impairments. Besides standard radiographic imaging modalities, MRI and electrophysiological tests should be added.

Mears defined a difficulty grading of late pelvic reconstruction from simple to demanding [43]:

- Isolated external rotation deformity
- Internal rotation deformity
- Sagittal/coronary rotational deformities
- Isolated posterior hemipelvic malunion
- Vertical displaced malunions/nonunions
- Vertical malunions/nonunions with additional rotational/translational malalignment

42.4 Treatment

Treatment of MU and NU is technically demanding due to the altered anatomy and the high risk of complications [44]. There are two main principal aims of treatment:

- Symmetric anatomical reconstruction of pelvic anatomy
- Recovery of quality of life

Conservative treatment has been tried to equalize the leg length difference and sitting imbalance. These include shoe raises and pelvic padding for sitting imbalance.

> Surgical correction is the treatment of choice [20]. Pennal et al. clearly stated that nonoperative management was associated with worse results [12].

Indications for surgery include pelvic pain, instability, and various symptomatic deformities [13], and nonunion-related and/or deformity-specific pain, while lumbosacral plexopathy-related pain should be excluded [13].

> Due to different MU localizations and types of pelvic NU, no universal treatment concept fulfills all possible treatment possibilities.

Kanakarsi et al. performed a literature review and stated that the combination of open reduction, internal fixation, and bone grafting was the preferred treatment method for pelvic MU and NU [8].

> A multistage procedure consisting of two or three stages (same anesthesia) was used in the majority of the patients [8].

Depending on the localization of the malunited apex, nonunion site, and/or joint instability, several treatment options were reported. Localization-dependent treatment options include:

1. Arthrodesis of the pubic symphysis
2. Arthrodesis of an SI joint
3. Anterior pubic rami nonunion treatment
4. Sacral nonunion treatment
5. Iliac nonunion treatment
6. Hemipelvic correction

42.5 Symphyseal Arthrodesis

NU at the anterior ring usually needs additional plate fixation of the fractures with bone grafting [20].

Symphyseal nonunion results in anterior ring instability, which can be painful. Additionally, posterior pain can be present. In the majority of cases, anterior standard plating is favored. Alternatively, Gautier recommended double plating in cases with previous implant failure or direct symphyseal arthrodesis [15].

Isolated internal (locked symphysis) and external rotation deformities can be approached through a single anterior incision [5, 20, 45]. Fang et al. recommended a single stage reconstruction even in severely displaced open book deformities [25].

Symphyseal fusion or arthrodesis is indicated when significant instability is present, especially when the posterior pelvic ring is involved.

The Pfannenstiel incision is proposed to expose the symphysis and the upper pubic rami. Additionally, the inferior pubic rami can be visualized intrapelvic using this approach. Today, the intrapelvic approach allows a more extended overview of the true pelvis.

In the supine position, after insertion of a Foley catheter, midline dissection is performed until reaching the retropubic space. For bladder protection, after mobilization, a malleable retractor is placed behind the symphysis into the space of Retzius. In severely contracted situations, the urinary bladder can be safely localized by trans-illumination via flexible cystoscopy [25].

Exposure of the pubic symphysis is performed by reflecting the rectus abdominis insertions from the midline. Direct curettage or drilling the fibrocartilaginous disk and hyaline cartilage is performed for symphyseal debridement until adequate cancellous bleeding bone is exposed. Standard reduction maneuvers are performed (see Chap. 23).

Olerud et al. proposed a wedge-shaped resection of the upper symphyseal part (nearly half of the entire symphysis) by resecting 7–8 mm bone on each side of the symphyseal cleft [46]. Here, a corresponding graft from the iliac crest, slightly superior in size to allow press-fit impaction, is inserted, and superior plate stabilization is performed with a specially designed six-hole superior plate. Retropubic cancellous grafts can support stability and healing.

Fang et al. used a tricortical strut graft to fuse the symphysis [25].

Single- or double-plate stabilization is the treatment of choice.

Cano-Luís et al. recommended additional iliosacral screw fixation in some cases to support the stability of the symphyseal arthrodesis [1].

Control of the vertical shear elements is often less successful [25].

42.6 SI Joint Arthrodesis

The classical anterolateral approach (first window of the ilio-inguinal approach) is performed for SI joint arthrodesis. Using this approach, direct visualization and debridement is possible and easier to achieve.

First, the anterior sacroiliac ligaments are released by dissection. Sharp dissection of these ligaments can be performed under direct visualization. The anterior anatomical structures have to be respected, e.g., the lumbosacral trunk, the S1 nerve root, and the superior gluteal vessels (Fig. 42.16). The lateral sacral shoulder is exposed by inserting Hohmann retractors into the bone, respecting the lumbosacral trunk. Alternatively, 2.5–3.0 mm K-wires can be introduced. The SI joint is then dissected superiorly. After opening the joint, a laminar spreader is inserted for joint visualization and excessive joint debridement (Fig. 42.17). Additionally, a supraacetabular femoral distractor or a laminar spreader allows lateral joint widening [25].

For further posterior dissection, an osteotome is inserted into the joint for releasing the interosseous ligaments (Fig. 42.17) up to the posterior ligaments to completely dis-

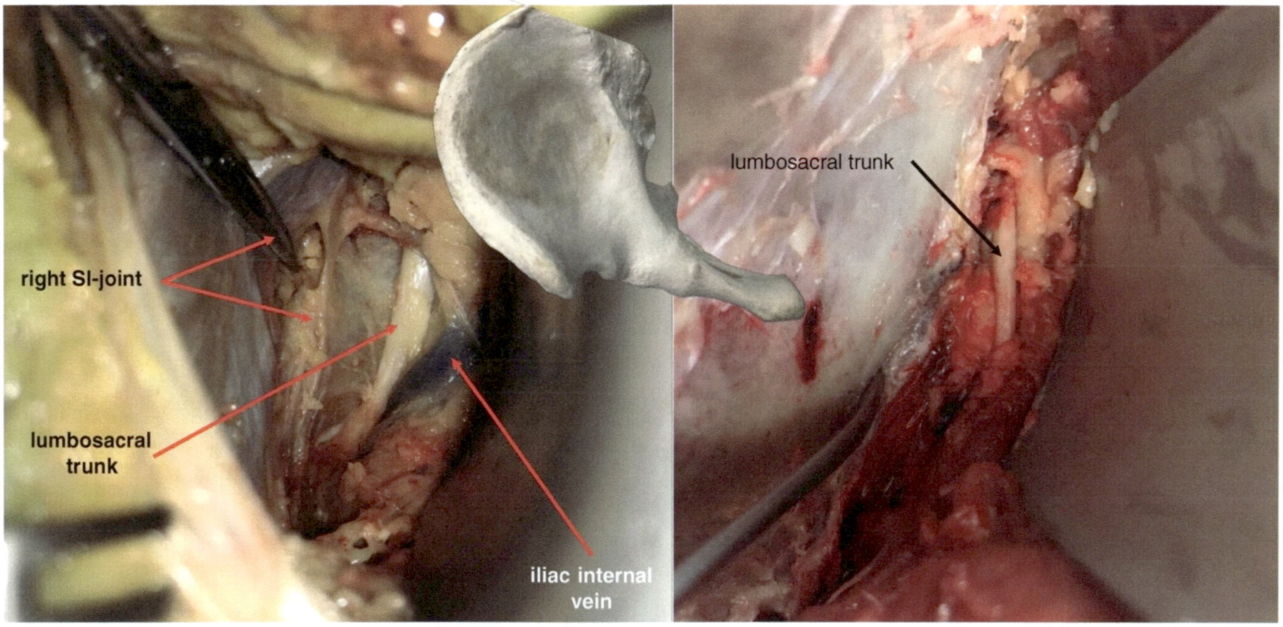

Fig. 42.16 Anterior neurovascular structures at risk during the anterior approach to the SI joint

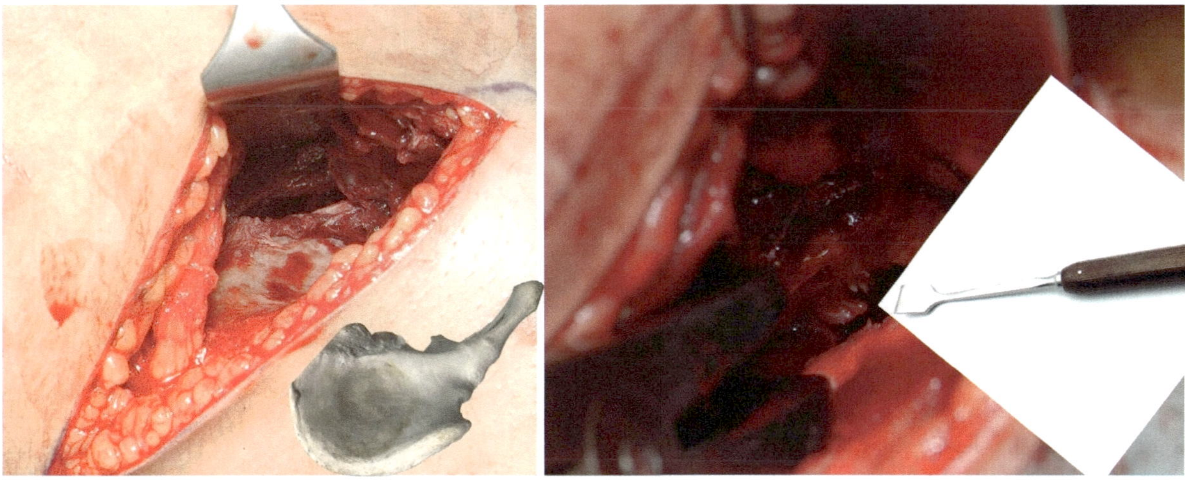

Fig. 42.17 Opening of the SI joint using a laminar spreader. Using a chisel or osteotome allows for dissection of the intraosseous and even posterior iliosacral ligaments

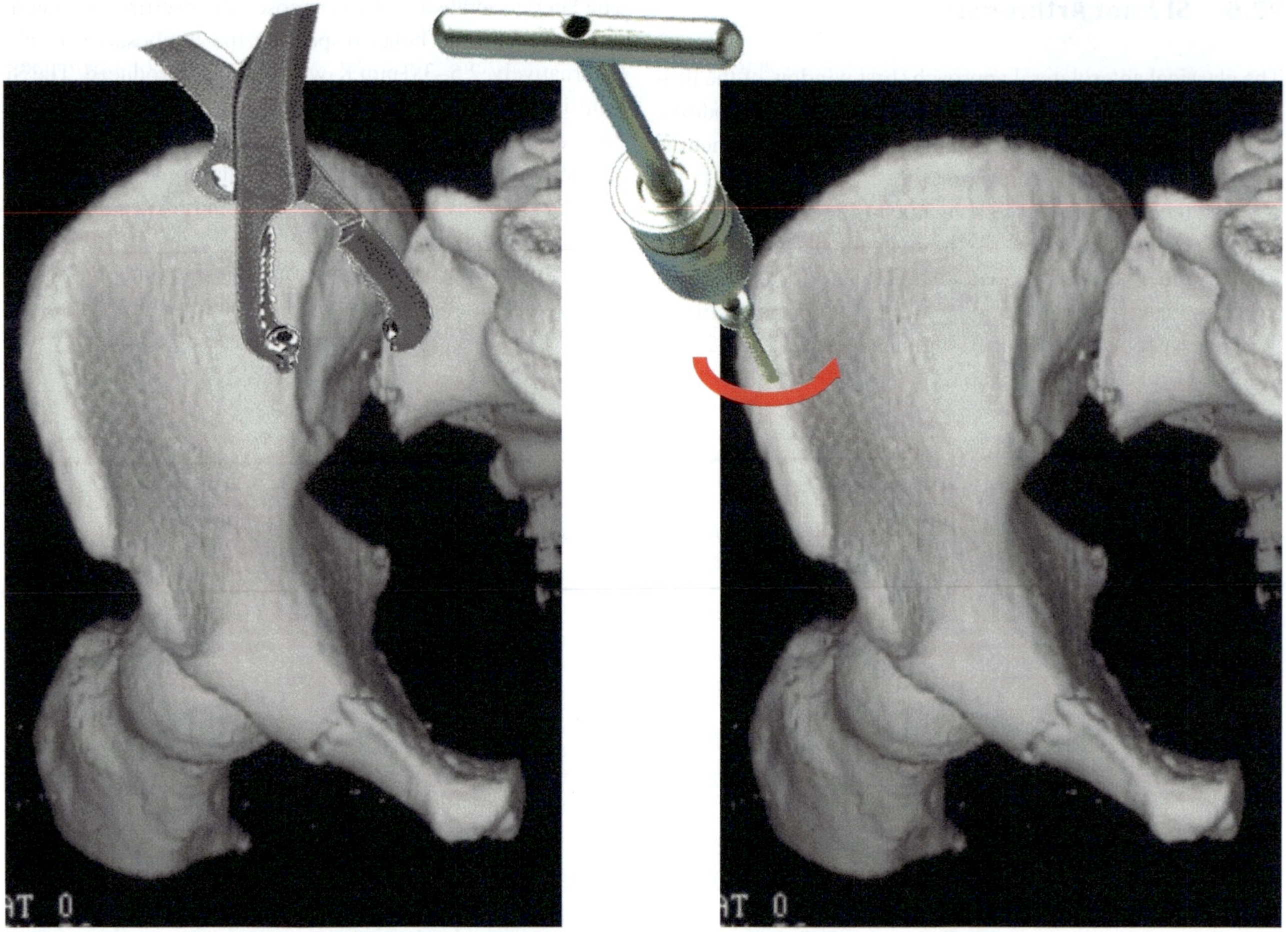

Fig. 42.18 SI joint reduction and compression using standard reduction maneuvers

sect the SI joint [25]. If necessary, the remaining iliolumbar ligaments have to be mobilized for full mobilization of the SI joint.

For preparing SI joint arthrodesis, drill holes are placed into the corresponding joint surfaces before reduction.

For SI joint reduction, several maneuvers can be used [25, 47]:

- Farabeuf or small Jungbluth clamps to control translation, posterior displacement, and to perform compression (Fig. 42.18)
- Iliac Schanz pins, supraacetabular external fixator/distractor or even pelvic C-clamps to control external rotation deformity (Fig. 42.18)

Before definitive stabilization of the SI joint, autologous cancellous bone and/or cortical bone blocks bone are inserted into the joint. Additionally, healing has been supported by bone morphogenic protein (BMP) sponges [25].

Fixation is performed by anterior SI joint plating and/or iliosacral screw fixation (Fig. 42.19) [1, 25].

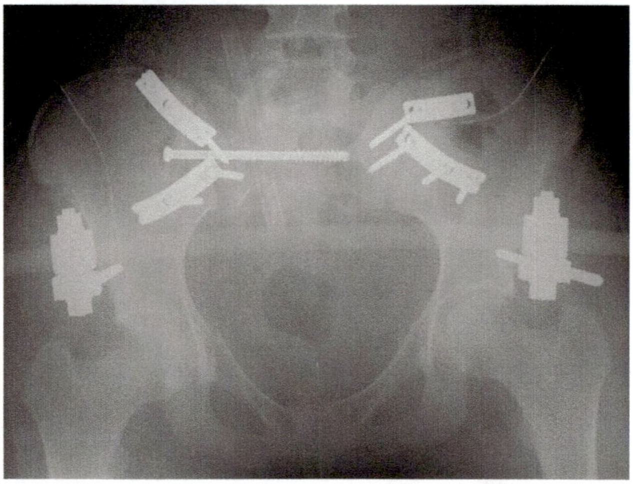

Fig. 42.19 Right anterior plating of the right SI joint with additional iliosacral screw fixation in an acute case

The SI joint can also be mobilized completely from posterior. Gautier et al. proposed this posterior fixation concept for SI joint nonunion [15]. He stated that only after nonanatomical reduction, primary anterior fusion is preferred.

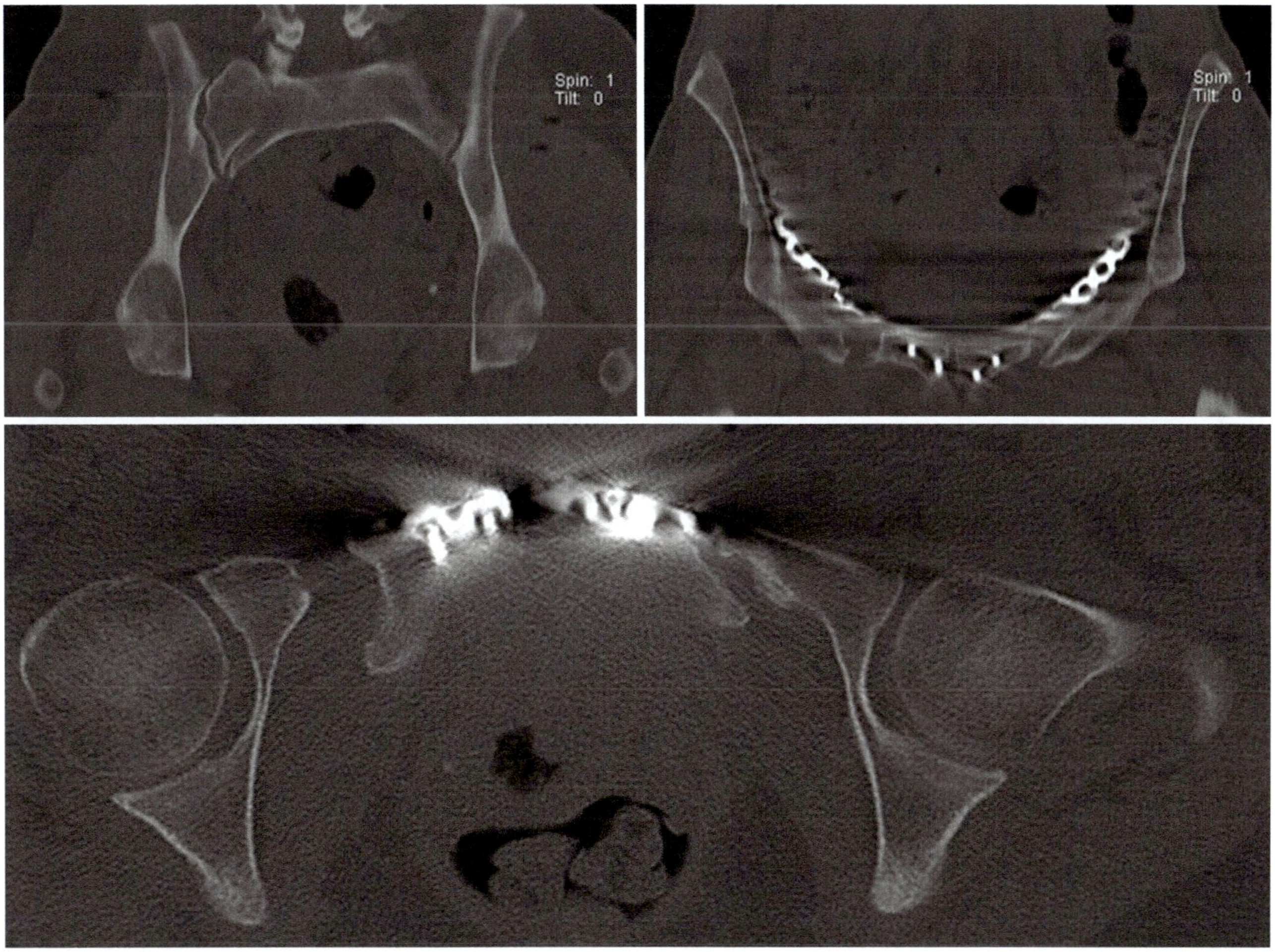

Fig. 42.20 Bilateral asymptomatic NU of the upper pubic ramus

In the prone position, a classical vertical posterior approach to the SI joint is used, slightly lateral to the iliac crest to avoid scar formation at the fulcrum. The SI joint is exposed by anterolateral mobilization of the gluteus maximus, starting at its junction to the erector spinae (see Chap. 29).

The SI joint is then dissected through the sacroiliac pit and the greater sciatic notch. The course of the gluteal neurovascular bundle has to be respected.

Frank et al. described a technique for SI joint arthrodesis using a nonvascularized autologous fibular strut graft [48]. In the prone position, a posterior approach to the SI joint was used for complete debridement of the SI joint. An iliosacral canal was developed using a 13 mm cannulated drill bit from a distal femoral nailing system. Two rows of 1.5 mm holes were created in the fibular graft. Press-fit insertion of the graft was performed by hammering the graft over a guide wire into the canal. Allogenic corticocancellous bone graft was used to fill remaining defects. For graft fixation, a screw inserted posteriorly was used. Neutralization plate osteosynthesis was performed with an ilioiliacal plate.

> The anterior approach for SI joint arthrodesis is preferred.

42.7 Anterior Pubic Rami Nonunion Treatment

Pubic rami nonunion may be completely asymptomatic if the posterior pelvic ring is healed and stable (Fig. 42.20) [49, 50]. Symptomatic nonunions of the superior ramus are treated by stable internal fixation with additional bone grafting. Atrophic nonunion is most often treated using plates [15].

If the pain is the main symptom and is attributable to nonunion, in situ fixation may be carried out [20, 51]. The standard approach is the intrapelvic approach [13], which allows adequate visualization of the entire superior pubic ramus for debridement of the nonunion site, approximation of the fracture ends, optional bone grafting of the gaps, and (supra)-

stable internal fixation, typically using a suprapectineal plate [13]. The inferior ramus is often atrophic and requires no additional treatment.

If necessary, the medial part of the inferior pubic ramus can be approached using the Pfannenstiel or intrapelvic incision, while for a more lateral exposure, an ischiopubic approach is chosen [43] or even the inferior part of the Kocher-Langenbeck approach.

Percutaneous retrograde superior pubic ramus screw fixation can be used for prolonged symptomatic NU of the superior pubic ramus [52, 53].

42.8 Sacral Nonunion

A posterior approach is favored for sacral nonunion treatment [15]. The classical direct posterior (median/paramedian) and the posterior-lateral approach according to Matta (Fig. 42.21) are both possible.

Additionally, preoperative evaluation should include analysis of ossifications between the L4 and L5 transverse processes and the iliac bone, which can clinically present in fixed lumbar spinal scoliosis [15].

The dissection technique as for sacral fractures is used to approach the nonunion site for debridement, decompression, and reduction (Fig. 42.21). Reduction techniques as described for sacral fractures and lumbopelvic fixations can be used to correct deformities.

Mobilization of the sacrotuberous and sacrospinal ligaments can be performed by direct dissection at the lateral sacral border for posterior pelvic release. The sacral nonunion is then cleaned until the anterior sacral aspect is reached. Sacral decompression is possible through the fracture line or by classical posterior laminectomy.

For stabilization of sacral NU, several options have been published:

- Lee et al. recommended 6.5 mm cannulated cancellous screw fixations after nonunion debridement and refreshing of the nonunion site. The excised bone was morselized and grafted. A supplementary anterior external fixator was additionally proposed [31].
- van den Bosch et al. published a case of sacral nonunion, which was exclusively treated by posterior percutaneous fixation using iliosacral lag screws [51].
- In another case, a transsacral fracture dislocation was fixed in the same way, without performing an arthrodesis of the SI joint. The disrupted symphysis was stabilized with two plates [51].

> Mechanical stability by compression stabilization can lead to uneventful healing, without nonunion debridement, when only minor malunion or LLD is present [51].

Additionally, partial hemilaminectomy, excision of the ligamentum flavum, and sacral nerve root decompression through the nonunion site are possible.

Kanezaki et al. reported on a young paraplegic patient with minor displaced bilateral sacral nonunion treated only with a transsacral bar and lumbopelvic fixation and observed bony healing within 1 year [54].

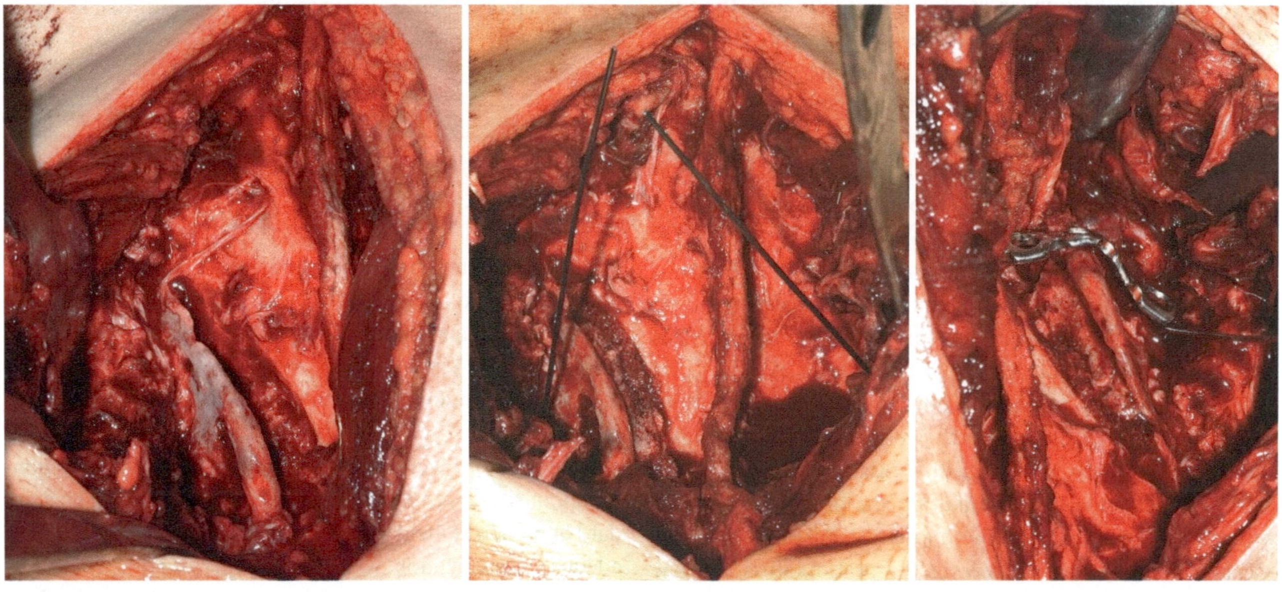

Fig. 42.21 Posterolateral approach (intraoperative): identification of the nonunion zone (left), bone grafting (middle), and iliosacral plate fixation bridging the right SI joint (right)

For sacral MU, Matta recommended an osteotomy lateral to the sacral foramina. Distraction can be achieved using an external fixator [11].

Corrective osteotomy of malunited sacral fractures with vertical displacement and associated heterotopic bone formation increases the risk of neurological complications, e.g., traction injuries of the lumbosacral nerve roots. Therefore, detailed nerve root neurolysis is recommended. Alternatively, an iliac osteotomy can be performed at the posterior part of the greater sciatic notch. Here, only neurolysis of the sciatic nerve is necessary [13].

42.8.1 Posterior L5 Nerve Root Decompression

The L5 nerve root can be affected in cranially displaced and malunited sacral fractures [55, 56].

Beside a detailed neurological examinations, preoperative diagnostics includes MRI of the lumbar or lumbosacral spine [55] or nerve root infiltration and CT radiculography [56].

Taguchi et al. treated a case with cranial displacement of a malunited sacral fracture with iliac bone osteotomy with decompression of the L5 nerve root through the opened osteotomy. Decompression was performed with lateral sacral bone debridement, until the nerve root was sufficiently free [56].

Alexander et al. reported on four patients with a persistent L5 nerve root lesion after malhealed sacral fractures [55]. Decompression of L5 was performed in the prone position using a standard midline approach (Figs. 42.19 and 42.20).

Typically, a median or slightly paramedian longitudinal incision is performed to address the posterior sacral surface. After classical dissection, the posterior sacral surface is identified until reaching the L5/S1 facet joint. The multifidus and longissimus muscles are mobilized laterally until reaching the posterior iliac crest.

The base of the L5 transverse process and the lateral aspect of the facet joint are digitally identified. Lateral to the L5–S1 facet joint, the posterior sacral border and the upper rim of the sacrum with the costal process are palpated. These structures are located deep in the surgical field.

From the authors' experience, relevant bleeding is often present during posterior decompression of the L5 nerve root, and, therefore, this approach is not favored.

After identification of these bony landmarks, Alexander et al. recommended high-speed drilling, which starts at the base of the superior S1 articular process (= medial wall of the paraarticular notch) and progresses superiorly. One third of the lateral facet joint can be removed without compromising joint stability (Fig. 42.22). Then, the inferior border of the medial L5 transverse process is removed to widen the usually, posttraumatic narrow interval between the sacral shoulder and the transverse process. The iliolumbar ligament is removed using a punch. The neurovascular bundle and the surrounding fat tissue are carefully dissected. Potential osteophytes from the vertebral body beneath the nerve are removed using curette, tamp, and/or mallets, until the L5 nerve root is clearly identified.

Anterior decompression of the lumbosacral trunk can more easily be performed using the first window of the ilioinguinal approach (Fig. 42.16) or using the pararectus approach [57].

42.9 Iliac Nonunion Treatment/Transiliac Osteotomy

The ilium is approached using the first window of the ilioinguinal approach or the posterior approach, depending on the localization of the nonunion site.

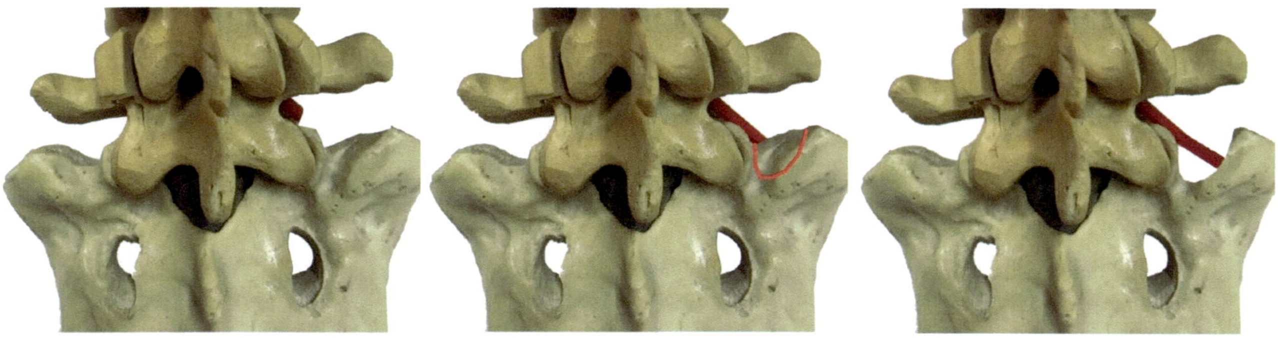

Fig. 42.22 L5/lumbosacral trunk decompression from posterior. After resection of the ligament between the L5 transverse process and the posterior sacrum, additionally, a small osteotomy of the posterior sacral ala can be performed to completely visualize the L5/lumbosacral trunk from posterior

Debridement of the NU is performed using standardized techniques until full mobility is achieved. In rare cases, both approaches can be necessary in a floppy lateral position of the patient.

In malhealed ilium fractures, an osteotomy should be considered. Lu et al. performed an iliac osteotomy in eight patients with malhealed type C injuries [4]. Preoperatively, the exact leg length difference has to be analyzed for defining the amount of necessary correction.

An iliac crest graft was taken using a Smith-Peterson incision (alternatively an ilioinguinal approach), slightly greater than the intended limb length correction. The osteotomy starts between the ASIS and AIIS and exits at the greater sciatic notch (Fig. 42.18). The osteotomy zone is distracted using a laminar spreader and/or by traction (Fig. 42.18). A traction table can be helpful to protect the contralateral hemipelvis. The iliac crest graft is inserted into the osteotomy zone by a press-fit technique, and the osteotomy gap is fixed with plates and screws.

42.10 Hemipelvic Correction

For hemipelvic correction, a combination of both anterior and posterior procedures is usually necessary. No clear concept can be advised from an analysis of the literature.

Matta, Mears, and Oransky highlighted a three-staged concept for treating pelvic NUs and MUs that can be either anterior-posterior-anterior or more commonly posterior-anterior-posterior [5, 11, 13].

Additionally, two-staged approaches and in some special situations even one-stage approaches can be used [1, 5, 11, 13, 58].

42.10.1 Concept Proposed by Cano-Luis

Cano-Luís et al. reported the above-mentioned classification, based on residual or complex instability, which also guides a treatment concept.

Parameters include pelvic ring deformity, pain localization, leg length discrepancy, sitting imbalance, and a stability testing [1].

42.10.1.1 Type I Reconstruction (Isolated Anterior Residual Instability)

In patients with residual instability of the anterior pelvic ring, two pathologies can be present: rotational instability due to instability of the pubic symphysis, or mal/nonunion of the pubic rami.

Arthrodesis of the pubic symphysis using an autologous bone block with single- or double-plate stabilization is the treatment of choice. Instabilities at the superior rami can be best treated by fracture/nonunion debridement, optional autologous cancellous bone grafting, and intrapelvic, suprapectineal plate stabilization. Additional iliosacral screw fixation was recommended in some cases to support symphyseal arthrodesis.

42.10.1.2 Type II Reconstruction (Isolated Posterior Residual Instability)

Isolated residual instability of the posterior pelvic ring can present as SI joint instability often with degenerative changes, and NUs of vertical sacral fractures with or without unilateral injury of the L5–S1 facet joint.

- SI joint problems can be addressed by anterior plate arthrodesis.
- Sacral NU can be treated by NU debridement, autologous cancellous bone grafting, or insertion of a bone block and osteosynthesis, dependent on fracture morphology, e.g., ilioiliacal stabilization techniques, sacral plating, or iliosacral screw fixation.
- Additional involvement of the L5/S1 facet joint can be treated by posterolateral arthrodesis with cancellous -cortical autograft and fixation with spinopelvic instrumentation.

42.10.1.3 Type III Reconstruction

Type III residual instability can result from more extended anterior-posterior compression injuries (APC II-III) or sacral nonunion with anterior and posterior instability:

- Rotational instability is treated by symphyseal arthrodesis stabilized with single or double plating and bone grafting, followed by SI joint arthrodesis; a combination of two different posterior types of osteosynthesis is recommended, e.g., anterior SI joint plating with additional iliosacral screw fixation; usually a one-stage reconstruction is favored.
- Sacral nonunion is usually treated using a two-stage procedure [59], first debridement, autografting, and osteosynthesis of the sacral nonunion is performed with two different stabilizations methods; after changing patient position, anterior stabilization is performed.

Whenever possible a two-stage procedure is preferred as three-stage procedures (first anterior mobilization in supine position, second posterior mobilization with new osteosynthesis and bone grafting, third anterior arthrodesis in supine position), were associated with higher blood loss and complication rates [5, 8, 11, 13, 16].

42.10.1.4 Complex Deformities

Complex deformities always require a staged surgery concept [1]. Intraoperative SEP monitoring is recommended during reduction maneuvers [15, 51].

42.10.1.5 Complex Type IA Instabilities (LLD <3 cm)

Type IA instabilities represent malhealed pelvic ring injuries associated with a LLD <3 cm. A sequential, usually three-staged treatment concept is favored [1]:

1. Anterior: supine, symphyseal mobilization or pubic rami osteotomy; iliac or SI joint osteotomy, rarely sacral osteotomy
2. Posterior: prone, traction table, or table-skeletal fixation system [60], dissection/mobilization pelvic floor and iliolumbar ligaments, complete removal of all callus/fibrous tissues; correction of LLD by spinopelvic reduction and fixation; correction of rotational and flexion deformity [5]; posterior osteosynthesis using combined stabilization systems
3. Anterior: supine position, osteosynthesis/arthrodesis anterior ring ± cancellous-cortical autograft

42.10.1.6 Complex Type IB Instabilities (LLD >3 cm)

Type IB instabilities represent malhealed pelvic ring injuries associated with a LLD >3 cm. A sequential, usually three-staged treatment concept is favored by Cano-Luís et al. [1]:

1. Anterior: supine, symphyseal mobilization, or pubic rami osteotomy; iliac or SI joint osteotomy, rarely sacral osteotomy
2. Progressive transcondylar skeletal traction over 7–10 days with increasing weight under regular neurovascular and radiological examinations
3. Posterior osteosynthesis/arthrodesis surgery: the healthy hemipelvis has to be secured to the operating table

NUs (type II instabilities) are treated comparable to type I lesions.

Persistent sitting imbalance can be addressed by palliative resection of the sciatic tuberosity on the healthy side [11, 13].

42.10.1.7 Concept Proposed by Guimarães

An anterior-posterior-anterior concept for SI joint injuries was proposed by Guimarães [58] for type C1.2 injuries with vertical and rotational hemipelvic deformities, circumferential ossification around the SI joint, and symphyseal diastasis:

1. Ilioinguinal approach: SI joint release with/without fixation of the anterior sacroiliac joint
2. Posterior SI joint approach: release and fixation of the posterior SI joint
3. Pfannenstiel approach: reduction and fixation of the pubic symphysis (double plating)

A posterior-anterior-posterior concept for SI joint injuries was proposed for type C1.2 injuries with vertical and rotational hemipelvic deformities, and predominant posterior ossification around the SI joint and symphyseal diastasis:

1. Posterior SI joint approach: release of the posterior SI joint
2. Pfannenstiel approach: reduction and fixation of the pubic symphysis (double plating)
3. Posterior SI joint approach: posterior fixation of the SI joint

Guimarães et al. presented a case with a posteriorly displaced SI joint in combination with a wide symphyseal diastasis treated with a posterior-anterior-posterior concept [58].

The SI joint area was first osteotomized posteriorly in the prone position from cranial to caudal in a 15° angulation lateral to the foraminal zone with thin osteotomes. At the anterior part of the joint, a thin bony layer remained intact to protect the neurovascular structures, which was then removed using a Kerrison punch Rongeur.

In the second surgical step, in the supine position, the displaced pubic symphysis was reduced, and an arthrodesis with a tricortical bone graft and double plating was performed.

The third step consisted of posterior reduction with a spinopelvic fixation system and posterior SI joint fusion with a bone graft in the prone position.

A two-staged anterior-posterior concept was sufficient for deformities with minimal vertical displacements and minimal opening of the pubic symphysis:

1. Ilioinguinal: anterior release of the SI joint, pubic symphysis stabilization
2. Posterior SI joint approach: posterior fixation of the SI joint

An isolated posterior stabilization concept is favored in cases with vertical and/or rotational deformities with only minimal opening of the pubic symphysis [58]. This deformity is present around a horizontal/vertical rotational axis at the pubic symphysis.

With a posterior SI joint approach, posterior release and fixation of the SI joint are performed.

An isolated anterior approach is possible for plate arthrodesis of the SI joint from anterior.

42.11 Other Recommendations

Due to the individuality of NU and MU treatments, several other recommendations were reported:

- Gautier recommended double plating of the symphysis in cases with previous implant failure or direct symphyseal arthrodesis and a posterior fixation concept for SI joint nonunions [15]. Only after nonanatomical reduction, primary anterior fusion was preferred.
- Indications for an isolated anterior approach (ilioinguinal, Pfannenstiel) are rotational deformities with integrity of the posterior SI joint structures and only anterior opening of the SI joint (type B1 deformities) [58]. When the SI joint is predominantly intact, only reduction and fixation of the pubic symphysis can be performed using the Pfannenstiel incision.
- A relevant intraoperative step is to release the contracted iliolumbar, anterior sacroiliac ligaments anteriorly [25].
- Simple nonunions without deformities may be addressed by a simple one- or two-staged procedure targeting the nonunion site [11].
- Rousseau et al. recommended a two-stage approach to address malhealing and nonunions after type B and C injuries [59].
- First, the posterior pelvis is addressed in the prone position for posterior SI joint and pelvic floor ligament release, followed by an ilioinguinal approach (most commonly only the first and third windows are in use) to address the pubic symphysis and/or the pubic rami. The anterior SI joint ligament release is performed anteriorly.
- Reduction is performed using axial traction on the traction table, and correction of malrotation is performed using several available reduction forceps.
- Fixation is performed with two percutaneous applied iliosacral screws and/or anterior plate, while the anterior pelvis is fixed with a plate. In case of posterior SI joint reconstruction, two symphyseal plates were preferred.
- Lee et al. proposed the ilioinguinal approach for anterior release and stabilization of anterior NU and MU [24].

42.12 General Recommendations

Some general statements can be gained from the literature dealing with pelvic NU or MU:

- In complex cases, multidisciplinary surgery is recommended including urologists, plastic surgeons, and gynecologists, especially when bladder mobilization, vaginopexy, urethrostomy, and reconstruction of the pelvic floor are necessary. Potentially, this has to be performed as a first step before secondary reconstruction of the bone ring [25].
- Neural monitoring using somatosensory-evoked potentials should be considered during NU and MU treatments [20].
- As a general rule, after hemipelvic mobilization, reduction is often easier to achieve using an anterior approach [43].
- BMP-7 application in pelvic nonunion treatments can support bone healing [61, 62].
- In pelvic MU, urinary tract symptoms can be addressed with bladder mobilization and excision of prominent bone, while a Foley catheter is in place [14].
- If leg length discrepancy is the major complaint, limb shortening is considered an option when no pelvic pain or deformity is present; if limb lengthening is required, distraction osteogenesis should be discussed and in complex situations, uni- or bilateral innominate osteotomy can solve this problem.

> Possibly due to high forces acting on late reduced deformities, combined fixation methods seem to be superior to standard osteosyntheses, e.g., double-plate stabilization of the symphysis and iliosacral screw fixation, and plate osteosynthesis of the SI joint or sacrum [1, 51].

42.13 Results

Matta reported results of 37 pelvic malunions and nonunions [11]. In 95% a three-staged reconstruction was performed either in a posterior-anterior-posterior or anterior-posterior-anterior sequence.

In the first step, osteotomy of malunions or mobilization of nonunions was performed followed by complete osteotomy and/or mobilization in the opposite way. The last step completed the reduction and fixation. Osteotomies were usually performed at the old injury sites. The mean operative time was 7 h (range, 1.5–10.4 h), and the mean observed blood loss was 1977 mL (range, 200–7200 mL).

Thirty-six patients presented with bony healing at an average of 3 years. Surgical complications included 8% neurologic injury and one vascular injury (3%). No surgical infections were observed. 32/37 patients showed adequate improvements of their clinical impairments.

Lindahl et al. reported on overall 37 delayed (between 22 and 42 days from injury) and late (>6 weeks from injury) reconstructions from a group of 401 pelvic ring injuries

(9.2%) [63]. Pelvic injuries consisted of 3 type A2 iliac wing fractures, 5 B1/B3-1 open book injuries, 3 B2/B3-2 lateral compression fractures, 26 C1–C3 fractures, and one H-type spinopelvic dissociation. In all type A and B injuries and in the case of spinopelvic dissociation, all patients had good to excellent clinical and radiological results. Vertical shear injuries were associated with 80.7% good and excellent radiological results. Loss of reduction occurred due to osteoporosis in two cases, a malunion with final displacement >10 mm was observed in 13%, anterior nonunion occurred in one patient, and one patient had signs of superficial wound infection while no deep wound infection was seen.

Mears et al. reported on 70 pelvic nonunions and 134 malalignments [13]. The mean follow-up was 8.7 years (2–20).

Overall, primary union was achieved in 96% and no persistent instability was present. Seventy-one percent reported no or only slight pain. 92.6% were satisfied with the result of the treatment. In contrast, pelvic malunions could be reconstructed anatomically in only 50%.

Undisplaced nonunions showed 100% satisfactory results. Patients with stable and united malalignment were associated with 98% satisfactory results and 90% adequate deformity correction.

Unstable, nonunited malalignment cases showed 87% satisfactory results and 89% adequate deformity correction.

Risk factors for worse results included unstable malalignments, present with ossifications. In these patients, the rate of inadequate reconstructions and neurological complications was increased.

Pelvic nonunions with local osteopenia and malalignment were best treated with fixation of all three columns.

Local resection of symptomatic bony prominences and in situ fixation of posterior nonunions were associated with adequate symptom relief but persistent low back pain.

Oransky et al. analyzed 55 patients with 44 malunions and 11 nonunions [5]. An anterior-posterior-anterior multistage procedure was performed. The mean duration of surgery was 6 h (range: 2–10 h), with a mean blood loss of 700 mL (range: 200–5000 mL). At a mean follow-up of 5.8 years, 54 patients presented with bony healing and a stable pelvis. Walking ability improved in all patients. Twenty-one percent had a nonanatomic pelvic ring reconstruction.

> Acceptable long-term results after pelvic MUs and NUs can be achieved in experienced hands (Figs. 42.22, 42.23, and 42.24).

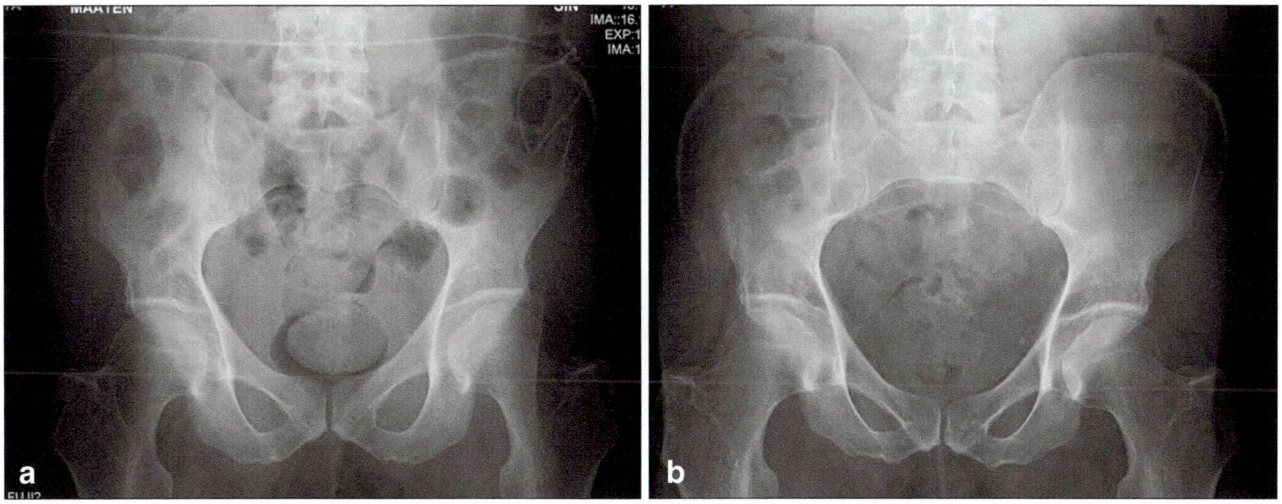

Fig. 42.23 Late reconstruction of nonunion of the right iliac wing fracture (A2) with malalignment. Initially, a 57-year-old male got a minimally displaced iliac wing fracture, which was treated nonoperatively (**a**). Two months later, some caudal displacement of the iliac crest fragment was seen, and the patient had anterior pelvic pain and irritation of the lateral femoral cutaneous nerve (**b**). After 10 months the patient was still symptomatic and the pelvic CT images showed non-united malunion (**c**–**e**). At that time late reconstruction was performed through the first window of ilioinguinal approach. (**f**) Nonunion debridement, autologous cancellous bone grafting, and 3.5 mm reconstruction plate and screw fixation was performed. Fracture healed within 3 months without any complications

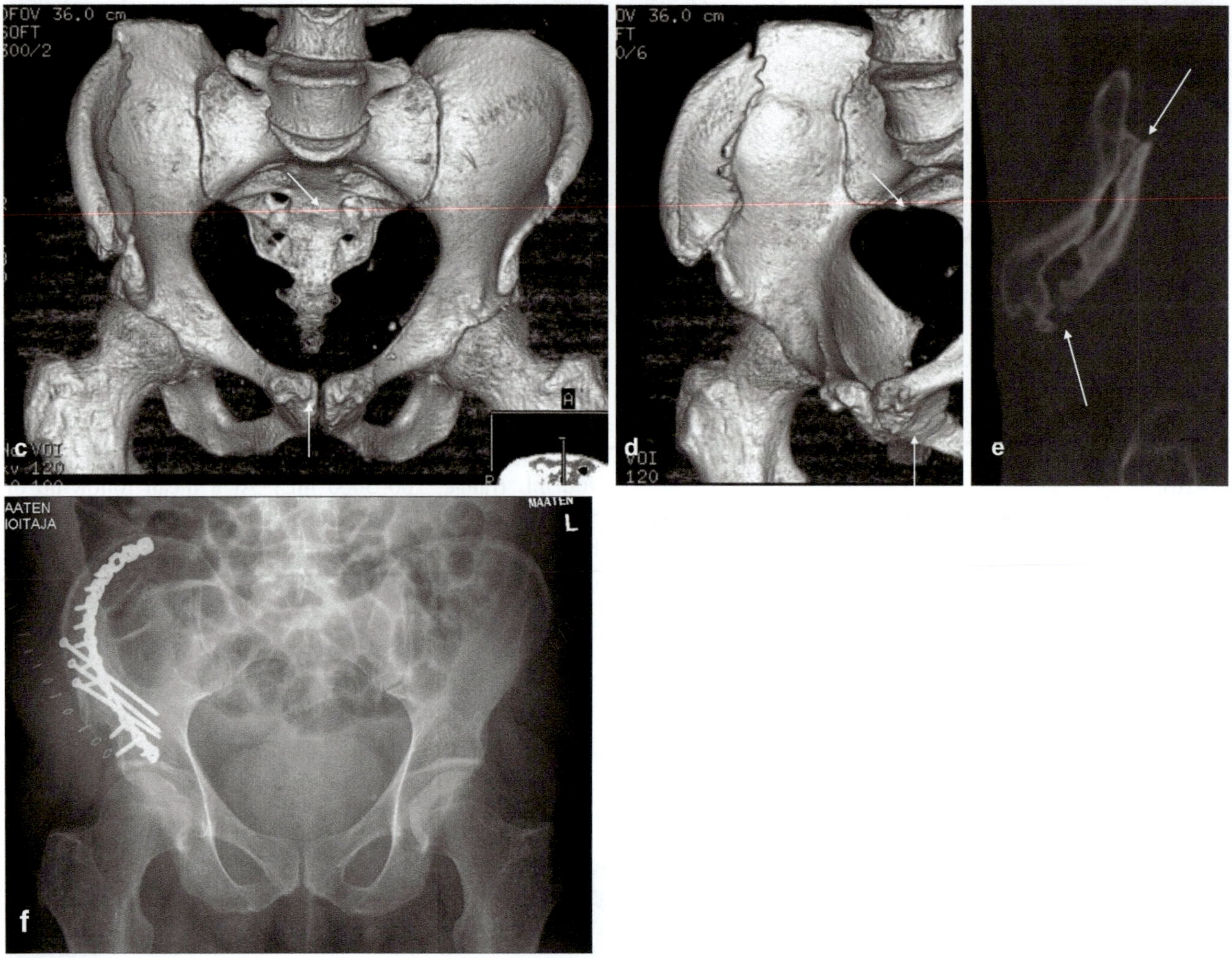

Fig. 42.23 (continued)

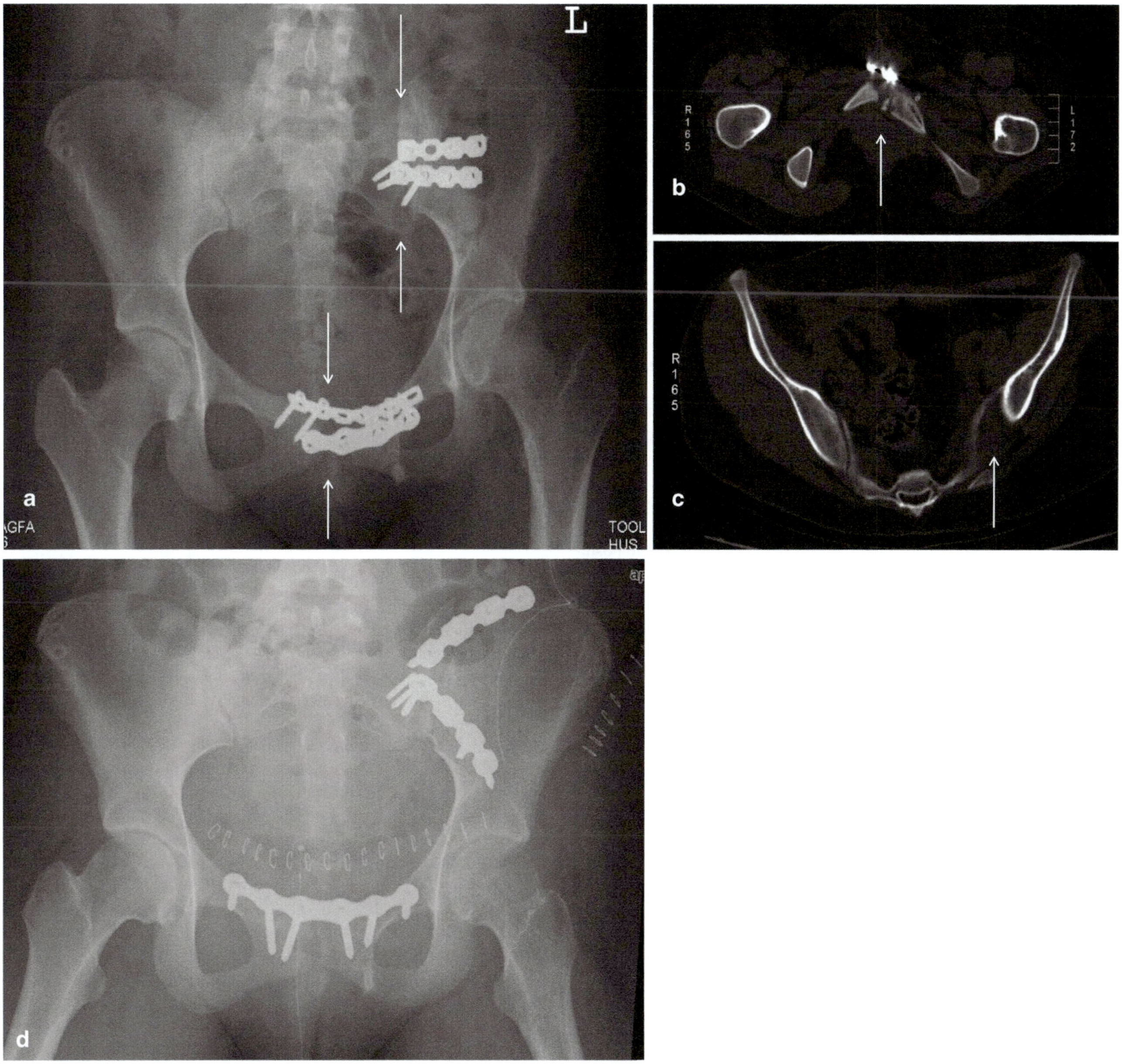

Fig. 42.24 One-stage reconstruction of vertically and rotationally unstable nonunited left hemipelvis with vertical and rotational malalignment. A 17-year-old female injured in a motorbike accident sustaining an AO/OTA type C1.2 injury to the left hemipelvis. The primary fixation of the left dislocated SI joint was performed through an anterior approach with two parallel 3.5 mm reconstruction plates and the disrupted symphysis pubis with two plates with 3.5 mm screws. (**a–c**) Loss of reduction and malalignment because of insufficient fixation was seen early. After 8 months the patient had severe pain in the posterior and anterior pelvis with difficulties to walk with crutches due to gait instability and leg length discrepancy. (**d**) At eighth month a late reconstruction was carried out by using simultaneous intrapelvic approach and approach along the iliac crest to reduce and stabilize both the posterior and anterior pelvic ring injuries. SI joint was stabilized with two 4.5 mm reconstruction plates positioned at nearly 90° angle to each other and the symphysis pubis with 4.5 mm symphyseal Matta plate. The end radiological and functional results were good

References

1. Cano-Luís P, Giráldez-Sánchez M, Andrés-Cano P. Pelvic post-traumatic asymmetry: assessment and sequenced treatment. EFORT Open Rev. 2018;3(5):335–46. https://doi.org/10.1302/2058-5241.3.170069.
2. Lindahl J, Hirvensalo E. Outcome of operatively treated type-C injuries of the pelvic ring. Acta Orthop. 2005;76:667–78.
3. Lindahl J, Hirvensalo E, Bostman O, Santavirta S. Failure of reduction with an external fixator in the management of injuries of the pelvic ring. Long-term evaluation of 110 patients. J Bone Joint Surg Br. 1999;81(6):955–62.
4. Lu S, Wu J, Fu B, Dong J, Yang Y, Xin M, Wang G, He T, Zhou D. Transiliac osteotomy in surgical management of pelvic post-traumatic malunions: a retrospective study. Medicine (Baltimore). 2016;95(13):e3144. https://doi.org/10.1097/MD.0000000000003144.
5. Oransky M, Tortora M. Nonunions and malunions after pelvic fractures: why they occur and what can be done? Injury. 2007;38:489–96.
6. Pohlemann T, Gänsslen A, Schellwald O, Culemann U, Tscherne H. Outcome after pelvic ring injuries. Injury. 1996;27(Suppl 2):S-B31–8.
7. Tornetta P, Matta J. Outcome of operatively treated unstable posterior pelvic ring disruptions. Clin Orthop. 1996;329:186–93.
8. Kanakaris N, Angoules A, Nikolaou V, Kontakis G, Giannoudis P. Treatment and outcomes of pelvic malunions and nonunions: a systematic review. Clin Orthop. 2009;467:2112–24.
9. Hundley J. Ununited unstable fractures of the pelvis. J Bone Joint Surg. 1966;48-A(5):1025.
10. Kellam J. The role of external fixation in pelvic disruptions. Clin Orthop. 1989;241:66–82.
11. Matta J, Dickson K, Markovich G. Surgical treatment of pelvic nonunions and malunions. Clin Orthop. 1996;329:199–206.
12. Pennal G, Massiah K. Nonunion and delayed union of fractures of the pelvis. Clin Orthop Relat Res. 1980;151:124–9.
13. Mears D, Velyvis J. Surgical reconstruction of late pelvic post-traumatic nonunion and malalignment. J Bone Joint Surg Br. 2003;85:21–30.
14. Tile M. Fractures of the pelvis and acetabulum. 2nd ed. Baltimore: Williams & Wilkins; 1995.
15. Gautier E, Rommens P, Matta J. Late reconstruction after pelvic ring injuries. Injury. 1996;27(Suppl 2):39–46.
16. Tripathy S, Goyal T, Sen R. Nonunions and malunions of the pelvis. Eur J Trauma Emerg Surg. 2015;41:335–42.
17. Herren C, Dienstknecht T, Siewe J, Kobbe P, Pape H, Hildebrand F. Chronic instability of the pubic symphysis: etiology, diagnostics and treatment management. Unfallchirurg. 2016;119:433–46.
18. Avilucea F, Whiting P, Mir H. Posterior fixation of APC-2 pelvic ring injuries decreases rates of anterior plate failure and malunion. J Bone Joint Surg. 2016;98-Am:944–51.
19. Isler B. Lumbosacral lesions associated with pelvic ring injuries. J Orthop Trauma. 1990;4(1):1–6.
20. Sen R, Goyal T, Tripathy S. Neglected pelvic fractures: an overview of literature. J Orthop Traumatol Rehabil. 2014;7:43–7.
21. Matta J, Saucedo T. Internal fixation of pelvic ring fractures. Clin Orthop. 1989;242:83–97.
22. Sagi H, Coniglione F, Stanford J. Examination under anesthetic for occult pelvic ring instability. J Orthop Trauma. 2011;25:529–36.
23. Whiting P, Auston D, Avilucea F, Ross D, Archdeacon M, Sciadini M, Collinge C, Sagi H, Mir H. Negative stress examination under anesthesia reliably predicts pelvic ring union without displacement. J Orthop Trauma. 2017;31:189–93.
24. Lee K, Min B, Oh G, Lee S. Surgical correction of pelvic malunion and nonunion. Clin Orthop Surg. 2015;7:396–401.
25. Fang C, Alabdulrahman H, Pfeifer R, Tarkin I, Pape H. Late reconstruction of severe open-book deformities of the pelvis—tips and tricks. Int Orthop. 2017;41:1777–84.
26. Ter-Grigorian A, Kasyan G, Pushkar D. Urogenital disorders after pelvic ring injuries. Cent Eur J Urol. 2013;66:352–6.
27. Pape HC, Pohlemann T, Gansslen A, Simon R, Koch C, Tscherne H. Pelvic fractures in pregnant multiple trauma patients. J Orthop Trauma. 2000;14(4):238–44.
28. Wright J, Nathens A, Rivara F, MacKenzie E, Wessells H. Specific fracture configurations predict sexual and excretory dysfunction in men and women 1 year after pelvic fracture. J Urol. 2006;176:1540–5.
29. Vallier H, Cureton B, Schubeck D. Pregnancy outcomes after pelvic ring injury. J Orthop Trauma. 2012;26:302–7.
30. Zhao J, Zhao C, Zhang L, Su X, Du H, Zhang L, Zhang L, Tang P. A computer aided measurement method for unstable pelvic fractures based on standardized radiographs. BMC Med Imaging. 2015;15:41. https://doi.org/10.1186/s12880-015-0084-x.
31. Lee S, Niikura T, Sakai Y, Miwa M, Nishida K, Kuroda R, Kurosaka M. Sacral fracture nonunion treated by bone grafting through a posterior approach. Case Rep Orthop. 2013;2013:932521. https://doi.org/10.1155/2013/932521.
32. Kurz S, Pieroh P, Lenk M, Josten C, Böhme J. Three-dimensional reduction and finite element analysis improves the treatment of pelvic malunion reconstructive surgery. A case report. Medicine (Baltimore). 2017;96:42.
33. Dickson K, Matta J. Surgical reduction and stabilization of pelvic nonunion and malunions. In: American Academy of Orthopedic Surgeons, 63rd Annual Meeting. Atlanta, USA. 1996.
34. Sponseller P, Bisson L, Gearhart J, Jeffs R, Magid D, Fishman E. The anatomy of the pelvis in the exstrophy complex. J Bone Joint Surg. 1995;77-Am:177–89.
35. Keshishyan R, Rozinov V, Malakhov O, Kuznetsov L, Strunin E, Chogovadze G, Tsukanov V. Pelvic polyfractures in children—radiographic diagnosis and treatment. Clin Orthop. 1995;320:28–33.
36. Stover M, Lack W. Malunion and nonunion of the pelvis: posttraumatic deformity. In: Tile, et al., editors. Fractures of the pelvis and acetabulum. AO Trauma. New York: Thieme; 2015. p. 415–24.
37. Stover M, Matta J. Malunion and nonunion of the pelvis: posttraumatic deformity. In: Tile, et al., editors. Fractures of the pelvis and acetabulum. 3rd ed. Philadelphia: Lippincott, Williams & Wilkins; 2003. p. 400–8.
38. Sagi H, Militano U, Caron T, Lindvall E. A comprehensive analysis with minimum 1-year follow-up of vertically unstable transforaminal sacral fractures treated with triangular osteosynthesis. J Orthop Trauma. 2009;23:313–9.
39. Lefaivre K, Blachut P, Starr A, Slobogean G, O'Brien P. Radiographic displacement in pelvic ring disruption: reliability of 3 previously described measurement techniques. J Orthop Trauma. 2014;28:160–6.
40. Nystrom L, McKinley T, Marsh J. Accuracy in radiographic assessment of pelvic ring fracture deformity: analysis of current methods. J Orthop Trauma. 2013;27:708–15.
41. Boontanapibul K, Harnroongroj T, Sudjai N, Harnroongroj T. Vertical pelvic ring displacement in pelvic ring injury: measurements in pelvic outlet radiograph and in cadavers. Indian J Orthop. 2015;49:425–8.
42. Nystrom L, McKinley T, Marsh J. Radiographic measurement of rotational deformity in pelvic fractures: a novel method with validity and reliability testing. J Orthop Trauma. 2015;29:365–9.
43. Mears D. Das Management von Beckenpseudarthrosen und Beckenfehlstellungen. Orthopade. 1996;25(5):441–9.
44. Taller S, Srám J, Lukás R, Krivohlávek M. [Nonunions or malunions of pelvic fractures]. Acta Chir Orthop Traumatol Cechoslov. 2009;76:121–7.

45. Frigon V, Dickson K. Open reduction internal fixation of a pelvic malunion through an anterior approach. J Orthop Trauma. 2001;15:519–24.
46. Olerud S, Walheim G. Symphysiodesis with a new compression plate. Acta Orthop Scand. 1984;55:315–8.
47. Gänsslen A, Pohlemann T, Krettek C. Internal fixation of sacroiliac joint disruption. Oper Orthop Traumatol. 2005;17:281–95.
48. Frank M, McCallum J, Dědek T. Fibular strut graft for posterior pelvic ring nonunion—a case report. Acta Chir Orthop Traumatol Cechoslov. 2017;84:211–4.
49. Leighton R. Nonunions and malunions of the pelvis. In: Chapman MW, editor. Operative orthopaedics. Philadelphia: Lippincott Company; 1988. p. 545–54.
50. Tile M. Fractures of the pelvis and acetabulum. Baltimore: Williams & Wilkins; 1984.
51. van den Bosch E, van der Kleyn R, Zwienen C, van Vugt A. Nonunion of unstable fractures of the pelvis. Eur J Trauma. 2002;2:100–3.
52. Akagi M, Ikeda N, Fukiage K, Nakamura T. A modification of the retrograde medullary screw for the treatment of bilateral pubic ramus nonunions: a case report. J Orthop Trauma. 2002;16:431–3.
53. Altman G, Altman D, Routt MJ. Symptomatic hypertrophic pubic ramus nonunion treated with a retrograde medullary screw. J Orthop Trauma. 2000;14:582–5.
54. Kanezaki S, Rommens P. Bilateral nonunion of the sacrum in a long-term paraplegic patient treated with trans-sacral bar and spinopelvic fixation. Arch Orthop Trauma Surg. 2015;135:345–9.
55. Alexander J, Brennan M, Rahm M. L5 nerve root decompression after malunion of surgically managed vertically unstable pelvic ring injuries. Am J Orthop. 2013;42:23–5.
56. Taguchi T, Kawai S, Kaneko K, Yugue D. Surgical treatment of old pelvic fractures. Int Orthop. 2000;24:28–32.
57. Keel M, Ecker T, Cullmann J, Bergmann M, Bonel H, Büchler L, Siebenrock K, Bastian J. The Pararectus approach for anterior intrapelvic management of acetabular fractures: an anatomical study and clinical evaluation. J Bone Joint Surg Br. 2012;94:405–11.
58. Guimarães J, Rocha V, Barcellos A. Posterior sacroiliac osteotomy: an alternative to the ilioinguinal approach for pelvic reconstruction in misalignment lesions. Rev Bras Ortop. 2017;52:63–8.
59. Rousseau M, Laude MF, Lazennec J, Saillant G, Catonné Y. Two-stage surgical procedure for treating pelvic malunions. Int Orthop. 2006;30:338–41.
60. Matta J, Yerasimides J. Table-skeletal fixation as an adjunct to pelvic ring reduction. J Orthop Trauma. 2007;21:647–56.
61. Giannoudis P, Psarakis S, Kanakaris N, Pape H. Biological enhancement of bone healing with Bone Morphogenetic Protein-7 at the clinical setting of pelvic girdle non-unions. Injury. 2007;38:43–8.
62. Nicodemo A, Capella M, Deregibus M, Massè A. Nonunion of a sacral fracture refractory to bone grafting: internal fixation and osteogenic protein-1 (BMP-7) application. Musculoskelet Surg. 2011;95:157–61.
63. Lindahl J. Delayed and late reconstructions of the pelvis. Finn Orthop Traumatol. 2011;34:43–8.

Outcome After Pelvic Ring Injuries

43

Axel Gänsslen and Jan Lindahl

In the literature, there is a lack of adequate long-term follow-up studies on pelvic ring fractures as the majority of reports are only dealing with emergency management and initial treatment, describing several techniques to treat these injuries and reporting on short-term results including surgery-related complications and quality of reduction.

> Additionally, there is a lack of adequate evaluation instruments. It is still today unclear which parameters should be analyzed or correlated with fracture types and treatment concepts.

For example, an analysis of results of symphyseal plating can be influenced by several parameters, including fracture type, performed posterior stabilization, type of posterior stabilization, type of plate, local soft-tissue injuries, accompanying intrapelvic organ injuries, concomitant whole body injuries etc.

It is generally accepted to distinguish pelvic ring injuries as stable, partially stable, or unstable according to Marvin Tile's classification or the AO/OTA classification.

Therefore, results should be analyzed regarding these fracture groups or even depending on the chosen stabilization method.

During the last decade, several reports were published regarding outcome evaluation after stabilization of vertically unstable type C injuries of the pelvic ring, whereas type B injuries were of minor interest.

A. Gänsslen (✉)
Department of Trauma Surgery, Orthopedics and Hand Surgery, Hospital Wolfsburg, Wolfsburg, Germany

J. Lindahl
Orthopaedics and Trauma Surgery, Helsinki University Hospital, Helsinki, Finland

43.1 Accepted Outcome Instruments

Outcome instruments can be used to get general data on functional and radiological outcome following pelvic ring injuries including an analysis of pain, return to work, urogenital complaints, neurological complaints, and to evaluate potential prognostic factors leading to inadequate long-term results.

Traditionally, evaluation of long-term results after bony injuries have focused on radiologic outcomes or nonvalidated measures of pain and function that did not facilitate comparison of results from one report to the next [1].

With the advent of validated measurement instruments, deficits in physical, social, and emotional functions subsequent to injury and disease now can be consistently quantified [2].

Several nonvalidated and validated outcome measures are used in describing the long-term results after pelvic ring fractures.

In 2012, Lefaivre et al. performed a systematic review on several outcome instruments used for evaluating long-term complaints after treatment of pelvic ring injuries [3].

Overall, their literature review found reported functional outcomes of 189 type A, 432 type B, and 727 type C injuries. The main disadvantage from these cases was the heterogeneity of treatment methods, with a predominance of surgically treated patients. No randomized studies were available for further analysis.

- *Generic outcome instruments*: Seven different instruments were used in 796 patients (SF-36 [4], Short Musculoskeletal Functional Assessment (SMFA) [5], EuroQol Quality of Life Score (EQ-5) [6], Sickness Impact Profile (SIP) [7], Functional Independence Measure (FIM) [8], Life Satisfaction Scale (Lis-AT 11) [9], and the Hamilton Depression Rating scale (HDARS) [10]).
- *Disease (pelvic)-specific instruments*: Six different instruments were used in 19 studies in a total of 978 patients,

A. Gänsslen et al. (eds.), *Pelvic Ring Fractures*, https://doi.org/10.1007/978-3-030-54730-1_43

with 1 questionnaire not further specified (Majeed Score [11], Iowa Pelvis Score (IPS) [12], Hannover Pelvic Score (POS) [13–15], Orlando Pelvic Score [16], and Merle d'Aubigné Score [17]).

Another rating scale, especially describing problems focused to the pelvic ring, is the Oswestry Lock Back Pain Scale [18]. Recently, the Pelvic Discomfort Index was developed and analyzed in different patient groups [19, 20].

Most authors use the validated 36-item short-form health survey SF-36 or the SMFA. Its main disadvantage is that they capture relevant impairments of the overall quality of life, but the individual importance of these limitations, localized to the pelvis, cannot sufficiently be analyzed [21].

43.2 Generic Outcome Instruments

43.2.1 Short-Form Health Survey SF-36

The SF-36 (Short-Form 36 Health Survey Questionnaire) (Table 43.1) is a short form of the 149-item Health Survey Questionnaire, which was developed in the 1960s and 1970s.

The SF-36 is the most common used validated outcome instrument for subjective self-assessment of mental health, physical, and social aspects [4]. It measures the subjective overall quality of life, but the relative individual importance of these limitations is not sufficiently analyzed. Thirty-six questions have to be answered, which are converted into eight health domain scales:

- Physical functioning (PF)
- Role limitations due to physical health (RP)
- Body pain (BP)
- General health perceptions (GH)
- Vitality (VT)
- Social functioning (SF)
- Role limitations due to emotional problems (RE)
- General mental health (MH)

Two component scores are summarized including different health domain scales:

- Physical Component Summary (PCS: PF, RP, BP, and GH)
- Mental Component Summary (MCS: VT, SF, RE, and MH)

The whole SF-36 Score ranges from 0 to 100, with higher scores indicating a better health state.

Recently, Laucis et al. analyzed the orthopedic literature. In fractures, the SF-36 was used only for general orthopedic trauma, isolated unstable ankle fractures, and acetabular fractures [22].

Bhandari et al. analyzed 215 patients after orthopedic trauma, with 54% sustaining lower extremity fractures. In 21%, psychological distress as a result of trauma was observed. Ongoing litigation and psychological symptoms were associated with PCS and MCS [23].

Borg et al. analyzed 129 patients after ORIF of acetabular fractures. Lower scores of all domains of the SF-36 were recorded during a 2-year evaluation [19].

Physical function and role physical improved over time, while perfect operative reduction of the acetabulum was associated with less reduction of overall quality of life.

Regarding pelvic ring injuries, several reports are available analyzing the SF-36 [16, 20, 24–41].

43.2.2 Musculoskeletal Function Assessment (MFA)

The MFA is a validated 101-item, self-reported health status questionnaire to detect differences in the functional status of patients who have a broad range of musculoskeletal disorders [42, 43].

Its short version (SMFA) is a two-part, 46-item, self-reported health status questionnaire (Table 43.2), which also can be used for clinical evaluation of impact of treatment in individual patients or patient groups after an injury [5]. It can be completed in about 10 min.

The main items are analysis of daily activities, general injury-related daily impairments, and injury-related impairments in daily activities including working abilities and

Table 43.1 Short-form 36 health survey questionnaire

SF-36

Please answer the 36 questions of the **Health Survey** completely, honestly, and without interruptions.

GENERAL HEALTH:

In general, would you say your health is:

☐ Excellent ☐ Very Good ☐ Good ☐ Fair ☐ Poor

Compared to one year ago, how would you rate your health in general now?

☐ Much better now than one year ago ☐ Somewhat better now than one year ago
☐ About the same ☐ Somewhat worse now than one year ago ☐ Much worse than one year ago

LIMITATIONS OF ACTIVITIES:

The following items are about activities you might do during a typical day. Does your health now limit you in these activities? If so, how much?

Vigorous activities, such as running, lifting heavy objects, participating in strenuous sports.

Yes, Limited a lot Yes, Limited a Little No, Not Limited at all

Moderate activities, such as moving a table, pushing a vacuum cleaner, bowling, or playing golf

☐ Yes, Limited a Lot ☐ Yes, Limited a Little ☐ No, Not Limited at all

Lifting or carrying groceries

☐ Yes, Limited a Lot ☐ Yes, Limited a Little ☐ No, Not Limited at all

Climbing several flights of stairs

☐ Yes, Limited a Lot ☐ Yes, Limited a Little ☐ No, Not Limited at all

Climbing one flight of stairs

☐ Yes, Limited a Lot ☐ Yes, Limited a Little ☐ No, Not Limited at all

Bending, kneeling, or stooping

☐ Yes, Limited a Lot ☐ Yes, Limited a Little ☐ No, Not Limited at all

Walking more than a mile

☐ Yes, Limited a Lot ☐ Yes, Limited a Little ☐ No, Not Limited at all

Walking several blocks

☐ Yes, Limited a Lot ☐ Yes, Limited a Little ☐ No, Not Limited at all

Walking one block

☐ Yes, Limited a Lot ☐ Yes, Limited a Little ☐ No, Not Limited at all

Bathing or dressing yourself

☐ Yes, Limited a Lot ☐ Yes, Limited a Little ☐ No, Not Limited at all

PHYSICAL HEALTH PROBLEMS:

During the past 4 weeks, have you had any of the following problems with your work or other regular daily activities as a result of your physical health?

Cut down the amount of time you spent on work or other activities ☐ Yes ☐ No

Accomplished less than you would like ☐ Yes ☐ No

Were limited in the kind of work or other activities ☐ Yes ☐ No

Had difficulty performing the work or other activities (for example, it took extra effort) ☐ Yes ☐ No

Table 43.1 (continued)

SF-36

EMOTIONAL HEALTH PROBLEMS:

During the past 4 weeks, have you had any of the following problems with your work or other regular daily activities as a result of any emotional problems (such as feeling depressed or anxious)?

Cut down the amount of time you spent on work or other activities □ Yes □ No

Accomplished less than you would like □ Yes □ No

Didn't do work or other activities as carefully asusual □ Yes □ No

SOCIAL ACTIVITIES:

Emotional problems interfered with your normal social activities with family, friends, neighbors, or groups?

□ Not at all □ Slightly □ Moderately □ Severe □ Very Severe

PAIN:

How much bodily pain have you had during the past 4 weeks?

□ Not at all □ Slightly □ Moderately □ Severe □ Very Severe

During the past 4 weeks, how much did pain interfere with your normal work (including both work outside the home and house work)?

□ Not at all □ Slightly □ Moderately □ Severe □ Very Severe

ENERGY AND EMOTIONS:

These questions are about how you feel and how things have been with you during the last 4 weeks. For each question, please give the answer that comes closest to the way you have been feeling.

Did you feel full of pep?

□ All of the time □ Most of the time □ A good Bit of the Time □ Some of the time □ A little bit of the time □ None of the Time

Have you been a very nervous person?

□ All of the time □ Most of the time □ A good Bit of the Time □ Some of the time □ A little bit of the time □ None of the Time

Have you felt so down in the dumps that nothing could cheer you up?

□ All of the time □ Most of the time □ A good Bit of the Time □ Some of the time □ A little bit of the time □ None of the Time

Have you felt calm and peaceful?

□ All of the time □ Most of the time □ A good Bit of the Time □ Some of the time □ A little bit of the time □ None of the Time

Did you have a lot of energy?

□ All of the time □ Most of the time □ A good Bit of the Time □ Some of the time □ A little bit of the time □ None of the Time

Have you felt down hearted and blue?

□ All of the time □ Most of the time □ A good Bit of the Time □ Some of the time □ A little bit of the time □ None of the Time

Did you feel worn out?

□ All of the time □ Most of the time □ A good Bit of the Time □ Some of the time □ A little bit of the time □ None of the Time

Have you been a happy person?

□ All of the time □ Most of the time □ A good Bit of the Time □ Some of the time □ A little bit of the time □ None of the Time

Did you feel tired?

□ All of the time □ Most of the time □ A good Bit of the Time □ Some of the time □ A little bit of the time □ None of the Time

Table 43.1 (continued)

SF-36

SOCIAL ACTIVITIES:

During the past 4 weeks, how much of the time has your physical health or emotional problems interfered with your social activities (like visiting with friends, relatives, etc.)?

☐ All of the time ☐ Most of the time ☐ A good Bit of the Time ☐ Some of the time ☐ A little bit of the time ☐ None of the Time

GENERAL HEALTH:

How true or false is each of the following statements for you?

I seem to get sick a little easier than other people

☐ Definitely true ☐ Mostly true ☐ Don't know ☐ Mostly false ☐ Definitely false

I am as healthy as anybody I know

☐ Definitely true ☐ Mostly true ☐ Don't know ☐ Mostly false ☐ Definitely false

I expect my health to get worse

☐ Definitely true ☐ Mostly true ☐ Don't know ☐ Mostly false ☐ Definitely false

My health is excellent

☐ Definitely true ☐ Mostly true ☐ Don't know ☐ Mostly false ☐ Definitely false

social status. As with the SF-36 an individual analysis of pelvic ring related impairments cannot be made and, therefore, only general functional impairments can be clearly distinguished.

The two parts of the SMFA questionnaire include the:

- Dysfunction index
- Bother index

The dysfunction index contains 34 items analyzing the overall functional performance of daily activities, emotional status, function of the arm and hand, and mobility, with each item graded on a Likert-type scale (1 point = good function, 5 points = poor function). The bother index includes 12 items analyzing recreation and leisure, sleep and rest, work, and family-related impairments (1 point = not at all bothered, 5 points = extremely bothered).

Unanswered items within a category are replaced with the individual's mean score for that category as long as more than 50% of the items in that category have been answered [4, 5]. Regarding pelvic ring injuries, the SMFA was rarely used [27, 38].

43.2.3 EuroQol Quality of Life Score

The EuroQoL5D analyses mobility, self-care, usual activities, pain/discomfort, and anxiety/depression using a questionnaire [6]. The patients can answer these questions as having (1) no problems, (2) slight, (3) moderate, (4) severe, or (5) extreme problems (Table 43.3).

Additionally, a visual analog scale (EQ VAS) is integrated for self-rating the patient's status with 100 points being optimal and 0 points being worse.

Table 43.2 Short musculoskeletal function assessment questionnaire

SHORT MUSCULOSKELETAL FUNCTION ASSESSMENT

Instructions

We are intersted in finding out how you are managing with your injury or arthritis this week, We would like to known about any problems you may be having with your daily activities because of your injury or arthritis.

Please answer each question by putting a check in thebox corresponding to the choice that best decribes you.

These questions are about how much difficulty you may be having this week with your daily activites because of your injury or arthritis.

	Not at All Difficult	A Little Difficult	Moderately Difficult	Very Difficult	Unable To Do
1. How difficults is it for you to get in or out of a low chair?	☐	☐	☐	☐	☐
2. How difficults is it for you to open medicine bottles or jars?	☐	☐	☐	☐	☐
3. How difficults is it for you to shop for groceries or other things?	☐	☐	☐	☐	☐
4. How difficults is it for you to climb stair?	☐	☐	☐	☐	☐
5. How difficults is it for you to make a tight fist?	☐	☐	☐	☐	☐
6. How difficults is it for you to get in or out of the bahutub or shower?	☐	☐	☐	☐	☐
7. How difficults is it for you to get comfortable to sleep?	☐	☐	☐	☐	☐
8. How difficults is it for you to band or kneel down?	☐	☐	☐	☐	☐
9. How difficults is it for you to use buttons, snaps, hooks, or zippers?	☐	☐	☐	☐	☐
10. How difficults is it for you to cut your own fingernails?	☐	☐	☐	☐	☐
11. How difficults is it for you to dress yourself?	☐	☐	☐	☐	☐
12. How difficults is it for you to walk?	☐	☐	☐	☐	☐
13. How difficults is it for you to get moving after you have been sitting or lying down	☐	☐	☐	☐	☐
14. How difficults is it for you to go out by yourself?	☐	☐	☐	☐	☐
15. How difficults is it for you to driver?	☐	☐	☐	☐	☐
16. How difficults is it for you to clean yourself after going to the bathroom?	☐	☐	☐	☐	☐
17. How difficults is it for you to trun knobs or levers (for exmaple, to open doors or to roll down car windows)?	☐	☐	☐	☐	☐
18. How difficults is it for you to write or type?	☐	☐	☐	☐	☐
19. How difficults is it for you to pivot?	☐	☐	☐	☐	☐
20. How difficults is it for you to do your usual physical recreational activities, such as bicycling, jogging, or walking?	☐	☐	☐	☐	☐
21. How difficults is it for you to do your usual leisure activities, such as hobbies, crafts, gardning, card-playing, or going out with friends?	☐	☐	☐	☐	☐
22. How much difficults are you having with sexual activity?	☐	☐	☐	☐	☐
23. How difficults is it for you to do light housework or yard work, such as dusting, washing dishes, or watering plants?	☐	☐	☐	☐	☐
24. How difficults is it for you to do heavy housework or yard work, such as washing floors, vacuuming, or mowing lawns?	☐	☐	☐	☐	☐
25. How difficults is it for you to do usual work, such as a paid job, housework, or volunteer activities?	☐	☐	☐	☐	☐

Table 43.2 (continued)

These next questions ask how often you are experiencing problems this <u>week</u> becasuse of your injury or arthritis.

	None of the Time	A Little of the time	Some of the TIme	Most of the Time	All of the Time
26. How often do you walk with a limp?	☐	☐	☐	☐	☐
27. How often do you avoid using your painful limb(s) or back?	☐	☐	☐	☐	☐
28. How often does your leg lock or give-way?	☐	☐	☐	☐	☐
29. How often do you have problems with concentration?	☐	☐	☐	☐	☐
30. How often does doing too much in one day affect what you do the next day?	☐	☐	☐	☐	☐
31. How often do you act irritable toward those around you (for example, snap at people, give sharp answers, or criticize easily)?	☐	☐	☐	☐	☐
32. How often are you tired?	☐	☐	☐	☐	☐
32. How often do you feel disabled?	☐	☐	☐	☐	☐
34. How often do you feel angry of frustrated that you have this injury or arthritis??	☐	☐	☐	☐	☐

These questions are about how much you are bothered by problems you are having <u>this week</u> because of your injury or arthritis.

	Not at All Bothered	A Little Bothered	Moderately Bothered	Very Bothered	Exteremely Bothered
35. How much are you bothered by problems using your hands, arms, or legs?	☐	☐	☐	☐	☐
36. How much are you bothered by problems using your back?	☐	☐	☐	☐	☐
37. How much are you bothered by problems doing work around your home?	☐	☐	☐	☐	☐
38. How much are you bothered by problems with bathing, dressing, toileting, or other personal care?	☐	☐	☐	☐	☐
39. How much are you bothered by problems with sleep and rest?	☐	☐	☐	☐	☐
40. How much are you bothered by problems with leisure or recreational activities?	☐	☐	☐	☐	☐
41. How much are you bothered by problems with your friends, family, or other important people in your life?	☐	☐	☐	☐	☐
42. How much are you bothered by problems with thinking concentrating, or remembering?	☐	☐	☐	☐	☐
43. How much are you bothered by problems adjusting or coping with your injury or arthritis?	☐	☐	☐	☐	☐
44. How much are you bothered by problems doing your usual work?	☐	☐	☐	☐	☐
45. How much are you bothered by problems with feeling dependent on others?	☐	☐	☐	☐	☐
46. How much are you bothered by problems with stiffness and pain?	☐	☐	☐	☐	☐

Table 43.3 EuroQol quality of life score

EQ-5D-5L

Under each heading, please tick the ONE box that best describes your health TODAY.

MOBILITY
☐ I have no problems in walking about
☐ I have slight problems in walking about
☐ I have moderate problems in walking about
☐ I have severe problems in walking about
☐ I am unable to walk about

SELF-CARE
☐ I have no problems washing or dressing myself
☐ I have slight problems washing or dressing myself
☐ I have moderate problems washing or dressing myself
☐ I have severe problems washing or dressing myself
☐ I am unable to wash or dress myself

USUAL ACTIVITIES (e.g. work, study, housework, family or leisure activities)
☐ I have no problems doing my usual activities
☐ I have slight problems doing my usual activities
☐ I have moderate problems doing my usual activities
☐ I have severe problems doing my usual activities
☐ I am unable to do my usual activities

PAIN / DISCOMFORT
☐ I have no pain or discomfort
☐ I have slight pain or discomfort
☐ I have moderate pain or discomfort
☐ I have severe pain or discomfort
☐ I have extreme pain or discomfort

ANXIETY / DEPRESSION
☐ I am not anxious or depressed
☐ I am slightly anxious or depressed
☐ I am moderately anxious or depressed
☐ I am severely anxious or depressed
☐ I am extremely anxious or depressed

We would like to know how good or bad your health is TODAY.

- Uase the scale on the right side. This scale is numbered from 0 to100.
- 100 means the best health you can imagine.
- 0 means the worst health you can imagine.
- Mark an X on the scale to indicate how your health is TODAY.
- Now, please write the number you marked on the scale in thebox.

YOUR HEALTH TODAY = ☐

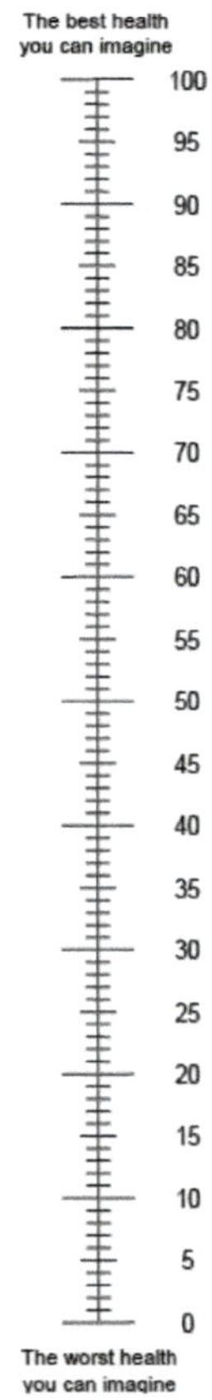

43.2.4 Sickness Impact Profile (SIP)

The sickness impact profile (SIP) measures the perceived health status [7]. The original version contains 136 items evaluating sleep and rest, eating, work, home management, recreation and pastimes, ambulation, mobility, body care and movement, social interaction, alertness behavior, emotional behavior, and communication.

The shorter SIP-68 version integrates analysis of somatic autonomy, mobility control, psychological autonomy and communication, social behavior, emotional stability, and mobility range [44].

The Functional Independence Measure (FIM) [8], Life Satisfaction Scale (Lis-AT 11) [9], and the Hamilton Depression Rating scale (HDARS) [10]) are further instruments of general health analysis. An overview of additional possible instruments is presented in the textbook *Encyclopedia of Clinical Neuropsychology*.

43.2.5 Oswestry Low Back Pain Disability Questionnaire

The Oswestry low back pain disability questionnaire as a region-specific validated score that measures the patient's permanent functional disability in the lumbosacral region (Table 43.4) [18]. Therefore, it can be helpful in analyzing posterior pelvic pain after unstable pelvic ring injuries. The resultant Oswestry Disability Index Score [18] consists of ten items with score values from 0 to 10%. The analyzed items include:

- Pain intensity
- General personal care (washing, dressing etc.)
- Weight lifting
- Walking ability
- Impairments while sitting
- Standing
- Sleeping
- Sexual impairments
- Social life
- Traveling

The score rates the disability into five categories:

- Minimal disability, 0–20%
- Moderate disability, 21–40%
- Severe disability, 41–60%
- Crippled disability, 61–80%
- >80% disability (bed bounded or symptom exaggerating)

The scoring of the items is performed on a six-point Likert scale (first answer = 0; last answer = 5). If all ten items are completed, a maximum score of 50 is possible. The score calculation is performed with the equation: total score/total possible score × 100.

If one section is not applicable, the following equation is used: total score/45 × 100.

43.3 Disease (Pelvic)-Specific Instruments

43.3.1 Majeed Score

The Majeed Score is a nonvalidated self-developed pelvic fracture specific functional assessment instrument with a maximum of 100 points for patients working before injury or 80 points for patients not working before injury [11] (Table 43.5).

The weighted score items include pain (30%), return to work (20%), sitting disturbances (10%), sexual impairments (4%), and walking ability (36%). The latter is subdivided into use of walking aids (12%), analysis of unaided gait (12%), and the walking distance (12%).

A score between 80 and 100 points is defined as the best result.

Patients who worked before injury are graded as:

- Excellent with a score >85
- Good with a score of 70–84
- Fair with a score of 55–69
- Poor with a score <55

Patient who did not work before injury are graded into:

- Excellent with a score >70
- Good with a score of 55–69
- Fair with a score of 45–54
- Poor with a score <45

The disadvantage of the Majeed Score is that neurological impairments, which have relevant prognostic influence, are not integrated and the score measures exclusively the functional component of the long-term pelvic injury.

A modification of Majeed Score has been used by Lindahl et al. [45, 46]. The ability to work was separated from this assessment giving a maximal total score of 80 points for each patient in order to compare the outcome of different types of fracture and subgroups. The total score for the functional outcome was also modified to take account of the outcome after the pelvic injury.

Table 43.4 Oswestry low back pain disability questionnaire

Instructions

This questionnaire has been designed to give information as to how your back or leg pain is affecting your ability to manage in everyday life. Please answer by checking ONE box in each section for the statement which best applies to you.

Personal care (washing, dressing etc)
☐ I can look after myself normally without causing extra pain
☐ I can look after myself normally but it causes extra pain
☐ It is painful to look after myself and I am slow and careful
☐ I need some help but manage most of my personal care
☐ I need help every day in most aspects of self-care
☐ I do not get dressed, I wash with difficulty and stay in bed

Pain intensity
☐ I have no pain at the moment
☐ The pain is very mild at the moment
☐ The pain is moderate at the moment
☐ The pain is fairly severe at the moment
☐ The pain is very severe at the moment
☐ The pain is the worst imaginable at the moment

Lifting
☐ I can lift heavy weights without extra pain
☐ I can lift heavy weights but it gives extra pain
☐ Pain prevents me from lifting heavy weights off the floor, but I can manage if they are conveniently placed eg. on a table
☐ Pain prevents me from lifting heavy weights, but I can manage light to medium weights if they are conveniently positioned
☐ I can lift very light weights
☐ I cannot lift or carry anything at all

Walking
☐ Pain does not prevent me walking any distance
☐ Pain prevents me from walking more than 2 km
☐ Pain prevents me from walking more than 1 km
☐ Pain prevents me from walking more than 500 m
☐ I can only walk using a stick or crutches
☐ I am in bed most of the time

Standing
☐ I can stand as long as I want without extra pain
☐ I can stand as long as I want but it gives me extra pain
☐ Pain prevents me from standing for more than 1 hour
☐ Pain prevents me from standing for more than 3 min
☐ Pain prevents me from standing for more than 10 min
☐ Pain prevents me from standing at all

Sitting
☐ I can sit in any chair as long as I like
☐ I can only sit in my favourite chair as long as I like
☐ Pain prevents me sitting more than one hour
☐ Pain prevents me from sitting more than 30 minutes
☐ Pain prevents me from sitting more than 10 minutes
☐ Pain prevents me from sitting at all

Sleeping
☐ My sleep is never disturbed by pain
☐ My sleep is occasionally disturbed by pain
☐ Because of pain I have less than 6 hours sleep
☐ Because of pain I have less than 4 hours sleep
☐ Because of pain I have less than 2 hours sleep
☐ Pain prevents me from sleeping at all

Travelling
☐ I can travel anywhere without pain
☐ I can travel anywhere but it gives me extra pain
☐ Pain is bad but I manage journeys over two hours
☐ Pain restricts me to journeys of less than one hour
☐ Pain restricts me to short necessary journeys under 30 min
☐ Pain prevents me from travelling except to receive treatment

Sex life (if applicable)
☐ My sex life is normal and causes no extra pain
☐ My sex life is normal but causes some extra pain
☐ My sex life is nearly normal but is very painful
☐ My sex life is severely restricted by pain
☐ My sex life is nearly absent because of pain
☐ Pain prevents any sex life at all treatment

Social life
☐ My social life is normal and gives me no extra pain
☐ My social life is normal but increases the degree of pain
☐ Pain has no significant effect on my social life apart from limiting my more energetic interests eg, sport
☐ Pain has restricted my social life and I do not go out as often
☐ Pain has restricted my social life to my home
☐ I have no social life because of pain

Fairbank JC, Pynsent PB. The Oswestry Disability Index. Spine 2000 Nov 15;25(22):2940-52

Table 43.5 Majeed pelvic score

Majeed Pelvic Score (MPS)

Pain	**30pt**	
	Intense, continuous at rest	0-5
	Intense with activity	10
	Tolerable, but limits activity	15
	With moderate activity, abolished by rest	20
	Pain Mild, intermittent, normal activity	25
	Slight, occasional or no pain	30
Work	**20pt**	
	No regular work	0-4
	Light wotk	8
	Change of job	12
	Same job, reduced performance	16
	Same job, same performance	20
Sitting	**10pt**	
	Painful	0-4
	Painful if prolonged or awkward	6
	Uncomfortable	8
	Free	10
Sexual Intercourse	**4 pt**	
	Painful	0-1
	Painful if prolonged or awkward	2
	Uncomfortable	3
	Free	4
Standing	**12pt Walking Aids**	
	Bedridden or almost	0-2
	Wheelchair	4
	Two crutches	6
	Two sticks	8
	One stick	10
	No stick	12
Standing	**12pt Gait unaided**	
	Cannot walk or almost	0-2
	Shuffling small steps	4
	Gross limp	6
	Moderate limp	8
	Slight limp	10
	Normal	12
Standing	**12pt Walking Distance**	
	Bedridden or few metres	0-2
	Very limited time and distance	4
	Limited with sticks, difficult without, prolonged standing	6
	One hour with stick limited without	8
	One hour without sticks, slight pain or limp	10
	Normal for age and general condition	12

The Majeed Pelvic Score. Adapted from: **Majeed SA.** Grading the outcome of pelvic fractures. *J Bone Joint Surg [Br]* 1989;71:304-6

The functional outcome was graded as:

- Excellent, 78–80 points
- Good, 70–77 points
- Fair, 60–69 points
- Poor, less than 60 points

43.4 Iowa Pelvis Score (IPS)

The Iowa Pelvic Score (IPS) consists of 25 items within 6 subscales [12] (Table 43.6), including:

- Activities of daily living (20 points)
- Work history (20 points)
- Pain (25 points)
- Limp (20 points)
- Visual pain line (10 points)
- Cosmesis (5 points)

Nepola et al. defined a grading scale [36]:

- Excellent: 85–100 points
- Good: 70–84 points
- Fair: 55–69 points
- Poor: <55 points

43.5 Hannover Pelvis Outcome Scale (POS)

The POS is a nonvalidated scale and consists of three items: clinical, radiological, and social integration criteria [13, 14, 45, 46] (Table 43.7).

- Clinical criteria include the subitems pain, functional impairments (limping, walking assistance), and persistent neurological and urogenital impairments.
- Radiological criteria focus on the reconstruction of the posterior pelvic ring and to a less relevant part on the integrity of the anterior pelvic ring.
- The social reintegration considers working ability, leisure activities, sporting activities, social activities, and necessity of external assistance.

To estimate the total result of the pelvic injury, the radiological (3 points) and clinical results (4 points) are summarized, and the resulting seven-point scale assesses the result of the pelvic injury as follows:

- 7 points for an excellent result
- 6 points for a good result
- 4 and 5 points for an adequate result
- 3 or 2 points for a poor result

43.6 Orlando Pelvic Score

The Orlando Pelvic Score (OPS) consists of 12 items within 6 subscales, 4 of which have to be completed by the patient [16]. The six subscales include (Table 43.8):

- Functional pain
- Subjective pain
- Narcotic use
- Activity status
- Physical examination
- Radiographic findings

43.7 Pelvic Trauma Questionnaire (PTQ)

The Pelvic Trauma Questionnaire (PTQ) is a further pelvic-specific analysis instrument (questionnaire with a six-level Likert scale based analysis from no discomfort to very severe discomfort), developed for estimation of pelvic discomfort [19, 20, 25].

Initially 11 closed questions (each with 6 responses) and 3 open questions were part of the questionnaire (Table 43.9). Statistical analysis revealed that four factors could explain 76% of the variance in the questionnaire responses [19]. This led to a reduction of relevant questions.

The six relevant questions focus on:

- Pain
- Walking
- Hip motion
- Sensation
- Pelvic scar tissue
- Sexual problems

A further factor analysis revealed that four factors could explain 92% of the variance of the 24 months results analyzing acetabular fracture patients. These included the hip region (pain, walking, and hip motion), peripheral neurology, sexual life, and operation scar.

For pelvic ring injuries, analysis of the 14-item questionnaire revealed that the two items, voiding bladder and bowel, had a very low frequency and, therefore, were excluded for analysis of the pelvic ring.

The same six questions were found to be relevant for patients after pelvic ring injuries.

Analysis of these data resulted in the development of the Pelvic Discomfort Index (PDI), a 0–100% scale of pelvic discomfort.

Using the PDI, patients with type B injuries had less discomfort than patients with type C injuries [20].

Lumsdaine et al. performed a systematic review on pelvic-specific outcome instruments (MPS, IPS, OPS) and the SF-36 [33].

Table 43.6 IOWA pelvic score

IOWA Pelvic Score (IPS)

ADL Questions (Activities of Daily Living)

- ☐ yes ☐ no Walk a mile
- ☐ yes ☐ no Stoop over a sink
- ☐ yes ☐ no Carry a bag of groceries
- ☐ yes ☐ no Make a bed
- ☐ yes ☐ no Ride in a car
- ☐ yes ☐ no Sit for a long period of time (eg. in a cinema)
- ☐ yes ☐ no Visit friends or relatives for an evening
- ☐ yes ☐ no Stand for an hour or more (eg. waiting in line)
- ☐ yes ☐ no Rake leaves or mow the lawn
- ☐ yes ☐ no Pick up small children
- ☐ yes ☐ no Sweep the floor with a broom
- ☐ yes ☐ no Dress without assistance
- ☐ yes ☐ no Cook a meal
- ☐ yes ☐ no Light Recreation (eg. bowling, dancing, etc)
- ☐ yes ☐ no Vigorous recreation (eg. jogging, tennis, etc)
- ☐ yes ☐ no Squat down
- ☐ yes ☐ no Walk up and down stairs normally (eg. foot over foot)
- ☐ yes ☐ no Walk up and down stairs (eg. one step at a time)
- ☐ yes ☐ no Activities that require reaching overhead
- ☐ yes ☐ no Sleep comfortably

IPS Evaluation

ADL's Score:	1 pt Per Question	(20 Pts)______
Work History:	No Change	(20 Pts)______
	Full Time, Change	(15 Pts)______
	Part Time	(10 Pts)______
	Unable	(5 Pts) ______
Pain:	None, Not Significant	(20 Pts)______
	Occasional Medication	(15 Pts)______
	Regular Medication	(10 Pts)______
	Hospitalization or Operation	(5 Pts) ______
Limp:	None	(20 Pts)______
	Yes	(15 Pts)______
	Ambulatory Aid	(10 Pts)______
	No Ambulation	(5 Pts) ______
Visual Pain Line:		(10 Pts)______
Cosmesis:	No Significant Change	(5 Pts) ______
	Significant Change	(0 Pts) ______
	TOTAL SCORE:	(100 Pts possible)_____

Templeman D, Goulet J, Duwelius PJ, Olson S, Davidson M. Internal fixation of displaced fractures of the sacrum. *Clin Orthop Rel Res* 1996;329:180-185

Table 43.7 Multicenter study group pelvis outcome scale (POS)

Clinical result	
4 points	no pain, no neurological or urological impairment, no functional limitation
3 points	pain only after severe effort, no analgesies required slight functional impainment (occasional limoing) slight neurological disturbance, not subjectively distressing
2 points	invariably pain after effort, occasional analgesics required significant impairment of function (limping, walking-stick required) Impairment of motor nerve function not regarded as a handicap and/or extensive sensory disturbance without loss protective reflexes micturition disrturbances without residual urine in bladder and/or partial erectile impotence, or other disturbances of sexual function not regardded as distressing
1 points	continous pain, pain at rest, analgesics frequently required permanent use of crutch or wheel chair required because of pelivic injury handicapped impairment of motor nerve function and/or sensoric deficits with loss of protective reflexes micturition disturbances, impotence/disturbances of sexual function, urinary or faecal incontinence
Radiological result	
3 points	posterior anatomical reconstruction residual displacement of the pubic symphysis < 5 mm and/or maximal residual displacement of the pubis/ischium < 10 mm
2 points	maximal posterior residual displacement 5 mm and/or residual displacement of the pubic symphysis 6–10 mm and/or maximal residual displacement of the pubis/ischium 10–15 mm
1 points	maximal posterior residual displacement > 5 mm and/or residual displacement of the pubic symphsis > 10 mm and/or maximal residual displacement of the pubis/ischium > 15 mm
Social reintergration	
3 points	same profession as before sports and free-time activities unchanged socail activites unchanged
2 points	limited employment in previous profession retraining being undertaken or completed reduced sporting activities occasional external support required
1 points	unable to work owing to accident or employment as handicapped person significantly reduced free-time activities, no sport socail life signicantly limted or socially withdrawn frequent external assistance required

It was concluded that "pelvic-specific tools produce similar results to the SF-36 and are potentially more sensitive in examining specific areas related to pelvic injuries and easier to perform and calculate than the SF-36."

43.8 Timing of Outcome Evaluation

On major concern while analyzing the outcome after pelvic ring injuries is to evaluate at which time follow-up studies should be performed.

Majeed et al. reported functional improvement during the first 18 months after trauma and then observed steady state stabilization [47]. In contrast, Kreder identified a functional plateau between 6 months and 1 year post injury [1].

Borg et al. analyzed the results of 73 consecutive patients with different types of pelvic ring type B and type C injuries after internal fixation and follow-up evaluation at 6, 12, and 24 months [20]. Using Pelvic Trauma Questionnaire (PTQ) during the 24 months period, the rate of none or slight discomfort increased from 6 to 12 and 24 months in the following categories:

- Pain: 42.1, 48.1, and 57.7%
- Walking: 45.6, 48.1, and 57.7%
- Hip motion: 43.9, 50, and 53.8%
- Leg sensation: 47.4, 46.2, and 51.9%
- Leg weakness: 36.8, 42.3, and 53.8%
- Sitting: 42.1, 50, and 59.6%
- Sexual life: 52.6, 57.7, and 61.5%

Table 43.8 Orlando pelvic score

Orlando Pelvic Score (OPS)

Functional Pain	Pain Secondary to physical activity	
	None	5
	Pain only with strenuous activity	4
	Mild pain with stair climbing, lifting, mowing, or other moderately strenuous activity	3
	Moderate pain with start up of activities and intermittent radicular pain	2
	Pain with sitting or standing longer than 1 hour, requires frequent position changes	1
Subjective Pain	**Average of resting and ambulation scores on a VAS scale**	
	0-2 points	4
	3-4 points	3
	5-6 points	2
	7-8 points	1
	9-10 points	0
Narcotic use	**>12 weeks postoperatively**	
	No	1
	Yes	0
Activity Status	**Ability to resume previous work, household, or recreational activities**	
	Without limitations	10
	With some discomfort	8
	With limitations such as tires more easily or cannot lift as much as before injury	6
	With marked limitations requiring change in work status to part time, sedentary, or with restrictions; requires assistance with household activities or avoids strenuous recreational activities	4
	Unable to resume any previous work, household, or recreational activities; cannot drive and requires assistance with stairs or with shopping	2
	Unable to resume any previous work, household, or recreational activities and requires assistance with activities of daily living	0
Physical Exam		
Gait	Normal gait	4
	Antalgic gait or limp	3
	Requires assistive device (cane)	2
	Requires assistive device (walker, occasionally uses wheelchair)	1
	Nonambulatory	0
Trendeleburg	Negative	1
	Positive	0
Tenderness	No sacral or pubic tenderness	2
	Sacral or pubic tenderness	1
	Sacral and pubic tenderness	0
muscle strength	Bilateral thigh flexion and extension = 5/5	1
	Thigh flexion/extension < 5/5	0
ab-/adduction	Bilateral thigh abduction and adduction = 5/5	1
	Thigh abduction/adduction < 5/5	0
ROM	Normal hip and trunk range of motion	1
	Trunk flexion <90°, hip flexion <90° or >20° difference in hip internal or external rotation when compared to contralateral side	0
Pelvic x-rays	**(AP, inlet and outlet views ; normal SI -joint width 4mm)**	
posterior	Displacement ≤ 0.5 cm without Sacroiliac joint reactive changes	6
	Displacement ≤ 0.5 cm with Sacroiliac joint reactive changes	5
	Displacement > 0.5 cm and ≤ 1.0 cm	4
	Displacement > 1.0 cm	2
	Nonunion	0
anterior	Displacement ≤ 0.5 cm	4
	Displacement > 0.5 cm and ≤ 1.0 cm	3
	Displacement > 1.0 cm and ≤ 2.0 cm	1
	Displacement > 2.0 cm	0

Table 43.9 Pelvic trauma questionnaire

Pelvic Trauma Questionnaire (PTQ)

Question no.	How much discomfort do you presently have	None	Very little	Little	Moderate	Severe	Very severe
1	Pain from the pelvis	☐	☐	☐	☐	☐	☐
2	From the pelvis when walking	☐	☐	☐	☐	☐	☐
3	Decreased mobility of the hips	☐	☐	☐	☐	☐	☐
4	Loss of sensation or numberss in the legs	☐	☐	☐	☐	☐	☐
5	Weakness in the legs	☐	☐	☐	☐	☐	☐
6	When sitting	☐	☐	☐	☐	☐	☐
7	In your sex life	☐	☐	☐	☐	☐	☐
8	From operation scars	☐	☐	☐	☐	☐	☐
9	When sleeping	☐	☐	☐	☐	☐	☐
10	When voiding your bladder	☐	☐	☐	☐	☐	☐
11	When voiding your bowels	☐	☐	☐	☐	☐	☐
A	Do you have other discomfort following the injured pelvis?	....					
B	Is there something you can no longer do that you could do before the pelvic injury?	....					
C	What are your major sources of disscomfort following the pelvic injury?	....					

How much discomfort do you presently have	None	Very little	Little	Moderate	Severe	Very severe
From pain in the pelvis?	☐	☐	☐	☐	☐	☐
From the pelvis when walking?	☐	☐	☐	☐	☐	☐
With decreased mobility of the hips?	☐	☐	☐	☐	☐	☐
From loss of sensation or numbness in the legs?	☐	☐	☐	☐	☐	☐
In your sexual life?	☐	☐	☐	☐	☐	☐
From operation scans?	☐	☐	☐	☐	☐	☐
How much are your activities of daily living affected by the pelvic injury?	☐	☐	☐	☐	☐	☐

- Sleep disturbances: 56.1, 55.8, and 80.8%
- Voiding urine: 71.9, 69.2, and 80.8%
- Voiding bowels: 70.1, 82.7, and 86.5%

Follow-up studies for pelvic ring injuries should have at least a minimal follow-up evaluation of 2 years.

43.9 Unselected Outcome Analyses After Pelvic Ring Injuries

Until recently, conflicting outcome data were reported in the literature after treatment of pelvic ring injuries:

- Type C injuries are associated with the most worse prognosis [46, 48, 49]
- No difference was observed between type B and C injuries [37]
- Analyzing type B injuries, type B1 fractures presented with the greatest degree of disability in contrast to type B2 and B3 fractures with the lowest degree of disability [1]

In a recent multicenter analysis, overall clinical results were excellent or good according to the Majeed Score in 85%. A decrease of these results was observed with increasing pelvic ring instability from type A to type C injuries. Neurological long-term sequelae increased with the type of pelvic ring injury with 4% after type A, 11% after type B, and 17% after type C injuries. Urological and sexual sequelae were both present in 8%, with highest rates after type C injuries (each 14%). Additionally, patients with less than 5 mm residual displacement showed best functional results with a Majeed Score of >90, whereas with increasing displacement significantly lower scores were observed [50].

Pavelka et al. found comparable results in their single-center analysis. Excellent and good clinical outcomes according to the Majeed Score were seen in 83% after type B and in 70% after type C fractures. The radiological result was excellent (<5 mm residual displacement) in 83% and 61%, respectively [51].

Ayvaz et al. analyzed 20 patients with unstable pelvic fractures, stabilized using percutaneous techniques using different outcome instruments after at least 2 years after initial trauma [24].

The mean Majeed Score was 93.3 points, indicating a near perfect result. The Iowa Pelvic Score had an average of 86 points. The mean Pelvic Outcome Score was 33/40 points. Overall, all patients presented with good and excellent results.

General health analysis using the SF-36 showed comparable results compared to the normal population with 3.3 points for body pain, 4.4 points for general health, and 7.9 points for social function. The average physical component score was 81.3, and the average mental component score 80.8. One of 14 patients had to change his job after trauma but was still working.

Lefaivre et al. analyzed 38 patients with type B and C injuries after a mean of 57 months [32]. Self-reported complaints in decreasing order included recreational/mobility difficulty, emotional stress and family strain, employment and financial difficulties, sleep disturbance and anxiety, and sexual function disturbances. Outcome instruments used for analysis of the long-term results were the Majeed Score, the IPS, the OPS, the Short Musculoskeletal Functional Assessment (SMFA), and the SF-36, respectively.

The Majeed Score, IPS, and OPS correlated with the PCS of the SF-36 and the subscales of the SMFA, while the MCS showed no correlation to the pelvic scores.

Lefaivre et al. concluded the "localized" pelvic outcome instruments were inadequate for analysis of psychologic distress, well-being, social functioning, and overall vitality.

Additionally, these scores showed a ceiling effect of 15–21%.

A difference between type B and type C injuries was observed. Type C injuries were associated with

- Lesser SF-36 PCS scores
- Lesser SF-36 MCS scores
- Higher SMFA Function scores
- Higher SMFA Bother scores
- Lesser Pelvic Scores (MPS, IPS, OPS)

indicating an association between pelvic instability (and, therefore, more extended soft-tissue involvement, including pelvic organ injuries) and more fair and poor results [32].

Ismail et al. analyzed 26 patients after the surgical stabilization of complex Tile type B or C pelvic fractures [52] at an average follow-up of 25 months. According to the Majeed Score, 78.6% had an excellent result after type B injuries and only 50% after type C injuries, but all patients were rated good or excellent. Additionally, the Hannover Pelvic Score showed 100% good and excellent results, while type C injuries had less excellent results in both scorings. Sexual dysfunction was independent of the fracture type but associated with urogenital injury. Type C injuries were associated with more chronic pain.

Kerschbaum et al. analyzed 60 patients after a mean follow-up of 60.5 months using the SF-36 and EQ-5D scores after sustaining different type B or C injuries treated by different posterior stabilization techniques [31]. The mean SF-36 PCS was 37.9 and the mean SF-36 MCS was 49.8. The mean EQ-5D VAS was 70.5.

Brouwers et al. analyzed the long-term results after a mean of 29 months of 195 patients after operative or conservative treatment of pelvic ring injuries performed by using the EQ-5D and the MPS [53]. The mean VAS EQ-5D for Tile type A, B, and C injuries was 74, 74, and 67, respectively. The mean EQ-5D index score was 0.81, 0.77, and 0.71. Relevant differences were present after usual activities and anxiety. Patient with type C injuries suffered from more pain.

The average Majeed Score showed highest differences between type A, B, and C injuries in patients <65 years of age: 86, 81, and 74, respectively, while small differences were observed in older patients (69, 68, 66 points).

Banierink et al. retrospectively compared the results of 192 patients with type A, B, and C injuries after a mean of 4.4 years using the SMFA and the EQ-D5. With increasing instability of the pelvis, more surgical stabilizations were performed without having data regarding type and localization of these osteosyntheses [54]. Analyzing the SMFA, type C injuries showed the worst results, followed by type B and type A injuries. No difference was observed between operatively and nonoperatively treated patients. A patient with a pelvic ring injury had a decreased physical function compared to the general population.

Hermans et al. analyzed 136 patients (55% surgical treatment) with different pelvic injuries after a median follow-up period of 8.7 years [55].

The mean MPS score was 85.1 points. The main complaint of the patients was sexual problems in almost 25%. There was difference of the scoring associated with the fracture type, while in patients with type C injuries a trend to more impairments was observed.

The EQ-5D-VAS score was 74–76 of 100, independent of the fracture type. The EQ-5D index score was highest (0.87) for Tile B patients, while after Tile A injuries this score was 0.81 and after type C injuries 0.82.

The mean score of the SMFA Function Index was 24 and the mean Bother Index score was 24. A minor trend to higher scores from type A to type C injuries was observed.

A multiple linear regression analysis revealed that after type B injuries better mobility results were observed compared to type C injuries.

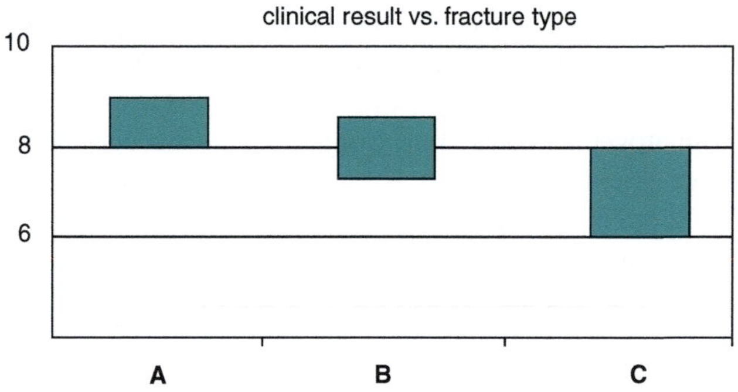

Fig. 43.1 Average discomfort at the pelvic region depending on the type of pelvic ring injury (acc. to Gänsslen et al., Acta Chir Orthop Traumatol Cech 2013)

A relevant ceiling effect was observed in about 1/3 of the patients.

Type C injuries are associated with more clinical long-term discomfort [56] (Fig. 43.1).

Therefore, outcome analyses should focus on fracture type specific results and results of different injury regions based on the type of stabilization in these different regions.

43.10 Unselected Outcome Analyses After Pelvic Ring Type B Injuries

Only few reports are available on long-term results after isolated type B injuries.

There is some data on SF-36 analysis after these injuries.

- In 11 patients with type B injuries at a mean follow-up of 2 years with a nonconsistent treatment concept, a reduced physical component score of 68.7 and a reduced mental component score of 72.2 was reported, which represents approximately 12% and 4% impairment compared with the U.S. normal population, respectively [37].
- Long-term results in 32 patients with type B injuries, which were treated by different treatment modalities including nonoperative treatment and several different stabilization concepts, showed a mean physical functional value of 75.8 and a pain value of 69.8 (4). This a reduction according to the normal U.S. population (in [37]) of 10.3% and 7.6%, respectively.
- Additionally, the results of 31 patients with type B injuries treated by external fixation in 60% and by nonoperative means in 40% with a follow-up of more than 5 years were within 2 standard deviations from established American populations norms and, therefore, showed no significant difference [35].
- The functional outcome of 32 patients with open book injuries was analyzed after a median follow-up time of 84 months using the SF-36 method [57]. All patients had initial anterior ring stabilization, and in approximately one fourth of the patients an additional iliosacral screw was applied. All values of the different SF-36 categories were lower compared to uninjured German and U.S. patients. The median level of physical functioning was 95%; no patient had role limitations and the median pain level using the VAS was 10%. Interestingly, patients treated by additional posterior iliosacral screw fixation showed a trend to worse results compared to patients with symphyseal stabilization alone.
- In an analysis of 30 patients with lateral compression pelvic ring fractures with extension into the anterior acetabulum, treated conservatively, after a mean follow-up of 4.2 years (2–6 years), SF-36 analysis showed functional deficits for mental and social functions compared to type B1 and type C injuries [58].
- Lefaivre et al. analyzed 23 patients with type B injuries after a mean of 57 months by self-reported complaint analysis, and the Majeed Score, the IPS, the OPS, the SMFA, and the SF-36. The SF-36 PCS was 45.01 and the SF-36 MCS was 48.76 [32]. The corresponding normative data from Canada [59] were 50.5 and 51.7, respectively, indicating a 10.9% and 5.7% impairment, respectively.

According to a validated outcome instrument (SF-36), there are only minor impairments after type B injuries compared to the normal population.

Some reports used nonvalidated outcome instruments to analyze the long-term result after type B injuries:

- In a multicenter analysis in Germany, the POS was used in 87 patients after isolated type B injuries without additional acetabular fractures. No consistent treatment regimen was documented, and follow-up evaluation was performed at 2 years [13].

  Of these patients, 79.3% reported no or slight pain in the pelvic region. Pain localization was reported to be solely anterior in 4.6% (symphyseal/pubic region), whereas 34.5% reported on single posterior pain, and 16.1% suffered from both ventral and dorsal pain.

  Functional limitations analyzed using the Merle d'Aubigné Score showed a mean value of 17 points, and 83% of the patients had bilateral identical scores or differences of a minimum of 1 point.

Leg length differences were exclusively the result of accompanying lower extremity injuries.

Radiological follow-up evaluation (at least an AP x-ray) was available in 78 patients (89.6%). Posterior anatomic healing was observed in 90%, whereas in 28% some anterior malhealing occurred.

A total of 88.5% of the patients offered a positive or neutral subjective assessment of their condition. Overall, 87% of the patients were still able to work. Seventy-four percent continued in their previous profession or remained in the same training program. Fourteen percent were at least partially able to work, and 13% of patients were unable to work as a result of the injury. Sixty-nine percent reported that their sporting activities had not been altered by the accident, and further 11% had only slight limitations. Ninety percent had no or only slight limitations regarding hobbies.

The total clinical result was assessed as excellent or good in 83.9% of the patients. A poor total clinical result was due to permanent urological and neurological disturbances or significant pelvic pain.

Overall pelvic outcome assessment revealed that 77.5% of the patients achieved a good or very good result after a type B injury [13].

- Using the Iowa Pelvic Score (IPS), the results in 31 patients with type B injuries treated by external fixation in 60% and by nonoperative means in 40% were analyzed after more than 5 years [35]:
  - 75% of patients returned to their previous occupation.
  - 73% had identical previous sexual activities.
  - 88% had an identical recreational level in light work.
  - 62% performed the same heavy work compared to the uninjured situation.
  - 27% suffered from sexual disturbances.

  35% reported significant persistent pain in the pelvic region.

  Overall, only 32% had no functional impairments [35].

- In an analysis of a mixed group of B1 and B2 injuries after ORIF of the anterior ring with a plate at least 1 year after trauma (12–84 months), full ambulation was possible in 96% but only 69% of these patients were pain free. Twenty-seven percent had pain with strenuous activity and overall 83% returned to work within 1 year after trauma, and 75% returned to their original jobs [60].
- In an analysis of 27 patients with type B injuries, all treated with ORIF, used the Majeed Score for functional evaluation and showed 81% good and excellent results. But only 48% of these patients were completely pain free at follow-up [61].
- Lefaivre et al. analyzed 23 patients with type B injuries after a mean of 57 months by self-reported complaint analysis, and the Majeed Score, the IPS and the OPS, respectively. The mean Majeed Score was 81.43 points,

In unselected patients with type B injuries a high radiological healing rate, approximately 30% long-term problems (pain, functional limitations), and an overall rate of 75–80% acceptable results can be expected [56].

43.11 Outcome Analyses After Pelvic Ring Type B1 "Open Book" Injuries

Type B1 injuries are supposed to be the most severe type B injuries with a potential risk of permanent disabilities. Available analyses show that different outcome instruments were used, making comparison of the results nearly impossible:

- In an analysis of nine patients with B1 injuries after ORIF using the Sickness Impact Profile (SIP) with a minimum follow-up of 1 year following injury, the mean SIP score was 12.4, indicating a moderate disability (<10 = slight disability, 10–30 = moderate disability, >30 = severe disability) (18). The total physical score was 11.1 with worst values for ambulation (20.2 points). The mean psychosocial score was 10.9 with emotional disability of 17 points. Sleep (16.6 points), working (25.7 points), home management (17.2 points), and recreation (24 points) showed moderate impairments.

  In a further analysis by this group, the Oswestry Back Pain Score (OBPS) was evaluated for the same study group. There was minimal to moderate disability related to low back pain [49].
- Twenty-two patients who were treated with symphyseal plating were analyzed at least 1 year posttrauma (range 1–9 years) using the POS [62]. Overall 41% of these patients reported some pelvic pain, even after anatomical reconstruction of the pelvic ring.
- In 15 patients after plate osteosynthesis of open book injury without additional complex pelvic trauma, reevaluation was performed 14–49 months postoperatively [63]. Using POS, 93.3% of these patients had an excellent or good functional result and all patients had anatomically healed pelves. Seventy-three percent were completely pain free.
- Using the Majeed Score, eight patients with open book injuries were analyzed after a mean of 4.1 years (1–11 years) [46]. All patients were treated with an anterior external fixation alone. Six of eight patients had a fair or poor radiological result at follow-up with >11 mm displacement at their injury site. Three of these patients had significant pelvic pain, and the functional results were graded fair or poor in 50%.

- In an analysis of 31 patients with B1 injuries which were treated by several stabilization techniques including external and ORIF techniques, good or excellent functional results were observed in 74% of these patients [64, 65]. Significant permanent pain was reported in 29%, and 36% of these had moderate to severe pelvic pain. In contrast, anatomical bony healing occurred in 93%.
- Recently, the functional outcome of 32 patients with open book injuries after a median follow-up time of 84 months using the SF-36 and the Majeed Score was analyzed [57]. All patients had initial anterior ring stabilization, and in approximately one fourth of the patients an additional iliosacral screw was applied. All values of the different SF-36 categories were lower compared to uninjured German and U.S. patients. The median level of physical functioning was 95%; no patient had role limitations and the median pain level using the VAS was 10%. Interestingly, patients who were treated by additional posterior iliosacral screw fixation showed a trend to worse results compared to patients with symphyseal stabilization alone. The average Majeed Score was high with 95.7 points.

After B1 injuries, moderate disability and 30–40% relevant persistent pain can be expected, despite a high rate of anatomical healing. The overall functional result is graded excellent and good in 70–90% when symphyseal plating was performed. Single external fixation seems to lead to worse results.

43.12 Outcome Analyses After Pelvic Ring Type B2 "Lateral Compression" Injuries

Some analyses evaluated the results of the more stable lateral compression injuries.

- In the analysis of 62 patients with lateral compression type B2 injuries treated by external fixation alone with a mean follow-up of 4.1 years (1–11 years) using the Majeed Score, 32.2% of these patients had a fair or poor radiological result with >11 mm displacement at their injury site but only 6.4% reported significant pelvic pain. The functional result was graded fair or poor in 25.8%. Especially when vertical pubic ramus displacement was >10 mm, significantly more patients had persistent pain or a worse functional result [46].
- In an analysis of 30 patients with lateral compression pelvic ring fractures with extension into the anterior acetabulum, treated conservatively in the majority of patients, follow-up was performed after a mean of 4.2 years (2–6 years), using the MFA and the SF-36 [58]. At follow-up, 93.3% of the pelves showed a maximum residual displacement of <10 mm. Functional deficits were observed for mental and social functions in the SF-36 compared to B1 and C injuries.
- Recently, Höch et al. compared 35 nonoperatively treated patients with B 2.1 injuries and 36 operatively treated patients using the SF-36 and the EQ5D after at least 1 year following trauma [29]. At a follow-up after a mean of 47 months, the mean VAC pain value was 2.8 and 2.6 after nonoperative vs. operative treatments, respectively. The mean SF-36 PCS was 44.8 points and the mean SF-36 MCS was 52.6 points, both lower than the normal German population. The EQ-5D was 89.5 and 91.8, and their mean VAS were 75.5 and 79.7, respectively. Operatively treated patients had a significantly higher complication rate. Thus, nonoperative treatment was recommended especially for younger patients.

After lateral compression type B2 injuries, a low rate of permanent pain (5–15%) can be expected despite anatomical healing of the pelvis in only 70–75%. An excellent or good overall functional result was observed in 75–90%.

43.13 Unselected Outcome Analyses After Pelvic Ring Type C Injuries

The majority of reports in the literature are dealing with completely unstable pelvic ring injuries, disrupting the anterior and posterior pelvic ring structures. Several reports have described the results of study groups with different types of type C injuries not distinguishing between classification, fracture types, fracture location, or treatment modalities [66–68].

There are some data available on SF-36 analysis after these injuries:

- In 24 patients with type C injuries at a mean follow-up of 2 years with a nonconsistent treatment, a reduced physical component score of 62.6 and a reduced mental component score of 69.3 was reported, which represents approximately 20% and 7.8% impairment compared with the U.S. normal population, respectively [37].
- Long-term results in 34 type C injuries, which were treated by anterior and posterior stabilization techniques, showed a mean physical functional value of 68.9 and a pain value of 60.1. This a reduction compared to the nor-

mal U.S. population (in [37]) of 12% and 16.8%, respectively.

- Additionally, 24 patients with type C injuries were treated with external fixation in 60% and by nonoperative means in 40% with a follow-up of more than 5 years. Eighty-one percent returned to their preinjury occupation level, but 42% had disturbances of their sexual activity [35]. These patients had the lowest rates of returning to their preinjury level of recreation. Persistent pain was present in 25 and 21% had a limited activity. Overall, only 17% showed no functional impairments.
- Distinguishing between posterior complete iliac fractures (type C.1.1), complete SI dislocations (type C.1.2), and unilateral type C sacral fractures (type C1.3), after anterior and posterior stabilization of the pelvis, mean SF-36 physical functional values of 63.8, 71.1, and 72.6 were reported, respectively, and the mean pain values were 54.5, 62.2, and 63.5, respectively. As complete iliac fractures and SI dislocation are more uncommon than sacral fractures, the long-term sequelae after unilateral sacral fractures seem to be better compared to other unilateral type C injuries [69].
- Lefaivre et al. analyzed 23 patients with type B injuries after a mean of 57 months by using the SF-36. The SF-36 PCS was 40.57, and the SF-36 MCS was 40.58 [32]. The corresponding normative data from Canada [59] were 50.5 and 51.7, respectively, indicating a 19.7% and 21.5% impairment, respectively.

According to a validated outcome instrument (SF-36), there are relevant impairments after type C injuries compared to the normal population. Operatively treated sacrum fractures showed better results than after pure SI joint dislocations.

Compared to type B injuries, a nearly twofold higher rate of impairments can be expected [35, 37, 69].

The majority of reports are dealing with nonvalidated outcome instruments to analyze the long-term result after type C injuries.

- Fifty-two patients with different unstable posterior pelvic ring injuries and operative treatment of the posterior pelvic ring were followed at 36 months (range 5–74 months). Ninety-eight percent showed bony union. In 88% the posterior pelvis healed within a maximal displacement of 5 mm. The pain level during rest using a VAS Scale was 28% on average and 41% for the ambulation pain score. An additional lumbosacral plexus injury leads to higher pain values. The overall rate of urinary complaints was 37%. Thirty percent of the male patients had signs of erectile dysfunction. The working status was identical to the preinjury level in 65 and 11% were partially integrated. The mean self-developed pelvic outcome score was 29 points. 28.8% had functional deficits related to associated injuries [16].
- In a further analysis of ORIF of with 46 patients with different unstable posterior pelvic ring injuries after at least 1 year after (mean 44 months, range, 12–101 months), 45.5% of the patients with sacral fractures were completely pain free, and further 18.2% had only slight pain, giving acceptable pain levels in 63.7% [70]. A persistent nerve deficit was present in 54.5% of these patients. 63.7% returned to their previous jobs. Despite a good radiological reduction, several patients reported on pain, indicating that the soft-tissue injury possibly contributes to the long-term clinical status.
- After pure sacroiliac dislocations, 61.5% had no and 7.7% had slight pain (69.2% acceptable pain level). Overall, 61.5% had a permanent lumbosacral plexus lesion. Previous occupational status could be reached by 46% of the patients. After sacroiliac fracture dislocations, 45.8% of patients were pain free and 12.5% had mild pain. After this injury type the lowest rate of acceptable pain levels (58.3%) were reported. A persistent nerve deficit was seen in 12.5% of the patients. The majority of patients (79.2%) was able to return to their previous jobs [70].
- In 40 patients treated with only anterior external fixation for type C injuries, the Majeed Score was used during follow-up after a mean of 4.1 years (1–11 years). Ninety-five percent had a fair or poor radiological result. 47.5% reported on significant pelvic pain, and the functional results were graded fair or poor in 85%. Posterior displacement of >10 mm was a bad prognostic indicator for functional impairments [46].
- In an analysis of 67 patients after type C injuries treated by different stabilization techniques including anterior and posterior techniques, the long-term functional result was graded excellent or good in 71.6% of the cases. Pain was frequent with 54% of patients having persistent pain. A permanent neurological deficit was observed in 13.4% [64].
- 101 patients with type C injuries treated by posterior fixation techniques in 98 patients, additional anterior fixation in 78 patients, and single anterior fixation in 3 patients had follow-up analysis at least 1 year after trauma with a mean of 23 months (range 12–85 months) [45]. The long-term radiological result was graded excellent (<5 mm residual displacement) in 65%, and good (5–10 mm residual displacement) in 24.8%. The Majeed Score was graded excellent or good in 83%. Despite this, late pain problems were common in 33.7% of patients, with the majority complaining of posterior pelvic pain. There was a strong correlation between the radiological and clinical

results. Additional analysis with the POS showed 80.2% good and excellent results for combination of the clinical and radiological results [45].

- In a further analysis of 11 patients with type C injuries, treated posteriorly with ORIF, the functional results were good and excellent in 73%, whereas 63.6% of these patients were completely pain free at follow-up [61].
- Moon et al. reviewed the results of 53 patients with different type C unstable pelvic injuries and different stabilization concepts [71]. The average Majeed Score was 86.2 with only two fair results. The type of stabilization did not influence the final result (isolated anterior, isolated posterior, and combined anteroposterior fixation). According to Matta and Saucedo, the radiological result of surgical treatment was graded excellent in 31 patients, good in 17, and bad in 5 patients. Worse results were associated with the presence of pelvis-related neurological injury.
- Lefaivre et al. analyzed 15 patients with type C injuries after a mean of 57 months by self-reported complaint analysis [32]. The mean Majeed Score was 66.26 points, the mean IPS was 72.86 points, and the mean OPS was 22.60.

In unselected patient groups with type C injuries, approximately 30–50% of patients suffer from significant persistent pain and have sexual or urogenital disturbances. An excellent or good overall functional result can be expected in 70–80%. The local soft-tissue injury at the posterior pelvis may influence the clinical long-term result. A rate of 65–90% healing with residual displacement<5 mm was observed, depending on the type of pelvic ring stabilization. Single external fixation is inadequate for treating these injuries. These studies support the concept of anterior and posterior stabilization in type C injuries.

43.14 Stabilization-Specific Outcome Analyses

It is of interest to analyze the results of different posterior pelvic ring stabilization techniques after type C injuries.

43.14.1 Iliosacral Screw Fixation of the Posterior Ring

Despite increasing reports on conventional and navigation-assisted techniques in stabilization of unstable sacral fractures, these studies predominantly focus on quality of reduction, safety of screw positioning, radiation exposure, and perioperative parameters [72, 73]. Only few reports focus on long-term results after this procedure.

In an analysis of 21 patients after iliosacral screw fixation, with a mean follow-up time of 31 months, only 33.3% of these patients had excellent or good clinical results in the POS. Removal of the screws led to an improvement of the functional results in 10 of 12 patients [74].

In a follow-up analysis at least 1 year postoperation (mean 32 months) of 71 patients with 10 type B and 61 type C injuries and pure SI dislocations or sacral fractures, 69 (97%) showed a satisfactory healing with a displacement <10 mm. In 21%, degenerative changes of the involved SI joint was seen at final follow-up [75]. The Majeed Score was used to grade the long-term functional result in 68 patients. Ninety-one percent of these patients had good or excellent results. Bad results were observed in patients with complex pelvic trauma or permanent lumbosacral plexus injury. Eighty-six percent of patients returned to their preinjury occupation and recreation levels.

Khaled et al. analyzed the results of 38 patients after a mean follow-up of 37.4 months [76]. After posterior stabilization of different posterior pelvic injuries with one screw, the mean Majeed Score was 92.76 points, while using two screws for posterior stabilization resulted in a mean Majeed Score of 84.14.

The long-term result after iliosacral screw fixation of posterior pelvic instabilities remains unclear. The functional result is potentially influenced by additional trauma to peripelvic soft tissues (urogenital, lumbosacral plexus, etc.). Secondary implant removal should be considered to optimize the result.

43.14.2 Anterior Plating of the Unstable SI Joint

Ragnarsson et al. were the first to analyze 21 patients with 23 type C injuries of the SI joint (OTA C1.2) [77]. In three patients, no anterior ring stabilization was performed (14%). At follow-up after a mean of 5 years (2–8 years), 47.6% of these patients were completely pain free, 14.3% reported slight pain, and 9.5% severe or disabling pain. Nineteen percent of these patients had moderate or severe limping, and in 14.3% walking support using a cane was necessary.

Additionally, 19% of the patients reported on problems while sitting, 14.3% had pain during sexual activity, and 1 patient had erectile dysfunction. Thirty-eight percent of these patients had persistent lumbosacral plexus injury. Seventy-one percent of the patients were partially or fully integrated in their previous occupations. According to the Harris Hip Score, the functional result was graded good or excellent in 85.7%.

Only one patient showed breakage of a plate screw. All others had identical x-rays compared to postoperative evaluation with anatomical healing in 81%. Overall, 57% of these patients showed relevant functional disability.

A further analysis only analyzed the radiological long-term result. Sixteen patients after anterior plating of a C1.2 injury were evaluated after a mean of 63.2 months (range 1–14 years). Anatomical healing was observed in 81%. The other patients showed some malalignment of 2–4 mm. In 10 patients with a follow-up CT scan, only 1 patient showed a "normal" SI joint. All others had degenerative changes at the SI joint (periarticular osteophytes, degenerative changes, and ankylosis) [78].

Anterior plating of the completely disrupted SI joint as part of a type C injury results in anatomical healing in 80%. Overall, approximately half of these patients can have relevant functional limitations.

43.14.3 Ilioiliacal Stabilization Techniques

Several techniques are described for posterior ilioiliacal stabilization of unstable pelvic ring lesions. These include sacral bar stabilization (extra- and intraosseous), application of an ilioiliacal internal fixator, and transiliac plate osteosynthesis. No study is available for long-term results after sacral bar stabilization.

- In 14 patients with unstable sacral fractures, posterior iliac reconstruction plate osteosynthesis was performed and no loss of reduction was observed. Overall, 57% of these patients reported pain [79].
- A comparable percutaneous technique with subfascial ilioiliacal plate osteosynthesis was analyzed in 25 patients with different posterior pelvic ring injuries after a mean of 17 months. Radiological analysis with POS criteria showed 64% anatomic reconstructions of the posterior pelvis (maximal displacement of the posterior pelvic ring <5 mm) and 32% with a good result (displacement 5–10 mm) [80].
- The same group reported the clinical results and the social reintegration in 23 patients after an average of 20 months (range 7–57 months) [81]. The clinical outcome (POS) was graded excellent or good in 73.9% of cases. 39.1% of the patients were complete socially integrated; further 43.5% had incomplete integration. A trend for better clinical results was observed after good bony reconstructions. The presence of lumbosacral plexus lesions and permanent urogenital complaints was associated with worse clinical results. The initial presence of polytrauma led to a worse social integration; for the clinical result only a trend could be observed.
- Stabilization of comminuted sacral fractures in 18 patients with ilioiliacal plate osteosynthesis showed 72.2% of the patients rated excellent or good using the Majeed Score with a mean score of 78.5 points. Radiographically, healing with displacement <5 mm occurred in 50%, and healing with displacement 5–10 mm in 38.9%. A persistent neurological deficit leads to significant lower scores [82].
- Results in 28 patients with SI dislocations or sacral fractures treated with a percutaneous technique of an ilioiliacal internal fixator showed after a mean of 2 years postoperation an overall rate of 62.5% excellent or good clinical results according to the POS [83]. All but two patients had posterior reconstructions with a residual displacement <5 mm. Patients with an additional pelvic complex trauma [84] showed worse clinical and radiological results and their social integration was impaired.

After percutaneous posterior ilioiliacal plating in type C injuries, 70–75% good to excellent clinical results can be expected. Healing with displacement <5 mm was observed in 50–80%. An additional peripelvic soft-tissue injury (complex pelvic trauma) may worsen long-term results.

43.14.4 Lumbopelvic Fixation

Lumbopelvic or spinopelvic stabilization techniques are of increasing popularity during the last years. Several different techniques are well described in the literature.

The basic concept is a connection of an internal fixator fixed in the distal lumbar spine pedicles to the sacrum and/or posterior ilium. Modifications include additional plate or iliosacral screw fixation.

A triangular lumbopelvic technique was used in unstable sacral fractures with complemented iliosacral screws or an ilioiliacal plate. Thirty-four patients had a follow-up examination at an average of 19 months postoperatively (range 8–52 months). All patients had unstable sacral fractures. No loss of reduction was observed, but clinical data were missing [85].

Using the same technique in 18 patients with SI dislocations and sacral fractures stated, after a mean follow-up time of 23 months (range 4–48 months) using the POS no patient was completely pain free. 66.7% had slight or occasional pain, 22.3% had moderate pain, and 11.1% had permanent severe pain. 11.1% of these patients required walking assistance (cane), and 61.1% had a normal gait [86].

A modification of the triangular technique was used in 20 patients with unstable sacral fractures, and follow-up was performed at a mean of 23 months (range 7–48 months). Ninety percent showed healing with a displacement of the sacrum <5 mm. The overall clinical result was graded excellent or good in 65% using the POS [87].

Unselected long-term results after lumbopelvic fixation in type C injuries show good to excellent clinical results in only 65% of these patients. The fixation concept shows adequate stability with low rates of loss of reduction.

43.14.5 Spinopelvic Fracture Dissociation Injuries After Lumbopelvic Fixation

As a special subgroup of type C injuries, spinopelvic fracture dislocation (dissociation) or "suicidal jumper's fractures" were evaluated by several authors. These injuries are extremely unstable as typically a longitudinal or oblique sacral fracture is associated with a transverse sacral component leading to flexion or extension displacement of the vertebral column with some part of the sacrum into the small pelvis.

The majority of these injuries are presently stabilized with a spinopelvic fixation construct. Only in minor displaced injuries, bilateral iliosacral screw fixation or even nonoperative treatment was recommended by some authors.

- Seventeen patients were treated with ORIF, sacral nerve root decompression, and lumbopelvic fixation. A bilateral lumbo-sacral-iliac internal fixator connected with a transverse bar was used. Twenty-six percent had wound complications. Follow-up was performed after at least 12 months. The kyphotic deformity could be reduced from an average of 43° to 20°. No loss of reduction was seen. Neurological recovery was observed in 83%, with full recovery of bowel and bladder function in 47% [88].
- In a first analysis of 15 patients, 67% good and excellent pelvic results using the POS and 67% good and excellent functional results using a modified Majeed Scale were stated [89].
- In an ongoing outcome study of 36 patients with a H-shaped sacral fracture, Lindahl et al. reported excellent (displacement ≤5 mm, 19 patients) or good (displacement ≤10 mm, 17 patients) radiological end results in all cases in the vertical sacral fractures [90]. Postoperatively there was no loss of sacral fracture reduction. Kyphosis in the transverse sacral fracture improved from a mean of 38° to 22°, and the translational displacement improved from a mean of 15 to 6 mm. Postoperatively, there was no loss of sacral fracture reduction. They found a significant association between the radiological and clinical outcomes. Patients with anatomical or near-anatomical reductions had a better clinical outcome than those with >5 mm residual displacement in the vertical sacral fracture lines. In addition, both the residual postoperative AP translation and kyphosis of the transverse sacral fracture were smaller in patients with good clinical outcomes than in those with poor outcomes. At least some neurological recovery was observed in 34 out of 35 patients with an associated sacral plexus injury. The only patient without any neurological improvement had T12 burst fracture with associated paraplegia. Seventeen of 29 patients (59%) with a cauda equina injury (Gibbons grade 4) had full recovery of their bladder and bowel functions. Of 36 patients, 7 (19%) underwent a full neurological recovery, 8 (22%) were left with sensory deficits, while 9 (25%) had motor and sensory deficits in the lower extremities, and 12 (33%) had permanent cauda equina deficits. An accurate reduction of all fracture components was associated with better clinical outcome. The functional outcome according to the modified Majeed Score was excellent or good in 62% with a primary lumbosacral plexus involvement in 95% of these cases.
- Ayoub followed up 28 patients with spinopelvic dissociation and sacral cauda equina syndrome treated with spinopelvic fixation [91]. In this series, 96% of cases had partial or complete neurological recovery. Nineteen patients (68%) had excellent or good clinical outcome according to the POS. However, no severe fall from height injuries were in this group.
- De Iure et al. analyzed long-term results of ten consecutive patients after lumboiliac fixation [92]. Three patients had significant discomfort.
- Tian et al. presented 18 consecutive patients who sustained a spinopelvic dissociation injury with a mean age of 33.1 years treated with lumbopelvic fixations and depending on neurological injury, simultaneous sacral canal decompression (6 cases) was performed [93]. In 16 cases a fall resulted in this injury, while in two cases a traffic accident caused the injury. Ten U-shaped fractures, six H-shaped fractures, and two Y-shaped fractures were observed, corresponding to 12 type II and 6 type III injuries of the Roy-Camille classification. There were 12 cases of type II and 6 cases of type III. At a mean follow-up of 32.4 months, all sacral fractures were healed. According to the Majeed Score, 12 cases were graded excellent, 4× good, and 2 cases as fair.

Spinopelvic dissociation injuries are associated with excellent and good results in <70% possibly due to the permanent nerve injury and a high pain rate, potentially due to permanent soft-tissue pain by the injury itself.

43.14.6 Results After Specific Posterior Pelvic Injury Types

The classical unilateral injuries to the posterior pelvic ring are complete iliac fractures (type C1.1), pure sacroiliac dislocations (SI dislocation, type C1.2), and sacral fractures (type C1.3). Only few data are available for analyzing these specific injuries.

43.14.7 Complete Iliac Fractures (Type C1.1)

Cole et al. treated four of these injuries by plate osteosynthesis. When comparing patients with different posterior fracture patterns, no statistical difference on outcome could be observed in this specific fracture type [16].

Another analysis using the SF-36 showed physical functional values of 63.8 and mean pain value of 54.5, indicating lower values than for the general population [69].

In conclusion, no clear data can be presented for this specific fracture type.

43.14.8 Pure SI Dislocations (Type C.1.2)

After ORIF of pure SI dislocations none or only slight pain was reported in 69.2%. The previous occupational status could be reached by only 46% of these patients [70].

Comparable results were found in 21 patients after anterior plating of the SI joint with no or slight pain in 61.9%. Additionally, 19% of these patients had moderate or severe limping and in 14.3% walking support using a cane was necessary. Nineteen percent of the patients reported on problems while sitting, 14.3% had pain during sexual activity, and 1 patient had erectile dysfunction. Thirty-eight percent of these patients had persistent lumbosacral plexus injury. Seventy-one percent of the patients were partially or fully integrated in their previous occupation. Overall, 57% of these patients showed relevant functional disability. Anatomical healing occurred in 81% [77].

Thus, between 30 and 40% of patients after ORIF of the SI joint reported persistent pain, and half of these patients have relevant functional impairments.

43.14.9 Sacral Fractures (Type C1.3)

After ORIF of 11 unstable sacral fractures, follow-up at least 1 year after the injury showed that 45.5% of the patients were completely pain free, and further 18.2% had only slight pain. 63.6% returned to their previous jobs [70].

Ilioiliacal reconstruction plate osteosynthesis in 14 patients showed no loss of reduction but 57% of these patients reported on pain [79].

The same technique was used in 18 patients in comminuted sacral fractures showing 72.2% excellent or good functional results with a mean Majeed Score of 78.5 points. Bony healing with residual displacement <5 mm occurred in only 50%. A persistent neurological deficit leads to significant lower scores [82].

Triangular stabilization in 20 patients resulted in bony healing with a displacement of the sacrum <5 mm in 90%. The POS showed excellent or good results in 65% [87].

Overall, more than 50% of patients after ORIF of sacral fractures report some pain at follow-up with an expected excellent or good functional result in 65–75%.

43.15 Prognostic Factors Influencing Long-Term Results

Several prognostic factors of worse clinical and functional outcomes after pelvic injuries are well described in the literature:

- Residual displacement
- Persistent nerve injury
- Additional pelvic soft-tissue injury (complex pelvic trauma)

43.15.1 Residual Displacement

A correlation between persistent vertical displacement of the posterior pelvic ring and body pain after treatment of unstable sacral fractures was early recorded [36].

The amount of displacement is potentially relevant. The German multicenter study analysis revealed that better functional results were observed with residual posterior displacement <5 mm in type C injuries [13].

Better functional results were found with residual posterior displacement <5 mm in type C injuries [48], whereas Tornetta et al. showed no difference in pain levels comparing patients with less or more than 4 mm posterior displacement after ORIF [70]. In contrast, a higher rate of urinary complaints was noted when more than 5 mm displacement persisted at the posterior pelvis [94].

In a recent analysis of 28 patients after ORIF of displaced sacral fractures and an 11-year follow-up, in 16/28 a residual displacement of ≥10 mm was present. Only eight patients reported no pain but no correlations between pain and radiological findings were found [95].

Optimal results should be expected only in patients with a residual posterior displacement of ≤5 mm.

43.15.2 Neurological Deficits

Many outcome analyses could confirm that a permanent lumbosacral plexus lesion is responsible for a worse clinical or functional result [16, 40, 75, 80, 81].

Even after type B and more often after type C injuries, persistent nerve deficits can be observed. Most severe nerve lesions were found in type C injuries, whereas after type B injuries only minor sensoric deficits were observed [14, 15, 45].

In a recent analysis on late nerve deficits, the lumbosacral plexus injury was one of the most common reason for an unsatisfactory functional result [96].

In a recent analysis on a late nerve deficit analysis, the lumbosacral plexus injury was identified as the mainly involved neurologic injury after pelvic trauma which has severe long-term implications regarding pain and gait outcome [97].

Recent data show acceptable rates of neurologic recovery between 30 and 70% [56]. Especially, unstable sacral fractures have the highest rates of additional nerve injury.

The combination of unstable sacral fractures or spinopelvic dissociations in combination with a lumbosacral plexus injury is of major negative prognostic value.

43.15.3 Additional Pelvic Soft-Tissue Trauma (Complex Pelvic Trauma)

Complex pelvic trauma is defined as a pelvic ring injury in combination with a significant peripelvic soft-tissue injury, e.g., open fractures, Morel-Levallé lesions, and additional urogenital or pelvic bowel injury as well as neurovascular injuries [84].

The relevance of an additional lumbosacral plexus lesion was already mentioned.

Open pelvic fractures led to reduced physical function scores and role physical scores of the SF-36 [26].

In a further analysis, nearly half of the patients with open pelvic injuries had long-term impairments in daily activities [98].

Urogenital long-term sequelae are of additional relevance.

In a comparable study of type B and type C injuries, higher rates of incontinence were observed after type C injuries, whereas after type B injuries a higher rate of micturition disturbances was observed. 12.5% of men had permanent erectile dysfunction after type C injuries [13–15]. In women 19% incidence of dyspareunia was reported [94]. In a literature overview, a rate of erectile dysfunction between 11% and 30% for all patients depending on the type of diagnostics and a rate of up to 42% in patients with additional injury to the urethra were found [99].

The relevance of the overall additional soft-tissue trauma could be confirmed as it was associated with decreased functional results, when a significant pelvic soft-tissue trauma was present [70, 83, 100].

Analysis of the German Multicenter Pelvis Study Group identified patients with severe pelvic pain as having a higher injury severity, a higher rate of unstable pelvic ring injuries and additional complex pelvic trauma, and a higher rate of neurological and urological long-term disturbances. Additionally, in patients with a poor clinical outcome more frequently additional peripelvic soft-tissue injuries were present [13].

An additional injury to relevant pelvic soft-tissues including pelvic organ injury influences the clinical and functional long-term results.

43.16 Results in Geriatric Patients

Schmitz et al. analyzed older patients (>60 years) after pelvic ring injuries (type A, B, and C) [39]. As expected, the overall complication rate was higher after surgical stabilization of the pelvis. Fifty-five patients were followed after 4.2 years. The mean SF-36 PCS was 33.6, and the mean SF-36 MCS was 45.3. The mean EQ-5D VAS reached 62.5.

These results were confirmed by Banierink et al. in an analysis of 153 patients with a mean age of 79 years [101]. Pelvic fractures in the elderly were significant risk factor of mortality:

- 20% at 30 days
- 27% at 1 year
- 41% at 3 years
- 100% after type C injuries

SMFA Function Index was 67.4 points and the Bother Index was 65.2 points. The mean EQ-5D Index score was 0.72.

Pelvic fractures in the elderly are associated with an expected substantially lower level of physical functioning and quality of life [101].

43.17 Summary

- No clear data are available as different treatment concepts are used, and the majority of published studies are not comparable regarding selected evaluation parameters.
- No well-accepted standardized measurement instrument is available to analyze the clinical and radiological results after pelvic ring injuries.
- More short-term evaluations with follow-up times of 1 year are available, while only few analyses present data on medium-term or long-term analyses.
- An increase of long-term sequelae can be expected from stable type A injuries to completely unstable type C injuries.
- Type B1 injuries lead to worse results than type B2 injuries.
- Concomitant injuries of other injury regions and associated local pelvic injuries (complex pelvic trauma) seem to influence the overall results.
- A sufficient pelvic outcome instrument which addresses relevant pelvic outcome parameters is missing.
- Results of treatment of specific fracture types are sparse as a wide range of different injury types and different treatment concepts are analyzed in the existing literature.
- Future evaluation of long-term results after pelvic ring injuries should include prospective, multicenter outcome studies.

References

1. Kreder H. Outcomes after pelvic ring injuries in adults. In: Tile M, Helfet DL, Kellam JF, editors. Fractures of the pelvis and acetabulum. 3rd ed. Philadelphia: Lippincott; 2003. p. 409–16.
2. Kreder H, Wright J, McLeod R. Outcome studies in surgical research. Surgery. 1997;121:223–5.
3. Lefaivre K, Slobogean G, Valeriote J, O'Brien P, Macadam S. Reporting and interpretation of the functional outcomes after the surgical treatment of disruptions of the pelvic ring: a systematic review. J Bone Joint Surg Br. 2012;94:549–55.
4. Ware J. SF-36 health survey: manual and interpretation guide. Boston: The Health Institute New England Medical Center; 1993.
5. Swiontkowski M, Engelberg R, Martin D, Agel J. Short musculoskeletal function assessment questionnaire: validity, reliability, and responsiveness. J Bone Joint Surg. 1999;81-A:1245–60.
6. Brazler J, Jones N, Kind P. Testing of validity of the EuroQol and comparing it to the SF-36 health survey questionnaire. Qual Life Res. 1993;2:169–80.
7. Jurkovich G, Mock C, Mackenzie E. The Sickness Impact Profile as a tool to evaluate functional outcome in trauma patients. J Trauma. 1995;39:625–32.
8. FIM. Guide for uniform data set for medical rehabilitation (Adult FIM), Version 4.0. Buffalo: State University of New York at Buffalo; 1993.
9. Fugl-Meyer A, Branholm I, Fugl-Meyer K. Happiness and domain specific life satisfaction in adult northern Swedes. Clin Rehabil. 1991;5:25–33.
10. Williams J. A structured interview guide to the Hamilton depression rating scale. Arch Gen Psychiatry. 1988;45:742–74.
11. Majeed SA. Grading the outcome of pelvic fractures. J Bone Joint Surg Br. 1989;71(2):304–6.
12. Templeman D, Goulet J, Duwelius P, Olson S, Davidson M. Internal fixation of displaced fractures of the sacrum. Clin Orthop. 1996;329:180–5.
13. Pohlemann T, Gänsslen A, Hartung S, für die Arbeitsgruppe Becken, H.T., H., Beckenverletzungen/Pelvic Injuries. Hefte zu "Der Unfallchirurg". Heft 266. 1998.
14. Pohlemann T, Gänsslen A, Schellwald O, Culemann U, Tscherne H. Outcome after pelvic ring injuries. Injury. 1996;27(Suppl 2):S-B31–8.
15. Pohlemann T, Tscherne H, Baumgärtel F, Egbers H, Euler E, Maurer F, Fell M, Mayr E, Quirini W, Schlickewei W, Weinberg A. Beckenverletzungen: Epidemiologie, Therapie und Langzeitverlauf. Übersicht über die multizentrische Studie der Arbeitsgruppe Becken. Unfallchirurg. 1996;99(3):160–7.
16. Cole J, Blum D, Ansel L. Outcome after fixation of unstable posterior pelvic ring injuries. Clin Orthop. 1996;329:160–79.
17. Merle d'Aubigné R, Postel M. Functional results of hip arthroplasty with acrylic prosthesis. J Bone Joint Surg. 1954;36-A:451–75.
18. Fairbank J, Pynsent P. The Oswestry disability index. Spine. 2000;25(22):2940–53.
19. Borg T, Berg P, Larsson S. Quality of life after operative fixation of displaced acetabular fractures. J Orthop Trauma. 2012;26:445–50.
20. Borg T, Hernefalk B, Carlsson M, Larsson S. Development of a pelvic discomfort index to evaluate outcome following fixation for pelvic ring injury. J Orthop Surg (Hong Kong). 2015;23:146–9.
21. Riemer B. Outcomes of pelvic ring injuries. Oper Tech Orthop. 1997;7(3):256–9.
22. Laucis NC, Hay R, Bhattacharyya T. Scoring the SF-36 in orthopaedics: a brief guide. J Bone Joint Surg. 2015;97-A:1628–34.
23. Bhandari M, Busse J, Hanson B, Leece P, Ayeni O, Schemitsch E. Psychological distress and quality of life after orthopedic trauma: an observational study. Can J Surg. 2008;51:15–22.
24. Ayvaz M, Cağlar O, Yılmaz G, Güvendik G, Acaroğlu R. Long-term outcome and quality of life of patients with unstable pelvic fractures treated by closed reduction and percutaneous fixation. Ulus Travma Acil Cerrahi Derg. 2011;17:261–6.
25. Borg T, Berg P, Fugl-Meyer K, Larsso S. Health-related quality of life and life satisfaction in patients following surgically treated pelvic ring fractures. A prospective observational study with two years follow-up. Injury. 2010;41:400–4.
26. Brenneman F, Katyal D, Boulanger B, Tile M, Redelmeier D. Long-term outcomes in open pelvic fractures. J Trauma. 1997;42(5):773–7.
27. Day A, Kinmont C, Bircher M, Kumar S. Crescent fracture-dislocation of the sacroiliac joint. A functional classification. J Bone Joint Surg. 2007;89-B:651–8.

28. Hernefalk B, Eriksson N, Borg T, Larsson S. Estimating pre-traumatic quality of life in patients with surgically treated acetabular fractures and pelvic ring injuries: does timing matter? Injury. 2016;47:389–94.
29. Höch A, Schneider I, Todd J, Josten C, Böhme J. Lateral compression type B 2-1 pelvic ring fractures in young patients do not require surgery. Eur J Trauma Emerg Surg. 2018;44:171–7.
30. Keating J, Werier J, Blachut P, Briekhuyse H, Meek R, O'Brian P. Early fixation of the vertically unstable pelvis—the role of iliosacral screw fixation of the posterior lesion. J Orthop Trauma. 1999;13(2):107–13.
31. Kerschbaum M, Hausmann N, Worlicek M, Pfeifer C, Nerlich M, Schmitz P. Patient-related outcome of unstable pelvic ring fractures stabilized with a minimal invasive screw-rod system. Health Qual Life Outcomes. 2017;15(1):248. https://doi.org/10.1186/s12955-017-0821-7.
32. Lefaivre K, Slobogean G, Ngai J, Broekhuyse H, O'Brien P. What outcomes are important for patients after pelvic trauma? Subjective responses and psychometric analysis of three published pelvic-specific outcome instruments. J Orthop Trauma. 2014;28:23–7.
33. Lumsdaine W, Weber D, Balogh Z. Pelvic fracture-specific scales versus general patient reported scales for pelvic fracture outcomes: a systematic review. ANZ J Surg. 2016;86:687–90.
34. McCarthy M, MacKenzie E, Bosse M, Copeland C, Hash C, Burgess A. Functional status following orthopaedic trauma in young women. J Trauma. 1995;39(5):828–36.
35. Miranda M, Riemer B, Butterfield S, Burke C. Pelvic ring injuries—a long term functional outcome study. Clin Orthop. 1996;329:152–9.
36. Nepola J, Trenhaile S, Miranda M, Butterfield S, Fredericks D, Riemer B. Vertical shear injuries: is there a relationship between residual displacement and functional outcome? J Trauma. 1999;46(6):1024–9.
37. Oliver C, Twaddle B, Agel J, Routt M. Outcome after pelvic ring fractures: evaluation using the medical outcomes short form SF-36. Injury. 1996;27(6):635–41.
38. Sagi H, Militano U, Caron T, Lindvall E. A comprehensive analysis with minimum 1-year follow-up of vertically unstable transforaminal sacral fractures treated with triangular osteosynthesis. J Orthop Trauma. 2009;23:313–21.
39. Schmitz P, Lüdeck S, Baumann F, Kretschmer R, Nerlich M, Kerschbaum M. Patient-related quality of life after pelvic ring fractures in elderly. Int Orthop. 2019;43:261–7.
40. Suzuki T, Shindo M, Soma K, Minehara H, Nakamura K, Uchino M, Itoman M. Long-term functional outcome after unstable pelvic ring fracture. J Trauma. 2007;63:884–8.
41. Van den Bosch EW, Van der Kleyn R, Hogervorst M, Van Vugt AB. Functional outcome of internal fixation for pelvic ring fractures. J Trauma. 1999;47(2):365–71.
42. Engelberg R, Martin D, Agel J, Swiontkowski M. Musculoskeletal Function Assessment: reference values for patient and non-patient samples. J Orthop Res. 1999;17:101–9.
43. Martin D, Engelberg R, Agel J, Snapp D, Swiontkowski M. Development of a musculoskeletal extremity health status instrument: the Musculoskeletal Function Assessment instrument. J Orthop Res. 1996;14:173–81.
44. de Bruin A, Buys M, de Witte L, Diederiks J. The sickness impact profile: SIP68, a short generic version. First evaluation of the reliability and reproducibility. J Clin Epidemiol. 1994;47:863–71.
45. Lindahl J, Hirvensalo E. Outcome of operatively treated type-C injuries of the pelvic ring. Acta Orthop Scand. 2005;76(5):667–78.
46. Lindahl J, Hirvensalo E, Bostman O, Santavirta S. Failure of reduction with an external fixator in the management of injuries of the pelvic ring. Long-term evaluation of 110 patients. J Bone Joint Surg Br. 1999;81(6):955–62.
47. Majeed SA. External fixation of the injured pelvis—the functional outcome. J Bone Joint Surg Br. 1990;72(4):612–4.
48. Dujardin FH, Hossenbaccus M, Duparc F, Biga N, Thomine JM. Long-term functional prognosis of posterior injuries in high-energy pelvic disruption. J Orthop Trauma. 1998;12(3):145–50; discussion 150–1.
49. Hakim R, Gruen G, Delitto A. Outcomes of patients with pelvic-ring fractures managed by open reduction internal fixation. Phys Ther. 1996;76(3):286–95.
50. Dzupa V, Chmelová J, Pavelka T, Obruba P, Wendsche P, Iimko P. Multicentrická studie pacientù s poranìním pánve: pøehled klinickπch vπsledkù a trvalπch následkù. Acta Chir Orthop Traumatol Cechoslov. 2011;78:120–5.
51. Pavelka T, Dzupa V, Tulík J, Grill R, Báca, Skála-Rosenbaum J. Vπsledky operaèní léèby nestabilního poranìní pánevního kruhu. Acta Chir Orthop Traumatol Cechoslov. 2007;74:19–28.
52. Ismail H, Lubis M, Djaja Y. The outcome of complex pelvic fracture after internal fixation surgery. Malays Orthop J. 2016;10:16–21.
53. Brouwers L, Lansink K, de Jongh M. Quality of life after pelvic ring fractures: a cross-sectional study. Injury. 2018;49:812–8.
54. Banierink H, Reininga I, Heineman E, Wendt K, Ten Duis K, IJpma F. Long-term physical functioning and quality of life after pelvic ring injuries. Arch Orthop Trauma Surg. 2019;139(9):1225–33. https://doi.org/10.1007/s00402-019-03170-2.
55. Hermans E, Brouwers L, van Gent T, Biert J, de Jongh M, Lansink K, Edwards M. Quality of life after pelvic ring fractures: long-term outcomes. A multicentre study. Injury. 2019;50:216–22.
56. Gänsslen A, Lindahl J. Evaluation tools and outcomes after osteosynthesis of unstable type B and C pelvic ring injuries. Acta Chir Orthop Traumatol Cechoslov. 2013;80:305–20.
57. van Loon P, Kuhn S, Hofmann A, Hessmann M, Rommens P. Radiological analysis, operative management and functional outcome of open book pelvic lesions: a 13-year cohort study. Injury. 2011;42:1012–9.
58. Laflamme G, Delisle J, Rouleau D, Uzel A, Leduc S. Lateral compression fractures of the superior pubic ramus with intra-articular extension. J Bone Joint Surg. 2009;91-B:1208–12.
59. Hopman W, Towheed T, Anastassiades T, Tenenhouse A, Poliquin S, Berger C, Joseph L, Brown J, Murray T, Adachi J, Hanley D, Papadimitropoulos E. Canadian normative data for the SF-36 health survey. Canadian Multicentre Osteoporosis Study Research Group. CMAJ. 2000;163:265–71.
60. Tornetta P, Dickson K, Matta J. Outcome of rotationally unstable pelvic ring injuries treated operatively. Clin Orthop. 1996;329:147–51.
61. Mardanpour K, Rahbar M. The functional outcome of surgically treated unstable pelvic ring fractures by open reduction, internal fixation. MJIRI. 2011;25(2):87–93.
62. Weber K, Vock B, Müller W, Wentzensen A. Rupture of the pubic symphysis. Diagnosis, treatment and outcome. Ann Saudi Med. 1999;19(6):544–6.
63. Pohlemann T, Gänsslen A. Die Operation der Symphysensprengung. Oper Orthop Traumatol. 1999;11:149–59.
64. Rommens P, Gercek E, Hansen M, Hessmann M. Mortalität, Morbidität und funktionelles Endergebnis nach open book Veletzungen und lateralen Kompressionsverletzungen des Beckenringes. Unfallchirurg. 2003;106(7):542–9.
65. Rommens PM, Hessmann MH. Staged reconstruction of pelvic ring disruption: differences in morbidity, mortality, radiologic results, and functional outcomes between B1, B2/B3, and C-type lesions. J Orthop Trauma. 2002;16(2):92–8.
66. Leutenegger A, von Planta A, Rüedi T. Epidemiologie und Nachuntersuchungsergebnisse operativ behandelter Beckenfrakturen. Swiss Surg. 1998;5:47–54.
67. Taguchi T, Kawai S, Kaneko K, Yugue D. Operative management of displaced fractures of the sacrum. J Orthop Sci. 1999;4:347–52.

68. Weber K, Vock B, Muller W, Wentzensen A. Quality of life after surgical treatment of pelvic ring fractures. Are long-term results predictable? Unfallchirurg. 2001;104(12):1162–7.
69. Cano-Luis P, Ricón-Recarey F, Lisón-Torres A, Marcos-Morales F. Treatment of pelvic fractures. Rev Ortop Traumatol. 2006;50:203–16.
70. Tornetta P, Matta J. Outcome of operatively treated unstable posterior pelvic ring disruptions. Clin Orthop. 1996;329:186–93.
71. Moon DH, Kim N, Won J, Choi J, Kim D. Outcome of surgical treatment of AO type C pelvic ring injury. Hip Pelvis. 2014;26:269–74.
72. Briem D, Windolf J, Rueger J. Percutaneous, 2D-fluoroscopic navigated iliosacral screw placement in the supine position: technique, possibilities, and limits. Unfallchirurg. 2007;110:393–401.
73. Zwingmann J, Konrad G, Kotter E, Südkamp N, Oberst M. Computer-navigated iliosacral screw insertion reduces malposition rate and radiation exposure. Clin Orthop. 2009;467:1833–8.
74. Yücel N, Lefering R, Tjardes T, Korenkov M, Schierholz J, Tiling T, Bouillon B, Rixen D. Ist die Entfernung des Osteosynthesematerials nach perkutaner iliosakraler Verschraubung bei iliosakraler Sprengung oder Sakrumfraktur indiziert? Unfallchirurg. 2004;107(6):468–74.
75. Schweitzer D, Zylberberg A, Córdova M, Gonzalez J. Closed reduction and iliosacral percutaneous fixation of unstable pelvic ring fractures. Injury. 2008;39:869–74.
76. Khaled S, Soliman O, Wahed M. Functional outcome of unstable pelvic ring injuries after iliosacral screw fixation: single versus two screw fixation. Eur J Trauma Emerg Surg. 2015;41:387–92.
77. Ragnarsson B, Olerud C, Olerud S. Anterior square-plate fixation of sacroiliac disruption. Acta Orthop Scand. 1993;64(2):138–42.
78. Gänsslen A, Pohlemann T, Krettek C. Internal fixation of sacroiliac joint disruption. Oper Orthop Traumatol. 2005;17:281–95.
79. Albert M, Miller M, MacNaughton M, Hutton W. Posterior pelvic fixation using a transiliac 4.5-mm reconstruction plate: a clinical and biomechanical study. J Orthop Trauma. 1993;7(3):226–32.
80. Dolati B, Krappinger D, Larndorfer R, Rosenberger R. Stabilisierung des dorsalen Beckenrings mit eingeschobener Platte. Oper Orthop Traumatol. 2007;19:16–31.
81. Krappinger D, Larndorfer R, Struve P, Rosenberger R, Arora R, Blauth M. Minimally invasive transiliac plate osteosynthesis for type C injuries of the pelvic ring. A clinical and radiological follow-up. J Orthop Trauma. 2007;21:595–602.
82. Suzuki T, Hak D, Ziran B, Adams S, Stahel P, Morgan S, Smith W. Outcome and complications of posterior transiliac plating for vertically unstable sacral fractures. Injury. 2009;40:405–9.
83. Füchtmeier B, Maghsudi M, Neumann C, Hente R, Roll C, Nerlich M. Die minimalinvasive Stabilisierung des dorsalen Beckenrings mit dem transiliakalen Fixateur interne (TIFI). Unfallchirurg. 2004;107:1142–51.
84. Bosch U, Pohlemann T, Haas N, Tscherne H. Klassifikation und Management des komplexen Beckentraumas. Unfallchirurg. 1992;95:189–96.
85. Schildhauer T, Josten C, Muhr G. Triangular osteosynthesis of vertically unstable sacrum fractures: a new concept allowing early weight bearing. J Orthop Trauma. 1998;12(5):307–14.
86. Thiemann A, Schmidt C, Josten C. Die trianguläre vetebropelvine Abstützung. Zentralbl Chir. 2003;128:202–8.
87. Nothofer W, Thonke N, Neugebauer R. Die Therapie instabiler Sakrumfrakturen bei Beckenringbrüchen mit dorsaler Sakrumdistanzosteosynthese. Unfallchirurg. 2004;107:118–28.
88. Schildhauer T, Bellabarba C, Nork S, Barei D, Routt M, Chapman J. Decompression and lumbopelvic fixation for sacral fracture-dislocations with spino-pelvic dissociation. J Orthop Trauma. 2006;20:447–57.
89. Lindahl J. Operative reduction and lumbopelvic fixation of spino-pelvic dissociation. Suomen Ortop Traumatol. 2008;31:48–51.
90. Lindahl J, Mäkinen T, Koskinen S, Söderlund T. Factors associated with outcome of spinopelvic dissociation treated with lumbopelvic fixation. Injury. 2014;45:1914–20.
91. Ayoub M. Displaced spinopelvic dissociation with sacral cauda equina syndrome: outcome of surgical decompression with a preliminary management algorithm. Eur Spine J. 2012;21:1815–25.
92. De Iure F, Cappuccio M, Palmisani M, Pascarella R, Commessatti M. Lumboiliac fixation in lumbosacral dislocation and associated injuries of the pelvis and lumbosacral junction: a long-term radiological and clinical follow-up. Injury. 2016;47:44–8.
93. Tian W, Chen W, Jia J. Traumatic spino-pelvic dissociation with bilateral triangular fixation. Orthop Surg. 2018;10:205–11.
94. Copeland C, Bosse M, McCarthy M, MacKenzie E, Guzinski G, Hash C, Burghess A. Effect of trauma and pelvic fracture on female genitourinary, sexual and reproductive function. J Orthop Trauma. 1997;11(2):73–81.
95. Adelved A, Tötterman A, Hellund J, FGlott T, Madsen J, Roise O. Radiological findings correlate with neuro,logical deficits but not with pain after operatiuvely treated sacral fractures. Acta Orthop Scand. 2014;85:408–14.
96. Lindahl J, Hirvensalo E. Surgical treatment of pelvic ring fractures. Suomen Ortop Traumatol. 2008;31(1):42–7.
97. Chiodo A. Neurologic injury associated with pelvic trauma: radiology and electrodiagnosis evaluation and their relationships to pain and gait outcome. Arch Phys Med Rehabil. 2007;88:1171–8.
98. Ferrera PC, Hill DA. Good outcomes of open pelvic fractures. Injury. 1999;30(3):187–90.
99. Harwood P, Grotz M, Eardley I, Giannoudis P. Erectile dysfunction after fracture of the pelvis. J Bone Joint Surg. 2005;87-B:281–90.
100. Gänsslen A, Pape H, Lehmann U, Lange U, Krettek C, Pohlemann T. Die operative Therapie von instabilen Sakrumfrakturen. Zentralbl Chir. 2003;128:40–5.
101. Banierink H, Ten Duis K, de Vries R, Wendt K, Heineman E, Reininga I, IJpma F. Pelvic ring injury in the elderly: fragile patients with substantial mortality rates and long-term physical impairment. PLoS One. 2019;14(5):e0216809. https://doi.org/10.1371/journal.pone.0216809.

GPSR Compliance

The European Union's (EU) General Product Safety Regulation (GPSR) is a set of rules that requires consumer products to be safe and our obligations to ensure this.

If you have any concerns about our products, you can contact us on ProductSafety@springernature.com

In case Publisher is established outside the EU, the EU authorized representative is:

Springer Nature Customer Service Center GmbH
Europaplatz 3
69115 Heidelberg, Germany

Batch number: 10731657

Printed by Printforce, the Netherlands